The ROAD to Critical Thinking

A new active-learning approach called **The ROAD to Critical Thinking** is included in this textbook in the ten chapters about psychiatric disorders. Each "ROAD" box presents a real person who has the disorder described in that chapter. The letters in the word "ROAD" form an acronym for the actions you will take to learn more about the person and the specific disorder:

- **Read** about the person at the beginning of the chapter and throughout.
- **Observe** the person in videos on the accompanying CD-ROM.
- **Assess** the person by answering the questions that follow the video.
- **Develop** a Care Plan on the CD-ROM and submit it to your instructor for homework.

Real People, Real Stories

Psychological problems happen to all types of people—people you know, people you see everyday, people like you. One of the best ways to understand psychiatric disorders is to see real people talk about how those disorders affects their lives.

In the **ROAD to Critical Thinking**, you will meet the people below who have opened their lives to help students like you become better psychiatric–mental health nurses.

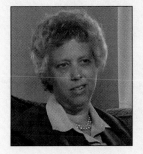

Ann
Paranoid Delusions
due to
Bipolar Disorder

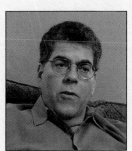

Steve
Anxiety Disorder

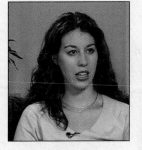

Jessica
Eating Disorder

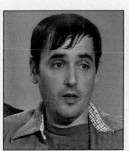

Josh
Bipolar Disorder

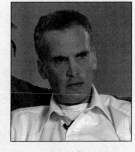

Larry
Paranoid
Schizophrenia
Disorder

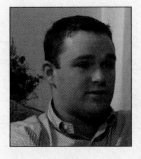

Chris
Substance-Related
Disorder

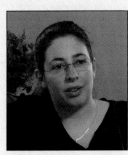

Kylie
Borderline Personality
Disorder

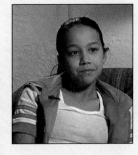

Ashley
Oppositional Defiant
Disorder and ADHD

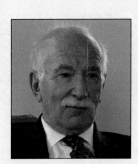

Everett
Suicidal Behavior

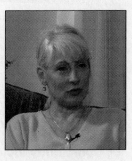

Sara
Interpersonal
Violence

CONTENTS IN BRIEF

Mental Health Nursing

Sixth Edition

Karen Lee Fontaine, RN, MSN, AASECT

Professor, Purdue University Calumet
Hammond, Indiana

PEARSON

Prentice
Hall

Upper Saddle River, New Jersey 07458

Library of Congress Cataloging-in-Publication Data

Fontaine, Karen Lee,
    Mental health nursing / Karen Lee Fontaine.—6th ed.
        p. ; cm.
    Includes bibliographical references and index.
    ISBN-13: 978-0-13-514655-2
    1. Psychiatric nursing.
    [DNLM: 1. Mental Disorders—nursing. 2. Psychiatric Nursing—methods. WY 160
F678m 2009] I. Title.
    RC440.E82 2009
    616.89'0231—dc22   2008015615

Publisher: *Julie Levin Alexander*
Assistant to Publisher: *Regina Bruno*
Editor-in-Chief: *Maura Connor*
Assistant to the Editor-in-Chief: *Marion Gottlieb*
Executive Acquisitions Editor: *Pamela Lappies*
Assistant to the Executive Acquisitions Editor: *Sarah Wrocklage*
Development Editor: *Stephanie Klein*
Editorial Art Manager: *Patrick Watson*
Media Product Manager: *John J. Jordan*
Director of Marketing: *Karen Allman*
Senior Marketing Manager: *Francisco del Castillo*
Marketing Coordinator: *Michael Sirinides*
Marketing Assistant: *Anca David*
Managing Editor, Production: *Patrick Walsh*
Production Editor: *Heather Willison, S4Carlisle*
Production Liaison: *Anne Garcia*
Media Project Manager: *Stephen Hartner*
Manufacturing Manager: *Ilene Sanford*
Senior Design Coordinator: *Maria Guglielmo*
Interior Design: *Wee Design Group*
Cover Design: *Wee Design Group*
Composition: *S4Carlisle Publishing Services*
Printer/Binder: *Courier/Kendallville*
Cover Printer: *Phoenix Color*

Pearson Education Ltd., London
Pearson Education Singapore, Pte. Ltd
Pearson Education Canada, Inc.
Pearson Education—Japan
Pearson Education Australia PTY, Limited
Pearson Education North Asia, Ltd., Hong Kong
Pearson Educación de Mexico, S.A. de C.V.
Pearson Education Malaysia, Pte. Ltd.
Pearson Education Upper Saddle River, New Jersey

Notice: Care has been taken to confirm the accuracy of information presented in this book. The authors, editors, and the publisher, however, cannot accept any responsibility for errors or omissions or for consequences from application of the information in this book and make no warranty, express or implied, with respect to its contents.

The authors and publisher have exerted every effort to ensure that drug selections and dosages set forth in this text are in accord with current recommendations and practice at time of publication. However, in view of ongoing research, changes in government regulations, and the constant flow of information relating to drug therapy and reactions, the reader is urged to check the package inserts of all drugs for any change in indications or dosage and for added warning and precautions. This is particularly important when the recommended agent is a new and/or infrequently employed drug.

DEDICATION

This book is dedicated to my new husband and long time paramour, Al Renslow, and to all my students who have stretched me to grow in many new and interesting ways.

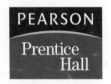

10 9 8 7 6 5 4 3 2 1

ISBN-13: 978-0-13-514655-2
ISBN: 0-13-514655-0

Karen Lee Fontaine received her bachelor's degree from Valparaiso University, Valparaiso, Indiana; a nursing degree from Lutheran Hospital in St. Louis, Missouri; and her master's degree in psychiatric nursing from Rush University, Chicago, Illinois. Karen is currently a Professor of Nursing at Purdue University Calumet, where she has been teaching for 26 years. She is also a certified sex therapist and maintains a private practice counseling individuals and couples.

Karen's publishing awards include the AJN Book of the Year Award 2000 for her text titled *Healing Practices: Alternative Therapies for Nursing*, Prentice Hall, and the Annual Nursing Book Review, Sigma Theta Tau 2000 award for *Mental Health Nursing*, Fourth Edition, Addison Wesley. Karen's distinguishing academic honors include the Outstanding Scholar for Purdue University Calumet for 2006–2007; Luther Christman Excellence in Published Writing Award, Gamma Phi Chapter, Sigma Theta Tau, Rush University, Chicago, Illinois, in 1997; and Distinguished Lecturer 1994–1995 from Sigma Theta Tau, International.

Karen is a frequent presenter at national and regional seminars covering psychiatric–mental health nursing practice, alternative therapies, sexuality, and sex therapy. She is a member of several professional associations, which include the International Society of Psychiatric–Mental Health Nurses, the National Alliance for the Mentally Ill (NAMI), National League for Nursing, and the American Association of Sex Educators, Counselors, and Therapists. Karen has also served on the Editorial Advisory Board for the *Journal of Couple and Relationship Therapy* since 2000.

Karen lives on a sand dune in Miller Beach with her new husband, Al, and their Greater Swiss Mountain dog, Whitney, and Great Dane, Roxie. She has three children, Jean-Marc, Simone, and Marcel, and three grandchildren, Danielle, Christopher, and Jaycee. Karen enjoys spending time with her family, art, reading, walking on the beach, and throwing "Goddess" parties with her friends.

THANK YOU!

I am most appreciative of the many professors who generously gave of their time and expertise to review chapters of this textbook. Without their valuable insights and suggestions, this book would not be what it is.

Reviewers for *Mental Health Nursing*, Sixth Edition

Kim Abel
Illinois Valley Community College
Oglesby, Illinois

Willie Mae Abel
Rowan-Cabarrus Community College
Salisbury, North Carolina

Canda Byrne
Northern Arizona University
Flagstaff, Arizona

Patricia A. Chin
California State University, Los Angeles
Los Angeles, California

Pattie G. Clark
Abraham Baldwin College
Tifton, Georgia

Susan Cohen
Broward Community College
Davie, Florida

Martha M. Colvin
Georgia College & State University
Milledgeville, Georgia

Rose E. Constantino
University of Pittsburgh
Pittsburgh, Pennsylvania

Lora Cruz
Davis & Elkins College
Elkins, West Virginia

Cindy Cunningham
Delaware Technical & Community College
Georgetown, Delaware

Susan Decker
University of Portland
Portland, Oregon

Leona F. Dempsey
University of Wisconsin
Oshkosh, Wisconsin

Barbara Fickley
Valencia Community College
Orlando, Florida

Shirley Lyon Garcia
McDowell Technical Community College
Marion, North Carolina

H. Lea Barbato Gaydos
University of Colorado, Colorado Springs
Colorado Springs, Colorado

Sandra Gustafson
Hibbing Community College
Hibbing, Minnesota

Paula Harrison
Miami University–Hamilton
Hamilton, Ohio

Evelyn L. Hoover
Randolph Community College
Asheboro, North Carolina

Katherine Purgatorio Howard
Charles E. Gregory School of Nursing
Raritan Bay Medical Center
Perth Amboy, New Jersey

Kim A. Jakopac
University of Louisiana at Lafayette
Lafayette, Louisiana

Dulcinea Kaufman
Great Bay Community College
Stratham, New Hampshire

Alice R. Kempe
Ursuline College
Pepper Pike, Ohio

Lynnette Kennison
Jacksonville University
Jacksonville, Florida

Laurinda Kettle
Pasadena City College
Pasadena, California

Karen Lipford
Chipola College
Marianna, Florida

Michael Landry
University of Louisiana at Lafayette
Lafayette, Louisiana

Maryjane LaRuffa
Erie Community College
Williamsville, New York

Michael Leaver
Samuel Merritt College
Oakland, California

Mary E. Malone
Jefferson Community & Technical College
Louisville, Kentucky

Michael W. Mangino
Suffolk County Community College
Selden, New York

Jeffrey Charles McManemy
St. Louis Community College
St. Louis, Missouri

Faye Mitchell
University of Southern Mississippi
Long Beach, Mississippi

CONTRIBUTORS

I am honored to have three contributors to the sixth edition of *Mental Health Nursing*. They are leaders in the profession and have long mentored, challenged, and supported me. This edition is enhanced by their expertise in nursing research, violence and disasters, and critical thinking. Thank you, Dee, Leslie, and Susan.

Dolores M. Huffman, RN, PhD
Associate Professor of Nursing
Purdue University Calumet
Hammond, Indiana
Using Research Evidence features

Leslie Rittenmeyer, PsyD, CNS, RN
Associate Professor of Nursing
Purdue University Calumet School of Nursing
Research Associate
Northwest Indiana Center for Evidence Based Practice

A Joanna Briggs Collaborating Center
Hammond, Indiana
Chapter 24: Community Violence
Chapter 25: Nursing Management of the Problems Associated With Exposure to Natural Disasters and Terrorism

Susan Siwinski-Hebel, RN, MSN, CCRC
Consultant
ROAD to Critical Thinking features

STUDENT AND INSTRUCTOR RESOURCE CONTRIBUTORS

Melissa Black
Greenville Technical College
Greenville, South Carolina

Jane Bostick
University of Missouri
Columbia, Missouri

Denice Davis
National Park Community College
Hot Springs, Arkansas

Susan Del Bene
Pace University
New York, New York

Patricia Freed
Saint Louis University
St. Louis, Missouri

Diane Gardner
University of West Florida
Pensacola, Florida

Rose Kutlenios
Wheeling Jesuit University
Wheeling, West Virginia

Dimitra Loukissa
North Park University
Chicago, Illinois

Marina Martinez-Kratz
Jackson Community College
Jackson, Mississippi

Virginia Osting
Radford University
Radford, Virginia

Patricia Posey-Goodwin
University of West Florida
Pensacola, Florida

Jean Rodgers
Hesston College
Hesston, Kansas

Cathy Weitzel, MSN, ARNP, BC
Wichita State University
Wichita, Kansas

Deborah Wilson
Howard University
Washington, DC

ACKNOWLEDGMENTS

I would like to express thanks to the many of those who have inspired, commented on, and in other ways assisted in the writing and publication of this book. On the publishing and production side at Prentice Hall, I was most fortunate to have an exceptional team of editors and support staff. My thanks go to Julie Alexander, Publisher, Pearson Health Sciences and Maura Connor, Editor-in-Chief. The Executive Acquisitions Editor, Pamela Lappies, and the Development Editor, Stephanie Klein, provided a great deal of support and guidance throughout this project. Thanks go to Sarah Wrocklage, Assistant to the Executive Acquisitions Editor, who was always willing to answer questions and find information. Thanks also go to Patrick Walsh, Managing Editor, Production; Anne Garcia, Production Liaison, and Maria Guglielmo, Senior Design Coordinator, for their commitment to the project and attention to detail. John J. Jordan, Media Product Manager, made a Herculean effort in integrating the video interviews and editing them for the ROAD videos on the CD-ROM. Heather Willison of S4Carlisle Publishing Services kept the book on schedule and brought these pages together.

I would like to extend a very special thanks to Catharine Sanderson and Rolfe Lawson, Expressive Arts Therapists at Four Winds–Saratoga. Their commitment, enthusiasm, generosity, senses of humor, and creative expertise, combined with the dedication and hard work of their Expressive Art therapy clients, are the result of the beautiful artwork and soulful poetry found in the part and chapter openers of this edition. Al Dodge, our photographer, worked his usual magic to capture this artwork and poetry in its greatest light and composition.

I am indebted to the past contributors for sharing their special knowledge of the discipline: Anita Finkleman, Carol Green-Nigro, Suzanne Beyea, Patriciann Brady, Brenda Lewis Cleary, Kathryn H. Kavanagh, Paula G. LeVeck, Pamela Marcus, Valerie Mattheisen, Susan F. Miller, Mary D. Moller, Ellen Marie Moore, Leslie Rittenmeyer, Mary J. Roehrig, Shirley Sennhauser, Joseph E. Smith, and Karen G. Vincent-Pounds. I give a special thanks to the reviewers for this sixth edition.

I appreciate the encouragement and support from many friends and family including Beata Halter, Sandy and Carl Werth, John Lee, Elaine and Jim Spicer, Patti Cleary, Brenda Ashley and Gary Johnson, Bill and Jean Robinson, Jack Rowe and Paul Vaclavik, George and MaryAnn McGuan, Matt and Geanie Dilts, Liz Locke, Fae Ann Meckelburg, Sue Eleuterio and Tom Sourlis, Terry and Bill Payonk, and Pam and Ken Shultz. I also thank my colleagues for inspiring me to continue: Leslie Rittenmeyer, Dee Huffman, Debby Kark, Lisa Hopp, and Ellen Moore. I could not have done it without you. Appreciation also goes to my immediate family: Al Renslow; Jean-Marc, Danielle, and Christopher Fontaine; Simone, Shawn, and Jaycee Hampton; Marcel and Jen Fontaine; and Jessie, Mandi, and Andrew Renslow.

Karen Lee Fontaine
Purdue University Calumet

Goals of *Mental Health Nursing*

Mental, behavioral, and social health problems are increasing throughout the world. According to recent world studies, neuropsychiatric conditions dominate the relatively short list of causes of years of life lived with a disability. In the United States, mental illnesses are the nation's second leading cause of disability, and mental illness has been classified as a public health crisis.

My goal is that nursing students and nurses in all professional practice specialties incorporate psychiatric nursing skills as they work with a variety of clients to improve the quality of life and achieve the highest possible level of functioning. Strong interpersonal and communication skills are critical to every area of practice. In addition, nurses encounter people with mental illnesses in inpatient, outpatient, and community sites including medical–surgical settings, intensive care units, emergency departments, obstetrics, and pediatrics. Thus, wherever nurses practice nursing, their mental health nursing skills will help them think critically and creatively as they empower clients by helping them restore their sense of value, strength, and ability to cope with life.

The sixth edition of *Mental Health Nursing* is designed to appeal to both traditional and nontraditional nursing students. The text is written in a user-friendly style for undergraduate students with the understanding that students and clients encompass a wide range of ages and ethnic groups, genders, and a variety of sexual identities. This diversity is reflected throughout the text.

The ROAD feature, new to this edition, is based on the acronym for four words: *Read, Observe, Assess,* and *Develop* a care plan. Appearing in 10 of the disorders chapters, it requires students to read about a person with a particular disorder in the chapter, view a video clip of the person on the CD-ROM that accompanies the book, assess the person by answering questions, and develop a care plan based on the assessment. By utilizing video with the nursing process and incorporating active learning, this new feature promotes understanding and stimulates critical thinking for students with various learning styles in an engaging, interactive manner.

This text is based on the belief that the practice of mental health nursing means taking time to be with clients and their families in deeply caring ways. To that end, nursing students are encouraged to engage in self-analysis in order to increase their self-understanding and self-acceptance. This is important because nurses who are able to clarify their own beliefs and values are less likely to be judgmental or to impose their own values and beliefs on clients.

Language is a powerful tool that reflects our beliefs and values. When we refer to someone with a disability by a label, we profess a belief that the disability is the most important feature about that person. This attitude is reflected when we label people as alcoholics, schizophrenics, or quadriplegics. In contrast, I use "people-first" language. I acknowledge the person first by saying, "a person with schizophrenia" or "a person who has a substance abuse problem." I believe these terms reflect people with options and choices who have the right to determine their own direction in life.

Philosophical and Theoretical Frameworks

Many theories and models are relevant to the practice of mental health nursing. It is the integration of these theories that creates the unique domain of mental health nursing as we respond to the social, cultural, environmental, and biological components of mental illness. It is important that we maintain the art of nursing which is being there, with another person or persons, in a context of caring. It involves compassion and sensitivity to each person within the context of her or his entire life.

The model basic to this text is one of competency. This is based on the belief that individuals and families are resourceful and have the capacity to grow and change. The competency model does not ignore pathology and dysfunction but emphasizes strengths and adaptation. The role of nursing is to empower people to respond and adapt to life circumstances. In this spirit, nurses develop collaborative partnerships with clients and families. The overall goal is to provide support, education, coping skills training, and advocacy necessary for successful living, learning, and working in the community. Client-sensitive nursing care helps people assume personal responsibility for where they are in their lives and for where they are going.

Traditional Strengths of *Mental Health Nursing*

In the sixth edition, *Mental Health Nursing* retains many of the strengths that have made it a popular "user-friendly" text for nursing students.

There is a heavy emphasis throughout the text on the development of effective communication skills. Each chapter in Unit 3, "Mental Disorders," features **Clinical Interactions,** illustrating a therapeutic interaction between a nurse and client. Chapter 7, "Illness Management: Communication and Psychoeducation," includes an example of a student–client interaction and an analysis thereof in the form of a process recording.

The nursing process is the organizing framework for chapters 11 through 25. This organizational consistency is extremely effective in helping students begin to assess, analyze, plan, implement, and evaluate in a systematic manner. **Focused Nursing Assessment** tables aid students in learning the type and range of assessment questions to ask particular clients. NANDA diagnoses are listed in tables. The planning and implementation of nursing care is described in detail in both text format and nursing care plan format. Goals and outcomes are specified for problems and diagnoses.

About the Artwork and Poetry

All of the artwork and corresponding descriptions at the opening of each unit and chapter are creative expressions of psychiatric clients involved in the Expressive Therapy program at Four Winds–Saratoga, Saratoga Springs, New York. In the Expressive Therapy groups, patients are encouraged to utilize a range of art media to depict and explore their internal landscapes, clarify and communicate their struggles, identify obstacles, as well as discover their strengths and create the ways to more effectively direct the journey toward a more gratifying life. Giving shape, form, and color to feelings promotes an increased sense of mastery over even the most painful affect. The communication through art then promotes the sharing of experiences in a safe and nonthreatening manner. The transformation of overwhelming feelings into the constructive communication embodied in the art object nurtures the clients' spontaneity and problem-solving skills in life, thereby promoting increased understanding of self and connection to others.

Submission of work for this book was voluntary and offered to clients at the end of each Expressive Therapy group over a period of 6 weeks. Once submitted, the appropriate legal releases of the work were secured from the individuals or their guardians, if under age 18. Many patients submitted work and were enthusiastic and appreciative of the invitation to contribute to the further education of professionals. By sharing their use of the modality of Expressive Therapy, they are sharing a very intimate dynamic expression of their search for direction, connection, strength, and hope in their individual healing process. Expressive Therapy makes manifest our belief that each individual is unique, as is his or her vision of life experience. To share that vision sparks our recognition of our common human experience. With that recognition comes the possibility of a society of greater benevolence, human dignity, and respect.

Catharine Sanderson, Expressive Arts Therapist, Four Winds–Saratoga

Focus Your Study for Success

Your textbook will help you learn and apply the concepts for your course as well as prepare you for your clinical experiences. This edition includes new and significantly updated material, new pedagogical features, and new emphases.

Chapter Introduction

Key Terms are listed to alert you to words used in the chapter that you should know. Next to the term is the page number where the definition is given.

Objectives point out the key concepts or knowledge that you will learn in the chapter.

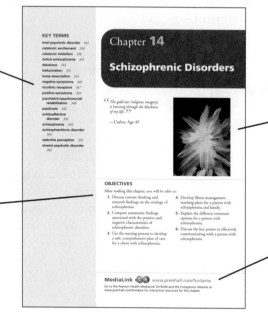

Art created by clients appears at the start of each chapter and unit. The artist's explanation of the artwork accompanies it.

MediaLink information mentions the CD-ROM and provides the Companion Website address, where you will find chapter-specific review questions, videos, case studies and more.

The ROAD to Critical Thinking

Your ability to learn, understand, and retain concepts improves when you put them to use. To help you make the most of your clinical experience, *Mental Health Nursing* presents the **ROAD to Critical Thinking**, an active-learning approach with real people who have been diagnosed with 10 psychiatric disorders. "ROAD" is an acronym for the following words that explain how to use this exercise in the 10 chapters with ROAD.

- **Read** about the client at the beginning of the chapter and throughout the chapter.

- **Observe** the client on the CD-ROM that accompanies this book.

- **Assess** the client by answering the questions at the end of the chapter in the book and that follow the video on the CD-ROM.

- **Develop a care plan** in the space provided on the CD-ROM. See Appendix C of the textbook for the completed ROAD care plan from Chapter 8 to use as a model. All the completed ROAD assessments and care plans are provided in the Instructor's Resource Manual and on the Instructor's Resource DVD-ROM.

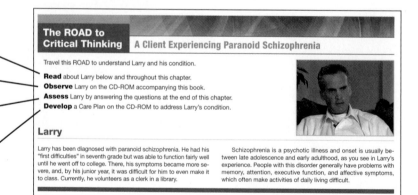

The ROAD to Critical Thinking

A Client Experiencing Paranoid Schizophrenia

Travel this ROAD to understand Larry and his condition.

Read about Larry below and throughout this chapter.
Observe Larry on the CD-ROM accompanying this book.
Assess Larry by answering the questions at the end of this chapter.
Develop a Care Plan on the CD-ROM to address Larry's condition.

Larry

Larry has been diagnosed with paranoid schizophrenia. He had his "first difficulties" in seventh grade but was able to function fairly well until he went off to college. There, his symptoms became more severe, and, by his junior year, it was difficult for him to even make it to class. Currently, he volunteers as a clerk in a library.

Schizophrenia is a psychotic illness and onset is usually between late adolescence and early adulthood, as you see in Larry's experience. People with this disorder generally have problems with memory, attention, executive function, and affective symptoms, which often make activities of daily living difficult.

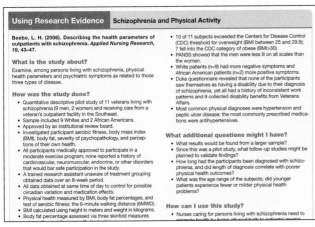

Using Research Evidence boxes present a specific study used to support nursing actions and show you how to read and evaluate it.

Focused Nursing Assessments aid students in learning the type and range of assessment questions to ask particular clients.

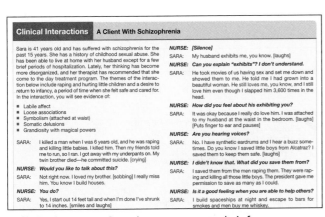

Clinical Interactions boxes present a brief client history and then provide clinical interactions between the client and nurse to promote effective therapeutic communication skills.

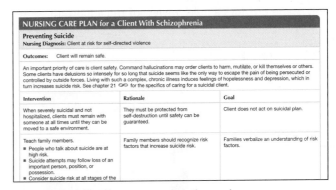

Nursing Care Plans appear at the end of the Nursing Process sections to help you see the outcomes, interventions, and short-term goals involved in nursing care.

Complementary/Alternative Therapies features describe the use of non-traditional treatments that can be used to enhance or replace medical treatments.

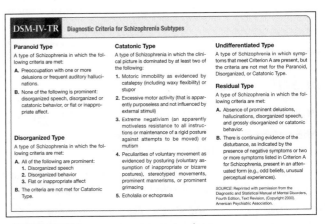

DSM-IV-TR boxes present up-to-date, complete DSM-IV-TR diagnostic criteria.

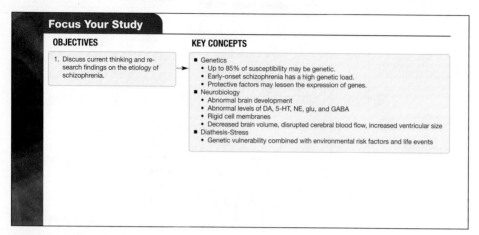

Focus Your Study diagrams at the end of each chapter link the learning objectives for the chapter to the key concepts that support them. This visual study guide provides a quick review of the important content from the chapter.

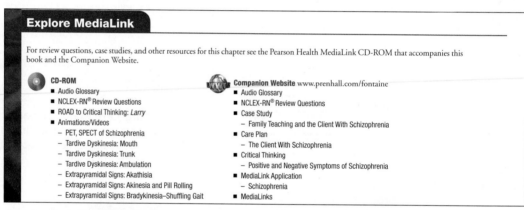

Explore MediaLink boxes conclude each chapter and list specific items that appear on the accompanying Pearson Health MediaLink CD-ROM and the Companion Website. MediaLink icons appear throughout the chapter to indicate topics in the textbook that are further explained on the accompanying media supplements.

Other Features

- **Nursing Process** sections walk you through the steps as they relate to the disorder.

- **Vignettes** throughout the book give insights into brief client scenarios and their applications relevant to chapter topics.

- **NCLEX-RN® Review Questions** at the end of each chapter help to identify areas needing further study. Answers appear in Appendix D.

- **Cross-reference icons** ∞ direct you to other chapters for related information.

RESOURCES FOR TEACHING AND LEARNING

To enhance the teaching and learning process, the following supplements have been developed in close correlation with the new edition of *Mental Health Nursing*.

Student Assessment...

Customized Study Plans...

The path to student success and nursing excellence in psychiatric mental-health nursing!

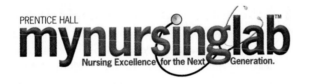

MyNursingLab is a user-friendly site that gives students the opportunity to test themselves on key concepts and skills in psychiatric mental health nursing. By using *MyNursingLab*, students can track their own progress through the course and use customized, media-rich, study plan activities to help them achieve success in the classroom, in clinical, and ultimately on the NCLEX-RN®. *MyNursingLab* can also help instructors monitor class progress as students move through the curriculum.

To take a tour and see the power of **mynursinglab** , go to *www.mynursinglab.com*.

Ask your Pearson Education sales representative for more information and packaging options for including *MyNursingLab* in your curriculum.

For Students

Pearson Health MediaLink CD-ROM.

The CD-ROM that accompanies this textbook contains all 10 ROAD features complete with video clips, assessment questions, and templates in which you will develop care plans. It also includes NCLEX-RN®-style questions with rationales, and videos and animations to help you understand and visualize more difficult concepts in mental health nursing care.

Companion Website. www.prenhall.com/fontaine

This chapter-specific, interactive online study guide includes modules for Objectives, Audio Glossary, NCLEX-RN®-style questions, Case Studies, Care Plans, Critical Thinking Exercises, and more. The Companion Website also offers two types of resource information relevant to the chapter topic: Books for Clients & Families and Community Resources.

For Instructors

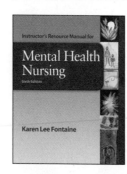

Instructor's Resource Manual.

This manual contains a wealth of material to help faculty plan and manage the Mental Health nursing course. It includes chapter overviews, PowerPoint Lecture Slides and Concepts for Lecture linked to chapter learning objectives, Classroom and Clinical Activities, and the entire test bank, complete with rationales and descriptors. Included are answers to all 10 ROAD features. The IRM also guides faculty in how to assign and use the resources on the Pearson Health MediaLink CD-ROM and Companion Website.

Instructor's Resource DVD-ROM.

This valuable resource provides an electronic test bank, comprehensive PowerPoint Lecture Slides, a collection of images from the textbook in PowerPoint format, and the same animations and videos that appear on the Pearson Health MediaLink CD-ROM that accompanies the textbook. In addition, the full-length ROAD videos are included for classroom use. This product is also available on CD-ROMs for those instructors who do not have access to a DVD drive.

Online Course Management Systems. This useful resource for online course learning and management is available in WebCT, Blackboard, Angel, Moodle, and other applications. Included are interactive modules with PowerPoint Lecture Slides, review questions, case studies, care plans, and more. For more information about adopting an online course management system to accompany *Mental Health Nursing,* please contact your Pearson Education sales representative or go online to *www.prenhall.com/demo.*

SPECIAL FEATURES

DETAILED CONTENTS

Unit 1

Foundations of Mental Health Nursing

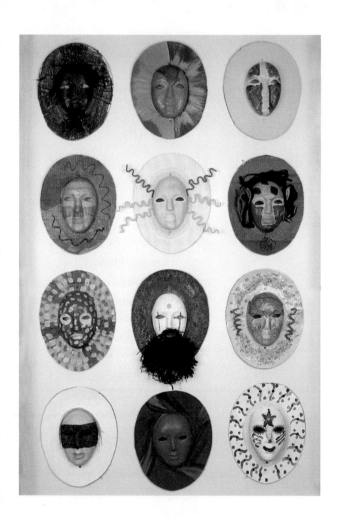

❝ The faces of many, together creating the courage to give vision and voice to their sense of self. ❞

—An artistic collaboration from several patients at Four Winds-Saratoga

Chapter 1

Introduction to Mental Health Nursing

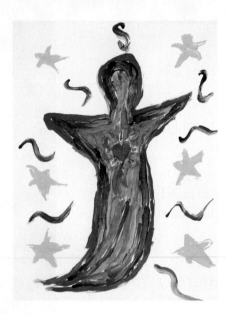

I am breaking out of the black ring of trauma that surrounds me. My inner core is secure.

—Sharon, Age 43

OBJECTIVES

After reading this chapter, you will be able to:

1. Describe the continuum from mental health to persistent and severe mental illness.
2. Compare and contrast the theoretical assumptions of neurobiological and prebiological models of mental disorders.
3. Apply the nursing process to mental health nursing.
4. Distinguish between the therapeutic relationship and the nursing process.
5. Discuss current issues in mental health nursing.

MediaLink www.prenhall.com/fontaine

Go to the Pearson Health MediaLink CD-ROM and the Companion Website at www.prenhall.com/fontaine for interactive resources for this chapter.

One of the first questions students ask at the beginning of their psychiatric nursing course is, "What is mental illness, or, for that matter, what is mental health?" It is not an easy question to answer. Cultural, family, and individual beliefs strongly influence what is defined as mental illness or mental health. For example, in one culture, seeing things others do not see (hallucinations) is a valued part of religious experience and is something to be desired. In another culture, hallucinating is evidence of insanity and is something to be avoided. Cultures, families, and individuals often define mental illness as behaviors, feelings, or ways of thinking that are unusual to them or not easily understood by them.

This lack of understanding often leads to negative moral judgments, or **stigma**, about people who are labeled "persistently and severely mentally ill." American attitudes toward, and stereotypes about, mental illness include the belief that persistently and severely mentally ill is incurable or that people are capable of bringing on or turning off mental illness at will, that it is caused by bad parenting or sinful behavior, and that people with mental illness are dangerous. These social attitudes determine how people with mental illness are treated. For example, if we believe someone is evil, we will punish her or him. If we believe someone is dangerous, we fear, avoid, or confine that person (Halter, 2004). Other examples of attitudes and resulting treatment are as follows:

Attitude	Treatment
Evil	Punish
Possessed	Exorcise
Inhuman	Abandon, disenfranchise
Bizarre	Avoid, degrade, isolate
Weak	Institutionalize
Sick	Medicate, hospitalize
Dangerous	Confine, control
Incompetent	Assume responsibility

Unfortunate stereotypes like these often keep people from seeking treatment or contribute to them feeling ashamed of needing treatment. The President's New Freedom Commission on Mental Health (2003; www.mentalhealthcommission.gov) stated that the stigma of mental illness prevents many people from seeking help for mental disorders. *Self-stigma* is agreeing with the stereotype and turning it against oneself. An example is, "People with mental illness are failures. I'm severely and persistently mentally ill; therefore I must be a failure. Why should I even try to work or go to school? I'm severely and persistently mentally ill and not capable of doing it."

Mental disorders are *brain disorders* that variably affect aspects of cognition, emotion, and behavior. The tragedy, however, is that these disorders continue to be cloaked in stigma and discrimination, the effects of which are often more damaging than the day-to-day struggles of living with an impairment. Another tragedy is that 25% of people with persistent and severe mental illness end up as *victims* of violent crime—more than 11 times the rate of the general population. Victimization can lead to anxiety or depression, complicating preexisting mental disorders (Teplin, McClelland, Abram, & Weiner, 2005).

As you begin the study of mental health nursing, you may believe many of society's myths and stereotypes about psychiatric clients. As you progress through your course, you will begin to realize that there is not a universally accepted definition of "normal" or "abnormal," nor are there clear parameters of mental health versus mental illness.

MENTAL HEALTH AND MENTAL ILLNESS

Mental health and mental illness can be viewed as end points on a *continuum*, with movement back and forth throughout life. You will study the continuum from several levels:

- Physical level, in the structure and function of the brain
- Personal level, in caring for and about the self
- Interpersonal level, in interactions with others
- Societal level, in social conditions and the cultural context

These levels interact in such a way that it is often difficult to separate the effect of each level. If a person's neurotransmitters do not function correctly, that person may have great difficulty organizing his or her thoughts. Disorganized thinking may interfere with the ability to perform activities of daily living. Because of poor hygiene and the inability to communicate clearly, others may shun the individual. As the person becomes more isolated, they may further lose contact with reality. If adequate community resources are not available, the person may become homeless.

In some cases, mental health disruption may begin at the cultural level. An example is the impact of sexism on the mental health of women in many parts of the world. Cultural sexism allows men to treat women as less worthy members of society. This treatment contributes to low self-esteem and potential depression. Disruptions can occur at any level; however, each level is so intertwined with the others, it is often difficult to pinpoint the original source of the distress. Personal, interpersonal, and cultural factors interact in ways that produce movement toward mental health or mental illness (Figure 1.1 ■). If more factors are on the mental illness side of the continuum, the balance will shift toward that end of the continuum. Likewise, the presence of more factors associated with mental health will shift the balance toward mental health.

MediaLink

MediaLink Application, Overcoming Stigma

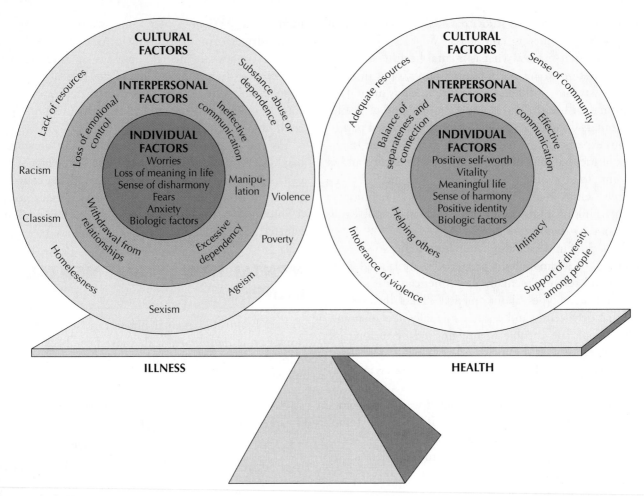

Figure 1.1 ■ Factors contributing to the mental health–mental illness continuum.

Mental Illness

Movement toward the **mental illness** end of the continuum may begin with a sense of disharmony with aspects of living that are distressing to the individual, family, friends, or community. Some aspects may be primarily distressing to the individual, such as feeling miserable, spending a great deal of time worrying, and suffering from multiple fears and anxieties. Other aspects may be distressing to family and friends, such as the individual's withdrawal from relationships, inability to communicate coherently, manipulation, and emotional outbursts. Other aspects are distressing to society, such as an individual's violence, substance abuse, and dependence. Contributing cultural factors include racism, classism, sexism, inadequate access to health care, and **disempowerment**, or the taking away of the power or authority of the self, of many individuals and groups. All these aspects are interdependent and interactive. They influence the development of disorders, the clinical signs and symptoms, the course and prognosis of the disorders, and the responses to therapeutic interventions.

People with mental illness are often disempowered in many societies, including the United States. This means that they have little voice or power in what happens to them, which results in inadequate and helpless feelings. In the past, many professionals had the idea that clients must be protected from real life and could not have jobs, careers, college degrees, apartments, or homes. Too often, client desires and preferences were simply ignored.

One goal of mental health nursing is to empower mental health clients by helping them restore their sense of value, strength, and ability to cope with life. **Empowerment** means that people have both the authority and the confidence to choose and act on options. The goal of empowerment is that clients regain or attain meaningful roles, relationships, and activities. Empowerment and recovery are covered in more detail in chapter 3 ∞. Unit 2 focuses on illness management and recovery to help clients move on with their lives.

Mental Health

Mental health is not a concrete goal; it is a lifelong process and includes a sense of harmony and balance for the individual, family, friends, and community. Mental health differs from the mere absence of a mental disorder in that it is a growing toward a potential, an inner feeling of aliveness. Movement toward the mental health end of the continuum brings with it a sense of harmony and balance, with a general feeling of vitality. Individual aspects may include a feeling of self-worth, a positive identity, and a sense of accomplishment. Aspects relating to family and friends may include a balance between separateness and connection, the ability to be intimate, and the desire or willingness to help others in need. Societal aspects may include tolerance for others who are different from oneself and the development of a sense of community. These aspects are also interdependent and interactive in the process of mental health.

One aspect of mental health is **social–emotional intelligence**. This idea puts emotions at the center of skills for living. Social–emotional intelligence encompasses the following six abilities (Goleman, 1995; Vaillant, 2003):

1. Recognizing emotions as they occur
2. Managing emotions internally
3. Emotional self-control
4. Recognizing emotions in others
5. Managing relationships
6. Delaying gratification to achieve a goal

We send and receive emotional signals in every interaction. *Emotional contagion* describes the tendency to automatically mimic the emotions we see in another person. This transmission of emotion is often subtle and outside of our awareness. Just seeing someone express an emotion can create that same feeling in us. Thus, seeing someone cry in great sorrow can bring tears to our own eyes.

Another aspect of mental health is that of **resilience**, or the ability to emerge relatively unscathed from negative life events. Resilience includes personality and temperament factors, along with specific skills and abilities that help people adapt and cope effectively. A resilient person adapts to changes, forms nurturing relationships, has good social skills, and is able to use the problem-solving process. Resilient people have a number of strengths or *coping styles*:

- *Insight:* They are able to ask themselves tough questions and give honest answers.
- *Anticipation:* They consider consequences of possible future events and consider alternative solutions.
- *Independence:* They recognize their own, and others', boundaries.
- *Relationships:* They develop intimate relationships that balance a mature regard for one's own needs with the capacity to give to someone else. They turn to others for support.
- *Initiative:* They take charge of and solve problems.
- *Creativity:* They find order and purpose in the midst of troubling experiences and painful feelings.
- *Humor:* They find the comical in the tragic.

- *Optimistic approach to life:* They expect the best outcome.
- *Morality:* They have an informed conscience that works toward a good personal life for themselves and all humankind.

To be healthy means to be whole, and to be whole has a spiritual quality to it. **Spirituality** is that part of us that deals with relationships and values and addresses questions of purpose and meaning in life. Spirituality unites people and is inclusive, not exclusive, in nature. It is not loyal to one group, continent, or religion. Although spirituality is not a religion, being involved in a particular religion is a way some people enhance their spirituality. Yet people can be very spiritual and not be religious. Spirituality involves individuals, family, friends, and community, as described in the following list.

- Individual
  - Moral values
  - Beliefs about the meaning and purpose of life and death
  - Provides a sense of identity
- Family and friends
  - Search for meaning through relationships
  - Feeling of connection with others
  - Feeling of connection with an external power often identified as God, a Supreme Being, or The Great Mystery
- Community
  - A sense of a common humanity
  - Belief in the fundamental sacredness and unity of all life
  - A sense of fairness and justice to all members of society

Our spiritual health is expressed through humor, compassion, faith, forgiveness, courage, and creativity. Spirituality enables us to develop healthy relationships based on acceptance, respect, and compassion.

Spiritual activities may include meditating or praying, religious activities, mystical experiences, self-help groups, caring for others, or enjoying nature. Health care professionals often consider spiritual problems those that question spiritual values, which may or may not be related to organized religion, the loss or questioning of faith, or problems associated with converting to a new faith (American Psychiatric Association [APA], 2000; North American Nursing Diagnosis Association [NANDA], 2003). In a broader sense, spiritual problems are related to fear, anger, greed, guilt, and worry. These barriers can be described as those daily problems that drain our energy and immobilize us. Left unresolved, they can prevent our development as healthy, spiritual beings (Pesut, 2004).

SIGNIFICANCE OF MENTAL DISORDERS

Mental, behavioral, and social health problems are increasing throughout the world. According to recent world studies, neuropsychiatric conditions dominate the relatively short list of causes of years of life lived with a disability. Hundreds of millions of women, men, and children suffer from mental illnesses; others experience distress from the consequences of violence, abuse, dislocation, poverty, and exploitation. The number of persons with major mental illnesses will continue to grow in the decades to come. One contributing factor is the increase in population, which brings a corresponding increase in the number of people with mental illness. Also, the rates of depression have increased worldwide in recent decades. Depression is now seen at younger ages and in greater frequency in countries as different as Lebanon, Taiwan, the United States, and countries of Western Europe (Mathers et al., 2004).

In the United States, mental illnesses are the nation's second leading cause of disability, and mental illness has been classified as a public health crisis. About half of all Americans will have a mental illness during their lifetime. Half of these cases start by age 14 and three fourths start by age 24 (Table 1.1 ■). Although a range of effective, well-documented treatments exist for most mental disorders, nearly 60% of all Americans who have a mental illness do not seek treatment. Of those who sought treatment, 23% saw a general medical provider, 16% saw a nonmedical mental health specialist (e.g., PhD, licensed psychologist), 12% went to a psychiatrist, 8% were treated by a human services provider, and 7% were treated by an alternative medical provider (treatment could be received by more than one source). Those treated in the general medical sector had fewer than two visits, whereas those treated in the mental health sector had more than seven visits. Most people in the United States are either untreated or poorly treated. Lack of coverage by insurance companies, stigma, the belief that disorders are under personal control, and the complexity of the mental health delivery system fail those in the United States who suffer from severe and persistent mental illness (Halter, 2004; Wang et al., 2005).

THEORIES OF MENTAL DISORDERS

Neurobiological Theory

Neurobiological theory focuses on genetic factors, neuroanatomy, neurophysiology, and biological rhythms as they relate to the cause, course, and prognosis of mental disorders. Chapter 6 ∞ presents neurobiology and behavior in detail. Additionally, genetic and neurobiological data are integrated into all chapters. The belief that mental illness is a brain disorder is basic to this text.

There is an increased understanding how mental disorders arise from neurodevelopmental or neurodegenerative processes; how life experiences intersect with these processes to help or hinder the development of disease processes; and how genes, molecules, and circuits interact dynamically in health and disease. Box 1.1 lists the various brain imaging techniques used to assess pathologic structure or function.

In the past, nurses have talked about psychological problems as separate from biological processes in the brain, as if the mind and the brain were separate entities. This mind–brain dualism argued that the processes and products of the mind had little to do with the processes and products of the brain. The new framework believes that all functions of the mind reflect functions of the brain. However, the details of the relationship between the brain and mental processes are still not understood. Kandel (1999) identifies *five principles* regarding the relationship of the mind to the brain:

1. All mental processes, including those conscious and unconscious, result from operations of the brain. Behavioral disorders are disturbances of brain function.
2. Genes are important determinants of how neurons function and thus exert significant control over behavior.

TABLE 1.1	Mental Disorders: Lifetime Prevalence and Age of Onset in the United States	
Disorder	**Lifetime Prevalence Estimates, %**	**Median Age of Onset, Years**
Anxiety disorders	28.8	11
Impulse control disorders	24.8	11
Mood disorders	20.8	30
Substance use disorders	14.6	20

SOURCE: Adapted from Kessler, R. C., Berglund, P., Demler, O., Jin, R., Merikangas, K. R., & Walters, E. E. (2005). Lifetime prevalence and age-of-onset distributions of DSM-IV disorders in the National Comorbidity Survey Replication. *Archives of General Psychiatry, 6297,* 590–592.

3. Social and developmental factors modify the expression of genes and thus the function of the neurons. All of nurture is ultimately expressed as nature.

4. Learning creates changes in neuronal connections. Abnormalities of behavior can be induced by social conditions.

BOX 1.1	Brain Imaging Techniques

Magnetic Resonance Imaging (MRI)

Distinguishes gray and white matter in three dimensions; identifies structural abnormalities.

Diffusion Tensor Imaging (DTI)

Looks deeper into the brain than an MRI; maps the fiber bundles under the brain's tissue.

Magnetic Resonance Spectroscopy (MRS)

Expands MRI readings by adding radioactive tracers; identifies structural abnormalities in three dimensions and physiological abnormalities.

Functional Magnetic Resonance Imaging (fMRI)

Locates metabolic changes associated with task performance throughout the brain.

Positron Emission Tomography (PET)

Uses radioactive tracers and measures physiological processes in the brain such as blood flow, metabolic functions based on glucose utilization, density of neurotransmitters, location of neuroreceptors, and intricate brain circuitry; much clearer than SPECT.

Single Photon Emission Computerized Tomography (SPECT)

Measures the same physiological processes as PET but costs less and is more widely available; measures brain blood flow based on distribution of a radiotracer; useful in monitoring the effects of medications on brain functions.

Magnetoencephalography (MEG)

Uses superconducting sensors to measure neuromagnetic fields generated by brain activity; provides information similar to EEG but is more accurate.

Xenon Computerized Tomography (Xe/CT)

Combines anatomic and blood flow imaging. CT is done before, during, and after inhalation of a mixture of xenon gas and oxygen. Low cost used primarily for brain bleeds; awaiting U.S. Food and Drug Administration approval.

Neurometrics

Measures the electrophysiology of the brain, especially increased or decreased beta, alpha, theta, and delta waves.

Cerebral Blood Flow (CBF)

Measures the circulation of blood in a given brain region; blood flow to gray matter and white matter can be determined.

Computer Electroencephalographic Tomography (CET)

Converts electrical signals into an electrical activity map of the brain; less accurate than PET but costs less and can be repeated without risk.

---

5. Counseling and therapy can create long-term changes through learning, which produces changes in gene expression.

Genomics

Research teams throughout the world are attempting to determine the causes of mental disorders. They hope not only to identify the genes in such diseases, but also to design therapies that can better treat or even cure. *Genetics* is the study of single genes and their effects. Genomics is the study of all the genes, including their function, their interaction, and their role in a variety of disorders. Box 1.2 lists organizations involved in genomics.

The **genome**, a word for the full complement of genetic information, is tightly packed into 23 pairs of chromosomes, each of which carries thousands of genes. All told, humans have about 30,000 genes. All genes are composed of just four different chemicals linked together in myriad combinations and lengths. Those chemicals, which scientists represent with the letters "A" (adenine), "C" (cytosine), "G" (guanine), and "T" (thymine), comprise a sort of genetic alphabet. Now that the Human Genome Project is complete (2003), we know that 99.9% of this sequence is shared among every human being. What we do not know is all the differences in the remaining 0.1% that make us individuals and, more importantly, which of those differences make us susceptible to disease.

This is the mystery that gene hunters are trying to solve. To do that, scientists compare the DNA of healthy and ill people. Using sophisticated technology to slowly sift through the 3.1 billion pairs of As, Cs, Gs, and Ts, they hope to identify the subtle differences that affect disease.

BOX 1.2	Organizations Involved with Genomics

International Society of Nurses in Genetics (ISONG)
121 Sunset Hills Road, Suite 130
Reston, Virginia 20190
703-437-4377
www.isong.org

Genomic Resource Centre
World Health Organization
Avenue Appia 20
CH-1211 Geneva 27
Switzerland
(41)-22-791-21-11
www.who.int/tenomics/en/

Cochrane Collaboration
PO Box 726
Oxford UK
OX2 7UX
44-1865-310138
www.cochrane.org/index0.htm

Genes determine *phenotype*—the structure, function, and other biological characteristics—of the cell in which genes are expressed. In any given cell, 80% to 90% of the genes are repressed or inactive. The 10% to 20% of the genes that are expressed, or active, make specific proteins that specify the character of that cell and determine, for example, whether the cell is a liver cell or a brain cell. Everything we do affects the activity of our genes in every cell and genes are turned on and off throughout life. Genes do not determine destiny. Genes set boundaries for behavior, but within the boundaries is immense room for variation determined by experience, choice, and chance.

Genes convey only *susceptibility* to mental disorders, not disease per se. It is also believed that multiple genes combine with one another and with environmental factors to cause mental illness. Given this, it is possible for people to have low, moderate, or high "doses" of the risk factors that predispose a person to mental illness. Using schizophrenia as an example, those with very high doses may experience the classic symptoms, such as disorganized thinking, bizarre behavior, inappropriate affect, hallucinations, and delusions. Other individuals with only moderate doses of the risk factors may merely demonstrate seemingly benign characteristics, such as odd speech, social dysfunction, or impaired attention. The more severe the psychopathology, the stronger the genetic loading for the disorder. Understanding the genetic contribution will allow us to redefine mental disorders. Currently, disorders are grouped by presenting symptoms. In the future, syndromes will be defined by genotype, which may be very different from the current classification (Insel & Collins, 2003).

Genetic anticipation may be apparent in some families. "Genetic anticipation" means that there is a progressively earlier onset of mental illness in successive generations or an increase in the severity of the disorder in successive generations, or both.

The *nature versus nurture* dilemma poses the question: Are we mainly products of our genes or of our environment? Both models are reductionistic and are based on very narrow theories. Those who say mental disorders are primarily caused by nature (neurobiology) fail to address the role of psychosocial precipitating factors. Those who say mental disorders are primarily caused by nurture (environment) oversimplify the role of stressors and do not address the interaction of environment with biology. Mental disorders are a result of the interaction between genes and environment.

The **diathesis–stress model** proposes that, in a biologically vulnerable person, when exposed to stressors or triggers, disease develops. It is as if there must be a second hit to convert genetic vulnerability into brain disorders. This second hit could be a perinatal injury, a toxin, and/or life experiences. Many of these stressors appear to be of normal intensity but they lead to catastrophic symptoms. Note that genetic influence is not static but rather reacts to and interacts with environmental experiences. Most people go through life with predispositions to mental disorders that are never expressed. The relationship between stress and mental disorders is nonspecific. That is, the same illness can be brought on by a variety of stressors, and the same stressors can bring on a wide variety of illnesses. In addition, the presence of an active mental disorder may lower the threshold for coping with stress (Day & Horton-Deutsch, 2004; Kendler, 2005).

Recent studies demonstrate that exposure to stressful life events is significantly influenced by genetic factors. In other words, people do not randomly experience stressful life events; rather, some people have a persistent tendency to put themselves into situations with a high probability of stressful outcomes. It is believed that this personality trait has a genetic basis (Kendler, Karkowski, & Prescott, 1999).

We must be careful not to equate the term *running in families* with hereditary causation. For example, if one of your parents is a nurse, there is a higher chance you will end up being a nurse. In this example, the simplistic and erroneous conclusion is that being a nurse is genetically determined. In studying the genetic factors in mental disorders, researchers must first establish that there is a higher than expected rate of incidence within families. The next step is to identify which parts are due to genetic factors and which parts are due to environmental factors. Studying monozygotic (identical) and dizygotic (fraternal) twins helps determine possible genetic influences. If the incidence of a mental disorder is greater among monozygotic twins than among dizygotic twins, there is at least some degree of genetic influence. However, environmental variables are also a factor, even with monozygotic twins. The best twin studies are those in which monozygotic twins have been separated at birth and reared separately. When these twins demonstrate a higher than expected incidence of a mental disorder, a strong degree of genetic influence is likely. It is important to understand genetic mapping because hereditary factors appear to play a role in the development of many mental disorders.

Research in *behavioral genetics* has lagged behind other research in understanding health and illness. Behavioral genetics looks at the contribution of genetic variability to behaviors. For example, the desire to engage in physical activity, the choice of intervals between meals, and a dietary preference for fats may have a genetic component that relates to a tendency toward thinness or obesity. Continuing research will better elucidate how genetically determined preferences interact with environmental factors. The degree to which certain behaviors are genetically or environmentally based may vary among individuals and among populations (Devlin, Yanovski, & Wilson, 2000).

The International HapMap Project is a multicountry effort to identify genes that affect health, disease, and individual responses to medications and environmental factors. It is hoped that this will enable the customization of medications to maximize effectiveness and minimize side effects, referred to as **pharmacogenomics**. Rather than the current trial-and-error method of figuring out which medications work best for a client, primary care providers will be able to examine each person's genomic information when making that determination. In addition, genome-based research will be critically important in the development of new drugs for mental illness.

Gender

Much of who we are, as female or male, is defined by brain differences, physiology, and hormones, as well as society's efforts at socialization into gender roles and expectations. Every human's personality is genetically driven and individually developed. The male brain is 10% larger than the female brain. The female brain has a larger corpus callosum, which connects both hemispheres. Female brains produce more serotonin (5-HT), the neurotransmitter that inhibits aggressive behavior. Males have much higher levels of testosterone and lower levels of 5-HT, creating more potential for aggressive behavior. We have much to learn regarding gender and brain organization and cognitive functioning. There are gender differences in prevalence of most mental disorders. We do not know why women and men are more vulnerable to different disorders (Kessler, Demler, et al., 2005).

Females

Anxiety disorders
Schizoaffective disorder
Depression
Dysthymic disorder
Eating disorders
Borderline, histrionic, dependent personality disorders
Alzheimer's disease

Males

Learning disorders
Autistic disorder
Asperger disorder
Attention deficit/hyperactivity disorder
Tourette syndrome
Conduct disorder
Substance use disorders
Schizophrenia
Antisocial, schizoid, schizotypal paranoid, narcissistic, obsessive–compulsive personality disorders
Vascular dementia

Both Genders

Bipolar disorder
Oppositional defiant disorder (after puberty)
Avoidant personality disorder

Neurotransmission

Theories of **neurotransmission** in mental disorders are concerned with the levels of biogenic amines (norepinephrine, serotonin, dopamine, acetylcholine), the amino acids (γ-aminobutyric acid, glutamate, and glycine), neuropeptides, neurohormones, and gases (nitric oxide and carbon monoxide) in the brain. As an electrical impulse travels to the nerve endings, neurotransmitters (chemical messengers) are released at the synaptic junction. These neurotransmitters react with the neuronal receptors, which allow the impulse to be conducted through the next nerve cell. Mental disorders are often related to a deficiency or an excess of neurotransmitters, an imbalance among the various neurotransmitters, or a modulation by neurotransmitters by one another. In other cases, there is a change in the sensitivity or the shape of the neuronal receptors, resulting in altered transmission of impulses. Neurotransmission is described in detail in chapter 6 ∞.

Biological Rhythms

Circadian rhythms are regular fluctuations of a variety of physiologic factors over a period of 24 hours. Temperature, energy, sleep, arousal, motor activity, appetite, hormones, and mood all demonstrate circadian rhythms. The biological clock is located in the suprachiasmatic nucleus in the hypothalamus and may be desynchronized by external or internal factors. An example of external desynchronization is jet lag: decreased energy level, reduced ability to concentrate, and mood variations resulting from rapid time zone changes. Internal desynchronization is demonstrated in some mental disorders when there are alterations in adrenal rhythm, temperature patterns, and sleep patterns. Chapter 6 ∞ provides further information on circadian rhythms.

Importance of the Neurobiological Model

Our understanding of mental disorders has been revolutionized by contemporary knowledge of the biological components of behavior, affect, cognition, and interpersonal relationships. Recognizing genetic factors in mental disorders minimizes the tendency to blame the victim or the family for the disorder. Mental disorders are no-fault disorders because none of us has a choice about the genes we get or the genes we give. In addition, problems in early attachment or trauma anytime in life lead to lack of integration among neural networks. When integration is disrupted, the networks of cognition, emotions, and behavior are disrupted. Understanding brain function helps you understand how neurobiology and psychotherapy converge. Neuroscientists believe that psychotherapy is effective to the extent that it contributes to change in physiologic processes in the brain. Psychotherapy can be viewed as an enriched environment designed to increase the growth of neurons and integrate neural networks. Psychotherapeutic experiences—such as interpretation, reality testing, expressing feelings, trying new behaviors, and connecting thoughts and feelings—stimulate the brain to develop new methods of processing and organizing information.

The breakthroughs in the Human Genome Project mean that we must be prepared to integrate genomic-based tests and therapies into nursing practice. As nurses' roles expand, nurses will be expected to complete a genetic family history assessment, teach clients about the genetic component of disease, counsel individuals and families before genetic testing, and help clients clarify their preferences for diagnosis and treatment (Jenkins, Grady, & Collins, 2005; Prows, Glass, Nicol, Skirton, & Williams, 2005).

Older Theories

The following theories and models focus on many different aspects of the person as a biopsychosocial being. Some focus on personality, others on behavior, and still others on learning. The theories are organized under the following headings, with representative theorists noted for each category: intrapersonal, social–interpersonal, behavioral, and cognitive. These nonbiological theories were favored during a time of limited understanding of neurobiology and limited medication options. The advances of genomics and neuroimaging technology are currently the major theories. Because the psychological and social aspects of mental illness are significant, we must be careful not to discard the older theories. Flaskerud and Wuerker (1999) summed this up well when they said: "Mental health nursing in the 21st century will have an expanding neuropsychiatric emphasis; it will, however, maintain its nursing focus, its caring, and its sensitivity to the human condition" (p. 15).

Intrapersonal Theory

Intrapersonal theory focuses on the behaviors, feelings, thoughts, and experiences of each person. Mental disorders are viewed as arising from within the individual. The intrapersonal theory of Sigmund Freud was the first to be developed. One of his great contributions was to identify components of the mind. Although there are many different versions than the original model, the concepts of consciousness, id, ego, superego, and defense mechanisms are widely used today. Erik Erikson expanded Freud's theory of psychosexual development to include the life cycle.

The most essential aspect of contemporary intrapersonal theory is the idea of the importance of early experience. Intrapersonal theorists believe that personality is more strongly shaped by events occurring in the earliest years of life than by those occurring later. It is believed that symptoms of mental disorders are rooted in events in the first 5 years of life.

Sigmund Freud Freud divided all aspects of consciousness into three categories: conscious, preconscious, and unconscious. The first category, **conscious**, includes thoughts, feelings, and experiences that are easily remembered, such as current addresses, phone numbers, anniversaries and birthdays, and recent enjoyable events. The second category, **preconscious** (sometimes called subconscious), includes thoughts, feelings, and experiences that have been forgotten but can easily be recalled, such as old phone numbers or addresses, the feeling a woman had during the birth of her first child, the name of a first girlfriend, and the animosity one felt toward a former boss. The third category, **unconscious**, encompasses thoughts, feelings, experiences, and dreams that cannot be brought to conscious thought or remembered (Freud, 1935).

Freud theorized that there are three components to the personality:

- The id
- The ego
- The superego

Each component has individualized functions, but the three are so closely interrelated it is difficult to separate their individual effects on a person's behavior.

The biological and psychological drives that a person is born with constitute the **id**. The id holds in reserve all psychic energy, which in turn furnishes the power for the ego and the superego. The id has no knowledge of outside reality and functions totally within its own subjective reality. The id is self-centered, and its major concern is instant gratification. The **ego** is the component of the personality that mediates the drives of the id with reality, in a way that promotes well-being and survival. The ego does not concern itself with moral values or societal taboos. The **superego** is the component of personality concerned with moral behavior. The structural relationship formed by the id, ego, and superego is the accumulation of societal rules and personal values as interpreted by individuals (Figure 1.2 ■). The superego emphasizes not reality, but the ideal, and its goal is perfection, as opposed to the id's pleasure or the ego's reality (Freud, 1935).

The id operates according to what Freud called the *pleasure principle*: the tendency to seek pleasure and avoid pain. Because this is not always possible, the demands of the id must be modified by the reality principle. The *reality principle* is a learned ego function by which people develop the capacity to delay the immediate achievement of pleasure. It also functions to manage the tension of not receiving immediate gratification until the person's needs are met.

Freud determined that the interplay between the three components of the personality have great significance in determining human behavior. He saw conflict arising because

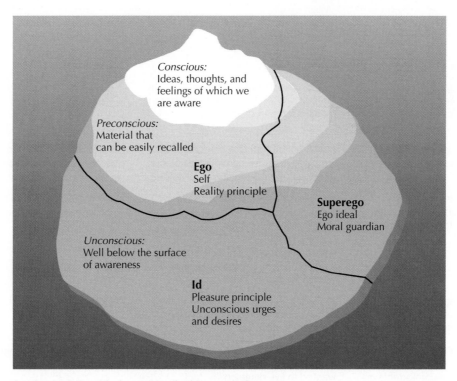

Figure 1.2 ■ The structural relationship formed by the id, ego, and superego.
SOURCE: Morris, C. G., & Maisto, A. A. (2001). *Understanding psychology* (5th ed). Upper Saddle River, NJ: Prentice Hall. Used with permission.

the components try to meet different goals—perfection, pleasure, or reality. Freud believed that the way people resolved this conflict determined the status of their mental health.

The concept of anxiety is a thread that runs consistently through Freud's intrapersonal theory. **Anxiety** is defined as a feeling of tension, distress, and discomfort produced by a perceived or threatened loss of inner control, rather than from external danger. The feelings brought about by anxiety are so uncomfortable that they force a person to take some type of corrective action. Anxiety is a warning of impending danger and a clear message to the ego that unless some palliative steps are taken, it is in danger of being overcome. The ego copes with anxiety by consistently applying rational measures to reduce feelings of discomfort. This process is often successful in healthy people, but there are times for all of us when the ego is unable to cope and resorts to less rational ways of handling anxiety. These processes are called **defense mechanisms**.

Defense mechanisms operate at an unconscious level and *alleviate anxiety* by denying, misinterpreting, or distorting reality. Defense mechanisms prevent painful feelings and ideas from entering conscious awareness. Not all defense mechanisms distort reality to the same degree (see Table 1.2 ■).

Freud called the process by which personality develops from birth to adolescence *psychosexual development* (see Table 1.3 ■). Each of five stages is differentiated by characteristic ways of achieving libidinal, or sexual, pleasure. The

psychosexual stages correspond to the maturational stages of the body:

■ Oral stage

■ Anal stage

■ Phallic stage

■ Latency stage

■ Genital stage

Readiness to move through each depends on how well the needs of the previous stage were met.

Erik Erikson Erik Erikson saw personality as developing throughout the life span rather than as stopping at adolescence. He differed with Freud in that he believed people could move backward to achieve developmental tasks that they were unable, for whatever reason, to achieve earlier. Erikson's perspective, the developmental theory of personality, offered the hope of achieving a healthy development pattern sometime during a life span.

Although Erikson accepted Freud's intrapersonal perspective of the importance of basic needs and drives in children, he believed personality was shaped more by conflict between needs and culture than by conflict among the id, ego, and superego. He based this philosophy on the assumption that drives are much the same from one child to another and that cultures differ from one part of the world to another. He also believed that cultures, like humans, are capable of developing.

TABLE 1.2	Defense Mechanisms	
Defense Mechanism	**Example(s)**	**Use/Purpose**
Compensation Covering up weaknesses by emphasizing a more desirable trait or by overachievement in a more comfortable area	A high school student too small to play football becomes the star long distance runner for the track team.	Allows a person to overcome weakness and achieve success
Denial An attempt to screen or ignore unacceptable realities by refusing to acknowledge them	A woman, though told her father has metastatic cancer, continues to plan a family reunion 18 months in advance.	Temporarily isolates a person from the full impact of a traumatic situation
Displacement The transferring or discharging of emotional reactions from one object or person to another object or person	A husband and wife are fighting, and the husband becomes so angry he hits a door instead of his wife. A student gets a C on a paper she worked hard on and goes home and yells at her family.	Allows for feelings to be expressed through or to less dangerous objects or people
Identification An attempt to manage anxiety by imitating the behavior of someone feared or respected	A student nurse imitates the nurturing behavior she observes one of her instructors using with clients.	Helps a person avoid self-devaluation
Intellectualization A mechanism by which an emotional response that normally would accompany an uncomfortable or painful incident is evaded by the use of rational explanations that remove from the incident any personal significance and feelings	The pain over a parent's sudden death is reduced by saying, "He wouldn't have wanted to live disabled."	Protects a person from pain and traumatic events
Introjection A form of identification that allows for the acceptance of others' norms and values into oneself, even when contrary to one's previous assumptions	A 7-year-old tells his little sister, "Don't talk to strangers." He has introjected this value from the instructions of parents and teachers.	Helps a person avoid social retaliation and punishment; particularly important for the child's development of superego
Minimization Not acknowledging the significance of one's behavior	A person says, "Don't believe everything my wife tells you. I wasn't so drunk I couldn't drive."	Allows a person to decrease responsibility for own behavior
Projection A process in which blame is attached to others or the environment for unacceptable desires, thoughts, shortcomings, and mistakes	A mother is told her child must repeat a grade in school, and she blames this on the teacher's poor instruction. A husband forgets to pay a bill and blames his wife for not giving it to him earlier.	Allows a person to deny the existence of shortcomings and mistakes; protects self-image
Rationalization justification of certain behaviors by faulty logic and ascription of motives that are socially acceptable but did not in fact inspire the behavior	A mother spanks her toddler too hard and says it was all right because he couldn't feel it through the diapers anyway.	Helps a person cope with the inability to meet goals or certain standards
Reaction formation A mechanism that causes people to act exactly opposite to the way they feel	An executive resents his bosses for calling in a consulting firm to make recommendations for change in his department but verbalizes complete support of the idea and is exceedingly polite and cooperative.	Aids in reinforcing repression by allowing feelings to be acted out in a more acceptable way
Regression Resorting to an earlier, more comfortable level of functioning that is characteristically less demanding and responsible	An adult throws a temper tantrum when he does not get his own way. A critically ill client allows the nurse to bathe and feed him.	Allows a person to return to a point in development when nurturing and dependency were needed and accepted with comfort
Repression An unconscious mechanism by which threatening thoughts, feelings, and desires are kept from becoming conscious; the repressed material is denied entry into consciousness	A teenager, seeing his best friend killed in a car accident, becomes amnesic about the circumstances surrounding the accident.	Protects a person from a traumatic experience until he or she has the resources to cope

TABLE 1.2	Defense Mechanisms *(continued)*		
Defense Mechanism	**Example(s)**	**Use/Purpose**	
Sublimation Displacement of energy associated with more primitive sexual or aggressive drives into socially acceptable activities	A person with excessive, primitive sexual drives invests psychic energy into a well-defined religious value system.	Protects a person from behaving in irrational, impulsive ways	
Substitution The replacement of a highly valued, unacceptable, or unavailable object by a less valuable, acceptable, or available object	A woman wants to marry a man exactly like her dead father and settles for someone who looks a little bit like him.	Helps a person achieve goals and minimizes frustration and disappointment	
Undoing An action or words designed to cancel some disapproved thoughts, impulses, or acts in which the person relieves guilt by making reparation	A father spanks his child and the next evening brings home a present for him. A teacher writes an examination that is far too easy, then constructs a grading curve that makes it difficult to earn a high grade.	Allows a person to appease guilty feelings and atone for mistakes	

Erikson believed that the ego is much more important than the id or superego in determining personality. He saw the ego as the mediating factor between the individual and society and felt that this relationship is at least as important as the influence of the basic drives. He also believed in the importance of social relationships in the development of individuals. Erikson expanded the determinants of personality development from merely instinctual and biological to social and cultural.

Erikson also expanded intrapersonal theory in his view of the future. Where Freud saw the most significance in past events, Erikson felt there was more significance in the future. He believed people's abilities to anticipate future events made a difference in the way they acted in the present. Many believe Erikson's theory is more hopeful and positive than Freud's theory. By expanding the intrapersonal perspective, Erikson acknowledged the chance to develop through the life span and to grow in a variety of ways.

According to Erikson, every person passes through eight developmental stages (see Table 1.4 ■ and Figure 1.3 ■). Each stage is characterized by conflicts and a set of tasks a person must accomplish before moving on to the next developmental stage. Erikson believed that people had difficulty developing normally if they were unable to accomplish the tasks of the previous stage. He believed that psychotherapy could help people return to a developmental task that had not been accomplished and relearn it (Erikson, 1963).

Social–Interpersonal Theory

The theories of Freud started a revolution in the field of psychology. During the late nineteenth century, other disciplines began to emerge and develop their own scientific bodies of knowledge. Sociologists and anthropologists started to believe that human development was more complex than previously thought, and it was not long before these beliefs started filtering into the knowledge gleaned

TABLE 1.3	Stages of Psychosexual Development According to Freud	
Stages of Development	**Period**	**Defining Characteristics**
Oral	Birth–18 months	Principal source of pleasure from mouth, lips, and tongue. Dependent on mother for care, so feelings of dependency are developed.
Anal	18 months–3 years	Focus on muscle control necessary to control urination and defecation. Expulsion of feces gives a sense of relief. Learns to postpone gratification by postponing the pleasure that comes from anal relief.
Phallic	3–6 years	Develops an awareness of the genital area. Sexual and aggressive feelings associated with functioning of the sexual organs are emphasized. Learns sexual identity during this stage. Masturbation and sexual fantasy are common.
Latency	6–12 years	Sexual development dormant. Focus of energy on cognitive development and intellectual pursuits.
Genital	12 years–early adulthood	Abundance of sexual drive. Primary goal is to develop satisfying relationships with members of the opposite sex.

TABLE 1.4	Stages of Social Growth and Development According to Erikson		
Stage of Development	**Period**	**Developmental Task**	**Defining Characteristics**
Sensory	Birth–1 year	Trust versus mistrust	Child learns to develop trusting relationships.
Muscular	1–2 years	Autonomy versus shame and doubt	Child starts the process of separation; starts learning to live autonomously.
Locomotor	3–5 years	Initiative versus guilt	Child learns about environmental influences; becomes more aware of own identity.
Latency	6–11 years	Industry versus inferiority	Energy is directed at accomplishments, creative activities, and learning.
Adolescent	12–19 years	Identity versus role confusion	Transitional period; movement toward adulthood. Adolescent starts incorporating beliefs and value systems that have been acquired previously.
Young adulthood	20s, 30s	Intimacy versus isolation	Person learns the ability to have intimate relationships.
Adulthood	40s, 50s	Generativity versus stagnation	Emphasis on maintaining intimate relationships. Movement toward developing a family.
Maturity	60 years and older	Integrity versus despair	Acceptance of life as it has been; acceptance of both good and bad aspects of past life. Maintaining a positive self-concept.

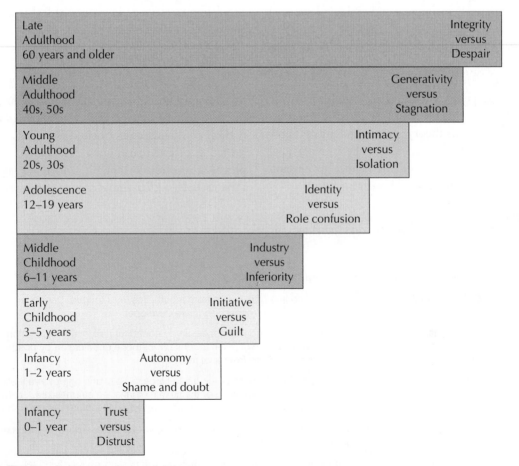

Figure 1.3 ■ Erikson's eight developmental stages.

SOURCE: Rice, F. P. (2001). *Human development* (4th ed). Upper Saddle River, NJ: Prentice Hall. Used with permission.

from advances in psychology. A number of theorists began to recognize the importance of the social context of personality development. The focus shifted away from forces within the individual to interpersonal relationships and events in the social context. Social–interpersonal theory was the result of this broader perspective.

Harry Stack Sullivan The work of Harry Stack Sullivan had its beginnings under the umbrella of the intrapersonal perspective. But Sullivan created a developmental system markedly different from that of Freud. Sullivan believed that personality was an abstraction that could not be observed apart from interpersonal relationships. Therefore, the unit of study for Sullivan was not the person alone but the person in the context of relationships. Sullivan described six stages of development from childhood through adolescence. These stages are explained in Table 1.5 ■. According to interpersonal theory, personality is manifested only in a person's interactions with another person or with a group. Sullivan acknowledged heredity and maturation as parts of development but placed far more emphasis on the organism as a social, rather than a biological, entity (Sullivan, 1953).

Although Sullivan saw personality more abstractly than Freud did, he still viewed it as the axis of human dynamics in the interpersonal sphere. He identified three principal components of this sphere: dynamisms, personifications, and cognitive processes.

A *dynamism* is a long-standing pattern of behavior. You may think of a dynamism as a habit. In Sullivan's theory, dynamisms highlight personality traits. For instance, a child who is mean can be said to have a dynamism of hostility. The important idea is that any habitual reaction of one person to another or to a situation constitutes a dynamism. Sullivan held that most dynamisms met the basic human needs of an individual by reducing anxiety.

Sullivan believed that an infant first feels anxiety as anxiety transferred from the mother. As a person grows older, anxiety is felt as a response to a threat to his or her security. Sullivan called the dynamism that develops to reduce anxiety the dynamism of the self, or the *self-system*. The self-system is the protector of one's security.

A *personification* is an image people have of themselves and others. Every person has many such images, made up of attitudes, feelings, and perceptions formed from experiences. For example, a child develops the personification of a good teacher by having the experience of being taught by one. Any relationship that leads to good experiences results in a favorable personification of a person involved in that relationship. Unfavorable personifications develop in response to bad experiences. Sullivan believed that personifications are formed early in life as a coping mechanism in interpersonal relationships. As a person gets older, however, rigid personifications can interfere with interpersonal relationships.

As the third component of the interpersonal sphere, **cognitive processes** are the development of the thinking process, from unconnected to causal to symbolic. Sullivan believed that cognitive processes, like personifications, are functions of experiences. He believed experiences could be classified into three types.

- A *protaxic* experience is an unconnected experience (not connected to one another—free flowing) that flows through consciousness. Examples are images, sensations, and feelings. Infants experience these most often, and protaxic experiences must occur before the other types.
- A *parataxic* experience is when a person sees a causal relationship between events that occur at about the same time but that are not logically related. Suppose, for example, a child tells his mother that he hates her and later she becomes ill. Parataxic thinking leads the

TABLE 1.5	Stages of Interpersonal Development According to Sullivan	
Stage of Development	**Period**	**Defining characteristics**
Infancy	Birth–18 months	Oral zone is the main means by which baby interacts with environment. Breastfeeding provides the first interpersonal experiences. Having needs met helps develop trust.
Childhood	18 months–6 years	Transition to this stage is achieved by child's learning to talk. Starts to see integration of self-concept. Gender development during this time. Child is learning delayed gratification.
Juvenile	6–9 years	This is a time for becoming social. Child learns social subordination to authority figures. Social relationships give a sense of belonging.
Preadolescence	9–12 years	Need for close relationships with peers of same sex. Learns to collaborate. This stage marks the beginning of the first genuine human relationships.
Early adolescence	12–14 years	Development of a pattern of heterosexual relationships. Searching for own identity. Ambiguity about dependence–independence issues.
Late adolescence	14–21 years	Prolonged introduction to society. Self-esteem becomes more stabilized. Will learn to achieve love relationships while maintaining self-identity.

child to conclude that every time the child tells his mother he hates her, she will become ill.

- *Syntaxic* experience, the highest cognitive level, involves the validation of symbols, particularly verbal symbols. These symbols become validated when a group of people understands them and agrees on their meaning. This level of cognition gives a logical order to experiences and enables people to communicate.

Abraham Maslow Abraham Maslow viewed personality as *self-actualizing*; that is, an ideal individual is at peak capacity for fulfilling his or her potential. However, before fulfillment can occur, certain needs must be met. Maslow devised a hierarchy of needs (see Figure 1.4 ■).

- *Basic needs* are physiologic, such as the need for food, water, and sleep.
- *Meta-needs* are growth related and include such things as love and belonging, esteem, and self-actualization.

Under most circumstances, basic needs take precedence over meta-needs. A person who is hungry is less concerned with truth and justice than a person who is not hungry, and whose basic needs have been met. Maslow felt that fulfilling meta-needs enables a person to rise above an animal level of existence. People who are unable to meet their growth needs, Maslow postulated, can become psychologically disturbed (Maslow, 1968).

Maslow looked primarily at the healthy, strong side of human nature. His is a *humanistic theory*, in which people

are defined holistically as dynamic combinations of physical, emotional, cognitive, and spiritual processes. Maslow emphasized health rather than illness, success rather than failure. He even viewed basic drives, such as the sex drive, as natural rather than as unhealthy urges to be controlled. Maslow believed that people have an inborn nature that is essentially good or, at worst, neutral.

Hildegard Peplau Hildegard Peplau is known as the mother of psychiatric nursing. She was one of the first nurses to analyze nursing action using an interpersonal theoretical model and published this theory in her 1952 book, *Interpersonal Relations in Nursing*. She defined nursing as a "significant therapeutic interpersonal process that makes health possible for individuals and groups" (p. xx, Preface). The major concepts of her theory include growth, development, communication, and roles.

Communication, described in detail in chapter 7 ∞, is a problem-solving process that takes place within the nurse–client relationship. Problem solving is a collaborative process in which the nurse may assume many roles in helping clients meet needs and continue their growth and development. As client conflicts and anxieties are resolved, personalities are strengthened. Peplau noted that nurses' and clients' culture, religion, ethnicity, education, experiences, and preconceived ideas influence interpersonal relationships.

Peplau believed that psychodynamic nursing liberated nurses from a tradition of being task oriented and gave them permission to focus on their excellent interpersonal

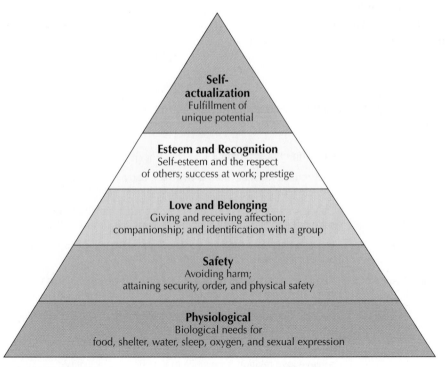

Figure 1.4 ■ Maslow's hierarchy of needs.

skills. Peplau's perspective is humane and compassionate, encouraging nurses to listen carefully and develop the empathy essential for the therapeutic relationship. Peplau's work continues to be the essence of psychiatric nursing.

Gender-Bias Theory Gender-bias theory has evolved out of a new focus on the events and themes important in the lives of females and males. For many years, there has been a double standard of mental health. Men and traditional male stereotypes were the model for a mentally healthy adult. Women and traditional female stereotypes were viewed as inadequate and mentally inferior. In fact, many thoughts, feelings, and behaviors of women are the result of social, political, economic, psychological, and physical oppression. The consequences of this oppression are low self-esteem, powerlessness, and general unhappiness.

Gender-bias theory examines how gender roles limit the psychological development of all people and inhibit the development of mutually satisfying and noncoercive intimacy. Gender-bias models of therapy strive to:

- Help people develop egalitarian rather than dominant–submissive relationships.
- Embrace the worth and dignity of all (children, women, men, and elderly persons).
- Listen to the stories of people's experiences.
- Implement social change through equality and justice for all groups of people.
- Eliminate the disparities in health status among groups in communities.
- Advocate change in social, political, economic, educational, and health services for a safer society.

(See the Gender section under Genomics earlier in this chapter for a list of gender differences in vulnerability to mental disorders.)

Crisis Theory Crisis theory provides another perspective for understanding people's responses to life events. A **crisis** is a turning point in a person's life, a point at which the usual resources and coping skills are no longer effective, and the person enters a state of disequilibrium. All people experience psychological trauma at some point. Neither stress nor an emergency necessarily constitutes a crisis. It is only when an event is perceived subjectively as a threat to fulfillment of need, safety, or a meaningful existence that the person enters a crisis state. A number of variables determine a person's potential for entering a crisis state (Aguiliera & Messick, 1990). These variables, known as *balancing factors*, include the following:

- How the person perceives the event
- The experience the person has had in coping with stress

- The person's usual coping abilities
- The support systems available to the person

To understand the development of a crisis state, you must be aware of the process of a crisis. Initially, people experience increased anxiety about the traumatic event and are unable to adapt to the situation. As their anxiety increases to high levels, they recognize the need to reach out for help. When inner resources and external support systems are inadequate, the person enters an active crisis state. During this time, the person has a short attention span and is unproductive and impulsive. People look to others to solve problems because they are consumed with feelings of going crazy or losing their mind. Often, interpersonal relationships deteriorate. Because a state of disequilibrium is so uncomfortable, a crisis is *self-limiting* and usually lasts about 4 to 6 weeks. It is during this time that people are most receptive to professional intervention. Because people in crisis are viewed as essentially healthy and capable of growth, changes may be made in a short period by focusing on the stressor and using the problem-solving process. The *minimum goal* of intervention is to help clients adapt and return to the precrisis level of functioning. The *maximum goal* is to help clients develop more constructive coping skills and move on to a higher level of functioning.

Behavioral Theory

The focus of behavioral theory is on a person's actions, not on her or his thoughts and feelings. Behavioral theorists believe that all behavior is learned and can therefore be modified by a system of rewards and punishment. They think that undesirable behavior occurs because it has been learned and reinforced and that it is possible for people to learn to replace undesirable behaviors with desirable ones.

B. F. Skinner Behavioral theory, particularly that of B. F. Skinner, had a major impact on the way scientists looked at personality development. Like the social–interpersonal theorists, Skinner rejected many of the conceptualizations of Freud and his followers. In addition, he questioned the validity of ideas such as instinctual drives and personality structure; he believed these could not be observed and therefore could not be studied scientifically.

The emphasis of Skinner's theory is functional analysis of behavior, which suggests looking at behavior pragmatically. What is causing a person to act in a particular way? What factors in the environment reinforce that behavior? Behavioral theory is less concerned with understanding behavior in relation to past events than with the immediate need to predict a trend in behavior and control it. Skinner did not attribute much importance to unconscious motivations, instincts, and feelings; he did attribute importance to a person's immediate actions.

Skinner thought a person's behavior could be controlled by rewards and punishment, that all behavior has specific consequences. He called consequences that lead to an increase in the behavior *reinforcements*, or *rewards*, and he called consequences that lead to a decrease in the behavior *punishments.*

One assumption of the behavioral perspective is that behavior is orderly and can be controlled. Skinner believed people become who they are through a learning process and by interacting with the environment. Further, he believed that personality problems are the result of faulty learning and can be corrected by new learning experiences that reinforce different behavior.

One major concept within Skinner's system is the *principle of reinforcement* (sometimes referred to as operant reinforcement theory). The ability to reinforce behavior is the ability to change the number of times a particular behavior occurs in the future. Skinner believed certain operations would decrease certain behaviors and increase other behaviors. According to the principle of reinforcement, a response is strengthened when reinforcement is given. Skinner referred to this as an *operant response*, that is, a response that works on the environment and changes it. An example of *operant conditioning* results when a nursing instructor teaches students that it is all right to hand in papers late by always accepting late papers. However, handing in papers late can be minimized if the instructor prohibits this behavior. Another way for the instructor to diminish the behavior is by handing out punishments for it; this is called a *punishing response* (Skinner, 1953).

Skinner's theories have been criticized by some and embraced by others. To some, the idea of controlling people's behavior by a systematically applied reward–punishment system is abhorrent. One argument in defense of the theory is that using punishment is not necessary to reinforce desirable behaviors. In other words, a systematic application of rewards can reinforce desirable behaviors, and punishment does not necessarily have to be part of the process.

Cognitive Theory

Cognitive theory gives us a blueprint for the process of learning. The ability to think and learn makes us human. It enables us to be rational, to make good judgments, to interpret the world around us, and to learn new skills. Without cognitive functions, we could not interpret our daily lives, adapt and make changes, and develop the insights to make those changes.

Jean Piaget Jean Piaget believed that intelligence grows by exposing children to the world around them. He hypothesized that children's experiences and perceptions are challenged by constantly changing stimuli, whereby they recognize discrepancies between their reality and the environment. Resolving these discrepancies helps children learn new relationships between objects and, therefore, develop a more mature understanding of the world (Piaget, 1972).

Piaget identified four major stages of cognitive development (Figure 1.5 ■):

- Sensorimotor stage
- Preoperational stage

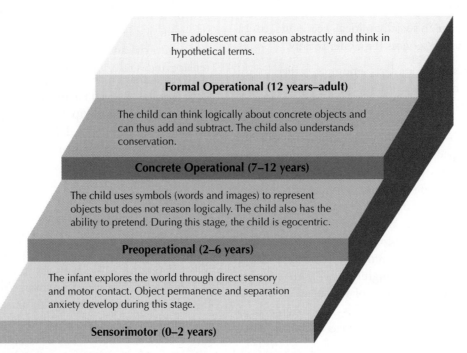

The adolescent can reason abstractly and think in hypothetical terms.

Formal Operational (12 years–adult)

The child can think logically about concrete objects and can thus add and subtract. The child also understands conservation.

Concrete Operational (7–12 years)

The child uses symbols (words and images) to represent objects but does not reason logically. The child also has the ability to pretend. During this stage, the child is egocentric.

Preoperational (2–6 years)

The infant explores the world through direct sensory and motor contact. Object permanence and separation anxiety develop during this stage.

Sensorimotor (0–2 years)

Figure 1.5 ■ Piaget's stages of cognitive development. Piaget portrayed development as a staircase in which the different steps, or stages, are distinguished by specific kinds of thinking.

SOURCE: Kassin, S. (2001). *Psychology* (3rd ed.). Upper Saddle River, NJ: Prentice Hall. Used with permission.

- Concrete operational stage
- Formal operational stage

Piaget emphasized the range of personal differences in rates of development. The speed by which a child moves through each period depends on biological, intrapersonal, and interpersonal factors.

Aaron Beck Cognitive theory, according to Aaron Beck, focuses not on what people do, but rather on how they view themselves and their world. He believed that much emotional upset and dysfunctional behavior is related to misperceptions and misinterpretations of experiences. Cognitive theory does not speak to ultimate causes of mental disorders but describes how negative thinking (*cognitions*) can be the first link in the chain of symptoms of mental disorders.

Two important constructs of Beck's cognitive theory are *schemas* and the *cognitive triad*. **Cognitive schemas** are personal controlling beliefs that influence the way people process data about themselves and others. For example, you may believe that you are unlovable. When your partner left for work this morning, he slammed the door. The way you processed this event was: "If John slams the door, it means he is angry with me. If he is angry with me, he will reject me. If he rejects me, I will be all alone. If I am all alone, I will not survive." In this example, your core belief led you to misinterpret the significance of the slamming door, which, in fact, was caused by a sudden gust of wind. It is thought that cognitive schemas become activated during depression, anxiety, panic attacks, and personality disorders. These distorted views of the self and the world appear to be reality to a person who is ill.

Cognitive schemas contribute to the development of Beck's cognitive triad. Included in this process is:

1. A view of the self as inadequate
2. A negative misinterpretation of current experiences
3. A negative view of the future

When clients become caught up in this process, a number of cognitive distortions may occur (Beck & Freeman, 1990).

- One type of distortion is *selective abstraction*, or focusing on certain information while ignoring contradictory information.
- Another distortion is *overgeneralization*, in which the person takes information or an impression from one event and attaches it to a wide variety of situations. Using such words as "always," "never," "everybody," and "nobody" indicates that the client is overgeneralizing.
- People who use *magnification* attribute a high level of importance to insignificant events.
- Through the distortion of *personalization*, or ideas of reference, clients believe that what occurs in the environment is related to them, even when no obvious relationship exists.
- There is also a tendency for *superstitious thinking*, in which the person believes that some unrelated action will magically influence a course of events.
- A further distortion is *dichotomous thinking*, an all-or-none type of reasoning that interferes with people's realistic perception of themselves. Dichotomous thinking involves opposite and mutually exclusive categories, such as all good or all bad, celibacy or promiscuity, depression or euphoria (see Table 1.6 ■).

Later chapters will discuss this topic in detail.

Personality

Personality is neither a model nor a theory of mental health nursing. It is a common concept in a variety of theories. The concept of personality can also illustrate the interconnections between the different theories.

Personality is perhaps the unique aspect of our individuality. **Personality** is the unique way we respond to the environment and it includes our patterns of behavior, emotion, and cognition that remain consistent from one situation to another. *Temperament*, or personality traits, is the behavioral disposition present at birth, such as social responsiveness, fear, irritability, or level of physical activity (e.g., some children are

TABLE 1.6	Examples of Cognitive Distortions
Distortion	**Example**
Selective abstraction	"Even though my husband says he loves me, I don't believe him. Look at how he never picks up his laundry."
Overgeneralization	"Women always turn mean after you marry them."
Magnification	"I know he saw the spot of coffee on my tie. Now I'll never get the job because he thinks I'm a slob."
Personalization	"I walked into the classroom and everyone stopped talking. I know they were talking about me."
Superstitious thinking	"If I never take off my wedding ring, my husband will never leave me."
Dichotomous thinking	"Either my life has to be absolutely perfect or I will commit suicide."

calm and slow moving, others are fast and perhaps anxious). Temperament is the inheritable component of personality.

There is much more to personality than just genetics. We are not robots shaped by our genes, nor are we infinitely adaptable to our environment. The interaction between temperament and social learning creates our personality. In some ways, we are who we learn to be. Parents reinforce behaviors and children imitate parental behaviors. Siblings may receive different treatment from parents or assume dissimilar niches in the family group. Children with different temperaments perceive the same environment differently. A child's temperament influences how others respond to that temperament, which in turn influences the quality of the child's environment. For example, temperamental excesses in children are amplified by the difficulties they create for the family, which may be one explanation why irritable or impulsive children are more likely to experience abuse and neglect in the family (Gabbard, 2004).

Nursing Research

A major aim of science is for theory to evolve. This is essential to a scientific discipline because theories draw together groups of concepts and relate them so meaning and understanding can be gleaned. These theories may then be used by practitioners to provide answers to questions and concerns. Because nursing is a practice discipline, theories are developed not only to name and explore concepts, but also to offer a prescription for practice and an ability to predict outcomes of that practice. The **nursing process** is a way to organize that scientific data to prescribe practice criteria. The nursing profession has chosen this vehicle to divide the abundant information into a workable system. Research and theories, by their nature, provide a great deal of information that can be applied in many different situations. Nurses are becoming more adept at using and applying research to particular practice situations.

All research endeavors have value. Societal, professional, and personal value can influence the outcomes of studies in the following ways:

- *Topic of study:* What is worth studying is a judgment on the value of something; attention is drawn to what is being studied and away from multiple other issues. Example: Studying stressors and the coping strategies of homeless individuals does not look at society's attitudes toward homeless people.
- *Unit of study:* Studying the individual, family, or community narrows the way issues are conceptualized. Example: Studying a family that has bipolar disorder does not speak to intrapersonal issues.
- *Definitions:* Determining which interactions are counted limits the behaviors studied. Example: Specific behaviors

define what is labeled as child abuse, and related behaviors are not studied.

- *Choice of variables:* The choice determines the selection of variables, such as age, income, and ethnic identity, used to organize the data. Example: Studying community violence in urban areas does not speak to community violence in rural areas.

The National Institute for Nursing Research has developed directions for psychiatric nursing research, including identifying biological–behavioral factors in mental disorders and testing biobehavioral interventions. In the words of Jacquelyn H. Flaskerud (2000), "Psychiatric nursing can lead the way in establishing research designs and methods that are truly reflective of the synthesis of biology, behavior, and environment that characterizes nursing science" (p. 2).

THE THERAPEUTIC RELATIONSHIP

Therapeutic relationships are established to help clients. The way you establish the relationship depends on your reactions to the clinical setting and how you are able to care for clients. In mental health nursing, you examine the relationship to ensure that it is goal directed and therapeutic.

Student Concerns

At the onset of your course in mental health nursing, you may be comfortable in the clinical setting, or you may experience uncertainties and concern relating to yourself and your clients. Your personal concerns may stem from being in an unfamiliar environment, not knowing what to talk about, believing you have nothing to offer, thinking you might say the wrong thing, or all of this. Your concerns about clients may be rooted in stereotypes of people with mental illness, your fear of rejection, your discomfort with anger, or your fear of being physically harmed by a client. Box 1.3 lists common student concerns and strategies for dealing with them.

Caring: the Art and Essence of Nursing

Caring is the essence of nursing and the foundation on which the nursing process is based. Caring is more than merely liking or comforting other people. It involves commitment and a binding of individuals in interpersonal connections. Before nurses can care for clients, they must first learn to value and care for themselves. As Keen (1991) states: "If we are unable to care first for ourselves as individuals, and then for our nursing colleagues, the caring we give to our patients is not as good as it could be" (p. 173).

BOX 1.3	Student Concerns and Strategies for Dealing with These Concerns

Stereotypical Ideas About People With Mental Health Problems

- Identify cultural stereotypes and discuss your expectations in the first clinical preconference.
- Identify specific concerns about clients and/or their families of origin or their current families.
- Approach the client as a person rather than as a diagnosis.
- Identify healthy aspects and resources of clients; they *are* able to cope effectively in many areas of life.

Fear of Not Knowing What to Talk About

- When first meeting a client, introduce yourself by name and position.
- Follow the client's lead in topics to be discussed in the initial interaction; pay attention to the client's nonverbal communication signals indicating comfort or discomfort.
- Give up the unrealistic expectation that you have to be absolutely right before you offer any observations to clients.
- Share your perceptions with clients and seek validation, by asking, for example, "Am I hearing you correctly, that you are very frustrated over this situation?" or "It sounds as if you are becoming more comfortable with being in the hospital."
- Using your nursing care plan, decide on specific topics and goals for your one-to-one interaction; be flexible if the client has different priorities.

Concern About Having Nothing to Offer

- Identify your own fears of inadequacy by listening to your self-statements: "How can I help this person when I don't know what's wrong with him?" "These clients are too sick/well, so how can I help them?"
- If clients question your qualifications, simply state why you are here and what your role is on the unit.
- Recognize that your knowledge and theory base will be increasing throughout the course.
- Identify the energy and enthusiasm you bring as a positive quality to be used therapeutically.
- Recognize that a positive interpersonal relationship is therapeutic because it increases self-esteem, develops interactional skills for clients, and promotes your own professional growth.
- Involve clients in the nursing process and work together as a team toward specific goals; solutions come from working *with* clients, not from doing something *to* clients.

Concern About Hurting Clients by Saying the Wrong Thing

- The quality of a caring relationship overcomes verbal mistakes; you will not destroy a client with a few ill-chosen words.

- Recognize that clinical experience is an opportunity to learn and that verbal mistakes will be made; opportunities for more appropriate interventions are seldom lost—they're just postponed.
- If you have made a mistake, apologize to the client and identify what would have been a more therapeutic response.
- Use process recordings or audiotapes to evaluate, improve, and increase your communication skills.

Concern About Rejection by the Client

- Identify your own characteristic response to rejection. Do you become angry? Feel hurt? Feel resigned to it? Withdraw from the person? In what other ways might you respond?
- Identify what is the worst thing that will happen to you if a client refuses to work with you.
- If a client is exhibiting behavior that indicates unwillingness to work with you, validate this behavior with her or him.
- Remember that you will have opportunities to work with other clients.

Concern About Client Anger

- Know and understand your own response to the feeling and expression of anger: "Nice people don't get angry," "It's okay to feel angry but it should be talked about calmly," "I'm uncomfortable if people shout when they are angry."
- Accept the client's right to be angry; feelings are real and cannot be discounted or ignored.
- Try to understand the meaning of the client's anger.
- Ask the client in what way you have contributed to the anger; help the client "own" the anger—do not assume responsibility for her or his feelings.
- Let clients talk about their anger.
- Listen to the client, and react as calmly as possible.
- After the interaction is completed, take time to process your feelings and your responses to the client with your peers and instructor.

Concern About Physical Harm From Clients

- Ask your instructor about the reality of this concern.
- Avoid being in a "trapped" position, e.g., isolated in a client's room.
- Recognize the early signs of an impending violent outburst.
- Seek help immediately from a staff member or instructor before a client gets out of control.
- If a client begins to act out physically, stay out of the staff members' way as they implement their plan of action.

One educational goal in mental health nursing might be discovering ways to provide self-care more effectively. Caring for yourself means reducing unnecessary stress, managing conflict more effectively, communicating with family and friends more clearly, and taking time out for oneself. Caring for your colleagues means respecting cultural differences, asking for collaboration, and responding to constructive criticism. Helpful books on this topic include *The Soul of the Caring Nurse, Stories and Resources for Revitalizing Profes-*

sional Passion (Henry & Henry, 2004) and *Callings: Finding and Following an Authentic Life* (Levoy, 1998).

The *art* of nursing is in being there, with another person or persons, in a context of caring. It is the capacity "to receive another human being's expression of feelings and to experience those feelings for oneself" (Chinn & Watson, 1994, p. xvi). Caring involves compassion and sensitivity to each person within the context of her or his entire life. Caring is the way we enter the world of our clients. In the past, nurses have been urged not to care too much or get too involved. However, caring, successful nurses do get involved with clients because they practice nursing as an art instead of nursing as just a day-to-day job. Clients have a right to competent nursing care, but they also desire a nurse who is committed to them. In many schools of nursing in the past 50 years, the art of nursing has been devalued and separated from the science of nursing. Consequently, caring has often been a minimal part of the curriculum. With client expectations and demand, nursing is beginning to restore its caring–healing art as the basis of nursing practice (George, 2002; Sieg, 2004).

As caring nurses, we are also keepers of *hope*. It is a privilege to be intimately present with other human souls at some of their darkest and brightest moments. With this privilege comes profound responsibility—to have a deep respect for that person who is our client. Hope is meaningfulness and dignity, even in the face of death. Hope is a way of relating to oneself and one's world. Hope is often attached to something or someone. Some people place hope in others, such as their primary care provider. Some people place hope in their own abilities, which is called self-confidence. Some people place hope in a higher power. Hope can be highly specific regarding a particular outcome. Hope implies openness to experience and possibilities. Hope is acting in spite of the circumstances.

Hope is also a way of being with our clients. Sometimes clients need to borrow our hope until they can regain their own. Nurses see clients not merely as they are, but as they can be. They need to hear about their own competence and about their ability to grow and change, especially in times of stress and discouragement.

The Nurse–Client Relationship

Throughout the text, the term *client* will be used to refer to individuals experiencing mental disorders and to their families and significant others. The nurse–client relationship is the key factor throughout the nursing process. It is the means by which nurses are able to assess clients accurately, formulate diagnoses, help clients establish outcomes, plan and implement interventions, and evaluate the effectiveness of the nursing process. The nurse–client relationship is therapeutic, not social. Social relationships are reciprocal in that both people expect their individual needs to be met as fully as possible. The therapeutic relationship, on the other hand, exists for clients, and the focus is on their needs. To minimize the possibility of client dependency, the nurse should not try to meet all the needs of every client; rather, the nurse should support them in meeting their own needs whenever possible. In the professional role, the nurse collaborates with the client as a team, forming a therapeutic alliance, with the goal being the client's growth and adaptation. The therapeutic relationship is client centered, goal specific, theory based, and open to supervision by peers, instructors, and supervising nurses.

In this era of sophisticated technology, managed care, and cost containment, the nurse–client relationship is often devalued. Health care is increasingly taking place outside of traditional institutions and moving into places where people live, work, and play. As the boundaries become more diffuse, health care is becoming less formal and demands greater attention to the relational dimensions of care. As you learn the art of mental health nursing, you will be in a unique position to bridge the gap between technology and therapeutic relationships (Krauss, 2004).

Nursing theorist Hildegard Peplau describes the nurse–client relationship as evolving through three phases: introductory, working, and termination. These phases are more easily identified in nurse–client relationships that last more than a few days. The phases often overlap and are thought of as interlocking. Goals are achieved in each phase of the relationship.

Introductory Phase

The introductory phase usually begins when the nurse initiates the therapeutic relationship with the client. Start by introducing yourself by name and position and explaining your role in helping the client identify problems and work toward resolving them. An acceptable agreement or contract is established to guide the relationship. This contract, which is typically verbal, should include the purpose of the relationship; the duration of the relationship; and where, when, and for how long you will meet. It is critical that the issue of confidentiality be discussed. (See chapter 5 ∞ for guidelines on confidentiality.)

Although client assessment continues throughout the therapeutic relationship, it is extremely important during the introductory phase. The introductory phase, which may last minutes to hours, ends with the development of preliminary diagnoses and outcomes identification.

Working Phase

The second phase of the therapeutic relationship is the working phase. The nursing process is dynamic; assessment, diagnosis, outcome identification, planning, implementation, and evaluation are continuous throughout this phase. Parts of the care plan are revised, expanded, or eliminated according to the individual client's needs. The conscious process of working together toward mutually established goals is referred to as the **therapeutic alliance**. The nurse identifies ineffective behaviors and thoughts as problems, and works together with clients to establish more effective ways of coping. During the working phase, the majority of client education and problem solving is accomplished.

Two phenomena that may occur during any phase of the relationship (but that are more likely to be noticed during the working phase) are transference and countertransference.

Transference is a client's unconscious displacement of feelings for significant people in the past onto the nurse in the current relationship. These displaced feelings can be positive or negative and may be highly emotional. Transference that is not identified and managed may decrease the effectiveness of the working phase because the meaning of the nurse–client relationship becomes misinterpreted. When transference occurs, the nurse and client must explore it and separate past relationships from the present one.

Sue, 20 years old, is working with Miguel, her nurse–therapist. Sue's father verbally abused her from early childhood until she left home at age 18. She constantly looks to Miguel, her nurse–therapist, for approval and acceptance. She is unable to disagree with him or challenge his interpretations. This is an automatic reaction, outside of Sue's awareness. Miguel verbalizes his observation and suggests that Sue observe herself when interacting with men in an effort to see how her fear of her father has been displaced onto other men.

Countertransference is the nurse's emotional reaction to the client based on significant relationships in the nurse's past. Countertransference may be conscious or unconscious, and the feelings may be positive or negative. Awareness of countertransference is critical because it could interfere with understanding the client and providing effective care. When nurses discuss feelings about their client with their instructor, it will help bring countertransference into conscious awareness.

Colleen's son was killed in an accident several years ago when he was 15 years old. Colleen is taking a course in psychiatric nursing and has been assigned to work with Brendan, who is 15 years old. Brendan is manipulative, and Colleen has difficulty setting limits on his behavior. Through the process of supervision with her instructor, Colleen begins to realize that her inability to recognize Brendan's manipulation is because he reminds her of her dead son. She has displaced her feelings about her son onto Brendan and has attributed to him positive qualities he really does not have.

Termination Phase

The third phase of the therapeutic relationship is the termination phase. Information about when and how this will occur is included in the introductory phase and discussed at times during the working phase. The primary goal of the termination phase is to reminisce about the relationship experiences in order to review the client's progress. Review plans with the client for the immediate future. Termination can be a traumatic experience for clients. Those who have had difficulty ending other relationships will likely have problems ending the therapeutic relationship. The nurse must understand their sense of loss and help them express and cope with their feelings. In an effort to continue the relationship, clients may introduce new problems or try to extend the relationship beyond the clinical setting. Here is an

example of part of the termination process between Colleen (the nurse) and Brendan (the client):

Brendan: "Colleen, I know this is your last day on the unit, and I'm going to be out of here next week. How about if you give me your phone number so I can call you sometime?"
Colleen: "Brendan, getting to know you has been very important to me. We can't continue our relationship once you are out of the hospital but I certainly will never forget you."
Brendan: "But Colleen, please, you really understand me. My own mother doesn't understand me. I just want to be able to call you if things get a little tough. Is that too much to ask?"
Colleen: "Yes, Brendan, it is. Let's talk about choices you do have if things get tough when you go home. I would also like to talk about feelings you're having right now as we are about to end our time together."

Components of the Relationship

The *physical component* of the nurse–client relationship includes all the procedures and technical skills that the nurse does with or for clients. This physical component is a large part of your early nursing education as you practice procedures and skills in the laboratory and in the hospital. As a student, you are praised and evaluated for tasks that can be observed, which reinforces the task orientation prevalent in the medical model of health care.

The *psychosocial component* of the nurse–client relationship, which is as important as the physical component, involves the nurse's response to the client as one human being to another. The nurse brings many qualities to these relationships: positive regard, a nonjudgmental attitude, acceptance, warmth, empathy, authenticity, and congruity of communication. (These attributes are discussed in further detail in chapter 7 ∞.) Nurses encourage clients to share their thoughts on how they perceive the world, their experiences and expectations, and their hopes and dreams for the future.

Together with the psychosocial component, the *spiritual component* of the nurse–client relationship comprises the caring relationship. The spiritual component is the feeling of connection between the nurse and the client. It is that inner sense of being a part of something more than yourself. It is respect for the client's cultural values and religious views. Spirituality is what allows us as nurses to connect with clients who may be very different from ourselves. We may not be able to see clearly the person who lives behind the mask of substance abuse or who is experiencing delusions or who has been forced into living on the streets, but responding to that person's spirit is what allows us to connect to them. Your role in providing spiritual care includes allowing clients to express important spiritual needs, such as the need for meaning in life, belief in God, or relief from fear, doubt, or loneliness. The important point is to recognize that spiritual needs are as diverse as our clients, their cultures, and their illnesses.

The *power component* of the nurse–client relationship is related to the nurse and her or his clients' beliefs in locus of control. People tend to ascribe their chances of success or failure to either internal or external causes. If the nurse reflects an **external locus of control**, the nurse expects the client to give up control to the staff, who then do "to" and "for" clients, stripping from them the right to choose their own healing journey and the quality of their life experiences. The focus of the nurse–client relationship has traditionally been one of curing, with health care professionals as the heroes. When clients have an external locus of control, they view their disease or disability as a thing that has been imposed on them and they believe they are not responsible for either the cause or the cure.

If the nurse believes in an **internal locus of control**, the nurse welcomes the clients' feelings, respects their wishes, and honors their needs for self-expression. The nurse's role is to empower clients by providing skills, information, and support as they choose options that are in their best interests. The relationship is built around clients' needs to shape and control their own lives as much as possible. Clients who have an internal locus of control feel powerful rather than victimized and are participants in their own healing process. They recognize behaviors, thoughts, and feelings that influence their own movement toward health or illness.

Boundaries of the Relationship

The boundaries of the nurse–client relationship are those edges that maintain a clear distinction between nurses and clients. Establishing clear boundaries creates an atmosphere of safety and predictability, within which the nursing process can be implemented. Nurses are in a position of power within the relationship because of their specialized skills, their access to private information about the client, and the client's vulnerability.

Violation of boundaries includes behaviors such as burdening the client with personal problems, spending excessive amounts of time with a client beyond that which is expected, exchanging gifts, or flirting with the client and acting secretive or defensive toward others in terms of the relationship. Much of the current concern about professional boundaries has grown out of a wish to prevent sexual misconduct by health care providers.

NURSING PROCESS IN MENTAL HEALTH NURSING

Critical Thinking

As nurses, we must be critical thinkers because of the nature of the discipline and the nature of our work. We are expected to solve client problems by performing critical analyses of the factors associated with the problems. This analytical process, or **critical thinking**, enables us to make better decisions. Thus, critical thinking, problem solving, and decision making are interrelated processes, and creativity enhances the result.

Because nursing decisions may profoundly affect the lives of clients and their families, nurses must think critically. But critical thinking is not limited to problem solving or decision making; nurses use critical thinking to make reliable observations, draw sound conclusions, create new ideas, evaluate lines of reasoning, and improve self-knowledge.

To think critically, you must have cognitive skills and be willing to use them. Critical-thinking attitudes provide the motivation to use cognitive skills. These attitudes are interrelated and integrated rather than used in isolation. For instance, it takes courage to acknowledge that you do not know something and to develop an inquiring attitude.

Characteristics of Critical Thinking

- *Thinking independently:* Critical thinking requires thinking for oneself. As we mature and acquire knowledge, we must evaluate beliefs we acquired as children, holding those we can rationally support and rejecting those we cannot.
- *Humility:* Intellectual humility means having an awareness of the limits of one's personal knowledge. As critical thinkers, we should be willing to admit what we do not know, to seek new information, and to rethink our conclusions in light of new knowledge.
- *Courage:* With an attitude of courage, nurses should be willing to consider and evaluate ideas or views fairly, especially those to which they may have a strongly negative reaction. This type of courage comes from recognizing that personally held beliefs are sometimes false, misleading, and prejudiced.
- *Integrity:* Intellectual integrity requires that nurses question their own knowledge and beliefs as quickly and as thoroughly as they would challenge those of another.
- *Perseverance:* As critical thinkers, we strive to find effective solutions to client and nursing problems. We resist the temptation to find a quick and easy answer. Important questions tend to be complex and therefore often require a great deal of thought and research.
- *Empathy:* It is easy to misinterpret the words or actions of a person from a different cultural, religious, or socioeconomic background. It is also difficult to understand the beliefs or actions of a person experiencing a situation one has never experienced. Empathy is the ability to see the world from another's perspective and to communicate this understanding and sensitivity for validation or correction.
- *Fair-mindedness:* As critical thinkers, we should be fair-minded, assessing all viewpoints with the same objectivity. Fair-mindedness helps us consider opposing points of view and work to understand new ideas before rejecting or accepting them (see Table 1.7 ■).

TABLE 1.7	Characteristics of Critical Thinking
Characteristic	**Description**
Rational	Based on logic rather than prejudice or fear
Reflective	Collect data; think through in disciplined manner
Inquiring	Examine claims; determine truth and validity
Analytical	Analyze issues for understanding; decide which authorities are credible
Objective	Attempt to remove bias from own and others' thinking; aware of own values and feelings
Evaluative	Evaluate arguments; decide on course of action; solve problems; use accepted standards

After gaining an idea of what it means to think critically, solve problems, and make decisions, you must become aware of your own thinking style and abilities. Acquiring critical-thinking skills and an attitude of inquiry then becomes a matter of practice. Critical thinking is not an either–or phenomenon; it exists on a continuum, along which people develop and use the process of inquiry. Solving problems and making decisions are risky. Sometimes the outcome is not what was desired. With effort, however, everyone can achieve some level of critical thinking in order to become effective problem solvers and decision makers (Kozier, Erb, Blais, Wilkinson, & Van Leuven, 2003).

The Nursing Process

The nursing process is the same in all clinical areas of professional practice. In the 2000 *Scope and Standards of Psychiatric–Mental Health Nursing Practice,* the American Nurses Association (ANA) delineates the standards to which nurses are held, both legally and ethically. These standards, based on the steps of the nursing process, are covered in Box 1.4. Such data can also be viewed on the American Nurses Association Web site.

Standard I: Assessment

Assessment in mental health nursing is based on the collection of data from multiple sources, such as the client, family and friends, other health care providers, medical records, and community agencies. The client's immediate condition or needs determine the order in which assessment data are collected. Clinical skills include observation, psychosocial history taking, neuropsychiatric assessment, and physical assessment. The assessment process provides the database for clinical decision making: diagnosis, outcomes, interventions, and evaluation.

Interview The interview is often the initial step in the assessment process. The setting for the interview and the length of time are determined by the client's mental and physical status. Prior to meeting the client, nurses should ask themselves: What assumptions do I have about this person, by virtue of her/his diagnosis, history, and lifestyle? Nurses must first recognize their assumptions and predictions in order to put them aside and be fully present to the situation and the individual.

All nurses, no matter which field they choose as a specialty, must be able to gain the client's cooperation and collaboration. Thus, one of the first goals of the initial interview is to establish and maintain rapport with clients. Clients should not feel as if they are "being interviewed" but rather that they are "talking to someone" who is sensitive and compassionate. As you gather information, you must constantly attend to rapport with the client.

Observation Careful, accurate observation is vital during the assessment process. Begin to observe the moment of meeting clients and their families. Observation involves all the senses, but seeing and hearing are the most critical. The chapters on disorders (units 4 and 5 ∞) discuss how to assess clients for the behavioral, affective, cognitive, sociocultural, and physiologic characteristics of each disorder. In general, here is how observations are used in each of those categories.

When observing clients *behaviorally*, answer the following questions:

- Where is the client, and what is she or he doing?
- Is the behavior appropriate to the setting (own home, public place)?
- Is the client dangerous to self or others?
- Is any bizarre or unusual behavior occurring?

When observing for *affective* characteristics, answer the following questions:

- Is there evidence of intense emotions, such as loud laughter, crying, yelling, or screaming?
- Is the affect appropriate to the situation?

When observing for *cognitive* characteristics, answer the following questions:

- Is the client going over and over the same topic (ruminating)?

BOX 1.4	Standards of Practice for Psychiatric-Mental Health Nursing

The six standards of practice describe a competent level of nursing care organized around the nursing process. Note that Standards SE, SF, and SG apply to advanced practice psychiatric mental health nurses only.

Standard 1. Assessment

The Psychiatric-Mental Health Registered Nurse collects comprehensive health data that is pertinent to the patient's health or situation.

Standard 2. Diagnosis

The Psychiatric-Mental Health Registered Nurse analyzes the assessment data to determine diagnoses or problems, including level of risk.

Standard 3. Outcomes Identification

The Psychiatric-Mental Health Registered Nurse identifies expected outcomes for a plan individualized to the patient or to the situation.

Standard 4. Planning

The Psychiatric-Mental Health Registered Nurse develops a plan that prescribes strategies and alternatives to attain expected outcomes.

Standard 5. Implementation

The Psychiatric-Mental Health Registered Nurse implements the identified plan.

Standard 5A: Coordination of Care

The Psychiatric-Mental Health Registered Nurse coordinates care delivery.

Standard 5B: Health Teaching and Health Promotion

The Psychiatric-Mental Health Registered Nurse employs strategies to promote health and a safe environment.

Standard 5C: Milieu Therapy

The Psychiatric-Mental Health Registered Nurse provides, structures, and maintains a safe and therapeutic environment in collaboration with patients, families, and other healthcare clinicians.

Standard 5D: Pharmacological, Biological, and Integrative Therapies

The Psychiatric-Mental Health Registered Nurse incorporates knowledge of pharmacological, biological, and complementary interventions with applied clinical skills to restore the patient's health and prevent further disability.

Standard 5E: Prescriptive Authority and Treatment (APRN only)

The Psychiatric-Mental Health Advanced Practice Registered Nurse uses prescriptive authority, procedures, referrals, treatments, and therapies in accordance with state and federal laws and regulations.

Standard 5F: Psychotherapy (APRN only)

The Psychiatric-Mental Health Advanced Practice Registered Nurse conducts individual, couples, group, and family psychotherapy using evidence-based psychotherapeutic frameworks and nurse-patient therapeutic relationships.

Standard 5G: Consultation (APRN only)

The Psychiatric-Mental Health Advanced Practice Registered Nurse provides a consultation to influence the identified plan, enhance the abilities of other clinicians to provide services for patients, and effect change.

Standard Evaluation

The Psychiatric-Mental Health Registered Nurse evaluates progress toward attainment of expected outcomes.

SOURCE: Reprinted with permission from American Nurses Association, American Psychiatric-Mental Health Nurses Association, & International Society of Psychiatric-Mental Health Nurses. *Psychiatric-mental health nursing: Scope and standards of practice,* ©2007. Silver Spring, MD: Nursebooks.org.

- Can you follow what the client is saying?
- Do themes recur during the interaction?

When observing for *sociocultural* characteristics, answer the following questions:

- Does the client interact with others? Who? Staff? Peers? Family?
- Is the client assertive or passive with others?
- Is the client having any problems in living at home, in a residential setting, or on the inpatient unit?
- How does the client manage conflict with others?

When observing for *physiologic* characteristics, answer the following questions:

- What is the client's motor behavior—for example, pacing, sitting in one position for a long period of time, foot swinging, teeth grinding?

- What does the client's nutritional status appear to be?
- Is the client sleeping at night? Taking naps during the day?
- Are there any physical complaints?

These question sets are general guidelines. As you learn about the mental disorders, you will gather information that is more specific to guide your observations.

Psychosocial Assessment Agencies often have specific forms to be completed as part of the psychosocial assessment. In general, the following information is gathered from the client and significant others:

- Client and family definition of present problem
- History of present problem, including health beliefs and practices
- Family history of psychiatric and medical illnesses
- Family interactions, including support systems and ethnic and cultural factors

- Social history, including communication skills, social networks, work/school roles, economic stressors, and legal stressors
- Living conditions, including availability of food and shelter
- Spiritual considerations, including beliefs, values, and religious concerns
- Strengths and competencies

The U.S. Department of Health and Human Services has launched a national public health campaign to encourage all American families to learn more about their family health history. Access this information and download for free the "My Family Health Portrait" tool at: www.hhs.gov/familyhistory.

Each chapter in units 4 and 5 contains a Focused Nursing Assessment table to help students learn the types of questions to ask and the particular characteristics to assess. Observing experienced nurses is a great way to learn basic interviewing skills, and see techniques that are more advanced. Be sure to discuss your observations with another nurse, and clarify anything that was unclear.

Neuropsychiatric Assessment The neuropsychiatric assessment provides information about the client's appearance, behavior, speech, emotional state, and cognitive functioning. See Box 1.5 for the neuropsychiatric assessment. Box 1.6 describes signs of disease when assessing client perceptions, forms of thought, and content of thought.

Physical Assessment Clinical skills include conducting a detailed physical assessment. In many community settings, psychiatric nurses are the only mental health care providers

---

BOX 1.5	Neuropsychiatric Assessment

General

- Age
- Relationship status
- Family composition
- Employment
- Living situation

Appearance

- General state of health
- Grooming and hygiene
- Posture

Activity

- Motor activity (appropriate; increased/decreased)
- Tremors, dystonias
- Hyperactivity (activity is purposeful)
- Agitation (activity is purposeless)

Speech and Language

- Fluency
- Comprehension
- Pace (fast, slow)
- Volume
- Tone (calm, hostile)

Emotional State

- Mood (sustained emotional state; what client describes; depression, anxiety, sadness, calmness, anger)
- Affect (immediate emotional expression; what others observe; appropriateness, intensity, lability, range of expression)

Perceptions

- Five senses: seeing, hearing, smelling, tasting, feeling

Cognitive Functioning

- Orientation (person, time, place)
- Concentration
- Memory (recent, remote)
- Intellectual functioning (general grasp of information, reasoning and judgment, insight)
- Form of thought
- Content of thought

BOX 1.6	Signs of Pathology

Perception

- Illusions (the misinterpretation of an environmental stimulus of sight, sound, touch, smell, or taste)
- Hallucination (occurrence of a sight, sound, touch, smell, or taste without any external stimulus)
- Depersonalization (feel sense of identity has been altered and therefore feel strange and unreal)
- Derealization (feel the environment has changed and is unreal)

Form of Thought

- Blocking (sudden stop in speech or train of thought)
- Circumstantiality (overly detailed, tedious; eventually reaches goal)
- Confabulation (unconsciously filling in memory gaps with imagined material)
- Derailment (speech is blocked and then begins again on unrelated topic)
- Flight of ideas (rapid, fragmented thoughts manifested in pressured speech)
- Loose association (disconnected thoughts)
- Neologism (making up new words; not understood by others)
- Tangential (thoughts veer from main idea and never get back to it)

Content of Thought

- Disorders range from transient preoccupations to intractable delusions
- Ruminations (recurring mood-congruent concerns usually related to anxiety or depression)
- Obsessions (unwanted, repetitive thoughts that lead to feelings of fear or guilt)
- Compulsions (thoughts or behaviors used to decrease the fear or guilt associated with obsessions)
- Delusions (grandiosity, persecution, control, sin and guilt; religious, erotomanic, somatic)
- Experiences of influence (ideas of reference, thought broadcasting, thought withdrawal, thought insertion)

prepared to complete a physical assessment. Details of physical assessment are not included in this text because those skills are learned in other courses in the curriculum.

Standard II: Diagnosis

Analysis of the significance of the assessment data results in formulation of nursing diagnoses.

Psychiatric Nursing Diagnosis Standardized labels are applied to client problems and responses to mental disorders. These standardized labels come from the list of approved nursing diagnoses accepted by the North American Nursing Diagnosis Association (NANDA). When we use standardized language to document the diagnoses of our clients, we can begin to build large databases that will expand nursing knowledge. Such data can also be viewed on the NANDA Web site.

In developing the nursing diagnoses further, it is necessary to describe the related or contributing factors. These include behavioral symptoms, affective changes, and disrupted cognitive patterns that accompany the mental disorders. Spiritually, people with mental illness often have difficulty with interpersonal relationships and may feel a lack of connectedness with others. Some people suffer from a lack of meaning in life, whereas others attempt to find meaning in their response to their mental disorder. Cultural pressures and expectations may be contributing factors to the development and prognosis of mental disorders. Signs and symptoms, referred to as *defining characteristics*, are subjective (symptoms) and objective (objective) data that support the nursing diagnosis. Defining characteristics are identified during the assessment process but are not usually written as part of the diagnostic statement. The following are examples of nursing diagnoses that might be used during the clinical experience:

- *Hopelessness* related to long-term effects of poverty and racism; dire expectations of the future
- *Self-Care Deficit:Bathing/Hygiene* related to low energy and decreased desire to care for self; distractibility in completing activities of daily living
- *Impaired Verbal Communication* related to retardation in flow of thought; flight of ideas; altered thought processes; obsessive thoughts; panic level of anxiety
- *Altered Family Processes* related to rigidity in functions and roles; enmeshed family system; demands of caring for a family member with dementia; use of violence to maintain family relationships

Nursing Diagnoses Versus DSM-IV-TR Diagnoses Mental disorders are classified in the *Diagnostic and Statistical Manual of Mental Disorders, 4th Edition* (*DSM-IV-TR*), published by the American Psychiatric Association. All members of the health care team use the DSM-IV-TR,

BOX 1.7	DSM-IV–TR Axes
Axis I:	Adult and child clinical disorders
	Conditions not attributable to a mental disorder that are a focus of clinical attention
Axis II:	Personality disorders
	Mental retardation
Axis III:	General medical conditions
Axis IV:	Psychosocial and environmental problems
Axis V:	Global assessment of functioning

SOURCE: Reprinted with permission from the *Diagnostic and Statistical Manual of Mental Disorders, Fourth Edition, Text Revision.* Copyright 2000 American Psychiatric Association.

which groups client information into five categories, called axes. (See Box 1.7 for a listing of the axes.) Axis I includes the majority of the mental disorders. Axis II lists long-lasting problems, including personality disorders and developmental disorders. Axis I and Axis II both describe the intrapersonal area of functioning. Axis III describes the physical problems of disorders that must be considered when planning the client's treatment program. If there are no physical problems, the diagnosis on Axis III will be stated as "none." Axis IV describes the psychosocial stressors (acute and long lasting) occurring in the past year that contributed to the current mental disorder. Nurses should be aware of how many stressors have occurred and how much change each stressor caused in the life of the client. Axis V rates the highest level of psychological, social, and occupational functioning the client has achieved in the past year, as well as the current level of functioning. It is especially important to be sensitive to cultural differences and expectations when rating clients on Axis V. Appendix A ∞ lists and describes the diagnostic categories of the DSM-IV-TR. Such data can also be viewed on the American Psychiatric Association Web site.

The bases of nursing diagnoses and DSM-IV-TR diagnoses evolve from problem solving, which begins with data collection. Data collection includes reviewing signs and symptoms exhibited by clients. With nursing diagnoses, those signs and symptoms are translated into related and contributing factors. With the DSM-IV-TR, the signs and symptoms are translated into diagnostic criteria, including the essential and associated features of specific mental disorders, and a differential diagnosis results.

There are some similarities between psychiatric nursing diagnoses and the DSM-IV-TR diagnoses. They both serve to guide practice by synthesizing data, leading to appropriate interventions. They are both communication tools basic to client care and research activities, and they are both international in scope. There are also significant differences between the two. DSM-IV-TR diagnoses are applicable only to individuals, whereas nursing diagnoses are applicable to individuals, families, groups, and communities. Nursing diagnoses are directed toward problems in daily living, whereas DSM-IV-TR diagnoses are oriented toward the "disease and cure" model.

Standard III: Outcome Identification

The widespread use of **NANDA nursing diagnoses** has increased awareness of the need for standardized classifications of nursing outcomes. Outcomes are positive or negative changes in health status that can be credited to nursing care. They allow us to evaluate the appropriateness of our decision-making process in selecting nursing interventions. Outcomes are important for the quality of nursing care and clinical evaluation research. **Nursing Outcomes Classification (NOC)** is a list of standardized measures that reflect the current status of clients. Outcomes are descriptive, on a continuum from the least desirable to the most desirable states or behaviors. Goals, on the other hand, are prescriptive—the state or behavior you want the client to achieve. Outcomes identify where the client is at any given moment, and goals identify where you want the client to end up (Johnson, Maas, & Moorhead, 2000; Gerolamo, 2004).

Once the outcomes are established, you and the client mutually identify *goals* for change. Mutual goal setting is the process of collaborating with clients to identify and prioritize care goals and develop a plan for achieving those goals. Underlying this process is respect for client cultural values. Begin by assessing the clients' degree of insight into their problems. If clients are too acutely ill to be actively involved in the initial goal formulation, or if they are in denial of mental health problems, they must at least be informed of the goals and given an opportunity to express their opinions (McCloskey & Bulechek, 1996), even if someone else will ultimately make the decision for them.

Clients are encouraged to identify strengths and abilities that they bring to this problem-solving process. The nurse helps them identify realistic, attainable goals and break down complex goals into small, manageable steps. After goals become manageable, work with clients on prioritization so they try to modify only one behavior at a time. Finally, help clients develop a plan to meet their goals, which includes identifying available resources, setting realistic time limits, and clarifying the roles of the nurse and the client. Establish regular review dates with clients and families to review progress toward outcomes and goals (McCloskey & Bulechek, 1996).

Standard IV: Planning

Once the nursing diagnoses, outcome criteria, and goals have been identified, the plan of care is developed to assist the client toward a higher level of functioning and im-proved mental health. Planning consists of establishing nursing care priorities, identifying interventions, and selecting appropriate nursing activities.

Priorities of Care In mental health nursing, safety needs are often more of a priority than physiologic needs. The nurse must be aware of many safety issues at all times. Frequently assess whether the client is in danger of the following:

- Exhaustion related to excessive exercise; lack of sleep; panic level of anxiety
- Inability to exercise good judgment related to problems in thinking or perceiving
- Self-mutilation based on past or current behavior
- Potential death related to toxic levels of medications, alcohol, or drugs
- Violence directed toward others based on past or current behavior
- Suicide related to hopelessness; command hallucinations

Interventions The widespread use of NANDA nursing diagnoses has increased awareness of the need for standardized classifications of nursing interventions or treatments. Until recently, there was no uniform way to define and document nursing care. The **Nursing Interventions Classification (NIC)** is the first comprehensive standardized classification of nursing interventions and is useful to nurses in all specialties and in all settings. Most of the interventions are for use with individuals, but many are for use with families, and a few are for use with entire communities (McCloskey & Bulechek, 1996).

Standard V: Implementation

Caring is a way of relating to people that enables them to grow toward their full potential. Nursing interventions should be implemented in a manner that recognizes the worth and dignity of people and considers the physical, emotional, social, cultural, and spiritual needs of clients and their families.

Roles of a Psychiatric Nurse No matter which mental disorder the client is experiencing, the nurse will assume several roles in helping the client grow and adapt. The appropriate role at any given time is determined by the planned interventions. The various roles of a nurse are described herein, most of which were described by Hildegard Peplau, the pioneer of psychiatric nursing.

Socializing Agent The nurse functions as a socializing agent with clients. Working one-to-one with your client, you will focus on difficulties the client may have in communicating thoughts and feelings to others. Socializing helps model appropriate interpersonal behavior. Informal conversations such as these give clients the opportunity to discuss nonstressful topics and provide some relief from anxiety.

Teacher Another nursing role is that of teacher. A great deal of teaching occurs in connection with the treatment plan (see chapter 7 ∞ for information on client and family education). Depending on client diagnoses, you may be involved in teaching activities of daily living. Some clients may need to learn basic cooking, laundry, or shopping skills to live independently. Those who have no diversions or hobbies may need help selecting appropriate activities and learning the skills associated with them. Some clients will need to learn and practice assertiveness skills, anger management skills, and/or conflict resolution strategies. The problem-solving process is discussed in detail in chapter 7 ∞.

Nurses will also teach clients and families about the purpose of medication, expected therapeutic effects, the length of time after taking the medication before a change, and the usual side effects. Clients must be informed about any dietary or activity restrictions related to their medications, as well as what to do if they forget to take a dose. Clients also must be instructed about any related blood testing or situations in which they should notify the physician immediately. In addition to oral instruction, written material (in the appropriate language) or pictures should be provided as a reference.

Model People learn by imitating models. Modeling enables clients to observe and experience alternative patterns of behavior. It helps clients clarify values and communicate openly and congruently. As a student nurse, you are a model for your clients, and you must not impose your own value system on impressionable individuals.

Advocate Nurses also act as advocates for clients. As an advocate, you will use a variety of communication techniques to reach clients in ways they can understand and to which they can respond. Nurse advocates serve as links between clients and other professionals or people in the community. As community members, nurses serve as advocates for all recipients of mental health care by striving to remove the stigma of mental illness.

Advocacy in nursing is based on a client's right to make decisions and a client's responsibility for the consequences of those decisions. Nurses must respect the decisions even when they disagree with them. However, if the decisions involve danger to self or others, the nurse must try to prevent the client from acting on the decision. As an advocate, you allow clients to express their feelings appropriately without censure or criticism. You teach responsible behavior of one person toward another, and you protect those clients temporarily unable to protect themselves.

Counselor Another nursing role is that of counselor. The counseling role is most typically assumed during regularly scheduled one-to-one sessions. The counseling interaction is directed toward specific goals and is based on the nursing care plan. As a counselor, you will create opportunities for clients to talk about thoughts, feelings, and behaviors that affect themselves and others. Effective verbal and nonverbal communication is modeled and practiced during the interactions. The effectiveness of counseling is seen when clients exhibit improved coping skills, increased self-esteem, and greater insight into and understanding of themselves.

Role-Player As role-players, nurses help clients recreate and enact specific past or future situations as if they were occurring in the present. You will create an environment in which new behaviors can be practiced in a nonthreatening way. Role-playing can strengthen a client's self-confidence in coping with problematic interactions, which in turn will increase the desire to implement what was learned in real-life situations. Through role-playing, you will help clients express themselves directly, clarify feelings, act out fears, and become more assertive. Clients who think at a concrete level, however, may not be able to transfer the role-playing experience to real-life situations. Role-playing is contraindicated with psychotic clients who are unable to comprehend "pretend" situations.

Milieu Manager Because of the round-the-clock contact with clients in some residential or hospital clinical settings, nurses have a unique opportunity to become milieu managers. The **therapeutic milieu** refers to the client's physical environment and all the interactions with staff members and other clients. The unit or facility is not just a place but is an active part of the treatment plan for each client, where there is a balance between the needs of individuals and the needs of the group. The environment influences client and staff behavior, and client and staff behavior changes the environment. The nurse must be aware of this interactive process at all times. Nurses must think about what they are doing and saying, and evaluate the impact on the therapeutic milieu.

The therapeutic milieu has many group activities and is as democratic as possible. In some settings, clients will elect officers from the client population. Community meetings provide opportunities for clients to solve problems related to living with a large group of people, to experience leadership, to help develop policies and rules, and to make decisions for themselves.

As milieu managers, nurses will provide clients with a safe environment in terms of avoiding self-mutilation, suicide, or violence to others. For some clients, nurses will have to set limits on behaviors that are not appropriate to the setting. Some clients require periods of privacy, whereas others need to be encouraged to socialize. Nurses manage the milieu by their presence and their contact with clients. To help clients learn new behaviors, nurses give support and direction and model appropriate behaviors.

The goal of a therapeutic milieu is to increase the client's sense of belonging; improve interpersonal skills, such as socialization or conflict management; and help clients recognize the impact of their own behavior on others and grow toward autonomy as much as possible. (Characteristics of the therapeutic milieu are covered further in chapter 9 ∞.)

Standard VI: Evaluation

The final step in the nursing process is evaluation. In this step, nurses evaluate and document client progress toward the outcome criteria and evaluate their own clinical practice.

Evaluation of Client Progress As you compare client behavior to previously established goals and outcome criteria, you should be able to answer the following questions:

1. Was the assessment adequate?
2. Were the nursing diagnoses accurate?
3. Was the client involved in setting goals? Were the goals appropriate? Were the goals attained?
4. Were the planned interventions effective?
5. Were the outcome criteria demonstrated?
6. What changes took place in the client's behavior?
7. Which nursing interventions were effective?
8. Which nursing interventions need revision?
9. Was the client satisfied with the nursing care?
10. What plans must be modified?
11. Are new care plans necessary?
12. Has adequate documentation of the client's progress been completed?

There are two types of evaluation: formative and summative. *Formative evaluation* is an ongoing process based on the client's responses to care. From the formative evaluation, the nurse maintains, modifies, or expands the nursing care plan. *Summative evaluation* is a terminal process and is used to determine whether the client has achieved the mutually set goals. Summative evaluations are done in the form of discharge summaries.

Documentation Documentation is a critical component of nursing practice. The general rule is: If it is not documented, it has not occurred. All steps of the nursing process pertinent to the client must be documented in the client's record. Documenting assessment includes recording psychosocial histories, focused nursing assessments, neuropsychiatric assessments, and client/family education

needs. Documenting diagnosis and planning is typically accomplished in one or more of the following formats: critical pathways, individual nursing care plans, standard nursing care plans, and multidisciplinary care plans. Further documentation includes specific plans for client/family education. Documenting implementation includes writing progress notes in the form of narrative and flow sheets. Inpatient agencies require that nursing progress notes be entered at specific times, such as once every shift or once every 24 hours. Any significant events must also be documented, as well as the client's participation in and influence on the therapeutic milieu. Some of the most critical documentation issues in inpatient nursing involve falls, and suicidal or violent behavior. Each clinical setting has specific routines and forms for close observation of these episodes. Documenting evaluation is done when progress toward the outcome criteria and goals is charted in the record. The client's level of knowledge achieved through the teaching plan must be included in the documentation. Discharge summaries are written when contact with the client has ended.

Self-Evaluation It is important for nurses to not only evaluate client progress, but also to evaluate themselves. Self-evaluation will increase nurses' self-understanding and improve their clinical practice. Nurses may use a variety of methods in this process, such as process recordings, one-to-one interactions with an instructor, and group supervision during preconferences and postconferences.

Dealing with client desires, needs, and emotions can lead to feelings of discomfort or burnout for mental health nurses. Therefore, beginning and experienced nurses both need support and supervision to maintain their effectiveness. Supervision is the process of having a peer, teacher, head nurse, clinical specialist, or mentor evaluate a nurse's clinical practice to increase his or her knowledge and competence. It is an opportunity for nurses to share feelings about themselves and their clients and to receive emotional support and guidance. From peers, nurses can determine the image they project and how others view them. Supervisors can assist in the process of self-evaluation by sharing their perceptions and offering suggestions for change.

MEETING THE CHALLENGES OF THE TWENTY-FIRST CENTURY

Evidence-Based Practice

Evidence-based practice bridges the gap that exists between clinical research and everyday practice. Nurses applying **evidence-based practice** use the best available research evidence, utilize their clinical expertise, and respect clients' choices, concerns, and values to arrive at the best client outcomes.

As students and beginning practitioners, you will need guidance from faculty and nursing researchers on how to obtain, interpret, and integrate the best available research as you develop your clinical expertise (Johnston & Fineout-Overholt, 2006).

When evidence-based practice is limited to double-blind randomized controlled trials, nursing loses its diverse theories and diverse types of evidence. In this narrow sense, evidence-based practice reduces and distorts nursing into a simplistic practice.

The Joanna Briggs Institute for Evidence-Based Nursing and Midwifery publishes Best Practice Information Sheets based on a systematic review that summarizes the current best evidence. These are available on the Joanna Briggs Web site. David Evans (2001) developed Best Practice. Music as an Intervention in Hospitals. The study populations were hospital patients awaiting treatment or recovering from treatment and patients who were undergoing unpleasant procedures at the time of the music intervention. Outcomes of the 19 studies included anxiety, pain, sedation, satisfaction, tolerance, mood, and physiological outcomes, such as heart and respiratory rate and blood pressure. Based on level 1 evidence (the highest level) the recommendation is that playing music to hospital patients reduces anxiety and improves mood but has little impact on blood pressure and heart rate. Music did *not* have any impact on patients undergoing unpleasant procedures. Bedside nurses can utilize this research information and teach patients that music may lower anxiety and improve mood. Those who choose to use music choose from a selection of musical styles such as classical, instrumental, relaxing, piano, and new age. This is an example of how evidence-based practice can be implanted in everyday nursing practice.

Psychiatric nurses use quantitative and qualitative research to support their decision-making process. To help nurses shift from traditional practice to evidence-based practice, Rosswurm and Larrabee (1999) developed the following model:

Step 1: Identify a Specific Problem With One Area of Nursing Practice.
- Involve nursing staff, other health care providers, administrators, and interested clients.
- Examine data that indicates a need for a change in practice.

Step 2: Link the Problem With Outcomes and Interventions.
- Use the language of standardized classifications: NANDA, NOC, and NIC.

Step 3: Synthesize Best Evidence.
- Using critical thinking skills, review the research to determine whether there is strong evidence to support a change in nursing practice.
- If the evidence is not strong enough to warrant a change in practice, assess the benefit versus risk factors to change.

Step 4: Design a Change in Practice.
- Develop a protocol or procedure, keeping the change as simple as possible to increase the chances that it will be accepted.
- Identify what resources are needed to make the change.
- Plan how change will occur.
- Define the outcomes of the change.

Step 5: Implement and Evaluate the Practice Change.
- Analyze the data and interpret the results.
- Decide to adopt, adapt, or reject the change based on results of research and feedback.

Step 6: Integrate and Maintain Change in Practice.
- Get people involved.
- Maintain open communication channels.
- Provide the necessary resources.
- Monitor process and outcomes.
- Reward quality performance with incentives.

Information Technology

There probably has not been a time of such rapid societal change as in the latter three or four decades of the twentieth century. In terms of nursing issues, there have been dramatic alterations in the way health care is organized and delivered: Technology has changed the way we practice our profession, and there have been massive changes in the number of ethical issues related to health care.

There have also been changes in nursing education. Computer knowledge is almost a prerequisite for taking nursing classes. Many courses use fiber optics and satellites to beam lessons to remote connections. Nursing students can acquire information using technologic advances, such as online search engines on the Internet, computerized reference databases, CD-ROMs, and video disks. Many nursing journals offer their issues online, and many electronic journals and books are available only online.

This explosion of knowledge shows no sign of diminishing. Technology allows nurses to access information, select and use the data obtained, make sound decisions about the appropriateness of the data, and create solutions that meet clients' needs.

Across the country, and the world, clients are learning about their own medical conditions and bringing that knowledge with them to their health care provider's office. The clients come with misinformation, however, because they are unable to evaluate the scientific quality of medical information on the Internet. As nurses, we are not only a resource for health information but we also help clients find sources of health information that are well researched. Many clients find online support groups invaluable because of the convenience, practical coping suggestions, and health care referrals. Online consumer health sites change frequently. The following are some respected sites that are likely to be around for some years:

Centers for Disease Control and Prevention, *www.cdc.gov*

U.S. Department of Health and Human Services, *www.healthfinder.gov*

Mayo Clinic Health Oasis, *www.mayohealth.org*

U.S. National Library of Medicine, *www.nlm.nih.gov*

Medscape, *www.medscape.com*

Mental Health Net, *www.mentalhelp.net*

Nursing Today

As nursing moved into the twenty-first century, it advanced beyond the Western biomedical model to incorporate many healing tools used by our Asian, Latino, Native American, African, and European ancestors. Some see this movement as a "return to our roots." Others believe it is a response to runaway health care costs, growing dissatisfaction with high-tech medicine, and increasing concern over the adverse effects and misuse of medications. The growth of consumer empowerment also fuels this movement.

The rise of chronic disease rates in Western society has motivated consumers to increasingly consider self-care approaches. As recently as the 1950s, we lived in a world of curable disease, largely infectious, where medical interventions were both appropriate and effective and only 30% of all disease was long term. Now, 80% of all disease is long term. Western medicine, with its focus on acute disorders, trauma, and surgery, is considered to be the best high-tech medical care in the world. Unfortunately, it cannot respond adequately to the current epidemic of long-term illness. As nurses, we must become active in reforming the current health care system to be able to meet the challenges that lie ahead.

MediaLink Community Resources

Focus Your Study

OBJECTIVES	KEY CONCEPTS
1. Describe the continuum from mental health to persistent and severe mental illness.	■ Each are end points on a continuum with movement back and forth throughout life. ■ Levels include physical (brain), personal (self-care), interpersonal (others), and societal (social and cultural context).
2. Compare and contrast the theoretical assumptions of neurobiological and prebiological models of mental disorders.	■ Mental disorders arise from neurodevelopmental or neurodegenerative processes ■ Life experiences help or hinder the development of mental disorders by modifying the expression of genes. ■ The diathesis–stress model proposes that when a biologically vulnerable person is exposed to triggers, they may develop a mental disorder. ■ The intrapersonal, social–interpersonal, behavioral, cognitive, gender-bias, and crisis theories focus on the psychological and social aspects of mental disorders.

3. Apply the nursing process to mental health nursing.	■ Assess clients using psychosocial assessment and neuropsychiatric assessment.
	  ■ Assessment by observation includes noting clients' behavior, affect, cognitions, interpersonal relationships, and physical condition.
	  ■ Psychosocial assessment includes history, family history, family interactions, social history, living conditions, and spiritual considerations, as well as strengths and competencies.
	  ■ Neuropsychiatric assessment provides information about clients' appearance, behavior, speech, emotional state, and cognitive function.

4. Distinguish between the therapeutic relationship and the nursing process.	■ The nursing process is a way to organize scientific data to prescribe practice criteria. ■ The therapeutic relationship is the means by which nurses are able to implement the nursing process. ■ Caring is the essence of the relationship. ■ The nursing process includes assessing clients accurately, formulating diagnoses, helping clients establish outcome, planning and implementing interventions, and evaluating the effectiveness of the plan of care.

continued

continued

5. Discuss current issues in mental health nursing.

→ ■ Critical thinking
■ Evidence-based practice
■ Information technology
■ Alternative therapies

Explore MediaLink

For review questions, case studies, and other resources for this chapter see the Pearson Health MediaLink CD-ROM that accompanies this book and the Companion Website.

CD-ROM
■ Audio Glossary
■ NCLEX-RN® Review Questions

Companion Website www.prenhall.com/fontaine
■ Audio Glossary
■ NCLEX-RN® Review Questions
■ Case Study
– Mentally Ill or Different?
■ Care Plan
– Managing Personal Anxiety
■ Critical Thinking
– People in Crisis: Applying Theory
■ MediaLink Applications
– Overcoming the Stigma
■ MediaLinks
– Books for Clients and Families
– Community Resources

NCLEX-RN® Review Questions

1-1. A nurse has received report on her assigned clients. Which of the following clients should the nurse see first? The client with:
1. Anorexia who has gained 2 pounds this week.
2. Alcohol withdrawal and a BP of 112/78.
3. Schizophrenia who is suspicious of staff.
4. Anxiety who is being discharged today.

1-2. A 57-year-old woman volunteers 3 days a week at a homeless shelter, assists grandmothers raising grandchildren, and reads to clients at a nursing home. According to Erickson's theories of personality development, this woman's behaviors are age appropriate for which developmental crisis?
1. Industry and inferiority
2. Intimacy and isolation
3. Trust and mistrust
4. Generativity and self-absorption

1-3. A nurse knows that professional nursing care is based on a theoretical framework. Those theories are:
1. Truths that can be validated.
2. Ideas and assumptions about behavior.
3. Anecdotal occurrences about phenomena.
4. Ideas that describe and explain phenomena.

1-4. In order for a nurse to effectively use Peplau's theory of interpersonal relations, the nurse must first:
1. Have a baccalaureate level of education.
2. Care about the client with problems.
3. Demonstrate comprehensive knowledge about therapeutic communication.
4. Deal effectively with personal feelings.

1-5. A registered nurse is asked to serve on a hospital committee that is planning to introduce evidence-based nursing practices. The nurse reads about evidence-based practice and finds that the committee should establish nursing practices based on:
1. Assumptions.
2. Historical methods.
3. Personal experience.
4. Research findings.

See Appendix D for answers.

References

Aguiliera, D. C., & Messick, J. M. (1990). *Crisis intervention: Theory and methodology* (6th ed.). St. Louis, MO: Mosby.

American Nurses Association. (2000). *Scope and standards of psychiatric–mental health nursing practice*. Washington, DC: American Psychiatric Nurses Association.

American Psychiatric Association. (2000). *Diagnostic and statistical manual of mental disorders* (4th ed., Text Revision). Washington, DC: Author.

Beck, A., & Freeman, A. (1990). *Cognitive therapy of personality disorders*. New York: Guilford Press.

Chinn, P. L., & Watson, J. (Eds.). (1994). *Art and aesthetics in nursing*. New York: NLN Press.

Day, P. O., & Horton-Deutsch, S. (2004). Using mindfulness-based therapeutic interventions in psychiatric nursing practice. *Archives of Psychiatric Nursing, 18*(5), 164–169.

Devlin, M. J., Yanovski, S. Z., & Wilson, G. T. (2000). Obesity: What mental health professionals need to know. *American Journal of Psychiatry, 157*(6), 854–866.

Erickson, E. H. (1963). *Childhood and society* (2nd ed.). New York: Norton.

Evans, D. (2001). Best practice: Music as an intervention in hospitals. *The Joanna Briggs Institute for Evidence Based Nursing and Midwifery, 5*(4): 1–6.

Flaskerud, J. H., & Wuerker, A. K. (1999). Mental health nursing in the 21st century. *Issues in Mental Health Nursing, 20*, 5–17.

Flaskerud, J. H. (2000). From the guest editor—Shifting paradigms to neuropsychiatric nursing. *Issues in Mental Health Nursing, 21*(1), 1–2.

Freud, S. (1935). *A general introduction to psychoanalysis*. New York: Simon & Schuster.

Gabbard, G. O. (2004). Reflective function, mentalization, and borderline personality disorder. In B. D. Beitman & J. Nair (Eds.), *Self-awareness deficits in psychiatric patients* (pp. 213–228). New York: W.W. Norton & Co.

George, T. B. (2002). Care meanings, expressions, and experiences of those with chronic mental illness. *Archives of Psychiatric Nursing, 16*(1), 25–31.

Gerolamo, A. M. (2004). State of the Science: Outcomes of acute inpatient psychiatric care. *Archives of Psychiatric Nursing, 18*(6), 203–214.

Goleman, D. (1995). *Emotional intelligence*. New York: Bantam Books.

Halter, M. J. (2004). The stigma of seeking care and depression. *Archives of Psychiatric Nursing, 18*(5), 178–184.

Henry, J., & Henry, L. (2004). *The soul of the caring nurse: Stories and resources for revitalizing professional passion*. New York: American Nurses Publishing.

Insel, T. R., & Collins, F. S. (2003). Psychiatry in the genomics era. *American Journal of Psychiatry, 160*(4), 616–620.

Jenkins, J., Grady, P. A., & Collins, F. S. (2005). Nurses and the genomic revolution. *Journal of Nursing Scholarship, 37*(2), 98–101.

Johnson, M., Maas, M., & Moorhead, S. (Eds.). (2000). *Nursing outcomes classification (NOC)* (2nd ed.). St. Louis, MO: Mosby.

Johnston, J., & Fineout-Overholt, E. (2006). Teaching EBP: The critical step of critically appraising the literature. *Worldviews on Evidence-Based Nursing*, First Quarter 2006, 44–46.

Kandel, E. R. (1999). Biology and the future of psychoanalysis: A new intellectual framework for psychiatry revisited. *American Journal of Psychiatry, 156*(4), 505–524.

Keen, P. (1991). Caring for ourselves. In R. M. Neil & R. Watts (Eds.), *Caring and nursing: Explorations in feminist perspective* (pp. 173–188), Pub. No. 14-2369. New York: NLN Press.

Kendler, K. S., Karkowski, L. M., & Prescott, C. A. (1999). Causal relationship between stressful life events and the onset of major depression. *American Journal of Psychiatry, 156*(6), 837–841.

Kendler, K. S. (2005). "A gene for . . .": The nature of gene action in psychiatric disorders. *American Journal of Psychiatry, 162*(7), 1243–1252.

Kessler, R. C., Berglund, P., Demler, O., Jin, R., Merikangas, K. R., & Walters, E. E. (2005). Lifetime prevalence and age-of-onset distributions of DSM-IV disorders in the National Comorbidity Survey Replication. *Archives of General Psychiatry, 62*(6), 593–602.

Kessler, R. C., Demler, O., Frank, R. G., Olfson, M., Pincus, H. A., Walters, E. E., et al. (2005). Prevalence and treatment of mental disorders. *New England Journal of Medicine, 352*(24), 2515–2523.

Kozier, B., Erb, G., Blais, K., Wilkinson, J., & Van Leuven, K. (2003). *Fundamentals of nursing* (7th ed.). Upper Saddle River, NJ: Prentice Hall.

Krauss, J. B. (2004). Promises, promises. *Archives of Psychiatric Nursing, 18*(1), 1–3.

Levoy, G. M. (1998). *Callings: Finding and following an authentic life*. New York: Three Rivers Press.

Maslow, A. (1968). *Toward a psychology of being* (2nd ed.). New York: Van Nostrand Reinhold.

Mathers, C. D., Bernard, C., Iburg, K. M., Inoue, M., Fat, D. M., Shibuya, K., et al. (2004). Global Burden of Disease in 2002. Paper No. 54. *World Health Organization*.

McCloskey, J., & Bulechek, G. M. (Eds.). (1996). *Nursing interventions classification (NIC)* (2nd ed.). St. Louis, MO: Mosby.

North American Nursing Diagnosis Association. (2003). *Nursing diagnoses, definitions and classification 2003–2004*. Philadelphia: Author.

Peplau, H. E. (1952). *Interpersonal relations in nursing*. New York: Putnam.

Pesut, D. J. (2004). Florence Nightingale: INTY at work. *Reflections on Nursing Leadership, 30*(3), 16–18.

Piaget, J. (1972). *The psychology of the child*. New York: Basic Books.

Prows, C. A., Glass, M., Nicol, M. J., Skirton, H., & Williams, J. (2005). Genomics in nursing education. *Journal of Nursing Scholarship, 37*(3), 196–202.

Rosswurm, M. A., & Larrabee, J. H. (1999). A model for change to evidence-based practice. *Image, 31*(4), 317–322.

Sieg, D. (2004). Lost your smile? *Reflections on Nursing LEADERSHIP, 30*(1), 36–38.

Skinner, B. F. (1953). *Science and human behavior*. Riverside, NJ: Macmillan.

Sullivan, H. S. (1953). *The interpersonal theory of psychiatry*. New York: Norton.

Teplin, L. A., McClelland, G. M., Abram, K. M., & Weiner, D. A. (2005). Crime victimization in adults with severe mental illness. *Archives of General Psychiatry, 62*(8), 911–921.

Vaillant, G. E. (2003). Mental health. *American Journal of Psychiatry, 160*(8), 1373–1384.

Wang, P. S., Lane, M., Olfson, M., Pincus, H. A., Wells, K. B., & Kessler, R. C. (2005). Twelve-month use of mental health services in the United States. *Archives of General Psychiatry, 62*(6), 590–592.

Chapter 2

The Family in Mental Health Nursing

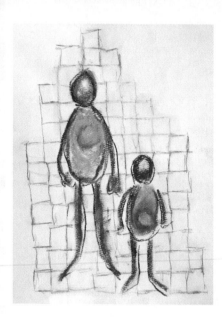

 Family

born into family
left to be rebuilt
when closets open

a new family
to be searched out
and discovered

a family
born of respect and love "

—Heather, Age 30

OBJECTIVES

After reading this chapter, you will be able to:

1. Outline the elements of the family system.
2. Discuss the impact of grief and loss on the family system.
3. Discuss the impact of persistent and severe mental illness on the family system.
4. Assess family functioning using the family competency model.
5. Characterize the roles of the mental health nurse in family nursing practice.
6. Design interventions to improve the functioning of clients and their families.

MediaLink www.prenhall.com/fontaine
Go to the Pearson Health Nursing MediaLink CD-ROM and the Companion Website at
www.prenhall.com/fontaine for interactive resources for this chapter.

This chapter provides an overview of family competency, uses grieving as a model to illustrate mental health and developmental issues, presents the impact of mental illness on the family system, and discusses mental disorders across the life span. The remainder of the chapter is devoted to family nursing practice.

For most of us, the family is our earliest and most enduring social relationship. Family is the fabric of our day-to-day lives and shapes the quality of our lives by influencing our outlook on life, our motivations, our strategies for achievement, and our styles for coping with adversity. It is within our families that we develop our sense of self and our capacity for intimacy. Through family interactions, we learn about relationships and roles and our expectations of others and ourselves. Each of us is simultaneously independent of and part of our families. We are individuals and family members both. We are part of our families and our families are part of us.

Family is defined as two or more persons related by birth, marriage, formal or informal adoption, or choice. This definition includes couples, traditional families, lesbian and gay families, communal families, families with cohabitating parents, extended families, multigenerational families, and even friends living together. Some families are protected by legal ties; others are not. A family is an intimate group with a shared past, present, and future. No one family form necessarily provides an environment that is better for people to live or raise children in.

Labels indicate how we view families, and labels tend to become a self-fulfilling prophecy. In the past, health care professionals have used a deficit model in looking at families. Families were labeled *functional* or *dysfunctional*, with the focus on fixing what needed repair. Psychiatric nursing has now moved to viewing families through a competency model. The **competency model** is based on the belief that all families are resourceful and have the capacity to grow and change. The model does not ignore pathology and dysfunction but emphasizes strengths, adaptation, and resources. The focus is one of building on competence rather than on correcting deficits. Focusing on family strengths and resources helps empower families to respond and adapt to life's circumstances (Mohr, Lafuze, & Mohr, 2000).

Family life becomes increasingly complex as the family responds to life events. Birth, death, and illness, such as severe and persistent mental illness, have a profound effect on family members and relationships. As nurses, it is important that we understand how a family relates to each person in the family and struggles with a variety of life issues. Each family has a unique story and each family makes sense. No matter how dysfunctional it may appear, each family has a finely tuned style of living and interacting among the members of the family. This does not mean that all families' ways of living are healthy, effective, or even enjoyable. But the family does make sense when seen as a whole.

FAMILY SYSTEMS

In understanding the complexity of family systems, consider how family members communicate, how they establish and maintain boundaries, how cohesive and flexible they are, and how emotionally available they are to others in the family. Understanding these interactions will provide a general idea of how well the family is able to adapt and function, both in everyday life and in the face of adversity, such as the occurrence of mental illness.

Family Communication

Family communication is measured by focusing on the family as a group with regard to its listening skills, speaking skills, self-disclosure, and tracking. In high-functioning families each person

- Listens—is empathetic and attentive.
- Speaks—speaks for oneself and does not speak for others.
- Self-discloses—shares personal feelings about oneself and others in the family.
- Tracks—stays on the topic at hand.

Families who communicate well are better able to adapt and cope. Families who find communication difficult may experience lower levels of expressiveness, vague requests to one another, an inability to comprehend each other's messages, frequent interruption of one another, speaking for others, and high levels of verbalized hostility.

Another aspect of family communication is the family's strategy to *resolve conflict*. The ability to resolve differences is based on the family's capacity to talk about areas of disagreement and its mutual willingness to negotiate and reach

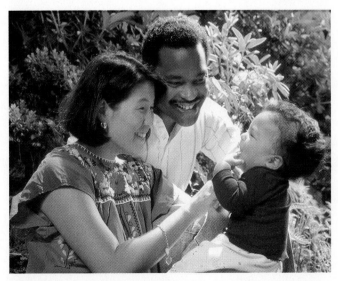

PHOTO 2.1 ■ Competent families have an emotional climate of intimacy and predictability.

SOURCE: Lawrence Migdale/Lawrence Migdale/Pix. Used with permission.

acceptable solutions. Problem-solving skills are critical to smooth family functioning. Without these skills, families seem to use strategies such as confrontation or avoidance, which are ineffective in reducing stress and do not resolve conflict satisfactorily.

Boundaries

Boundaries are the invisible lines that define the amount and kind of contact allowable among members of the family and between the family and outside systems. Boundaries determine the patterns of how, when, and to whom family members relate. Boundaries define the divisions among the spousal, parental, and sibling subsystems.

- *Clear boundaries:* Firm yet flexible; family members are supported and nurtured but also allowed a certain degree of autonomy.
- *Rigid boundaries:* Family members are isolated from one another and there is little room for negotiation and individual development.
- *Diffuse boundaries:* Everyone is into everyone else's business; there is little distinction between family members and there is too much negotiation, resulting in a loss of autonomy.

In the modern Western nuclear family, competent families have clear hierarchical boundaries between generations in terms of power, authority, and responsibility. Competent adult leadership provides an emotional climate that considers everyone's needs and provides a sense of security. Members spend time apart, as well as time together. Mutual respect is also a boundary issue. Competent families respect and value the individual's opinions and feelings. The family system tolerates individual differences and honors differing opinions.

Boundaries are a social construction and, as such, are culturally determined. What appears to be a boundary violation in one culture may be acceptable in another culture. For example, how family members respect privacy in regard to toileting, bathing, changing clothes, and sleeping arrangements varies by culture. Multigenerational boundaries in terms of power and authority vary from culture to culture.

Family Cohesion

Family cohesion is defined as the emotional bonding that family members have toward one another. There are four levels of cohesion (Figure 2.1■):

1. Disengaged (very low)
2. Separated (low to moderate)
3. Connected (moderate to high)
4. Enmeshed (very high)

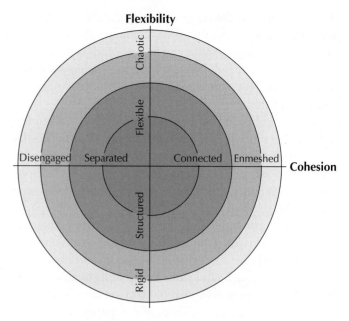

Figure 2.1 ■ Circumplex model.

In Western, developed societies, it is believed that the central ranges of cohesion (separated and connected) contribute to optimal family competency. The extremes (disengaged or enmeshed) are seen as less adaptive. Disengaged families seem almost like a group of strangers who happen to be living together. There is little loyalty or closeness. Members of enmeshed families cannot develop a separate identity, and each person must yield autonomy to belong to the family. Uniqueness is experienced as distance, and individuality is viewed as alienation and disloyalty (Olson, 1996). See Box 2.1 for characteristics of family cohesion.

BOX 2.1	Characteristics of Family Cohesion

Disengaged

- Little closeness
- Little loyalty
- High independence

Separated

- Low-moderate closeness
- Some loyalty
- Interdependent with more independence than dependence

Connected

- Moderate-high closeness
- High loyalty
- Interdependent with more dependence than independence

Enmeshed

- Very high closeness
- Very high loyalty
- High dependency

Family Flexibility

Family flexibility is the amount of change in a family's leadership, role relationships, and relationship rules. Flexibility also refers to the family's ability to respond to stress. There are four levels of flexibility (see Figure 2.1):

1. Rigid (very low)
2. Structured (low to moderate)
3. Flexible (moderate to high)
4. Chaotic (very high)

As with cohesion, it is believed that the central ranges (structured and flexible) are more conducive to family adaptation, with the extremes (rigid and chaotic) less competent (Olson, 1996). See Box 2.2 for characteristics of family flexibility.

Rules determine appropriate roles and relationship patterns within the family. Rules express the family's values and form a boundary around each family, which then screens outside information for compatibility with the family's value system. If the message is not congruent with the family's values, such statements as, "That is not the way we do things in this family" or "I don't care what Marc is allowed to do; in this family, we . . ." will appear. To understand rules more clearly, reflect for a moment on the family in which you grew up. There were certain things that you just did, that you knew were expected. Other things were not permitted. For purposes of assessing a few of the rules in your family of origin, complete the statements in Box 2.3.

BOX 2.2	Characteristics of Family Flexibility

Chaotic

- Lack of leadership
- Dramatic role shifts
- Erratic discipline
- Too much change

Flexible

- Shared leadership
- Democratic discipline
- Role-sharing change
- Change when necessary

Structured

- Leadership sometimes shared
- Somewhat democratic discipline
- Roles stable
- Change when demanded

Rigid

- Authoritarian leadership
- Strict discipline
- Roles seldom change
- Too little change

BOX 2.3	Assessing Rules in Your Family of Origin

In my family, we were never allowed to . . .

In my family, we were always expected to . . .

In my family, girls were required to . . .

In my family, girls were allowed to . . .

In my family, girls were forbidden to . . .

In my family, boys were required to . . .

In my family, boys were allowed to . . .

In my family, boys were forbidden to . . .

In my family, household responsibilities were determined by . . .

In my family, we handled conflict by . . .

In my family, the most important thing in life for women is . . .

In my family, the most important thing in life for men is . . .

Emotional Availability

Families who cope well encourage the members within the family to express a wide variety of feelings. The emotional climate is one of intimacy and predictability. In other families, the emotional climate may be angry, cold, or distant and unpredictable.

Emotional availability is another way to describe the quality of parent–child interactions. Areas for assessment include parental sensitivity, structuring, nonintrusiveness, and nonhostility. *Parental sensitivity* is assessed by how parents pick up on children's emotional signals and how appropriately they express their own emotions. *Parental structuring* refers to the ability of parents to support learning and exploration without overwhelming the child's autonomy. *Parental nonintrusiveness* refers to the ability to be available to the child without being interfering, overprotective, or overwhelming. *Nonhostility* refers to ways of interacting with the child that are patient and pleasant. When angry, parents express the anger in an appropriately controlled manner (Biringen, 2000).

Family Competency

Competency is found in a diversity of family arrangements. More important than the form or type of family are the family's relational resources and adaptive abilities. The most distinctive trait of competent families is the ability to productively manage stress. Simply put, adaptive families evolve and shift with changing situations. This is often referred to as *resiliency*. Walsh (1998) describes family resiliency as the "process of coming to terms with all that has happened, reaching new emotional and relational equilibrium with changed circumstances, and becoming more resourceful in facing whatever lies ahead" (p. 75). Life crises and developmental transitions can stimulate family growth and transformation. Resilient families make it through crises such as disability and death with a renewed sense of confidence and purpose.

Death and the Family System

Death is a choiceless event that leads to chaos and disorder for survivors. Coming to terms with death is the most difficult task families confront. We live, die, grieve, and survive within a family context. Prior experiences with death and loss in the family influence how we grieve. Families teach us the cultural norms of how to behave when someone close to us dies.

Grief

Bereavement is the feelings, thoughts, and responses that loved ones experience following the death of a person with whom they have shared a significant relationship. **Grief**, or mourning, is the active process of learning to adapt to the loved one's death. *Mourning* is a progression through a series of phases that includes recognition and acceptance of the death, the experience of emotional and physical pain, and the rebuilding of a life without the loved one. Grieving also occurs with any significant loss and is a person's process of learning to live with feelings as she or he struggles to reestablish self-esteem or self-confidence in the face of these personal losses. The process of grieving is essential for mental and physical health because it allows people to cope with loss gradually and to accept it as part of reality. Families, religious beliefs, and cultural customs influence mourning and grieving. It is a social process and is best shared and carried out with the help of others. No one grieves predictably or uniformly. As caring nurses, we must always respect individuality in the way persons grieve and mourn.

Family gender roles also affect reactions at times of loss. In North America, women are often the ones who grieve outwardly in the form of tears and sorrow, whereas men are expected to "be strong" and show minimal emotion during grief. Men may choose strategies such as logical reasoning, as opposed to emotional expression, or diversional activities to manage their unacknowledged feelings. Families' spiritual beliefs and religious practices influence how people react to loss and death and their resulting behavior. Most religious groups have customs and practices, which can help survivors with the process of grieving.

Family systems, like individuals, experience symptoms of grief, including changes in family structure and changes in relationships outside the family. The death of a family member radically disrupts the family system. The first priority in managing grief is to reestablish a stable equilibrium, which is necessary to support ongoing family development.

This requires the resources of the individual, extended family, friends, and community.

In response to death, family *structure* often changes temporarily. All family members play roles within and outside the family. When a family member dies, those roles she or he played are temporarily unfulfilled. Realignment of roles is a necessary function of grieving, and the process of recovery includes redistribution of role functions. Roles may be reassigned based on achievement and interest or on the basis of gender and age. Individuals must adapt and adjust to the new roles and the absence of the deceased member. A more flexible family typically will be more successful. Like individuals, families are unique in their mourning processes. What is effective for one family may not be effective for another.

Relationships with people outside the family often change because death disrupts established patterns of interaction. Some families are able to reach out to others, but some withdraw from their friends and other support networks. At times, families may be overprotective toward some or all members, effectively isolating these individuals.

Children experience the same emotions of grief as adults but are less likely to show acute grief in the initial phase and are more likely to experience the process over a much longer period. At each developmental level, children rework the meaning of a family member's death from a more mature cognitive and emotional functioning level.

- Preverbal children are very sensitive to the emotional climate created by their grieving family members.

- Preschoolers believe death to be reversible and that the person could come back. They may regress to an earlier stage of development and use play to cope with feelings.

- School-age children tend to avoid speaking of their grief more than either preschoolers or teens. This

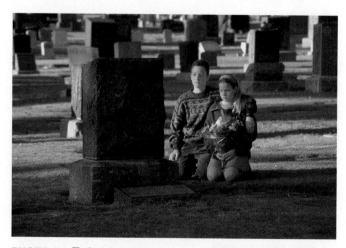

PHOTO 2.2 ■ Children experience the same emotions of grief as adults.

SOURCE: David Young–Wolff/PhotoEdit, Inc. Used with permission.

gives the impression of unconcern. School-age children may develop school problems.

- Typically, 8- to 9-year-old children begin to understand the finality of death and may find this very frightening. They equate death with abandonment, which makes them especially vulnerable to depression, anxiety, self-blame, and low self-esteem for months.
- Adolescents cognitively understand death in adult terms. As they strive for their independence in the midst of this tragedy, some may become closer to the family, whereas others may act out.

Homicide of a family member has a devastating effect on the family. Few people are prepared for this unexpected tragedy. Their loved ones may have been killed during a domestic quarrel, a robbery, a mass murder, or a terrorist attack. The ensuing legal processes, which may take years to resolve, complicate the family's ability to grieve and heal (Vessier-Batchen & Douglas, 2006).

Disenfranchised Grief

Every culture establishes grieving norms and denies such emotions to people deemed to have insignificant losses. Insignificant losses are not acknowledged or validated by others, and the survivors are deprived of their right to grieve. **Disenfranchised grief** means that the loss cannot be openly acknowledged, socially validated, or publicly mourned. Typically, there are three categories of disenfranchised grief:

- The relationship is not recognized.
- The loss is not recognized.
- The griever is not recognized.

Often, the significance of the loss is not recognized when the connections are loose or informal. These might include friends, neighbors, or coworkers. Some people negate the loss of relationships that are not socially sanctioned, such as nontraditional relationships, extramarital affairs, or same-gender relationships. Relationships that existed primarily in the past often are not recognized as needing to be grieved over, such as former friends, past lovers, or ex-spouses. Some losses are not recognized socially. These include elective abortions, perinatal deaths, giving up a child for adoption, and even the loss of a beloved pet.

In the instance of grievers who are not recognized, the person is socially defined by the culture as not touched by grief. The very old, who are thought to be too frail and fragile to cope with loss, and the very young, who are thought to be oblivious to loss, are often excluded from discussions and rituals. Sometimes it is assumed that people who are developmentally disabled are incapable of understanding death and have no need to mourn. As nurses, we must remember that people exist in multiple relationships and form meaningful

and significant attachments in different kinds of relationships. The dominant culture often ignores these in favor of the nuclear family, which is given a monopoly on mourning. Past relationships, such as an ex-spouse, may still hold a degree of attachment and there may be grief. When the promise of unborn children is broken, parents experience grief. In modern society, significant pet–human bonds develop, and there is grief when the pet dies. People are capable of a great capacity for attachments, so they are vulnerable to grief when these attachments are ended. Problems result when that fact is forgotten and the grief is minimized or ignored.

Complicated Grief

The boundaries between normal and **complicated grief** are unclear. The judgment that a person's grief is complicated is based not only on the individual, but also on the range and tolerance of differences in grieving allowed by the culture. Complicated grief is generally considered the presence of unremitting and incapacitating distress for at least 6 months and is associated with the presence of mental disorders. See Box 2.4 for factors that contribute to increased distress or to a good outcome during mourning.

It is unclear how complicated grief may be related to incidents of mass violence or terrorism. When violence is sudden and there are a number of deaths and injuries, survivors are at high risk for posttraumatic stress disorder (PTSD). The media brings these events into the lives of millions more individuals who may also develop PTSD. Survivors of homicide and suicide victims experience more stigma, guilt, and rejection than those whose loved ones died through illness or accidents and are at higher risk for PTSD. Future

BOX 2.4	Factors Influencing Outcomes in Mourning

Increased Psychological Distress

- Predeath psychiatric disorder—coping with changes is especially difficult
- Manner of death—sudden, unexpected death more difficult to manage
- Family life cycle—loss of spouse for young parent with children
- Dysfunctional relationship with deceased person
- Constricted capacity to express feelings
- Financial problems

Increased Ability to Cope

- Sense of optimism
- Belief system that helps deal with death
- Self-sufficient
- Experience with loss
- Competent family interactions
- Supportive social network
- Adequate financial resources

TABLE 2.1	Differences Between Depression and Grief	
Trait	**Depression**	**Grief**
Trigger	Specific trigger not necessary	Trigger usually loss or multiple losses
Active/passive	Passive behavior tends to keep them "stuck" in sadness	Actively feel their emotional pain and emptiness
Emotions	Generalized feeling of helplessness, hopelessness	Experience a range of emotions that are usually intense
Ability to laugh	Likely to be humorless and incapable of being happy or even temporarily cheered up; likely to resist support	Sometimes will be able to laugh and enjoy humor, more likely to accept support
Activities	Lack of interest in previously enjoyed activities	Can be persuaded to participate in activities, especially as they begin to heal
Self-esteem	Low self-esteem, low self-confidence; feels like a failure	Self-esteem usually remains intact; does not feel like a failure unless it relates directly to the loss
Feeling of the failure	May dwell on past failures, catastrophize	Any self-blame or guilt relates directly to loss; feelings resolve as they progress toward healing

research will help us understand how complicated grief relates to these situations (Gray & Prigerson, 2004; Vessier-Batchen & Douglas, 2006).

Complicated grief may include symptoms of intrusive images, severe feelings of emptiness, and neglect of activities at home and at work. Other symptoms include preoccupation with thoughts of the deceased person, yearning and searching for her or him, inability to accept the death, auditory and visual hallucinations of the person, bitterness and survivor guilt over the death, and symptoms of identification—such as having pain in the same part of the body as the deceased person. These disturbances cause significant impairment in social, occupational, and family functioning.

Individuals who experience complicated grief are at a higher risk for a variety of health problems. In American culture, grief is considered complicated when there are enormous social, psychological, and medical problems. Psychiatric complications include depressive episodes, anxiety-related symptoms and disorders, suicidal ideation, or psychotic denial of the death (see Table 2.1■). Medical problems include hypertension, cardiac problems, impaired immune function, and cancer. Some people develop chronic illness behavior and hypochondriasis, which leads to a preoccupation with health and an inability to reinvest energy or interest in social relationships (Raphael & Wooding, 2004).

SEVERE MENTAL ILLNESS AND THE FAMILY SYSTEM

Family members of individuals with mental illness often share in the many losses that accompany the illness. Families are the major source of support and rehabilitation for their loved ones. Of clients discharged from acute care, 65% return to their families. At any given time, 40% to 50% of the 48 million Americans who are severely and persistently mentally ill live with their families on a regular basis. Even when clients do not live at home, their families are often the only source of support. Care for the mentally ill has become as much family based as community based in the United States. This situation can result in overwhelming emotional and economic stress on the family system (Rose, Mallinson, & Gerson, 2006).

In an ideal world, family members would be supportive and effective in dealing with an ill family member. The person with the mental disorder (client) would not act out (or threaten to act out). In reality, family relationships can be conflicted. When clients try to assert their autonomy, families worry about what will happen and become critical or try to control the situation. As families struggle with guilt and fear, clients feel rejected and abandoned. Clients may also experience a sense of shame over being mistrusted and monitored.

Family Burden

Families have important needs of their own in response to their loved one's mental illness. Severe and persistent mental illness often puts the family under catastrophic levels of stress. As families respond to the grief and trauma, they need empathy and support from health care professionals.

Family burden is the overall level of distress experienced as a result of the mental illness. The **objective family burden** is related to the actual, identifiable family problems associated with the person's mental illness. One burden the family must manage relates to *symptomatic behaviors*. Their loved ones' deficit behaviors—such as lack of motivation, difficulty in completing tasks, isolation from others, inability to manage money, poor grooming and personal care, and poor eating and sleeping behavior—can be of great concern to families. Intrusive or acting-out behaviors—such as lack of consideration for others, excessive arguing, conflicts with neighbors and friends, damaging material possessions, inappropriate sexual behavior, suicide attempts, substance abuse, and violent outbursts—are very disturbing to family members. These behaviors may be more episodic than the deficit behaviors but may have more severe immediate consequences. This family burden may lead to loss of independence and increased responsibility as families try to cope with day-to-day living. This burden includes disruption in household functioning, restriction of social activities, and financial hardship due to medical bills and the cost of their loved one's economic burden.

Another objective burden related to family problems is *caregiving*. Families may find that community services are not always available and not always satisfactory. Inadequate funding results in lack of treatment programs and lack of services for families themselves. Families also find themselves negotiating with the legal and criminal justice system. With few long-term psychiatric facilities available, many people who would have previously been cared for in state hospitals now find themselves in jails and prisons. Often, the "crimes" with which they are charged are misdemeanors resulting from their symptoms of mental illness, such as disorderly conduct, trespassing, and drunkenness.

Families must also cope with the burden of **stigma**, which is a collection of negative attitudes and beliefs that lead people to fear, reject, avoid, and discriminate against people with mental illness. In response to stigma, people with mental disorders internalize these attitudes and become ashamed of themselves and their illness. People with mental illness continue to be ostracized from mainstream society. Families may become isolated as they avoid others who misunderstand the illness. When a family member has cancer or heart disease, other people respond with kindness. When a family member has a mental disorder, the response is often avoidance because there is a perception of unpredictability and

danger. Thus, stigma severely limits support from extended family and friends. As they and their loved one face multiple discriminations, families may feel isolated and shameful, may lose self-esteem, and may run the risk of self-stigmatization (Rose, Mallinson, & Gerson, 2006; Stengler-Wenzke, Trosbach, Dietrich, & Angermeyer, 2004).

The **subjective family burden** is defined as the psychological distress of the family members in relation to the objective burden. They often experience frustration, anxiety, depression, hopelessness, and helplessness. Families also experience intense feelings of grief and loss. They must mourn for the person they knew before the onset of the illness and the potential loss of hopes, dreams, and expectations. They live with a sense of chronic sorrow for those loved ones who experience periods of remission and relapse. There is also a sense of empathetic pain as they watch their family member become a victim of the illness. Living with and caring for a person with mental illness can have a tremendous impact on the family. Some families cope fairly well, whereas others are easily exhausted and give up (Jungbauer, Wittmund, Dietrich, & Angermeyer, 2003). See Table 2.2 ■ for descriptions of the language of family pain.

Family Recovery

Stage 1 of family recovery involves discovery and denial. Family members are often the first to notice that another member is exhibiting unusual behavior. The family's initial response may range from minimizing (it's not so serious) to denial (it's just a phase). This response is a temporary, rather than maladaptive, reaction to avoid a painful reality. As the family attempts to explain the changes to others, they may attribute the changes to something more socially acceptable than mental illness. For example, they might tell others that the person is suffering from exhaustion or an endocrine problem or that stress at school or work is causing the difficulties. Others' prejudice and the family's avoidance of stigma can lead to family isolation and loss of relationships outside the immediate family system.

TABLE 2.2	The Language of Family Pain

Catastrophe: Watching as your loved one slips away. This is like a horror movie, in which the hero/heroine (loved one) is utterly transformed by some unseen, monstrous force.

Torture: The agony of watching a loved one experience relentless pain and suffering without being able to make it stop. The absolute panic when he or she refuses your assistance, rejects your help, resists your protection at the time when it is most needed.

Anguish: The pain of having loved ones turn on those who are trying to help them, attack them angrily, or blame them for their difficulties.

Horror/fear: A dread that the ill person will do something terrible to self or others.

Nightmare: Rejection, labeling, and ostracism by the mental health system when we are trying to help.

SOURCE: Reprinted with permission from Burland, J. (1999). *NAMI provided education program*. Arlington, VA: National Alliance for the Mentally Ill.

Stage 2 of family recovery involves recognition and acceptance. As it becomes more evident that there is a significant problem, the family begins to search for reasons and solutions by gathering available information. Families begin to develop their own image of the disease process and expectations of mental health professionals. Many families also hope for what was in the past and for what might be in the future. It is very sad to lose a close family member to the world of mental illness. Many people do not believe that mental illness is a brain disease. If the disorder begins in childhood, it is easier to think that it is a result of bad parenting because that means good parenting should fix it. That is like telling parents of a child with leukemia that if they were better parents they could stop those white cells from growing. When a person experiences a mental disorder, expectations and dreams may necessitate alteration. Some clients come through the experience of mental illness able to develop meaningful and productive lives. Others, who do not respond to current treatment strategies, may have to grieve the loss of their hopes and dreams (Tweedell, Forchuk, Jewell, & Steinnagel, 2004).

Stage 3 of family recovery involves coping and competence. This includes day-to-day efforts to cope with all the changes in the family. When people become persistently and severely mentally ill, they may have difficulty carrying out their family roles and responsibilities. In this case, other family members must assume those roles and come to terms with an altered family lifestyle. Family members develop cognitive, emotional, and behavioral coping strategies to live with their loved one who is experiencing a mental disorder. As they take stock of the challenges, constraints, and resources, they are better able to make the most of their options.

Coping strategies protect the affected family member and maintain the stability of family functioning. Some of these strategies include expressing affection, suggesting alternatives, reducing conflict, seeking social support, and trying to make the best of their experiences by focusing on the positive parts of the relationship with the ill family member.

Rose (1997) describes four family support sources:

- Professional support
- Friend support
- Family support
- Spiritual support

Professional support includes a nonblaming and respectful attitude toward families, and providing information on how to respond to symptoms and help in locating community resources, such as housing or vocational training. *Friend support* comes from non–family members, such as close friends and coworkers. Friend support is most valued

when the concern is genuine and stigma is minimized. *Family support* often comes in the way of tangible assistance, such as respite care for family members and physical presence in times of crisis. Many families find emotional strength from their religious faith. They find *spiritual support* as they search for meaning through relationships and feeling connected with others. Supportive relationships build and sustain courage, helping families make the best of their difficult lives.

As families learn to cope effectively, the intense focus on the ill family member lightens up as other members begin to focus on taking care of themselves and reconnecting with others outside the family as they move through the process of adjustment. The family adapts to its changed circumstances and continues to function successfully.

The final stage of family recovery is personal and political advocacy. This stage involves working with the mental health system to obtain treatment. Family members want to be seen as partners in treatment and do not want to be excluded from discussions and treatment recommendations. Ideally, professionals, clients, and families all work together in joint problem solving. At times, the issue of client confidentiality is raised. Family members generally respect confidentiality but do need information about treatments, medications, resources, and ways to cope with certain behaviors.

Some families go on to educate the public about mental illness and lobby for improved public policy and legislation, often through the National Alliance on Mental Illness (NAMI), an organization composed of clients, families, and professionals. NAMI actively lobbies for improved legislation and improved health care benefits at local, state, and federal levels.

MENTAL DISORDERS ACROSS THE LIFE SPAN

Youth

An estimated 12% to 20% of children in the United States have a serious emotional disturbance and substantial functional impairment, nearly 50% of which lead to serious disability. Children with mental disorders are more likely to drop out of school and be marginalized members of society in adulthood. Few young children are identified with mental disorders and most do not receive appropriate and timely treatment (Gerkensmeyer, Austin, & Miller, 2006).

When a child or adolescent experiences a mental disorder, the entire family system is strained. When primary responsibility for caregiving falls to one person, the parental system is stressed, which often leads to increased conflict and a greater likelihood of parental separation. The siblings are often excluded, leading to confusion or misunderstanding of the problem. Sibling feelings may range from shame to protectiveness. At times, they may feel superior for not having "problems," while at other times they may feel neglected if the child with the disorder receives more parental attention. Families often become socially isolated because they are too fearful or ashamed to bring the child to social gatherings. The financial strain can be tremendous because mental illness is usually covered inadequately by health insurance. The cost of specialized child care may be prohibitive, which may force a parent to decrease or discontinue outside employment (Fristad & Goldberg-Arnold, 2003).

Family turmoil can trigger the onset of a disorder in a biologically and genetically predisposed child. The emotional and affective styles of families may be a factor in the onset. The parent–child relationship is often severely strained due to stressors related to a child's mental disorder. Some parents respond in ways that foster dependence, which contributes to separation/individuation problems or boundary issues. Some parents may reject and be critical of a child with a disorder. Other parents alternate between overprotection/overcontrol and rejection. Other families learn to adapt in ways that foster the growth and development of all the children. Remember that family patterns are not the primary cause of childhood mental disorders; mental disorders have multiple etiologies, including the interaction of biological, genetic, psychological, and social factors.

Many children live in homes in which one or both parents have a mental disorder. Some of these children develop mental disorders themselves because of the factors described in the next sections. Others seem to be resilient and thrive despite their adverse experiences. It is unclear how children become resilient, but some factors may be the need to assume diverse roles within the family, the presence of a healthy adult in the home, personality traits, relationship with a parent substitute, and the use of external support systems (Mordoch & Hall, 2002).

Pregnancy

Pregnancy and childbirth are major issues for most women. For a severely and persistently mentally ill woman who already has problems in adjustment and coping, pregnancy can be a sufficient strain and exacerbate symptoms of the mental illness. Women with a history of mental illness must be monitored closely throughout pregnancy. Although 10% to 15% of pregnant women meet the criteria for depression, they often remain undiagnosed because the symptoms of depression are similar to the somatic changes of pregnancy. For many women, the postpartum period is associated with mental health problems, including postpartum blues in as many as 80% of new mothers, postpartum depression in 13% of new mothers, and postpartum psychosis in 1 to 2 in 1,000 women (Beck, 2003; Ugarriza, 2004). (See chapter 13 ∞ for more information on postpartum depression.)

In the general U.S. population, 50% of pregnancies are unplanned; the rate is higher among women who are severely and persistently mentally ill. For women with bipolar disorder whose manic episodes increase their sexual activity and impair their judgment, the risk of unplanned pregnancy is high. It is not uncommon for women and their families to be unaware of a pregnancy until the pregnancy is far advanced, which places both the woman and the fetus at risk. Other problems may include a diminished ability to comply with prenatal care, an inability to plan realistically for the newborn, an increased risk of substance abuse during the pregnancy, and poor nutrition. Others look forward to impending motherhood and are well able to care for themselves and their unborn babies during the pregnancy. Family members and friends can be of great support during the pregnancy and as coaches during labor and delivery. If the woman is pregnant and is taking psychotropic medications, the primary health care provider must weigh the risk of fetal anomalies against the exacerbation of the illness, which may present a danger to the mother and others, including the fetus. All effective mood-stabilizing agents pose risks during pregnancy. Tegretol (carbamazepine) and Depakote (valproic acid) are associated with increased risk for neural tube defects, craniofacial defects, and developmental delay. Lamictal (lamotigine) is safer than the other anticonvulsants. The main pregnancy risks with lithium are polyhydramnios, premature labor, neonatal toxicity, and neonatal hypothyroidism. Antipsychotic and antianxiety medications are often used because they cause fewer fetal anomalies and problems with pregnancy. Electroconvulsive therapy (ECT) is an effective and relatively safe treatment for some clients because uterine muscle does not contract as part of the generalized tonic–clonic seizure (Valdivia & Rossy, 2004; Yonkers, Wisner, Stowe, Leibenluft, Cohen, Miller, et al., 2004).

In the future, when disease-related genes are identified for mental disorders, it will be possible to develop prenatal tests for these diseases. Individuals at high risk for passing on a disorder will have the option to take such tests and to abort an affected fetus. Serious ethical considerations are involved with such options, and appropriate guidelines must be developed for the eventual genetic testing for mental disorders. Health care professionals must never make those decisions for clients and must be extremely careful not to accuse parents of perpetuating mental disorders.

Parenting

It is estimated that, in North America, 50% of adults with mental disorders have children living with them. Severe and persistent mental illness among parents of newborns and young children may be troublesome for the family. If the parent is acutely ill at the time of the birth, she or he may be separated from the newborn, which may slow the bonding process. Periodic relapses of acute illness lead to disruption of the family system because children endure repeated separations. Parents may be physically and emotionally unavailable during these times of acute illness. With support from family, friends, and community many parents with mental illness are well able to nurture and care for their children. In fact, the process of parenting may contribute to a sense of well-being and competency (Montgomery, 2005).

Nursing interventions for young families include helping the family develop a social support system and use community resources. Programs such as Head Start, day care centers, and recreational programs can stimulate the children and provide a time of respite for the parent. Teaching includes providing information about normal growth and development, stress-management techniques, time-management skills, and problem-solving skills. Collaborating with the extended family may minimize the impact of mental illness on the primary family.

Couples

Most people who become severely ill at a fairly young age remain single. Their social functioning is so limited that they are unable to sustain a relationship. In contrast, research suggests that people with depression may be able to be part of a couple. Studies indicate, however, that as many as 50% of individuals with depression report serious couple difficulties and hope to resolve these relationship problems in therapy. In addition, couples who are experiencing relationship distress are at higher risk for depression.

In some relationships, the person with the disorder demands that the partner keep silent about the problem. The well partner has no one to confide in, which increases stress. The couple presents a facade of health and must cover up episodes of illness or hospitalization. In addition, the family of origin of the ill partner may blame the well partner for the disorder (Stengler-Wenzke et al. 2004).

One of the hallmarks of relationship distress is poor communication. Depressed partners behave in ways that discourage social interaction and increase relationship conflict. They are less skillful socially and more withdrawn; they seem to express more hostility and criticism of themselves and others; they may engage in long and hateful arguments; and they often express dissatisfaction with sexual activity. Living with a depressed person can also increase the nondepressed partner's susceptibility to depression. The goals of relationship therapy are to decrease conflict, to increase the degree of intimacy and relationship satisfaction, and to enhance effective coping and social competence.

Adult Children

The current focus of mental health care is returning clients to their communities to live in the least restrictive yet realistic environment. As a result, at least half of the severely and persistently mentally ill adult population is living with their families on a regular basis. Professionals are beginning to look at and respond to the burden of family caregivers. Some problems that families of these adult children face are the need for daily caretaking, lack of freedom, emotional drain, stress of the unexpected, and financial strain. Parents often struggle to find a balance between supporting their adult child with an illness as a dependent and fostering her or his independence to the greatest extent. This balance involves both the person with the disability and the caregiving parent.

Symptoms of client illness, such as inappropriate behavior, labile emotions, hallucinations, delusions, and outbursts of rage, are often difficult for families to manage. Other symptoms that strain the family are dependency, poor social skills and outlets, and difficulty finding employment. Financial considerations may force the parents to delay their expected retirement. They are often concerned about the welfare of their child after their death. Siblings, too, worry about assuming the responsibility when the parents are no longer able to be caretakers through disability or death. Family caregivers need support and practical knowledge to enhance their ability to cope and their ability to support their loved one (Brady & McCain, 2005).

Older Adults

With the increase in the number of older adults, family care for this population is very important. By the age of 65 years, 12% of people have limitations on activities of daily living. By the age of 85 years, this percentage jumps to 38%. These individuals often depend on family to keep them living in the community. Those with mental disorders often have three or four medical problems complicating the situation. Caregivers of older people with mental disorders are themselves more likely to be depressed than caregivers of those who have physical disorders. This may be related to stigma, misunderstanding, and low social support (Jeon, Brodaty, & Chesterson, 2005).

FAMILY NURSING PRACTICE

Until recently, family members were sometimes a source of information about their ill members but were rarely involved in treatment, psychoeducation, or family therapy, and the idea of the family as a unit of care was controversial. With environments that are less restrictive, shorter hospital stays, and fewer community programs, nurses must now develop a collaborative partnership with clients and their families. This collaborative relationship means that the family is viewed as the unit of care and as partners in treatment and rehabilitation. Therefore, programs must be in place to provide support, education, training for coping skills, social network development, and family therapy. It is critical that family nurses take the time to be with families in deeply caring ways. As we share our ideas and our strengths our goal is to help families develop as more balanced and caring systems.

Family Assessment

As nurses, we must focus our attention on the family, both as the context for the individual and as the unit of care. It is important to assess and involve families because they are in a position to be affected by and to influence the course of an individual's problems. The questions we ask influence how we view the family. For example, if we ask only questions regarding problems, we are likely to "find" problems in the family. On the other hand, if we also include questions about resourcefulness, we have an increased chance of discovering *family competency*. Questions shape our experience of and our interactions with clients and families. The following questions are examples of assessing the resourcefulness of the family system:

- What do you hope for in the future?
- How will your life be different when your concerns are no longer problems?
- What strengths, resources, and knowledge do you have to deal with the problems?

Assessment includes gathering information on how partners, parents, and children in the family experience or react to the client's symptoms. Nurses must learn how others are affected by problems and how they have attempted to cope with problems. If we want to know the family, we must listen to its story. The family's story will tell us who the members are and what is meaningful to them. Telling their stories also allows families to make sense of any confusion.

Family nurse therapists often use one or more of the following three tools for family history assessment (McGuinness, Noonan, & Dyer, 2005):

- **Genograms** are three generational maps of the family system. They consider family structure and relationships and the degree of cohesion and flexibility within the various groups. Genograms help identify family strengths and deficits and tailor interventions specific to each family.
- **Ecomaps** view the family system as it relates to the larger community. Using the genogram as a center point, ecomaps identify interactions between the family and the neighborhood, work, school, social groups, and religious systems, to name a few. Ecomaps provide further information on family strengths and weaknesses to help individualize nursing care.

- The third tool, a **pedigree analysis**, is a three-generational family tree specific to biological and medical histories. All major medical and psychiatric illnesses and significant health behaviors are identified for each individual. For those deceased, age and cause of death are recorded.

Together, clients, families, and nurses collaborate to identify the family's strengths, resources, and social support and try to identify problems that might cause stress for any of the family members. Factors in assessing clients and their families include family communication, conflict resolution, boundaries, cohesion, flexibility, emotional availability, leadership patterns, and overall family functionality.

Assessing Relapse Vulnerability

Understandably, families are very concerned with their loved one's vulnerability to relapse. Although families should not be blamed for mental disorders, their interactions may influence the course of the disorder. Relapse is less common in families who see the client as ill (rather than as lazy or manipulative) and who provide support to one another. Relapse is more common in families that are highly critical, highly anxious, and preoccupied with their problems. Researchers have studied two family patterns: family **expressed emotion (EE)** and family **affective style (AS)**. EE and AS are measures of the family's emotional climate. Families rated as high EE tend to be hostile, critical, and emotionally enmeshed with each member. They are also less flexible, less tolerant, and lower in empathy and achievement than low EE families. Families rated as high AS are intrusive and make guilt-inducing remarks during emotionally charged family discussions. High EE and AS families both are predictors of relapse for people with severe and persistent mental illness. Twenty-five studies found that the 1-year relapse rate in high EE families averaged 50.1%, compared with low EE families for which it was 21.1% (Murray-Swank & Dixon, 2005). Families are more likely to be excessively critical or overinvolved when they lack information about the disorder and when they believe the symptoms are under the client's control. Family members who do not understand the nature of severe and persistent mental illness may mistake the negative symptoms as laziness. (See chapter 14 ∞ for further information on negative symptoms.) High EE families may not be a factor in relapse among American minority groups. Research shows high EE as a risk factor for Euro-American, Israeli, and Japanese families but not for Mexican American families. Further research is necessary to discover the reasons for the differences (Barrowclough & Hooley, 2003; Brady & McCain, 2005).

Noncompliance with medication regimens and substance abuse are other changeable factors related to relapse. Noncompliance with medication regimens is linked to lack of insight into the disorder, medication side effects, medication cost, missed outpatient appointments, and negative client/family attitudes toward medication. Mental health status is further compromised by the use of alcohol or drugs.

Other social–environmental stressors related to relapse include alcohol/drug use, family crises, vocational stress, and interpersonal conflict. Inconsistent daily routines and sleep deprivation are also factors.

It is important that the nurse assess the family for protective factors in regard to relapse. These include monitoring moods and triggers for fluctuations, maintaining consistent daily and nightly routines, relying on family and social supports, taking medications as prescribed, and participating in psychosocial treatment programs.

Cultural Assessment

A person's culture shapes her or his concept of self. One way to look at the cultural self is along a continuum between egocentric and sociocentric orientations. The **egocentric self**, usually found in Western industrialized societies, exhibits characteristics such as individualism, separateness, autonomy, competition, and mastery of and control over one's environment. The **sociocentric self**, found in many non-Western societies, is interdependent and interconnected and values cooperation, cohesiveness, group identity, and harmony with one's environment. The person is defined by kinship and is seen in relationship terms.

Africans, Asians, Latin Americans, and their descendents in North America, as well as Native Americans, tend toward sociocentric orientations. There is a high value on interpersonal relationships, group membership, and cohesiveness. Relationships to others, family, and community are central to one's sense of well-being. An extensive kin network provides economic and emotional support to its members. Severe and persistent mental illness is often viewed as a family affair because it affects all family members. These families express greater hope, optimism, and faith about long-term outcomes of their family member's mental illness. Siblings of severely ill persons are more likely to be involved in caregiving and less likely to find their involvement burdensome than are Euro-American siblings. See Box 2.5 for examples of family orientations in various cultures.

Generalizations about ethnic groups increase our level of awareness and alert us to the possibility of differences. It is very important, however, that nurses never assume that ethnic group generalizations accurately describe the family with whom they are working. How a problem is viewed and how distress is handled vary with different family and cultural norms. Nurses must also recognize and understand that differences are not disease or dysfunction but simply another way of life. Nurses must take the families as they are, help them achieve their goals, and facilitate health in the way that is most useful for them. (See chapter 4 ∞ for additional information on the role of cultural diversity.)

BOX 2.5	Family Orientations
Arab	Hierarchical and patriarchal structure with regard to sex and age; extended family very important; very loyal to kin and consider them part of the family
Greece	Extended family lives nearby; child-centered perception of marriage and the family; in younger couples there is more of a focus on adult relationships; family cohesion is important
India	Varies according to religion, community, castes, and urbanization; multigenerational families are hierarchical with male preference; family dignity and status are important
Israel	Similar to Western societies; repeated wars, terrorist acts, and other security-related problems compound family stress
Japan	Family boundaries are rigid; family keeps secrets about negative aspects of family life, such as mental illness, suicide, and divorce; most important relationship is between parent and child
Nigeria	Yoruba of Nigeria love children and women; family stability very important; traditional healers provide family counseling and guidance in problem solving
Russia	Very few nuclear families living away from family of origin—usually three generations are living together; family roles and functions are intertwined; family ties are highly valued and individualism is practically nonexistent
South America	Family unity, religious commitment, and respect for each other is important; strong sense of family commitment, obligation, and mutual responsibility; have to manage political oppression, social isolation, and immigration issues
Western Societies	Clear generational boundaries; most important relationship is between adult partners; self-control, self-reliance, and independence are highly valued

SOURCES: Adekson, M. (2003). Indigenous family work in Nigeria. In K. S. Ng (Ed.), *Global perspectives in family therapy* (pp. 147–160). New York: Brunner-Routledge. Lavee, Y. (2003). Family therapy in a multicultural society: The case of Israel. In K. S. Ng (Ed.), *Global perspectives in family therapy* (pp. 175–194). New York: Brunner-Routledge. Prabhu, R. (2003). The beginning of family therapy in India. In K. S. Ng (Ed.), *Global perspectives in family therapy* (pp. 57–69). New York: Brunner-Routledge. Softas-Nall, B. (2003). Reflections on forty years of family therapy, research, and systemic thinking in Greece. In K. S. Ng (Ed.), *Global perspectives in family therapy* (pp. 125–145). New York: Brunner-Routledge. Tamura, T. (2003). The development of family therapy and the experience of fatherhood in the Japanese context. In K. S. Ng (Ed.), *Global perspectives in family therapy* (pp. 19–30). New York: Brunner-Routledge. Varga, A. (2003). Family therapy and family life cycle in Russia. In K. S. Ng (Ed.), *Global perspectives in family therapy* (pp. 105–114). New York: Brunner-Routledge.

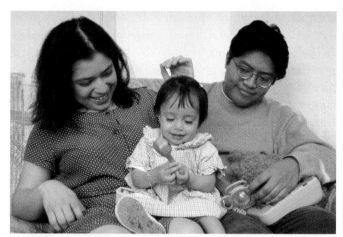

PHOTO 2.3 ■ Cultural differences exert a profound influence on how parents and children relate to one another.

SOURCE: Michael Newman/PhotoEdit, Inc. Used with permission.

The Nurse as Educator

Psychoeducation has proven to be an important aspect of family nursing. (See chapter 7 ∞ for more detailed information on psychoeducation.) Nurses must be able to answer questions, help families identify feelings and reactions, help them adopt more flexible beliefs about the nature of their loved one's problems, and encourage their coping efforts. Research shows that psychoeducation programs must be at least 9 months in duration to be effective (Murray-Swank & Dixon, 2005).

Families need information about severe and persistent mental illness and service delivery programs. Illness education occurs in the context of the basic family unit and with multifamily groups. Information should be provided about the:

■ Diathesis stress model of mental disorders

■ Symptoms, using the client as the expert

■ Treatment choices

■ Social and environmental stressors

■ Protective factors

■ Early warning signs of relapse specific to client

■ Community resources

Families also need skills to cope with the illness. Nurses help families identify problems and work out solutions that fit the family's current patterns of living. Family education programs include:

■ Conflict-management skills

■ Problem-solving strategies

■ Crisis plans

■ Communication skills

■ Assertiveness training

■ Responses to stigmatization and discrimination

■ Stress-management techniques, such as relaxation exercises, visualization, affirmations, meditation, and physical exercise. (Information on alternative therapies is found in chapter 9 ∞, as well as integrated throughout the text.)

As educators, we realize we cannot make decisions for others' lives. Clients and families know more about their lives and are the best judges for future direction. Through education, nurses enhance the strengths and creativity of the family system and assist members in making changes and developing the lives they choose.

The Nurse as Life Coach

The primary goal of coaching a family is to improve its challenging situations. The nurse must listen carefully to all family members, acknowledge the difficulties they are experiencing, and affirm the strengths and resources they bring to the situation. Basic to life coaching is building rapport while focusing on a collaborative relationship. Every family deserves a consistent one-to-one relationship with a primary health care provider, and that person is often a nurse. Communication with professionals is the greatest need identified by caregivers. This means that the professional not only returns phone calls, but also initiates contact to evaluate progress toward goals and modify strategies that are less effective. Because many mental disorders begin in childhood, parents may need some help with parenting skills. Help them find a way to agree on parenting tasks. The children's behavior may be unpredictable and, at times, dangerous. When this occurs, children should not be allowed to blame the illness for their behavior. The expectation is that they must learn to manage themselves with parental support. The family expectation for all members is that no one hurts any other with words or actions. Consequences are established for violating this norm. Parents must also make time for the children who do not have the disorder so that they do not get lost in times of crisis (Fristad & Goldberg-Arnold, 2003).

As a life coach, discuss and role-model ways to enhance family communication. As families learn new ways of talking and listening, they will experience a reduction in stress and an improvement in relationships. These skills are:

■ Active listening (e.g., asking clarifying questions, summarizing other's statements)

■ Giving praise and positive feedback whenever it is legitimate

■ Giving criticism in a calm voice

■ Using positive requests (e.g., "I would like you to...")

■ Monitoring nonverbal communication

■ Refraining from arguing with someone who is severely agitated or psychotic

Family members must also find time to care for themselves. Strategies for managing stress are:

- Establishing good sleep habits
- Initiating healthy eating
- Balancing work and play
- Establishing expectations for household chores
- Avoiding overload on time and energy
- Utilizing support systems
- Seeking respite with assistance from supportive friends/family
- Using specific stress-reducing techniques

Most of these strategies can be integrated into the family problem-solving process. As the family becomes efficient in problem solving, it will better manage particular problems as they occur.

The Nurse as Referral Agent

Because families often feel stigmatized and alone, referrals to support groups are helpful. Networking with other families that are struggling with similar issues normalizes the family's experiences.

Family nurses act as referral agents in making an effort to facilitate the transaction between family and community. As family advocates, nurses must be familiar with local community resources, such as crisis centers, community mental health centers, telephone hotlines, support groups, religious institutions, acute care facilities, and specific names of mental health professionals. The goal is to provide opportunities for people who are severely and persistently mentally ill to maximize their ability to live, work, socialize, and learn in communities of their choice. Working together, clients, families, and health care providers can develop strategies to help clients achieve lives of value, meaning, and better health and become contributing members of their communities. (See chapter 3 ∞ for detailed information on community resources.)

NAMI is a grassroots, self-help, support and advocacy organization of people with mental illness and their families and friends. The NAMI mission is to eradicate mental illness and to improve the quality of life for those who have these brain diseases. Local self-help support groups enable members to share concerns, learn about mental disorders, and receive practical advice on treatment and community resources. NAMI provides the Family-to-Family Education Program, which is led by trained volunteers from families of people with mental illness. NAMI provides up-to-date scientific information through publications, the Helpline, and an annual Mental Illness Awareness Week campaign. At federal, state, and local levels, NAMI demands improved services for people who are severely and persistently mentally ill, such as greater access to treatment, housing, and employment and better health insurance. NAMI actively supports increased federal and private funding for research into causes and treatments of persistent and severe mental illnesses.

Mental health nurses are expected to systematically assess families; identify their structure, development, communication, and decision-making patterns; and recognize and refer multi-stressed families to family therapy. Family therapists should be specially educated in the practice of family therapy. An increasing number of psychiatric nurse practitioners and clinical specialists are being prepared in graduate programs that provide theory and supervised clinical practice in this specialized area. Although undergraduate nursing programs focus on the importance of family nursing, they do not prepare nurses as family therapists. (See chapter 9 ∞ for more information on family therapy.)

The Nurse as Spiritual Caregiver

Any serious illness, but perhaps especially a severe and persistent mental illness, is really a disease process. Both the illness and the associated stigma eat away at people's spirits, and they often feel beaten and broken. They begin to believe that their worth and value as a human being is diminished. Nurses must respond to the whole person, who is at once spirit, mind, and body. People who are severely and persistently mentally ill are entitled to dignified and meaningful lives.

Many people who have severe and persistent mental illness use religious beliefs or activities to cope with daily problems or frustrations. Specific activities include prayer and reading holy scriptures. Attending religious services may decrease feelings of loneliness and disconnectedness. It is important to ask clients about the role of spirituality and religion in their lives

Spiritual care includes developing caring and thoughtful relationships. Nurses must foster family attitudes that arise from people's spiritual dimensions, such as love, forgiveness, hopefulness, and acceptance. Spiritual caregiving includes helping "patients" stop being patients and instead become active clients and collaborators. Supporting individuals and families who seek ways to heal and achieve balance in their lives is an important aspect of spiritual nursing care.

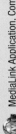

Focus Your Study

OBJECTIVES	KEY CONCEPTS

1. Outline the elements of the family system.

- Communication—good communication to better adapt and cope
- Boundaries—amount and kind of contact allowed
- Emotional availability—range of expression of feelings
- Competency—relational resources and adaptive abilities

2. Discuss the impact of grief and loss on the family system.

- Children:
  - Preverbal: death as separation; sensitive to survivor's emotions
  - Preschool: death is reversible; may regress in behavior
  - School-age: understand finality of death; avoid talking; self-blame
  - Teens: acknowledge reality; impact normal individuation from family
- Family structure:
  - Role realignment
  - Relationships with people outside the family

3. Discuss the impact of severe and persistent mental illness on the family system.

- Family burden:
  - Objective: problems associated with behaviors, caregiving, and stigma
  - Subjective: psychological stress related to objective burden
- Youth:
  - Between 2% to 20% of children have a serious emotional disturbance.
  - The entire family system is strained.
- Pregnancy:
  - May be unplanned.
  - Need to balance need for medications with impact on fetus.
- Parenting:
  - Many children live in a home where one or both parents have a mental disorder.
  - Parents may be physically and emotionally unavailable during acute illness.
- Couples:
  - Mental disorders put a strain on the couple relationship.
- Adult children:
  - Half of the persistently and severely mentally ill adult population live with their families.
  - Client symptoms are often difficult for families to manage.
- Older adults:
  - Older adults with mental disorders often have medical problems that complicate the situation.

4. Assess family functioning using the family competency model.

- Flexibility—leadership
  - Rigid
  - Chaotic
- Cohesion—emotional bonding
  - Disengaged
  - Enmeshed

5. Characterize the roles of the mental health nurse in family nursing practice.

- Educator
- Life coach
- Referral agent
- Spiritual caregiver

6. Design interventions to improve the functioning of clients and their families.

- Help the family develop a social support system and use community resources.
- Help family members decrease conflict, enhance effective coping, improve communication, manage stress, and increase the degree of relationship satisfaction.
- Help those families who have high EE and AS moderate their expression of emotion and their affective style.
- Teach about mental illness—causes, symptoms, treatment choices, stressors, protective factors, and early signs of relapse.
- Encourage networking with other families.
- Provide spiritual care by supporting religious beliefs and activities; fostering family love, forgiveness, and acceptance; and encouraging clients to become active in their own care.

Explore MediaLink

For review questions, case studies, and other resources for this chapter see the Pearson Health Nursing MediaLink CD-ROM that accompanies this book and the Companion Website.

 CD-ROM
- Audio Glossary
- NCLEX-RN® Review Questions

 Companion Website www.prenhall.com/fontaine
- Audio Glossary
- NCLEX-RN® Review Questions
- Case Study
  - Family Education and Intervention
- Care Plan
  - Family Dysfunction
- Critical Thinking
  - Boundaries Within Families
- MediaLink Application
  - Psychiatric Families
- MediaLinks
  - Books for Clients and Families
  - Community Resources

NCLEX-RN® Review Questions

2-1. An elderly client is admitted to the hospital. He is accompanied by his wife. The client is most tearful and agitated. The client states, "I am fine. I have no worries." The nurse recognizes the client's behavior as:
   1. An aggressive state.
   2. A self-reflective state.
   3. Incongruous between his verbal and nonverbal communication.
   4. Protective of his wife.

2-2. What is the first step the nurse should take to assist a family who recently experienced the loss of a family member?
   1. Assess the family's coping stage.
   2. Teach the family the steps of the grieving process.
   3. Establish support systems outside of the family.
   4. Assist the process of reordering the family structure.

2-3. The family of a client with schizophrenia is struggling to cope with the effects of the clients' illness on family function. Which of the following treatments is the most helpful to the family as it deals with a family member with psychiatric disability?
   1. Counseling for each of the family members
   2. Medication management for the client with schizophrenia
   3. A family member talking with the pastor about the family's spiritual needs
   4. Family education groups

2-4. Two married clients and their three children are attending a family therapy group. The 13-year-old son tells the nurse therapist that his father doesn't understand him, and his mother is the only one who cares about him. The father states, "My wife lets him do whatever he wants to do. His grades are poor and when I try to correct him, my wife contradicts everything I tell my son." The nurse's initial assessment should be:
   1. Conflicted communication patterns between the mother and the son.
   2. Conflicted communication between the mother and the father.
   3. Blurred communication patterns.
   4. Transparent communication patterns.

2-5. An advance practice psychiatric nurse and a basic level nurse are caring for families in the mental health clinic. Which of the following nursing interventions can be implemented only by the advanced practice nurse?
   1. Counseling.
   2. Case management
   3. Health teaching
   4. Psychotherapy

2-6. A psychiatric nurse is conducting a group for couples over 65 years old. The nurse is planning to review successful methods for meeting the developmental tasks using Erikson's eight stages of development. Which of the following psychosocial crises should be the main focus for this group?
   1. Identity versus role confusion
   2. Intimacy versus isolation
   3. Generativity versus self-absorption
   4. Integrity versus despair

See Appendix D for answers.

References

Barrowclough, C., & Hooley, J. M. (2003). Attributions and expressed emotion: A review. *Clinical Psychology Review, 23*(6), 849–880.

Beck, C. T. (2003). Recognizing and screening for postpartum depression in mothers of NICU infants. *Advances in Neonatal Care, 3*(1), 37–46.

Biringen, Z. (2000). Emotional availability: Conceptualization and research findings. *American Journal of Orthopsychiatry, 70*(1), 104–114.

Brady, N., & McCain, G. C. (2005). Living with schizophrenia: A family perspective. *Online Journal of Issues in Nursing, 10*(1), 1–22.

Fristad, M. A., & Goldberg-Arnold, J. S. (2003). Family interventions for early-onset bipolar disorder. In G. Geller & M. P. Delbello (Eds.), *Bipolar disorder in childhood and early adolescence* (pp. 295–313). New York: Guilford Press.

Gerkensmeyer, J. E., Austin, J. K., & Miller, T. K. (2006). Model testing: Examining parent satisfaction. *Archives of Psychiatric Nursing, 20*(2), 65–75.

Gray, M. J., & Prigerson, H. G. (2004). Conceptual and definitional issues in complicated grief. In B. T. Litz (Ed.), *Early intervention for trauma and traumatic loss* (pp. 65–84). New York: Guilford Press.

Jeon, Y. H., Brodaty, H., & Chesterson, J. (2005). Respite care for caregivers and people with severe mental illness: Literature review. *Journal of Advanced Nursing, 49*(3), 297–306.

Jungbauer, J., Wittmund, B., Dietrich, S., & Angermeyer, M. C. (2003). Subjective burden over 12 months in parents of patients with schizophrenia. *Archives of Psychiatric Nursing, 17*(3), 126–134.

McGuinness, T. M., Noonan, P., & Dyer, J. G. (2005). Family history as a tool for psychiatric nurses. *Archives of Psychiatric Nursing, 19*(3), 116–124.

Mohr, W. K., Lafuze, J. E., & Mohr, B. D. (2000). Opening caregiver minds: National Alliance on Mental Illness' (NAMI) Provider Education Program. *Archives of Psychiatric Nursing, 14*(5), 235–243.

Montgomery, P. (2005). Mothers with a serious mental illness: A critical review of the literature. *Archives of Psychiatric Nursing, 19*(5), 226-235.

Mordoch, E., & Hall, W. A. (2002). Children living with a parent who has a mental illness. *Archives of Psychiatric Nursing, 16*(5), 208–216.

Murray-Swank, A., & Dixon, L. (2005). Evidence-based practices for families of individuals with severe mental illness. In R. E. Drake, M. R. Merrens, & D. W. Lynde (Eds.), *Evidence-based mental health practice* (pp. 425–452). New York: W.W. Norton.

Olson, D. H. (1996). Clinical assessment and treatment interventions using the family circumplex model. In F. W. Kaslow (Ed.), *Handbook of relational diagnosis and dysfunctional family patterns* (pp. 59–77). New York: John Wiley & Sons.

Raphael, B., & Wooding, S. (2004). Early mental health intervention for traumatic loss in adults. In B. T. Litz (Ed.), *Early intervention for trauma and traumatic loss* (pp. 147–178). New York: Guilford Press.

Rose, L. E. (1997). Caring for caregivers: Perceptions of social support. *Journal of Psychosocial Nursing, 35*(2), 17–24.

Rose, L. E., Mallinson, R. K., & Gerson, L. D. (2006). Mastery, burden and areas of concern among family caregivers of mentally ill persons. *Archives of Psychiatric Nursing, 20*(1), 41–51.

Stengler-Wenzke, K., Trosbach, J., Dietrich, S., & Angermeyer, M. C. (2004). Experience of stigmatization of relatives of patients with obsessive compulsive disorder. *Archives of Psychiatric Nursing, 18*(3), 88–96.

Tweedell, D., Forchuk, C., Jewell, J., & Steinnagel, L. (2004). Families' experience during recovery of nonrecovery from psychosis. *Archives of Psychiatric Nursing, 18*(1), 17–25.

Ugarriza, D. N. (2004). Group therapy and its barriers for women suffering from postpartum depression. *Archives of Psychiatric Nursing, 18*(2), 39–48.

Valdivia, I., & Rossy, N. (2004). Brief treatment strategies for major depressive disorder. *Topics in Advanced Practice Nursing eJournal, 4*(1), 1–12.

Vessier-Batchen, M., & Douglas, D. (2006). Coping and complicated grief in survivors of homicide and suicide. *Journal of Forensic Nursing, 2*(1), 25–32.

Walsh, F. (1998). Beliefs, spirituality, and transcendence. In M. McGoldrick (Ed.), *Re-visiting family therapy* (pp. 62–77). New York: Guilford Press.

Yonkers, K. A., Wisner, K. L., Stowe, Z., Leibenluft, E., Cohen, L., Miller, L., et al. (2004). Management of bipolar disorder during pregnancy and the postpartum period. *American Journal of Psychiatry, 161*(4), 608–620.

Chapter 3

The Community in Mental Health Nursing

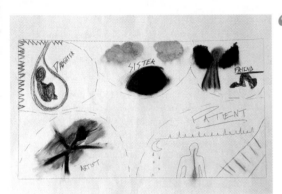

66 *Roles*

Daughter: Created to become a creator

Sister: A rock to weather life's turmoil

Friend: The duty to protect and the comfort of protection

Artist: The gift of making an ugly world tolerable

Patient: To live a life of night scares, starvation, and mutilation 99

—Kate, Age 19

OBJECTIVES

After reading this chapter, you will be able to:

1. Describe the current community mental health system.
2. Distinguish between levels of care available in different community mental health settings.
3. Outline the available community mental health services.
4. Describe the impact of severe and persistent mental illness on members of disenfranchised populations.
5. Develop appropriate interventions using community mental health services.
6. Describe the qualities of a transformed mental health system.

MediaLink www.prenhall.com/fontaine

Go to the Pearson Health MediaLink CD-ROM and the Companion Website at www.prenhall.com/fontaine for interactive resources for this chapter.

The developing model of community mental health is one of competency. It is based on the belief that individuals and families are resourceful and have the capacity to grow and change. The goal of community mental health nursing is to promote health and provide opportunities for clients to maximize their ability to live, work, socialize, and learn in the communities of their choice. Expanding client "voice" and choice is the major focus for nurses working in the community. Successful support means that clients of mental health services will be able to achieve lives of value and become contributing members of their communities.

Community-based nurses have distinct advantages in providing care, including a firsthand opportunity to observe clients and their families in a natural setting. These nurses are able to more accurately assess clients and intervene when they understand the problems that are troublesome to people in daily living in the community. Because they understand the social context of specific stressors, nurses can also identify possible pitfalls to effective interventions. In addition, community-based nurses focus on the problems identified by clients as most important in daily life.

THE MENTAL HEALTH SYSTEM

History

Ideas about where and how treatment is rendered to clients in need of mental health care have changed drastically during the past five decades. Prior to the 1960s, most clients with mental disorders were institutionalized in long-term care facilities, some never leaving the institution in their lifetime. In 1955, the U.S. government established a commission to create a comprehensive plan for meeting the population's mental health care needs. In 1963, Congress passed an act that was the beginning of the community mental health movement. This act was based on the philosophy that individuals would receive better care if they remained in their local communities and were not separated from their families and friends. The general plan was to make an array of community-based services available to all people seeking mental health care. Each community mental health center was expected to provide five basic services to the community: inpatient care, outpatient care, emergency care, partial hospitalization, and consultation and education. In addition to mental health centers, aftercare programs, halfway houses, and foster care were included in the plan.

With the passage of the Americans with Disabilities Act (ADA) in 1990, society made it a priority to promote the full participation of people with psychiatric disabilities in the economic and social mainstream. To accomplish this goal, mental health services changed the focus from inpatient care to family and community care. In the past, professionals greatly underestimated the clients' abilities to make choices for themselves and determine the course of their lives. Through stressing the importance of client choice, the self-help and mental health client movements have demonstrated that individuals with severe and persistent mental illness can live successfully in local communities when given appropriate support.

Current System

The mental health system in the United States is in disarray. Sadly, almost two decades since the passage of the ADA, the impact of the ADA on people with mental disorders is negligible. The rate of unemployment—85% to 90%—remains the same. The majority of people with mental disorders is impoverished, with 71% reporting an annual income of $20,000 or less and nearly 20% reporting less than $5,000. Those who live solely on disability benefits cannot afford even a modest efficiency apartment. As a result, those with severe and persistent mental illness may be homeless, live in shelters, or have rooms in cheap boarding hotels (Gruttadaro, 2005; Hall, 2003).

Unfortunately, services for those with severe and persistent mental illness are often disorganized and poorly funded. People who are severely ill are frequently unable to cope with the complex public system of care. When one's thoughts are disorganized, it is difficult and frustrating to try to locate appropriate help. At times, they may be brought to an acute care setting by case managers or the police. After being stabilized by medication, they are discharged back into the community, only to begin the vicious cycle over again. If individuals are a danger to themselves or others, they may be referred or court-ordered to a public long-term care facility. There is usually a waiting list for these facilities, and there is often inadequate funding for quality care. Following long-term treatment, clients are once again discharged back into the community. What was designed to be less restrictive is, in fact, often inhumane.

In 2001, President George W. Bush appointed a commission to study the problems and gaps in the mental health system and make recommendations for change. In the report (New Freedom Commission on Mental Health, 2003), the members confirmed that there are many unmet needs and many obstacles to care. The commission also developed specific strategies to transform the system. Unfortunately, the initiative has yet to be funded and, therefore, adequate mental health care remains a dream.

Obstacles to Care

There are a number of obstacles to receiving adequate mental health care in the community. Around 80% of the country's employers provide less health insurance coverage for mental health than for physical health services. Mental health care is delivered through a variety of federal, state, and local programs, all of which have different criteria and different funding, making it a very fragmented delivery system (Gruttadaro, 2005). Following are other obstacles to receiving adequate mental health care in the community:

- Stigma that surrounds mental illness
- Extreme shortage of mental health providers, especially for children and adolescents
- Lack of community-based services
- Cutbacks of psychiatric inpatient beds
- Geographic barriers
- Failure to prioritize mental illness as worthy of taxpayer support

COMMUNITY MENTAL HEALTH

Principles

Several principles help guide how community mental health care is provided to clients. The principle of **normalization** affirms that people with disabilities should be able to lead as normal a life as possible. This involves making modifications to both the physical environment, such as housing options, and the social environment, such as family respite care, community education, and employment opportunities. One goal of normalization is integration into the mainstream community. Integration is not simply physically housing severely ill individuals within the community; it includes teaching necessary social skills to clients and educating members of the community at large. With real integration comes the destigmatization of those who are severely and persistently mentally ill. Another goal of normalization is independence. This means creating opportunities for clients to develop their own senses of autonomy and self-help. Professionals and family members do not "do for" clients but rather help them with doing.

Another principle of community mental health care is that of **contextualization**, or maintaining clients in their context. This means that clients are kept in as close contact as possible with their usual surroundings, both geographic and interpersonal. There may be temporary displacements, such as utilizing a transitional residential facility, but the long-range goal is living in their desired community. Another principle is **choice**. Client choice is critical to community mental health care. Having choices helps people cope with stressful situations and increases feelings of competence. The principle of **self-advocacy** arises from the belief that those who are most affected by decisions should have the greatest influence on those decisions. This means advocating for client involvement when setting treatment goals and determining their own care. As clients are empowered they move ahead with their lives and regain or attain meaningful roles, relationships, and activities.

Recently, the relationship has shifted between mental health nurses and those who use their services. This shift is reflected in commonly used terms: Once it was *patients* and now it is *clients*. This change in language demonstrates an increasing awareness of persons with mental illness as autonomous individuals who have preferences and who make choices (Pratt & Gill, 2005).

Treatment Settings and Services

Clients of mental health services may receive care in a variety of settings. The types of services offered in these settings vary: the amount of support, structure, and restrictiveness and the hours of operation. Community treatment for those who are severely and persistently mentally ill should focus on helping them learn the basic coping skills necessary to live autonomously and in the least restrictive environment possible. The **least restrictive environment** is defined as referring or placing a client in the therapeutic setting that will provide *safe* care while allowing maximum freedom. The least restrictive environment can vary, from clients living on their own to being hospitalized in a locked unit. The determination is always made based on the level of protection needed to keep the client safe at that moment in time.

Hospitals

A small group of clients require long-term hospitalization for their own safety and for the protection of family and the community. These individuals profit most from treatment programs that emphasize highly structured behavioral interventions, such as a token economy, point systems, and skills training that can improve their level of functioning.

Treatment in an acute care hospital provides a safe, structured, and supervised environment, lowering the stress on clients and family members. In some situations, inpatient care is the preferred setting:

- For clients who are a danger to themselves or others, such as those who are acutely suicidal or homicidal
- For those who are acutely psychotic and thus a serious danger to themselves because of confusion and disorganization
- For treatment of acute intoxicated states and withdrawal from alcohol or drugs

Hospital stays have been reduced to 3 to 8 days. Hospitalization allows the health care team to closely monitor the level of symptoms and reaction to treatments.

Day hospitalization can be used as an alternative to inpatient care or following a brief hospitalization. Day hospitalization is less disruptive to the person's life than inpatient care and treatment is given in a less restrictive environment. The person should not be at risk of harming him- or herself or others and should be able to cooperate minimally in treatment. People participating in day hospitalization programs typically attend the program for 6 to 8 hours a day and are at home, work, or school the other hours. Services include medication administration and monitoring; group, individual, and expressive therapies; and opportunities for recreation and socialization.

Outpatient Services

Clients are not likely to be successful in making the transition from highly structured inpatient or day treatment programs until there are support systems within the home or the community. *Day treatment programs* provide ongoing supportive care and are usually not time limited. They provide structure and programs to help prevent relapse and to improve social and vocational functioning. They may also provide family therapy. The type of structured activities encountered in a full day of employment is introduced gradually. Clients may be employed part-time while in the program. Day treatment programs have low staff-to-client ratios and minimal or no nursing staff.

Medication clinics are part of a more comprehensive program. They are helpful to clients who cannot manage their medications on their own. Nurses administer medications and monitor for side effects. Client education is a major focus of these clinics. Because the severely ill may not be able to afford psychotropic medications, nurses often must be creative in locating funding sources, which may include research programs or financial assistance from drug companies.

Psychosocial clubhouses are therapeutic communities where staff members function as coaches whose roles are to encourage decision making and socialization by the "members" of the club. Clubhouses exist primarily to improve the quality of life of their members. Members are accepted without regard to their symptoms, and they can stay as long as they like. Club activities focus on recreational, vocational, and residential functions. The approach is transitional, with individuals gradually assuming more responsibility and privileges.

Housing

Supportive housing is a program used for clients who do not live on their own or with their families and who would benefit from some degree of assistance in self-care and self-management. These programs can increase social and vocational functioning, improve quality of life, and decrease homelessness and the need for repeat hospitalization. Alternative housing often enables people with disabilities to increase their independence and develop the capacity to live as independently as possible.

Most clients with mental illness prefer their own residence and want autonomy over their housing choices. Most clients prefer an apartment or a house that allows them to

---

BOX 3.1	Types of Residential Facilities

Transitional Halfway Houses

- Provide room and board until suitable housing is available

Long-Term Group Residences

- On-site staff
- Appropriate for persistently and severely mentally ill person
- Length of stay is indefinite

Cooperative Apartments/Supported Housing

- No on-site staff
- Staff members make regular visits to assist residents

Intensive Care or Crisis Community Residences

- Used to help prevent hospitalization or shorten length of hospitalization
- On-site nursing staff and counseling staff

Foster or Family Care

- In private homes
- Close supervision of foster family to ensure a therapeutic environment

Nursing Homes

- Appropriate for some psychiatric clients who are geriatric or medically disabled
- Psychiatric clients may have facilities or units separate from residents without a history of mental illness
- Activity programs and psychiatric supervision

---

live independently. Clients who live in transitional housing often see these arrangements as stepping stones to greater independence. See Box 3.1 for types of residential facilities.

Residential crisis services are a new alternative to hospitalization and are provided in neighborhood homes that are staffed and organized to treat acutely ill clients. Clients include adolescents with psychiatric problems, people experiencing an acute psychiatric emergency resulting from a life crisis, or other individuals going through acute psychiatric episodes. The residential crisis service offers a respite from their current living situation, which may be stressful or unsatisfactory, and provides intensive treatment in a program that uses medication, milieu therapy, and other forms of therapy.

Studies have shown that perceived choice over one's living arrangements is important to physical and psychological well-being. Having choice over housing can reduce the stress of repeated moves. Stable housing is the foundation of long-term recovery. When basic housing needs are met, clients can begin to focus on other goals, such as employment, making friends, and participating in community activities.

The goal of client choice in supported housing has not yet been achieved. Many clients believe that they have little or no choice and that their choices are highly or completely influenced by others. People who are severely mentally ill may be living on SSI (supplemental security income) or SSDI (Social Security Disability Insurance), which are inadequate to rent even "affordable housing" in the United States. The majority receive $617 per month for total living expenses, which includes supplements provided by most programs to help pay rent. The average rent for a small apartment is $676 a month, or 109% of their income. As nurses, we must become advocates at community, state, and federal levels to secure decent and affordable housing of choice in communities that clients can call home (Kidd, 2007).

Schools

Nationwide, only one third of the children who need mental health services actually receive it. The main barriers to care are availability, accessibility, and affordability. In some cases, services may not be available; in other cases, families may be unaware of the available services. There may also be cultural barriers, such as language differences or a poor ethnic match between clients and care providers. Access is a major problem for children because they are unable to seek mental health services for themselves and are dependent on adults, such as parents or teachers, to recognize this need and to initiate contact. Other accessibility problems are transportation, day care, and parental schedules. Many children and families cannot afford services and are unaware that care may be available at adjusted rates or even at no cost (Evans, 2006; Gruttadaro, 2005).

Children with mental illness and emotional disturbances are covered under the Individuals with Disabilities Education Act (IDEA). The IDEA has not been very effective, similar to the ADA. Compared with students with other disabilities, children with mental illness have the lowest academic achievement and the highest dropout and failure rates (Gruttadaro, 2005; Schainker & Grant, 2003). Teachers and support staff often do not understand mental illness and are unaware of appropriate and positive behavioral intervention for this population. The National Alliance on Mental Illness (NAMI) has developed a number of programs for school systems. Some are directed to students (Breaking the Silence, Hope for Tomorrow) and some are directed to teachers and parents (Hand-to-Hand, Hope for Tomorrow, Parents and Teachers as Allies).

In a few locations, mental health services have teamed up with schools to provide services to behaviorally and emotionally disordered children. Services integrated into the school setting seem more natural for children and parents and improve access and limit barriers. Teachers often know the child and family well and are able to provide valuable information regarding strengths and weaknesses. The community mental health nurse is able to observe the child in the classroom, in the lunchroom, and on the playground, which provides a broader and more useful picture of problems and assets. As communities broaden outreach into the school system, the mental health needs of more children with a wide range of psychiatric and behavioral problems will be met, regardless of the family's ability to afford or access mental health care.

Home Care

Providing mental health services to clients and their families in their homes is a fairly new initiative in the mental health field. There are some distinct advantages of home care treatment. Direct observation of family interactions leads to more accurate evaluation of strengths and limitations. (See chapter 2 ∞ for family assessment.) Home visits facilitate the participation of all family members, including young children. Because the family is in their own home and the nurse is a guest, family members often feel more in control and empowered in the relationship. Clients and families report more communication with staff, increased participation in treatment decisions, and receiving care with dignity and respect. Other advantages are that daily routines are less disrupted, relationships are less restricted, and levels of anxiety are minimized.

Home treatment may be an alternative to inpatient treatment during the acute phase of a mental illness. Acute home care treatment involves providing intensive support through home visits by nurses, social workers, psychiatrists, and homemakers. Staff members are available 24 hours a day and provide services such as medication management, interpersonal support for clients and caregivers, behavioral management, housing maintenance, assistance with activities of daily living (ADLs), reality orientation, and social/recreational activities. Once clients stabilize, they return to their case manager team for continuing support (Fagin, 2001; McNab, Smith, & Minardi, 2006).

Home health care nurses must always consider their own safety. If possible, they should call ahead and let the client know their arrival time. Family members or friends may be called on to escort the nurse from the car to the home if there are concerns about neighborhood safety. Portable phones should be turned on and programmed to speed dial 911 in case of emergency. Once in the home, nurses must be alert to situations that might be risky, such as agitation, suspicious thinking, hostility, and threats. If calmness and nonthreatening support are ineffective in deescalating the threatening behaviors, it may be necessary to call for emergency assistance (Clark, 2003).

Disenfranchised Populations
Rural Communities

Increases in community-based services are needed in rural and urban areas both. Rural communities, however, face more severe challenges in meeting the mental health needs of their residents than do urban communities. Groups at greater risk for mental disorders—that is, those who are chronically ill, the poor, the dependent, and the elderly—are disproportionately represented in rural areas. Studies have consistently identified many rural services as fragmented, costly, and often ineffective. Poverty, inadequate transportation, and limited economic opportunities restrict treatment alternatives to the already insufficient numbers of mental health care providers. Stigma, religious values, and a belief that emotional problems are the domain of healers and family contribute to poor utilization of available services. Women in rural areas have a much higher rate of major depressive disorder: 41% compared with 13% to 20% of urban women (Farrell & McKinnon, 2003; Hauenstein, 2003; Patterson, 2003).

The cost of services is a major barrier. Many of the newer psychotropic medications are very expensive. Rural clients may not be able to travel the distances needed to obtain the medication. Of those individuals who have medical insurance, many lack coverage for psychotherapy even if they can find a therapist. Lack of quality inpatient care for acutely ill people is another problem in rural areas. These clients are often hospitalized far from family and friends. Once discharged back into the community, psychosocial rehabilitation services are limited, which frequently leads to repeat hospitalizations.

Although there are significant problems facing clients who live in rural settings, there are also considerable community strengths in rural settings. Generally, rural communities have a strong loyalty to family, church, and community. This loyalty results in a higher degree of tolerance for perceived "abnormal behavior" among community members and a willingness to help those who are less fortunate. Depending on the rural community, there are indigenous care providers, ranging from companion/aid to confidant/therapist to healer/shaman. These natural helpers within the community may complement professional mental health providers and may also serve as a "bridge" between clients and professionals.

Homeless Populations

On any given night, 800,000 Americans are **homeless**, living on streets or in woods, and, if they are lucky, sleeping in emergency shelters each night. The homeless include people of every race, ethnic background, and educational level. Men are more likely to be homeless than women. The ethnic group at highest risk is African Americans, followed by Euro-Americans. Latinos and Asian Americans are at significantly less risk. It is difficult to estimate the number of homeless people with mental illness, but it is believed that one third has severe and persistent mental illness and up to one half of the one third has a concurrent substance use disorder. This is a deeply disad-

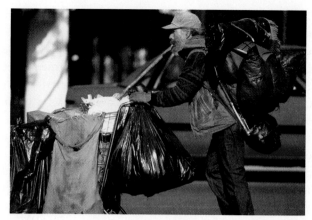

PHOTO 3.1 ■ Lacking adequate funding and staff, mental hospitals frequently failed to provide adequate treatment to their residents. Beginning in the 1950s and 1960s, the policy of deinstitutionalization led to the release of many individuals, who, without proper follow-up care, ended up living on the streets. Although not all homeless people are mentally ill, estimates suggest that between 30% and 50% of homeless persons have some type of mental disorder.

SOURCE: Tom Prettyman/PhotoEdit, Inc. Used with permission.

vantaged and difficult-to-reach-and-treat population (Folsom et al., 2005; Practice Guideline, 2004).

Chronic substance abusers may end up with no home if they are abandoned by family and friends. If the disease has interfered with the ability to maintain a job, the person may be forced to live on the streets. If these people are actively using substances, they are turned away from supportive housing programs.

Families now constitute 36% of the homeless population. Many homeless families are headed by women who take their children and flee from an abusive husband or partner. Homeless families may lose their sense of identity as a family; parents lose their sense of competence; and children lose the idea of home. Some of these families are on waiting lists for subsidized housing (National Health Care for the Homeless Council, 2005).

Many adolescents find themselves living on their own as a consequence of running away from home or being thrown out by their families. Some have been physically or sexually abused in their homes. In other situations, parents of adolescents who are acting out may force the teenager out of the home as a way to gain control in their own lives. Adolescents also become homeless because of family conflict, chaotic family systems, and unsuccessful foster care situations.

American society has been minimally responsive to the homeless population. In addition, societal issues such as unemployment, low wages, lack of affordable housing, lack of health insurance, and limitations of public funding are contributing factors (National Health Care for the Homeless Council, 2005).

MediaLink   Care Plan, Mobile Emergency Services

Nurses help the homeless population through outreach, social support groups, case management, and provision of transitional housing. Outreach to homeless people includes advertising in missions and shelters, using former "street people" as liaison staff, and using mobile crisis services. The purpose of outreach is to explain the available services and help homeless clients negotiate the system.

Nurse-managed outreach clinics often provide care to homeless people. This is an appropriate setting because homelessness contributes to multiple health problems, such as respiratory infections, tuberculosis, trauma, hypertension, and peripheral vascular disease. Vulnerability to infection places this population at higher risk for HIV and hepatitis B and C infections. Homeless persons tend to go without care until relatively minor problems become urgent medical emergencies. Lack of access for good hygiene practice can lead to dental problems and skin problems, such as lice, scabies, and impetigo. The inability to meet their self-care needs contributes to sustained feelings of despair and hopelessness (National Health Care for the Homeless Council, 2005).

Social support groups are set up in shelters, soup kitchens, drop-in centers, transitional housing units, and single-room-occupancy (SRO) houses. Through these groups, nurses can empower clients, increase their problem-solving skills, help them develop self-confidence, and support their identity with a group of people.

Through case management, nurses can help clients negotiate appointments and services from a variety of agencies. Nurses may also monitor compliance with medication, assist with ADLs, find appropriate shelter, and assist with developing support systems.

Correctional Systems

The number of severely and persistently mentally ill people in correctional settings continues to increase. With few long-term psychiatric facilities, many people who were previously cared for in state hospitals are now found in jails and prisons. People with severe and persistent mental illness are almost five times more likely to be jailed rather than hospitalized. The increase in numbers is also related to a lack of support in the community for those with severe and persistent mental illness. It is believed that more than 300,000 inmates in U.S. jails and prisons have serious mental illness. Thousands of mentally ill American children, some as young as 7, are locked up in juvenile detention centers because there is no other place for them to go. Jails, prison, and juvenile detention centers are ill-equipped to meet the mental health needs of these individuals (Honberg, 2005; Monahan, Swartz, & Bonnie, 2003). See chapter 6 ∞ for more information on this topic.

COMMUNITY MENTAL HEALTH SERVICES

Community-based services for diverse populations must be *culturally appropriate*. The egocentric orientation of Western cultures values independent action with the goal of psychosocial rehabilitation being one of autonomy and self-sufficiency. Those cultures with sociocentric orientations, however, typically reflect interdependence and family orientation. The rehabilitation goal of independence may not be culturally appropriate with these individuals. Thus, it is critically important that nursing interventions be relative to the culture of the clients.

Di, a 28-year-old Japanese American, came to the United States with his family when he was a teenager. He has continued to live at home while finishing college and starting his career. Having recently lost all his money and his job due to compulsive gambling, Di attempted suicide. He states that he cannot go back home because he has brought shame to his family, nor can he live apart from his family, as he is unmarried.

Screening Programs

Community screening programs help provide early identification of mental health problems. Screening tests are used because it is not readily apparent to people that they have a disorder, because the disorder is prevalent in the population and is treatable, and because early intervention will make a difference in the outcome. There must also be an accurate and cost-effective screening tool. A number of physical conditions meet these requirements, such as hypertension, breast cancer, lead poisoning, and stroke. Screening for mental disorders is relatively new. National Depression Screening Day, begun in 1991, was the first national, community-based, voluntary screening program for mental illness. Research suggests that the program has been effective in bringing individuals with depression into treatment. Those clients who do not comply with screening recommendations to seek treatment often have misinformation about their disorder or lack financial means or insurance to seek additional evaluation and intervention. Other at-risk groups that would benefit from screening programs include single parents with young children, children and adolescents, teen parents, victims of family and community violence, and older adults living alone. Community outreach must be increased to ensure that those who are at risk for or who have mental disorders receive appropriate and adequate assistance.

Case Managment

The theory behind case management is effective collaboration among nursing, medicine, home care, ambulatory care, and administration. The goals are to increase appropriate use of resources, encourage collaborative team practice, facilitate continuity of care, and decrease duration of need for services to promote quality and cost-effective outcomes. Case managers are employed in almost every imaginable health care setting, including acute care hospitals, rehabilitation facilities, community centers, outpatient clinics, and home care. Case managers are responsible for a number of activities (Woodside & McClam, 2006):

- Identify clients and determine whose needs are congruent with available services and resources.
- Assess individual needs and strengths.
- Work with other providers to determine the best way to meet needs and support skills and strengths.
- Link clients to available services by helping them meet qualifying criteria.
- Create access to services.
- Advocate by negotiating with agencies and policy makers to gain resources for clients.
- Ensure that service is provided in a consistent manner.
- Provide direct care in the form of a therapeutic relationship, supportive psychotherapy, and crisis response.

This planning determines linkage, which is the next step in treatment. The case manager links clients to available services by helping them meet the qualifying criteria. If services are inaccessible, case managers may broker for services; that is, they create access to services. They also serve as advocates by negotiating with agencies and policy makers to gain resources for clients. Coordination ensures that providers deliver service in a consistent manner. Almost all case managers also provide *direct care* in the form of a therapeutic relationship, supportive psychotherapy, and crisis response.

Crisis Response Services

In the traditional mental health system, the hospital is used to stabilize acute illness, but staff may have limited ability to help clients adapt to the real world after discharge. Severely and persistently mentally ill clients often cannot or will not follow up with services at a clinic, resulting in relapse into acute illness. Family or police bring them to the emergency department, where they are admitted to the acute care setting. This perpetuates the cycle of crisis–hospitalization– discharge–crisis. Some people go into crisis because they are unable to understand their everyday problems and are unable to participate in a complex treatment plan. Some are unable to access their own care because the services are limited, expensive, and often inconvenient. Some go into crisis due to lack of housing, an absence of a social group, or relapse with drugs or alcohol. These problems result in feelings of shame, humiliation, and guilt. One person in crisis has an impact on the lives of others in the community—friends, family, neighbors, coworkers, and passersby. Those around the individual in crisis can be fearful, rejecting, or even hostile.

Many acutely mentally ill people can be evaluated, treated, and stabilized by bringing therapists directly to clients in crisis. *Mobile emergency treatment* services bridge the gap between inpatient, outpatient, and family-based care. Some clients are too anxious, fearful, agitated, or depressed to come to traditional treatment settings. Visiting clients in their own environment helps the professional maximize clients' home and community resources. Emergency services must be available when clients' coping skills are overwhelmed or when mental illness worsens and clients begin to experience dangerous symptoms.

Mobile crisis services are staffed by interdisciplinary teams of psychiatrists, nurses, social workers, psychologists, and counselors. The team is available 24 hours a day, 365 days a year. The mobile team may be called to private homes, group homes, shelters, hotels, street corners, malls, public buildings, recreational areas, police stations, or anywhere in the entire community. In the majority of requests for mobile assistance, professionals are at little risk, if any. However, if the situation is potentially dangerous—an assaultive person, one who is suicidal, or a homicidal person with a weapon—the team members attempt to calm and support the client over the phone before or during their ride to the client's location. In this type of situation, the police are always asked to accompany the treatment team. The client must be informed that the police will be coming along and that the police will leave once everything is under control. If clients are not manageable in the community setting, the team will bring them to the hospital. See Box 3.2 for intervention guidelines.

Bridging Strategies

Almost two thirds of clients discharged from acute care facilities fail to keep outpatient referral appointments. Failure to engage in outpatient services increases the probability of relapse and repeat hospitalization. Nurses can use several strategies to help people readjust to community living. These bridging strategies include sessions that make the family a part of the treatment team, linking family/friends to support services, improving communication regarding discharge plans between inpatient and outpatient staff, and enabling clients to begin outpatient programs before discharge. Successful community living requires adequate discharge preparation and linking the client to the appropriate community services. In the Transitional Discharge Model, originating in Canada and Scotland, staff from the acute care setting continue to see discharged clients while they establish a relationship with a health care professional in the community. The program also includes formal linkage with peers as a supportive social network Research

BOX 3.2	Intervention Guidelines for Mobile Crisis Services

Control Behavior

- Use the approach that is least restrictive but that maximizes safety for everyone.
- Make sure you are not alone, especially in a closed-in area.
- Remain calm and be observant as you approach the client.
- Remove items that could become harmful, such as ties, necklaces, large or dangly earrings, pens, and pencils. Stop about 6 feet away.
- Introduce yourself and address client by last name. Ask permission to use client's first name.
- If you do not feel endangered, ask whether client will shake hands with you.
- Explain procedures using simple, ordinary language, for example, "I need to check your blood pressure."

Assess Quickly

- Rule out a potentially life-threatening process that could be causing client's psychiatric signs and symptoms, such as hypoglycemia, head injury, or neurological illness.
- Look for Med-Alert bracelet, signs of injury.

Treat Specifically

- Psychotic and agitated behavior must be treated vigorously by ensuring a safe environment. Restraints are used only as a last resort.
- Appropriate medication will decrease violent symptoms and rapidly decrease the danger to self and others.

demonstrates shorter stays in the acute care setting with fewer readmissions (Forchuk, Reynolds, Sharkey, Martin, & Jensen, 2007; Mojtabai, Herman, Susser, Sohler, Craig, Lavelle et al. 2005).

Support Services

Assertive community treatment (ACT) allows clients to live in their own communities while they receive the individual assistance needed for everyday life and managing their illness. ACT teams include a psychiatrist, nurses, social workers, peer specialists, a substance abuse specialist, and a vocational specialist. The team goes out to meet and work with the client, who does not have to make and keep office appointments. Team members help individuals find and keep housing and employment and manage everything from their medication to their money. Together, the ACT team and the client work to achieve the client's goals.

Psychogeriatric Assessment and Treatment in City Housing (PATCH) is an outreach program, in some areas of the country, for elderly public-housing residents who need mental health care. Diagnosis and treatment of mental illness are less likely to occur among the older population because of such factors as withdrawal, fearfulness, cognitive impairment, stigma, and decreased mobility. The PATCH team consists of two psychiatric nurses who are the service

providers and two part-time psychiatrists who serve as consultants. PATCH has an extensive outreach program to identify individuals in need of care who are then provided with an in-home assessment by psychiatric nurses. Nurses serve as case managers and also provide direct care to the elderly residents. The program also has an educational arm geared toward lessening the stigma of mental illness and facilitating individuals' access to community services.

Psychosocial Rehabilitation

The field of psychosocial rehabilitation grew out of a need to create opportunities for people with severe and persistent mental illness. **Psychosocial rehabilitation** is the development of skills and supports necessary for successful living, learning, and working in the community. This approach creates collaborative partnerships with all interested people—clients, families, friends, and mental health care providers. **Recovery**, a facet of rehabilitation, refers to incorporating the disability as part of reality, modifying dreams and aspirations, exploring new ideas, and eventually adapting to the disease. Each person's road to recovery is unique. It is assumed that the client will be "in charge" with regard to setting goals for where and how to live, work, learn, socialize, and recreate. Rehabilitation is a process, not a quick fix. This approach is different from the traditional approach to long-term clients in which the assumption was that decisions must be made for people with severe and persistent mental illness.

People with mental illness differ little from the general population. They want meaningful and self-enhancing work and the opportunity to socialize with others. Psychosocial rehabilitation is anchored in the values of *hope* and optimism that people can grow, learn, and make changes in their lives. One essential element is *power*. People who have mental disorders need power and control in their relationships with professionals, in their own lives, and in the way resources are allocated. This allows them to take personal responsibility for where they are in their lives and where they are going.

NAMI has developed a nationwide Peer-to-Peer Recovery Education Course. Courses are taught by teams of three mentors and are free to persons who live with mental illness. For 2 hours a week, over 9 weeks, mentors help individuals create a relapse prevention plan, formulate an advance directive for psychiatric care, and practice stress management and other coping strategies. Part of recovery is being around people who see mental disorders not as permanent, but as an illness from which they can take increasing control of their lives.

Nurses not only provide care, but also work with clients to make decisions about treatment and about daily life. Recovery is about providing temporary support during hard times while working with clients to take responsibility for their own wellness. Box 3.3 lists guidelines for recovery-oriented nursing interventions.

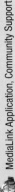

MediaLink MediaLink Application, Community Support

Recovery is a personal choice. When a nurse finds resistance and apathy to recovery, he or she may feel frustrated. It is important to recognize that severity of symptoms, motivation, and personality type can affect a person's ability to work toward recovery. Some people work at it intensely, whereas others approach it more slowly. It is not up to you to determine when a person is ready to make progress—it is up to the person. Box 3.4 lists the key aspects of recovery.

Social support has an effect on physical and mental status. Research indicates that people with more social resources or networks are better able to adapt to change and are in better health. Unfortunately, people who have severe mental illness have fewer social networks and weaker support systems than people without mental illness. This restricted network may not be able to provide the amount and type of support necessary for clients to live in the community. Nurses can provide an important service: the enhancement of social support networks. This is accomplished by reinforcing existing ties, improving family ties, and building new ties.

Social network interventions are designed to improve the relationships within the client's social network. These interventions include peer client support, connection with indigenous healers, volunteer matching, family education and support, social skills training groups, and linkage with community resources. As networks increase in size and strength, clients will be more able to remain in their communities of choice.

Individuals who are severely mentally ill may need *social skills training* to enable them to live successfully in the community. Social skills training includes such things as personal hygiene and grooming skills, self-care, communication, time management, handling money, leisure activities, meal preparation, use of resources, problem-solving skills, and conflict management. Clients learn to interact appropriately with strangers, family members, and friends, both at work and at school. Social skills training fosters their ability to live and work in their communities just like anyone else. (See chapter 9 ∞ for further information on social skills training.)

Education

The 1990 IDEA mandates support for people with disabilities in educational settings. With the onset of a major mental illness in childhood or adolescence, educational programs are individualized to improve clients' level of academic functioning, with the goal of enhancing quality of life and developing career options. There are three types of supported postsecondary education programs. In the *self-contained classroom*, all the students have disabilities and the focus of the curriculum is on career planning and skill building. This is the least integrated model of the three. The *on-site support model* is the most common, with the goal of assisting students in utilizing resources that already exist within the school community. Services are provided through the disabled student services or through student counseling services. The *mobile support model* involves staff from the local mental health center as supports for individual students.

Employment

The unemployment rate of people with psychiatric disabilities is 85% to 90% (Gruttadaro, 2005). Many of these individuals would, however, benefit from work because work can provide needed daily structure, an opportunity for socialization and

---

BOX 3.3	Guidelines for Recovery-Oriented Nursing Interventions

- Treat the person as an adult partner in care with the capacity and responsibility to learn, change, and make life decisions no matter how severe the symptoms.
- Make planning and treatment a truly collaborative process, with personal choice being most important.
- Accept that a person's life path is up to him or her.
- Never scold, threaten, punish, patronize, judge, or condescend to the person.
- Rather than focusing on a diagnosis or a label, concentrate on how the person feels, what the person is experiencing, and what the person wants.
- Limit the sharing of ideas. One idea a day or per visit is plenty. Avoid overwhelming the person.
- Pay close attention to individual needs and preferences.
- Implement evidence-based practice by learning about "best practices" based on scientific studies.

SOURCES: Adapted from Lehman, A. F. (2000). Putting recovery into practice. *Community Mental Health Journal, 36*(3), 329–331; and Mead, S., & Copeland, M. E. (2000). What recovery means to us: Consumers' perspectives. *Community Mental Health Journal, 36*(3), 315–328. With kind permission from Springer Science and Business Media.

BOX 3.4	Key Aspects of Client Recovery

Hope

- Eliminate internalized dire predictions.
- Offer help as well as receive help.
- Take positive risks.

Self-Responsibility

- Work to heal oneself.
- Wellness is up to each individual.

Self-Advocacy

- Learn to see self as worthwhile and unique.
- Make treatment choices for self.
- Refuse treatments that are not in your best interests.
- Create your own advance directive.
- Create the life of your choice.

SOURCES: Adapted from Mead, S., & Copeland, M. E. (2000). What recovery means to us: Consumers' perspectives. *Community Mental Health Journal, 36*(3), 315–328; with kind permission from Springer Science and Business Media and Pratt, C. W., Gill, K. J., Barrett, N. M., & Roberts, M. M. (1999). *Psychiatric rehabilitation.* San Diego: Academic Press, with permission from Pratt.

meaningful activity, and self-sufficiency. Severe mental illness and the accompanying unemployment, poverty, social stigma, hospitalizations, symptoms, and medication side effects contribute to lower quality of life. Being fired from a job or being persistently unemployed contributes to feelings of inadequacy and low self-esteem.

Not all clients want to be employed, but many desire to work and may need support in locating positions, filling out applications, role-playing interviews, and learning job expectations and behaviors. A Thinking Skills for Work program assesses how cognitive problems have interfered with past job performance. Clients then engage in cognitive remediation and compensatory strategies through 24 computer-based sessions over 12 weeks. Employment specialists may be consulted to manage any further difficulties. Supported employment (SE), according to the Rehabilitation Act Amendments of 1998, means that ongoing support services are provided according to the needs of each individual. Some community mental health centers provide job coaches if necessary; these coaches work alongside clients on the job until they can gradually become self-sufficient in the job. These programs work because they help people find work quickly and provide them with ongoing support as long as necessary. Unfortunately, the programs have not been widely implemented because of problems with long-term funding. See Box 3.5 for vocational services.

The financial disincentives to employment have yet to be addressed. Individuals receiving SSI or SSDI funds risk losing this financial assistance when they become employed, even in entry-level, low-wage positions. People who even take part-time work lose entitlement income, including food stamps and rent subsidies, which amounts to an effective tax of 64% on their earnings. The greatest fear clients have is the loss of medical coverage. A way must be found to encourage employment while providing enough support to maintain community living and health care protection.

Telehealth

Telehealth is the use of electronic information and telecommunications technologies to support long-distance clinical health care and client and professional health-related education. This technology shows promise in overcoming the obstacles in the delivery of mental health services to underserved locations and disenfranchised populations. Telehealth may decrease travel time for clients, increase access to care, maximize the use of resources, reduce disparities in service, reduce stigma, enable specialty consultation, and improve professional knowledge. The technologies and tools used in telehealth include videoconferencing, telephones, videophones, the Internet, articles, chat rooms, support groups, newsletters, resource links, and e-mail discussion for professionals. As telehealth becomes more widespread, research is needed in the areas of clinical outcomes, best practices, predictors of satisfaction, costs, and educational outcomes (Farrell & McKinnon, 2003; Hilty, Marks, Urness, Yellowlees, & Nesbitt, 2004).

TRANSFORMING THE MENTAL HEALTH SYSTEM

The president's New Freedom Commission on Mental Health has made recommendations regarding the transformation of the mental health system in the United States. As it states, "In a transformed system, clients and family members will have access to timely and accurate information that promotes learning, self-monitoring, and accountability. Health care providers will rely on up-to-date knowledge to provide optimum care for the best outcome . . . . The highest quality of care and information will be available to clients and families, regardless of their race, gender, ethnicity, language, age, or place of residence" (New Freedom Commission on Mental Health, 2003, p. 6). Box 3.6 describes the six goals of the transformed system.

| BOX 3.5 | Vocational Services |

Transitional Employment

- Program of time-limited jobs in regular work settings
- Regular pay
- Agency staff provide training and support for that job.
- When specified time of employment is over, job is filled by another client.

Job Club

- Structure and resources to assist members in own job search
- May not provide enough support for severely ill clients.

Sheltered Workshops

- Workshop solicits manufacturing jobs from local business to provide work for people with disabilities.
- May be a permanent placement or a step to competitive employment

Affirmative Industries

- Businesses are owned, managed, and operated by mental health agencies ranging from cleaning services to landscaping to bakeries and caterers.
- Clients are supervised by agency staff and paid by agency.

Supported Employment

- Based on the philosophy that, given adequate supports, most people are capable of competitive employment.
- Agency provides support services for people who are severely disabled.

BOX 3.6	Goals in a Transformed Mental Health System

Goal 1: Create an understanding in America that mental health is essential to overall health.

- Stigma will be reduced and eliminated.
- Education campaigns will target rural Americans, racial and ethnic minority groups, and people for whom English is a second language.
- Treatments will be more readily available and focused on recovery.

Goal 2: Mental health care is client and family driven.

- Clients and families will actively participate in designing and developing the systems of care in which they are involved.
- Basic to this goal is access to health care, gainful employment opportunities, adequate and affordable housing, and the assurance of not being unjustly incarcerated.

Goal 3: Eliminate disparities in mental health services.

- Tailor services for culturally diverse populations.
- Improve access to quality care in rural areas.

Goal 4: Early mental health screening, assessment, and referral to services are common practice.

- Quality screening and early intervention will occur in readily accessible, low-stigma settings.
- Improve and expand school mental health programs.

Goal 5: Deliver and accelerate excellent mental health care.

- Provide evidence-based mental health services.
- Expand research in four understudy areas: mental health disparities, long-term effects of medications, trauma, and acute care.

Goal 6: Use technology to access mental health care and information.

- Empower clients and families through advanced communication and information.
- Use telehealth to improve access and coordination of mental health care.

SOURCE: New Freedom Commission on Mental Health. (2003). *Achieving the promise: Transforming mental health care in America. Final report.* (DHHS Publication No. SMA-03-3832). Rockville, MD: Author.

Focus Your Study

OBJECTIVES	KEY CONCEPTS
1. Describe the current community mental health system.	- Many unmet needs - Many obstacles to care - Inadequate funding - Inadequate insurance coverage - Shortage of providers
2. Distinguish between levels of care available in different community mental health settings.	- Acute care hospitalization - Day hospitalization or treatment programs - Medication clinics - Psychosocial clubhouses - Supportive housing - Residential crisis services - School programs - Home treatment
3. Outline the available community mental health services.	- Screening—early identification - Case management—identify clients, assess needs/strengths, find services, direct care - Crisis response—mobile emergency services - Bridging—involves family/friends, discharge planning, link to services - School—IDEA - Employment—supported employment, transitional jobs, job club, sheltered workshops, affirmative industries - Support services—ACT, PATCH - Telehealth—long-distance health care education

continued

continued

4. Describe the impact of severe and persistent mental illness on members of disenfranchised populations.	■ Clients unable to cope with a complex system of care ■ Clients often in a cycle of hospitalization, return to community, hospitalization ■ Waiting lists for long term care facilities ■ Inadequate services in rural areas ■ Cost of services is prohibitive ■ Few services for the homeless population
5. Develop appropriate interventions using community mental health services.	■ Reach out to the rural population through nurse-managed clinics and telehealth programs. ■ Reach out to the homeless population through nurse-managed outreach clinics, social support groups, case management, provision of transitional housing. ■ Establish screening programs throughout communities. ■ Provide social network interventions.
6. Describe the qualities of a trans-formed mental health system.	■ Stigma eliminated ■ Screening/early intervention ■ Treatment available and accessible ■ Clients/family actively involved ■ Disparities eliminated ■ Gainful employment ■ Adequate, affordable housing ■ Improved/expanded school programs ■ Research/evidence-based services

Explore MediaLink

For review questions, case studies, and other resources for this chapter see the Pearson Health MediaLink CD-ROM that accompanies this book and the Companion Website.

CD-ROM
- Audio Glossary
- NCLEX-RN® Review Questions

Companion Website www.prenhall.com/fontaine
- Audio Glossary
- NCLEX-RN® Review Questions
- Case Study
  – Use of Mobile Emergency Services
- Care Plan
  – A Client with Mental Illness in a Homeless Shelter
- Critical Thinking
  – Rural Mental Health Services
- MediaLink Application
  – Community Support
- MediaLinks
  – Books for Clients and Families
  – Community Resources

NCLEX-RN® Review Questions

3-1. The psychiatric community nurse is working with clients who have substance abuse issues. Many clients in the group have had relapses. The group is multicultural and comprised of young adults. The most appropriate nursing intervention in dealing with these clients is to:
  1. Provide confidence so that the clients have the ability to deal with the triggers that cause them to repeat their behaviors.
  2. Demonstrate an authoritarian attitude that the clients have a weakness in character.
  3. Provide reassurance that the problem will resolve itself in time.
  4. Work collaboratively with the clients in developing new coping strategies.

3-2. A nurse is providing secondary crisis care to clients in the community. The nurse recognizes that which of the following clients is experiencing an adventitious crisis?
  1. A man who has lost his job
  2. The family who has lost a child
  3. The couple having marital problems
  4. A woman attending a rock concert where rioting resulted in many injuries

3-3. A 17-year-old client comes to the community crisis clinic. She has multiple superficial cuts on her wrists. She is crying uncontrollability and states that her boyfriend has left her and she doesn't want to live without him. The nurse's initial response should be:
  1. "Let's set some boundaries on your behavior here."
  2. "Many boyfriends change their minds about relationships."
  3. "Don't worry, at your age you will find another boyfriend."
  4. "I know that you are feeling anxious. I will stay with you until you feel better."

3-4. The community psychiatric nurse conducts weekly education groups for clients in a senior citizen day care center. The nurse suspects that one of the clients is in an abusive environment. The client has bruises on her body and tells the nurse she often falls in the home. The priority care plan for this client is for the nurse to:
  1. Make an immediate appointment to visit the home.
  2. Disregard the client because she is confused.
  3. Alert the doctor.
  4. Wait a few weeks to assess additional bruises.

3-5. The mobile crisis unit of a large metropolitan city receives an emergency call from a teenage client who states, "My life is worthless. I do not want to live anymore." The mobile crisis unit is on the way to the home. The nurse's first response is to:
  1. Attempt to calm and support the client.
  2. Provide reassurance that life is not that bad.
  3. Ask the teenager if she felt like this before.
  4. Do not tell the client that the police will accompany the crisis team.

3-6. A nurse is developing skills to ensure provision of culturally competent care in the community. Which of the following actions is the most important for the nurse?
  1. Encourage acculturation.
  2. Encourage assimilation.
  3. Identify the nurse's own attitudes and biases.
  4. Work only with cultural groups that the nurse has prior knowledge.

See Appendix D for answers.

References

Clark, M. J. (2003). *Community health nursing* (4th ed.). Upper Saddle River, NJ: Prentice Hall.

Evans, M. E. (2006). Integrating nursing care into systems of care for children with emotional and behavioral disorders. *Journal of Child and Adolescent Psychiatric Nursing, 19*(2), 62–68.

Fagin, C. M. (2001). Revisiting treatment in the home. *Archives of Psychiatric Nursing, 15*(1), 3–9.

Farrell, S. P., & McKinnon, C. R. (2003). Technology and rural mental health. *Archives of Psychiatric Nursing, 17*(1), 20–26.

Folsom, D. P., Hawthorne, W., Lindamer, L., Gilmer, T., Bailey, A., Golshan, S., et al. (2005). Prevalence and risk factors for homelessness and utilization of mental health services among 10,340 patients with serious mental illness in a large public mental health system. *American Journal of Psychiatry, 162*(2), 370–376.

Forchuk, C., Reynolds, W., Sharkey, S., Martin, M. L., & Jensen, E. (2007). Transitional discharge based on therapeutic relationships: State of the art. *Archives of Psychiatric Nursing, 21*(2), 80–86.

Gruttadaro, D. (2005). Consumer- and family-driven care in a transformed mental health delivery system. *NAMI Advocate, 3*(1), 12–13.

Hall, L. L. (2003). NAMI members across the nation report on "shattered lives." *NAMI Advocate, 1*(4), 6.

Hauenstein, E. J. (2003). No comfort in the rural south: Women living depressed. *Archives of Psychiatric Nursing, 17*(1), 3–11.

Hilty, D. M., Marks, S. L., Urness, D., Yellowlees, P. M., & Nesbitt, T. S. (2004). Clinical and educational telepsychiatry applications. *Canadian Journal of Psychiatry, 49*(1), 1–3.

Honberg, R. (2005). Decriminalizing mental illness. *NAMI Advocate, 3*(1), 4–5.

Kidd, L. I. (2007). The test of our progress: Affordable housing for seriously mentally ill clients. *Archives of Psychiatric Nursing, 21*(2), 117–119.

McNab, L., Smith, B., & Minardi, H. A. (2006). A new service in the intermediate care of older adults with mental health problems. *Nursing Older People, 18*(3), 22–26.

Mojtabai, R., Herman, D., Susser, E. S., Sohler, N., Craig, T. C., Lavelle, J., et al. (2005). Service use and outcomes of first-admission patients with psychotic disorders in the Suffolk county mental health project. *American Journal of Psychiatry, 162*(7), 1291–1298.

Monahan, J., Swartz, M., & Bonnie, R. J. (2003). Mandated treatment in the community for people with mental disorders. *Health Affairs, 22*(5), 28–38.

National Health Care for the Homeless Council. (2005). The basis of homelessness. Retrieved August 4, 2005, from http://www.nhchc.org/Publications/basics_of_homelessness.html.

New Freedom Commission on Mental Health. (2003). *Achieving the promise: Transforming mental health care in America. Final report.* (DHHS Publication No. SMA-03-3832). Rockville, MD: Author.

Patterson, S. M. (2003). Metropolitan–nonmetropolitan differences in amount and type of mental health treatment. *Archives of Psychiatric Nursing, 17*(1), 12–19.

Practice Guideline. (2004). For treatment of patients with schizophrenia (2nd ed.). *American Journal of Psychiatry, 161*(2 Suppl), 1–56.

Pratt, C. W., & Gill, K. J. (2005). What are community mental health services? In R. E. Drake, M. R. Merrens, & D. W. Lynde (Eds.), *Evidence-based mental health practice* (pp. 21–41). New York: W. W. Norton.

Schainker, E., & Grant, L. (2003). Medical home meets educational home: How you can make the most of school health services. *Contemporary Pediatrics, 20*(3), 55–81.

Woodside, M., & McClam, T. (2006). *Generalist case management* (3rd ed.). Pacific Grove, CA: Thomson/Brooks/Cole.

Chapter 4
The Role of Cultural Diversity in Mental Health Nursing

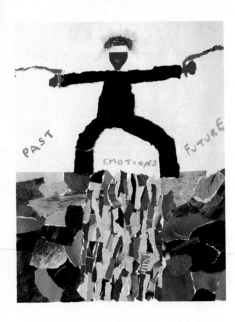

Bridging different aspects of identity

—Kate, Age 19

OBJECTIVES

After reading this chapter, you will be able to:

1. Analyze the impact of culture on mental health.
2. Analyze the impact of predominant American values on nursing practice.
3. Outline the skills necessary for culturally competent nursing care.
4. Utilize culturally congruent methods of assessment and intervention.

MediaLink www.prenhall.com/fontaine

Go to the Pearson Health MediaLink CD-ROM and the Companion Website at www.prenhall.com/fontaine for interactive resources for this chapter.

As a nation, the United States continues to change. Currently non–Euro-Americans comprise 29% of the U.S. population. By the year 2050, almost half the U.S. residents will trace their ancestry to Africa, Asia, the Pacific Islands, or the Hispanic or Arab worlds, rather than to Europe. That is a radical change for a country in which Euro-Americans have been the majority and have held the bulk of power, status, and wealth for several hundred years. In fact, even the term *minority status* is linked to powerlessness. In 1988, Canada became the first nation to pass a multiculturalism act with the goal of providing equal opportunities to all citizens, despite their race, ethnicity, language, or religion (Schim, Doorenbos, & Borse, 2005).

Some people find the trend toward increased ethnic and racial diversity threatening. Others view it as an opportunity and a challenge to make the United States the type of democracy that it has idealized but has not achieved. In any event, this transition, referred to as *the browning of America,* is occurring. Nurses must be prepared to care for this diverse population, just as members of those diverse groups must be prepared to become nurses (Coffman, Shellman, & Bernal, 2004).

The United States has more than 100 ethnic groups, whose members have thousands of beliefs and practices related to health and illness. There are more than 562 American Indians and native Alaskan tribes and nations alone, plus dozens of different Asian and Pacific Island cultures. Various subgroups of African Americans live in the United States, as do different Black cultures from Africa, the Caribbean, and other parts of the world. Although they are not identified in the national census by ethnicity, it is estimated that 1 million Roma live in the United States. There are also numerous Euro-American groups, each with its own ethnicity. The fastest growing ethnic populations in the United States are Asian Pacific Americans, who make up more than 43 distinct ethnic groups, and Latino (also known as Hispanic), composed of diverse nationalities. Each of these major categories is so diverse that differences within groups may be as great as, or greater than, those between different groups. For instance, differences in the world views and experiences of Oglala Sioux and Lumbee Indians, or of Puerto Rican persons and Bolivian individuals, or of African American people who are poor and those who are middle class are often greater than differences between such visibly dissimilar groups as African Americans and Euro-Americans. In addition, many Americans cross group lines and have blended the identities of more than one racial or ethnic group. Therefore, it is simply not realistic to assume that nurses can know everything about groups that number in the millions and have great internal variation. However, we can educate ourselves to become culturally competent nurses.

Culture is a pattern of learned behavior based on values, beliefs, and perceptions of the world. Our culture teaches us how to view the world, how to experience it emotionally, and how to behave in relation to nature, higher powers, and other people. More important than a specific behavior are the underlying values, beliefs, and perceptions that encourage or discourage a particular behavior. Culture is taught and shared by members of a group or society. It is always in process and constantly changing. In contemporary social science, ethnic or national groups are loosely grouped together under the classification of modern or industrialized versus traditional or Western versus non-Western cultures.

A **subculture** is a smaller group within a large cultural group that shares values, beliefs, behaviors, and language. Although it is part of the larger group, a subculture is somewhat different. Nursing students may remember when they were members of the teenage subculture. What they valued, what they believed in, and how they viewed the world may have been very different from their parents' subculture of adulthood. Their development and use of specific words, or informal language, may not have been understood by their parents. At the same time, they and their families belonged to the larger cultural group with which they identified.

Ethnicity is ethnic affiliation and a sense of belonging to a particular cultural group. Culture is so much a part of everyday life that it is taken for granted. We tend to assume that others share our perspective, including those for whom we care. When we believe that our own culture is more important than, and preferable to, any other culture, we are expressing **ethnocentrism**. It is impossible to provide sensitive nursing care from an ethnocentric position.

Nursing must change to meet the needs of an increasingly diverse population. **Diversity** refers to variation among people. Customs and lifestyles that may seem strange to those outside a client's cultural group may be very important to that client. Valuing diversity in the practice of nursing means helping clients reach their full potential, preserving their ways of doing things, and helping them change only those patterns that are harmful (Spector, 2004).

As people throughout the world become more mobile, both in traveling and in resettling, nurses increasingly are faced with the prospect of caring for people of a culture different from their own. More than ever, there is a need for nursing care that is designed around unique cultural beliefs and the values and practices of clients. Therefore, understanding and respecting cultural diversity is basic to the individualization of nursing care through **cultural competence**.

A main reason for being flexible in handling diversity is that culture is only one way in which people differ. There are also differences in ethnicity, age, health status, experience, gender, sexual orientation, and other aspects of social and economic position. The same person might be Methodist, diabetic, Japanese American, Democrat, a student, a sheet-metal worker, a bowler, and a parent. None of these characteristics describes the person's sex, family connections (being a son or daughter, sister or brother, cousin, etc.), educational level, socioeconomic status, or health status. Yet, just as each characteristic is part of this person, each is worthy of recognition, and each has a potential impact on his or her mental health situation.

CULTURE AND MENTAL HEALTH

Ideas about mental health, mental illness, psychiatric problems, and treatments are based on cultural values and understanding. These ideas, called *explanatory models*, make sense out of illness as individual members of different groups understand it. Models delineate what is considered normal and abnormal in a particular population, explain how things happen, shape clinical presentations of mental disorders, and determine culturally patterned ways in which mental disorders are recognized, labeled, explained, and treated by other members of that group. By talking with clients, a nurse can learn, for example, whether mental illness in their culture is considered psychologic, emotional, spiritual, physical, or a combination of these categories. Many cultural groups do not view the body and mind as separate, but as one (Spector, 2004).

What is considered normal or abnormal depends on the specific viewpoint. The same behavior may be seen as positive in one situation and pathologic in another. Hallucinations, for instance, are typically viewed as abnormal by psychiatric standards but are normal and even encouraged by certain Native American tribes as symbolic spiritual experiences, called *vision quests*. Knowing about values and patterns of behavior helps nurses minimize the potential for imposing their expectations on people who come from different backgrounds and have different needs and goals.

Although most cultures believe that mental illness is not contagious, they also believe that those with mental illness should be avoided. Many beliefs about the cause of psychiatric disability exist worldwide:

- Punishment for wrongdoing
  - Eating a taboo food
  - Killing a relative
  - Offending ancestors, gods, and goddesses
- Being "witched"
  - Those offended put a sign or hex on the person who is at fault
  - This person then goes "crazy"
- Passed down through the family
  - Passed only through the mother, since she is the one who gives birth to the child

Problems Related to Culture
Immigration

Immigrants to North America are a diverse group of people, varying from highly educated professionals who speak English fluently to people who are illiterate and speak no English. Most immigrants are somewhere between these two extremes. Some immigrants are forced out of their homeland by war, terrorism, natural disasters, or famine. They may have spent significant time in refugee camps where they may have been further traumatized. The greater the difference between one's culture of origin and the new environment, the greater the degree of culture shock. *Culture shock* is anxiety and disorientation as people try to adjust to the new culture. It can be overwhelming to learn a new language and new ways of interacting with others. Gender roles may change and cause conflict. There is often a significant degree of discrimination. Those who are undocumented immigrants live in constant fear of discovery.

The ideal cultural transition is one of biculturalism or multiculturalism that validates and reaffirms a person's identity by two or more cultures. Traditional values and new cultural competencies are equally valued. The goal is helping people become flexible and open to different cultural perspectives.

Alienation From Group

Psychosocial problems can include problems related to culture. People can become alienated from their cultural group for any number of reasons, including geographic moves or marriage into a different group. They may also be expelled from their religious or ethnic associations for many reasons such as sexual orientation, interracial marriage, or other violations of cultural norms. These types of problems result in loss of social status and self-esteem. Accurate assessment of culture-related factors is important in providing holistic care to clients and their families.

Socioeconomic Status

In the United States, the highest rates of mental disorders and psychologic distress are found among groups with the lowest socioeconomic status (SES). One reason is that all major psychosocial risk factors for mental illness are more prevalent in lower SES levels. These include short- and long-term stress, lack of community support services, lack of economic resources, and lack of control and mastery over one's life. Poverty has a powerful influence on mental disorders. For example, although poverty does not cause schizophrenia, it is strongly related to the experience of those who have schizophrenia. The added stress of poverty may influence the rate of exacerbation and even the likelihood of recovery. With very limited community resources, many people with schizophrenia and who live in poverty find themselves homeless. Access to health care varies for them according to health insurance status, geographic area, and the availability of bilingual professionals. Research suggests that people in lower SES levels receive less mental health treatment, that is, fewer sessions, nonprofessional therapists, and less medication. All of these factors increase the severity of the experience of mental illness (*Morbidity and Mortality Weekly Report*, 2004; Siegel, Haugland, & Schore, 2005).

Culture-Specific Syndromes

Certain forms of mental illness are restricted to specific areas or cultures. These well-defined syndromes occur in response to certain situations in a particular culture. These syndromes form a heterogeneous group that can be further subdivided into three groups. **True syndromes** are illnesses with specific symptoms. **Illnesses of attribution** have a pre-sumed cause but no specific signs and symptoms. An example in Western medicine might be an illness classified only as *infectious disease.* **Idioms of distress** occur in people who are especially vulnerable to stressful life events. This vulnerability makes them susceptible to a wide variety of physical and mental illnesses. See Box 4.1 for information on culture-specific syndromes (Paniagua, 2001).

BOX 4.1	Culture-Specific Syndromes

True Syndromes—Dissociative Phenomena

Amok	Characterized by homicidal frenzy followed by amnesia; many different cultures
Falling Out	Sudden collapse in which the eyes are open but the person cannot see or move; southern United States and Caribbean
Latah	Hypersensitivity to sudden fright with trancelike behavior; Malaysia
Pibloktoq	Abrupt episodes of extreme excitement followed by seizures, transient coma, and amnesia; Eskimo
Grisi Siknis	Victim believes she is being attacked by devils and runs through the village; Nicaragua and Honduras
Shin-Byung	Anxiety and somatic complaints followed by dissociation caused from possession by ancestral spirits; Korea

True Syndromes—Anxiety States

Ataque de Nervios	Shaking, palpitations, flushing, and shouting or striking out; Latin America
Dhat	Extreme anxiety associated with discharge of semen, which is thought to lead to depletion of physical and mental energy; Asia
Koro	Man believes his penis is retracting into his body and that this will end in death; Asia
Kayak Angst	Intense anxiety associated with fear of capsizing and drowning when going out to the open sea in a kayak; Eskimo
Taijin Kyofusho	Intense anxiety about possibly offending, embarrassing, or displeasing others; Japan

True Syndromes—Affective/Somatoform Disorders

Brain Fag	Pressure in the head, difficulty concentrating, anxiety, and visual complaints believed to result from too much thinking; West Africa
Shenjing Shuairuo	Physical and mental exhaustion, difficulty concentrating, memory loss, sleeping and appetite problems, and irritability; China
Anorexia Nervosa	Obsessive preoccupation with weight loss and delusional body image; Western cultures

True Syndromes—Psychotic States

Boufee Delirante	Sudden outburst of aggressive behavior, confusion, agitation, paranoid ideation, and auditory and visual hallucinations; West Africa and Haiti

Illnesses of Attribution—Induced by Anger

Bilis, Colera	Tension, somatic expressions, and fatigue; Latin America
Hwa-Byung	Suppression of anger leads to indigestion, fatigue, fearfulness, and general dysphoria; Korea

Illnesses of Attribution—Induced by Fright

Susto	Sudden fright believed to cause the soul to leave the body, leading to many physical and emotional symptoms; Latin America

Illnesses of Attribution—Induced by Witchcraft

Ghost Sickness	An illness believed to be induced by witches, with symptoms such as delirium, nightmares, terror, anxiety, and confusion; Native American
Voodoo	Illness ascribed to hexing, witchcraft, or the evil influence of another person; believed to cause a variety of symptoms and even death; Caribbean, Southern United States, Latin America
Evil Eye	A fixed stare by an adult is believed capable of causing illness in a child or another adult; Mediterranean, Latin America

Idioms of Distress

Nervios/ Nevra	A term describing people who are vulnerable to stress and who display a wide variety of physical and emotional illnesses; Latin America, Greece
Locura	The most severe form of chronic mental illness; victim is incoherent, agitated, unpredictable, and possibly violent; Latin America

SOURCES: American Psychiatric Association. (2000). *Diagnostic and statistical manual of mental disorders (4th ed., Text Revision).* Washington, DC: Author; Guarnaccia, P. J., & Rogler, L. H. (1999). Research on culture-bound syndromes. *American Journal of Psychiatry, 156*(9), 1322–1327; and Levine, R. E., & Gaw, A. C. (1995). Culture-bound syndromes. *Psychiatric Clinics of North America, 18*(3), 523–536.

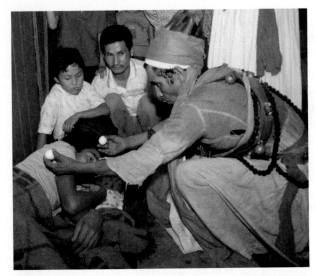

PHOTO 4.1 ■ This Nepalese shaman, known as Jhankari, treats a patient by holding eggs over his head to ward off evil spirits.

SOURCE: Earl & Nazima Kowall/Corbis/Bettmann. Used with permission.

VALUES

Values are a set of personal beliefs about what is meaningful and significant in life. Values provide general guidelines for behavior; they are standards of conduct that people or groups of people believe in. Values are the frame of reference through which people integrate, explain, and evaluate new ideas, situations, and relationships. Values may be *intrinsic*, internalized from a person's particular situation and experience, or *extrinsic*, derived from the culture's standards of right and wrong.

Value Orientations

It has long been recognized that, in every society, basic values emphasize shared ideals about the relationship between humans and nature, the relationship between humans and the universe, a sense of time, a sense of productivity and activity, and interpersonal relationships.

Humans and Nature

Values about the relationship between humans and nature fall along a continuum, as do values about each of the other subjects. The model relationship between humans and nature may be seen as predetermined, perhaps by God, or fate, or genetics, implying that some aspect of nature controls people. It may also be viewed as independent, with people controlling nature.

Humans and the Universe

Relationships with nature tend to reflect those between humans and the universe in being close and personal or distant and impersonal. Both orientations affect attitudes toward illness prevention and health care. For example, if a person believes her or his fate is predetermined, that person has little motivation for preventive strategies, such as proper nutrition and immunization. In contrast, the more familiar value in the United States is mastery over the universe, the attitude that nature can be conquered and controlled if a person learns enough about it. This attitude has led to the development of extensive technology focused on health care, along with the assumption that it is appropriate to intervene in what were traditionally viewed as natural phenomena—disease and death.

Sense of Time

Societies have values regarding time. People tend to be oriented toward the past, the present, or the future. They may emulate history and reclaim the *past*, such as through believing in ancestral spirits. If people focus too much on the past, they may have little awareness of their present problems or joys and remain preoccupied with what has already happened. Others may live in the *present*. Living in the present allows a person to be open to the possibilities of each moment as it unfolds. Living only in the present also has the potential for problems. Olympic contenders were asked, if there were a magic pill that would guarantee a gold medal but would kill them within a year, would they take it? The 50% who said they would take the pill live only in the present moment, with little consideration for the future. On the same continuum is an orientation toward the *future* that encourages people to save money, to get an education and qualify for a career, and to set other long-range goals, such as preventing disease. Some people become preoccupied with the future and many spend hours upon hours worrying about future events.

The healthiest approach for most individuals is a *balance* of past, present, and future, with an awareness of exactly what they are doing in and with their lives and the effects their actions and thoughts have on what they do, and do not do.

Productivity

Likewise, attitudes toward productivity are varied. For some, it is enough to exist; it is not necessary to accomplish great things to feel worthwhile. For others, a desire to develop the self is its own reward and requires no outside recognition. For still others, there is a belief that hard work will pay off materially as well as psychologically. As a result of attitude toward productivity in life, people are relatively passive or active.

Interpersonal Relationships

Values about interpersonal relationships also exist on a continuum. One parameter is *dependency versus autonomy*. Certain cultures, for example, think that some people are born followers and others are born leaders. This belief implies that the follower need not assume responsibility for the self and can and should rely on others, such as health care professionals. Other cultures believe that all people have equal rights and should control their own destinies, become assertive, and take the lead, at least over their own lives. Between those two extremes are people who take their problems to close friends or family members, sharing the problem but keeping responsibility for it within a close personal group.

Values about interpersonal relationships are also reflected in the ideas people have about being individuals and members of groups. In some cultures, *interdependence*, affiliation, and loyalty to the family and community are more highly valued than individuality and personal achievement. The individual is inseparable from her or his status within the family and community, and many decisions of consequence are made in reference to the immediate social group. Thus, shame becomes a driving force in these groups. Denial of the self for the sake of others is common in Indian, Asian, Arab, African, and Latin American cultures.

Scandinavian, European, and American cultures tend to value *individualism* highly, with members of families or communities being a secondary priority. Autonomy and individuality are highly valued and people are perceived as being responsible for their own fate. Hard work is the basis for financial gain and personal advancement. Thus, guilt is a driving force in these groups. Interestingly, ethnic minorities and women in the United States are more likely to define themselves in interdependent terms than are men or members of the Euro-American majority.

Each of these sets of values exists along a continuum that illustrates wide human variation. No values are implicitly right or wrong; they simply shape ideas and responses. It is dangerously misleading to assume that all clients share a given orientation.

Predominant American Values

The most prominent values in the United States are reflected in the health care system, but those values tend to represent the dominant groups (Euro-American, middle class, Judeo-Christian, and male) and not the numerous and diverse subgroups within the country. The dominant set of values is oriented toward individuals, who are viewed as accountable for decision making, self-care, and many other self-oriented tasks. Hard work is regarded as the basis for personal achievement and financial gain. Privacy rights and personal freedom are based on the value of individualism. In many American subcultures, however, being individualistic is not a primary value.

Parrillo (2002) has created a useful list of values that predominate in the United States, as shown in Box 4.2. Consider ways each of these values is promoted not only in society in general, but also in nursing practice.

Nursing Values

Nursing reflects the society in which it exists. Nursing would not be accepted and used if it did not reflect the cul-

---

BOX 4.2	Predominant American Values

Personal Achievement and Success

The emphasis is on competition, power, status, and wealth. What is good for the individual may be more important than what is good for the larger group, such as the community.

Activity and Work

People who do not work hard are considered lazy. It is assumed that hard work will be rewarded. Little consideration is given to people who have not had the same opportunities for success.

Moral Orientation

There is a tendency to moralize and to see the world in absolutes of right or wrong, good or bad. This pattern reinforces the inclination to stereotype.

Humanitarian Mores

Although quick to respond with charity and crisis aid, Americans often use these to limit deeper involvement with issues. Even professional "caring" relationships are typically kept impersonal.

Efficiency and Practicality

Solutions to problems are often based on short-term rather than long-term results.

Progress

Change is often seen as progress in which technology is highly valued and the focus is on the future rather than the present.

Material Comfort

The United States is a consumer-oriented society with a high standard of living.

Personal Freedom and Individualism

Individual rights are valued above the good of the group.

Equality

Personal freedom is a stronger value than equality, especially when there is competition for resources or opportunities.

External Conformity

Despite the value of personal freedom, there is pressure to conform to the Euro-American, middle-class, Judeo-Christian, and male values that predominate. Those differing are labeled deviant.

Science and Rationality

The medicalization of society has led to high expectations for "quick fixes," technology, and the efficiency of scientific medicine.

SOURCES: Parrillo, V. N. (2002). *Strangers to these shores: Race and ethnic relations in the United States* (7th ed.). Thousand Oaks, CA: Sage Publications; Paniagua, F. A. (2001). *Diagnosis in a Multicultural Context.* Thousand Oaks, CA: Sage Publications.

---

tural values and social norms that predominate. Although American values generally reflect those of the dominant culture, in reality, many cultural subgroups have quite different values and norms. Nursing as a discipline tends to have the same values as middle-class Americans of Euro-American background. Yet nurses must be flexible enough to meet the needs expressed by a diverse population with widely varying values. In other words, standard nursing practice exhibits less diversity than clients or nurses possess. Nurses must be aware of the standard values and avoid assuming that they apply to everyone.

Attitudes and Perceptions

Being knowledgeable about diversity includes understanding the attitudes and perceptions that perpetuate social equality and inequality. Attitudes and perceptions are formed from biases. Paul and Elder (2002) describe two different types of bias. The first type is **natural bias**, which refers simply to how a person's point of view causes her or him to notice some things and not others. The second type is **negative bias,** a refusal to recognize that there are other points of view. Natural and negative biases come into play when nurses organize or process information in such a way that they develop attitudes of open-mindedness or discrimination. Nurses must always be open-minded—learn what their natural and negative biases are and change those that prevent them from seeing and understanding the perspectives of other people.

Generalizations, Stereotypes, and Prejudice

We all work with huge amounts of information every day. To make it more manageable, we organize information into categories. One way we organize is through descriptive generalizations. **Generalizations**, which arise from our natural biases, are changeable starting places for comparing typical behavioral patterns with what is actually observed. When we use generalizations to process information, we are more likely to remain open-minded—to develop open relationships with our clients, to understand their point of view, and to provide culturally competent nursing care.

Another way to organize information is by using stereotypes, which arise from negative biases. **Stereotypes** are images frozen in time that cause people to see what they expect to see, even when the facts differ from their expectations. Stereotypes often capture characteristics that are real and common to a group. However, stereotypes may also be out of date and dangerously limited. They are particularly dangerous when they involve negative beliefs about a person or group, leading to prejudgment (or prejudice) that ignores actual evidence.

Prejudice is a negative feeling about people who are different. Prejudicial attitudes are based on limited knowledge, limited contact, and emotional responses rather than on careful observation and thought. They are beliefs, opinions, or points of view that are formed before the facts are known, or in spite of them.

Stereotypes can be favorable as well as unfavorable, although even favorable ones disregard facts and rely on preconceived notions. For example, Asian American students are often expected to excel in mathematics because of the stereotype that associates Asian Americans with technical accomplishments. Because every group has some individuals who do well in math and others who do not, Asian Americans who struggle with math must contend with a sense of failure. The same process occurs in many forms: A child is expected to do well because his or her older siblings did; people with glasses read a lot of books; all African Americans are good dancers or athletes. Although these are not negative stereotypes, they are potentially harmful because they impose unrealistic expectations.

There are two pathways of information processing: one leading to open-mindedness; the other leading to discrimination (Figure 4.1 ■).

Discrimination

Several types of prejudice are commonly observed in health care settings and can lead to discriminatory behavior. **Discrimination** is prejudice that is expressed behaviorally. Racism is one example of discrimination. Differentiating people according to racial characteristics has always been a pervasive social process in the United States. Despite nurses' extensive knowledge of biology, incorrect ideas about race are left unchallenged.

We are all members of the human race. Nonetheless, we use racial terms to divide and separate people. People often refer to skin color to group other people into different races. Imagine somehow lining up the more than 6 billion people on this planet, starting on one end with the darkest skinned and ending with the lightest skinned. The very dark individuals would seem quite different from the very light, yet the majority would be in between, in every shade of brown. Based on skin color, no one would be able to tell where one race ends and the next begins.

The time when African Americans, Asian Americans, Latinos, and American Indians were prevented from enter-

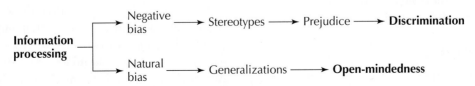

Figure 4.1 ■ Pathways to open-mindedness and discrimination.

ing the social and economic mainstream is officially over. However, despite formal integration, stereotypes and prejudices associated with White versus non-White status remain. For instance, negative stereotypes that associate African Americans with poverty, drugs, and violence ignore the fact that most African Americans are not poor and have nothing to do with either drugs or violence. Assuming that a client is on welfare because he or she is African American or that substance abuse exists or physical aggression is likely may result in treatment different from that given to clients who are not African American.

Racism is defined as excessive and irrational beliefs regarding the superiority of a given group. Racism can traumatize, hurt, humiliate, enrage, and ultimately prevent the optimal mental health of individuals and communities. Racism affects all people, including dominant and nondominant group members. People who are targets of discrimination experience unsolicited and unwarranted violence, whether physical or mental and covert or overt. Such experiences are significant stressors that interfere with

mental, social, and physical adjustment. This is evidenced in part by the reality that one leading cause of death of African Americans is stress-related disease (Breslau, Kendler, Su, Gaxiola-Aguilar, & Kessler, 2005).

Likewise, those individuals of the dominant group who hold racist views have difficulty making a healthy adaptation to an increasingly multicultural society. They project blame on the victims in an effort to maintain a system of denial. Early on, they learn to feel justified in continuing the oppression of others. Continued projection and denial lead to maladaptive behaviors and poorer mental health. Harrell (2000) identified ways in which racism increases stress and affects well-being. Anxiety, depression, and hypertension are just a few of the many negative outcomes (see Table 4.1 ■).

A number of other forms of discrimination may be observed in health care settings. These patterns of interaction have acquired the label *isms* (pronounced iz-ums) because of their common word ending. Each ism involves a tendency to judge others according to similarity to or dissimilarity to a

---

TABLE 4.1	Racism-related Stress Factors

Racism-Related Life Events

- Experiences are relatively time limited
- Occur in various settings/situations such as neighborhood, work, education, legal, health care
- Examples: being discriminated against in the emergency department, being harassed by the police, being rejected for a loan

Vicarious Racism Experiences

- Occur through observation and report
- Create a heightened sense of danger/vulnerability, anger, sadness
- May happen to family, friends, or strangers
- Example: the dragging death of James Byrd in Texas

Daily Racism Microstressors

- Subtle putdowns that are daily reminders that something racist can happen at any moment
- These slights and exclusions may be intentional or unintentional
- Experiences can feel demoralizing, disrespectful, or objectifying
- Examples: poor service in public accommodations, being followed by a store detective, being mistaken for someone who serves others (e.g., a maid, a janitor)

Chronic–Contextual Stress

- Political and institutional racism
- Unequal distribution of and access to resources
- Examples: lack of ethnoculturally diverse mental health service providers, out-of-date textbooks in schools, unchecked community violence

Collective Experiences

- Experiences of racism at the group level
- Examples: lack of political representation, stereotypic portrayals in the media

Transgenerational Transmission

- Historical context of the group and wider American society
- Examples: stories that are passed down through generations such as the slavery of African people, the internment of Japanese Americans during World War II, the removal of Native People from their tribal lands

SOURCE: Adapted with permission from Harrell, S. P. (2000). A multidimensional conceptualization of racism-related stress: Implications for the well-being of people of color. *American Journal of Orthopsychiatry, 70*(1), 42–55.

TABLE 4.2	Forms of Discrimination	
Form	**Description**	**Example**
Ableism	The assumption that the able-bodied and sound of mind are superior to those who are physically or mentally ill	A person who is mentally ill is not offered treatment choices.
Adultism	The assumption that adults are superior to youths	Children are ignored and not given opportunities to learn decision making.
Ageism	The assumption that members of one age group are superior to those of other age groups	Older people are assumed to be senile and incompetent.
Classism	The assumption that certain people are superior because of their socioeconomic status or position in a group or organization	A poorly dressed high school dropout is not offered the same treatment facility as a well-dressed college graduate.
Egocentrism	The assumption that one is superior to others	A person who has never experienced a mental illness thinks he or she is better than those who are diagnosed with a mental disorder.
Ethnocentrism	The assumption that one's own cultural or ethnic group is superior to that of others	Everyone is expected to speak English and to know the rules for living in America.
Heterosexism	The assumption that everyone is or should be heterosexual	When gays or lesbians experience a mental disorder, the cause is assumed to be their sexual orientation.
Racism	The assumption that members of one race are superior to those of another	The color of one's skin determines educational and career opportunities.
Sexism	The assumption that members of one gender are superior to those of the other	Women are viewed as less rational and more emotional, and therefore more likely to have a mental illness, than men.
Sizism	The assumption that people of one body size are superior to those of other shapes and sizes	Obese people have fewer job opportunities and advancements.
Sociocentrism	The assumption that one society's way of knowing or doing is superior to that of others	Biomedicine is expected to be effective, while folk medicine is discounted.

standard considered ideal or normal. Isms are shaped by personal or group judgment. For example, focusing on oneself is known as egocentrism. When an entire society promotes one way of behaving or thinking as the best way, it is called *sociocentrism*, as in Eurocentric or Afrocentric education. We frequently hear about ethnocentrism. Nearly every ethnic group sees itself as best. However, in a society composed of multiple groups, such biases, or "isms," must be counteracted to prevent discrimination and social injustice. Table 4.2 ■ can also be applied to victims of other forms of discrimination.

There is considerable evidence that, even when the intent is to treat people fairly, people may be approached in ways that indicate subtle prejudice. In health care settings, one group tends to be treated well and another may receive less attention, fewer choices, and generally less vigorous care. This unequal treatment is a reflection of the traits that society values. The *YAVIS* are **Y**oung, **A**ttractive, **V**erbal, **I**ntelligent, and **S**uccessful (or appear potentially successful). The *QUOIDS*, by contrast, are **Q**uiet, **U**gly, **O**ld, **I**ndigent (poor), **D**issimilar (in lifestyle, language, or culture), and thought to be **S**tupid. Although someone carefully observing interactions in health care settings may readily discern preferential patterns involving YAVIS and QUOIDS, those who work there may be unaware of how their biases lead to discriminatory behavior.

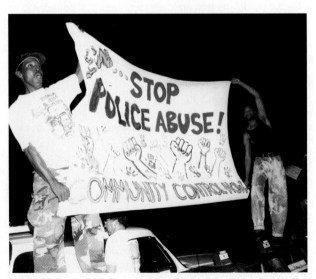

PHOTO 4.2 ■ Demonstrators protest the police acquittal in the Rodney King case in 1992.
SOURCE: Nick Ut/AP Wide World Photos. Used with permission.

MediaLink

Case Study, Cultural Competence

CARING FOR A DIVERSE POPULATION

To understand and care for diverse clients, the nurse must learn to understand and appreciate multiple interpretations of events and behaviors. There are thousands of cultures and subcultures, and we cannot possibly know all there is to know about each one. Personal and group identities are complex. Many people are exposed to or have been raised in more than one culture. Many others have altered their traditional cultural orientation to adapt to American society or specific life circumstances.

In 2003 the International Society of Psychiatric Nurses (ISPN) approved a *Position Statement on Diversity, Cultural Competence, and Access to Mental Health Care.* The goal of the position statement is to support psychiatric nurses in their quest to become culturally competent nurses. Since there is a dearth of psychiatrists in rural areas, the ISPN encourages advanced-practice psychiatric nurses to provide care to these underserved areas (Yearwood, Hines-Martin, Dato, & Malone, 2006).

We often hear about the importance of sensitivity to cultural differences. However, being only sensitive can leave you frustrated and powerless. You must also learn to become an advocate for diverse populations. **Advocacy** is supporting and defending people's rights to their beliefs, attitudes, and values. Effective advocacy depends on a balance of knowledge, sensitivity, and skills.

Cultural Knowledge

The first step in building knowledge is getting to know ourselves. We cannot expect to understand others and help them achieve their full potential if we do not first develop an understanding of who we are as people and as nurses. This is not always simple, and it is an ongoing, never-ending process. When we identify our own attitudes, values, and prejudices we help ourselves understand our feelings about people who are different. It helps us be nonjudgmental and may prevent us from exhibiting discriminating behavior when interacting with clients from a different cultural or subcultural group. For us to confront our own ethnocentrism takes careful attention to our thoughts and behaviors. Self-understanding is enhanced when we, as nurses, ask for and listen carefully to feedback from clients, peers, faculty members, and supervisors. There is no easy way to acquire a depth of knowledge about cultural groups different from our own. Wherever we practice nursing, we must assume responsibility for learning about the culture of our clients. This can be done through reading, by talking to and listening to clients, and by attending workshops about diverse cultural groups. This begins the process of giving culturally competent nursing care. The list of community resources at the end of this chapter provides information sites for increasing your knowledge.

Cultural Sensitivity

It is critical for nurses to know themselves to become sensitive nurses. Once we become aware of our own attitudes, values, and prejudices, we must evaluate how those attitudes, values, and prejudices affect our nursing practice. Nurses should ask: Do I pay more attention to clients who have a background similar to mine? Do I approach clients from a different background with initial suspicion or distrust? Does my body language change when I interact with someone from a different background? What stereotypes do I have of people from various cultures? When I do not understand a client's behavior, do I ask for clarification or do I make assumptions about that behavior? Am I open to learning about alternative healing practices? Do I penalize clients whose values or behaviors are different from mine?

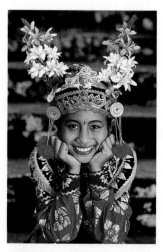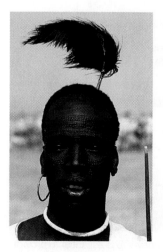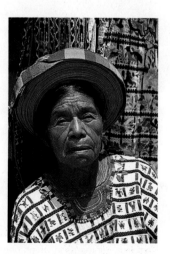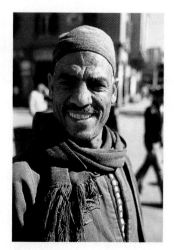

PHOTO 4.3 ■ To understand human behavior fully, nurses must appreciate the diversity of human beings throughout the world.
SOURCE: Steve Vidler/SuperStock; Robert Caputo/Stock Boston; Arvind Garg/Getty Images, Inc.—Liaison; Frank Siteman/Photolibrary.com.

Skills in Culturally Congruent Nursing Care

Knowledge empowers us to understand cultural differences. Sensitivity enables us to respect and honor differences. Sensitivity and knowledge must be combined with skills for appropriate and culturally congruent nursing care.

Communication is crucial to all nursing care, but it is especially important when caring for mental health clients from diverse backgrounds. To establish contact, you should present yourself in a confident way without acting superior. Shake hands, if appropriate. Allow clients to choose their comfortable personal space. Respect their version of acceptable eye contact. Ask how they prefer to be addressed. Most people are pleased when others show sincere interest in them. Small things can often communicate acceptance. Making a setting comfortable by considering seating arrangements, background noises, and other environmental variables helps clients feel welcome and recognized.

Talk with clients to determine their level of fluency in English, and arrange for an interpreter if needed. Speak directly to the client even if an interpreter is present. Choose a style of speech that promotes understanding and demonstrates respect for each client. Avoid the tendency to speak louder as if it will increase understanding or fluency. Avoid jargon, slang, complex sentences, and body language that may be offensive or misunderstood.

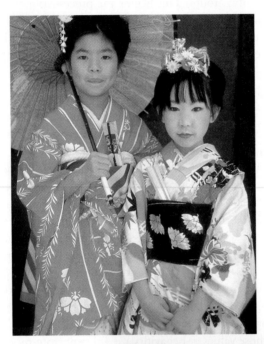

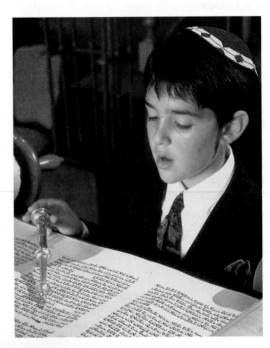

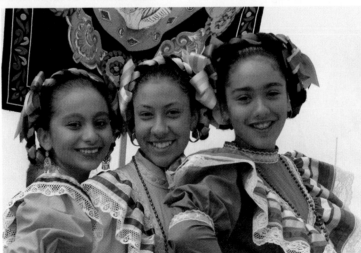

PHOTO 4.4 ■ Acknowledging the diverse environments in which people develop is essential to providing culturally competent care.

SOURCE: Photo Researchers, Inc. (top); Skjold Photographs (bottom). Used with permission.

Before using any written materials, ask clients whether they can read English. They may feel defensive about their reading ability. Softening the question can help. For example, asking "Are you comfortable reading this or would you prefer I read it to you?" avoids the issue of ability and allows clients to say that they prefer to have printed materials read to them. The ability to read varies widely, and many people who speak English do not read it. Medications and the symptoms of mental disorders can also interfere with the ability and motivation to read.

To obtain information, use open-ended questions or questions phrased in several ways. Allow plenty of time for answers. Be aware that some people consider only open-ended questions to be acceptable, such as "How do you manage your job when you feel sick?" Others prefer closed-ended questions, such as "Do you sleep a lot when you feel sick?" Still others (members of certain Native American, Pacific Island, and African groups, for example) consider direct questions impolite. They may expect inquiries to be presented like a story, as in "One client told me that when he feels really bad, he wears a special shirt. I guess we all have things we do at certain times."

You may need to learn to use certain indirect styles of communication and wait to see if and how the client responds. Observe how the client communicates with others to learn what style is most appropriate. Ask family members or significant others whether they can help with this information. It is important to avoid forcing clients to conform to communication patterns with which they are not comfortable.

Several different frameworks have been developed for assessment when planning health care services or programs within any multicultural group. The Heritage Assessment Tool (Box 4.3) is a practical and useful way to investigate a client's ethnic, cultural, and religious heritage (Spector, 2004).

Storytelling is a valuable approach to sharing views. Inviting clients to share stories about themselves and their problems is an excellent way to find out what is important to them and how they view their situations. "Can you tell me a story about when you were growing up?" "Would you tell me a story about coming to the hospital?" Communication is most productive when you acknowledge that clients know more about their personal situation than you do. Having clients tell the story of their life and of their illness often provides information that will help you understand their experiences and views. Although this approach requires good listening skills and adequate amounts of time, it forms the core of effective care and treatment in many societies.

Client values, beliefs, and practices do not have to change simply because they are different from those of health care providers. You can help people recognize what

to change and what not to change. To provide care that is knowledgeable and sensitive, it is essential to identify the following (Leininger, 2001):

- Those aspects of the client's life that mean a lot, are valuable just as they are, and should be understood and preserved without change
- Those aspects that can be partially preserved but need some adjustment, to be negotiated with the client
- Those aspects that require change and repatterning

Analysis of the situation to clarify what is happening, and the probable consequences of each type of intervention, helps you make informed decisions. If your relationship with the client is reciprocated and communication lines are open, it may quickly become clear that the client's value orientation can be maintained or will require only minor alteration. Lack of knowledge and insensitivity often leads to the conclusion that a client's approach is wrong and requires radical overhauling. To gain the client's cooperation, preserve the integrity of the client's view by being flexible, sensitive, knowledgeable, and skillful.

On the other hand, at times you must take a stand for substantive change, as in cases of illegal or injurious behavior. It may be appropriate to consult the client's family or friends to help articulate a particular point of view. Many communities have rosters of organizations and individuals who will share information about the populations they represent. Getting help from these people is especially important when language or value differences create barriers between you and your clients.

Becoming competent and confident in managing diversity requires expertise and practice. Implementing knowledge, sensitivity, and skills in psychiatric nursing settings requires considerable time and energy. These efforts are rewarded, however, when difficult situations are handled as openly, jointly, and respectfully as possible and by seeing clients respond favorably to such humanistic treatment.

DIVERSITY WITHIN THE PROFESSION

The challenge is not only to learn how to understand and uphold the cultures of clients. Nurses must do the same with their coworkers so that cultural diversity is a positive force that enhances the nursing team. It is important that you take time to learn about those with whom you work through open dialogue, over time, and in a positive environment.

Because nondominant group members are underrepresented in all health professions, including nursing, it is important that nurses achieve greater representation in the

MediaLink

MediaLink Application, Cultural Competence

BOX 4.3	Heritage Assessment Tool

This set of questions is to be used to describe a given client's—or your own—ethnic, cultural, and religious background. In performing a *heritage assessment*, it is helpful to determine how deeply a given person identifies with his or her traditional heritage. This tool is most useful in setting the stage for assessing and understanding a person's traditional health and illness beliefs and practices and in helping to determine the community resources that will be appropriate to target for support when necessary. The greater the number of positive responses, the greater the degree to which the person may identify with his or her traditional heritage. The one exception to positive answers is the question about whether or not a person's name was changed.

1. Where was your mother born? _____

2. Where was your father born? _____

3. Where were your grandparents born? _____

   a. Your mother's mother? _____

   b. Your mother's father? _____

   c. Your father's mother? _____

   d. Your father's father? _____

4. How many brothers _____ and sisters _____ do you have?

5. What setting did you grow up in? Urban _____ Rural _____

6. What country did your parents grow up in?

   Father _____

   Mother _____

7. How old were you when you came to the United States? _____

8. How old were your parents when they came to the United States? _____

   Mother _____

   Father _____

9. When you were growing up, who lived with you? _____

10. Have you maintained contact with _____

   a. Aunts, uncles, cousins?   (1) Yes _____   (2) No _____

   b. Brothers and sisters?   (1) Yes _____   (2) No _____

   c. Parents?   (1) Yes _____   (2) No _____

   d. Your own children?   (1) Yes _____   (2) No _____

11. Did most of your aunts, uncles, and/or cousins live near your home?

   (1) Yes _____   (2) No _____

12. Approximately how often did you visit family members who lived outside of your home?

   (1) Daily _____   (2) Weekly _____   (3) Monthly _____

   (4) Once a year or less _____   (5) Never _____

13. Was your original family name changed?

   (1) Yes _____   (2) No _____

14. What is your religious preference?

   (1) Catholic _____   (2) Jewish _____

   (3) Protestant Denomination _____

   (4) Other _____   (5) None

15. Is your spouse the same religion as you?

   (1) Yes _____   (2) No _____

16. Is your spouse the same ethnic background as you?

   (1) Yes _____   (2) No _____

17. What kind of school did you go to?

   (1) Public _____   (2) Private _____   (3) Parochial _____

BOX 4.3	Heritage Assessment Tool *(continued)*

18. As an adult, do you live in a neighborhood where the neighbors are the same religion and ethnic background as yourself?

    (1) Yes _____   (2) No _____

19. Do you belong to a religious institution?

    (1) Yes _____   (2) No _____

20. Would you describe yourself as an active member?

    (1) Yes _____   (2) No _____

21. How often do you attend your religious institution?

    (1) More than once a week _____   (2) Weekly _____

    (3) Monthly _____   (4) Special holidays only _____

    (5) Never

22. Do you practice your religion in your home?

    (1) Yes _____   (2) No _____ (if yes, please specify)

    (3) Praying _____   (4) Bible reading _____   (5) Diet _____

    (6) Celebrating religious holidays _____

23. Do you prepare foods special to your ethnic background?

    (1) Yes _____   (2) No _____

24. Do you participate in ethnic activities?

    (1) Yes _____   (2) No _____   (if yes, please specify)

    (3) Singing _____   (4) Holiday celebrations _____

    (5) Dancing _____   (6) Festivals _____

    (7) Costumes _____   (8) Other _____

25. Are your friends from the same religious background as you?

    (1) Yes _____   (2) No _____

26. Are your friends from the same ethnic background as you?

    (1) Yes _____   (2) No _____

27. What is your native language? _____

28. Do you speak this language?

    (1) Prefer _____   (2) Occasionally _____   (3) Rarely _____

29. Do you read your native language?

    (1) Yes _____   (2) No _____

SOURCE: Spector, R. E. (2003). *Cultural diversity in health and illness* (6th ed.). Upper Saddle River, NJ: Prentice Hall. Used with permission.

nursing profession. Although minorities comprise 29% of the overall population, they account for only 12% of nurses. American Indian individuals are the least represented of all minority groups, including men, in the nursing profession. This lack of diversity in the nursing workforce is potentially harmful to the profession and the population it serves. Nursing programs must continue efforts to recruit minorities into the field. This means that faculty must evaluate their programs for barriers to success and support programs that enhance student–faculty communication and student academic success. Programs such as RAIN (Recruitment and Retention of American Indian Nurses) work to attract and support minority students in nursing (Nardi & Siwinski-Hebel, 2005).

Focus Your Study

OBJECTIVES	KEY CONCEPTS
1. Analyze the impact of culture on mental health.	■ Ideas about mental health, mental illness, psychiatric problems, and treatments are based on cultural values and understanding. ■ What is normal or abnormal depends on the cultural viewpoint. ■ People become alienated from their cultural group for any number of reasons. This often results in stress and loss of social status and self-esteem. ■ Certain forms of mental illness are restricted to specific areas or cultures.
2. Analyze the impact of predominant American values on nursing practice.	■ Nursing reflects the society in which it exists. ■ Nurses must learn what their natural and negative biases are and change those that prevent them from understanding the perspectives of other people.
3. Outline the skills necessary for culturally competent nursing care.	■ Identify personal values and prejudices. ■ Assess own verbal and nonverbal communication. ■ Gain knowledge of clients' cultures. ■ Adapt communication style as appropriate. ■ Support clients' values and traditions. ■ Serve as an advocate for clients. ■ Help clients reach their full potential. ■ Actively support diversity in the profession.

4. Utilize culturally congruent methods of assessment and intervention.	■ Determine clients' level of fluency in English and arrange for an interpreter if needed.
	■ Choose a style of speech that demonstrates respect for each client.
	■ Assess ability to read English before using any written materials.
	■ Use open-ended or closed-ended questions depending on clients' cultural preferences.
	■ Ask clients to tell stories about themselves and their problems.
	■ Utilize the Heritage Assessment tool to guide nursing practice.
	■ Help clients recognize what values, beliefs, and practices to change and what not to change.
	  – Those aspects that mean a lot, are valuable just as they are, and should be understood and preserved without change
	  – Those aspects that can be partially preserved but need some adjustment, to be negotiated with clients
	  – Those aspects that require change and repatterning

Explore MediaLink

For review questions, case studies, and other resources for this chapter see the Pearson Health MediaLink CD-ROM that accompanies this book and the Companion Website.

CD-ROM
■ Audio Glossary
■ NCLEX-RN® Review Questions

Companion Website www.prenhall.com/fontaine
■ Audio Glossary
■ NCLEX-RN® Review Questions
■ Case Study
  – Cultural Competence
■ Care Plan
  – Cultural Communication
■ Critical Thinking
  – Cultural Congruence
■ MediaLink Application
  – Cultural Competence
■ MediaLinks
  – Books for Clients and Families
  – Community Resources

NCLEX-RN® Review Questions

4-1. A nurse therapist conducts group counseling for young homeless women. The leading cause of death for these young women is acquired immunodeficiency syndrome (AIDS). To meet the priority needs for this group the nurse should:
1. Determine the women's knowledge level about AIDS and the factors that contribute to the high incidence in this city.
2. Identify the strengths and weaknesses of the members of the family of these women.
3. Determine that the clients will not practice safe sex even though they are instructed about the perils of unprotected sex.
4. Identify the list of sexual partners of the clients and call them on the telephone to discuss safe sex practices.

4-2. A 45-year-old Haitian male is admitted to the hospital with a diagnosis of hypertension. The client lives in a low socioeconomic area of a large metropolitan city. He eats at fast-food restaurants and works two jobs to support his family. This is the client's third admission to the hospital because his hypertension is uncontrolled. What is the priority nursing action for this client?
1. Determine the client's level of knowledge about the relationship of hypertension and lifestyle choices.
2. Identify health practices used in the family.
3. Classify the expected outcome criteria for this client.
4. Determine the client's level of anxiety.

4-3. The nurse therapist working with minority women teaches a class on acquired immunodeficiency syndrome (AIDS). After four sessions, what would be an indication that the nurse has accomplished the outcome established for the clients?

1. The clients still are involved in unprotected sex but have discussed the possibility in the future to change their behavior patterns.
2. The clients have gained an increase of knowledge about the disease and the consequences of the disease.
3. Some of the clients have broken up their relationship with their former boyfriends but are now in new relationships.
4. The clients state, "It is difficult to find boyfriends in the community."

4-4. A group for minority women meets monthly. In one of the sessions, a client tells the group, "My boyfriend tells me I don't love him if he needs to practice safe sex." The response of the nurse should be:
1. "Why do you think he will not love you?"
2. "Do you really believe a man loves you only for unprotected sex?"
3. "Tell me what you mean about not loving him?"
4. "Let us ask the group about your boyfriend."

4-5. The treatment team conducted a meeting to discuss intervention strategies for a client, an 8-year-old girl who drew a picture of a child in the water alone. The priority strategy for this client is:
1. Ignore the drawing and monitor her for 6 months.
2. Coax the child to add things to the picture that could help the child.
3. Discuss with the child why she placed the child in the water alone.
4. Discuss with the doctor on the team about prescribing possible medication for the child.

See Appendix D for answers.

References

Breslau, J., Kendler, K. S., Su, M., Gaxiola-Aguilar, S., & Kessler, R. C. (2005). Lifetime risk and persistence of psychiatric disorders across ethnic groups in the United States. *Psychological Medicine, 35*(3), 317–327.

Coffman, M. J., Shellman, J., & Bernal, H. (2004). An integrative review of American nurses' perceived cultural self-efficacy. *Journal of Nursing Scholarship, 36*(2), 180–185.

Harrell, S. P. (2000). A multidimensional conceptualization of racism-related stress: Implications for the well-being of people of color. *American Journal of Orthopsychiatry, 70*(1), 42–55.

Leininger, M. M. (Ed.). (2001). *Culture, care, diversity, and universality: A theory of nursing.* Sudbury, MA: Jones & Bartlett.

Morbidity and Mortality Weekly Report (2004, December 2). CDC Surveillance Summaries. Self-reported frequent mental distress among adults—United States, 1993–2001. Atlanta, GA: Centers for Disease Control and Prevention.

Nardi, D. A., & Siwinski-Hebel, S. (2005, May 23). Cultural issues in home care. *ADVANCE for Nurses, 7*(12), 21–25.

Paniagua, F. A. (2001). *Diagnosis in a multicultural context.* Thousand Oaks, CA: Sage Publications.

Parrillo, V. N. (2002). *Strangers to these shores: Race and ethnic relations in the United States* (7th ed.). Riverside, NJ: Macmillan.

Paul, R. W., & Elder, L. (2002). *Critical thinking: Tools for taking charge of your professional and personal life.* Upper Saddle River, NJ: Financial Times Prentice Hall.

Schim, S. M., Doorenbos, A. Z., & Borse, N. N. (2005). Cultural competence among Ontario and Michigan healthcare providers. *Journal of Nursing Scholarship, 37*(4), 354–360.

Siegel, C., Haugland, G., & Schore. R. (2005). The interface of cultural competency and evidence-based practices. In R. E. Drake, M. R. Merrens, & D. W. Lynde (Eds.), *Evidence-based mental health practice* (pp. 273–299). New York: W.W. Norton.

Spector, R. E. (2004). *Cultural diversity in health & illness* (6th ed.). Upper Saddle River, NJ: Prentice Hall.

Yearwood, E. L., Hines-Martin, V., Dato, C., & Malone, M. (2006). Creating an organizational diversity vision. *Archives of Psychiatric Nursing, 290*(3), 152–156.

Chapter 5

Legal and Ethical Issues

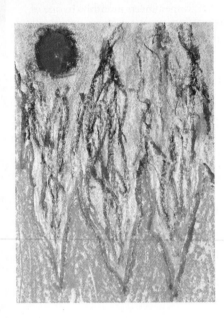

" *Spectacular frustration* **"**

—Brian, Age 19

OBJECTIVES

After reading this chapter, you will be able to:

1. Discuss the issues involved in the involuntary admission process.
2. Explain the rights of a client receiving mental health services.
3. Identify the exceptions to a client's right to confidentiality.
4. Analyze the role competency plays in mental health treatment and research.
5. Discuss the relationship between mental illness and the criminal justice system.
6. Outline the elements of ethical nursing practice.

MediaLink www.prenhall.com/fontaine

Go to the Pearson Health MediaLink CD-ROM and the Companion Website at
www.prenhall.com/fontaine for interactive resources for this chapter.

Laws and ethical principles affect many decisions that nurses must make each day. It is important to be familiar with federal and state laws pertaining to nursing practice in general and with those that have implications for the practice of psychiatric nursing in particular.

Mental disorders sometimes affect a person's ability to make decisions about health and well-being. Whenever possible, client autonomy and liberty must be ensured by treatment in the *least restrictive setting* and by active client participation in treatment decisions. The challenge for nurses is maintaining the client's personal freedom in situations in which public welfare or the client's best interests are threatened.

TYPES OF ADMISSION

Voluntary admission occurs when a client, for the purpose of assessment and treatment of a mental disorder, consents to hospitalization and signs a document indicating this. If clients choose to leave the hospital, they must give written notice of their intention to leave the facility. The number of hours or days between notice of intention and actual discharge is determined by individual states. This notification period provides the health care team with time to complete discharge arrangements or seek authorization for further hospitalization through the court system.

Parents can sign commitment papers requesting psychiatric treatment for their child. In most states, when the individual is 18 or 21 years of age, she or he is considered an adult. An adolescent who has lived away from home for a certain period may be legally regarded as an emancipated minor. If the young adult or emancipated minor refuses hospitalization or treatment, the only recourse the parents have is to seek an involuntary admission.

Commitment, or **involuntary admission**—detaining a client in a psychiatric facility against his or her will—may be requested in most states on the basis of being dangerous to self or others. A few states have altered their laws by including the criterion of preventing significant physical or mental deterioration. Some groups are lobbying for additions such as *grave disability* (people are unable to provide for their basic needs such as food and shelter), *need for treatment*, and *lack of capacity* (people are unable to fully understand and make an informed decision regarding the need for treatment). Mandatory outpatient treatment refers to court-ordered outpatient treatment for those who have not been able or willing to participate in a voluntary clinic and who are in serious need of treatment for their mental disorder.

In most states, adults can be held temporarily on an *emergency basis* until there is a court hearing. At the judicial hearing, which is a civil procedure, the health care team must present clear and convincing evidence of dangerousness or need for treatment. Commitment is for a specific period, which varies by state. Commitment may be for inpatient or outpatient treatment, and the decision is made by the committing judge. Outpatient commitment is designed to be a less restrictive alterative to involuntary hospitalization. At the end of the specified time, the health care team must discharge the client or petition the court for continued hospitalization.

Commitment is a controversial issue. In the United States, people have a fundamental right to make important decisions about their treatment. At the same time, an individual may not be able to make treatment decisions when experiencing an acute episode of a mental disorder. There are legitimate concerns on both sides of the issue (Salize & Dressing, 2005; Swartz, Swanson, Wagner, Hannon, Burns, & Shumway, 2003).

Following are some of the reasons for commitment:

- Intervention will ease suffering and, in some cases, save lives.
- Commitment will alleviate embarrassment and rejection by the general public when grossly disturbing behaviors affect others.
- Commitment may reduce the duration of a crisis, and this reduction seems to improve the prognosis for long-term recovery.
- In many instances, commitment is the only way to obtain treatment from the public mental health care system.
- In some cases, the family must protect itself against actual or threatened violence.
- The family may not be able to care for an acutely ill member and may see commitment as the only option.
- Outpatient commitment may reduce victimization by reducing homelessness, improving judgment, diminishing hostility, and increasing self-control.
- Outpatient commitment provides increased access to effective community resources.

Commitment is a very serious action because it restricts the freedom of someone who has not engaged in criminal activity. Following are some of the arguments against commitment:

- Commitment hearings are often perfunctory, and even though clients are entitled by law to an attorney, they often do not have one. Clients may not even be allowed to hear what is being said against them.
- The implicit promise of commitment is that the environment will be therapeutic, but many institutions dehumanize, degrade, and abuse clients.
- Coercion in mental health treatment does more harm than good, causing clients to distrust mental health caregivers.

MediaLink Case Study, Involuntary Admission

■ Commitment reinforces the stigma that mentally ill people are dangerous and unpredictable.

■ It is a socioeconomic issue in that most clients who are committed are poor and undereducated.

■ If the family has requested commitment, the process damages trust among family members.

■ Outpatient commitment ignores the real issue, which is the lack of appropriate, accessible, and acceptable community services.

Commitment must never be viewed as a permanent or long-term solution. Alternatives must be explored. In some areas, mobile crisis teams or client-run services are offered as a substitute for hospital treatment. (See chapter 3 ∞ for further information on alternative treatments and treatment settings.)

Because severe and persistent mental illness is often cyclical, stabilized clients may sign an **advance directive** indicating permission for treatment in the case of future incompetence. This legal document is formulated between acute episodes and assists family and caregivers who must make decisions for clients when they are unable to make decisions for themselves. Advance directives empower clients who have severe and persistent mental illness. Health care providers are given important information about the client's preferences for treatment. Family and friends experience less conflict and guilt during times of psychiatric crises. Templates for advance directives can be obtained online from the Judge David L. Bazelon Center for Mental Health Law.

The advance directive plan is initiated by the client and allows the person to:

■ Describe symptoms indicating the inability to make decisions at this time.

■ Name an individual who will make decisions and give consent on the person's behalf.

■ Provide instructions about treatment preferences, including selecting a psychiatrist/psychotherapist, hospitalization, alternatives to hospitalization, medications, electroconvulsive therapy, emergency interventions, and experimental studies or drug trials.

■ List who should be notified when hospitalized, who should be prohibited from visiting, and who should have temporary custody of children.

COMPETENCY

Competency is a legal determination that a client can make reasonable judgments and decisions about medical or nursing treatment and other significant areas of personal life. The principle is one of **autonomy** or self-determination. Autonomy is the freedom to choose and the ability to assume

responsibility for one's acts—in others words, freedom from pressures of any kind and the ability to govern one's life. Clients are considered legally competent unless legally judged incompetent or temporarily incapacitated by a medical condition. When a court rules an adult incompetent, it appoints a guardian or a surrogate to make decisions on that person's behalf. Commitment is not a determination of incompetence. Clients who are committed for treatment are still capable of participating in health care decisions.

CLIENT RIGHTS

Clients do not lose constitutional, legal, or ethical rights when they receive treatment for a mental disorder. See Box 5.1 for a list of clients' rights.

Confidentiality and Privacy

The primary reason for confidentiality is to encourage clients to be honest and open, to facilitate accurate diagnosis and effective treatment. Nurses have a legal and ethical duty to protect client confidentiality. **Confidentiality** ensures that health care professionals, including nursing students, do not talk about clients with anyone who is not involved in their care. It is a serious breach of confidentiality to go home and tell family members about clients and what happened on the unit. Discussing clients while in the hospital elevator or the cafeteria also breaches confidentiality. Nursing schools and hospitals have regulations regarding confidentiality. Breach of confidentiality is considered unprofessional conduct and is grounds for discipline by the state licensing board.

In order for mental health clients to discuss their illness with health care professionals, they must be assured of *privacy* because the information is highly personal, possibly embarrassing, and potentially damaging. This has become more difficult in a climate of government monitoring of care, demands by private insurers and managed care companies for access to client records, and the rapid computerization of medical record keeping. Nurses must be extremely careful to protect client privacy when using e-mail, cell

BOX 5.1	Client Rights

■ Right to confidentiality and privacy
■ Right to informed consent
■ Right to treatment
■ Right to refuse treatment
■ Right to least restrictive environment
■ Right to communicate with others
■ Right to freedom from unnecessary restraints and seclusion
■ Right to participate in legal matters
■ Right to religious freedom
■ Right to consensual sexual relationships

phones, voice mail, and other communications technologies. The American Nurses Association (ANA Position Statement, 2001) supports the following principles of privacy and confidentiality:

- Individuals have the right to decide to whom and under what circumstances their identifiable health information will be disclosed.
- Clients have the right to access their health information and the right to supplement or correct this information.
- Clients must be told how their health records are used.
- If client consent has not been obtained, health information may be shared if the person's life is endangered, if there is a threat to the public, or if there is a compelling law enforcement need.
- There should be severe consequences for violations of privacy and confidentiality.

Under some circumstances, the nurse has a legal and ethical duty *not* to protect client confidentiality and privacy. These circumstances include the following:

- The client is a danger to self or others.
- The client is a minor, elderly, or disabled and is believed to be a victim of abuse.
- Disclosures are needed to other professionals or supervisors directly involved in the treatment.
- A therapist is appointed by the court to evaluate the client, and this therapist requires disclosure of information.
- A court order or other legal proceedings or laws requires disclosure of information.

When working with clients, the subject of confidentiality must be discussed. Explain to clients that what is discussed is shared only with the staff and the instructor. If the client is known from outside the hospital, reassure the client that his or her presence on the unit is confidential. In this situation, you should not provide care for this person or read the chart.

There are federal regulations regarding chemical dependence (CD) programs. Everyone, including professionals and visitors, must sign a confidentiality statement before entering a CD unit. Staff members are not allowed to disclose any admission or discharge information. They cannot even acknowledge whether the client is in the treatment facility.

Legally, a child does not have the right to confidentiality. In most cases, the parents, as legal guardians for the child, have the right to know what is going on in treatment. Parents usually desire information and some level of involvement in their child's treatment plan. They often seek advice about how to cope with the day-to-day challenges, what they might expect in the future, and sources of community support.

Most states have laws regarding when HIV test results or the diagnosis of AIDS may be disclosed. In many states, this information cannot even be put in the medical record without the client's written consent. In some states, clients must give written consent before HIV tests can be performed, whereas in other states, oral consent is sufficient. However, because oral consent is difficult to prove, most institutions require written consent. A large proportion of people infected with HIV are adolescents. It is unclear, however, if adolescents have the right to consent to HIV testing and treatment. Each state is responsible for determining a minor's capacity to consent to health care. All 50 states require the reporting of AIDS cases to the Centers for Disease Control and Prevention without client consent (Grusky et al., 2005; Ho, Brandfield, Retkin, & Laraque, 2005).

Informed Consent

Informed consent is the client's right to receive enough information to make a decision about treatment and to communicate the decision to others. For consent to be given, the health care professional must inform the client of the objective, the benefit, and the risks of the proposed treatment. The client must also be told about any possible alternative interventions. The client must understand the information and be able to apply it to her or his personal situation. The purpose of informed consent is to ensure that clients are not abused and that they are acknowledged as independent, responsible persons whose rights and private space must be respected.

Right to Treatment

Although there is a belief in the right to treatment, there is often not adequate provision for clients. Services are not always accessible or appropriate. Every mental health client has the right to fully participate in and approve a treatment plan and to decide which services to accept. Our mental health care systems must expand to ensure this right.

Right to Refuse Treatment

Clients may not be touched or treated without consent. If treatment is given without consent, the health care provider is held responsible for battery or offensive touching according to the law. In the event of an emergency, with no time to obtain consent without endangering health or safety, a client may be treated without legal liability. Clients must be informed of the potential risks of psychotropic medications or treatments. Competent adults have the right to refuse medication. When client values are different than those of

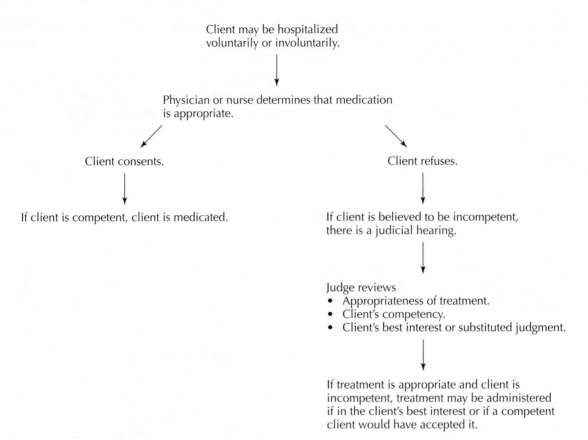

Figure 5.1 ■ Outcomes of client medication decisions.

SOURCE: Adapted with permission from Applebaum, P. S. (1988). The right to refuse treatment with antipsychotic medications. *American Journal of Psychiatry, 145*(1), 145–146.

health professionals, the professional's responsibility is to respect and facilitate client self-determination in regard to health care decisions.

If a client refuses medication or other treatments and the physician believes it is essential for effective treatment, the physician may take the case to the courts for a decision (see Figure 5.1 ■).

Least Restrictive Environment

Clients have the right to treatment with the least restrictive environment, which means clients are referred to or placed in the therapeutic setting that will provide *safe* care while allowing maximum freedom. The least restrictive environment ranges from clients living on their own to being hospitalized in a locked unit, based on the individual client's needs. The determination is always made based on the level of protection needed to keep the client safe at that moment in time.

The Right to Communicate With Others

Clients have the right to send and receive mail, the right to telephone contact, and the right to visitors when hospitalized. The facility may have some regulations such as no

phone calls during scheduled therapy sessions and times for visiting hours.

The Right to Freedom From Unnecessary Restraints or Seclusion

The use of involuntary seclusion or mechanical or human restraints is justified only as an emergency safety measure against imminent danger to oneself or others and only after less restrictive methods have been inadequate to prevent injury. Seclusion and restraints are not treatment interventions but security measures; these are extreme measures that are very controversial in mental health care. See chapter 9 ∞ for a more detailed discussion on the negative impact of restraints and seclusion.

The Right to Participate in Legal Matters

Mental health clients do not lose their legal rights. They can marry or divorce, sell or buy property, sign contracts, and make a will. In spite of the fact that clients do not lose their legal rights, 26 states restrict voting rights for people with mental illness. This is further evidence of the stigma that remains part of American society. Many states prohibit voting by people who have been declared *incompetent* and have a guardian. Some states prohibit voting by *idiots, lunatics,* or *the insane* without specifying how the condition is supposed to be determined. The National Alliance on Mental Illness (NAMI) has begun a campaign to educate representatives throughout the country on this denial of rights of citizenship (Burley, 2004).

Right to Consensual Sexual Relationships

Adult mental health clients have the right to consensual sexual relationships. This has been a problem for staff in long-term facilities, acute care facilities, and group homes. In addition, family members have often tried to restrict the sexual activity of their loved ones. Sexual relationships are part of life. The staff must provide privacy for consenting adults and safety for those who choose not to engage in sex or who lack the ability to give consent (Dobal & Torkelson, 2004).

REPORTING LAWS

All states make it mandatory for nurses to report suspected cases of child abuse or neglect. Failure to report these cases subjects the nurse to criminal penalties and civil liability. Reporting protects the nurse from being sued by the parents or guardian. Many states have enacted adult abuse laws similar to child abuse reporting laws. It is important that nurses know the laws for their state.

Duty to Disclose/Protect

The **duty to disclose/protect** is the health care professional's obligation to warn identified individuals if a client has made a credible threat to kill them. In some states, the duty to disclose also includes threats against property. In the 1970s, a client told his psychiatrist that he would kill his girlfriend. When the client murdered his girlfriend, her parents sued the psychiatrist for wrongful death. The courts upheld the case, stating that the physician had a duty to warn the victim. In 1980, the duty to disclose was clarified to mean that the potential victim was someone who could be readily identified (Guido, 2006).

When a client threatens violence, mental health providers have a special responsibility to evaluate the person's dangerousness and to take appropriate action to protect others from the danger. Studies show that many of the targets of client threats are family members, spouses, boyfriends, or girlfriends. The duty to disclose supersedes the client's right to confidentiality. Prevention of violent criminal actions is more important than confidentiality. The general rule is to warn identified persons and the local police of believable threats when the client is not confined to the hospital.

In 1997, the duty to disclose was extended to staff members. The attending physician must inform nurses of any clients who are aggressive and dangerous. Furthermore, safety measures must be instituted for the staff's protection. These measures may include medications, seclusion, or transfer to a more secure setting (Guido, 2006).

LEAVING AGAINST MEDICAL ADVICE

Clients who have been voluntarily admitted to a restrictive hospital setting may wish to exercise the right to liberty and leave the facility, or leave against medical advice (LAMA). A client who is competent and who is no danger to self or others cannot be prevented from leaving. If a client is a danger to himself or herself or others, the staff must make a decision between safety and the right to refuse treatment. If necessary, commitment proceedings are initiated. Some of the more common reasons people seek discharge against medical advice include (Guido, 2006):

- Family concerns, such as the care of young children or dependent elderly relatives
- Financial reasons, such as wanting to conserve lifetime benefits for mental health care
- A need to return to work
- Disagreement with staff that the duration of hospitalization is necessary for treatment goals
- Uncomfortable withdrawal symptoms from substance abuse

Some clients simply walk out of the facility without notifying staff. This is often called **elopement**, and the eloper might be either a voluntary admission or committed to the facility. When staff believe that a client may attempt to leave the facility, *elopement precautions* are instituted. Frequent checks on the client's location are a standard elopement precaution. The nurse should take some basic precautions if assigned to a locked unit. When entering or leaving the unit, look around and be aware of clients very near the door. These clients may slip out when the door is opened. If you leave the unit with other students, make sure that a client has not joined the group. If a client asks you to accompany him or her off the unit, you should check with the staff on each client's status for off-unit privileges.

When a client successfully elopes, the staff notifies the physician, the hospital administration, and the family. If it is determined that the client is dangerous to self or others, local police are informed. A hospital can be sued when clients who elope commit suicide, are injured or killed in accidents, or injure or kill others while away from the hospital. Liability is determined on the basis of two elements.

MediaLink Care Plan, Duty to Warn

The first element is how much the staff knew or should have known about the level of danger to self or others. The second element is the appropriateness of precautions taken to prevent LAMA in light of that knowledge.

CLIENTS WITH LEGAL CHARGES

Some clients admitted to the psychiatric unit may have pending legal charges. It may be difficult to work with these clients when the behavior that resulted in the legal charges is in conflict with personal values. Examples include a client admitted for severe depression with legal charges of sexually molesting his child, and a client admitted to a substance abuse program who hit a pedestrian while driving under the influence. When ethical dilemmas arise, the nurse must identify personal feelings and seek peer or supervisor advice in managing the situation and avoiding punitive reactions. Confidentiality is extremely important in such circumstances. Clients must also be informed that the court may request medical records and that staff members may be required to testify in court.

THE MENTALLY ILL IN CORRECTIONAL SETTINGS

The number of severely and persistently mentally ill people in correctional settings has increased over the past 30 years. Studies indicate that 10% to 18% of prison inmates have a major mental disorder. With few long-term psychiatric facilities, many people who were previously cared for in state hospitals are now found in jails and prisons. The increase in number is also related to a lack of support in the community for the severely and persistently mentally ill population. About one third of these individuals are homeless and victims of a cycle of mental hospitals, the street, and jail as a way of life over which they have no control. They may be jailed because no other agencies are available to respond to their psychiatric emergency. The jail has become the mental hospital that cannot say *no*. Often, the crimes with which they are charged are misdemeanors resulting from symptoms of mental illness, such as disorderly conduct, trespassing, camping out, and public intoxication. This *criminalization* of mental illness is one of the most disturbing trends in our nation and must be stopped. Under the 14th Amendment of the Constitution, mentally ill jail detainees have a right to mental health services. The reality is that psychiatric evaluation and intervention is haphazard. Mental health treatment is primarily centered on decreasing the symptoms through medication (Brugha et al., 2005; Honberg, 2005).

The prison subculture makes those who are severely and persistently mentally ill more vulnerable to abuse and victimization by inmates and guards because those who

are mentally ill hold low status. Women prisoners are sexually vulnerable to a largely male correctional force. Many mentally ill people suffer cruelty and abuse by other inmates, including torment, beatings, and rape. When an inmate needs someone to take the blame or punishment, a mentally ill inmate is easily manipulated into this position. Guards often place severely mentally ill prisoners in solitary confinement for misbehavior that is a product of their mental illness. Symptoms worsen with the prolonged social isolation, sensory deprivation, excessive use of force by guards, use of restraints as punishment, and inadequate medical care. Solitary confinement is no place for a seriously mentally ill patient (O'Connor, Lovell, & Brown, 2002).

The suicide rate among jail inmates is eight times that of the U.S. population, and hanging is the most common method. The first 24 hours following an arrest is the period of highest risk because people with mental illness are put in cells and abandoned and ignored during an extremely stressful period. Adolescents may be especially vulnerable due to feelings of fear, humiliation, and isolation from their peer group. People charged with murder may be at highest risk due to a generalized impulsivity (Way, Miraglia, Sawyer, Beer, & Eddy, 2005).

Thousands of mentally ill American children, some as young as 8 years old, are locked up in juvenile detention centers because there is nowhere else for them to go. More than half the juvenile detainees meet the criteria for mental disorders and, of those, 24% have a very high level of symptoms. In addition, nearly three fourths of this population has substance use disorders. Juvenile detention centers are designed to care for children who have been charged with crimes and those who are awaiting court hearings or placement. They lack the resources, education, and staff to care for children with mental disorders (Abram, Teplin, McClelland, & Dulcan, 2003; McClelland, Elkington, Teplin, & Abram, 2004; Thomas, Gourley, & Mele, 2004).

Congress is examining strategies to create local *mental health courts*. These programs would provide supervision of offenders with mental illness or mental retardation who are charged with nonviolent crimes. It is hoped that there will be provision for life-skills training, housing placement, vocational training, education, job placement, health care, and relapse prevention for each participant. The goal of these programs would be to create alternatives to incarceration.

People with severe and persistent mental illness are at high risk of police contact, the outcome of which is largely determined by police actions. As a result, more communities are providing crisis intervention programs to police, probation, parole, and correctional personnel to help them recognize a psychiatric emergency and intervene in a safe manner for all concerned.

CARING: A PREREQUISITE TO ETHICAL BEHAVIOR

Caring is the essence of nursing and the foundation for ethical behavior. People who are in a caring relationship are likely to behave in an ethical manner toward each other. Caring involves compassion and sensitivity to each person within the context of her or his entire life. Caring is being respectful of people's choices as to the best course of action. Caring is accepting people as they are and envisioning what they may become. Caring is honoring each person's wholeness of being—mind, body, emotions, and spirit.

NURSING ETHICS

Ethics refers to a system of morals or rules of behavior. It is the evaluation of right or wrong behavior in any given culture. Ethics are the principles that govern human behavior. The term *ethics* is also used to describe the study of standards governing the practice of professional nurses. Nursing, like many disciplines, has identified guidelines for ethical behavior.

Principalism

Nursing is a value-laden practice. Nurses are required to make numerous ethical decisions every day. Traditionally, nurses have been taught ethics from the perspective of *principalism*. This is based on the belief that there are universal, objective principles that ought to govern the moral behavior of people. The principles are autonomy, beneficence, nonmaleficence, veracity, fidelity, and justice. *Autonomy* is the right to make decisions for oneself. Nurses support client rights to make these decisions even if they disagree with the decision. Clients do not have the right, however, to endanger others by their decisions. *Beneficence* is performing good acts that benefit others. The nurse may encourage clients to take medications or consider electroconvulsive therapy if these interventions will improve the quality of life. In contrast is *nonmaleficence*, which is not acting in a way that would cause pain or suffering to self or others. *Veracity* is telling the truth. Nurses follow this principle when they provide psychoeducation to clients and families. *Fidelity* is keeping promises. Fidelity is critically important in the nurse–client relationship. The principle of *justice* states that people should be treated equally and people should be recognized for responsible behavior. The problem with the perspective of principalism is that socioeconomic and cultural contexts are ignored. They are also far too abstract to have any practical application in clinical practice (Demarco, 2005; Guido, 2006).

Values

Values are personal beliefs about what is right or wrong and give direction to everyday life. Values develop from the norms of the culture, families, and religion and are classified as personal, professional, or societal values. Caring for clients whose values and lifestyles are similar to your own does not challenge you to make the choice to accept the client's inherent worth. As society becomes more ethnically diverse and multicultural, the potential for rising ethical conflicts increases. When values and lifestyles are dissimilar, we are challenged to make caring, ethical decisions.

Nurses have the most difficulty when situations involve both ethics and the law. Consider how each of the following clients might pose an ethical dilemma when admitted to a mental health care facility: a known drug pusher; a mother who has killed her baby through physical abuse; a teenager who has sexually molested his sister; an adult daughter who has physically abused her elderly father; an accused rapist. We must be able to respect the humanness of every client in spite of differences in values and lifestyles.

Competent Care

The expectation that nurses will deliver competent care is fundamental to the notion of professional nursing practice. This is evidenced by the ANA Nursing Code of Ethics described in Box 5.2. Competence is both *knowing what* and *knowing how*. It is not a permanent state achieved when obtaining a nursing license but rather a continuing process of improving and refining skills and knowledge. Competence is education and attitude. Education is the academic program a student is enrolled in and continuing education throughout her or his years of practice. Attitude includes being open to criticism by colleagues and a willingness to admit to lack of knowledge or error when appropriate. Competence is the recognition of one's limitations as well as one's strengths and skills. With the explosion of scientific information, competent nurses must stay current with developments in their areas of practice. Competent nurses who apply evidence-based practice use the best available research evidence, use their clinical expertise, and respect clients' choices, concerns, and values to arrive at the best client outcomes. The ANA Code of Ethics can be viewed online by accessing the ANA Web site, which can be retrieved through a resource link on the Companion Web site for this book.

Research

An ethical dimension exists in mental illness as it relates to clients and their participation in nursing research. This is especially true for people with the more debilitating mental illnesses such as schizophrenia and bipolar disorder. When problems with cognition, emotion, motivation, and memory

---

BOX 5.2	ANA Code of Ethics for Nurses

1. The nurse, in all professional relationships, practices with compassion and respect for the inherent dignity, worth, and uniqueness of every individual, unrestricted by considerations of social or economic status, personal attributes, or the nature of health problems.
2. The nurse's primary commitment is to the patient, whether an individual, family, group, or community.
3. The nurse promotes, advocates for, and strives to protect the health, safety, and rights of the patient.
4. The nurse is responsible and accountable for individual nursing practice and determines the appropriate delegation of tasks consistent with the nurse's obligation to provide optimum patient care.
5. The nurse owes the same duties to self as to others, including the responsibility to preserve integrity and safety, to maintain competence, and to continue personal and professional growth.
6. The nurse participates in establishing, maintaining, and improving health care environments and conditions of employment conducive to the provision of quality health care and consistent with the values of the profession through individual and collective action.
7. The nurse participates in the advancement of the profession through contributions to practice, education, administration, and knowledge development.
8. The nurse collaborates with other health professionals and the public in promoting community, national, and international efforts to meet health needs.
9. The profession of nursing, as represented by associations and their members, is responsible for articulating nursing values, for maintaining the integrity of the profession and its practice, and for shaping social policy.

SOURCE: Reprinted with permission from American Nurses Association. Code of Ethics for Nurses with Interpretive Statements, © 2001 American Nurses Publishing, American Nurses Foundation/American Nurses Association, Washington, DC.

---

are combined with symptoms such as delusions and hallucinations, these impairments might limit the client's ability to understand, appreciate, and reason about the choices in regard to research.

Clients who are considering participation in research, along with their caregiving family members, must be fully aware of what the protocols involve, what risks they will face, what options they have, and who they should contact with questions or issues. Nurses must not mistakenly assume that impaired capacity necessarily implies that potential research subjects cannot give informed consent. Often, individuals may just have a harder time grasping the content of the disclosure. Approaches to this problem include repetitive disclosure of information, group sessions to answer questions, and the involvement of family members.

Research involving people with mental disorders is essential if nurses are to better understand the underlying causes of these illnesses, how individuals and families cope, and which interventions are most effective. There are also

rewards for individuals participating in nursing research. Rewards may include the pride that comes from altruistic behavior, the hope that they might benefit from the results of the study at some point in the future, and the more immediate possibility that they may have access through the study to therapeutic approaches that would not otherwise be available to them (Rice & Broome, 2004).

The challenge for nurses is to continue to work with volunteers who have mental disorders to discover and develop better nursing interventions while doing all that can be done to protect the rights and well-being of those who participate in research.

Ethics of Care

Nursing is based on ethics of care. Nurses use many perspectives in the process of ethical decision making, which can be summarized in four categories: medical indications, client preferences, quality of life, and contextual factors. *Medical indications* include the diagnosis, prognosis, and treatment options with probable outcomes. *Client preferences* relate to an individual's values and goals for life and advance directives when acutely ill. *Quality of life* involves client perceptions about their lives and what they would like life to be. *Contextual factors* include social and environmental details about the problem and how these affect treatment options

The *International Council of Nurses Code of Ethics for Nurses* (2000) identifies four fundamental responsibilities:

- Promoting health
- Preventing illness
- Restoring health
- Alleviating suffering

The nursing profession places a high value on client autonomy and the client's right to participate in treatment planning and implementation, as reflected in the *Nursing Code of Ethics for Nurses* (2000). This code implies that one of the primary functions of the nurse is to be an *advocate* for the client's wishes. At times, the nurse may function much in the same way as an advance directive. The Patient Self-Determination Act became federal law in 1990. This law states that clients have a right to participate in their own care. In addition, health care professionals are required to inform clients of the right to accept or refuse medical care, including medication.

Ethics is more a process than a set of answers. At the heart of every ethical dilemma is the potential for conflict—conflict within oneself, conflict between nurse and client, or conflict among professionals. Nurses must confront difficult ethical problems and arrive at options that best support the client's values and wishes.

Focus Your Study

OBJECTIVES

KEY CONCEPTS

1. Discuss the issues involved in the involuntary admission process.

- Reasons for commitment:
  - Obtain treatment to decrease suffering
  - Limit rejection by general public
  - Protect from threatened or actual violence
- Arguments against commitment:
  - Absence of criminal activity
  - Dehumanization of clients
  - Coercion contributing to distrust
  - Continuation of stigma of mental illness

2. Explain the rights of a client receiving mental health services.

- Confidentiality and privacy:
  - Right to decide to whom, and under what circumstances, their health information will be disclosed
  - Right to access own health information and to supplement or correct this information
  - Right to be told how health records are used
  - All professionals and visitors to chemical dependence programs must sign a confidentiality statement before entering the unit.

3. Identify the exceptions to a client's right to confidentiality.

- The client's life is endangered, the client is a threat to the public, or if there is a compelling law enforcement need
- Client is a minor, an elderly person, or disabled and is thought to be a victim of abuse
- Disclosures to other professionals directly involved in the treatment, or legal proceedings that require disclosure of information
- Duty to disclose

4. Analyze the role competency plays in mental health treatment and research.

- Competency is the legal determination that a client can make reasonable judgments and decisions about medical care and other significant areas of personal life.
- Clients are considered legally competent unless legally judged incompetent or temporarily incapacitated by a medical condition.
- Informed consent is the client's right to receive enough information to make a decision about treatment and to communicate the decision to others. This information includes the objective, the benefit, the risks, and any alternative interventions of the proposed treatment.
- Clients considering participation in research must be fully aware of what the protocols involve, what risks they will face, what options they have, and who they should contact with questions or issues.

5. Discuss the relationship between mental illness and the criminal justice system.

- With few long-term psychiatric facilities, jails and prisons have become the mental hospital that cannot say "no." This criminalization of mental illness is one of the most disturbing trends in the United States and must be stopped.
- Treatment for mental illness in correctional settings is haphazard or nonexistent.
- Mentally ill people in correctional settings are vulnerable to abuse and victimization by inmates and guards.
- Thousands of mentally ill American children are locked up in juvenile detention centers because there is nowhere else for them to go.

6. Outline the elements of ethical nursing practice.

- The International Code of Ethics for Nurses identifies four fundamental responsibilities:
  - Promoting health
  - Preventing illness
  - Restoring health
  - Alleviating suffering
- Encourage client autonomy and right to participate in treatment planning and implementation.
- Act as an advocate for clients' wishes.

Explore MediaLink

For review questions, case studies, and other resources for this chapter see the Pearson Health MediaLink CD-ROM that accompanies this book and the Companion Website.

CD-ROM
- Audio Glossary
- NCLEX-RN® Review Questions

Companion Website www.prenhall.com/fontaine
- Audio Glossary
- NCLEX-RN® Review Questions
- Case Study
  - Involuntary Admission
- Care Plan
  - Duty to Warn
- Critical Thinking
  - Client Rights
- MediaLink Application
  - Smoking Bans
- MediaLinks
  - Books for Clients and Families
  - Community Resources

NCLEX-RN® Review Questions

5-1. A psychiatric treatment team is planning care for a client who was involuntarily admitted for treatment of depression and suicide ideation. One understanding utilized in planning client care is that the client is:
1. Able to refuse medication.
2. Able to demand and obtain release.
3. In need of a guardian.
4. Considered to be incompetent.

5-2. The health care provider is discussing a new treatment that requires an informed consent with a client. Which of the following does the client receive before signing a statement of informed consent? (Select all that apply.)
1. Guarantee of safe outcome from the treatment
2. Objective of the treatment
3. Benefits of the treatment
4. Risks of the treatment
5. Names of others who have had the treatment
6. Any alternatives to the treatment

5-3. A client with a history of aggression and violence is admitted to the hospital. Which of the following principles guide the health care provider to inform nurses about the client's danger to them?
1. Patient Self-Determination Act
2. Adult abuse laws
3. Right to confidentiality
4. Duty to disclose/protect

5-4. A client was admitted for treatment of the symptoms of bipolar disorder. The court decided that this client was not able to understand the consequences of the decisions that he was making. Which of the following terms describe the status of this client?
1. Admitted with consent
2. Emergency involuntary admission
3. Competent
4. Legally incompetent

5-5. A homeless person with schizophrenia is yelling obscenities at those who pass by. The nurse should first take this client to which of the following locations?
1. Religious shelter
2. Crisis center
3. Jail
4. Mental hospital

5-6. After 3 days on the unit a client says to the nurse, "I would like to date you; tell me how I can reach you outside of the hospital." Which response by the nurse is most appropriate?
1. "It is against hospital policy for me to date you."
2. "I can date you after you leave the hospital."
3. "I would like to date you. Give me your phone number."
4. "My relationship with you is professional and not social."

See Appendix D for answers.

References

Abram, K. M., Teplin, L. A., McClelland, G. M., & Dulcan, M. K. (2003). Comorbid psychiatric disorders in youth in juvenile detention. *Archives of General Psychiatry, 60*(11), 1097–1100.

American Nurses Association. (2001). *Code for nurses with interpretative statements.* Washington, DC: Author.

Brugha, T., Singleton, N., Meltzer, H., Bebbington, P., Farrell, M., Jenkins, R., et al. (2005). Psychosis in the community and in prisons. *American Journal of Psychiatry, 162*(4), 774–780.

Burley, C. (2004). Legal advocates challenge Missouri voter practices. *Bazelon Center for Mental Health Law.* Retrieved August 11, 2005, from www.bazelon.org/newsroom/10-7-04mo_voting.htm.

Demarco, J. P. (2005). Principalism and moral dilemmas. *Journal of Medical Ethics, 31*(2), 101–105.

Dobal, M. T., & Torkelson, D. J. (2004). Making decisions about sexual rights in psychiatric facilities. *Archives of Psychiatric Nursing, 18*(2), 68–74.

Grusky, O., Roberts, K. J., Swanson, A. N., Joniak, E., Leich, J., McEvoy, G., et al. (2005). Anonymous versus confidential HIV testing. *AIDS Patient Care and STDS, 19*(3), 157–166.

Guido, G. W. (2006). *Legal and ethical issues in nursing.* Upper Saddle River, NJ: Prentice Hall.

Ho, W. W., Brandfield, J., Retkin, R., & Laraque, D. (2005). Complexities in HIV consent in adolescents. *Clinical Pediatrics, 44*(6), 473–478.

Honberg, R. (2005). Decriminalizing mental illness. *NAMI Advocate, 3*(1), 4–7.

International Council of Nurses. (2000). *The ICN code of ethics for nurses.* Geneva, Switzerland: Author.

McClelland, G. M., Elkington, K. S., Teplin, L. A., & Abram, K. M. (2004). Multiple substance use disorders in juvenile detainees. *Journal of the American Academy of Child and Adolescent Psychiatry, 43*(10), 1215–1224.

O'Connor, R. W., Lovell, D., & Brown, L. (2002). Implementing residential treatment for prison inmates with mental illness. *Archives of Psychiatric Nursing, 16*(5), 232–238.

Rice, M., & Broome, M. E. (2004). Incentives for children in research. *Journal of Nursing Scholarship, 36*(2), 167–172.

Salize, H. J., & Dressing, H. (2005). Coercion, involuntary treatment and quality of mental health care. *Current Opinions in Psychiatry, 18*(5), 576–584.

Swartz, M. S., Swanson, J. W., Wagner, H. R., Hannon, M. J., Burns, B. J., & Shumway, M. (2003). Assessment of four stakeholder groups' preferences concerning outpatient commitment for persons with schizophrenia. *American Journal of Psychiatry, 160*(6), 1139–1146.

Thomas, J., Gourley, G. K., & Mele, N. (2004). The impact of managed behavioral health care on youth in the juvenile justice system. *Archives of Psychiatric Nursing, 18*(4), 135–142.

Way, B. B., Miraglia, R., Sawyer, D. A., Beer R., & Eddy, J. (2005). Factors related to suicide in New York state prisons. *International Journal of Law and Psychiatry, 28*(3), 207–221.

Chapter 6

Neurobiology and Behavior

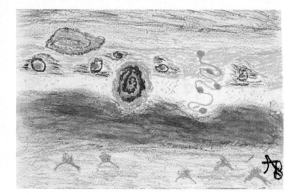

66 *Free-floating connections* 99

—Anthony, Age 17

OBJECTIVES

After reading this chapter, you will be able to:

1. Describe the development of the brain over the life span.
2. Relate the functions of the brain to its major anatomical features.
3. Describe the functions of the different neurotransmitters.
4. Outline the mental health symptoms that can occur with disruptions in neuroanatomy and neurophysiology.
5. Discuss the relationship between stress and the immune system.
6. Discuss the impact of nutrition on brain functioning.

MediaLink www.prenhall.com/fontaine

Go to the Pearson Health MediaLink CD-ROM and the Companion Website at www.prenhall.com/fontaine for interactive resources for this chapter.

The human brain is among the most complicated objects in the universe. This dynamic ecosystem adapts to internal and external environments and responds to use or disuse. The brain has 100 billion neurons, 1,000 billion other cells, multiple levels of organization, and thousands of genes that construct it and permit it to function properly. Each neuron may have from 1 to 150,000 synaptic connections to other neurons. No brain is perfect, no two brains are alike, and each brain is continually changing.

The **mind** is a property of brain activity; that is, it is a process, not a thing. Though we cannot see the mind, it is as real as the processes of other organs. Psychophysiological processes such as perception, thinking, emotion, memory, motivation, behavior, and conscious experience reflect the activation of complex networks of neurons throughout the brain and illustrate how the brain and the mind are a unified process. In addition, the mind grows in response to life experiences and interpersonal interactions.

Historically, lack of understanding of brain function led to separation of mental disorders from other serious illnesses and to stigmatization of those who were suffering. Problems were blamed on childhood trauma or bad parenting. Mental disorders are now understood as brain deficits, and neuropsychiatric science now focuses on the etiology and treatment of these mental disorders. Biological psychiatry encompasses neuroanatomy, neurophysiology, neurochemistry, neurogenetics, neuroimmunology, neuropsychology, neuroendocrinology, neuroimaging, and neurocomputational sciences. Researchers hope to learn how the brains of those affected by mental disorders are different from the brains of those who are not. There is still much to understand regarding how they occur, but it is known that mental disorders are serious brain disorders, much like strokes and brain tumors are.

What this means for the nursing student is that, in addition to principles from nursing, sociology, and psychology, nursing care of clients with mental disorders also includes principles from the biological sciences.

DEVELOPMENT OF THE BRAIN

Genes and Environment

Mental health and mental illness both involve complex interactions of genes and environments, from conception through the end of life. *Genes* give direction for initial development and provide the broad outline of development. Although they are the basic building blocks, genes do not determine destiny. The term *environment* refers to the multiple factors that turn genes on or off, causing cells to differentiate, divide, sprout new connections, or strengthen others. For a given nerve cell, these environments may be the number, rate, and firing patterns of neighboring neurons; hormonal factors within the brain; stress hormones passed within the mother's breast milk; trauma to specific nerve cells; and events and experiences perceived by the brain. For the developing brain, environment refers to factors ranging from obstetric complications, intrauterine infections, and early nutrition to exposure to stressful life experiences such as community violence. As knowledge about the brain increases, it is known that some disorders, such as autism, are disorders of brain development; whereas others, such as posttraumatic stress disorder, result from traumatic experiences that affect the brain's structure and function.

Genes and environment interact continually from the moment of conception to death. In some situations, genes are more important and, in others, environment is more important. Our brain changes every second of our lives in response to everything we perceive, think, feel, and do. It is safe to say that the brain is the most interactive organ. (Genetics are covered in more detail in chapter 1 ∞.)

Fetal Brain

Fetal brain development is a highly regulated process under the control of a large number of genes, many of which remain to be discovered. It proceeds in a sequence of steps, and each step is strongly dependent on those that precede it.

During the third and fourth week after fertilization, the *neural tube* develops, which will give rise to the brain and the spinal cord. The first major step in the development of the brain is generation of a large number of nerve cells. Complications during this period are usually fatal to the fetus.

The second major step occurs during the second trimester as these cells migrate and differentiate. After a cell is born, it *migrates* to where it is genetically programmed to go. Nerve cells destined for the brain migrate over considerable distances, following guides provided by other cells. When the cell gets to its predetermined location, it starts to *differentiate* and *communicate* with other neurons. Trauma or disruption during this process affects a neuron's ability to communicate with other neurons. Problems in neuronal communication ultimately affect overall brain function. For example, it is believed that alcohol causes faulty brain cell migration during fetal development. Fetal alcohol syndrome is the third leading cause of birth defects in the United States. During the third trimester the neurotransmitter glutamate (glu) must be regulated within very narrow bounds. Too much or too little glu leads to neurodegeneration. Alcohol interferes with the release of glu, another contributing mechanism to fetal alcohol syndrome (Dowling, 2004; Farber & Newcomer, 2003). More detailed information on intrauterine substance exposure is covered in chapter 15 ∞.

The third major step, the *brain growth spurt*, begins in the third trimester, reaches peak acceleration prior to term, and continues at a gradually decreasing rate until the age of 2.

Once neurons have differentiated they never divide again, which explains why the brain initially overproduces neurons.

Infant Brain

The newborn infant has an incompletely developed central nervous system. There are as many as 12 growth spurts between birth and the early 20s when brain development is finally completed. The infant's brain contains twice as many neurons as the adult brain, but there are relatively few synapses. Synapses develop in the context of experiences with caregivers, and synaptic density peaks during childhood. By age 1 or 2 years, there are twice as many synapses as in the adult brain. This production then levels off for several years, and begins a gradual reduction around age 8 years.

As the infant grows, weak or unused neurons are *pruned* away. This means the environment in early years can have an incredible impact. In many cases there is a window of time during which a person must have a particular experience in order to keep particular neurons. For example, in an infant born with cataracts vision neurons are not stimulated. If the problem is not corrected by 6 months of age, the vision neurons are eliminated because they are not being used. In this situation, the child will never gain sight, even when the cataracts are removed (Teicher, Andersen, Navalta, Polcari, & Kim, 2004).

Childhood Brain

As the left cerebral hemisphere undergoes a growth spurt in the first 2 years, children develop what is referred to as the *conscious, linguistic self.* They become conscious of the world around them and curiously explore their environments. They also experience a spurt of language comprehension and expression. A growth spurt occurs at the same time in the right hemisphere, resulting in the *physical, emotional self.* Physical coordination advances and children learn to crawl and walk. At this age they begin to learn regulation of their emotions (Cozolino, 2002).

Myelination, the progressive covering of axons with layers of myelin or a lipid protein sheath, insulates the axons, making them more functional and efficient. As more myelin is produced, primitive reflexes give way to voluntary movements followed by improved gross and fine motor skills and refined hand–eye coordination.

In the first 3 to 5 years, there is an increase in glial and other supporting cells as well as an increase in blood vessels. Neuron cell bodies grow in size and extend more dendrites, which grow larger and go longer distances.

During childhood, a second dramatic elimination phase occurs. Between 7 and 15 years of age, the synapses overproduced in earlier years are pruned back by almost 40%. There are seven excitatory synapses to each inhibitory synapse.

Teenage Brain

The teenage brain is a work in progress. Millions of synapses are lost and a million are connected. The shift is to fewer and faster connections, increasing the efficiency of brain function. The ratio of excitatory synapses to inhibitory synapses drops to 4:1 in late adolescence, which results in a calmer brain and better inhibition control. Initially, gray matter overproduces and thickens and then there is an enormous loss (7% to 10%) of gray matter, thinning the cortex to adult levels.

The teenage brain continues to develop myelin especially in the hippocampus, which sorts out memories, and in the cingulated gyrus, which is related to emotions. Therefore, in early adolescence, emotional experiences are not well integrated with cognition, which explains the impulsive behavior often seen in this age group. Executive functions, such as reasoning, motivation, and judgment, develop slowly throughout adolescence. Teens want to be adults but they do not have the adult prefrontal cortex to regulate their behavior. Simultaneously the body's hormones are surging, which contributes to quick anger and impulsive behavior (Giedd et al., 2006).

Prior to adolescence, girls and boys experience similar levels of aggression and mood disorders. This changes during adolescence, when girls are more likely than boys to be depressed and boys are more likely than girls to be aggressive. It is important to remember that hormones alter gene expression and subsequent brain development, especially during adolescence (Pihl & Benkelfat, 2005).

The cortex is very susceptible to critical and long-lasting damage. The teen years may be the worst time to expose the brain to drugs, alcohol, or even a steady dose of violent video games. The period of greatest risk for traumatic brain injuries is from the mid teens through the mid 20s, when the cortex is most vulnerable to damage (Strauch, 2003). See chapter 20 ∞ for further information on traumatic brain injury.

Adult Brain

In adulthood, the frontal lobes attain their stable adult state. The major site of neuroplasticity seems to be the cortex. Neurons continue to sprout new dendrites and form new synapses. Neurons are different from other cells in the body in that they have an absolute requirement for oxygen. Without oxygen, neurons die in a few minutes. Other cells can break down glucose to produce enough energy to keep going and survive much longer. Therefore, people who experience cardiac arrest and are placed on life support systems may experience permanent brain damage, but their other organs recover completely.

Compared to the brain, many other parts of the body produce new cells. For example, when the skin is cut, new cells are generated and fill in the defect. It was long thought that no neurons were produced in the brain and that only new glial cells could be generated. Very recently, stem cells have been discovered in a part of the hippocampus and the olfactory bulb, and these stem cells generate new neurons. The number of new neurons produced decreases with age and the new neurons only last for a few weeks. If there are stem cells in other parts of the brain and if these stem cells can be induced to produce enough new neurons, neurodegenerative disorders such as Alzheimer disease, Parkinson disease, and the disabilities that accompany trauma and brain attacks may be treated (Dowling, 2004).

Aging Brain

Until recently, it was thought that brain cells die off by the millions throughout life, resulting in a poorly functioning brain in old age. New research shows that, although the cells function less efficiently, there is no devastating loss of function in *healthy aging brains*. The reductions in brain dopamine (DA) activity that occur as part of aging are associated with changes in motor activity and cognitive changes in the speed of processing information and memory retrieval. Aging causes a slowdown in the communication network of the brain rather than a massive death of brain cells (Smith et al., 2006).

Some of the normal changes of aging can be slowed down through active use of your brain. Intellectual activity stimulates brain cells to develop new dendrites, creating millions of new synapses between neurons. The brain is like a muscle—using it leads to growth, whereas disuse causes atrophy. Mental stimulation builds many more synapses between neurons, which appears to make brains more resistant to deterioration and Alzheimer disease.

Gender Differences

Scientists have found convincing evidence that the brains of women and men are different in overall size, size of certain brain structures, cerebral blood flow, and glucose metabolism. In the XY fetus, the testes secrete testosterone, which masculinizes the reproductive tract and the brain of male fetuses. The female fetal brain is not exposed to testosterone and develops in a female pattern. These disparities may help to explain *gender-related differences* in behavior. A consistent finding is that men perform better than women in spatial and motor-targeting tasks, whereas women have greater verbal fluency and fine motor skills than men. The same emotion might trigger a man to fight and a woman to react with words, facial expressions, and gestures. Women are more vulnerable to mood disorders and Alzheimer disease, whereas men are more vulnerable to schizophrenia. Therefore, the adult brain has been shaped in part by its hormonal environment.

Neuroplasticity

The brain is extraordinarily plastic, which means that it spends much of its life improving itself, refining structures, and responding to internal and external changes. **Neuroplasticity** illustrates the unity of our internal and external worlds and the interaction of nature and nurture. Dendrites grow and retract, the number of synapses may increase or decrease, the release of neurotransmitters changes, and receptors may alter their shape. Research has shown that even in old age, new synaptic connections form. The fact that most people are able to learn new skills and remember new information is evidence for ongoing neuroplasticity. Figure 6.1 ■ illustrates neuroplasticity.

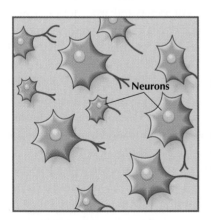

A At birth, the infant's brain has a complete set of neurons but not very many synaptic connections.

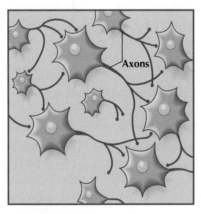

B During the first year, the axons grow longer, the dendrites increase in number, and a surplus of new connections is formed.

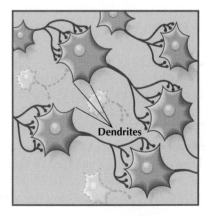

C Over the next few years, active connections are strengthened, while unused connections atrophy.

Figure 6.1 ■ The developing brain. At birth, the infant's brain has a complete set of neurons but relatively few synaptic connections.
SOURCE: Kassin, S. (2001). *Psychology* (3rd ed.). Upper Saddle River, NJ: Prentice Hall. Used with permission.

Brain Repair

Throughout life, all cells, including brain cells, are bombarded by attacks from unstable chemicals called *oxygen free radicals*. As the body goes through its normal processes and oxygen is used to provide cellular fuel, some of the oxygen molecules lose one of their pair of electrons. When this happens, the formerly stable oxygen molecules become dangerous free radicals that try to stabilize themselves by stealing another electron from stable molecules, thus damaging them and creating more free radicals. All organs and tissues are subject to damage from free radicals, but the brain is extremely vulnerable because it uses so much oxygen in producing vast amounts of energy to fire millions of neurons. In addition, as enzymes in the brain synthesize neurotransmitters, more oxygen free radicals are formed.

Free radicals are normally kept under control through the production of **antioxidants**, enzymes that act as free radical scavengers to search out and neutralize dangerous free radicals. These antioxidants are vitamin E, vitamin C, glutathione, coenzyme Q10, and lipoic acid. An antioxidant donates an electron to a free radical, thus neutralizing it. As a result, the antioxidant itself becomes unstable but harmless. Antioxidants work together as a team when another antioxidant donates an electron for rehabilitating the first one, ensuring continued survival of the antioxidants (Fontaine, 2005).

Antioxidants manage to repair at least 99% of the free radical damage to cells. The amount of permanent brain damage depends on the strength of the antioxidant defenses. As people age, they produce more free radicals and fewer antioxidants. The more free radical damage, the more likely people are to age prematurely and experience chronic diseases. Many people believe the best way to avoid these age-related changes is to boost the intake of antioxidants.

Research suggests that regular *physical exercise* makes the body more adept at delivering oxygen and nutrients to the brain. The brain is a hungry machine that comprises just 2% of the body weight but consumes 20% of the total oxygen and glucose stores. It functions best when arteries are kept clear, which is more likely to happen with exercise. People who exercise regularly have increased connections between neurons in the cingulated gyrus and the superior parietal lobe. This improvement in the efficiency of these circuits increased subjects' ability to focus on goals and maintain attention. Ultimately, genetics and lifestyle both have a significant impact on the aging process of the entire body, including the brain (McAuley, Kramer, & Colcombe, 2004).

NEUROANATOMY

The brain is regionally specialized; that is, different regions do different things. This is in contrast to functionally homogeneous organs like the liver in which any section can more or less substitute for another. Every area of the brain is directly or indirectly interconnected with every other area.

Brain Cells

The most abundant cells in the brain are the *glial cells*. There are 10 glial cells for every neuron. They are embedded in a matrix that contains growth factors, sugars, and proteins. Growth factors regulate dendrite and axon branching and cell death. There are four types of glial cells: astrocytes, oligodendroglia, ependyma, and microglia. *Astrocytes* regulate groups of neurons by controlling the concentration of neurotransmitters and ions. They even release their own neurotransmitters, causing dramatic changes in nearby neurons. Astrocytes are also responsible for the blood–brain barrier. *Oligodendroglia* coat the axon with a fatty substance called *myelin*, which protects the axon and controls the speed of impulses in the axon. The *ependymal cells* produce cerebrospinal fluid, and the *microglial cells* are responsible for phagocytosis, cleaning up dead neurons (Dowling, 2004).

There are as many as 100 billion individual *neurons*. Each neuron has a small, rounded body with short, dense branches called *dendrites* and a single, long nerve fiber called an *axon*. Dendrites are the way neurons get information, and axons are the way neurons pass on information. Dendrites are covered with receptors that receive incoming signals from other neurons. **Receptors** are proteins in the cell membrane that combine with a hormone, chemical transmitter, or a drug to alter the function of the cell. The *synapse* is the space between the end of the axon of one cell and the dendrites of other cells. Each neuron may have a direct synaptic connection with as many as 10,000 other neurons. All neurons, directly or indirectly, talk to each other, relay information, and network in ways we are only beginning to understand. There are at least 50 different kinds of neurons, varying in lengths and branching patterns of dendrites and axons. Even then, no two cells are alike. From day to day, some synaptic connections are not likely to remain exactly the same. Some will have retracted their dendrites or axons; others will have extended new ones; and certain others will have died, depending on the individual's experiences. It is through strengthening or weakening these connections that most development and learning occurs. This is part of the neuroplasticity previously discussed (Cozolino, 2002).

Individual cells are effective only in a group working together toward a single goal. *Ganglia* are dense collections of nerve cells with common functions. Ganglia may have as few as 50 neurons or as many as 10,000 neurons. There may be as many as 100 million ganglia in the brain.

Nerve Tracts

Nerve tracts are groups of nerve fibers that carry signals to and from the same area. The two main nerve tracts are the corpus callosum and the cingulate gyrus. The *corpus callosum* is composed of 200 million nerve fibers that connect the left and right cerebral hemispheres and relays sensory information between the two. The *cingulate gyrus*, part of the limbic system, encircles the hippocampus and other limbic structures. The cingulate gyrus is the main information highway of emotion. It integrates emotions with thinking in order to send a coherent message to the hypothalamus.

The brain is divided into three main areas: the brain stem, the cerebellum, and the cerebrum. They are all interconnected and work as an integrated unit.

Brain Stem

The *brain stem*, consisting of the midbrain, pons, and medulla, forms the stalk from which the cerebral hemispheres and the cerebellum sprout (Figure 6.2 ■). The brain stem is the location of functions vital to sustaining life. Such functions include the central processing of respiration, heart rate, balance, and blood pressure. It is the part of the brain that is most important to life. A person can survive damage to the cerebrum and cerebellum, but damage to the brain stem usually means rapid death. The brain stem is also the home of the 12 *cranial nerves*, which carry sensory and motor information to and from higher brain regions.

Three tiny structures in the brain stem—the raphe nuclei, the locus coeruleus, and the substantia nigra—are the focus of great interest to neuroscientists. The *raphe nuclei* are the primary source for serotonin (5-HT) in the brain and the spinal cord. Clusters of serotonergic neurons lie along the midline of the brain stem, from the midbrain to the medulla, and project to all levels of the brain. The *locus coeruleus*, located in the pons and with connections to almost every part of the brain, is the primary source of norepinephrine. Stimulation of the locus coeruleus creates an instant fear response in humans and animals. The locus coeruleus and the raphe nuclei are part of the *reticular activating system* (RAS). The RAS controls inhibitory and excitatory functions both by receiving impulses from all over the body and relaying them to the cortex. It is the central structure in the brain responsible for arousal, wakefulness, consciousness, sleep regulation, and learning. It may influence whether a person's behavior is aggressive or passive. The relationship between RAS dysfunction and mental disorders is not well understood at this time (Dowling, 2004).

The *substantia nigra* is a major source of dopamine for the brain. It projects axons to the striatum, which is involved in the initiation of voluntary movement. This area of the brain is black because cells contain the pigment melanin, which is a product of the breakdown of DA. Degeneration of the DA cells in the substantia nigra produces the motor disorders of Parkinson disease. Many antipsychotic medications are potent DA receptor blockers, resulting in side effects such as movement disorders (Dowling, 2004).

Cerebellum

The cerebellum, which wraps around the brain stem, has a unique appearance and has several lobes. This part of the brain is the least heritable, as seen by the greatest differences in monozygotic (identical) twins as they interact with the environment. It is 14% larger in adolescent boys than in adolescent girls (Strauch, 2003).

The cerebellum helps coordinate the planning, timing, and patterning of skeletal muscle contractions during movement. For example, the cerebellum enables a person to grasp a glass on the first try and walk in an upright manner. It maintains posture and equilibrium by receiving input about balance from the inner ear. The cerebellum is responsible for the storage, retrieval, and use of procedural memory. Procedural memory impairments include difficulty performing normally habitual tasks, such as brushing teeth and getting dressed.

Just as the cerebellum coordinates physical movement, it also coordinates the movement of thoughts. It plays a role in a person's ability to visualize his or her favorite beach or plan the sequence of an argument. It was recently discovered that the cerebellum also sets the timing and rhythm of brain function by delaying or speeding up the coordination of stimuli, memories, and thoughts. The cerebellum is involved in recognizing social cues and eases participation in social interactions. It has become clear that the cerebellum plays a more complex role in brain functions than previously thought.

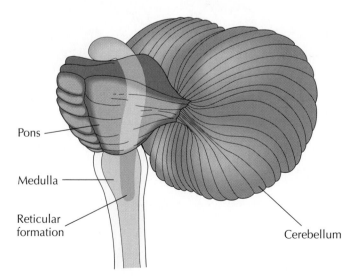

Pons
Medulla
Reticular formation
Cerebellum

Figure 6.2 ■ The brain stem. The brain stem is the most primitive structure of the brain. Resting atop the spinal cord, it contains the medulla, pons, and reticular formation and is attached to the cerebellum.

SOURCE: Kassin, S. (2001). *Psychology* (3rd ed.). Upper Saddle River, NJ: Prentice Hall. Used with permission.

TABLE 6.1	Functions of the Left and Right Hemispheres

Left Hemisphere	Right Hemisphere
Conscious coping	Heavily wired to the limbic system
Problem solving	Comprehends emotionally laden language
Processes information in a linear, sequential manner	Evaluates emotional facial expressions
Brain's basic instinct to explain things it cannot understand	Nonverbal aspect of communication Appraises safety and danger
Confabulation—filling in gaps in memory or making a guess at what happened	Visual–spatial and musical abilities: Intuition, feelings, fantasy, visual images

Mental disorders associated with cerebellum dysfunction include autism, Asperger disorder, attention deficit hyperactivity disorder, mood disorders, and schizophrenia (Ramnani, 2006; Vogel, 2005).

Cerebrum

The cerebrum, sitting on top of and surrounding the brain stem, comprises 80% of the weight of the brain. The cerebrum is divided into two hemispheres—right and left. Each of the hemispheres has separate and unique functions. See Table 6.1 ■ for the functions of each hemisphere. *Mental health* is the balance of activation, inhibition, and integration of left and right hemisphere control. Yet if one hemisphere is damaged, the other hemisphere seems to be able to take on some of its functions.

Each hemisphere is divided into the *cortex* (the highly convoluted matter on the outside) and the *subcortical structures* (buried within). In fresh tissue, the outer surface of the cortex appears gray due to the presence of cell bodies and dendrites mostly, hence the term *gray matter*. Underneath the gray matter, the tissue appears white due to the presence of large numbers of axons covered in myelin, hence the term *white matter*. The role of the brain in chronic pain conditions is not clearly understood. Twenty-six people with chronic back pain showed 5% to 11% less gray matter volume than their matched control subjects. The amount of this decrease is equivalent to the gray matter volume lost in 10 to 20 years of normal aging. These results imply that chronic pain causes long-term changes in the brain (Apkarian et al., 2004).

The cortex is further divided into four lobes: frontal, parietal, temporal, and occipital (Figure 6.3 ■). The subcortical structures of the cerebrum include the limbic system and the basal ganglia.

Frontal Lobe

The *frontal lobe* is the site of a person's ability to think and plan, and is partially responsible for executive functions, which are discussed later in this chapter. The frontal lobe regulates emotions and behavior and stability of the personality and inhibits primitive emotional responses. It also controls general motor ability and the motor aspects of spoken and written speech. It participates with other brain regions in aspects of learning and memory, attention, and motivation.

The *prefrontal cortex*, right behind the forehead, comprehends the beliefs, intentions, and perspective of others. Damage to the prefrontal cortex in childhood results in problems with empathy for others. The prefrontal cortex is responsible for the emotional component of decision making, especially in the context of interpersonal relationships. Feelings are an important part of decision making, in that feelings point one in the right direction. *Gut* feelings distinguish humans from inanimate computers in the decision-making process.

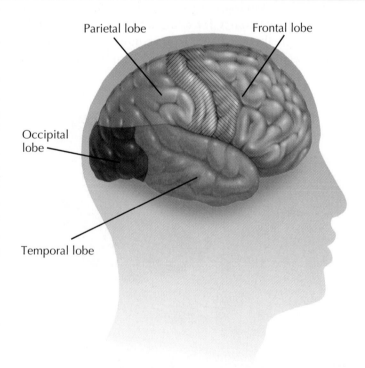

Figure 6.3 ■ The four lobes of the cerebral cortex. Deep fissures in the cortex separate these areas or lobes.

SOURCE: Morris, C. G., & Maisto, A. A. (2001). *Understanding psychology* (5th ed.). Upper Saddle River, NJ: Prentice Hall. Used with permission.

The prefrontal cortex is linked to motivation and the ability to recognize important or desirable things. It is a key brain area involved in the craving of food and addictive drugs. Activity in this brain area peaks in anticipation of a reward, such as when cocaine addicts see white powder or non–drug addicts see and smell the foods they crave (Galvan, Hare, Davidson, Spicer, Glover, & Casey, 2005).

Mental disorders related to frontal lobe problems include schizophrenia, depression, obsessive–compulsive disorder, and substance use disorders.

Parietal Lobe

The parietal lobe is the site of the sensory functions of touch, taste, and temperature and the perception of pain. Additional sensory functions include receptive speech and the ability to envision written words (e.g., to read the word *tree* and visualize a tree).

A significant function of the parietal lobe is **proprioception,** the ability to know where one's body is in time and space (position sense). An example of disordered proprioception sometimes reported by people with mental disorders is the inability to see in three dimensions. This impairment may contribute to difficulty dressing, eating, and drinking in an organized manner.

The parietal lobe also regulates the ability to evaluate muscular activity. This lobe may control a person's capacity to sit motionless for hours or to hold a single body part in one position for long periods of time. Another function of the parietal lobe is the ability to associate the memory of primary sensory experiences with more complex memories. Dysregulation of this function may result in repeating the same mistake over and over.

Temporal Lobe

The temporal lobe is the site of the complex processes of memory, judgment, and learning. It processes the world of sight and sound into meaningful information. The temporal lobe is the site for abnormal perceptions (illusions) and auditory hallucinations. Déjà vu (the sensation of having been somewhere before when one has not been there) and jamais vu (not recognizing familiar places) result from disturbances in the temporal lobe.

The dominant side, usually the left, is involved in understanding and processing language, complex memory, and emotional stability. Increased or decreased activity may contribute to labile moods, intense violent thoughts, aggression, and homicidal or suicidal behavior. Abnormal activity in the nondominant side leads to social skill problems and the inability to recognize facial expression.

The temporal lobe connects with the limbic system to allow for memory and the expression of emotions. Another temporal lobe function is gender identity, the sense of being

female or male. Do not confuse gender identity with sexual orientation, the site of which is deep inside the brain in the anterior hypothalamus (Kassin, 2004).

Occipital Lobe

Unlike the other lobes, which have multiple functions, the occipital lobe has only one function—vision. It is responsible for sight and the ability to understand written words. It is also involved in producing visual hallucinations.

Subcortical Structures
Limbic System

The limbic system is often referred to as *the emotional brain.* Emotional responses such as anger, fear, anxiety, pleasure, sorrow, and sexual feelings are generated in the limbic system but are interpreted in the frontal lobe. The limbic system is the reward center of the brain, which is what motivates people to do something or learn something so they feel satisfied. Another function of the limbic system is the interpretation of our most basic and primitive sense: the sense of smell. The limbic system is thought to be the site of olfactory hallucinations. The ability to interpret sensations from the internal organs, referred to as *visceral reflexes,* also resides in this region.

The limbic system consists of portions of the frontal, parietal, and temporal lobes that form a continuous band of cortex in a ringlike formation around the top of the brain stem. Other structures of the limbic system are the amygdala, the hippocampus, the cingulate gyrus, the nucleus accumbens, the thalamus, and the hypothalamus (See Figure 6.4 ■).

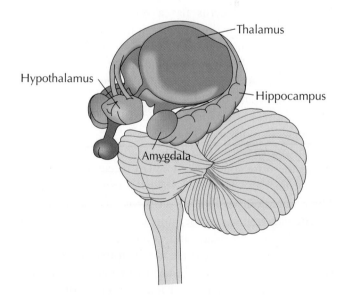

Figure 6.4 ■ The limbic system. Just above the inner core, yet surrounded by the cerebral cortex, the limbic system plays a role in motivation, emotion, and memory. As shown, this system is composed of many structures, including the thalamus, amygdala, hippocampus, and hypothalamus.

SOURCE: Kassin, S. (2001). *Psychology* (3rd ed.). Upper Saddle River, NJ: Prentice Hall. Used with permission.

The *amygdala* coordinates the actions of the autonomic nervous system and the endocrine system and is involved in the control of emotions. It is essential to nurturing behavior and fear conditioning. When something scares or upsets a person, the amygdala stamps that moment in memory. From then on, when something seems to resemble that original moment of distress, the amygdala recognizes the similarity and dictates that person's response in a few 100ths of a second, even before the stimulus reaches the cognitive centers of the person's brain. Dysfunction in the amygdala contributes to inappropriate rage and fear, anxiety, posttraumatic stress disorder (PTSD), and attention deficit/hyperactivity disorder (ADHD) (Sinha, Mohlman, & Gorman, 2004).

The *hippocampus* is the critical information processing station between the parts of the brain that receive sensory experiences and the parts of the brain that translate these experiences into action. It channels sensory input to the appropriate brain area and regulates the resulting motor output pathways. The hippocampus responds to more complex fear cues than does the amygdala, but they act together in generating anxiety.

The hippocampus is intricately involved in regulating the immune system and in collating memories stored in other parts of the brain. Damage or incomplete formation of the hippocampus results in declarative memory impairment. People with hippocampal dysfunction appear to resist learning and may be perceived as lazy or unmotivated, when in fact they are unable to recall previously learned information.

The cingulate gyrus has a role in regulating stress through changes in the autonomic nervous system. It receives more input from the thalamus than any other cortical region. It is also responsible for regulating the emotional content of physical pain. The cingulate gyrus is the executive organizer and directs a person's attention and decides what information gets into the frontal lobes. It is also the link between motivation and behavior.

The *nucleus accumbens* is the reward center of the brain. When there are abnormally low DA receptors in this area, the person has a decreased ability to experience pleasure. Much attention has focused on the nucleus accumbens as the site of action of cocaine, amphetamines, nicotine, marijuana, alcohol, chocolate, and carbohydrates. Levels of DA in the nucleus accumbens are also increased through high-risk behaviors. High-risk behaviors demand increased attention and concentration for long periods of time, which forces an increase in the release of DA. This understanding has led to the identification of a new syndrome—the **reward deficiency syndrome**. The decreased ability to experience pleasure drives the person to seek external forms of gratification through the use of substances, pathological gambling, or other high-risk behaviors.

The *thalamus* enables us to have impressions of agreeableness or disagreeableness in response to sensations. It monitors sensory input and acts as a relay station in processing nearly all sensory and motor information coming from the spinal cord, brain stem, and cerebellum. Pain sensations travel from the spinal cord through the brain stem to the thalamus, which then sends the pain signals to the parietal lobe. Dysfunction within the thalamus makes it difficult for people to sense or interpret pain. The thalamus is thought to regulate levels of awareness and emotional aspects of sensory experiences by exerting a wide variety of effects on the cortex.

Thalamic dysfunction is involved in obsessive–compulsive disorder, schizophrenia, and mood disorders, and contributes to the similarity in symptoms experienced by people diagnosed with various mental disorders.

The *hypothalamus* is a neuroendocrine (neurons that produce hormones) group of nuclei vital to homeostasis. As an integration center, the hypothalamus converts thinking and feeling into hormones, causing physical changes throughout the body via the autonomic nervous system. With the *pituitary gland*, the hypothalamus helps regulate the autonomic nervous system by assisting with the vital functions of water balance, blood pressure, sleep, appetite, temperature, and carbohydrate and fat metabolism. Dysregulation of the hypothalamus can lead to excessive thirst and insatiable hunger. The hypothalamus may be involved in anorexia nervosa and bulimia nervosa. As one of the main concentration sites of the neurotransmitter dopamine, the hypothalamus is implicated in many of the common side effects of psychotropic medications that influence dopamine transmission.

The *suprachiasmatic* nuclei (SCN) in the hypothalamus are responsible for circadian rhythms, which are discussed later in this chapter. Almost all the neurons in the SCN use gamma-aminobutyric acid (GABA) as their primary neurotransmitter. It is not clear how the SCN sets the timing of many important behaviors.

Basal Ganglia

The basal ganglia are areas of brain nuclei that lie in the center of each cerebral hemisphere deep in the temporal lobe (Figure 6.5 ■). The basal ganglia consist of the cau-

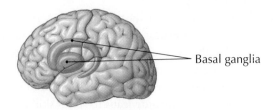

Figure 6.5 ■ Location of the basal ganglia.

SOURCE: Smock, T. K. (1999). *Physiological psychology: A neuroscience approach.* Upper Saddle River, NJ: Prentice Hall. Used with permission.

date, the putamen, and the globus pallidus. The caudate and putamen together are called the *striatum*, which has an important role in the control of movement. The main stimuli to the basal ganglia come from the amygdala, hippocampus, thalamus, and cortex. The basal ganglia participate in many higher brain functions in concert with the cerebral cortex. The purpose of the basal ganglia is to organize complex patterns of thought and movement under the influence of emotional tone (Table 6.2 ■) for brain structures, functions, and dysfunctions.

TABLE 6.2	Major Brain Structures: Functions and Dysfunctions	
Structure	**Functions**	**Effects of Dysfunction**
Frontal lobe	Ability to think and plan	Difficulty with abstract thinking, attention, concentration; lack of motivation
	Insight	Inability for self-evaluation
	Stability of personality	Instability of personality
	Inhibition of primitive emotional responses	Labile affect, irritability; impulsiveness; inappropriate behavior
	Motor aspects of written speech	Unintelligible and illogical writing
	Motor aspects of spoken speech	Words are garbled and difficult to understand
Parietal lobe	Receiving and identifying sensory information	Inability to recognize sensations such as pain, touch, temperature; inability to sense pain from an uncomfortable body position
	Memory association	Inability to learn from past
	Proprioception	Inability to recognize the body in relation to the environment
		Difficulty dressing, eating, etc. in an organized manner
	Sensory speech	Inability to recognize spoken or written words
Temporal lobe	Hearing	Auditory hallucinations
	Complex memory	Memory impairment; difficulty learning
	Emotion	Difficulty recognizing own emotions and controlling sexual and aggressive drives
	Gender identity	Confusion about masculinity and femininity
	Production of speech	Types of aphasia
	Analysis of speech	Difficulty attaching meaning to spoken words
Occipital lobe	Vision	Visual hallucinations; loss of visual memory
	Visual speech	Inability to understand the meaning of written words
Limbic system	Regulation of emotional responses	Excessive emotional responses; inability to recognize own emotions; decreased ability of cognition to affect emotions
	Interpretation of smell	Olfactory hallucinations; inability to interpret smell
	Memory collation	Difficulty with declarative memory
		Working and long-term memory problems; difficulty learning
	Impressions of agreeableness or disagreeableness of sensations	Hypersensitivity or hyposensitivity to pain
	Regulation of autonomic nervous system	Increased thirst; insatiable hunger
Reticular activating system (RAS)	Receiving of impulses from entire body and relaying to cortex	Sedation and loss of consciousness; difficulty controlling aggression; may contribute to passivity
Cerebellum	Coordination of skeletal muscles during movement	Difficulty learning motor skills; problems regulating the force and range of movements
	Maintenance of equilibrium	Problems with balance
	Maintenance of posture	Difficulty walking upright
	Procedural memory	Difficulty performing tasks
	Reward center	Decreased ability to experience pleasure
		Reward deficiency syndrome

Ventricles

There are two large ventricles on either side of the cerebral hemispheres called the lateral ventricles. A smaller one in the center is called the third ventricle, and, in the brain stem, a fourth ventricle communicates with the central canal of the spinal cord. The fluid in the ventricles is called cerebrospinal fluid (CSF), which circulates slowly through the brain and the spinal cord, cushioning the brain from physical shocks. CSF has an excretory function and regulates the chemical environment of the central nervous system. It also acts as a channel for chemical communication within the brain. Neurochemicals secreted by nearby neurons cross into the CSF, circulate, and cross back into the brain at any given point, facilitating communication between different areas of the brain.

Blood–Brain Barrier

The **blood–brain barrier** is a highly regulated membranous barrier of brain capillaries that segregate the central nervous system from systemic blood circulation. Unlike capillaries throughout the rest of the body, brain capillary pores are specialized and do not allow free movement of substances. This permeable barrier serves to protect the brain. The first function is to import critical nutrients and hormones, while exporting metabolic waste products. The second function is to protect the brain against foreign circulating chemicals, thereby protecting it from exposure to potential toxins.

NEUROPHYSIOLOGY

Knowledge of brain physiology is incredibly incomplete in many areas. The current technology used to evaluate brain function has many limitations. It is likely that whatever models are present today will be replaced by more advanced models as understanding expands.

Everyone is subject to fluctuations in brain chemistry. The structures of the brain depend on hundreds of chemicals—glucose, vitamins, minerals, amino acids, and neurotransmitters—to carry out their functions. As a person's brain chemistry fluctuates, he or she experiences episodic problems with speech patterns, memory recall, spontaneous decision making, and any or all of the executive functions. People who experience more severe disruptions in brain chemistry may exhibit symptoms of mental disorders.

Interestingly, during rapid eye movement (REM) sleep, everyone experiences symptoms of mental illness. Nurses can think about their own experiences to help them understand clients' experiences. Box 6.1 describes what happens when a person sleeps.

NEUROENDOCRINE FUNCTION

When a person perceives a stressful event, the limbic–hypothalamus–pituitary–adrenal (LHPA) axis responds. The limbic system alerts the hypothalamus to increase production of corticotropin-releasing factor (CRF), which stimulates the pituitary gland to release adrenocorticotropic hormone (ACTH). ACTH enters the general circulation and travels to the adrenal cortex where it stimulates cortisol release. Cortisol acts throughout the body to mobilize energy reserves in an effort to manage stress. Cortisol, which readily crosses the blood–brain barrier, interacts with specific receptors in the hypothalamus and other parts of the brain, completing the feedback cycle. Problems in neuroendocrine function have been

---

BOX 6.1	How the Brain Goes Out of Its Mind

Every 80–90 minutes, during REM sleep, we become completely psychotic.

Experience	Psychiatric Label
We see things that are not there.	Hallucinations
We believe things that could not possibly be true.	Delusions, magical thinking
We become confused about times, places, and persons.	Disorientation
Scenes simply appear and thoughts come and go.	Attention deficit
We think we are awake even though we are doing and seeing impossible things.	Lack of insight
We experience wildly fluctuating emotions.	Labile affect
We invent implausible narratives.	Confabulation, loose association
We forget almost everything on awakening.	Amnesia

This nocturnal madness is not only normal but probably essential to our health. Deprived of REM sleep, we become anxious and irritable and have trouble concentrating. Understanding this normal delirium may help you become more empathetic with persons experiencing those same symptoms while awake.

SOURCE: LaBerge, S., & Rheingold, H. (1990). *Exploring the world of lucid dreaming.* New York: Ballantine Books.

linked to depression, postpartum psychosis, schizophrenia, panic disorder, obsessive–compulsive disorder, and anorexia.

NEUROTRANSMISSION

Neurotransmission is the electrochemical process that allows nerve signals to pass from one cell to another at the synapse, the microscopic area where two neurons meet. As the impulse travels through the axon of a neuron, storage vesicles release a small amount of stored neurotransmitters, which diffuse across the synapse and latch on to *receptor proteins* embedded in the postsynaptic, or second, neuron. Receptors are specific to one neurotransmitter, much like a lock and key. No matter how much of a neurotransmitter is released, if it does not have a perfect fit, the receptors will not be activated. Binding of the neurotransmitter to the receptor triggers the activation of the second cell. Once the transmitter completes its function, the receptor releases it back into the synapse. At this point, one of two things happens: an enzyme deactivates the transmitter or *transporters* take the transmitter back into the presynaptic terminal (reuptake). Transporters allow the body to recycle previously used transmitters so they do not have to be replaced by biosynthesis (Figure 6.6 ■).

Neuromodulators are chemicals that alter the threshold to the flow of information but do not necessarily alter the nature of the signal. They act as filters, allowing information to be processed, more or less.

The term **ligand** is used to describe any substance that binds to the receptors. Ligands can be subdivided into two categories. **Agonists** bind to and activate the receptor and are described as having weak or strong potency. Agonists include neurotransmitters and hormones as well as drugs. **Antagonists** block the action of a neurotransmitter at its receptors. Once an antagonist occupies the receptor, agonists can no longer bind and neurotransmission is blocked (Figure 6.7 ■).

Neurotransmitters may be deactivated or returned to the presynaptic terminal before they reach the receptors. The postsynaptic neuron can be temporarily deactivated so it fails to respond to the stimulus. Neurotransmitters can act together to enhance transmission of impulses, and at other times they act as antagonists—with one neurotransmitter inhibiting the action of another. Other factors such as hydration, electrolyte balance, overall metabolic demand, and glial cell influences affect the readiness of the

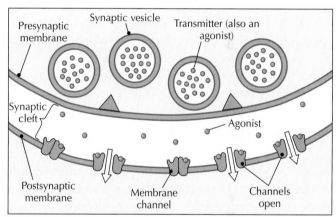

(A) Strong agonist activates receptors without transmission.

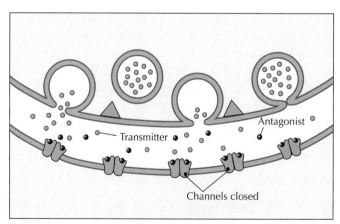

(B) Antagonist blocks receptors. Agonist cannot act.

Figure 6.7 ■ Ligands: Agonists and antagonists. Agonists and antagonists bind to the same binding site as transmitter. An agonist has potency so it activates the cell biologically (A). Antagonists bind and have no potency (B). An antagonist produces its effect by blocking the binding site, preventing a transmitter from binding, and producing its biological effect.

SOURCE: Smock, T. K. (1999). *Physiological psychology: A neuroscience approach.* Upper Saddle River, NJ: Prentice Hall. Used with permission.

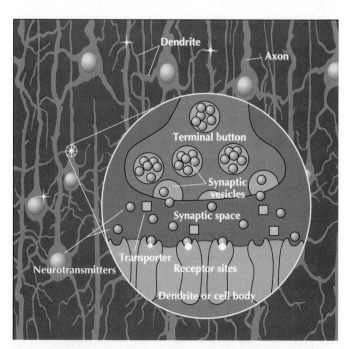

Figure 6.6 ■ Neurotransmission: How neurons communicate.

SOURCE: Morris, C. G., & Maisto, A. A. (2001). *Understanding psychology* (5th ed.). Upper Saddle River, NJ: Prentice Hall. Used with permission.

BOX 6.2	Factors Influencing Rate of Neurotransmission

Speed Up Neurotransmission

- High level of precursors
- Increased synthesis of transmitters
- More transmitters in storage sites
- More transmitters released
- Greater number of receptors
- Slower reuptake process
- Fewer transmitters deactivated

Slow Down Neurotransmission

- Low level of precursors
- Decreased synthesis of transmitters
- Fewer transmitters in storage sites
- Fewer transmitters released
- Not enough receptors
- Faster reuptake process
- Too many transmitters deactivated

neuron to fire. It is evident the process of neurotransmission is complicated, with potential for errors at many points along the way. Box 6.2 shows factors influencing the rate of neurotransmission.

Neurotransmitters

Neurotransmitters are the key information molecules of the brain. We know of at least 50 to 100 possible neurotransmitters, representing diverse chemical *classes*, including the biogenic amines, amino acids, peptides, neurohormones, and gases. **Neurotransmitters** act, as the word implies, to transmit signals from one neuron to another. They can facilitate, activate, or inhibit postsynaptic neurons. Smaller molecule neurotransmitters, such as the biogenic amines, are usually *rapid acting* and generate the most dramatic responses in the brain. The larger and *slower acting* molecules, such as the peptides, have less dramatic effects but cause more long-term alterations at the receptor sites by changing the number or sizes of the synapses. These effects can persist for days.

Neurons in different parts of the brain contain different neurotransmitters. Most neurons have numerous receptor types for a variety of neurotransmitters, enabling each neuron to receive many different signals. In addition, there are several types of receptor sites for each neurotransmitter. For example, there are 5 dopamine receptor types and 18 serotonin receptor types.

It is difficult to fully appreciate the role of neurotransmitters; entire textbooks are devoted to each of them. Neurotransmitters do not operate in isolation. Much like a symphonic orchestra, they interact with each other and function as a group. It is believed that when dysfunctions occur with some neurotransmitters, others adapt and compensate for the dysfunction. See Table 6.3 ▪ for neurotrans-

mitter functions and dysfunctions. You may want to read the principles of psychopharmacology in chapter 10 ∞ after reading this section, as each category of medication affects one or more of the neurotransmitters.

Biogenic Amines

The biogenic amines are more often implicated in the psychobiology of mental disorders. There are six biogenic amine neurotransmitters: dopamine, serotonin, norepinephrine and epinephrine, acetylcholine, and histamine, which are synthesized in neurons. Dopamine, norepinephrine, and epinephrine are synthesized from the same dietary amino acid called *tyrosine*. Serotonin is synthesized from the dietary amino acid called *tryptophan*.

Dopamine Dopamine is the grandparent of neurotransmitters. It is a catecholamine from which norepinephrine and epinephrine are metabolized. An excess or deficit of DA affects the levels of these other neurotransmitters.

DA plays an important role in motor activity, motivation, and reward. High levels of DA are reflected in sharper thinking, focused attention, and formation of long-term memory. It is often referred to as the *learning neurotransmitter*.

DA also provides the motivation to act and find what is needed for survival. When a need is perceived, DA directs the motor system to move the body to get it. DA is also what makes a person smile and feel alert and energetic. It drives one to seek pleasure and rewards and provides an emotional high. DA is the *gotta have it* neurotransmitter, the facilitator, and the motivator. If DA reaches levels that are too high, hypomania or even mania can result (Hunt, 2006).

Dopamine deficiency interferes with learning, memory, and motivation. Antipsychotic drugs, used to treat hallucinations and delusions, block DA receptors, which decreases the ability to feel pleasure. People who are chronically deficient in DA (reward-deficient individuals) often engage in dopamine-boosting activities, such as addictions that range from cigarettes to drug abuse to hypersexuality. Other reward deficiency syndromes include attention deficit/hyperactivity disorder (ADHD) and Tourette syndrome (see chapter 17 ∞). Activities that provide instant reward become more important than long-term goals (Pihl & Benkelfat, 2005).

Serotonin Serotonin (5-HT) plays an important role in mood and emotional behavior. In contrast to DA, 5-HT is the soother, the constrainer, and the anti-impulsive neurotransmitter. The neurotransmitter 5-HT acts to balance DA. It decreases a person's focus and the flow of information. It is what a person needs when she or he is feeling overwhelmed and prevents the person from getting out of control from fear or worry. This neurotransmitter is calming and elevates mood and self-esteem. Abnormally low levels of 5-HT, when combined with other genetic factors and

TABLE 6.3	Neurotransmitters: Functions and Dysfunctions		
Neurotransmitter	**Functions**	**Effects of Excess**	**Effects of Deficit**
Dopamine (DA)	Abstract thinking, decision making Pleasure and reward system Integration of thoughts and emotions Increase in sex drive, facilitation of orgasm	Mild: Enhanced creativity and problem solving; ability to generalize situations; good spatial ability; premature ejaculation Severe: Disorganized thinking, loose associations; disabling compulsions; tics; stereotypic behaviors	Mild: Poor impulse control; poor spatial ability; inability to think abstractly; no joy, no anticipation of pleasure Severe: Parkinson disease; endocrine changes; movement disorders
Norepinephrine (NE) Epinephrine (E)	Alertness, ability to focus attention, ability to be oriented Necessary for learning and memory Primes nervous system for fight or flight	Hyperalertness; anxiety, panic Paranoia Loss of appetite Increased sensation-seeking behaviors	Dullness, low energy Depression
Serotonin (5-HT)	Inhibition of activity; calmness, contentedness Regulation of temperature of sleep cycle Pain perception Precursor to melatonin, which plays a role in circadian rhythms	Sedation; decreased anxiety Increased sleep Decreased sex drive; decreased orgasms Indecision Craving for sweets and carbohydrates If greatly increased, may have hallucinations	Irritability, hostility; increased aggresssion Decreased impulse control; increased suicidal tendencies Insomnia Increased sex drive
Acetylcholine (ACh)	Preparation for action; stimulation of parasympathetic system Emotional regulation Social play, exploration Control of muscle tone by balance with DA	Self-consciousness, excessive inhibition; anxiety Somatic complaints Depression	Lack of inhibition; euphoria Poor short-term memory Antisocial behaviors Parkinson disease
GABA	Calmness, contentedness Reduction of aggression	Sedation Impaired recent memory Anticonvulsant	Irritability Lack of coordination Seizures

environmental stressors, may result in decreased impulse control, aggression, and violence (Pihl & Benkelfat, 2005).

The neurotransmitter 5-HT is the *got it* neurotransmitter, which allows a person to stop a particular behavior when the person achieves what she or he needs. For example, when a person is hungry DA drives the person to search for food and 5-HT lets the person know when she or he has had enough to eat. Without 5-HT, the person would be unable to stop eating once she or he found food.

Due to its broad range of functions, 5-HT is quickly becoming the most widely researched neurotransmitter. It tends to control the activity of other neurotransmitters and is the key player in all brain functions related to circadian

rhythms. It is synthesized from the dietary amino acid tryptophan.

A significant research finding relevant to mental health nursing is that isolation reduces 5-HT levels. This finding helps to explain some of the devastating effects of seclusion on many clients. The converse is also true. Spending time in the company of people who are trusted can raise 5-HT levels. Cocaine, alcohol, and nicotine are known to reduce 5-HT levels. Newer antidepressants are selective inhibitors of 5-HT reuptake, keeping more 5-HT available in the synapse.

Norepinephrine and Epinephrine Norepinephrine (NE) and epinephrine (E) are derived from dopamine and are the

MediaLink Care Plan, Genetic Links

adrenaline of the brain. Although NE accounts for only 1% of all available neurotransmitter content, people are very sensitive to even the smallest fluctuations. NE is the primary neurotransmitter mediating the sympathetic nervous system and is the key component of the emergency fight–flight system of the brain. NE increases attention and decreases pain sensitivity. It also serves to enhance memory for stressful and traumatic events. Individuals who take antidepressants that increase NE may experience side effects of agitation and irritability (Hunt, 2006; Sinha, Mohlman, & Gorman, 2004).

Acetylcholine Acetylcholine (ACh) is found in abundance in the brain and is the "guardian angel" of the parasympathetic nervous system. ACh continually strives to keep the sympathetic nervous system in check. DA and ACh function in relative balance. ACh is thought to greatly influence learning and memory; it may also be involved in mood and sleep disorders. Other effects include emotional regulation, social play, exploration, thermoregulation, water intake, and motor function.

There are two types of ACh receptors: muscarinic and nicotinic. Blockage of the muscarinic receptors results in the anticholinergic side effects of many of the psychotropic medications. Nicotine acts at the nicotinic ACh receptors, causing widespread effects on the central and peripheral nervous systems. Nicotine enhances cognition, improves attention, decreases stress, and regulates weight. These effects contribute to tobacco dependence. The medication succinylcholine (Anectine) is a nicotinic receptor antagonist that is given to clients receiving electroconvulsive therapy to induce muscle relaxation and prevent injury-producing muscle contractions.

ACh and glutamate also act on the glia and increase the production of *nerve growth factor* (NGF). NGF accelerates nerve fiber growth necessary for synapse formation and strengthens synapses.

Histamine Little is known about the functions of histamine as a neurotransmitter. We do know that histamine is involved in allergic reactions and may be involved in the medication side effects of sedation and hypotension. Recent research has suggested that histamine plays a role in sexual behavior.

Amino Acids

The major inhibitory amino acid neurotransmitters are GABA and glycine. The major excitatory amino acid neurotransmitters are glutamate and aspartate. Glycine and aspartate appear to be particularly active in the spinal cord.

Gamma-Aminobutyric Acid Gamma-aminobutyric acid is the principal inhibitory neurotransmitter and is present in 25% to 40% of the synapses. GABA regulates anxiety and influences muscular coordination. Deficiencies can cause a high level of tension and anxiety, a lack of coordination, and expression of epileptic seizures. GABA may play a role in cognition, memory, and aggressive behavior. It is also one of the neurotransmitters involved in antianxiety medication dependence. Antianxiety medications partially fill the receptor sites normally filled by GABA, and the normal production of GABA is reduced. Over time, the brain becomes reliant on the exogenous antianxiety agents to fill the receptor sites, and dependency results.

Glutamate Glutamate is one of the most abundant neurotransmitters; it is stored in large quantities, and is the main excitatory neurotransmitter. Glu excites neurons and makes them fire. Without glu, brain neurons could not communicate. Glu is important to learning and memory as well as to the development and strengthening of synapses. Blockage of glu receptors stimulates symptoms of schizophrenia.

Too much glu in the brain can lead to a number of brain diseases and even death. Glu-induced cell death is seen in stroke, epilepsy, brain damage due to hypoglycemia, brain trauma, Alzheimer disease, and amyotrophic lateral sclerosis. Damage to neurons releases toxic levels of glu, which rapidly kill neurons by overexciting them, a process called **excitotoxicity**. The administration of glu antagonists appears to prevent cell death. The same process seems to occur in situations of uncontrolled neuron firing, such as during repeated seizures. The process is less clear in Alzheimer disease in which destruction of certain brain areas is responsible for the devastating memory loss. When the same brain area is treated with excitotoxins in animals, they exhibit characteristic memory deficits and plaques and tangles (Farber & Newcomer, 2003).

Faulty functioning of glu receptors leads to an increase in the release of glu. Glu overstimulation contributes to disinhibition symptoms in cognition and behavior. Lamictal (lamotrigine), a mood-stabilizing anticonvulsant medication, inhibits excessive release of glu.

Neuropeptides

Neuropeptides include substance P, neurotensin, L-tryptophan (L-T), neuropeptide Y (NPY), vasoactive intestinal polypeptide (VIP), galanin, cholecystokinin (CCK), and orexins. These neurotransmitters were discovered only recently and their functions are just being understood. Neuropeptides are large molecules stored in and released from secretory granules in axon terminals. Because peptides are often found in the same neuron with other neurotransmitters, they may serve as modulators for other transmitters, the neuroendocrine system, and the autonomic system.

Galanin can affect memory, mood, learning, epilepsy, and weight. Too little may lead to increased pain and seizures. Too much may cause memory loss, depression, and obesity. Researchers are hopeful that galanin may be the foundation for the next era of psychotropic medications.

CCK has a high density in the brain areas that mediate anxiety and is linked to panic attacks. CCK produces anxiety by itself and in conjunction with other neurotransmitters. CCK also has a role in inhibiting food intake in adults (Weller, 2006).

Orexins are produced in the hypothalamus. Orexins affect sleep and arousal and are implicated in narcolepsy. It is believed that they play a role in hunger and satiation by interacting with other hypothalamic peptides. They may also affect cardiovascular function via sympathetic nervous activity. There is a strong indication that orexins are involved with reward and motivation (Kotz, 2006; Samson, Taylor, & Ferguson, 2005).

Neurohormones

Hormones are chemical substances produced by cells within an organ or gland. Hormones are manufactured and stored in the cells. When the cells receive the appropriate signal, usually from the nervous system, they release an appropriate amount of the stored hormone into the circulatory system. Neurohormones are those hormones that act as neurotransmitters or modify the actions of neurotransmitters. Neurohormone examples that relate to mental disorders are endorphin and enkephalin, dehydroepiandrosterone (DHEA), oxytocin, vasopressin, phenylethylamine (PEA), estrogen, and androgens.

Endorphin and Enkephalin Endorphin and enkephalin are opioids that are produced in the brain from a complex chain of amino acids. They play a significant role in the ability to experience pleasure and protect from pain perception. Being touched and stroked by another person increases the amount of endorphin in the brain. Endorphin also increases when a person smiles and when a person thinks positive thoughts. We may smile because we are experiencing a surge of endorphin or we may get a surge of endorphin when we smile.

DHEA There is more DHEA in our bodies than any other hormone. It could be called the parent of all hormones because most of our other hormones are derived from it. Although most of our DHEA is produced by the adrenals, our brain can make its own. DHEA improves cognition, protects the immune system, decreases cholesterol, promotes bone growth, and serves as an antidepressant. As the precursor of pheromones, it influences who we find attractive and who is attracted to us. DHEA serves as a natural aphrodisiac and increases in the brain during orgasm.

Oxytocin Oxytocin is secreted from the pituitary gland and travels to receptor sites in various parts of the brain and to the reproductive tract. It increases DA, 5-HT, estrogen, testosterone, prolactin, and vasopressin. Oxytocin promotes touching and touching produces more oxytocin. Oxytocin is instrumental in the bonding between mates and between parents and children. It decreases cognition and impairs memory.

Vasopressin Vasopressin balances the influence of oxytocin. It improves cognition through enhancing attention and alertness while reducing emotional extremes. One benefit of vasopressin is its influence on how we think. It focuses us on the present and helps us pay attention to what we are doing. It is an antidote for anxiety and depression. Increased levels of vasopressin may be related to higher levels of aggression. Serotonin may be a balancing factor by inhibiting vasopressin-induced anger by stopping its release in the hypothalamus.

PEA PEA is a natural form of amphetamine produced in the brain and fluctuates according to thoughts, feelings, and experiences. It is believed that PEA is the *hormone of love*, rising to high levels during romantic times and is possibly involved in "love at first sight." Low levels of PEA have been associated with depression, and high levels may contribute to psychotic symptoms.

Estrogen and Testosterone There are receptors for estrogen and testosterone all over the brain. These hormones influence everything from emotions to cognition and memory. These hormones can make brain cells and dendrites grow or disappear, can create neurotransmitters, and can turn genes on or off. Estrogen also serves as an antioxidant, destroying destructive free radicals.

During early puberty, the hypothalamus stimulates the pituitary to secrete follicle stimulating hormone (FSH). FSH in turn stimulates the ovaries to produce estrogen and the testes to produce testosterone. Women have 10 times as much estrogen as men and men have 10 times as much androgen as women. In males, androgen can be turned into estrogen. Estrogen levels change on a monthly schedule. Testosterone levels change many times during the day, by as much as 150%. Testosterone levels are lowest at noon. When a man is faced with a challenge, the levels rise abruptly. In contrast, when a man experiences a competitive loss, such as a team sport, there is an abrupt drop in the level of testosterone (Strauch, 2003).

Melatonin Melatonin, originally discovered as a hormone of the pineal gland, is also synthesized in the immune system. Melatonin serves as an immunostimulator agent in infection, inflammation, and autoimmunity. There may be a future role in melatonin preventing the progression of neurodegenerative diseases (Carrillo-Vico, Guerrero, Lardone, & Reiter, 2005; Poeggeler, 2005).

Melatonin also regulates the sleep–wake cycle and other biological rhythms. A shift in sleep timing occurs at puberty. Adolescents start to secrete melatonin 2 hours later than when they were younger. The impact of the melatonin also lingers longer in the morning hours. Therefore, teens stay up late, sleep late in the morning, and most need 9 hours of sleep a night (Strauch, 2003).

Gases In the brain, *nitric oxide* (NO) is formed in the neurons in response to the release of other neurotransmitters. As a gas, it cannot, however, be stored in the synaptic vesicles. NO is a neurotransmitter involved in vasodilation of blood vessels in the brain. Low levels of NO lead to chronic vasoconstriction, brain hypoperfusion, and eventual neuronal death. NO stimulates the DA receptors involved in memory and learning (Keilhoff, 2005; Pak, Cadet, Mantione, & Stefano, 2005).

Similar to NO, *carbon monoxide* (CO) is a gas that is active in the brain. CO inhibits platelet aggregation, thus preventing excessive clotting and diminished blood flow. CO works with NO in vasodilation.

Cyclic Patterns

The daily lives of all living things are filled with various changes that take place in cyclic patterns. **Circadian rhythms** are regular fluctuations of a variety of physiological factors over 24 hours. These include adrenal, thyroid, and growth hormone–secreting patterns, as well as temperature, sleep, arousal, energy, appetite, and motor activity patterns. *Ultradian rhythms* are regular fluctuations shorter than 24 hours and repeat more than once a day. An example of an ultradian rhythm is the 90-minute REM/non-REM sleep cycle. *Infradian rhythms* are regular fluctuations over periods longer than 24 hours, such as the menstrual cycle.

The biological clock, or internal pacemaker, is located in the suprachiasmatic nuclei in the hypothalamus. Neurons in the SCN are sensitive to light, which coordinates sleeping and waking with light–dark cycles. It is not yet clear how the SCN sets the timing of so many important behaviors.

Rhythms may be desynchronized by external or internal factors. An example of external desynchronization is jet lag, in which rapid time zone changes result in decreased energy levels and ability to concentrate, as well as mood variations. In some individuals, internal desynchronization may result in depression or manic episodes. The tendency toward internal desynchronization is probably inherited, but stresses, lifestyle, and normal aging also influence it.

FUNCTIONS OF THE BRAIN

The brain is the site of all nonconscious and conscious processing. Most of the brain's work is done *nonconsciously*, that is, by automatic selection of perceptual, cognitive, and behavioral routines that are appropriate to the situation. This type of processing is fast and efficient, which is critically important. The lowest levels of the brain are specialized for

the quick and automatic handling of routine tasks, such as reflexes, eye movements, and basic perceptions that do not require deliberate processing. Simple tasks like talking and walking become automatic early in childhood. Nonconscious processing allows a person to devote her or his limited *conscious processing* capacity to higher level activities, such as self-monitoring, planning, and organizing actions. This awareness of oneself and the outside world occurs at higher brain levels. In a well-functioning brain, nonconscious and conscious processes work in tandem.

The brain relies on complex feedback and "feedforward" systems for the regulation of activity. **Feedback** dynamics allow for modification of a behavior while it is in progress. For example, a toddler has just stepped into the busy street. In running toward the child, perceptual input is assimilated—obstacles in the way, how close the cars are to the child—as the person is running. **Feedforward** is the prediction of what is about to occur without waiting for feedback. Thus, behavior—running toward the child—is begun before the situation is fully understood. Feedback and feedforward work together. Feedback provides more precise control of behavior but also requires more processing, which is slower. Feed-forward quickly takes the person to the needed area or initiates the necessary response.

Executive Functions

Executive functions of the brain are complex cognitive abilities that include interpreting, analyzing, sorting, and retrieving information about internal and external environments. It also includes the ability to assess one's strengths and weaknesses, plan ahead, and problem solve. The executive brain makes decisions and acts on those decisions. *Insight* is the ability to observe oneself and come to an understanding of the motivation for one's behavior. Nurses will find that some of their clients lack insight; that is, the clients have little or no ability to observe their own behavior or determine if it is appropriate for the situation. The ability to *regulate behavior* is another executive function. This allows a person to stop purposeless or inappropriate behavior and to initiate and complete goal-directed activity. Problems in regulating behavior result in either distractibility or apathy. Clients who are *distractible* find it difficult or impossible to inhibit their responses to a wide range of internal and external stimuli and are unable to focus their attention. Clients who are *apathetic* are unable to start or follow through with even simple self-care activities without being told to do so.

Memory

Learning is the gathering of new knowledge, and **memory** is the retention of that knowledge for future use. Memory is not static but changes over time and involves a variety of brain systems. Without memory, you would be unable to read this sentence or find your way to school tomorrow or recognize family members. Memory provides the foundation for learning throughout life. Every thought a person has, every word a person speaks, a person's very sense of self and her or his sense of connectedness to others, is owed to memory, to the ability of the brain to record and store experiences. It is why the loss of memory due to Alzheimer disease or accidents is so profound.

Working/Short-Term Memory

Two types of memory exist: *working,* or *short-term, memory* and long-term memory. Working memory, lasting minutes to hours, causes temporary changes in the function of neurons. If the memory is to last longer, it must be transferred

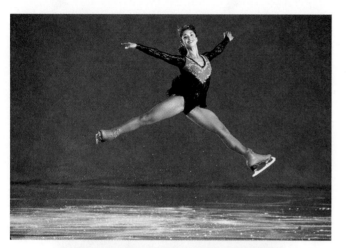

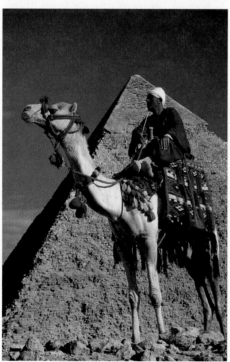

PHOTO 6.1 ■ There are two types of long-term memory. Procedural memory contains knowledge of various skills, such as how to figure skate. Declarative memory contains knowledge of facts, for example, what a pyramid is or where it can be found.

Source: William R. Sallaz/PCN Photography; © Dave Bartruff/Danita Delimont.com. Used with permission.

into a long-term memory store. Working memory allows us to ignore distractions so that we can make sense out of what we experience at any given moment. It is a place for briefly holding on to information such as a telephone number. It also allows us to make judgments, anticipate consequences, and take responsibility.

Long-Term Memory

Long-term memory is activated only if the stimulation is strong and repetitive (Figure 6.8 ■). So yes, it would pay to read this chapter more than once before the exam! In general, events that cause great joy or pain are easier to recall. Bits and pieces of a single memory are stored in different neuronal groups all around the brain. It is believed that the hippocampus brings these pieces together when it is time to recall that memory. Rather than storing memories, the hippocampus collates memories (Pelham & Lovell, 2005).

The REM stage of sleep is important to human memory. Brain wave activity in the hippocampus during REM sleep consolidates experiences into long-term memory. This is evidenced by experiments interrupting either REM sleep or non-REM sleep 60 times a night. When REM sleep is interrupted, there is a complete block of learning, while interruption of non-REM sleep appears to have no effect on learning. It is believed, therefore, that REM sleep is critical for organizing the pieces for long-term memory.

Memories are imperfect and suggestible. The act of imagining an event makes it familiar, and this familiarity later gets mistakenly remembered as a past experience. Memory is modified each time it is remembered. We write and rewrite the stories of ourselves by editing and changing memories. Keep in mind that memory is vulnerable to the power of suggestion and that memory cannot be taken as truth. For example, a therapist may believe that a client was abused as a child and shares this perspective with the client. Unconsciously, the client then fabricates a memory of abuse and then comes to believe the abuse is true. Thus, false memories reflect an error in reconstructing past experiences (Laney & Loftus, 2005). Long-term memory is divided into two types: declarative and procedural memory. *Declarative memory* is memory for people and facts, is consciously accessible, and can be verbally expressed (i.e., can be declared). The hippocampus and the medial temporal lobes are the seat of declarative memory. But the process of capturing and recalling information spreads throughout the brain, often in milliseconds. Each memory seems to be a compilation of tiny bits of information stored in a vast network of different cells. Just the simple ability to recall a phone number is believed to involve the activation of several thousand neurons throughout the brain. *Procedural memory* (knowing how) does not require conscious awareness and involves the memory of motor skills and procedures, such as riding a bicycle or typing a paper. The basal ganglia are involved in procedural memory.

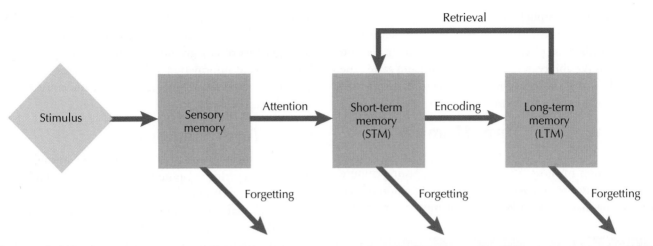

Figure 6.8 ■ An information-processing model of memory. Many stimuli register in sensory memory. Those that are noticed are briefly stored in short-term memory, and those that are encoded are transferred to a more permanent facility. As shown, forgetting may be caused by failures of attention, encoding, or retrieval.

SOURCE: Kassin, S. (2001). *Psychology* (3rd ed.). Upper Saddle River, NJ: Prentice Hall. Used with permission.

Cognition and Language

People with mental disorders may have noticeable problems in the form and content of their thinking and speech. *Abstract thinking* is the ability to generalize information, make predictions, build on prior memory, and evaluate the consequences of decisions. It is also the ability to appreciate nuances in meaning and use metaphors and allegories. In the absence of abstract thought, thinking becomes concrete. *Concrete thinking* is characterized by a focus on facts and details, a literal interpretation of messages, and an inability to generalize. Concrete thinking is a significant problem in people with mental disorders because it results in impulsiveness, instant need gratification, egocentricity, and an inability to follow a multiple-stage command. An example of a concrete response to an abstract question is as follows:

Nurse: "You said you spend a lot of time taking care of your mom and the house. Do you have any outside interests?"

Client: "Yes, I cut the grass."

When there is no apparent relationship between thoughts, the person is said to have *loose association*. A person appears to have *illogical thinking* when expressed ideas are inconsistent, irrational, or self-contradictory. Some people exhibit *tangential speech* when thoughts veer from the main idea and never get back to it. *Circumstantial speech* occurs when the person includes many unnecessary and insignificant details before arriving at the main idea. A person is said to have *pressured speech* when her or his speech is rapid, tense, strained, and difficult to interrupt.

Language functions are distributed throughout the brain more than previously thought. The sound of a word may be in one area and the meaning of that word may be in another area. Language is primarily in the left hemisphere in 90% of the population, in the right hemisphere in 5% of the population, and split evenly in 5% of the population. The emotional aspect of language is located in the right hemisphere for most of us. The left inferior frontal cortex is involved in the production of audible speech and also where we engage in *self-talk*. Self-talk is part of problem solving as we think of solutions, consider consequences, and make decisions. Self-talk is indispensable for the development of empathy, understanding, and cooperation, which are basic to human social interaction.

Emotion

Emotions are responses evoked by environmental stimuli and are the result of multiple brain and body systems working together. When an emotional stimulus enters the brain, it goes through two pathways. One pathway is for a body reaction via the limbic system. The stimulus goes to the amygdala for motor responses, the anterior cingulate for autonomic nervous system responses, the hypothalamus for endocrine responses, and the brain stem for heart rate and breathing responses. The other pathway is to the cerebral cortex where a cognitive assessment is made. For example, when we see a growling dog (stimulus), our body prepares for fight or flight and we begin to run away (body reaction) even before our brain registers that we are afraid (cognitive assessment) (See Figure 6.9 ■).

Negative emotions motivate people to withdraw from or avoid situations. Positive emotions motivate people to approach situations. Highly arousing situations create more intense physiologic reactions and allow people to direct energy toward those situations most crucial to survival.

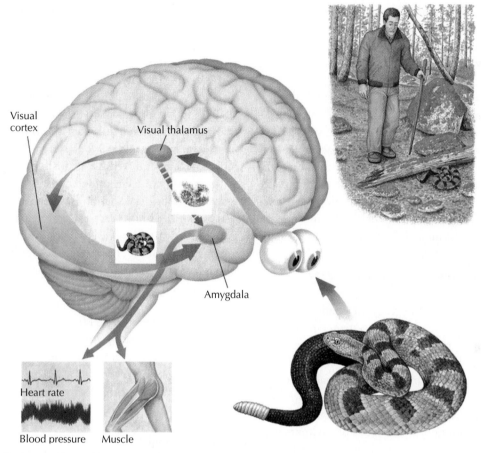

Figure 6.9 ■ Pathway of fear without "thought."
SOURCE: Kassin, S. (2001). *Psychology* (3rd ed.). Upper Saddle River, NJ: Prentice Hall. Used with permission.

There are four basic emotions: fear, anger, sadness, and joy, although some researchers would add surprise, disgust, and guilt. All other emotions are combinations of these four.

Fear is the fastest physical reaction possible as the body is flooded with adrenaline. As just described, the most rapid pathway is through the limbic system, which provides a fast but less accurate assessment of the danger. The pathway to the frontal cortex is slower but provides a more accurate assessment of the danger.

It is important that all social animals, including humans, be able to control their *anger* and aggression. When the frontal lobes are underactive and executive function is compromised, anger may turn to aggression. Frontal lobe activity is necessary to restrict impulses.

Sadness ranges from feeling blue to uncontrollable crying. Sadness allows us to regroup and process what we are experiencing. Sadness may also be motivation to change. When a person is feeling sad, activity in the left amygdala and right frontal cortex is increased and activity in the right amygdala and left frontal cortex is decreased. When a person is sad for long periods of time, the store of neurotransmitters is depleted and the person enters a state of depression or emotional numbness.

Joy is its own incentive. DA and endorphins play an important role in the nucleus accumbens. One of the side effects of medications that block DA is a sense of unhappiness and lack of motivation. When DA levels are too high, euphoric, disorganized, and psychotic behavior may be seen.

Mood is more difficult to define than emotions. **Mood** is the pervasive and sustained quality of a person's emotional tone. Mood, compared with emotions, is less clearly related to environmental stimuli, more long-lasting, more diffuse, and more subjective. It is believed that people have an inborn set point for mood. This means that people have a steady, overall sense of happiness or sadness. Although mood may change with life circumstances, it will inevitably return to the base level (Bhangoo, Deveney, & Leibenluft (2003).

Motivation

Motivation is not an emotion per se, but ties emotion to action. **Motivation** is an inner state that energizes us to create goals and guides goal-directed behavior. It is what drives us to act. Motivation is adaptive, allowing flexible responses to ever-changing contexts. It allows goals and values to influence both perception and action. In any context, there is an infinite range of possible actions or responses. If we had to sort through all the possibilities, we would get bogged down. The motivational system quickly inhibits irrelevant actions and narrows the field of possible actions to a short list (Marin & Chakravosty, 2005).

The cingulate gyrus, part of the limbic system, is the link between motivation and behavior. Outputs to the basal ganglia cause a motor reaction, outputs to the brain stem lead to physiological arousal, and outputs to the hippocampus contribute to memory formation. Disorders of motivation include impulse control disorders and obsessive–compulsive disorder. *Apathy* is a dysfunction of motivation or a malfunction of the motivation circuits of the brain and is a symptom in a number of mental disorders.

PSYCHONEUROIMMUNOLOGY

Psychoneuroimmunology is the study of relationships between the environment, the hormonal system, the immune system, and the central nervous system. Today we recognize that the highly complex immune system interacts with an equally complex nervous system in a bidirectional manner.

Stress is an aversive state of arousal triggered by the perception that an event threatens a person's ability to cope effectively. Stress includes not only a wide range of environmental events, but also reactions to nerve-wracking life events. The field of psychoneuroimmunology is now providing evidence about the ways in which stressors, and the negative emotions that they generate, can be translated into physiologic changes.

Acute stressors are minor disturbances that often are insignificant in terms of general health. Acute stressors may affect health, however, when people are already at risk because of high long-term or severe stress, such as chronic pain, long-term job stress, or severe relationship difficulties. In this situation, a moderate acute stressor can change the balance and contribute to illness. *Chronic stressors* may also affect health. The effect of daily, repeating stress is more pronounced than the effect of a major life event such as death or divorce. More important than the number of daily stressors is the person's sense of control over stressors in terms of immune response (Glaser & Kiecolt-Glaser, 2005).

The *immune system* is a surveillance system that protects the body. The immune system responds to a person's internal and external environments. It must distinguish between normal cells and malignant cells and identify and destroy foreign and disease-causing organisms.

Cytokines are the chemical messengers of the immune system. They coordinate antibody and T-cell immune interactions; they include interferons, lymphokines, and interleukins. Because cytokines are closely associated with neurotransmitters and because stress stimulates cytokine production, researchers are beginning to investigate a possible role for cytokines in major mental disorders such as depression, schizophrenia, and Alzheimer disease (Starkweather, Witek-Janusek, & Mathews, 2005).

The central nervous system and the immune system work as an integrated whole to maintain a state of healthy balance within the body. Dysregulation in one induces change in the other. The pathways of communication are the autonomic nervous system and the neuroendocrine system. The autonomic nervous system innervates all the immune tissue and releases transmitters that activate the immune system. The other communication pathway involves hormone production by the hypothalamus and pituitary gland. These hormones are capable of altering the function of virtually every type of immune cell. The release of many of these hormones is significantly related to thoughts and feelings. Each thought and feeling has a chemical consequence within the brain relating to the production of neurotransmitters and neurohormones by the limbic system (Motzer & Hretig, 2004).

Cognitive and sociocultural stimuli are among the most potent factors in activating the biological responses to stress. An example is the effect of bereavement on a person's health. After the death of a spouse, the surviving spouse's risk for death is especially high during the first six months. This increased risk is thought to be related to a depressed immune system.

NUTRITIONAL NEUROSCIENCE

Nutritional neuroscience is a new research area regarding ways to keep the brain functioning at a peak level with supplements, diet, and other lifestyle changes.

Glucose is needed for neurotransmitter synthesis and secretion. Other necessary nutrients are amino acids, vitamins, minerals, and essential fatty acids. For example, brain cells need tryptophan to create 5-HT and choline to synthesize ACh. The B vitamins are necessary for synthesis of 5-HT and GABA, and copper and tyrosine are needed for DA synthesis. Carnitine promotes cognition, magnesium is involved in sleep, and vitamin C is needed to cope with stress. Cholesterol is necessary to make myelin that surrounds and protects nerve fibers. Rapidly lowered cholesterol levels are associated with depression, anxiety, panic disorder, violence, and suicide. Memory loss, confusion, depression, and other mental problems in the elderly, once thought to be part of normal aging, can result from a poor diet.

Omega-3-type fish oil is necessary to keep the brain in top shape. It is composed of two specific fatty acids: DHA (docosahexaenoic acid) and EPA (eicosapentaenoic acid). Essential fatty acids maintain pliability of neurons and synthesize neurotransmitters and molecules of the immune system. Fatty acids must be supplied from the diet and are found in omega-3-rich seafood, green leafy vegetables, flax seed, canola oil, walnuts, Brazil nuts, seaweed, and algae. Although the brain needs a continuous supply throughout life, there are two particularly sensitive periods—infancy and aging. Fatty acid deficiency during infancy delays brain development and in aging will accelerate deterioration of brain functions (Yehuda, Rabinovitz, & Mostofsky, 2005).

Oxidative damage may play a key role in the pathology of neurodegenerative diseases such as Alzheimer disease and Parkinson disease. *Antioxidants* are critically important for optimal brain function, as discussed earlier in the chapter. It is often necessary to take antioxidant vitamins such as vitamin A, thiamine, folic acid, vitamin C, vitamin E, and coenzyme Q10 in supplemental form because most Western diets do not contain high enough levels. Vitamin A acts as an antioxidant and is closely related to the carotenoids, including beta-carotene, alpha-carotene, lycopene, lutein, and xeazanthin. These are found in deeply colored fruits and vegetables. Flavonoids, found in citrus fruits and berries, are also antioxidants. Nutrients with the highest levels of antioxidants are prunes, raisins, blueberries, blackberries, garlic, kale, cranberries, strawberries, spinach, raspberries, and tomatoes, as well as black and green tea and red wine. Vitamin C is an antioxidant required for tissue growth and repair. It also aids in the production of interferon, which enhances immunity. Vitamin E inhibits the oxidation of lipids and the formation of free radicals. It also aids in the utilization of vitamin A. Coenzyme Q10 may be an even more powerful antioxidant than vitamin E. It has also been used to improve mental function in people with schizophrenia and Alzheimer disease (Beal, 2004; Fontaine, 2005; Shults, 2005).

DYSREGULATION

The ability to function and problem solve in everyday life depends on how the brain functions and processes information. Dysregulation of the brain, regardless of the cause, results in disruption of the ability to process information. There are four main causes of brain dysregulation: anatomical abnormalities or damage, lack of oxygen or glucose, electrolyte imbalance, and neurotransmitter dysfunction (see Table 6.4 ■). It is important to understand the current information in biological psychiatry in order to respond to the client as a bio-psycho-social-spiritual being.

It is essential to understand the contribution of neurobiology to mental illness. For example, it is important to teach clients and families about neurotransmitter imbalances and the rationale for biochemical treatment (medications). It is hoped that when society recognizes that mental disorders are brain diseases, the current level of stigma will decrease or go away.

TABLE 6.4	Causes of Brain Dysregulation	
Cause	**Source**	**Clinical Implications**
Anatomical abnormalities	Trauma Brain tumors Problems in brain development	Difficulty in information processing and coping with daily life stressors
Lack of oxygen and/or glucose	Blood flow to brain slowed Lack of oxygen in blood Insufficient food intake	Symptoms of dementia, delirium, and schizophrenia
Alteration in electrolytes	Insufficient food intake Disordered electrolyte balance	Behavior may be stuporous or manic Hallucinations and delusions may occur Anxiety may be experienced
Neurotransmitter dysfunction	Substance abuse Diets high in sugar and fat Genetic influence	Symptoms of depression, bipolar disorder, schizophrenia, and panic disorder; difficulty in information processing and coping with daily life stressors

Focus Your Study

OBJECTIVES

KEY CONCEPTS

1. Describe the development of the brain over the life span.

- Genes and environment interact from conception to death.
- Genes give direction for initial brain development and provide the broad outline of development.
- Environmental factors turn genes on or off, causing cells to differentiate, divide, sprout new connections, or strengthen other connections.
- The infant's brain has twice as many neurons as the adult brain, but relatively few synapses; weak or unused neurons are pruned away.
- By 2 years of age, there are twice as many synapses as in the adult brain; between the ages of 7 and 15 years they are pruned back by almost 40%.
- Teens do not have the fully developed prefrontal cortex to regulate their impulsive behavior and quick emotions.
- The aging brain processes information more slowly. Mental stimulation builds more synapses, which appears to make brains more resistant to deterioration.
- Neuroplasticity allows the brain to improve itself, refine structures, and respond to internal and external changes.

2. Relate the functions of the brain to its major anatomical features.

- The brain stem is responsible for vital functions such as respiration, heart rate, and blood pressure. It is also the home of the 12 cranial nerves.
- The cerebellum is responsible for posture, equilibrium, skeletal movement, and procedural memory. It is also involved in timing and rhythm of brain function and recognizing social cues.
- The frontal lobe is responsible for thinking and planning, regulating emotions, stability of personality, regulating motor activity, and the motor aspects of spoken and written speech. It participates with other regions in learning, memory, attention, and motivation.
- The parietal lobe is the site of the sensory functions of touch, taste, temperature, and pain. It is also the site for receptive speech, the ability to envision written words, and proprioception.
- The temporal lobe is involved in complex memory, analysis and production of speech, emotional stability, and gender identity.
- The occipital lobe has only one function, which is vision.
- The limbic system is involved in regulating emotions, collating memories, interpreting smell, and regulating the autonomic nervous system; the reward center of the brain is located here.

3. Describe the functions of the different neurotransmitters.

- Dopamine is involved in motor activity, motivation, reward, abstract thinking, and decision making.
- Serotonin elevates mood and self-esteem and induces a sense of calm.
- Norepinephrine and epinephrine are necessary for learning and memory; they also focus attention and prepare the nervous system for fight or flight.
- Acetylcholine stimulates the parasympathetic nervous system, influences learning and memory, and helps regulate emotions.
- GABA is the primary inhibitory neurotransmitter and regulates anxiety and muscular coordination.
- Glutamate is the primary excitatory neurotransmitter that allows brain neurons to communicate.

4. Outline the mental health symptoms that can occur with disruptions in neuroanatomy and neurophysiology.

- Disorders associated with cerebellum dysfunction include Asperger disorder, ADHD, mood disorders, and schizophrenia.
- Disorders associated with frontal lobe dysfunction include schizophrenia, depression, obsessive–compulsive disorder, and substance use disorders.
- Dysregulation of the parietal lobe may result in repeating the same mistake over and over and the inability to recognize sensations.
- Dysfunction of the temporal lobe may result in auditory hallucinations, memory impairment, problems with aggression, difficulty understanding spoken words, and types of aphasia.
- Dysfunction of the occipital lobe includes visual hallucinations, loss of visual memory, and the inability to understand written words.
- Dysfunction of the limbic system includes excessive emotional responses, reward deficiency syndrome, olfactory hallucinations, problems with declarative memory, and difficulty learning.

5. Discuss the relationship between stress and the immune system.

→

- Acute or chronic stressors may affect health when people are already under long-term stress such as chronic pain, long-term job stress, or severe relationship difficulties. Acute stress can change the balance of the immune system and contribute to illness.
- The individual's sense of control over stressors is very critical in terms of immune response.
- The central nervous system and the immune system work as an integrated whole to maintain a state of health balance in the body.

6. Discuss the impact of nutrition on brain functioning.

→

- Supplements, diet, and lifestyle changes are areas for study in optimal brain function.
- Necessary nutrients for brain functioning are glucose, amino acids, minerals, essential fatty acids in omega-3-type fish oil, and antioxidants.

Explore MediaLink

For review questions, case studies, and other resources for this chapter see the Pearson Health MediaLink CD-ROM that accompanies this book and the Companion Website.

CD-ROM
- Audio Glossary
- NCLEX-RN® Review Questions
- Animations/Videos
  - Neurological Synapse
  - Serotonin Reuptake Inhibition
  - Occupation of Receptor Sites by Agonists/Antagonists
  - Seizures
  - Complex Seizure
  - Grand Mal

Companion Website www.prenhall.com/fontaine
- Audio Glossary
- NCLEX-RN® Review Questions
- Case Study
  - Neurobiology
- Care Plan
  - Genetic Links
- Critical Thinking
  - Neurotransmitter Intervention
- MediaLink Applications
  - Schizophrenia—Related Gene
- MediaLinks
  - Books for Clients and Families
  - Community Resources

NCLEX-RN® Review Questions

6-1. Executive functions such as reasoning, motivation, and judgment develop differently throughout adolescence. The adolescent's hormones are surging, which contributes to anger and impulsive behavior. The nurse is aware that:
1. Girls are less likely to be depressed than boys.
2. Boys are less likely to be depressed than girls.
3. There are no differences in depression between the sexes.
4. Girls are more likely to be aggressive than boys.

6-2. The nurse is caring for a 16-year-old client with a history of anorexia nervosa. The nurse is aware of the theories that suggest a specific area of brain is involved in anorexia nervosa. Which of the following areas of the brain does the nurse know influences a person's eating and drinking?
1. Thalmus
2. Hypothalmus
3. Pineal gland
4. Midbrain

6-3. The admitting note describes a client on the psychiatric unit as having anhedonia and anergia. The nurse knows that increasing the levels of the neurotransmitter serotonin will have a positive effect on this client. Which of the following activities should the nurse plan to meet the goal of increasing the client's serotonin level?
1. Daily exercise
2. Reminiscence group
3. Individual counseling
4. Group therapy

6-4. Clients with disordered proprioception have the potential for difficulty in:
1. Dressing, eating, and drinking in an organized manner.
2. Memory retention and the ability to reach short-term events.
3. Loss of vision.
4. Limited expression of emotion.

6-5. An older client has experienced the death of his spouse. They were married for 50 years and the client depended on his wife for simple activities of daily living. The nurse, assessing him for depression, is aware that:
1. The client's risk for illness is relatively high.
2. The client's risk of morbidity remains the same as before the spouse's death.
3. The client should be advised to relocate after the death of his spouse.
4. The client's pessimism will not have an impact on his health.

6-6. The nurse is conducting a client education group about the effects of nutrition on healthy daily living. A client asks, "What is one vitamin or mineral I should take to help my mental functioning? Which vitamin should the nurse suggest that the client take to enhance mental function?
1. Vitamin A
2. Vitamin B
3. Vitamin C
4. Vitamin D

See Appendix D for answers.

References

Apkarian, A. V., Sosa, Y., Sonty, S., Levy, R. M., Harden, R. N., Parrish, T. B., et al. (2004). Chronic back pain is associated with decreased prefrontal and thalamic gray matter density. *Journal of Neuroscience, 24*(46), 10410–10415.

Beal, M. F. (2004). Mitochondrial dysfunction and oxidative damage in Alzheimer's and Parkinson's diseases and coenzyme Q10 as a potential treatment. *Journal of Bioenergetics and Biomembranes, 36*(4), 381–386.

Bhangoo, R. K., Deveney, C. M., & Leibenluft, E. (2003). Affective neuroscience and the pathophysiology of bipolar disorder. In B. Geller & M. P. Delbello (Eds). *Bipolar disorder in childhood and early adolescence* (pp. 175–192). New York: Guilford Press.

Carrillo-Vico, A., Guerrero, J. M., Lardone, P. J., & Reiter, R. J. (2005). A review of the multiple actions of melatonin on the immune system. *Endocrine, 27*(2), 189–200.

Cozolino, L. J. (2002). *The neuroscience of psychotherapy.* New York: WW Norton.

Dowling, J. E. (2004). *The great brain debate: Nature or nurture?* Washington, DC: Joseph Henry Press.

Farber, N. B., & Newcomer, J. W. (2003). The role of NMDA receptor hypofunction in idiopathic psychotic disorders. In B. Geller & M. P. Delbello (Eds), *Bipolar disorder in childhood and early adolescence* (pp. 130–157). New York: Guilford Press.

Fontaine, K. L. (2005). *Complementary & alternative therapies for nursing* (2nd ed.). Upper Saddle River, NJ: Prentice Hall.

Galvan, A., Hare, T. A., Davidson, M., Spicer, J., Glover, G., & Casey, B. J. (2005). The role of ventral frontostriatal circuitry in reward-based learning in humans. *Journal of Neuroscience, 25*(38), 8650–8656.

Giedd, J. N., Clasen, L. S., Lenroot, R., Greenstein, D., Wallace, G. L., Ordaz, S., et al. (2006, July 25). Puberty-related influences on brain development. *Molecular and Cellular Endocrinology, Jul 25,* 154–162, 254–255.

Glaser, R., & Kiecolt-Glaser, J. K. (2005). Stress-induced immune dysfunction. *Nature Reviews Immunology, 5*(3), 243–251.

Hunt, R. D. (2006). Functional roles of norepinephrine and dopamine in ADHD. *Medscape Psychiatry & Mental Health, 11*(1), 1–6.

Kassin, S. (2004). *Psychology* (4th ed.). Upper Saddle River, NJ: Prentice Hall.

Keilhoff, G. (2005). Foreword basic research on nitric oxide. *Cellular and Molecular Biology, 51*(3), 245.

Kotz, C. M. (2006). Integration of feeding and spontaneous physical activity: Role for orexin. *Physiology & Behavior, 88*(3), 294–301.

Laney, C., & Loftus, E. F. (2005). Traumatic memories are not necessarily accurate memories. *Canadian Journal of Psychiatry, 50*(13), 823–828.

Marin, R. S., & Chakravosty, S. (2005). Disorders of diminished motivation. In J. M. Silver, T. W. McAllister, & S. C. Yudofsky (Eds.), *Textbook of traumatic brain injury* (pp. 337–352). Washington, DC: American Psychiatric Press.

McAuley, E., Kramer, A. F., & Colcombe, S. J. (2004). Cardiovascular fitness and neurocognitive function in older adults. *Brain, Behavior, and Immunity, 18*(3), 214–220.

Motzer, S. A., & Hretig, V. (2004). Stress, stress response, and health. *Nursing Clinics of North America, 39*(1), 1–17.

Pak, T., Cadet, P., Mantione, K. J., & Stefano, G. B. (2005). Morphine via nitric oxide modulates beta-amyloid metabolism. *Medical Science Monitor, 11*(10), 357–366.

Pelham, M. F., & Lovell, M. R. (2005). Issues in neuropsychological assessment. In J. M. Silver, T. W. McAllister, & S. C. Yudofsky (Eds.), *Textbook of traumatic brain injury* (pp. 159–172). Washington, DC: American Psychiatric Press.

Pihl, R. O., & Benkelfat, C. (2005). Neuromodulators in the development and expression of inhibition and aggression. In R. E. Tremblay, W. W. Hartup, & J. Archer (Eds.), *Developmental origins of aggression* (pp. 261–280). New York: Guilford Press.

Poeggeler, B. (2005). Melatonin, aging, and age-related diseases. *Endocrine, 27*(2), 201–212.

Samson, W. K., Taylor, M. M., & Ferguson, A. V. (2005). Non-sleep effects of hypocretin/orexin. *Sleep Medicine Review, 9*(4), 243–252.

Ramnani, N. (2006). The primate cortico-cerebellar system. *Nature Reviews: Neuroscience, 7*(7), 511–522.

Shults, C. W. (2005). Therapeutic role of coenzyme Q(10) in Parkinson's disease. *Pharmacology & Therapeutics, 107*(1), 120–130.

Sinha, S. S., Mohlman, J., & Gorman, J. M. (2004). Neurobiology. In R. G. Heimberg, C. L. Turk, & D. S. Mennin (Eds.), *Generalized anxiety disorder* (pp. 187–216). New York: Guilford Press.

Smith, C. D., Chebrolu, H., Wekstein, D. R., Schmitt, F. A., & Markesbery, W. R. (2006). Age and gender effects on human brain anatomy: A voxel-based morphometric study in healthy elderly. *Neurobiology of Aging, 28*(7), 1075–1087.

Starkweather, A., Witek-Janusek, L., & Mathews, H. L. (2005). Applying the psychoneuroimmunology framework to nursing research. *Journal of Neuroscience Nursing, 7*(1), 56–62.

Strauch, B. (2003). *The primal teen.* New York: Doubleday.

Teicher, M. H., Andersen, S. L., Navalta, C. P., Polcari, A., & Kim, D. (2004). Neuropsychiatric disorders of childhood and adolescence. In S. C. Yudofsky & R. E. Hales (Eds.), *Essentials of neuropsychiatry and clinical neuroscience* (pp. 535–606). Washington, DC: American Psychiatric Press.

Vogel, M. (2005). The cerebellum. *American Journal of Psychiatry, 162*(7), 1253.

Weller, A. (2006). The ontogeny of postingestive inhibitory stimuli. *Developmental Psychobiology, 48*(5), 368–379.

Yehuda, S., Rabinovitz, S., & Mostofsky, D. I. (2005). Essential fatty acids and the brain. *Neurobiology of Aging, 26*(Suppl 1), 98–102.

Unit 2
Illness Management and Recovery

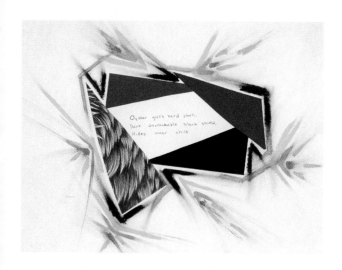

❝ *Oyster girl's hard shell.*
Dark uncrackable black shield.
Hides inner child. ❞

—Kate, Age 19

Chapter 7
Illness Management: Communication and Psychoeducation

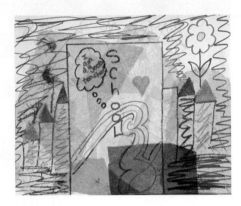

" I will be a good teacher and help kids and be there for them. "

—Crystal, Age 12

OBJECTIVES

After reading this chapter, you will be able to:

1. Explain the factors involved in developing a therapeutic relationship with a client.

2. Analyze communication in yourself, individuals, families, and groups.

3. Differentiate between effective and ineffective communication techniques.

4. Utilize the nursing process to educate clients and significant others about issues regarding mental illness.

5. Help clients and families implement the problem-solving process.

MediaLink www.prenhall.com/fontaine

Go to the Pearson Health MediaLink CD-ROM and the Companion Website at www.prenhall.com/fontaine for interactive resources for this chapter.

The art of nursing is caring, and it is the foundation on which the nursing process is based. This is true for any setting in which the profession of nursing is practiced. The fundamental components of *therapeutic support* are rapport and relating, communicating, educating, and problem solving. Your experiences in mental health nursing help you fine tune and incorporate these caring skills into your professional practice.

RELATING

The ability to relate to clients effectively depends to some extent on the nurse's ability to translate caring into nursing action. Caring implies compassion and sensitivity to each person within the context of her or his entire life. Caring involves a deep respect for the individual who is the client. Caring is also the way nurses enter the world of their client.

Therapeutic nurse–client relationships have a sense of harmony and understanding, which is referred to as **rapport**. Rapport is also about connection. From the introductory phase through the termination phase, the relationship evolves as the client experiences the nurse's caring approach.

Characteristics of Caring Helpers

The ability to integrate the characteristics of caring helpers into nursing practice will increase growth and satisfaction for both you and your clients. These interpersonal qualities and skills are critical to the therapeutic relationship through which nursing interventions are implemented. Used in isolation from the nursing process, they become characteristics of a social rather than a professional relationship.

Nonjudgmental Approach

One characteristic of caring nurses is a nonjudgmental approach to clients. It may be impossible for you to be completely nonjudgmental about clients. You make cognitive judgments when you assess clients and formulate reasonable plans of care. Emotional judgments are evidenced by such statements as "I really like her" or "He frightens me." Clients are also judged within the social context of appropriate or inappropriate behavior. Spiritual judgments include moral approval or condemnation of another person. Cultural judgments include being critical of behaviors, beliefs, and values that are different from yours.

A nonjudgmental approach to clients means that you are not harshly critical of them. Develop sufficient self-awareness to identify pejorative thoughts and feelings about particular clients. With this insight, you can avoid acting on negative judgments. Nonjudgmental nurses allow clients to talk about thoughts and feelings, and they respect clients as responsible people capable of making their own decisions.

Acceptance

Acceptance of clients is another characteristic of caring nurses. Acceptance is affirming people as they are and recognizing that clients have the right to emotional expression. Accepting nurses respect clients' thoughts and emotions and help them achieve self-understanding. As internal responses to one's perception of others and the environment, feelings are genuine and cannot be criticized, argued with, or denounced. To tell clients how they should or should not feel is to discount their past experiences, present state, and future potential. Being uncomfortable with one's own feelings often leads to discrediting the feelings of others.

Unless it is detrimental to the client or to others, accept client behavior. Certain behavior, such as masturbating in public, causes social embarrassment and discomfort to others and may later be a source of shame for the person. Protect clients by providing them with private space and time for this normal human activity. Set limits on activities that will lead to a client's complete exhaustion. Do not accept a client's violence toward self or others.

In determining whether a behavior is acceptable, first assess the probable consequences of the behavior. If you think it will be detrimental to the client or others, formulate a plan for intervention. Remember that if a client is incapable of changing behavior or chooses not to change it, physical force may be necessary. Ask the following questions during assessment: "Is this behavior detrimental, or is it just a source of irritation to me?" "Are the rules and regulations of the unit more important than the client's rights and dignity?" "Is this behavior dangerous enough to use physical force to stop it?" "Am I willing and able to use physical force to change the behavior?" The following examples illustrate this process.

Maria is a nurse in the emergency department. She is assigned to a client, Tom, whom the police arrested for intoxication and disorderly conduct. He has been placed in a room designed to be safe for this type of client. When Maria enters the room, she finds Tom smoking a cigarette, which is against the rules of the department. When he ignores her requests to put out the cigarette, she attempts to take it away from him forcefully. Tom strikes out in anger and Maria ends up with a facial cut that requires stitches.

Connie is a nurse on the psychiatric unit. She has been attempting to intervene with Roberta, a client who has become very angry with another client. When it is obvious that Roberta is losing control, Connie calls for help from other staff members, and they quickly formulate a plan for intervention. As Roberta picks up a chair and threatens the other client, three staff members surround her and firmly take the chair away from her. She is then escorted to her room, where two staff members remain with her until she has better control over her behavior.

It is apparent that Maria attempted to enforce the rules of the department without pausing to plan and prioritize.

Since Tom was in a room by himself where there was no danger of fire, his smoking a cigarette did not constitute a fire hazard. Maria might have made the decision to remain with him while he finished his cigarette, to prevent any accidents with the smoking material, but using physical force to stop the behavior was inappropriate because the incident was not dangerous. If Maria was determined to stop Tom's behavior, she should have sought help and thought of a plan to accomplish this outcome.

In contrast, Connie identified that Roberta's behavior was unacceptable because there was the danger of another client being injured. Connie and her staff members formulated and implemented a plan so that no one on the unit was injured, and Roberta was given the opportunity to talk about the feelings underlying her unacceptable behavior.

Warmth

Another characteristic of caring nurses is warmth, the manner in which concern for and interest in clients is expressed. This does not mean that you should be effusive with clients or attempt to be their buddy. Warmth is primarily expressed nonverbally, by a positive demeanor, a friendly tone, and an engaging smile. Simply leaning forward and establishing eye contact are expressions of warmth, as is physical touch, as long as it is acceptable and not frightening to the client.

Empathy

Much has been written about empathy as a necessary characteristic of caring nurses. Empathy is the ability to see another's perception of the world and it is accepting how clients see themselves, what they are feeling, and what they are striving to become. Empathy is a two-step process of understanding and validating. The first step is careful consideration of the meaning of what clients are communicating and the feelings being expressed. The second step is for nurses to verbally communicate understanding so that clients are able to validate or correct your perceptions. Most clients are not searching for a person who feels as they do. Rather, they are searching for someone who is trying to understand what they feel. Empathy can facilitate therapeutic collaboration and help clients experience and understand themselves more fully.

Authenticity

To be a caring nurse means to rely on personal authenticity—be genuinely and naturally yourself in therapeutic relationships. When you make a commitment to clients, you take on a professional role. This is different from "playing" the professional role, which makes a pretense of helping clients. When you are more concerned about how you appear than what you are and do, you erect a façade of helping and are incapable of being authentic with clients, peers, and supervisors.

Congruency

Nurses are genuine when their verbal and nonverbal behavior indicates congruency. Clients can quickly sense when others are incongruent, saying one thing verbally and another thing nonverbally. Congruency is a necessary ingredient to building trust.

It is Steve's first day on the psychiatric unit as a nursing student. He is in the day room interacting with a group of clients and two other students. He appears tense, with upright body posture, clenched hands, and a swinging foot. His voice is pitched higher than normal. One of the clients jokingly asks him, "What's the matter? Are you afraid of us crazies?" Steve quickly replies, "No, I'm not afraid. I like being here." The clients respond to him with looks of disbelief and change their focus to the other two students. Steve seeks out his instructor for help with this problem. The two of them discuss how his verbal and nonverbal communication did not match and the effect this incongruity had on the clients.

Several weeks later, Steve finds himself becoming increasingly frustrated with a client who has consistently refused to participate in any unit activities. This time he is able to be congruent and express his frustration directly to the client rather than trying to cover up his feelings.

Patience

It is essential that you have patience with clients, to give them the opportunity to grow and develop. Patience is not passive waiting, but active listening and responding. By allowing them to grow according to their own timetables, patience gives clients room to feel, think, and plan what changes need to be made. You must also be patient with yourself. Look for opportunities to develop self-awareness and gain new knowledge. Moreover, recognize that professional competence is not simply a goal; it is a long-term process of learning and developing as a nurse.

Respect

Respect for clients is another characteristic of caring nurses. Respect includes consideration for clients, commitment to protecting them and others from harm, and confidence in their ability to participate actively in solving their own problems. Do not let the nurse–client relationship become a dependent, parent–child relationship.

Trustworthiness

Trustworthiness is a characteristic of caring nurses toward which all the preceding characteristics build. By using good interpersonal skills, nurses help clients attach to them emotionally, which in turn helps build trust. This therapeutic attachment is facilitated through the nursing process. When you are trustworthy, you are dependable and responsible. You adhere to time commitments, keep promises, and are consistent in your attitude. Clients learn they can rely on you. Trust is also built when you demonstrate your willingness to continue working with clients who show little progress.

Trustworthy nurses respect the confidentiality of the nurse–client relationship. Client privacy must be protected because of the stigma associated with mental disorders. Reassure clients that information will not go beyond the health care team. Because you and your clients may live in the same community, some clients may fear that people will learn they are receiving mental health care. To minimize this fear, emphasize the issue of confidentiality. (Confidentiality is covered further in chapter 5 ∞.)

Distrust may develop when clients are denied access to the information in their records. Clients have the right to read their records; this right protects them by ensuring that all viewpoints, including their own, are represented. Sharing nursing notes can be beneficial in that further discussion can develop from your initial observations and interpretations. Every clinical agency has regulations for sharing record information with clients, and you must adhere to these rules.

Self-Disclosure

Trust develops when nurses offer appropriate self-disclosure. To establish trust and openness, beginning students often believe they should be no more than passive, nonjudgmental listeners. But trust cannot be achieved if you withhold your own thoughts and feelings. Only when relationships are open and active can real progress be made. Appropriate self-disclosure is always goal directed and determined by the client's needs, not yours. Nurses frequently ask clients to talk about their feelings as a therapeutic intervention. For clients who have minimal interpersonal skills, however, it is equally important to teach them how to perceive other people's feelings and to validate this perception. Through your self-disclosure, clients can improve their interpersonal relationships. For clients, self-disclosure can lead to further self-exploration; they are often reassured that their feelings are real and shared by others.

Joe, a nursing student, is talking with Sara about how she copes with loss. They are using the recent death of Sara's dog as an example.

Sara: "I don't know how to feel. I mean it's a dog, not a person."

Joe: "You had her for 10 years, ever since she was a puppy—right?"

Sara: "Right. But my mother told me to just get over it and get on with my life."

Joe: "I remember when my dog died when I was a teenager. I felt really sad for a few weeks. Pets are often very important to the people who live with them."

Self-disclosure is not always appropriate. Clients who are acutely ill may not be able to see themselves as separate individuals from the staff. Self-disclosure in this situation may be a source of confusion because these clients may believe that you are talking about them. Self-disclosure about personal details is often inappropriate and should be avoided. If clients ask for information about your personal life, simply express your discomfort with sharing that information, and refocus the conversation on the client's issues.

Berta, a nursing student, is having a one-to-one session with Jim, her client of 1 week.

Jim: "I notice you don't have a wedding band on. Does that mean you aren't married?"

Berta: "That's right."

Jim: "Do you have a boyfriend, or are you dating anyone right now?"

Berta: "Jim, I'm not comfortable talking about my private life. We were just discussing your recent divorce. Could we go back to that topic, please?"

Jim: "I just want to know if you're available, that's all. I mean, maybe we could go out for dinner sometime after I get out of here."

Berta: "Jim, you know that our relationship is a professional one and is limited to my time here in the clinic with you. It is not possible to continue it after your discharge."

Jim: "Well, I'm so lonesome since my wife left me, and you seem so nice and friendly."

Berta: "Let's talk about your loneliness and see if we can find more appropriate ways to deal with this problem."

Humor

Humor is a useful tool in effective nurse–client relationships. Some nurses erroneously consider humor to be unprofessional. Healthy humor must be distinguished from harmful humor. Harmful humor ridicules other people by laughing at them. Humor is also potentially harmful if it is used to avoid resolving genuine problems. Healthy humor, on the other hand, is a way to elicit laughter. It occurs when laughing with other people. Healthful humor is appropriate to the situation and protects a person's dignity. A good sense of humor is a mature coping mechanism and can help people adapt to difficult situations.

Humor creates and invites laughter; as such, it is a communication process. Humor is a cognitive communication that creates an affective response, such as delight or pleasure, followed by a behavioral response, such as smiling or laughing. Humor reduces anxiety and fear. It diffuses painful emotions, which the person cannot experience when laughing, and decreases stress and tension. Humor may also be a safety valve for the energy generated by anger. If people are able to look at an irritating situation and laugh rather than explode in anger, the energy is discharged in an adaptive manner (Christie & Moore, 2005).

The diagnosis of a terminal disease is incredibly stressful. Nurses often use humor to ease the pain and help everyone cope. It is not unusual for clients to use humor to temporarily lighten the mood of a serious situation. When used sensitively, humor can build connection among clients, families, and nurses (Dean & Gregory, 2005). Nurses in Taiwan have developed a "Chinese Humor Scale" with the goal of studying the use of humor in nursing (Hsieh, Hsiao, Liu, & Chang, 2005).

Jean's oncology physician explained that her hair loss would occur everywhere except on her legs. Jean joked with all her friends over the irony of losing all her hair except for that on her legs, which would have been her first choice of loss. Even though she will be bald as a cue ball, she will still have to shave her legs!

Bill, age 85, enjoys old-age infirmity jokes. One of his favorite jokes is: The doctor comes in and tells the patient that he has some bad news and some really bad news. The patient asks for the bad news first. The doctor responds, "You have Alzheimer's. And the really bad news? You have cancer." The patient replies, "Well, at least I don't have cancer."

There are cultural differences in expressing humor. All people laugh, and people of all cultures have a sense of humor. The greatest difference between cultural groups is the content of humor. For example, the Irish make jokes about drinking, whereas the Israelis do not. American humor tends to have sexual and aggressive themes, which are not present in Japanese humor. People from so-called pioneer countries, such as the United States, Australia, and Israel, express humor with exaggeration and tall tales; in contrast, British humor is understated and intellectual. Jews and Britons tell many jokes revolving around self-mockery (Provine, 2001).

A client's sense of humor may be a diagnostic cue for you. Changes in patterns of laughter may indicate other difficulties in adaptation. Clients who are depressed retain a cognitive sense of humor, but they receive no pleasure and are unable to laugh. Clients who are in a manic phase find everything funny, but because of their lack of judgment, their humor can turn into sarcastic wit and be potentially harmful to others. Those experiencing suspicious thoughts cannot laugh about their situation and are so frightened that they view humor as evidence of a personal attack. Clients who have difficulty with abstract thinking have

problems understanding jokes. The influence of alcohol or other drugs may reduce a person's inhibitions so that nearly all stimuli in the environment appear funny. In assessing clients, it is appropriate to ask, "What is your favorite joke?" Responses to this question will provide an indication of the client's sense of humor.

COMMUNICATING

Communication is the foundation of interpersonal relationships and is a key factor in the nursing process. The purpose of communication is twofold: to give and receive information, and to make contact between people. Students in mental health nursing use communication to assess clients and families and to implement the plan of care (giving and receiving information). Communication is also the means by which you initiate and establish relationships with clients (interpersonal contact). Clients use communication to share their feelings, express their thoughts, and talk about their lives. Through interpersonal contact with you, clients and families learn more effective and adaptive ways of communicating with others.

The Nature of Communication

People often assume that communication is merely one person giving information to another person. However, communication is much more complex than the transfer of information. Communication takes place in the context of the people involved. To analyze communication, consider all aspects: spoken words, paralanguage (sounds), the thinking process, emotions, nonverbal behavior, and the culture of the person who is sending the message. How the message is heard depends on the listening skills, analysis of the message, emotions, and culture of the person who is receiving the message (see Figure 7.1 ■).

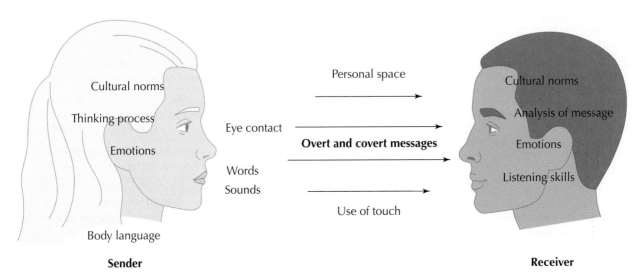

Figure 7.1 ■ The communication process.

Effective communicators analyze their communication and others' in terms of the behavioral, affective, and cognitive messages implied in the transfer of information. *Behavioral analysis* considers how accompanying nonverbal actions modify or enhance the verbal message. *Affective analysis* includes understanding the emotions involved in the communication, which are imparted both verbally and nonverbally. *Cognitive analysis* involves comprehension of the stated words and the thinking process of the person communicating. The cognitive component is communicated verbally or in writing.

Analysis of **paralanguage,** or sounds, provides additional information about the message being transmitted: the rate of speech, tone of voice, and loudness of the voice. Paralanguage also includes sounds that are not words, such as laughing, sobbing, snorting, and clicking of the tongue. You must also analyze how *culture* influences communication. Much of our communication is influenced by our cultural norms, for example, the use of personal space, acceptable body language, the amount of eye contact, and the types of paralanguage.

Nonverbal Communication

Because two thirds of communication is considered *nonverbal,* it is critical that you observe, understand, and respond to clients' nonverbal cues (see Table 7.1 ■). You must also be a *self-observer,* and pay attention to the messages they are communicating nonverbally. **Body language** includes your position, posture, and movements. Sitting face to face with a person will encourage more interaction than sitting side by side. Removing barriers, such as desks or tables, will facilitate communication. Standing over a client who is sitting is a dominating or intimidating position and will often interfere with effective communication. A rigid body posture may express anger or fear, while a relaxed body posture expresses openness and a feeling of

safety. Leaning back may convey a message of distance and withdrawal; learning forward indicates warmth and receptivity. People who sit with their arms and legs tightly crossed appear to be protecting themselves from some real or perceived danger. A person whose body seems to be pulling in on itself may be experiencing depression and low self-esteem. Body movements such as finger tapping, leg swinging, and nail biting may signal frustration, anxiety, anger, or embarrassment. Gestures such as pointing fingers, hands on hips, and shoulder shrugs are all aspects of communication.

Eye contact is extremely important in initiating, encouraging, and terminating communication. The listener usually maintains more eye contact than the speaker. Raised eyebrows may indicate interest, while frowning eyes may express disagreement. Suspicion is often communicated with narrowed eyes. Increased eye contact may be a cue that a person is anxious. Minimal eye contact may be evidence of shyness, low self-esteem, or boredom with the interaction.

Remember that different cultural and subcultural groups have varying patterns of nonverbal communication. Validate impressions and inferences with clients during the observing and interviewing processes. This is even more important when you and your clients are from different cultural backgrounds. For example, in some cultures, minimal eye contact does not indicate low self-esteem or boredom but is considered polite and respectful.

Personal space and *boundaries* are culturally determined and may range anywhere from 2 inches to 2 feet (5–61 cm). In mental health nursing, it is essential to respect client boundaries and their need for personal space. This respect includes how closely you sit with clients, how much space you give them when walking together, and asking for permission before entering their room.

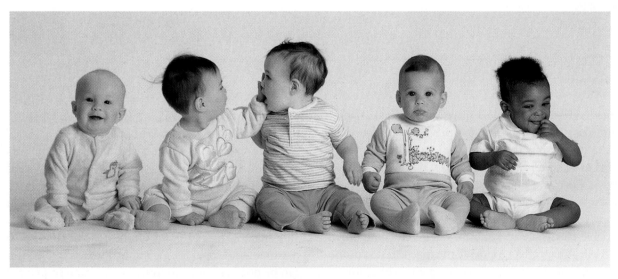

PHOTO 7.1 ■ Infants communicate with body language long before they speak.
SOURCE: Barbara Campbell/Getty Images, Inc.—Liaison. Used with permission.

TABLE 7.1	Forms of Nonverbal Communication

Behavior	Possible Meaning
Standing	
At beginning or end of the interaction	Initiation or termination of the interaction
Over other person while talking	Intimidation or domination
Sitting	
Face to face	Interest
Side by side	Neutrality
Turned away	Termination of the interaction
At the edge of the chair	Anxiety or eagerness
Body posture	
Relaxed	Friendliness, warmth
Rigid or tense	Fear or anger
Leaning back	Withdrawal, distance
Leaning forward	Interest, friendliness
Arms and/or legs tightly crossed	Self-protection, withdrawal
Shrinking in	Depression, low self-esteem
Turned away	Distance, withdrawal
Gestures	
Leg or foot shaking, finger tapping	Anxiety, frustration, anger
Fidgety, restless movements	Anxiety, embarrassment
Finger shaking, hands on hips	Authority, intimidation
Hiding hands	Shyness, insecurity
Fist-clenching	Anger, frustration
Wringing hands	Hopelessness, helplessness
Eyes	
Frequent eye contact	Interest, honesty
Minimal eye contact	Low self-esteem, shyness, boredom
Rapidly shifting eye contact	Confusion
Frequent blinking	Anxiety
Touch	
Touching arm or hand	Interest, concern

Touch is related to personal space and boundaries and is determined by cultural norms and previous experiences. In mental health nursing, the use of touch must be well thought out, so as to avoid misunderstandings. You must think about if, how, or when you might use touch with each client. It is usually better to ask the client whether you may touch her or his hands, for example, than to make assumptions as to how comfortable clients are with touch. Before touching others, ask yourself: What is the purpose of the touch? Is it appropriate? How might this person interpret the touch? With this kind of analysis, touch can be another form of nonverbal communication. (Table 7.2 ■ gives clues to what might be the reasons behind certain cultural behaviors.)

Mirroring clients' verbal and nonverbal communication is very effective in building rapport. Mirroring verbal communication involves using language similar to theirs. Mirroring body language involves using body movements that look like the mirror image of clients' movements. It is amazing how powerful this can be. Clients feel "heard," understood, and cared for. A simple illustration of this process can be done at home. Sit quietly with a loved one and consciously time your breathing to match the other's breathing.

TABLE 7.2	Nonverbal Communication of Major Ethnic Groups in the United States
Group	**Nonverbal Patterns**
African	Touch is common with family, extended family members; close personal space
Chinese	Not accustomed to being touched by strangers; avoid direct eye contact when listening; distant personal space
Eastern Indian	Handshakes between men only; direct eye contact considered disrespectful
Europeans	Eye contact acceptable; noncontact people; distant personal space; Southern countries have closer contact and touch
Filipino	Touch is stressed; some may fear eye contact; if eye contact is established, it should be maintained
Iraqi	Touch and embrace on arrival and departure
Israeli	Touch is demonstrative
Japanese	Handshakes acceptable; not accustomed to physical contact; distant personal space; direct eye contact shows lack of respect
Mexican	Touch often used, especially between those of same sex; close personal space
Native American	Periods of silence during communication shows respect; eye contact very limited; close personal space—no boundaries
Saudi	Male may touch only females in family; handholding by men acceptable

SOURCES: Shea, S. C. (1998). *Psychiatric interviewing: The art of understanding* (2nd ed.). Philadelphia: Saunders; and Spector, R. E. (2003). *Cultural diversity in health and illness* (6th ed.). Upper Saddle River, NJ: Prentice Hall.

It is not necessary to explain what you are doing. Pay attention to the sense of connectedness that begins to build as you continue synchronized breathing. In the same way, mirroring communication builds a sense of connectedness for clients. It may seem a bit awkward at first, but it soon becomes an unconscious process of building rapport.

Marcel is telling his nurse, Dani, about his impending divorce. As his feelings intensify, he leans forward with his arms on his thighs. At that moment, Dani purposefully leans forward with her arms in the same position. By mirroring Marcel's position, Dani expresses her interest and close attention to what he is saying.

Sometimes it is not appropriate to mirror clients' communication, such as with clients who are extremely anxious, agitated, or angry. Mirroring this behavior would only serve to escalate the clients' behavior. In these situations, communicate calmness and control with a relaxed body posture and a low, measured speech pattern. The goal is to de-escalate client behavior as they follow and mirror your verbal and nonverbal communication.

Listening

The art of nursing is the art of good **listening.** Good nurses listen for more than what is said by words alone. Every sentence has a meaning beyond the words. Successful communication occurs when you hear what people *mean*, not just what they say.

If you are rehearsing what you are going to say next when the other person is talking, you are not listening. Many people think they are good listeners, but more often than not, people talk too much. Often, we talk too much because we think we are supposed to "make things better" for our clients. We cannot solve people's problems for them. It is egocentric to think we can instantaneously analyze problems and fix them on the spot. It is important to realize the other person is not really looking for an answer. They are seeking empathy, sensitivity, and understanding.

To listen well, we must interrupt our preoccupation with ourselves and enter into the experience of the other person. Listening well is often silent but it is never passive. Listening means paying attention to what the person is saying, acknowledging feelings, holding back on speaking, avoiding interruption, and controlling the urge to give advice.

Better listening does not start with a set of techniques. It starts with making a sincere effort to pay attention to what is going on in the other person's experience. Listeners who pretend interest do not fool anyone for long—except, perhaps, themselves. Practice listening whenever your partner, family member, or friend speaks to you. Listen with the sole intention of understanding what that person is trying to express. Listen to yourself; get to know something about your own ways of communicating. Self-understanding will enable you to relate more effectively to other people.

Failure to be heard and understood is painful. Everyone has the need to communicate what it feels like in their own private world of experience. The importance of listening, as a part of communication, cannot be overestimated. Being listened to means that one is taken seriously, and the gift of someone else's attention and understanding makes one feel validated and valued. In opposition, not being listened to makes one feel ignored, unappreciated, cut off, and alone.

Levels of Messages

Listen to overt and covert levels of the message being transmitted in order to understand clients' experiences. **Overt messages** are conveyed by spoken words and are heard in the context of the person's feelings. Tone of voice, rate of speech, body posture, gestures, eye contact, and facial expression convey **covert messages,** which clarify or modify the overt message. For example, 2 hours ago, Jorge, age 22 years, was admitted for the first time to an acute care psychiatric facility. He asks the nurse, "What time are visiting hours?" The overt message is a simple request for information. If his words are spoken angrily and loudly or if his body posture is visibly tense, Jorge may be trying to assume some degree of control in an environment in which he feels uncomfortably dependent. If he speaks those same words in a frightened tone of voice, he may be terrified at being separated from his loved ones. Problems in communication can arise not from a lack of technical communication skills but from insensitivity to covert messages.

Communication Difficulties

Listening You will be more effective if you focus on listening and understanding clients' communication rather than trying to plan your reponses. A common concern of nursing students is: What am I going to say next, and what is the client going to say then? Beginning students frequently focus on trying to say the "right thing" or use the "right technique" and may appear either distant or oversupportive. It is more beneficial to clients to simply be yourself. As you become more comfortable with communication skills, saying the right thing will become secondary to listening and understanding.

Be aware of the pitfalls of being merely a polite listener, in which the listener goes through the motions of listening without truly hearing or understanding. Often seen in social interactions, this pattern can extend to nurse–client interactions. This may occur if one fears being regarded as inadequate or unintelligent. The polite listener is bored or impatient, and more interested in talking than in listening.

Nurses often assume that most of their communication has been listened to and understood by clients. However, feelings such as anxiety and anger may interfere with a client's ability to listen. Nurses should frequently ask yourself: Has the client listened to and understood what I have said? If you suspect that a client has not understood you, ask questions such as: "Could you tell me what you heard me saying?" or "I'm not sure I said that very clearly. What did you hear?"

Questioning Nurses are taught to ask many questions during the history-taking and assessment processes. When this continues into the implementation phase, difficulties will usually develop. The nurse and client become simply questioner and questioned. The relationship becomes *unequal* because the questioner has the power to determine the course of the interaction. There is a tacit understanding that the questioner is the authority figure and the questioned must be submissive. A clue that you are asking too many questions is when clients give short answers or seldom take the initiative during interactions.

Silence One of the most difficult aspects of communication is periods of silence. Students often feel uncomfortable with silence because of a belief that they should always have something therapeutic to say. With silent clients, the tendency among anxious students is to be excessively verbal. Silence has many meanings. Among them are:

- I am too tired to talk right now.
- I don't want to talk to you.
- I can't hear you; I'm listening to the voices.
- I don't know what you want from me.
- I'm lost and don't know what to say next.
- I don't know where this discussion is going.
- I would like to think about what was just said.
- I'm comfortable just being with you and not talking.

To respond appropriately, try to understand the reason for the client's silence. An observation such as "I've noticed that you have become very quiet. Could you tell me something about that quietness?" may encourage clients to share more.

Verbosity Verbose clients may also pose problems. Just as students tend to be verbal with silent clients, they tend to be passive with talkative ones. You may be reluctant to interrupt for fear of being thought disrespectful or feeling inadequate in the face of such unrelenting talk. You may also feel a sense of relief that clients are finally talking to you. Some students mistakenly interpret clients' incessant verbalizing as evidence that the interactions are therapeutic. It is difficult to understand nonstop talk for more than 30 seconds. Interrupting will allow you to focus on the concerns being expressed and to convey a sense of involvement with the client's problems. Here are some examples of helpful interruptions:

- "You are bringing up a number of concerns. Could we discuss them one at a time?"
- "Let me interrupt you for a minute to make sure I understand what you are saying."

- "I don't want to stop you, but I need you to slow down so that I can understand better."

Deafness Of the 20 million hearing-impaired people in the United States, about 10% are profoundly deaf. Significant hearing loss impairs language and communication. Those who use American Sign Language (ASL) or English Sign Language (ESL) may have difficulty with spoken English. Deaf individuals often learn mental health terminology from deaf friends, family, or reading. They may recognize concepts such as *depression* or *addiction* but are less likely to understand the concept of *psychosis*. Since language fluency is essential for psychotherapy, interpreters may be necessary. The use of an interpreter then raises concerns about confidentiality. When an interpreter is used, that person should sit next to you and across from the client. This makes it easier for the client to read facial expressions, which are critical to sign language. Group therapy may also become a problem when several people speak at the same time and the deaf person, being able to follow only one speaker at a time, misses much (McAleer, 2006).

The Americans with Disabilities Act prohibits discrimination against people who are deaf. Health care facilities must provide deaf clients with the means to communicate clearly with the staff. All hearing-impaired clients should be asked about their preferred communication approach, such as lip reading, writing notes, sign language, an interpreter, or a telecommunication device for the deaf. All staff must then be alerted to the form of communication the client and family prefer.

Effective Communication

Effective communication is not an inborn skill but a learned process. Many instructors have their nursing students write up their one-to-one interactions (1:1) with clients—called process recordings—in order to analyze the communication process. This type of evaluation will help you understand yourself and your clients. The consistent use of analysis, along with input from peers and supervisors, will heighten your level of expertise (see Table 7.3 ■).

Questions Questions can be closed ended or open ended. *Closed-ended questions* can be answered with a yes, a no, or a simple fact. They are useful for finding out exact information or for helping a client focus on a topic more clearly. Clients who are experiencing a high level of anxiety or disorganized thinking respond more easily to closed-ended questions. Examples are: "How long have you been married?" "Are you still living with your wife?" "Are you hearing voices right now?" *Open-ended questions* cannot be answered in a few short words. They are useful for increasing the client's participation in the interaction and for encouraging the client to continue the discussion. Examples are: "Would you tell me more about your relationship prob-

lems?" "How is that similar to your family when you were growing up?" Use open-ended and closed-ended questions both during interactions, but use open-ended questions whenever possible or appropriate. If several closed-ended questions are asked in succession, the interaction takes on an atmosphere of cross-examination, and the client may become reluctant to continue.

Questions beginning with *What* are generally used to evoke facts. Examples are: "What kind of work do you do?" "What do you argue about?" Questions beginning with *How* lead to a discussion of feelings and may elicit a client's personal view of a situation. Examples are: "How did you feel when he gave you that ultimatum?" "How do you think your work should be supervised?" Questions beginning with *Could* allow the client to have some control over the interaction and are the most open-ended of questions. Examples are: "Could you give me an example of how he mistreats you?" "Could you tell me, what is the most important problem to focus on today?" Questions beginning with *Why* lead to a discussion of reasons and often put clients on the defensive. *Why* questions do not typically help clients understand their situation more clearly but rather force them to explain and justify their behavior. Examples are: "Why did you skip group today?" and "Why did you say that to your husband?"

Questioning is basic to critical thinking, problem solving, and creativity. Skillful questioning is basically an interactive process. Asking the right questions can help clients move beyond their usual patterns of thinking and responding. Questions can be used for *gathering information*. As stated earlier, you must be careful not to overuse this type of questioning. Nurses formulate their questions on the basis of their theoretical framework (Goldberg, 1998). See chapter 1 ∞ for assessment questions using specific theoretical models. Consider the following interaction as the nurse gathers information:

Sonja: "I am so tired of being depressed. I just don't want to be depressed anymore."

Nurse: "Tell me, how will you know when you are no longer depressed?"

Sonja: "I'll be happy."

Nurse: "But I'm not sure how you will know when you are happy. Give me a word picture of what you will be like when you are happy."

Sonja: "Well, I would play with my daughter, I would smile and laugh more, I would enjoy my garden, and I would visit with my friends."

Nurse: "What are you going to do to get started?"

Sonja: "Maybe I will try to play a little bit with my daughter this afternoon."

Questions can also be used as *interventions*. When nurses pose these types of questions, they invite the client to gain

MediaLink

Case Study, Developing a Therapeutic Relationship with Clients insight and explore new possibilities. These types of questions often center on choices people make throughout their lives. Examples of questions as interventions include: "Where do you hope to be in 6 months? 1 year? 5 years?" "In what way could you make your relationship more satisfying?" "Could you help me understand more about your reasons for making that decision?" "In thinking back, what might you have done differently?" "What do you think might happen if you did?"

TABLE 7.3	Process Recording of Client Interview With a Student Nurse		
Jeff is in the process of divorce. He is unemployed and homeless. He has made threats to kill his wife and daughter, believing that if all 3 of them die, "it will be a better ending to the story." The one-to-one time began with Jeff saying he is stressed and has many problems.			
Client's Communication	**Analysis of Client's Response**	**Student's Communication**	**Analysis of Student's Response**
My wife and I are getting a divorce, I don't have a job or a home, and the FBI is after me.	*Seems calm when discussing these rather upsetting topics. Wonder whether he is trying to distance himself from the pain through detachment.*	The FBI is looking for you?	*Restatement. This allows Jeff to elaborate on the topic.*
(Nods) Yeah, there were some guys at my work who were constantly around me; they were from the FBI. They didn't think I knew, but I did, that's why I quit. I told them I was quitting because I was going to be moving since I'm getting a divorce. (Shrugs). Haven't seen those guys since.	*Delusions of persecution. If he was having problems at work, they could be the fault of these harmful others. A drastic and self-defeating response to the delusions. Still enough in touch with reality to create a story that his boss would understand. Believes quitting was an effective solution.*	Help me understand what you think the FBI wanted from you.	*Clarifying. Want to understand his delusion without feeding into it.*
They have all of these charges against me, but I didn't do anything. I think the cops who were at my house that one night my wife and I were having an argument got the FBI after me. They didn't like me very much. (Good eye contact)	*Jeff has spent some time thinking about the delusion. Wonder whether this ties into the fact that there is a restraining order against him. This may feed into his paranoid thinking.*	Help me understand what happened that evening.	*Clarifying. Want to know the context of his thinking.*
(Rolling eyes). Yeah, she called them up when things started heating up. I was trying to talk to her about all the problems that are going on and all she ever wanted to do was yell. Then when I got frustrated and raised my voice, she called the cops and told them I was being aggressive toward her and our daughter.	*I know from the chart that Jeff believes his real wife died 3 months ago when he left, and now someone from the FBI is posing as her. He believes the situation was a set up—he would get mad at his wife, become aggressive, and the cops could arrest him.*	It sounds like you were feeling fairly helpless in that situation.	*Reflection of feelings.*
Yeah. And now I can't see my daugher because they got a restraining order against me. But she doesn't mind it. She likes that I can't see her.	*Jeff is certain that his daughter wants nothing to do with him. This could be accurate or more paranoid thinking.*	Has she said that to you?	*Clarifying. I was not sure whether he is assuming or whether she had told him this.*
She calls me stupid. I always go into situations with her thinking I will stay calm and be the strong one—but she just aggravates me so much, I lose it.	*Jeff expects the situation to improve even though he does nothing to change things. External locus of control—he's not responsible for his behavior.*	Have you thought of alternative ways to approach these situations?	*Encouraging formulation of a plan of action. Want to see whether he has started problem solving*
Jeff goes on to discuss his problems with his wife and daughter and his inability to control his anger. We began the problem-solving process around anger management for the rest of the one-to-one time.			

SOURCE: Contributed by Jaimie Rzab, Purdue University Calumet.

Skillful use of questions helps guide clients through the problem-solving process. Clients become empowered as they learn from situations they have encountered. Questions also help clients assume responsibility for their own actions.

Facilitating Techniques Effective communication techniques communicate your listening, understanding, and caring. The nurse must analyze the behavioral, affective, and cognitive components of communication in order to respond to overt and covert messages. Effective communication also encourages clients to examine feelings, explore problems in more depth, build on existing strengths, and develop new coping strategies (see Table 7.4 ■).

TABLE 7.4	Effective Communication Techniques
Technique	**Examples**
Broad opening	"What would you like to work on today?"
	"What is one of the best things that happened to you this week?"
Giving recognition	"I notice you're wearing a new dress. You look very nice."
	"What a marvelous afghan that is going to be when you finish."
Minimal encouragement	"Go on."
	"Ummm."
	"Uh-huh."
Offering self	"I'll sit with you until it's time for your family session."
	"I have at least 30 minutes I can spend with you right now."
Accepting	"I can imagine how that might feel."
	"I'm with you on that [nodding]."
Making observations	"Mr. Robinson, you seem on edge. You are clenching your fist and grinding your teeth."
	"I'm puzzled. You're smiling, but you sound so resentful."
Validating perceptions	"This is what I heard you say. . . . Is that correct?"
	"It sounds like you are talking about sad feelings. Is that correct?"
Exploring	"How does your girlfriend feel about your being in the hospital?"
	"Tell me about what was happening at home just before you came in the hospital."
Clarifying	"Could you explain more about that to me?"
	"I'm having some difficulty. Could you help me understand?"
Placing the event in time or sequence	"Which came first . . . ?"
	"When did you first notice . . . ?"
Focusing	"Could we continue talking about you and your dad right now?"
	"Rather than talking about what your husband thinks, I would like to hear how you're feeling right now."
Encouraging the formulation of a plan of action	"What do you think you can do the next time you feel that way?"
	"How might you handle your anger in a nonthreatening way?"
Suggesting collaboration	"Perhaps together we can figure out. . . ."
	"Let's try using the problem-solving process that was presented in group yesterday."
Restatement	*Client:* "Do you think going home will be difficult?"
	Nurse: "How difficult do you think going home will be?"
Reflection	*Client:* "I keep thinking about what all my friends are doing right now."
	Nurse: "You're worried that they aren't missing you?"
	Client: "He laughed at me. My boss just sat there and laughed at me. I felt like such a fool."
	Nurse: "You felt humiliated?"
Summarizing	"So far we have talked about . . . ."
	"Our time is up. Let's see, we have discussed your family problems, their effect on your schoolwork, and your need to find a way to decrease family conflict."

Broad openings are open-ended questions or statements. The purpose of a broad opening is to acknowledge clients and to let them know you are listening and are concerned about their interests. But the overuse of broad openings will force the relationship to remain on a superficial level.

Giving recognition is noting something that is occurring at the present moment for clients. It is a fairly superficial level of communication but indicates attention to and caring for individuals.

Minimal encouragements are verbal and nonverbal reinforcements that indicate active listening to and interest in what clients are saying. They prompt clients to continue with what is being said.

Offering self is a way of informing clients of care and concern. It is used to offer emotional and moral support.

Accepting lets clients know that the nurse comprehends their thoughts and feelings. It is one way to express empathy.

Making observations moves the interaction to a deeper therapeutic level. It involves paying very close attention to the behavioral component of communication and connecting it to the affective and cognitive components. When communication is incongruous, you can comment on the inconsistency and, with the client, explore the underlying meaning of the mixed messages. Clients experiencing disorganized thinking may be unable to take part in this process.

Validating perceptions gives clients an opportunity to validate or correct your understanding of what is being communicated. Using this technique will decrease confusion and affirm your genuine interest in understanding your clients.

Exploring helps clients feel free to talk and examine issues in more depth. As they organize their thoughts and focus on particular problems, their understanding of themselves and others increases.

Clarifying is useful when you are confused about clients' thoughts or feelings. It is appropriate to acknowledge your confusion and ask clients to rephrase what they just said.

Placing the event in time or sequence helps clients sort out what happened to them in what order. The goal is to help them understand the progression of events.

Focusing allows clients to stay with specifics and analyze problems without jumping from topic to topic. You may choose to focus on the main theme, to facilitate exploring the problem in more depth. Clients are often unaware of how they contributed to and participated in the development of their problems. By focusing on their feelings, thoughts, and behaviors, you pave the way for increased understanding and responsibility. Clients with disorganized thinking usually need help in staying focused.

Encouraging the formulation of a plan of action is the process of helping clients decide how they plan to proceed. Avoid telling clients what they should do. Instead, asking them what they will or might do will reinforce that they are in control of and responsible for themselves. If they are unable to formulate a plan of action, implement the problem-solving process. If clients are highly anxious or experiencing disorganized thinking, they may be unable to problem solve or make appropriate judgments.

Suggesting collaboration is one technique of introducing the problem-solving process. It is an offer to help clients work through each step of the process and to brainstorm alternative solutions to their problems. Suggesting collaboration stresses the nurse–client team effort to develop more adaptive coping skills.

Restatement is the use of newer and fewer words to paraphrase the basic content of client messages. Restatement focuses on the cognitive component of communication and creates an opportunity to explore facts or reinforce something important clients have said.

Reflection involves understanding the affective component of communication and reflecting these feelings back to clients without repeating their exact words. Reflection helps clients focus on feelings and allows the nurse to communicate empathy.

Summarizing is the systematic synthesis of important ideas discussed by clients during interactions. The goal is to help them explore significant content and emotional themes. Summarizing may also be used to move from one phase of the interaction to the next, to conclude the interaction, or to begin the interaction by reviewing the previous session. (See Table 7.5 ■ for use of clarifying techniques when clients use unclear or nonspecific language.)

Techniques That Contribute to Ineffective Communication

Nurses who worry about what they are going to say next, who do not listen carefully, and who do not focus on trying to understand what clients are attempting to say are often ineffective communicators. Ineffective communication is also described as communication that avoids underlying feelings, remains on a superficial level, tells people what to do, or moralizes and expresses judgment (see Table 7.6 ■).

Stereotypical comments indicate that the nurse cares little about the individual experiences of clients and is relying on folklore and proverbs to communicate. Additional problems occur for clients whose thinking is concrete because many stereotypical comments rely on abstract understanding. Stereotypical comments are culture specific and therefore make little sense to people with different cultural backgrounds.

Parroting is simply repeating back to clients the words they have used. When you merely repeat what clients have said, the communication becomes circular; clients do not progress in understanding; the interaction grinds to a halt.

TABLE 7.5	Unclear, Nonspecific Communication		
Common Problem	**Meaning**	**Verbal Example**	**Clarifying Technique**
Deleting	Object of the verb is left out	"I'm afraid."	Inquire: "Afraid of what in particular?"
		"I'm really uncomfortable."	"What is making you uncomfortable?"
Unspecified verbs	Verbs in which the action needs to be more specific	"He really frustrates me."	Inquire: "How, exactly, does he frustrate you?"
		"They ignored me."	"In what way did they ignore you?"
Universal qualifiers	Words that generalize a few experiences to a multitude of experiences (all, every, never, always, nobody, only)	"I never do anything right."	Inquire: "Has there ever been a time that you did do something right?"
		"You always hurt me."	"Has there ever been a situation in which I haven't hurt you?"
Necessity and possibility	Statements that identify rules or limits to a person's behavior and that often indicate no choice (have to, must, can't, no one can, not possible, unable)	"I have to take care of other people."	Inquire: "What would happen if you didn't take care of other people?"
		"No one can get me out of this mess."	"What would happen if you got out of this mess?"
		"I can't do it."	"What stops you from doing it?"
		"It's not possible."	"What do you need?" "What will have to happen so it is possible?"

Changing the topic occurs when you introduce topics that might be of interest to you but are not relevant to the client. This technique can be a way of avoiding topics that make you uncomfortable. If you change the topic often, clients will begin to feel that what they are trying to say is not important. Clients may also change the topic if they are highly anxious about the topic being discussed or if their thinking is disorganized.

Disagreeing with clients' ideas and emotions denies them the right to think and feel as they do. Disagreeing provides clients with no opportunity to increase self-understanding.

Challenging clients forces them to defend themselves from what appears to be an attack by you. When you challenge clients, they are forced to offer reasons for their feelings, thoughts, or behaviors.

Requesting an explanation is similar to challenging and usually begins with *Why.* The implication is that the client should not be behaving a certain way or experiencing a particular feeling.

False reassurance is another way of telling clients how to feel and ignoring their distress. Clients feel condescended to when you act as if you know better and more than they do.

Belittling expressed feelings gives the message that you have not listened carefully, that you are ignoring the importance of their problems.

Probing occurs when you fail to respect clients' decisions regarding privacy of feelings and thoughts. Probing implicitly accuses them of keeping secrets and blames them for not progressing in treatment.

Advising occurs when you tell clients what to do, preventing them from exploring problems and using the prob-lem-solving process to find solutions. Advising makes you, rather than the client, responsible for the outcome.

Imposing values is demanding that clients share your biases and prejudices. It is preaching and moralizing rather than accurately understanding their values.

Double/multiple questions are ineffective because they tend to confuse clients. When asked a series of questions with no opportunity to respond, clients may end up feeling bewildered or cross-examined.

Communicating with Families and Groups

Nurses are involved with a variety of family systems, as well as informal and formal groups, in every clinical setting. Communication within families and communication within groups are presented together here because they are similar. To help people become more effective communicators, you must be able to analyze communication patterns.

The overall process in understanding family and group communication is as follows:

- What do I see and hear? (perception of nonverbal and verbal communication)
- How do the members feel? How do I feel? (affective analysis)
- What does this mean? (cognitive interpretation)
- Is my assessment correct? (validation by asking others, gathering more information)
- How shall I respond? (interventions based on your assessment)

TABLE 7.6	Ineffective Communication Techniques
Technique	**Examples**
Stereotypical comments	"What's the matter, cat got your tongue?" "Still waters run deep."
Parroting	*Client*: "I'm so sad." *Nurse*: "You're so sad."
Changing the topic	*Client*: "I was so afraid I was going to have another panic attack." *Nurse*: "What does your husband think about your panic attacks?"
Disagreeing	"I don't see any reason for you to feel that way." "No, I think that is a silly response to your mother."
Challenging	"Is that a valid reason to become angry?" "You weren't really serious, were you?"
Requesting an explanation	"Why did you react that way?" "Why can't you just leave home?"
False reassurance	"Don't worry anymore." "I doubt that your mother will be angry about your failing math."
Belittling expressed feelings	"That was four years ago. It shouldn't bother you now." "You shouldn't feel that all men are bad." "It's wrong to even think of your mother like that."
Probing	"I'm here to listen. I can't help you if you won't tell me everything." "Tell me what secrets you keep from your wife."
Advising	"You sound worried. I think you'd better talk to your doctor or your rabbi." "I think you should divorce your husband."
Imposing values	*Client*: [With head down and low tone of voice] "I was going to go on the cruise, but my mother is coming to stay with me." *Nurse*: "You must be looking forward to her arrival."
Double/multiple questions	"What makes you feel that you should stay? How would you get along if you left? Would you rent an apartment or move in with a friend?"

The *significance of nonverbal communication* must always be considered. When working with families or groups, consider the following questions, and then interpret the significance of the answers:

- How close together do people sit?
- Are some members physically isolated from others?
- Can each person see the other members fairly easily?
- Do members look at the person who is speaking?
- Do members behave in a distracting manner while a person is speaking?
- How is touch used within the group?
- Are nonverbal behaviors directed toward a particular member or the entire group?
- How do facial expressions change throughout the interaction?

- What kinds of gestures are used?
- Are there changes in voice tone?

Another consideration is the *significance of verbal communication.* Consider the following questions, and interpret the significance of the answers:

- Is somebody refusing to talk?
- Who speaks to whom, about what, and when?
- Are there individuals who are speaking for others?
- Who interrupts others?
- Who is talkative?
- Who contributes little?
- Who asks questions?
- Who gives the answers?
- Who gives opinions?

- Who tries to clarify misunderstandings?
- Who initiates problem solving?
- If English is not the native language, how fluent are various family members?
- Are one or two members expected to interpret for others?

Affective expression among family and group members can be analyzed by answering these questions:

- To what extent is the communication of feelings encouraged?
- Are feelings expressed directly or indirectly?
- What happens when a member breaks the group's "rules" about expressing feelings?
- How much does the group encourage members to be sensitive to each other's feelings and to communicate this awareness?
- What feelings underlie the members' communication with one another?
- Who is helpful and friendly?

As a nurse, you help members improve their listening skills and their ability to be congruent in their communication by modeling and teaching effective communication. As the members gain more adaptive skills, they will be better able to cope with individual, family, and group problems.

Communicating with Children and Adolescents

Communicating therapeutically with a child or an adolescent can be bewildering. You should answer the following questions as a first step toward communicating effectively with children and adolescents:

- What do I say?
- How can I get this person to talk to me?
- How do I feel?
- In what context have I interacted with people in this age group before? What emotions does this child or teen stir in me?
- What is my role when working with children or adolescents? Am I there to guide, direct, teach, advise, or protect?

Rather than probing for details, listen for feelings. It is more important to help children learn how to interact effectively than to gather particulars. Children easily fall into superficially answering adults' questions and simply waiting for the next one. In this routine way, the nurse sets the pattern of a question-and-answer session. There are two prob-

lems with this pattern: The child will provide only short answers and not expand on the topic, and you will be frustrated when you run out of questions and have not achieved any therapeutic purpose.

You will learn more by listening than by questioning. Use an open-ended format to obtain information. For example, rather than asking, "Do you have friends?" say, "Tell me about the friends you like to do things with." Respect the children's periods of silence. They may need this time to sort out thoughts and feelings and will be unable to do so if you bombard them with questions. Children soon discover whether you are a good listener. Some children do not respond to "talking" therapy because they have never experienced an adult really listening to them, they may not have been encouraged or allowed to express feelings, or they may not have the cognitive development to express their problems.

Children and adolescents recognize fake sentiments and insincere platitudes. They want to know that you are genuine, trustworthy, and your word is good. Explain what you expect of the child and what the child can expect from you. The clients you work with may have heard mixed messages throughout their lives and probably have learned to expect that adults make promises they do not keep. Working with young clients provides an opportunity to model honest, adult behavior.

Communicating with Older Adults

Nurses can use knowledge of their own personal experience of being children and adolescents themselves when communicating with children and adolescents. Thus, you have some understanding of appropriate conversation. When communicating with older adults, you have not had that developmental experience to enrich your understanding, and in some ways it is new territory.

Older adults are sometimes the targets of patronizing speech, such as extremely slow speech, simple sentences, concrete vocabulary, and demeaning emotional tone. Some health care professionals even use baby talk, especially with elderly persons who live in nursing homes. Patronizing speech implies that there is a question regarding the competence of the older person; this communicates a lack of respect that undermines self-esteem and dignity.

Condescending speech is the result of age-related stereotypes. Some of these negative beliefs are that older adults are feeble, egocentric, incompetent, or abrasive. It is important that you evaluate your beliefs about older people and how they communicate. You must also examine how you talk to older individuals. Ask for feedback from others in order to examine your communication skills.

Older people take longer to decode and encode messages and therefore take longer to react during conversation.

At times, they may also have difficulties in word retrieval and name recall. The key to interacting in this situation is patience. People's senses play an important role in communication with others. Loss of hearing can make interactions more difficult. You should not cover your mouth or chew gum when you speak, since many older adults rely on lip reading to clarify what is being spoken. Since lip reading is 45% accurate at best, hearing-impaired adults may guess at what was said. If people respond inappropriately, it may be that they did not hear any or part of the message. It is helpful to speak more slowly. Consider the external environment when interacting with people who are hearing impaired since external noise is very distracting when struggling to listen to speech. Eyesight also has an important role in conversation. Nonverbal cues that expand on the spoken message may be missed by those whose vision is impaired (Nussbaum, Pecchioni, Robinson, & Thompson, 2000).

EDUCATING

Education of clients and families is basic to nursing care. Knowledge empowers people to make informed decisions regarding their health status, to plan for maintaining wellness, and to make choices regarding illness care. Communication is the most important skill in effective education of psychiatric clients and their families. Good communication contributes to thorough assessment and accurate diagnosis of learning needs, and it is the major tool for implementing the teaching plan. You evaluate your teaching through verbal and (sometimes) written communication with your clients. Documentation is the written communication in records.

Education in the mental health care setting involves more than giving information to passive people. Education is an active process that is done with people, not to people. The steps of the nursing process are used in the educational process: assessing the learning needs, diagnosing the knowledge deficit with contributing factors, planning content, implementing the most effective methods of education, evaluating the effectiveness of the teaching, and documenting the entire process.

Assessment

The first step in the client/family teaching process is assessment. It is important to understand the client's views of psychiatric illness. Clients and families often believe cultural stereotypes—mental illness means being possessed by a demon, mental illness occurs only in people who are "bad," or families cause mental illness. These stereotypes must be countered with factual data. Through assessment, determine what clients have learned in previous contact with mental health professionals. If you have the erroneous

view that people with severe and persistent mental illness cannot possibly understand their disorders and their medications, you will be surprised to learn how much these people do know.

Assessment also involves determining what clients want and think they need to know. Ask what they consider their most important problems at this time. Little progress will be made if you assume authority for prioritizing their problems. People are not likely to be open to learning about difficulties they consider unimportant; they will only learn material that is meaningful to them. You may need to help some individuals to be specific if they have described their problems in vague terms.

Max has been readmitted to the psychiatric unit because he stopped taking his medication 6 months ago. Ryan, his nurse, has determined that Max needs to learn why it is important to keep taking his medication. Max says the reason he doesn't do it is that his wife is always nagging him to take it. He believes if she would just leave him alone, he would not have a problem taking it. It is more important for Max to learn skills that will help him get along with and communicate better with his wife than to learn the facts about how his medication works.

Diagnosis

The nursing diagnosis often used in client/family education is "Deficient Knowledge." There are, however, any number of other diagnoses that can be used, such as "ineffective individual coping," "ineffective management of therapeutic regimen," or "altered role performance." When forming a nursing diagnosis, specify exactly what people need to learn and what the related factors may be. Examples are:

- Deficient Knowledge: Lithium Therapy related to initiation of the drug
- Deficient Knowledge: Basic Cooking Skills related to mother doing all the cooking and her recent death
- Ineffective Individual Coping related to work stress that is contributing to high levels of anxiety and increased conflict at work
- Ineffective Management of Therapeutic Regimen related to noncompliance with medications
- Altered Role Performance related to recent divorce and becoming a single parent

Diagnosis also includes specifying what barriers exist, if any, that might hinder the teaching and learning process. Clients experiencing a great deal of anxiety have a very short attention span, an extremely narrowed perceptual field, and very little capacity to learn. Attempting to teach clients when they are in a manic phase, delusional, or experiencing hallucinations may not be practical. Disorganized thinking, obsessive thoughts, and other cognitive impairments make it very difficult for clients to learn. Those who are depressed and who feel hopeless and helpless about the present and future may have no motivation to learn. Clients or family members who are angry and hostile must find a way to manage their emotions before effective learning can take place. People who deny the reality of mental disorders will not be open to increasing their knowledge or improving their coping skills.

Planning

Preparing clients for as much self-care as possible to live in the least restrictive setting is both the focus and the goal of client/family teaching. Design planning to meet the specific needs of the client and family. Direct the educational plan not only toward increasing knowledge but also toward improved problem solving and more adaptive coping skills. Helping clients learn from their situations and take responsibility for the results of their actions is empowering. Develop outcome criteria to evaluate the behavioral, affective, and cognitive changes resulting from effective teaching and learning.

To help people learn to cope with their problems, emphasize the present: Change is possible only in the here and now. The past and future are also important, but only as perspectives on the present. Meanings attached to the past and expectations of the future influence present perceptions. But it is in the present that one evaluates the past, anticipates the future, and changes behavior. People who brood over past problems and pain without attending to the present are in danger of accepting the problems as permanent, with no hope for change. People who have dire future expectations and ignore the present potential for change will probably see their expectations fulfilled.

Implementation

Two of the most important skills to bring to client/family education are the ability to *communicate clearly* and the capacity to develop a *relationship* that is warm and caring. A humanistic approach has proven more successful than a technical approach in terms of client/family understanding and their willingness to participate in the process.

Education is both formal and informal. Examples of *formal teaching* are psychoeducational groups and audiovisual tools. The effectiveness of group education depends on a group leader with a high level of skill. Carefully assess clients for appropriateness to the group. Those whose thinking is disorganized and those who are hyperactive, highly anxious, or hallucinating may not be appropriate for an educational group. One advantage of the group format is the ability to reach more people in a limited amount of time. Another advantage is that clients interact with others who have similar problems and concerns. Sharing solutions to problems and coping behaviors can foster the learning process. The group should not have so many members that individuals have little opportunity to ask questions and provide answers. The best physical arrangement is a circle of chairs, to encourage a sense of connectedness.

Probably the most effective education format is the *informal process*. Every interaction with clients and their families is an opportunity to facilitate their learning. Informal teaching is when you discover a learning need and respond to it immediately. Examples are explaining the need for a new medication and helping a client control anger in response to an immediate situation.

General Areas of Learning

Client and family education may be the single most important factor in promoting healthy lifestyles. There are six general areas of learning to consider when implementing teaching plans. The first area relates to *knowledge of the mental disorder*. Clients and families who have struggled to live with severe and persistent mental illness may be very knowledgeable in this area, in contrast with those experiencing disorders for the first time. Topics typically discussed are an explanation of the diagnosis, myths and folklore surrounding the disorder, goals of treatment, and the overall treatment plan. Clients and their families should also learn the signs and symptoms of relapse and know when to call the physician.

The second general area of learning is *medications*. Most clients and families are able to understand basic neurotransmission, which helps them understand how the medication works and why they need it. If they are caring for themselves, they should know when to take each medication and have a system for accurate administration at home. Teach them about the possible side effects and how to manage them. If there are special precautions for a particular medication, emphasize them. General medication teaching principles are covered in chapter 8 ∞.

Some clients will need to learn activities relating to *managing activities of daily living* (ADLs). They may never have had the opportunity to learn how to shop for groceries, plan menus, prepare food, and do laundry. Some clients benefit from grooming groups, which reinforce basic hygiene, teach makeup and hair care, and help clients plan appropriate clothing, such as for job interviews and leisure activities. Some clients will need to learn how to use public transportation. Teach clients about available community resources for leisure activities, support groups, and religious expression.

Many clients and families need to learn the basics of *interpersonal communication*. They must be able to identify and express their own feelings and respect and listen to those of others. Family conferences and family therapy provide opportunities to help family members learn to communicate more effectively.

Clients often need to learn more effective skills for *coping with life*, including family, social, and vocational aspects. It is helpful if clients can identify how their illness has affected their lives and move on to a discussion of what the future might look like. Clients need to learn stress-avoidance and stress-management techniques and how to manage any symptoms they may be experiencing. Ask clients what goals they have that they have not been able to achieve because of their illness. Help them identify a goal in specific behavioral terms, identify subgoals, and list behavioral steps to achieve their goals. Clients often need to learn assertiveness skills and the problem-solving process. Some will need to develop a plan to avoid social isolation. More detailed teaching is included in each of the disorders chapters.

Another area of general learning is *community resources*. Types of programs are intermediate care facilities, partial-hospital programs, outpatient centers, respite care, transport resources, financial aid, pharmacies, and food programs. Self-help and support groups exist in most communities.

Some useful general information Web sites for you, your client, and his or her families include:

- National Library of Medicine http://www.nln.nih.gov
- Mayo Health Clinic http://www.mayohealth.org
- Medscape http://www.medscape.com

The Problem-Solving Process

The *most important process* for clients and families to learn is how to solve problems. As they become increasingly skilled at problem solving, they will expand their coping skills and enhance the quality of their lives. In teaching the problem-solving process, focus on one problem at a time, and measure progress by observing small changes.

Because all problems are connected, changes in one problem will cause changes in others. Remind people that in the past they have done their best to deal with problems, and that, now, new solutions may be found. The nurse's role is to listen, observe, encourage, and evaluate. More effective coping behavior will be the ultimate result of the problem-solving process. But before the process can begin, you must help identify the problem. Identification includes the person's definition of the problem, the significance of the problem, and the influence of the past and future. Box 7.1 describes the steps in problem identification.

Throughout the problem-solving process, it is extremely helpful to have clients keep a written list of all the ideas generated. The list can be modified as time goes on.

After problem identification, the steps of the problem-solving process consist of the following:

1. Identifying the solutions that have been attempted
2. Listing alternative solutions

BOX 7.1	Steps in Problem Identification

1. Client definition
   - How would you describe the problem?
   - For whom is this a problem? You? Family members? Employer? Community?
2. Significance of the problem
   - When did this problem begin?
   - What are the factors that cause this problem to continue?
3. Past and future influence
   - What past events have influenced the current problem?
   - What are your future expectations and hopes concerning this problem?
   - What is the most you hope for when this problem is resolved?
   - What is the least you will settle for to resolve this problem?
4. Concrete problem definition
   - Is there more than one problem here?
   - Which part of the overall problem is most important to deal with first?

---

3. Predicting the probable consequences of each alternative
4. Choosing the best alternative to implement
5. Implementing the chosen alternative in a real-life or practice situation
6. Evaluating outcomes

Box 7.2 lists sample questions for each step. The first step is identifying what solutions have been tried thus far. Items that must be clarified include the specifics of the attempts, how the attempts were implemented, and what occurred as a result. Because the problem continues to exist, these solutions were not effective, so they should be either modified or discarded.

The second step is having the client list alternative ways of solving the problem. Frequently, the client will have only one or two ideas. The nurse can propose brainstorming sessions to increase creativity in problem solving. All possible solutions, even those that are unrealistic or absurd, are written down. Thinking of absurd solutions often opens the mind to other creative, realistic solutions to the problem. Finally, after the client has listed all his or her ideas for solving the problem, you can add your own suggestions.

The third step is predicting the probable consequences of each alternative, which helps clients anticipate outcomes of behavior.

After thorough discussion, the nurse and the client go on to the fourth step: choosing the best alternative to implement. Do not make this decision for clients; doing so would undermine the process by placing them in a child-like, dependent position. Using action-oriented terms, develop the selected solution further, as concretely and specifically as possible. At the same time, formulate measurable outcomes to use in evaluating the process.

BOX 7.2	Steps in the Problem-Solving Process

1. Identify attempted solutions
   - What have you done to try to solve the problem thus far?
   - How exactly did you do this?
   - What happened when you tried this?
2. List alternatives
   - What other ideas do you think you could try?
   - What might be some absurd solutions to this problem?
   - What else might be effective?
   - Have you thought about . . . ?
3. Predict consequences
   - What might happen if you tried the first idea?
   - Is there anything else that might happen?
   - What might happen if you tried the second idea (etc.)?
4. Choose the best alternative
   - Which alternative seems like the best decision at this time?
   - What specific behaviors are you going to try with this alternative?
   - Specifically, how will things be different if you are successful?
5. Implement the alternative
   - With whom are you going to attempt this solution?
   - When are you going to practice this new behavior?
   - Is there anything you need from me to help you try this out?
6. Evaluate
   - What was the result of your attempted solution?
   - Were your expectations met successfully?
   - Is there anything that needs to be modified?
   - If you were not successful, what other alternative idea from the list could you try?

The fifth step is implementing the proposed solution in either a practice or a real-life situation. Clients must be allowed to make mistakes during this step. If you rescue them, you are giving the message that the clients are incapable of taking charge of their lives.

Evaluation is the sixth step in the problem-solving process. Review the outcomes, and determine the degree of success or failure. Achieving an outcome means that the solution was effective and that it can continue to be implemented. Failing to achieve an outcome means you and your client must analyze how and why the solution was ineffective. Then return to step 4, and either select a new solution or modify the old one.

As clients experience the steps of the problem-solving process, they increase their skills, which then can be applied to other problematic areas of life. With an improved ability to make and assume responsibility for decisions, they develop an internal locus of control, leading to competence and self-esteem.

When clients are acutely ill and unable to think logically, the problem-solving process is not an appropriate intervention. The following interaction illustrates the problem-solving process in action with a nurse and client.

Beth, a 25-year-old graduate student, has been seeing Miyuki, a nurse therapist, for several months. Beth has been in a long-term relationship with a married man who has been physically and emotionally abusive to her.

Beth: "It's really time to end the relationship. I've known for a long time that it's not good for me to stay with Todd. I just don't know how to do it."
Miyuki: "What have you tried to do so far in ending the relationship?"
Beth: "In the past 2 years, I've told Todd several times that I don't want to see him anymore. Then he doesn't call me for a month and I start to miss him, so I give in when he finally calls me."
Miyuki: "So, when you say no to Todd, he punishes you by not calling, with the end result that he manipulates you into going back to him."
Beth: "Yes, I guess that's what happens. What's really unbelievable is that I don't even like him very much anymore. What I really miss is the sex after a while. So I just give in because of the sex."
Miyuki: "If you really want to end this relationship, how might you go about doing it differently since just telling him hasn't seemed to work?"
Beth: "All my friends have been telling me to dump Todd. I guess I could tell some of them that I'm finally going to do it."
Miyuki: "What might happen if you did that?"
Beth: "Well, when I would be tempted to go back to Todd, I could call them up for some moral support not to go back. I guess I would have to tell them ahead of time that's what I'd want them to do."
Miyuki: "Are there some friends who would be better than others to depend on in this situation?"
Beth: "I think Carmela and Grace would be the best. They would try and help me, but they also wouldn't make me feel like a fool if I failed again. Leslie and Eva would just yell at me and be very critical."
Miyuki: "What else might help you break up with Todd?"
Beth: "I suppose I could try and do things with different friends. I always sit at home waiting for Todd to call me. I haven't gone out much with my friends in a long time."
Miyuki: "How would that help you not go back to Todd?"
Beth: "At least I wouldn't be so lonesome. Maybe it's the loneliness as much as the sex that makes me go back to him."
Miyuki: "What are some of the things that might get in the way of your staying away from Todd?"
Beth: "He has told me for years that no one else would want me because I'm fat and ugly and the only thing I'm good for is sex. I guess I really believe that after hearing it for so long. What if no one else will ever love me for the rest of my life?"
Miyuki: "It's understandable how you believe what he has told you. Men who are abusive undermine their victim's self-esteem to prevent the victim from leaving. It seems to me that is another aspect of the problem we should also try to solve. Let's finish discussing the loneliness and friends issues first, and then move on to your self-esteem issue."

Since problem solving stresses autonomy, teaching the process is not always *culturally* appropriate. When assessing cultural norms you may find that (Paniagua, 2001):

- American Indians value group consensus in establishing individual goals. Problem solving must be modified to include group consensus.

- Hispanic culture expects men to make decisions in families, excluding women and children from the process.
- People of Asian ancestry value the process of negotiation rather than confrontation.

Family Education

Family and friends often have questions about the disorder and want to know how they can best help. Including supportive others in education may improve the rehabilitative process because the living environment often affects the course of many mental disorders. Unless clients are acutely agitated or psychotic, they should be actively involved in the process of family education. Things to consider when planning family/friends/caregiver teaching include:

- Mental illnesses are no-fault disorders; people do not get to choose the genes they get or the genes they give; mental illness is a brain disorder.
- Manage responsibilities of care giving, such as stigma and symptomatic behaviors.
- Identify triggers to symptoms.
- Locate and utilize community resources.
- Find a balance between overprotecting the loved one and ignoring problematic behavior.
- Establish a regularity to family life and developing healthy lifestyles.
- Identify adaptive and maladaptive responses.
- Communicate effectively with one another.
- Recognize early prodromal symptoms to minimize the risk of relapse.
- Develop an action plan for responding to relapse situations.

More specific family teaching information is found in chapter 3 ∞ and in the chapters covering the various mental disorders. Teaching in a group setting is presented in chapter 10 ∞.

Evaluation

Client and family education is effective if the outcome criteria are met. The only way to discover what people have learned is through evaluation. Evaluation must be measurable; that is, people must be able to hear or see evidence that they did or did not meet the outcome criteria. If criteria were not met, look for where the problem might be. The difficulty could be in any of the steps of the nursing process. Box 7.3 describes common problems that prevent meeting the outcome criteria. Use this box as a guide for lo-

---

BOX 7.3	Problems in Client Education

Assessment

- Teaching material was not meaningful to the client.

Diagnosis

- Barriers to learning were not identified.

Planning

- Areas of learning were stated in vague terms.
- Outcome criteria were vague and unmeasurable.
- The focus remained on the past rather than on present problems.

Implementation

- Communication skills were ineffective.
- The nurse displayed a distant, uncaring attitude toward the client.
- The family and significant others were not included.
- The teaching methods and tools were not appropriate for the client.

Evaluation

- Areas of learning were no longer appropriate for the client's circumstances.

---

cating problems in education. Revise teaching according to evidence from the evaluation.

Evaluation can be done in a number of ways. One way is to have people verbalize attitudes, values, feelings, and facts. Written tests may be appropriate for cognitive information. Interpersonal skill achievement can be evaluated by role-playing. Psychomotor skill achievement can be evaluated by having the learner demonstrate the skill. This final step of the nursing process is critical to effective education.

Documentation

Documentation is an important step in the process of education. Communication between all members of the multidisciplinary team is essential to the effectiveness of the process. Much of that communication is through documentation. Documentation also provides legal protection for the staff. The rule is the same as with any other nursing activity: If it is not written down in the chart, it did not happen.

Documentation should include areas of learning, what has been taught, client/family response to the teaching, degree of success in meeting the outcome criteria, and what further areas of teaching are required. Any one of a number of forms may be used to document education, including narrative notes and teaching flow sheets. It is the nurses' responsibility to document all phases of client education in which they are involved.

Focus Your Study

OBJECTIVES	KEY CONCEPTS

OBJECTIVES

1. Explain the factors involved in developing a therapeutic relationship with a client.

KEY CONCEPTS

- Characteristics of caring helpers:
  - Trustworthy
  - Nonjudgmental
  - Accepting
  - Empathetic
  - Authentic
  - Warm
  - Respectful
  - Congruent
  - Sense of humor
  - Appropriate self-disclosure
- Communication

---

2. Analyze communication in yourself, individuals, families, and groups.

- Behavioral analysis:
  - How accompanying nonverbal actions modify or enhance verbal message
- Affective analysis:
  - Understanding the emotions involved in the communication
- Cognitive analysis:
  - Comprehending the stated words
  - Thinking process of persons communicating
- Analysis of paralanguage:
  - Sounds that provide additional information
- Cultural context:
  - Personal space
  - Acceptable body language
  - Eye contact
  - Types of paralanguage
  - Use of touch

---

3. Differentiate between effective and ineffective communication techniques.

- Effective communication techniques:
  - Listening well is critical to the nurse–client relationship.
  - Analyze overt and covert messages when listening to clients.
  - Open-ended questions encourage clients to talk about themselves.
  - Facilitating techniques include broad openings, giving recognition, minimal encouragement, offering self, accepting, making observations, validating perceptions, exploring, clarifying, placing the event in time or sequence, focusing, encouraging the formulation of a plan of action, suggesting collaboration, restatement, reflection, and summarizing.
  - When working with children and adolescents, you will learn more by listening than by questioning.
  - When communicating with older adults, give them a longer time to react during a conversation, make certain they are able to hear and see you, and avoid patronizing speech.
  - Communication is the most important skill in effective client and family education.
- Ineffective communication techniques:
  - Too many questions when intervening with clients
  - Avoids underlying feelings, remains on a superficial level, tells people what to do, or moralizes and judges clients.
  - Ineffective techniques include stereotypical comments, parroting, changing the topic, disagreeing, challenging, requesting an explanation, false reassurance, probing, advising, imposing values, and multiple questions.

(continued)

(continued)

4. Utilize the nursing process to educate clients and significant others about issues regarding mental illness.

→
- Assess client's and family's areas of learning.
- What is their view of psychiatric illness?
- What do they want and need to know?
- What do they need to make informed decisions regarding their health status, to plan for maintaining wellness, and to make choices regarding illness care?

5. Help clients and families implement the problem-solving process.

→
- Problem identification includes the client's and family's definition of the problem, the significance of the problem, and the influence of the past and future.
- Teach clients and families the steps of the problem-solving process which are identifying solutions that have been attempted, listing alternative solutions, predicting the probable consequences of each alternative, choosing the best alternative to implement, putting this alternative into action, and evaluating the outcomes.

Explore MediaLink

For review questions, case studies, and other resources for this chapter see the Pearson Health MediaLink CD-ROM that accompanies this book and the Companion Website.

CD-ROM
- Audio Glossary
- NCLEX-RN® Review Questions

Companion Website www.prenhall.com/fontaine
- Audio Glossary
- NCLEX-RN® Review Questions
- Case Study
  – Developing a Therapeutic Relationship With Clients
- Care Plan
  – Therapeutic Communication and the Use of Self
- Critical Thinking
  – Communicating With Clients
- MediaLink Application
  – Nonverbal Communication: Interpreting Gestures From Different Cultures
- MediaLinks
  – Books for Clients and Families
  – Community Resources

NCLEX-RN® Review Questions

7-1. The nurse is caring for a client who attempted suicide 2 weeks ago. The client states, "Sometimes I wish I could die and not feel the pain anymore." Which of the following responses by the nurse demonstrates empathy?
1. "I feel that way sometimes, but I would never do anything to hurt my family."
2. "It sounds like you're in a lot of pain and you don't have much hope for the future."
3. "Maybe you should talk to your psychiatrist and tell him how you feel."
4. "Are you planning to harm yourself again?"

7-2. During an interaction with a female client, several of the nurse's nonverbal messages are hindering the conversa-

tion. Which of the following nonverbal behaviors by the nurse would effectively facilitate the interaction? (Select all that apply.)
1. Make frequent brief eye contact with the client.
2. Sit back with legs crossed at the ankles as the client leans forward.
3. Smile as the client begins to discuss her latest alien abduction.
4. Rub the client's shoulders when her eyes begin to well up.
5. Glance over at the clock on the wall as the lunch cart is wheeled into the room.
6. Remain seated as the client inches her chair in the opposite direction.

7-3. The client is discussing recent marital problems and asks the nurse, "Do you think I should ask for a divorce?" Which of the following questions by the nurse are examples of an effective response? (Select all that apply.)

1. "What other options besides asking for a divorce have you considered?"
2. "How would you feel about asking for a divorce?"
3. "Why do you want to file for a divorce?"
4. "Could you explain to me some of the reasons you want a divorce?"
5. "Yes, I think you should ask for a divorce."
6. "Have you tried marital counseling or talked to a lawyer or considered a trial separation?"

7-4. The client has been attending an anger management workshop and is discussing the changes he has made in his behavior. Which one of the following statements demonstrates an effective outcome?

1. "I feel like a new man. All my anger is completely gone."
2. "I never knew I was such a bully. I don't hate anyone anymore."
3. "I know that I'll feel angry at times, but I can control my response now."
4. "I just walk away from the situation and forget about it."

7-5. Questions that guide the client through the six steps of the problem-solving process are provided in the list below. Arrange these questions in the correct sequence. All options must be used.

1. "Which of these stress management methods would work best for you?"
2. "How would you rate your stress level since you've been meditating?"
3. "I see you've been practicing meditation this week, haven't you?"
4. "Meditation is a good idea. What would happen if you tried it?"
5. "What are some other ways you could manage your stress?"
6. "How have you coped with stress in the past?"

See Appendix D for answers.

References

Christie, W., & Moore, C. (2005). The impact of humor on patients with cancer. *Clinical Journal of Oncology Nursing, 9*(2), 211–218.

Dean, R. A., & Gregory, D. M. (2005). More than trivial: Strategies for using humor in palliative care. *Cancer Nursing, 28*(4), 292–300.

Goldberg, M. C. (1998). *The art of the question.* New York: John Wiley & Sons.

Hsieh, C. J., Hsiao, Y. L., Liu, S. J., & Chang, C. (2005). Positive psychological measure: Constructing and evaluating the reliability and validity of a Chinese Humor Scale applicable to professional nursing. *Journal of Nursing Research, 13*(3), 206–215.

McAleer, M. (2006). Communicating effectively with deaf patients. *Nursing Standard, 20*(19), 51–54.

Nussbaum, J. F., Pecchioni, L. L., Robinson, J. D., & Thompson, T. L. (2000). *Communication and aging* (2nd ed.). Mahwah, NJ: Lawrence Erlbaum.

Paniagua, F. A. (2001). *Diagnosis in a multicultural context.* Thousand Oaks, CA: Sage Publication.

Provine, R. (2001). *Laughter: A scientific investigation.* London: Penguin Books.

Shea, S. C. (1998). *Psychiatric interviewing: The art of understanding* (2nd ed.). Philadelphia: WB Saunders.

Spector, R. E. (2003). *Cultural diversity in health and illness* (6th ed.). Upper Saddle River, NJ: Prentice Hall.

Chapter 8
Illness Management: Common Clinical Behaviors

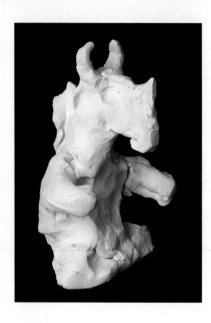

66 *This represents my anger as a Giant Dragon, 20 feet tall. It's taller than any human, it screeches and hurts your ears and it will try and eat you. To control it, find a magic stone. I am still looking for that stone.* 99

—Anthony, Age 14

OBJECTIVES

After reading this chapter, you will be able to:

1. Differentiate between the parts of the brain implicated in common clinical behaviors.

2. Compare and contrast the assessment process for different common clinical behaviors.

3. Outline interventions for common clinical behaviors.

MediaLink www.prenhall.com/fontaine

Go to the Pearson Health MediaLink CD-ROM and the Companion Website at
www.prenhall.com/fontaine for interactive resources for this chapter.

The ROAD to Critical Thinking

A Client Experiencing Paranoid Delusions

Travel this ROAD to understand Ann and her condition.

Read about Ann below and throughout this chapter.

Observe Ann on the CD-ROM accompanying this book.

Assess Ann by answering the questions at the end of this chapter.

Develop a Care Plan on the CD-ROM to address Ann's condition.

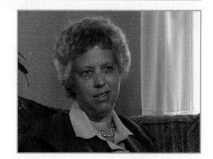

Ann

The onset of Ann's bipolar disorder occurred 6 months after giving birth to her first child. Prior to this, Ann was a successful professional woman with an MBA and a PhD and taught at Harvard Business School. During her manic episode, Ann suffered from paranoid delusions and ideas of reference. With no medical treatment, over the next 6 years she divorced, lost her job, and temporarily lost custody of her daughter.

One woman in a thousand experiences postpartum psychosis. Although the symptoms usually begin shortly after delivery of the infant, the disorder may begin anytime during the first year after the birth. Postpartum psychosis may be accompanied by delusions, which are false beliefs that cannot be changed by logical reasoning or evidence. They may be fixed in the person's mind only for a few weeks or months or may fluctuate over time. Delusions of persecution involve beliefs that someone is trying to harm the person. Delusions can become so intrusive that they disrupt the individual's entire life with severe consequences for the quality of life.

During your clinical rotation in mental health nursing, you will encounter certain common problems. These problems occur in a variety of settings, including inpatient units, residential care programs, outpatient settings, and the home. Not necessarily related to a specific disorder, these problems may be symptoms of a number of mental disorders.

Hallucinations and delusions often accompany **psychosis,** a state in which a person is unable to comprehend reality and has difficulty communicating and relating to others. Psychosis is a nonspecific indicator for severe mental illness and is usually characterized by hallucinations, delusions, or gross disorganization of thought or behavior. Hallucinations may trigger violent episodes if voices command people to hurt themselves or others. Delusions may lead to dangerous situations, such as jumping from high places because of the belief that one can fly.

Hallucinations and delusions may be considered normal in one culture and abnormal in another culture. Fears of evil attacks by spirits may be a part of local beliefs. Some people hear voices in religious ceremonies. Some Native Americans encourage hallucinations as symbolic spiritual experiences, called vision quests. It is not unusual for individuals who are grieving the loss of a loved one to experience visual and auditory hallucinations of that person. Knowing about values and patterns of behavior prevents us from mislabeling these experiences as pathological.

Violence against oneself, such as self-mutilation, and aggression against others are two problems needing immediate intervention. These behaviors are often impulsive.

Impulsivity is the failure to resist an impulse or urge or to respond after a period of reflection. Impulsive behavior is related to low levels of *serotonin* (5-HT), hyperactivity of the *limbic system,* or inadequate control by the *cortex.* Any verbal or nonverbal force meant to harm or abuse another person is referred to as **aggression.**

CLIENTS EXPERIENCING HALLUCINATIONS

An **hallucination** is the occurrence of a sight, sound, touch, smell, or taste without any external stimulus to the sensory organs. The experience is real to the person. These perceptual changes are often early symptoms in mental disorders. **Illusions** are simply one or more of a person's five senses playing tricks on the person. They are a sensory *misperception* of environmental stimuli. An example of an illusion is looking at a cord on the floor and thinking one is seeing a snake. A common illusion is seeing heat rising from highway pavement and believing there is a large pool of water on the pavement.

Although hallucinations are most commonly associated with schizophrenic disorders, only 70% of clients with schizophrenia experience them. Hallucinations also occur in the manic phase of bipolar disorder, severe depression, substance dependence, and substance withdrawal. Hallucinations represent a complex interaction between brain physiology, environmental stimuli, and the person's perception of the world.

Studies have shown that 90% of people who experience hallucinations also experience delusions (Papolos & Papolos, 2002).

Types of Hallucinations

Auditory hallucinations, which account for 70% of hallucinations, are thought to be caused by dysfunction in the language centers of the cerebral cortex, located in the *temporal lobes* of the brain. These sounds can fluctuate from a simple noise or voice to a voice talking about the client, to a voice talking about what the client is thinking, to complete conversations between two or more people. Most people say the hallucinations are distressing. The voices may make derogatory remarks and try to get clients to do or say something that is potentially harmful to themselves or to others.

Some people continue to hallucinate during periods of remission, but voices are usually different during these times. These voices appear to be similar to the self-talk most people engage in. Self-talk is part of problem solving as people think of solutions, consider consequences, and make decisions. In a similar way the voices help people plan their daily activities, solve problems, give advice, and provide feedback regarding behavior. In this situation, the voices are considered helpful and adaptive (England, Tripp-Reimer, & Rubenstein, 2005).

Visual hallucinations are thought to be caused by dysfunction in the *occipital lobes* of the brain. They can fluctuate from flashes of light or geometric figures to cartoon figures to elaborate and complex scenes or visions. Visual hallucinations are often accompanied by auditory hallucinations.

Gustatory and *olfactory hallucinations* typically consist of putrid, foul, and rancid tastes or repulsive smells. *Tactile hallucinations* involve the sense of touch. People may verbalize feeling electrical sensations coming from the ground or inanimate objects or feel like "they are being touched by others" when there is no one around. *Kinesthetic hallucinations* involve the feeling of body processes such as blood pulsing through the veins, food digesting, or urine forming. These types of hallucinations are typically associated with *organic changes* such as those that occur in a stroke, brain tumor, seizures, substance dependence, and substance withdrawal (Papolos & Papolos, 2002).

A *command hallucination* is a special type of auditory hallucination that is potentially dangerous. Occasionally, the command can be to do something useful, such as calling the doctor. More typically, the voice orders the person to do something that is frightening and may cause harm, such as cutting off a body part or striking out at someone. Fear from command hallucinations can also cause dangerous behavior, such as jumping out a window to escape a person who is trying to intervene.

Nikki describes her experience. "I left home without anyone knowing. I went to the public and took my clothes off. I had to take my clothes off because there is a bad God and a good God, so the bad God told me to take my clothes off. I heard him say it and I had to listen to him."

Assessment

Hallucinations are very real to the person having them. In people experiencing psychosis, hallucinations are symptoms that need to be assessed in the same manner as any other symptoms. Left unattended, hallucinations will continue and may escalate. Talking about one's hallucinations is a reassuring and self-validating experience. Such a discussion can take place only in an atmosphere of genuine interest and concern.

Nurses may ask themselves: How can I tell whether my client is actually experiencing hallucinations? Behaviors often perceived as inappropriate may be a response to hallucinations. These behaviors include inappropriate laughter, conversations with an unseen person, difficulty paying attention to the task at hand, and a slow verbal response. In the case of severe hallucinations, the person may be unable to respond to anything in the external environment. See Table 8.1 ■ for behavioral clues to hallucinations.

Assessment of auditory hallucinations includes the frequency, duration, disruption, severity, loudness, intensity, and location of the voices. Other assessment criteria include how distressful the voices are, the extent of negative or derogatory content, and the person's belief about the origin of the voices (England, Tripp-Reimer, & Rubenstein, 2005).

Hallucinations serve as a useful indicator in the ongoing assessment of a client's level of functioning. If the client is in remission, the voices may be a positive, adaptive presence. At other times, hallucinations are a symptom of psychosis. In this case they may interfere with activities of daily living (ADLs) to the point of complete withdrawal, depending on the level of intrusiveness. Assessment of the level of functioning provides direction for nursing interventions.

Interventions

Intervening with clients experiencing disruptive hallucinations requires patience and the ability to spend time with them. Clients consistently report the following three interventions as most helpful during the acute phase of hallucinations:

- Having someone with them
- Hearing a real person talk
- Being able to see the person who is talking

Clients experiencing hallucinations have no voluntary control over the neurobiological dysfunction causing the

TABLE 8.1	Hallucinations and Client Behaviors
Sense	**Observable Client Behaviors**
Auditory	Moving eyes back and forth as if looking for someone
	Listening intently to a person who is not speaking
	Engaging in conversation with an invisible person
	Grinning or laughter that seems inappropriate
	Slowed verbal responses as if preoccupied
Visual	Suddenly appearing startled, frightened, or terrified by another person or object or by no apparent stimulus
	Suddenly running into another room
Olfactory	Wrinkling nose as if smelling something horrible
	Smelling parts of the body
	Smelling the air while walking toward another person
	Responding to an odor with terror
Gustatory	Spitting out food or beverage
	Refusing to eat, drink, or take medications
Tactile	Slapping self as if putting out a fire
	Trying to brush invisible things, like bugs, off the body
	Jumping up and down on the floor as if avoiding pain or other stimuli to feet
Kinesthetic	Verbalizing and/or obsessing about body processes
	Refusing to complete a task that may require a part of the body the client believes is not working

SOURCE: Adapted with permission from Moller, M. D., Rice, M. J., & Murphy, M. F. (1998). *Psychiatric protocols for family nurse practitioners.* Philadelphia, PA: Saunders.

hallucinations. Hallucinations cannot be simply willed or talked away. It is crucial that the nurse stay with clients during this intense and often frightening experience. Isolating clients during this time of sensory confusion often exacerbates the hallucinations. Remain nearby because having a real person to talk and listen to will help clients return to reality.

When you *talk to clients*, you may need to talk slightly louder than usual, but use very short and simple phrases. Maintain friendly eye contact, and use the client's preferred name. If the hallucinations are being caused by abnormalities in the temporal lobes, clients may not be able to hear you but will see that your mouth is moving and have a sense that you are real. Perceiving that someone real is talking and calling them by name validates that they are alive. Even if they may not be able to respond to you, they are aware of your presence.

Ask the client to describe what is happening. Talking about the hallucination gives the person permission not to continue to try and hide the experience. Look around the immediate area and *identify* any possible environmental *triggers*. Objects that are reflective or cause glare, such as television screens, photographs behind glass, and fluorescent lights, can contribute to visual hallucinations.

Encourage the client to *describe feelings* related to the hallucinations. If the client asks whether she or he is experienc-

ing the hallucination, you should simply point out that they are not experiencing the hallucination. Do not argue about what is or is not occurring. The client is usually seeking validation and may be grateful to learn that you are not experiencing the same phenomenon.

Teaching clients self-management techniques will assist those who experience ongoing hallucinations to cope better. These strategies involve focusing, reducing anxiety, and distraction. Box 8.1 provides detailed information to include in the psychoeducation process.

CLIENTS EXPERIENCING DELUSIONS

Delusions are false beliefs that cannot be changed by logical reasoning or evidence; they result from misunderstanding reality. These thoughts are so firmly fixed that providing evidence to the contrary does nothing to change the false belief. It is important to realize that a delusion does not always last. It may be fixed in the person's mind only for a few weeks or months or may fluctuate over time. Many clients have reported relief when they realized the belief was a delusion and not a reality.

Delusions can be a single thought, or they can pervade the person's cognitive process. When there is an extensively

BOX 8.1	Hallucinations and Self-Help Strategies

Self-Monitor

- Keep a journal of when each hallucination occurred and what was happening at the time.
- Develop a list of what makes a hallucination better or worse.

Read Aloud/Talk With Someone

- Speaking may reduce the loudness, clarity, and duration of auditory hallucinations.
- Reality orientation may reduce fear associated with hallucinations.

Increase Physiological Arousal Level

- Walking or jogging may distract from hallucinations.
- Doing housework or yard work may distract from hallucinations.
- Go to a crowded place.

Decrease Physiological Arousal Level

- Listening to music or a relaxation tape with headphones decreases anxiety and shifts attention away from hallucinations.
- Wearing earplugs may decrease environmental triggers.
- Take PRN medication.

Talk Back to/Ignore the Voices

- Responding to the voices may make them go away.
- Saying "stop and go away" aloud is a thought-stopping technique to reduce auditory hallucinations.
- Naming environmental objects aloud may block the auditory input of the voices.

Participate in Structured Activities

- Hallucinations decrease in situations with more structure such as playing games, participating in groups, and so on.

SOURCES: Biccheri, R., Trygstad, L., Kanas, N., & Dowling, G. (1997). Symptom management of auditory hallucinations in schizophrenia. *Journal of Psychosocial Nursing, 35*(12), 20–28; Sayer, J., Ritter, S., & Gournay, K. (2000). Beliefs about voices and their effects on coping strategies. *Journal of Advanced Nursing, 31*(5), 1199–1205; Tsai, Y. F., & Ku, Y. C. (2005). Self-care symptom management strategies for auditory hallucinations among inpatients with schizophrenia at a veterans' hospital in Taiwan. *Archives of Psychiatric Nursing, 19*(4), 194–199.

developed central delusional theme from which conclusions are deduced, the delusions are called *systematized.* Of people experiencing delusions, 90% have concurrent hallucinations.

Delusions are believed to be caused by dysfunction in the information-processing circuits within and between the brain's two hemispheres. Studies demonstrate a positive correlation between the degree of reality distortion and activity in the *medial temporal* and *ventral limbic* areas. Delusions occur in schizophrenia, delusional disorder, depression with psychotic features, bipolar disorder, anorexia, obsessive–compulsive disorder, body dysmorphic disorder, hypochondriasis, and dementia. As with hallucinations, the severity of delusions can be a valuable indicator in monitoring the course of a mental disorder (Blackwood et al., 2001).

Types of Delusions

There are a number of delusional types. *Grandiosity,* also known as *delusions of grandeur,* is an exaggerated sense of importance or self-worth. It is often accompanied by beliefs of magical thinking, when a person believes that thinking about a possible occurrence can make it happen. Delusions *of control* occur when the person believes that feelings, impulses, thoughts, or actions are not one's own but are being imposed by some external force. *Erotomanic delusions* are beliefs that a person, usually someone famous and of higher status, is in love with the person. *Somatic delusions* occur when people believe something abnormal and dangerous is happening to their bodies. *Ideas of reference* are remarks or actions by someone else that in no way refer to the person but that are interpreted as related to her or him. *Thought broadcasting* occurs when people believe that others can hear their thoughts. *Thought withdrawal* is the belief that others are able to remove thoughts from one's mind. *Thought insertion* is the belief that others are able to put thoughts into one's mind.

Ann:

❝ "I thought I was under investigation by the CIA and I was getting messages from the TV and the newspaper. I would bring the newspaper into work and read it for a couple of hours a day, trying to decipher the messages. ❞

Religious delusions involve false beliefs with religious or spiritual themes. Religious ideas that may appear delusional in one culture may be commonly held in another. It is important that the nurse distinguish religious beliefs and experiences from delusional psychotic symptoms. Delusions in psychotic episodes:

- Are more intense than usual experiences in a person's religious community
- Are often terrifying for the person
- Involve obsessional preoccupation with the delusion
- Are associated with deterioration of self-care and social skills
- Often involve special messages from religious figures

Delusions of persecution involve beliefs that someone is trying to harm the person. These delusions are preoccupying, obtrusive, and distressing to the client. The danger is that clients will act on their delusional beliefs, harming others in an attempt to protect themselves. People with persecutory delusions are hypervigilant to threat-related stimuli. When things are going well for them, clients are convinced it is their own doing. When things go badly, they are convinced that it is the fault of other people who are "out to get them." They are preoccupied with the intentions of others. It is hypothe-

TABLE 8.2	Types of Delusions
Delusion	**Example**
Grandiosity (delusions of grandeur)	"I've been a member of the President's cabinet since the Reagan years. No president can do without me. If it weren't for me, we would probably be in World War IV by now."
Persecution	"The CIA and the FBI are both out to get me. I am constantly being followed. One of the other patients in here is really a CIA agent and is here to spy on me."
Control	"I have this wire in my head, and my family controls me with it. They make me wake up and make me go to sleep. They control everything I say. I can't do anything on my own."
Religious	"As long as I wear these 10 religious medals and keep all these pictures of Jesus pinned to my clothes, nothing bad can happen to me. No one can hurt me as long as I do this."
Erotomanic	"Julia Roberts is really my wife. We got married last week. She adores me and will be here soon to visit."
Sin and guilt	"I know I often hurt my parents' feelings when I was growing up. That's why I can't ever keep a job. When I get a job and start doing good, I have to quit it to make up for my bad behavior."
Somatic	"My esophagus is being torn apart. I have this rat in my stomach, and sometimes he comes all the way up to my throat. He's eating at my esophagus. Look in my throat now—you can probably see the rat."
Ideas of reference	"People on TV last night told me I was in charge of saving the environment. That's why I'm telling everyone to stop using their cars. It's my job because that's what they told me last night."
Thought broadcasting	"I'm afraid to think anything. I know you can read my mind and know exactly what I'm thinking."
Thought withdrawal	"I can't tell you what I'm thinking. Somebody just stole my thoughts."
Thought insertion	"You think what I'm telling you is what I'm thinking, but it isn't. My father keeps putting all these thoughts in my head. They are not my thoughts."

sized that excessive amygdala activity underlies persecutory delusions since the amygdala is important in the processing of threatening stimuli and the social meaning of that stimuli. See Table 8.2 ■ for examples of the various types of delusions.

Michelle is very distressed, thinking that people in the neighborhood are out to get her. She often shows up at the police station, thinking she has an appointment with a detective who will take care of her problem. She believes one neighbor is stealing her mail and trying to put a block on her phone. She states she was riding her bike yesterday when she felt another neighbor following her in the car trying to run her over. She believes her neighbors are jealous of her.

Ann:

❝I went to the Dean of the Harvard Business School and I said, 'The place is under electronic surveillance. Please bring the police in.' And it happened to be the same time that the spaceship Challenger exploded. So then I thought I had a role in blowing up the Challenger.❞

As Internet technology becomes more widespread in society, Internet delusions are becoming more common. It does not seem to matter whether the client is computer literate. This is an example of how culture influences delusional content. Compton (2003) reports the following examples:

A middle-aged woman believes that the Internet has been controlling her and her home for the past 3 years. When she is walking around and she bumps the furniture, she thinks the Internet is controlling her. She also believes the Internet turns the appliances on and off, changes channels on the television, and causes her to burn herself on the stove.

A young woman takes all her clothes off at home because she believes that microchips have been implanted in her body and put in her clothes to record her actions. She believes that these recordings are being broadcast on the Internet.

An older woman has a complex delusion regarding the "www people" (referring to the World Wide Web). She believes the www people have wired her house, follow her around when she leaves her house, and secretly tape conversations. Having no familiarity with computers, she said she learned about the www people on the television and radio.

Assessment

Delusions are very real to the person having them. They are symptoms that need to be assessed in the same manner as any other symptoms. Nurses may ask themselves: How can I tell whether my client is experiencing delusions? Behaviors often perceived as inappropriate may be a response to delusional thoughts. The kinds of assessment questions appropriate for delusional clients are:

- What kinds of thoughts bother you the most?
- Do you feel that anyone is trying to harm you?
- Do you feel that anyone is controlling you?

- Do you believe that you are someone very important?
- Have you ever thought that you have special powers that other people do not have?
- Do you think about religion a lot?
- Do you believe that you are very guilty for something you have done?
- Do you think anything abnormal is happening to your body?
- Do you think people are talking about you often?
- Do you believe others can hear your thoughts?
- Do you believe others can take away your thoughts?
- Do you believe others can put thoughts into your head?
- Do you have thoughts of harming yourself? Harming others?

Delusions are a useful indicator in the ongoing assessment of a client's level of functioning. It is important to identify delusions as a symptom of psychosis. Assessing the level of functioning provides direction for nursing interventions.

Interventions

Delusions are often very frightening. *Providing an opportunity to discuss delusions* may lessen the fear. Provide comfort and *reassurance of safety*. After listening and reassuring, refocus the conversation to another topic to provide distraction from the troubling thoughts. If possible, help the client identify situations in which it is socially unacceptable to discuss delusions to prevent further public rejection and social isolation.

It is important to *monitor delusions for content*. Identifying beliefs that may be harmful to self or harmful to others is necessary to protect the client and others from behaviors that may be unsafe. Encourage clients to verbalize delusions to caregivers before impulsively acting on them.

If asked, simply point out that you, yourself do not experience the delusion. Always present reality, but do it gently, without implying that the client is wrong. Do not attempt to reason, argue, or challenge the delusion because that puts the client on the defensive. Do not attempt to logically explain the delusion. Only the client understands the logic behind the delusional content.

Identify triggers of the delusion. Focus on the underlying feelings since unexpressed feelings can trigger delusions. Once triggers have been identified, assist the client in problem solving to avoid or eliminate stressors that precipitate delusions.

Teach coping techniques that reinforce and focus on reality. Talk about real people and real events. Recreational and diversional activities that require attention and skill provide temporary relief from disturbing delusions.

CLIENTS WHO SELF-MUTILATE

Self-mutilation is the deliberate destruction of body tissue without conscious intent of suicide. Other terms used to describe self-mutilation include deliberate self-harm, self-injurious behavior, and aggression against the self. Understanding this behavior, recognizing the warning signs, and managing ongoing risk is an important challenge to mental health nurses.

Some studies have found that females are more likely than males to self-mutilate and other studies have found no gender differences. Self-mutilation usually begins in adolescence although it can begin as young as 7 years of age. Self-mutilation affects people of all ethnic backgrounds in the United States. Every year as many as 2 million Americans deliberately cut, burn, or hurt themselves in other ways, which is 30 times the rate of suicide attempts (Klonsky, Oltmanns, & Turkheimer, 2003).

Self-mutilative behavior may occur once or sporadically, or it may become repetitive. Some behaviors are not premeditated but occur because of an inability for the person to control his/her temper in response to an argument. This form of impulsive behavior is more common among males. Self-mutilation occurs in an estimated 24% to 40% of mental health clients. It is a symptom associated with childhood sexual and physical abuse, borderline personality disorder, eating disorders, cognitive impairment disorders, obsessive–compulsive disorder, posttraumatic stress disorder, dissociative identity disorder, and cognitive impairment. Self-mutilation may occur in response to delusions, command hallucinations, and substance abuse or dependence (Specht, Singer, & Henry, 2005).

Juan goes to a specialized school for emotionally handicapped students. One of the ways he "copes" with stress is through self-mutilation. One morning at breakfast he got into a verbal confrontation with a peer that escalated into a pushing match. Juan threw his breakfast tray at the other boy, who then started hitting Juan. They were separated by staff and went to the classroom for school activities. The teacher noticed that Juan was exhibiting increasing signs of anxiety and could not concentrate on school work. Juan began to stare into space and started rubbing the inside of his eyelids with his finger, which progressed to using the sharp end of a pencil on his inner eyelids. The teacher sat down directly in front of Juan and talked to him in a low, calm voice. Within a short period of time, Juan was able to leave his dissociative state and stop his self-mutilative behavior.

The Internet has served as a mechanism to enable and abstain from self-mutilation. There are chat rooms in which individuals discuss how to self-mutilate and there are even group times to engage in the activity. There are also Internet sites that seek to prevent self-mutilation through chat room support. Because many parents are unaware of what their children are doing, you should encourage them to monitor their children's use of the Internet.

Forms of Self-mutilation

People who self-mutilate often use multiple methods of self-harm. The most common forms are *superficial* to *moderate* self-mutilation behaviors, including skin cutting (the most common form), skin carving (words, designs, symbols), skin burning, severe skin scratching, needle sticking, self-hitting, tearing out hair, inserting dangerous objects into the vagina or rectum, ingesting sharp objects, bone breaking, and interfering with wound healing. Most individuals use more than one form of self-mutilation. Occasionally, *severe* acts of self-mutilation occur, such as eye enucleation, castration, and amputation of fingers, toes, or limbs. Psychosis is a major factor in severe self-mutilation, often related to delusions and command hallucinations.

Stereotypic self-mutilation occurs in fixed patterns that are often rhythmic, such as head banging and finger biting. This behavior occurs most often in people who are institutionalized for cognitive impairment (Paul, Schroeter, Dahme, & Nutzinger, 2002). Box 8.2 describes the stages of self-mutilation.

Biological studies have found that the neurotransmitters *dopamine* (DA) and *serotonin* (5-HT) influence self-mutilative behavior. DA and 5-HT dysfunction are related to impulsive and aggressive behaviors. Dysphoria may be lessened as endorphins are released in response to the physical pain. Since the frontal lobes in adolescents are not yet fully developed, teens have some difficulty with self-awareness, emotional control, impulse restraint, and rational decision making—all of which may factor into self-mutilation (Cerdorian, 2005).

BOX 8.2	Stages of Self-mutilation

Stage 1: Precipitating Event

- This may include events such as the loss of a significant relationship or the perception or threat of an imminent loss.

Stage 2: Intensification of Feelings

- Unpleasant feelings such as anxiety, anger, helplessness, hopelessness, emptiness, and despair increase to high levels.

Stage 3: Attempts to Cope

- Client tries to delay the act of self-inflicted violence.

Stage 4: Action

- Client "gives in" to internal demand to self-mutilate.
- Acts of self-mutilation occur in private; unless medical attention is required, the behavior is often not discovered.

Stage 5: Aftermath

- Client may experience feelings of relief from tension or feelings of shame, guilt, or sense of failure.

SOURCES: Faye, P. (1995). Addictive characteristics of the behavior of self-mutilation. *Journal of Psychosocial Nursing, 33*(6), 36–39; and Strong, M. (1998). *A bright red scream: Self-mutilation and the language of pain.* New York: Viking.

Tori describes her self-mutilation: "I feel so sad and zoned out all the time. It gets to the point that I feel numb inside and cutting makes me feel alive. I hate crying, so now the blood has become my tears. It feels like I have some control in my life."

Assessment

Self-mutilating behavior is generally impulsive, and the onset is often linked to a stressful situation. As one client described her experience, "I thought I needed to be punished, that I was bad. I'd cut myself and get relief. I got relief from seeing my own blood; it was like my feelings were flowing out." Self-mutilation has great meaning, often hidden from others, for those who do it. One of the purposes of client assessment is to understand the unique meaning of the behavior for each client. Only when the meaning is understood can nursing interventions be designed. Some of the many possible meanings of or reasons for self-mutilation are:

- Ending a dissociative experience
- Reorienting from flashbacks
- Reenacting childhood trauma
- Reconnecting to a feeling of being real and alive
- Seeking distraction from emotional pain
- Feeling something other than despair
- Releasing tension or rage
- Punishing oneself
- Requesting nurturance
- Crying for help
- Feeling powerful and in control
- Influencing others

Sheri describes her experience: "I start to feel tense and then I feel overwhelmed with hopelessness and failure. I know I should talk about it but I can't get it out. I cut when I feel this way."

Slajana states: "I feel numb. The pain lets me know I'm alive. I feel so much emotional pain, the physical pain relieves it. The other night the nurse gave me an injection and it felt really good feeling the pain without inflicting it myself, so I didn't feel guilty."

Interventions

It is very important to establish a *trusting relationship* with clients who self-mutilate. They have probably experienced much criticism and little understanding regarding their self-injurious behavior. Let them know that you understand what they are going through as a way to validate their personhood. Victims often have been told that they should just stop the behavior and have been scolded for not being competent enough. Under these conditions, the failure to stop the self-harm leads to even greater shame and concealment.

People who self-mutilate respond best to a *nonjudgmental* and accepting attitude, a caring approach, and limit setting to minimize the potential for physical injury. It is a delicate balance between keeping these individuals safe versus giving them as much control as possible over their lives. It is also understandable that staff members may react with frustration and even guilt when clients choose to harm themselves despite well-planned interventions and a caring approach (Livesley, 2003; Weber, 2002).

There are three basic goals in helping clients manage their self-harmful behavior. The first goal is to *encourage communication* about self-injury since clients are often secretive and shameful about the behavior. Supportive listening may help them communicate and thus feel less isolated. The second goal is to *improve the related quality of life*, such as through reducing their shame and isolation, decreasing their self-criticism, and ensuring that they receive adequate medical attention. The nurse's ability to respond without blame or shame may help clients begin the process of self-healing. The third goal is to *diminish or extinguish the use of self-mutilation* as a coping tool. As client understanding of their own experiences grows, they will improve their ability to manage, live with, or cease their behavior.

Box 8.3 describes appropriate nursing interventions when intervening with people who self-mutilate. Finding alternatives to self-harming behaviors is a critical step for people who wish to stop hurting themselves. Sometimes this means learning new skills in the areas of problem solving or relaxation and anxiety reduction. *Teaching* clients alternative coping skills is an appropriate intervention. Box 8.4 lists noninjurious alternatives clients may wish to consider.

BOX 8.4 — Alternatives to Self-mutilation

Nonharmful Symbolic Enactments

- Draw the "blood" or "cuts" on paper.
- "Injure" a toy or stuffed animal.
- Make marks with red marker or crayon on your skin.

Physical Awareness

- Breathe slowly and mentally scan each part of the body.
- Stroke your arm or leg, place ice on your skin, snap a rubber band on your wrist.

Distraction

- Promise yourself to wait 5 to 10 minutes before self-injuring.
- Read a book, watch a video, go to a movie.

Interpersonal Contact

- Call a friend; talk about the impulse toward self-harm.
- Call a support group member.

Physical Activity, Tension Reduction

- Exercise, dance, play a physical game.

Art and Writing Activities

- Draw the feeling or the memory.
- Write about your feelings; write a letter to a significant person.

Expressive Anger Activities

- Pound a tennis racket on a bed; pound pillows.
- Break old dishes or glasses in safe ways; throw ice cubes; smash aluminum cans.

SOURCES: Loughrey, L. (1997). Patient self-mutilation: When nursing becomes a nightmare. *Journal of Psychosocial Nursing, 35*(4), 30–34; and Strong, M. (1998). *A bright red scream: Self-mutilation and the language of pain.* New York: Viking.

BOX 8.3 — Behavior Management: Self-harm

Identify the Functions of the Behavior

- In a nonjudgmental manner, ask, "How does this help you?" or "What does this do for you?" This will increase clients' self-understanding and decrease feelings of shame.

Identify the Triggers

- Have clients keep a journal describing the stressors preceding the behavior, situations in which the behavior occurs, and the effect on others.

Use Behavioral Contracts

- Contracts focus on the fact that clients are responsible for their own behavior and they have to live with the consequences of their behavior.
- Contracts include a clear understanding of treatment goals and mutual expectations of behavioral change.

SOURCES: McCloskey, J. C., & Bulechek, G. M. (1996). *Nursing interventions classification (NIC)* (2nd ed.). St. Louis, MO: Mosby; and Strong, M. (1998). *A bright red scream: Self-mutilation and the language of pain.* New York: Viking.

CLIENTS WHO ARE AGGRESSIVE

Physical aggression and destruction of property are among the most severe and frightening client behaviors, which occur in treatment settings, as well as in the home. Violence is often directed at family members, friends, and acquaintances and may result in physical injuries. When violence occurs in treatment settings, professionals or other clients are often the victims. Aggression affects every person in the environment in which it occurs. A violent client may be injured directly from the aggressive behavior or during a restraining procedure. Other clients and staff members may be purposefully or accidentally injured. Studies show that nurses are threatened, verbally abused, and physically assaulted at higher rates than other professionals. Psychiatric nurses are at the highest risk of violence compared with other hospital nurses. Out-of-control behavior frightens everyone, and violence disrupts the unit or home environment (Chen, Hwu, & Williams, 2005; Kindy, Petersen, & Parkhurst, 2005).

Aggressive behavior is a complex phenomenon that may occur in clients with schizophrenia, mood disorders, borderline personality disorder, conduct disorder, and substance use disorders. Aggression may be related to a lower level of activity in the *cingulate gyrus* and the *frontal cortex*, resulting in an underactive executive system. The result is a lack of inhibition messages and an inability to moderate aggressive thoughts and behaviors. Reduced activity of *serotonin* (5-HT), either genetically (50% of the cases) or because of early brain injury (prenatal alcohol exposure), is a risk factor in aggression but is not enough by itself. When low 5-HT is combined with other genetic factors and environmental stressors, impulsiveness and aggression may be triggered. With the onset of environmental stressors, there is a rapid release of *norepinepherine* (NE), resulting in increased arousal and attention. This may also contribute to an increase in aggressive behavior. Some people taking antidepressant medication that increases NE may experience agitation and irritability as a side effect (Frankle et al., 2005; Perusse & Gendreau, 2005; Pihl & Benkelfat, 2005).

When an individual learns that acting on aggressive impulses brings a kind of relief, that person can get "addicted" to aggression as a way to solve problems and relieve frustrations. This makes it very difficult for she or he to control angry outbursts, even when they want to. Other factors related to societal violence include personal pressures such as lack of social support, employment difficulties, or financial problems; an easy access to weapons; and the tendency in U.S. culture to condone violence as a solution to problems (Woodside & McClum, 2006).

Explosive behavior may be the result of organic disease, such as temporal lobe epilepsy, dementia, delirium, hypoxia, or hypoglycemia. Explosive behavior may also be related to substance use, substance withdrawal, and antisocial personality disorder. In these situations, the diagnosis of intermittent explosive disorder is not appropriate.

Intermittent explosive disorder (IED) is a DSM-IV-TR diagnosis. The affected person has episodes of aggressive impulses that result in serious assaultive acts or destruction of property. The degree of aggressiveness is grossly out of proportion with the associated stress. Clients may experience rage and increased energy during the episode, and depressed mood, fatigue, and remorse after the acts. This disorder results in severe psychosocial and legal consequences. It may begin as early as childhood or as late as the 20s. Among young people, IED is on the increase, and it may set the stage for the onset of other mental disorders. Two things generally set these people off: perceived threats and frustrating situations. For some people it is a temporary condition, while for others it has a long-term course (American Psychiatric Association, 2000; Kessler et al., 2006).

Triggers to Aggression

Violence may be a consequence of poor frustration tolerance, ineffective individual coping, impulsivity, and real or imagined threats to the person's territory, body space, or life. In residential and day programs and inpatient settings, aggression and violence have been related to staff provocation. Violence occurs at a higher rate in settings in which staff members have an authoritarian or controlling approach to clients. Telling clients what they can or cannot do, detaining them against their will, and forcing them to take medication contribute to staff–client conflicts. When these actions are used with people who are accustomed to controlling their environment through aggression and violence, one can predict an escalation of violent behavior.

Curtis, age 17, lives in a residential setting for severely emotionally handicapped adolescents. He was physically and emotionally abused as a child, and his family environment is chaotic. He has a cyclical pattern of aggressive and passive behaviors. Curtis talked to his mother by phone earlier in the day. At the time he was supposed to be in group therapy, he was in the kitchen with the staff. The staff told him to leave the kitchen and go to the group room. Curtis refused. As they repeated their directions, he began to posture aggressively, stare without blinking, and refused to move. More staff members were called to the kitchen to defuse the situation. One staff member took the lead and began talking to Curtis in a calm, nonthreatening manner, while the other staff members remained in the background. The staff member helped him identify his feelings of abandonment that resurfaced following the phone conversation with his mother. After a period of time, the intervention was successful and Curtis was able to join the group for the remainder of the therapy session. Shortly after Curtis's violent episode, an intervention and contract were initiated. He had to reflect on and respond in writing to these topics:

1. Reflect on the facts of the situation.
2. Identify what he was feeling at the time.
3. List alternative behaviors that he could have chosen.
4. Identify consequences, such as loss of privileges, for skipping group therapy.

It is believed that the increase in violence is related to increased substance abuse by people with mental disorders. Silver, Yudofsky, and Anderson (2005) describe the relationship of violence to substance use:

- Direct effect of the substance on the brain—especially crack cocaine and amphetamines, which are associated with irritability, impulsiveness, and paranoid delusional thinking

- Exposure to a dangerous environment, such as drug dealing and crack houses

- Activities, such as robbery and prostitution, by which money is obtained for drugs

Assessment

Aggressive behavior can range from slaps, pushes, or shoves in play to serious attempts to hurt another person. The threat of imminent violence is very frightening to staff, other clients, and, indeed, to the aggressive person him- or herself. The best predictor of future violence in a client is a *history of violent behavior*. In assessing for the potential, keep in mind the following situations in which violence is more likely to occur:

- The person may not have been completely evaluated and treatment may not have begun (first 1 or 2 days after admission)
- Auditory hallucinations: telling person to strike out
- Visual hallucinations: protecting self from what is being seen

- Tactile hallucinations: disengages self from what is being felt
- Delusions: may perceive violence as the only option; may believe she/he is fighting for her/his life
- Affective dysfunction: motivated by fear, frustration, or rage
- Poor impulse control: in response to limit setting by caregivers
- Drugs or alcohol: intoxication can contribute to aggressive behavior
- Secondary gains: motivated by power and control

TABLE 8.3	Phases of Aggression
Phase 1: Triggering Phase	
Feeling	Anxiety
Behavior	Agitation, pacing, avoiding contact
Nurse's response	Identify triggering factors, decrease anxiety, problem solve if possible.
Phase 2: Transition Phase	
Feeling	Anger
Behavior	Increased agitation
Nurse's response	Do not match anger with anger; keep talking; set limits and give directions; negotiate compromise; explore consequences; get help.
Phase 3: Crisis	
Feeling	Increased anger and aggression
Behavior	Agitation, threatening gestures, invasion of personal space; profanity; shouting
Nurse's response	Continue phase 2 interventions; increase personal space; warn (do not threaten) of consequences; try to maintain communication.
Phase 4: Destructive Behavior	
Feeling	Rage
Behavior	Assault; destruction
Nurse's response	Protect other clients; escape; perform physical restraint.
Phase 5: Descent Phase	
Feeling	Aggression
Behavior	Stopping of overtly destructive behavior; reduction in level of arousal
Nurse's response	Remain vigilant as new violent behavior is still possible; avoid retaliation or revenge.
Phase 6: Transition Phase	
Feeling	Anger
Behavior	Agitation, pacing
Nurse's response	Resume focus on problem solving.

SOURCE: Adapted with permission from Leadbetter, D., & Paterson, B. (1995). De-escalating aggressive behaviour. In B. Kidd & C. Stark (Eds.), *Management of violence and aggression in health care* (pp. 49–84). London: Gaskell.

- Environmental cues: violence may be reinforced through encouragement by peer group
- Poor impulse control: overreact to intrusions or insults from other clients
- Alzheimer's disease: aggression usually unplanned and reactive; often during ADLs
- General medical problems triggering aggression: hypoglycemia, acute febrile illness, temporal lobe epilepsy, head trauma

It is important to continually assess for ongoing signs of escalation of aggressive behavior. If nurses assess accurately and respond early and appropriately, they may be able to halt the progression of aggressive behavior. Table 8.3 ■ describes the phases of aggression.

Warning signs of aggression include:

- Speaking more quickly with subtly angry tone of voice
- Sarcastic comments or challenges such as "You think you're a big shot, don't you!"
- Pacing, refusing to sit down
- Rapid and jerky gestures
- Lengthy, intense staring
- Threatening gestures such as vigorously pointing a finger at the nurse
- Clenching fists, raising of closed fist, pounding fist into opposite palm

Interventions

Prevention

It is much better for all people involved to prevent out-of-control behavior than to manage it. In some instances, no matter what preventative actions are undertaken, aggression will erupt. The goal is to decrease the likelihood of this happening.

An effective intervention is to teach *nonviolent coping strategies*. This is done at a time when the client is not angry or tense. Assist the client in identifying the source of the anger or frustration. Following that, you can help identify the function that anger, frustration, and rage serve for the client. Teach the client to develop appropriate methods to express feelings, such as assertiveness and "I" feeling statements. Together you can plan strategies to prevent inappropriate expression of anger. Some clients may find physical outlets helpful, such as vigorous exercise, lifting weights, strenuous cleaning or gardening, throwing light foam balls, or other nondestructive physical activities. Others may find that time-outs help decrease feelings of hostility. You may also role-play potentially frustrating situations at a time when the client is feeling calm and in control. Box 8.5 describes anger management techniques.

BOX 8.5	Anger Management

Teaching

- Nature and function of anger
- Healthy anger is that which leads to desirable, productive change.
- Unhealthy anger is that which is too intense and leads to problems with other people.
- Types of aggression: verbal and physical

Signals

- Personal triggers to anger
- Recognizing cues of escalating anger
- Stop before you react.

Calming Strategies

- Controlled breathing
- Distraction or refocusing—drawing, listening to music, talking with someone, time with a pet
- Counting backward
- Leaving the situation

Problem Solving

- Explore the relationship between thinking, feeling, and acting.
- Identify the problem, consider options, predict consequences, select best response, enact response, evaluate outcomes.
- Changing thoughts and actions will change feelings.

SOURCES: Adapted with permission from Geller, B., & Debello, M. P. (2003). *Bipolar disorder in childhood and early adolescence.* New York: Guilford Press; and Larson, J. (2005). *Think first: Addressing aggressive behavior in secondary schools.* New York: Guilford Press.

A *behavioral contract* is often a very effective way to prevent violence. It is one way to present the rules of the milieu and help the client become engaged in the treatment process. Understanding that there are consequences, perhaps legal consequences, to violent acts may help clients gain control of their impulses. The contract also enables clients to feel like they have some input into the treatment plan and, thus, responsibility for carrying out the plan.

Interpersonal Skills

The way that the nurse interacts may decrease or increase violent behavior. A *calm*, professional, confident approach often diffuses hostility. In an impending aggressive situation, it is important not to lose sight of the client as a unique individual with unique needs and who is deserving of respect. Acknowledging that you are trying to understand the situation helps individuals respond without violence. When people are treated with dignity, they often deescalate their aggression.

The cultural background of the client is also a consideration. Concepts of respect and disrespect vary, as do boundaries, personal space, and gender roles. You must understand these cultural variations so that you do not

MediaLink

Care Plan, Common Clinical Behaviors

Jorge, age 37, has been admitted to an acute care setting with the diagnosis of schizoaffective disorder, bipolar type. He has received psychiatric care for 22 years. His mood is labile, he is easily distracted, and he has a very short attention span. The nurse is meeting Jorge for the first time to begin the assessment. Their interaction will show evidence of:

- His hallucinations
- His delusions
- His disorganized thinking

NURSE: *"What happened to bring you into the hospital?"*

JORGE: "Well, there were three killings in my house and then I heard voices outside on my front lawn and they were distracting me."

NURSE: *"Tell me more about the killings."*

JORGE: "There were two killings and when I came down the stairs I accidentally crushed Angelina Jolie. Then there were three killings."

NURSE: *"That sounds like a scary experience. What about the voices?"*

JORGE: "The voices outside were Saddam and Gorbachev from a different planet. When I came outside they blew their heads off and disappeared."

NURSE: *"How did you react to that?"*

JORGE: "I thought I was responsible for the killings, so I called the police and asked them to bring a gun to my house to kill me. But they never brought it and that made me angry."

NURSE: *"What happened next?"*

JORGE: "I went to the clinic and they sawed off my legs and arms but they stuck together because I'm innocent."

Tsai, Y. F., & Ku, Y. C. (2005). Self-care symptom management strategies for auditory hallucinations among inpatients with schizophrenia at a veterans' hospital in Taiwan. *Archives of Psychiatric Nursing, 19*(4), 194–199.

What is the study about?

Persistent auditory hallucinations (AHs) are very stressful for persons living with schizophrenia and have been related to anxiety, depression, and suicidal behavior. Therefore, this study explored how inpatients living with schizophrenia managed AHs via self-care strategies.

How was the study done?

This quantitative, descriptive exploratory study used a convenience sample of 200 men and women living in a veterans' hospital in eastern Taiwan. This study was approved by the veterans' hospital. Participants met the diagnostic criteria for schizophrenia of the *Diagnostic and Statistical Manual of Mental Disorders*, 4th edition, and willingly provided information about AHs they had experienced on a daily basis for a minimum of 6 months. In addition, participants were residents of a subacute or chronic unit for psychiatric care for more than 3 months, and did not have severe cognitive deficits that would bar them from answering questions about AHs.

Data were obtained through self-report and designed semi-structured questionnaires. These participants were first asked to rate their AHs, on a 1–10 scale, for severity and level of interference. Next they were asked to identify three self-care strategies they frequently used to gain relief from their AHs, rate each strategy's effectiveness, and identify its source. The resulting data were analyzed quantitatively for frequencies, means, and standard deviations. Content analysis was used to categorize the strategies. Trustworthiness of the content analyses was established by having two clients, the principal investigator, and the research assistant arrive at a mutual agreement of the findings.

What were the results of the study?

The AHs were, on average, moderately severe (5.6 on a scale of 10) and moderately interfering (5.8 on a scale of 10). The self-care management strategies fell into three categories: physiological, cognitive, and behavioral. Physiological strategies and reported frequencies were: listen to music (17), exercise (11), smoke cigarettes (11), sleep (4), take extra medication (4), walk (3), lie down (1), rest (1), and drink alcohol (1). Cognitive activities and frequencies were: reduce attention to voices (124), ignore voices (124), accept voices (47), verify voices (27), ask self to calm down (23), argue with voices (21), accept and stay with voices peacefully (10), do as voices say (8), and talk to voices (6). Behavioral strategies and related frequencies were: cover ears (55), watch television (37), seek help from the nurse (28), talk to others (16), pray or read Buddhist scripture (15), do things to shift attention (15), seek help from the doctor (13), sing (10), go to a crowded place (7), read a book or a magazine (5), isolate self (4), cry (4), masturbate (3), go to a quiet place (2), meditate (2), hurt self (1), be wakeful (1), play cards (1), and shake head (1).

What additional questions might I have?

How do these findings compare with those from persons living in Western culture and experiencing AHs? Are preferences for self-care management strategies for AHs influenced by culture? Are the results relevant to both clients living in a psychiatric residential center and those living in the community? Did the use of psychiatric medications influence the selection of positive or self-harming coping strategies?

How can I use this study?

Nurses need to assist persons living with schizophrenia and experiencing AHs to develop positive self-care management techniques such as listening to music. However, nurses must be cognizant that some of the coping strategies used with AHs may harm the individuals. Nurses should inform clients about the hazards associated with some strategies and help them develop safe and effective self-management strategies for AHs.

SOURCE: Contributed by Dolores Huffman, PhD, RN, Associate Professor of Nursing, Purdue University Calumet, Hammond, Indiana.

unwittingly behave in some way that would offend or threaten a client from a different culture.

Nonverbal Communication Skills

Nonverbal behavior is very important when interacting with clients who are aggressive. Aggression is a two-person process. The nurse's nonverbal behavior may inadvertently cause the behavior of an already agitated client to escalate. Approach the client in a *nonauthoritarian manner.* Stand in front, at an angle; give enough interpersonal space; and do not attempt to touch the person. Maintain normal eye contact. Prolonged eye contact is perceived as aggressive and avoidance of eye contact implies fear or lack of interest. Avoid using threatening body language such as clenched fists, hands on hips, or crossed arms. If the client says, "Get away from me!" move away in a slow manner that is respectful of the communication but that does not show fear.

Verbal Communication Skills

The immediate goal is to gain some time and help the person regain self-control. At all times, nurses should be aware of how their verbal messages are delivered; that is, the tone, loudness, and pitch of their voice. The nurse's voice should be normal, unhurried, and assertive. Do not speak in an authoritarian manner or make antagonistic remarks that would likely escalate the hostility. Use clear, appropriate language and short sentences in a nonthreatening manner. Do not overreact or talk too much. Paraphrase what the client is saying.

Telling people what they can do is more effective than stating what is not allowed. "Put the chair by the table" may work better than "Don't pick that chair up." Telling people what they cannot do may set up power struggles. Losing control can be equally as frightening to clients as to staff. Another approach is to give clients choices. "There are two quieter places you may go to: your room or the deck. Which one would you like?" Each time a choice is given, the person will pause and consider the option. Each pause decreases the amount of energy behind the anger. Giving choices also helps people feel they have some control in the situation.

Talking down is another effective approach. For the time being, agree with what the client is saying. Avoid arguing so that you do not get stuck on the content of the client's communication. At this point, it does not matter whether all nurses are uncaring, whether you should go jump in the lake, or who your ancestors were. None of that matters. What matters is that you help the behavior deescalate by not arguing and not giving the person a reason to continue to be angry. Continue to speak in a soft voice and give the person choices.

Medication may be necessary to help people regain control of themselves. The use of medications to prevent psychosis or violent behavior is covered in chapter 10 ∞. Ziprasidone (Geodon) and aripiprazole (Abilify) are second-generation antipsychotic agents that can be given intramuscularly (IM) for the control and short-term management of clients who are acutely psychotic and agitated. They produce less sedation than other medications and are effective within 30 to 60 minutes. Haloperidol (Haldol) administered IM is effective in controlling aggressive behavior usually within 30 minutes. Lorazepam (Ativan) administered IM is frequently used for the immediate control of psychotic disruptive behavior. It may also be given at the same time as haloperidol to decrease the side effects of akathisia and acute dystonias. Unfortunately, this means two injections since lorazepam cannot be mixed in the same syringe with any other medication.

Seclusion and Restraints

Some clients find it helpful to go to the "quiet room" when they feel they are going to lose control. This should be a room under close staff supervision where the person can be comfortable and away from other clients. The client should be free to come and go as desired.

In rare instances, when medications and other interventions may not work rapidly enough to protect clients and staff, seclusion or restraints may be necessary. Become familiar with the state laws regarding their use. Most clients experience restraint as traumatic, dehumanizing, or humiliating. Use of restraints requires physical force that increases the risk of injury to the client and staff. Use of physical force with clients reinforces their perception that violence is a valid method of gaining control. It also reinforces the client's self-image as a tough person and increases the likelihood of future violent confrontations. Unfortunately, these methods do not teach clients coping skills to help them avoid using aggression in the future. Because clients often view restraints as punishment, this method fosters distrust of, and malice toward, staff members. See chapter 9 ∞ for further discussion on problems regarding the use of restraints.

Critical Incident Review

After a serious assault, staff members are angry and apprehensive; the aggressive client is humiliated, angry, and fearful; and other clients who witnessed the event are intimidated and terrified. After everyone's safety is ensured, all staff members participate in a critical incident review. The goal of this review is to understand what happened prior to and during the assault. There is a discussion of measures that were taken to calm the client and ensure everyone's safety. Precipitants to the hostility are identified, as well as client behaviors that indicated escalating aggression. Any necessary revisions to the treatment plan will be made. The main questions are: "What did we do to deescalate the behavior?" "Was the person treated with respect?" "How can we help this person learn nonviolent means of coping with stress?"

These common clinical behaviors—hallucinations, delusions, self-mutilation, and aggression—occur in a variety of settings among clients with a variety of mental disorders. Recognize that these problematic behaviors are not limited to a specific diagnosis. This recognition allows the nurse to respond to the individual with the problem rather than be limited by the diagnostic category.

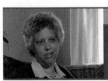

ROAD Assessment: Critical Thinking Questions

Go to the CD-ROM to assess Ann by answering the following critical-thinking questions based on what you have **R**ead about Ann and **O**bserved on the videos.

1. Based on your understanding of what can trigger altered thought processes and mania in bipolar disorder, what would have been important to assess in Ann's postpartum visits after the birth of her daughter? Provide the rationale for your answers. (Hint: Refer to chapter 13 in the textbook for additional information that will help you in formulating your answers.)

2. What type of delusion is Ann describing during her interview on the video clip? Provide the rationale for your answers.

3. When Ann states that she was terrified she would be assassinated by the CIA, what additional assessment questions would it have been important to ask? Provide the rationale for your answers.

4. Ann has been hospitalized for an increase in delusions that put her at risk for harming others. It is 6 hours after her admission to an open, adult unit. As you are walking out of another client's room, you hear Ann curse a client. She accuses the client of taking her picture with an invisible camera in a book and working with the CIA to assassinate her while she's in the hospital. During the past 6 hours since admission, Ann has been avoiding contact with staff and clients. Slamming her door, she returns to her room. What phase of escalating aggression is Ann displaying? Give specific examples of nursing and staff responses that can be offered to Ann. Provide the rationale for your answers.

5. Ann's agitated behavior continues. While staff members collaborate to implement nonpharmacological interventions that assist Ann in managing her anxiety and anger, you reflect, wondering whether the physician has ordered the needed medication. Which IM pharmacological agent would you expect to see on the medication sheet and why? Provide the rationale for your answers.

ROAD: DEVELOP A CARE PLAN

Go to the CD-ROM to Develop a care plan based on your assessment of Ann. Identify nursing diagnoses, outcomes, goals, and interventions.
SOURCE: Contributed by Susan Siwinski-Hebel, RN, MSN.

Focus Your Study

OBJECTIVES

1. Differentiate between the parts of the brain implicated in common clinical behaviors.

KEY CONCEPTS

- Auditory hallucinations:
  - Dysfunction in the language center in the temporal lobes
- Visual hallucinations:
  - Dysfunction in the occipital lobes
- Delusions:
  - Dysfunction in the information-processing circuits within and between the brain's two hemispheres:
  - Medical temporal area
  - Ventral limbic area
- Self-mutilation:
  - Dopamine (DA) and serotonin (5-HT) dysfunction
- Impulsive behavior is related to:
  - Low levels of serotonin (5-HT)
  - Hyperactivity of the limbic system
  - Inadequate control by the cortex

2. Compare and contrast the assessment process for different common clinical behaviors.

→

- Assess for the presence of hallucinations:
  - Frequency, duration, disruption, severity, loudness, intensity, and location
  - Client's belief regarding the origin of the hallucinations
  - Inappropriate laughter
  - Conversations with an unseen person
  - Difficulty paying attention to the task at hand
  - Slow verbal response
  - Inability to respond to anything in the external environment
- Assess for the presence of delusions:
  - What kinds of thoughts bother you the most?
  - Do you feel that anyone is trying to harm you?
  - Do you feel that anyone is controlling you?
  - Do you believe that you are someone very important?
  - Have you ever thought that you have special powers that other people do not have?
  - Do you think about religion a lot?
  - Do you believe that you are very guilty for something you have done?
  - Do you think anything abnormal is happening to your body?
  - Do you think people are talking about you often?
  - Do you believe others can hear your thoughts?
  - Do you believe others can take away your thoughts?
  - Do you believe others can put thoughts into your head?
  - Do you have thoughts of harming yourself? Harming others?
- Assess the functions of self-mutilating behaviors for individual clients:
  - Ending dissociative experiences
  - Reorienting from flashbacks
  - Reenacting childhood trauma
  - Reconnecting to a feeling of being real and alive
  - Seeking distraction from emotional pain
  - Feeling something other than despair
  - Releasing tension or rage
  - Punishing oneself
  - Requesting nurturance
  - Crying for help
  - Feeling powerful and in control
  - Influencing others
- Assess for signs of escalating aggression:
  - The best predictor of future violence in a client is a history of violent behavior.
  - Speaking more quickly with subtly angry tone of voice
  - Sarcastic comments
  - Pacing, refusing to sit down
  - Rapid and jerky gestures
  - Lengthy, intense staring
  - Threatening gestures
  - Clenching fists, raising closed fist, pounding fist into opposite palm

3. Outline interventions for common clinical behaviors.

→

- Hallucinations:
  - Stay with clients during this frightening experience.
  - Talk to clients with short, simple phrases using preferred name.
  - Identify any environmental triggers.
  - Ask clients to describe what is happening and how they are feeling.
  - Self-help strategies include journaling, talking with others, physical exercise, relaxation techniques, talking back to the voices, talking aloud to block the voices, and participation in structured activities.
- Delusions:
  - Give clients opportunities to discuss delusions and monitor for content.
  - Gently present reality without implying that clients are wrong.
  - Avoid arguing or challenging the delusion.
  - Reassure of safety
  - Identify triggers
  - Provide distracting activities

(continued)

(continued)

3. Outline interventions for common clinical behaviors. →

- Self-mutilation:
  - Validate clients' sense of self.
  - Establish a trusting, nonjudgmental, caring relationship.
  - Encourage communication about self-injury to decrease shameful feelings.
  - Reduce isolation and self-criticism to improve the quality of their lives.
  - Formulate a non–self-injury contract.
  - Diminish or extinguish the use of self-mutilation as a coping tool.
  - Self-help strategies include journaling, nonharmful symbolic enactments, increasing body awareness, distraction techniques, talking with others, physical exercise, writing or drawing the pain, and safe expression of angry feelings.
- Aggression:
  - Preventing aggression includes teaching nonviolent coping strategies and formulating a behavioral contract.
  - Professional behavior to prevent violence includes a calm, confident, and nonauthoritarian approach, and a respect for boundaries and cultural roles.
  - When clients are angry, take care to avoid escalating the hostility. Remain assertive and unhurried.
  - Give clients safe choices for their behavior.
  - Medication may be necessary to help people regain control.
  - Seclusion and restraints are only used in rare and dangerous situations.
  - Self-help strategies include identifying personal triggers to anger, recognizing cues to escalating anger, calming strategies, and utilizing the problem-solving process.

Explore MediaLink

For review questions, case studies, and other resources for this chapter see the Pearson Health MediaLink CD-ROM that accompanies this book and the Companion Website.

CD-ROM
- Audio Glossary
- NCLEX-RN® Review Questions
- Road to Critical Thinking: *Ann*

Companion Website www.prenhall.com/fontaine
- Audio Glossary
- NCLEX-RN® Review Questions
- Case Study
  - Intermittent Explosive Disorder
- Care Plan
  - Common Clinical Behaviors
- Critical Thinking
  - Interventions for Clients With Common Clinical Behaviors
- MediaLink Application
  - Bipolar Youths' Misreading Faces May be Risk Marker for Illness
- MediaLinks
  - Books for Clients and Families
  - Community Resources

Review Questions

8-1. The nurse is teaching family members about the brain's connection to behaviors commonly seen in mental illnesses. The nurse is using the term *neurotransmitter*. The nurse should explain that a neurotransmitter is:
1. A specific location in the brain.
2. A chemical that is released in the brain.
3. A nerve that transmits impulses in the brain.
4. A hormone in the brain.

8-2. During the initial assessment, the client exhibits pressured speech and launches into a lengthy explanation of her ability to read "the writing on the wall." She points to certain patterns on the wallpaper and says, "This is Hurricane Katrina and this is 9/11. Thousands of people died because I read the writing. I should never have read the writing; it was my fault." When documenting the client's behaviors in the nursing assessment, which of the following words should the nurse use?
1. Illusion
2. Hallucination
3. Ideas of reference
4. Religious delusion

8-3. A client is sitting in the day room and is laughing out loud, shaking his head, and whispering behind his hand. Suddenly he begins banging his head against the wall violently and repeatedly. Which of the following interventions is most appropriate?

1. Calmly walk over to the client and say, "Tell me what's going on."
2. Stand in the doorway and say, "I'll have to put you in restraints if you don't stop that."
3. Call the operator and page the emergency response team immediately to the unit.
4. Approach the client and say, "You need to write your feelings down in your journal."

8-4. A female client with a history of being sexually abused is hospitalized for depression after a recent suicide attempt. She states that she often cuts her body in hidden places as punishment. "When I see the blood I feel better because then I know I'm alive." Which of the following nursing diagnoses should have the highest priority?

1. Self-mutilation: Cutting related to feelings of guilt and low self-esteem
2. Risk for Suicide related to shame and self-doubt
3. Powerlessness related to history of sexual abuse
4. Ineffective Coping related to recent suicide attempt

8-5. A client has been pacing up and down the hallway for the last hour. He stares at others without blinking, clenches his fists, and mutters to himself. Another client walks down the hall and accidentally bumps into the first client. The first client punches the second client in the face and pulls his hair. The team acts quickly to restrain the first client and moves him safely to the seclusion room. During a staff review of this critical incident, several alternatives are discussed. Which of the following actions should be taken to prevent a similar incident? (Select all that apply.)

1. Quietly and calmly ask the client if he would rather go to the quiet room or the exercise room.
2. Offer the client a PRN dose of ziprasidone (Geodon) by mouth.
3. Restrict other clients from going down the hallway while the client is pacing.
4. Call the assault response team to the unit as soon as the client starts pacing.
5. Assign a staff member to stand at the open end of the hallway as soon as the client starts pacing.

See Appendix D for answers.

References

American Psychiatric Association. (2000). *Diagnostic and statistical manual of mental disorders* (4th ed., Text Revision). Washington, DC: Author.

Biccheri, R., Trygstad, L., Kanas, N., & Dowling, G. (1997). Symptom management of auditory hallucinations in schizophrenia. *Journal of Psychosocial Nursing, 35*(12), 20–28; Sayer, J., Ritter, S., & Gournay, K. (2000). Beliefs about voices and their effects on coping strategies. *Journal of Advanced Nursing, 31*(5), 1199–1205; Tsai, Y. F., & Ku, Y. C. (2005). Self-care symptom management strategies for auditory hallucinations among inpatients with schizophrenia at a veterans' hospital in Taiwan. *Archives of Psychiatric Nursing, 19*(4), 194–199.

Blackwood, N. J., Howard, R. J., Bentall, R. P., & Murray, R. M. (2001). Cognitive neuropsychiatric models of persecutory delusions. *American Journal of Psychiatry, 158*(4), 527–539.

Cerdorian, K. (2005). The needs of adolescent girls who self-harm. *Journal of Psychosocial Nursing and Mental Health Services, 43*(8), 40–46.

Chen, S. C., Hwu, H. G., & Williams, R. A. (2005). Psychiatric nurses' anxiety and cognition in managing psychiatric patients' aggression. *Archives of Psychiatric Nursing, 19*(3), 141–149.

Compton, M. T. (2003). Internet delusions. *Southern Medical Journal, 96*(1), 61–63.

England, M., Tripp-Reimer, T., & Rubenstein, L. (2005). Exploration of the psychometric properties of an inventory of voice experiences. *Archives of Psychiatric Nursing, 19*(2), 58–69.

Frankle, W. G., Lombardo, I., New, A. S., Goodman, M., Talbot, P. S., Huang, Y., et al. (2005). Brain serotonin transporter distribution in subject with impulsive aggressivity. *American Journal of Psychiatry, 162*(5), 915–923.

Kessler, R. C., Coccaro, E. F., Fava, M., Jaeger, S., Jin, R., & Walters, E. (2006). The prevalence and correlates of DSM-IV intermittent explosive disorder in the National Comorbidity Survey Replication. *Archives of General Psychiatry, 63*(6), 669–678.

Kindy, D., Petersen, S., & Parkhurst, D. (2005). Perilous work: Nurses' experiences in psychiatric units with high risks of assault. *Archives of Psychiatric Nursing, 19*(4), 169–175.

Klonsky, E. D., Oltmanns, T. F., & Turkheimer, E. (2003). Deliberate self-harm in a nonclinical population. *American Journal of Psychiatry, 160*(8), 1501–1508.

Livesley, W. J. (2003). *Practical management of personality disorder.* New York: Guilford Press.

Papolos, D., & Papolos, J. (2002). *The bipolar child.* New York: Broadway Books.

Paul, T., Schroeter, K., Dahme, B., & Nutzinger, D. O. (2002). Self-injurious behavior in women with eating disorders. *American Journal of Psychiatry, 159*(3), 408–411.

Perusse, D., & Gendreau, P. L. (2005). Genetics and the development of aggression. In R. E. Trembly, W. W. Hartup, & J. Archer (Eds), *Developmental origins of aggression* (pp. 223–241). New York: Guilford Press.

Pihl, R. O., & Benkelfat, C. (2005). Neuromodulators in the development and expression of inhibition and aggression. In R. E. Trembly, W. W. Hartup, & J. Archer (Eds.), *Developmental origins of aggression* (pp. 261–280). New York: Guilford Press.

Silver, J. M., Yudofsky, S. C., & Anderson, K. E. (2005). Aggressive disorders. In J. M. Silver, T. W. McAllister, & S. C. Yudofsky (Eds.), *Textbook of traumatic brain injury* (pp. 259–277). Washington, DC: American Psychiatric Press.

Specht, J., Singer, A. J., & Henry, M. C. (2005). Self-inflicted injuries in adolescents presenting to a suburban emergency department. *Journal of Forensic Nursing, 1*(1), 20–22.

Tsai, Y. F., & Ku, Y. C. (2005). Self-care symptom management strategies for auditory hallucinations among inpatients with schizophrenia at a veterans' hospital in Taiwan. *Archives of Psychiatric Nursing, 19*(4), 194–199.

Weber, M. T. (2002). Triggers for self-abuse: A qualitative study. *Archives of Psychiatric Nursing, 16*(3), 118–124.

Woodside, M., & McClum, T. (2006). *Generalist case management* (3rd ed.). Pacific Grove, CA: Thomson/Brooks/Cole.

Chapter 9

Illness Management: Treatment Decisions

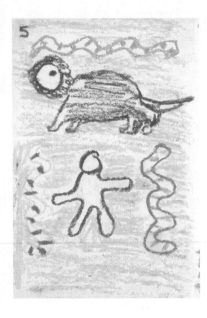

Danger in the jungle

—Sandy, Age 32
Young mother who lost her child in a motor vehicle accident—she was driving.

OBJECTIVES

After reading this chapter, you will be able to:

1. Differentiate between the professional roles that exist in mental health settings.
2. Describe characteristics of milieu therapy.
3. Outline psychosocial nursing interventions.
4. Describe the key points in assessment and intervention in crisis situations.
5. Compare and contrast different forms of psychological and biological therapies.
6. Describe the different roles nurses play in group settings.
7. Discuss the use of alternative therapies in mental health settings.

MediaLink www.prenhall.com/fontaine

Go to the Pearson Health MediaLink CD-ROM and the Companion Website at www.prenhall.com/fontaine for interactive resources for this chapter.

KEY TERMS

advanced practice nurse (APN) *166*

behavioral therapy *175*

civil rights protection *165*

client *165*

cognitive–behavioral therapy *174*

collaboration *167*

complementary/alternative therapies *184*

crisis intervention *172*

deep brain stimulation (DBS) *183*

electroconvulsive therapy (ECT) *181*

family therapy *176*

gene therapy *184*

group therapy *178*

individual psychotherapy *176*

magnetic seizure therapy (MST) *183*

milieu *168*

nursing informatics *166*

psychiatric consultation liaison nursing (PCLN) *166*

psychosurgery *183*

repetitive transcranial magnetic stimulation (rTMS) *182*

social skills training *169*

twelve-step programs *180*

vagus nerve stimulation (VNS) *183*

MENTAL HEALTH CARE CLIENTS

For decades, people with mental disorders were shut away in psychiatric institutions and effectively barred from demanding better treatment while their families were blamed and shamed into silence. That is changing. People with mental disorders and their families are fighting for **civil rights protection** and more government services. One in two adult Americans meets the criteria for a mental disorder at some point during her or his lifetime. Half of these start by age 14 and three fourths by age 24. **Clients**, those people who utilize mental health services, are children, adolescents, adults, and older adults, and they come from all segments of society. They need a wide variety of services: individual therapy, crisis intervention, family therapy, group therapy, residential services, short-term or long-term inpatient services, rehabilitative services, partial-hospitalization programs, and home care programs. Figure 9.1 ■ illustrates these pathways to change (Wang, Lane, Olfson, Pincus, Wells, & Kessler, 2005).

Increasingly, psychiatric nurses are supporting *client-sensitive health care goals* and programs. Mental health care should be client centered, based on and responsive to the needs, values, and desires of the clients rather than of the mental health system or the needs of the professionals. Clients have the right to the fullest possible control over their own lives and should be actively involved in treatment-planning decisions, including selecting:

- The services and therapies they want and need
- The setting of care
- Who will provide the care

Clients have the right to humane treatment; to personal privacy; to be free from excessive medication, physical restraint, and isolation; to exercise the right to refuse treatment; and to be free from retaliation. Box 9.1 provides a list of mental health care clients' rights, as established by Congress.

BOX 9.1	Mental Health Care Clients' Rights

1. Right to appropriate treatment supportive of a person's personal liberty
2. Right to an individualized, written treatment plan and its appropriate periodic review and reassessment
3. Right to ongoing participation in the treatment plan and a reasonable explanation of the plan
4. Right not to receive treatment, except in an emergency situation
5. Right not to participate in experimentation without informed, voluntary, written consent
6. Right to freedom from restraint or seclusion
7. Right to a humane treatment environment
8. Right to confidentiality of records
9. Right of access to one's mental health care records
10. Right of access to telephone, mail, and visitors
11. Right to be informed of these rights
12. Right to assert grievances based on the infringement of these rights
13. Right of access to a qualified advocate to protect these rights
14. Right to exercise these rights without reprisal
15. Right to referral to other mental health services on discharge

SOURCE: Adapted with permission from Mental Health Systems Act Report, 1980.

You will meet mental health clients in a variety of clinical settings—in emergency rooms, in the general hospital, in clinics, in homes, and in shelters. Even if psychiatric nursing is not your specialty, there are standards of care all nurses are expected to provide. You must be able to relate to these clients in a therapeutic manner and foster a caring relationship. You must be able to provide basic mental health nursing care and collaborate with a variety of professionals.

A variety of treatment options are available to clients. The choice may be dictated by the setting of care, as in milieu therapy, or by the people involved, as in family therapy. Clients often participate in several therapies during the course of their disease. This chapter describes the more common treatment methods.

MENTAL HEALTH CARE PROFESSIONALS

Many different professional groups provide services to clients experiencing mental health problems. All professional groups are educated according to the philosophical and theoretical beliefs of their particular discipline, which gives them specific skills. In reality, the functions and responsibilities of the various professionals often overlap. Professionals from the various disciplines work together in what is referred to as the *multidisciplinary team*.

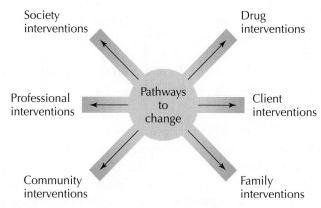

Figure 9.1 ■ Pathways to change.

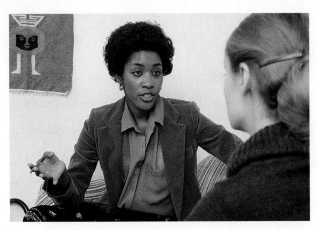

PHOTO 9.1 ■ Psychiatric–mental health nurses perform a wide variety of roles as staff nurse, educator, case manager, nurse manager, therapist, and researcher.

SOURCE: Michal Heron/Michal Heron Photography. Used with permission.

Nurses

According to the American Psychiatric Nurses Association (2005), psychiatric–mental health nursing focuses on the "promotion of optimal mental health, the prevention of mental illness, health maintenance, management of and/or referral of mental and physical health problems, the diagnosis and treatment of mental disorders and their sequelae, and rehabilitation" (www.apna.org/resources/positionpapers/psychiatric).

Working with individuals, families, groups, and communities, nurses gather assessment data for the purpose of diagnosing, planning, implementing, and evaluating nursing care. Because they spend more time with clients than any other staff members do, they often have the most information about a client's day-to-day level of functioning. With this knowledge base, nurses act as the liaison between other members of the multidisciplinary team.

Nurses also assume responsibility for the physiological integrity of clients. Aside from psychiatrists, nurses are the only other members of the team who have the education and skill to perform physiological assessments. While other team members may not understand the significance of physical problems, nurses are expected to identify potential or actual problems and follow up with the appropriate action.

Client education about health is another area of expertise nurses bring to the psychiatric setting. Empowering clients with knowledge about their illness and prescribed treatments is very important.

Basic Level of Practice

Nurses assume a wide variety of roles within the mental health care system. Specific roles are determined by educational level and specialized preparation. Nurses with a bachelor's or associate degree practice at the *basic level* as staff nurses, case man-

agers, and nurse managers. They provide primary mental health services to individuals, families, groups, and communities. Practice includes health promotion, intake screening and evaluation, case management, milieu therapy, promotion of self-care activities, psychobiological interventions, health teaching, counseling, crisis care, and psychiatric rehabilitation. Interventions are "based on scientific, theoretical knowledge, and are designed to address behavioral change and assist patients in their response to health experiences" (McCabe, 2002, p. 57).

Advanced Practice

Advanced practice nurses (APNs) with a doctorate or master's degree in mental health nursing are found in all settings, including private practices, home health care, schools, community centers, acute care hospitals, and prisons. They focus on health promotion, illness prevention, education, and psychotherapy. APNs are well educated in individual and group therapy and may have taken advanced preparation in other areas such as family therapy, sex therapy, or substance abuse therapy. They also have prescriptive authority, provide consultation, and design and implement research activities. They provide leadership to improve care and advance nursing practice and health care delivery systems. APNs are accountable for using evidence-based practice research and implementing the results in direct client care. APNs throughout the world improve access to mental health services (Fisher, 2005; Heitkemper & Bond, 2004; Wortans, Happell, & Johnstone, 2006).

Consultation

Psychiatric consultation liaison nursing (PCLN) is an advanced practice subspecialty. The focus of practice is with clients who are physically ill or disabled and their families. Care is provided in nonpsychiatric care settings such as hospitals, rehabilitation centers, extended care facilities, clinics, and home settings. PCLN nurses have expertise in medical–surgical nursing and psychiatric–mental health nursing. Their concentration is "psychophysiological interrelationships and their impact on wellness, physical illness, and recovery" (Minarik & Neese, 2002, p. 3). They bridge the gap between mental health and medical–surgical nursing care by providing short-term, crisis interventions (Sharrock, Grigg, Happell, Keeble-Devlin, & Jennings, 2006).

Nurse Informaticists

One of the most recent advanced practice subspecialties is **nursing informatics**, which is the integration of "nursing science, computer science, and information science to manage and communicate data, information, and knowledge in nursing practice" (American Nurses Association, 2001,

p. vii). Informaticists work in hospitals, the corporate level of health care systems, and consulting firms. They develop, customize, or update computer information and clinical documentation systems. They also train and support users in the role of liaison (Sensmeier, West, & Horowitz, 2004).

Psychiatrists

Psychiatrists are physicians who have completed a residency program in psychiatry. They are able to admit clients to the inpatient setting and order the necessary diagnostic and laboratory tests. Psychiatrists are responsible for diagnosing mental disorders and prescribing medications and other somatic therapies. While most focus on the biochemical treatment of mental illness, some are well educated in psychotherapy. Subspecialties within psychiatry include work with children and adolescents, work with older adults, and work with special types of problems such as eating disorders, substance abuse, and crisis situations.

Psychologists

Psychologists practice in all areas of the mental health care system. People with a bachelor's degree in psychology are frequently hired as mental health technicians in inpatient and residential settings. Those with a master's degree in psychology are often employed in community mental health centers. Those with a doctorate in psychology (clinical psychologists) usually maintain a private practice or contract their services to an agency.

Most clinical psychologists are educated in psychotherapy and conduct individual, couples, family, and group sessions. One characteristic that distinguishes them from other professionals is their expertise in psychological testing. Psychologists administer and interpret all psychological tests that aid in the diagnosis and treatment of clients. Some common tests include the Minnesota Multiphasic Personality Inventory-2 (MMPI-2), Psychological Screening Inventory (PSI), Sentence Completion Test, Thematic Apperception Test (TAT), and the Rorschach test.

Psychiatric Social Workers

Psychiatric social workers have earned a master's degree in social work. They are found on inpatient units, in community mental health centers, and in private practice. Many states require the presence of a psychiatric social worker to perform social histories and arrange placement for clients. These trained professionals are the best informed about referral resources for clients. Many are educated in psychotherapy and provide individual, couples, family, and group sessions. People with a bachelor's degree in social work may be hired as mental health technicians for inpatients or as case managers for outpatients.

Occupational Therapists

Occupational therapists have either a bachelor's or a master's degree in occupational therapy. Usually employed on inpatient units or in partial-hospitalization programs, they are responsible for providing activities that help clients increase their attention span, improve their motor skills, expand their socialization skills, and improve their ability to perform activities of daily living (ADLs). Through goal-directed activities, occupational therapists create situations in which clients can feel a sense of accomplishment.

Recreational Therapists

Recreational therapists usually have a bachelor's degree. They are responsible for providing group diversional activities that allow clients to engage in appropriate social and physical functions on inpatient units or in partial-hospitalization programs.

Specialists

The mental health care system often includes therapists with specialized expertise. These specialists may be skilled in the use of dance, art, music, and play to help clients communicate their thoughts, feelings, and needs in creative ways.

Clergy

Pastoral counselors and healers from various cultural and religious groups are also part of the multidisciplinary team in many clinical settings. People with emotional problems often turn to clergy or healers because they know them, there is less of a stigma in visiting them, and the service is often free. Clergy may refer people to mental health professionals, just as mental health professionals may refer clients to clergy. Clergy respond to the religious issues that arise for people with mental disorders. The spiritual focus is especially helpful for those who are dealing with issues related to meaning and purpose in life. Alternatively, people may seek the help of a religious leader who includes healing practices in her or his religious practice. Nurses, regardless of personal belief, must recognize that religion or spirituality is often an essential part of the life of those entrusted to their care (Milstein, 2003).

Collaboration

Nurses collaborate with clients and families of mental health care. **Collaboration** involves people who have mental illnesses, their family members, and professionals, all working together to improve quality of life and achieve the highest level of functioning. Nurses help clients acquire new knowledge and skills for basic living, learning, and working in the community and in developing new resources for success. Clients must be treated with dignity and respect. They have the same needs, aspirations, rights, and responsibilities as other people. They have the right to access the opportunities and supports everyone needs, as well as a variety of mental health services.

The current challenge to all mental health care professionals is to learn how to collaborate with other professionals to ensure the best possible care for all clients. Mental health professionals must give up their "What's in it for me?" attitude and become team players. It is necessary to develop cooperative relationships based on trust, communication, and commitment to quality care. Building on each other's ideas and goals will help all mental health professionals develop new strategies for mental health care delivery.

MILIEU THERAPY

In its earliest conception, milieu was a word that described a scientifically planned community. Research efforts focused on defining the types of environments that would be most therapeutic for specifically diagnosed psychiatric clients. The work of Cummings and Cummings (1962) suggested that the environment (milieu) itself might be a strong force in bringing about changes in client behavior.

Kraft (1966) defined the idea of **milieu** more precisely as a therapeutic community in which the entire social structure of the unit or residence is designed to be part of the helping process. Kraft's idea of a therapeutic community emphasized the social and interpersonal interactions that become the therapeutic tools influencing change in client behavior. This view differed somewhat from the pure idea of milieu therapy, in which the emphasis was on "manipulation" of the environment to effect therapeutic change.

Hildegard Peplau (1952), the mother of psychiatric nursing theory, described the roles of the nurse in the therapeutic milieu. Peplau also described the *therapeutic use of self;* that is, using one's personhood to provide psychiatric nursing care. Within the nurse–client relationship, nurses use their personalities, beliefs, values, feelings, cognitions, and perceptions as they implement holistic nursing practice. (These roles are discussed in detail in chapter 1 ∞.)

Milieu therapy has certain basic goals, whether the setting is a group home, a community center, a day program, or an inpatient unit. These goals include an emphasis on:

- Clients as responsible people
- Group and social interaction
- Client rights to choose and participate in a variety of treatments
- Informality of relationships with health care professionals

Characteristics of the Therapeutic Milieu
Clear Communication

Communication between all people in the milieu is open, honest, and appropriate. Clients are encouraged to express their thoughts and feelings without retaliation, and staff members have a responsibility to hear what clients are saying without feeling threatened. Communication skills are role-modeled by staff members, helping clients learn the positive effects of therapeutic communication. Respect for the dignity of each person in the milieu is emphasized through the communication process.

Safe Environment

Policies, procedures, and rules of the residence, center, or unit are designed to ensure the safety of all members of the therapeutic milieu. All members of the community are informed of the rules. Structures and controls are provided for clients who are confused, anxious, suicidal, homicidal, or out of control to ensure their safety and the safety of those around them.

Activity Schedule With Therapeutic Goals

In short-term acute care settings, clients are usually at different levels of functioning. In most therapeutic communities, clients are assigned to specific groups for activities. This assignment usually depends on the client's level of functioning at the time of admission and is changed as the client's level of functioning improves. Level of functioning can be determined by asking questions such as:

- Does the client have some insight into the illness? Little insight? No insight?
- How well does the client understand the goals of treatment? Well? Only slightly? Not at all?
- Is the client in contact with reality?
- How motivated is the client?

It is common to see high-functioning groups, moderate-functioning groups, and low-functioning groups in the same setting. Activities are then planned to meet the individual needs, interests, and skills of clients in that group.

Group activities are balanced to provide clients with different types of experiences. Everyone needs balance between work, sleep, and play—a fact that is frequently overlooked in the psychiatric setting. Even a well-functioning person would have difficulty with 6 hours of intense therapy in one day. Therefore, the activity schedule is varied, with daily therapeutic community meetings, group therapy, ADL training, some type of physical activity such as sports or movement therapy, art therapy, play therapy, medication teaching and other educational groups, reality orientation groups, periods of rest and relaxation, time for one-to-one interactions, free time, and mealtime.

Support Network

Clients will begin to feel a sense of support from the therapeutic community or milieu. Through the process of group therapy and other support groups, clients begin to feel a sense of commonality with other clients. Clients often value treatment that helps them feel some control over crisis and a sense of social connectedness. One of the greatest benefits of the therapeutic community is that it is one of the few places where clients may feel safe, secure, and supported.

Because, in many settings, nurses spend more time with clients than do any other staff members, they often have the most influence on the effectiveness of the milieu. As a nurse, you can help establish the milieu as an open, confirming, and dignified place for people to be ill and to get well. Individuals who are severely mentally ill have problems relating to others. When clients have been conditioned to a life of loneliness and stigma, nurses may find it takes a great deal of time to establish the trusting relationship necessary for successful treatment. As nurses, we are healers, and through the milieu we create an atmosphere of nurturance and protection that removes the pressure to "cure" and allows the sometimes slow process of healing to take place.

PSYCHOSOCIAL NURSING INTERVENTIONS

One of the goals of mental health nursing is to empower clients by helping them restore their sense of value, strength, and the ability to cope with life. Empowerment means that people have both the authority and the confidence to choose and act on options. The goal of empowerment is that clients regain or attain meaningful roles, relationships, and activities. Chapter 3 ∞ has further details under psychosocial rehabilitation.

Social Skills Training

Individuals with severe mental illness often benefit from **social skills training**. Community treatment focuses primarily on teaching basic coping skills necessary to live as autonomously as possible in the community. In the past, inadequate social and vocational skills forced clients to remain in institutional settings. That is rapidly changing, as the focus is on independent living with the highest possible quality of life. Social skills training to overcome disabilities is repetitive and lengthy and is measured in months or years. Clients must also have opportunities and encouragement to practice the skills in real life and reinforcement for the use of the skills in community life.

Social skills training can be done in individual or group sessions. Clients have individualized behavioral goals to guide them as they empower themselves to adapt to community living. Steps in teaching social skills are as follows:

1. Provide a rationale for learning the skill.
2. Break the skill into component steps.
3. Model the skill through role-playing.
4. Review with clients what they observed in the role-playing.
5. Role-play with clients to practice the skill.
6. Provide positive feedback about components that were performed well.
7. Provide corrective feedback on how the skill could be done better.
8. Help clients role-play the skill with other clients.
9. Encourage clients to practice the skill at home/work.

Activities of Daily Living Skills

Activities of daily living and instrumental activities of daily living (IADL) skills include grooming and personal hygiene, room upkeep, laundry upkeep, cooking, shopping, eating at restaurants, budgeting, use of public transportation, and time management. Clients who are severely ill benefit from being taught in their own setting. For instance, laundry upkeep is most effectively taught in the client's neighborhood self-service laundry; cooking, on her or his own stove; and room cleaning, in her or his own home. The inability to perform several of these basic ADLs or IADLs for a length of time can create enormous frustration and stress, which may contribute to relapse.

Vocational Skills

Severely mentally ill clients may lack not only specific work skills, but also job-seeking abilities and good work habits. Being persistently unemployed contributes to feelings of inadequacy and low self-esteem. Clients may need support in locating positions, filling out applications, role-playing interviews, and learning job expectations and behaviors. Some community mental health centers provide job coaches if necessary; these coaches work alongside clients on the job until they can gradually be self-sufficient in the job.

Leisure-Time Skills

Some clients lack either the interest or the necessary skills to fill their free time in a satisfying manner. When clients spend the majority of their free time in solitary television viewing, they are susceptible to increasing withdrawal, with accompanying loneliness and depression often leading to gradual decompensation. Clients are encouraged to find leisure and social activities that are enjoyable and involve interaction with others. Discover meaningful activities for each individual and their preferences for activities. Help them choose activities consistent with their physical, psychological, and social capabilities. Focus on skills they have rather than on deficits. Discuss with clients the scheduling of specific periods for leisure activity into their daily routine. As with ADLs, leisure-time activities should be carried out in the client's own neighborhood. Teach clients about available community resources for leisure activities (YMCA, YWCA, community center, local bowling alley, swimming pool, gym), support groups, and religious expression.

Communication Skills

With less than adequate communication skills, it is difficult to implement many of the activities just mentioned. Some individuals will need assistance with verbal and nonverbal communication. Discuss facial expressions, eye contact, posture, gestures, and interpersonal distance. Keep in mind that nonverbal communication is culturally determined; teach within those cultural expectations. Give examples of how being aware of nonverbal communication helps build relationships. Ask clients to demonstrate a thought or feeling without words, such as happiness, anger, or frustration. The goal is to increase clients' awareness of their nonverbal communication and that of others.

Conversation is another social skill. Discuss volume, tone, and rate of speech. Model taking turns in speaking and not interrupting. Have clients practice skills such as initiating conversations, asking questions, making appropriate self-disclosures, and ending conversations gracefully.

Assertiveness training is appropriate for clients who are either passive or aggressive in their style of relating to others. Assertive people are able to say no to activities in which they do not wish to participate and to unreasonable demands. They are able to express positive and negative feelings in an appropriate manner and accept constructive criticism and praise from other people. Assertiveness may be inappropriate in some cultures, especially those in which children or teens are not allowed to disagree with parents or those in which women are to be obedient and submissive to men.

Conflict-Management Skills

Everyone has disagreements with other people. It is critical that clients know how to manage conflict when it occurs, without resorting to verbal or physical aggression. Conflict management involves learning compromise and negotiation skills so that disagreements with others can be worked out in a satisfactory manner. Specific skills include:

- Anger management techniques (covered in chapter 8 ∞)
- Clear communication
- Accepting responsibility for one's behavior
- Apologizing for wrongdoing
- Respecting the opinions of others

- Accepting "no" for an answer
- Compromising on issues
- Problem solving to find mutually acceptable solutions

Nurses can take advantage of incidental learning in which naturally occurring behaviors or events are used to teach and reinforce appropriate conflict resolution. Role-playing with feedback is also effective. Outcomes of effective conflict management include fewer coercive interactions, more cooperative behavior, improved acceptance of differences, and less rejection by others.

Self-esteem Interventions

Self-esteem involves two components: the cognitive judgment of one's abilities or appearance and the emotional reaction to that judgment. People with high self-esteem have more positive evaluations of themselves, whereas those who have low self-esteem have more negative self-evaluation. Before the age of 6 or 7 years, young children are not able to accurately rate their own abilities. For example, young children will say they are very capable of doing almost any activity you can name. After age 6 or 7 years, children become more aware of their abilities and rate themselves in terms of academic performance, physical abilities, physical appearance, and social relationships. A person's self-esteem becomes fairly well established by middle childhood (Ball & Bindler, 2006).

Mental disorders often have a devastating effect on an individual's self-esteem. Negative social, educational, and vocational experiences influence how clients see themselves and their "problems." Carrying the burden of low self-esteem can hinder a sense of well-being and even contribute to relapse.

Clients improve their self-esteem when they feel good about themselves, know their good points, are satisfied with themselves, and forgive themselves. Their self-esteem also improves when they take care of themselves, take calculated risks, accept failures, and learn from their mistakes. Box 9.2 lists

BOX 9.2	Self-esteem for All

1. Be patient, kind, and understanding with yourself.
2. Acknowledge your strengths.
3. Accept compliments.
4. Do not accept put-downs.
5. Set achievable realistic goals and work to accomplish them.
6. Visualize change. Imagine the person you want to become 6 months from now.
7. Take time to be pleased when you achieve something good. Reward yourself for your successes.
8. Don't blame yourself out of all proportion if something doesn't go the way you had planned.
9. Take up a new hobby or interest, join a new group, or try volunteering.
10. Counteract negative thoughts with positive thoughts.
11. Think of yourself as a lovable and capable person.

ideas for discussion with clients who wish to improve their self-esteem. Additional nursing interventions regarding self-esteem issues are presented in chapters 11 through 18 ∞.

Remotivation Therapy

Remotivation therapy focuses on people's abilities rather than their problems. It encourages an attitude of hope and enthusiasm. Nurses may see this in hospitals, long-term care settings, day care programs, social clubs, group homes, and even prisons. Remotivation groups usually meet once a week for 30 to 60 minutes and are led by a certified remotivation therapist who may be a nurse, a social worker, an occupational therapist, or a volunteer.

Bierma (2005a, p. 43) describes motivation as measured by a "person's voluntary, intrinsic desire to do something and perform the action without either internal or external rewards or punishments." In other words, motivation is what creates and guides one's goal-directed behavior. See chapter 6 ∞ for information on motivation and the brain. Motivational therapy is based on client autonomy and the concept of acceptance. Internal motivation is facilitated by giving people relevant information, choice, and acknowledgment of their perspective. Expected outcomes of this therapy include increased interaction with others, increased ability to accomplish ADLs and IADLs, active involvement in treatment decisions, improved self-esteem, and increased feelings of belonging to a group (Herlihy-Chevalier, 2005).

Bierma (2005a) looked at 13 studies from 1965 through 1992 that included people with mental disorders, cognitively impaired children, and geriatric populations. In evaluating these studies for evidence-based efficacy he found that people accepted more responsibility for a change in their behavior when they had internal motivation rather than external motivation. In looking at other studies, Bierma (2005b) also found evidence that therapists and programs that support client autonomy and choices have better and longer lasting outcomes in smoking cessation, weight loss, substance abuse treatment, HIV risk behaviors, diabetes, schizophrenia, and medication compliance.

Reminiscence Therapy

Reminiscence is a guided recollection in which older clients are encouraged to remember the past and share their memories with family, peers, or staff. Life review is a normal developmental process especially as elderly people approach the end of their lives. Reminiscence focuses on strengths and does not encourage people to dwell on losses. It can raise self-esteem and help people gain self-awareness and self-understanding, adapt to stress, and see their part in the larger historical and cultural context. Reminiscence therapy establishes group cohesiveness and increases social intimacy and is one of the most popular psychosocial interventions

for people with dementia (Hsieh & Wang, 2003; Woods, Spector, Jones, Orrell, & Davies, 2005).

The best way to conduct reminiscence therapy is to choose a comfortable setting and set aside adequate time. You may begin the session with questions such as: "Tell me about your home when you were a child," "What was one of your favorite toys when you were a child?" or "What memories do you have of your early school years?" Encourage verbal expression of feelings of past events. In an empathic manner, comment on the feelings that accompany the memories. Use direct questions to refocus on life events if clients digress.

By encouraging older adults to talk about their lives, you can learn about where they have been and where they would like to go. In listening, you will learn about hope, grief, achievement, and loss. It is a way that you can communicate caring while helping clients maintain their sense of identity.

Physical Exercise

People who have severe mental illness tend to have high rates of physical illness, poor general fitness, poor cardiovascular fitness, obesity, and low energy. Often, their main activities are sedentary, such as watching television, listening to music, or reading. The physical benefits of exercise are well known in regard to heart disease, diabetes, colon cancer, sleep, and bone density. Exercise increases the number and density of blood vessels in the motor cortex and cerebellum. Exercise that involves learning complex movements, such as dance, basketball, or t'ai chi, strengthens the neural networks in our brain.

There have been a few studies on the psychological benefits of exercise. These studies show that there is less depression and anxiety and better self-esteem when both the well and the client population engage in exercise. Exercise also appears to have a positive effect on self-concept, mastery, self-sufficiency, body image, cognitive processing, and attention to the here-and-now. It has been found that 10 minutes of moderate intensity exercise provides some short-term relief from alcohol urges; 15 to 20 minutes of low intensity walking diminishes the urge to smoke for at least 20 more minutes. Thus, exercise is an important component of drug treatment programs (Ussher, Sampuran, Doshi, West, & Drummond, 2004).

Clients should have health clearance before beginning an exercise program. You must also assess the client's readiness for exercise. It may be difficult for people with depression to summon the energy to exercise. They often say, "I'll exercise when I feel better." An appropriate response by the nurse is, "You'll feel better when you exercise." Other barriers to exercise are medication side effects such as sedation, weight gain, and fear of being mugged in urban areas. Often, people are more consistent if they have an exercise partner, perhaps a friend or family member (McDevitt, Snyder, Miller, & Wilbur, 2006).

Clients taking psychotropic medications should begin with a low intensity of exercise. Side effects such as muscle rigidity, dehydration, muscle weakness, fatigue, and impaired coordination should be considered when designing the program. Help clients monitor short- and long-term benefits with regard to mood, energy, well-being, and weight control. If clients are to maintain an exercise program, the activity must be enjoyable and there must be positive reinforcement.

CRISIS INTERVENTION

There are many definitions of crisis, most of which concur that a *crisis* is a turning point in a person's life—a point at which usual resources and coping skills are no longer effective. Two symbols in the Chinese language communicate the meaning of crisis: the symbol for *danger* and the symbol for *opportunity*. This text views crisis as both a danger and an opportunity.

Throughout life, people experience events to which they must respond. Many of these events are expected life changes that are anticipated at particular ages—such as graduation, employment, marriage or partnership, and parenthood. Depending on individual circumstances, these expected life changes may evoke crisis states referred to as *maturational crises*. Because of individual differences, not all people choose or have the opportunity to experience all the expected life changes. Unexpected life changes—such as divorce, serious illness, or death—may result in *situational crises*. It is only when the expected or unexpected event is perceived subjectively as a threat to need fulfillment, safety, or a meaningful existence that the person enters a maturational or situational crisis state. The inability to maintain emotional equilibrium is an important feature of a crisis. This state of disequilibrium usually lasts 4 to 6 weeks. Typically, the high level of anxiety during this short period forces the individual to do one of the following:

- Adapt and return to the previous level of functioning
- Develop more constructive coping skills
- Decompensate to a lower level of functioning

It is during this time that people are most receptive to professional intervention. A thorough assessment of supports and previous coping behaviors includes an evaluation of the client's self-destructive feelings and behavior. If there is considerable threat to client safety, inpatient intervention may be necessary. Table 9.1 ■ describes crisis assessment from an individual, family, and community perspective.

The primary goal of **crisis intervention** is to assist the client in resolving the immediate problem and regaining emotional equilibrium. The minimum goal of intervention is to help clients adapt and return to the precrisis level of functioning. The maximum goal is to help clients develop more constructive coping skills and move on to a higher level of functioning. Assisting the client in crisis resolution will, hopefully, lead to better use of coping mechanisms when dealing with future stressful life events.

The nurse's role in crisis intervention is one of active participation in solving the problem. It is important for nurses to point out that they do *not* take over and make decisions for clients unless clients are suicidal or homicidal. The primary point of crisis intervention is self-help on the part of the client, with assistance from the nurse.

There are behavioral, affective, spiritual, cognitive, and psychosocial skills that people can draw on or learn so they can adapt to a crisis state. The relative importance of these skills varies with each person and each crisis. Most likely, they are used in various combinations, with the effectiveness of specific skills depending on the specific event.

Behavioral skills involve seeking information as the first step in the problem-solving process. Nurses help the individual identify alternative ways of resolving the crisis and predict probable consequences for each of the alternatives. The next step is choosing an alternative and taking concrete action. The final step is an evaluation of the consequences, and, if necessary, a return to finding solutions. (See chapter 7 ∞ for more detail on the problem-solving process.) During the crisis state the client is more receptive to trying a variety of coping behaviors to decrease anxiety. You must remember to continually reinforce the client's strengths by reviewing the crisis event, the coping effectiveness, and new methods of problem solving that have been learned.

Beth has come to the mental health center seeking crisis intervention. Jill, her partner of 5 years, has abruptly left her, saying that she (Jill) could not take Beth's passivity any more. For example, Jill told Beth that she never had a personal opinion about anything, never made an independent decision, and never voiced her preference for social activities. As you work through the problem-solving process with Beth, you want to keep in mind that assertiveness training might be an option for Beth. If she does not list this as a possible new coping strategy, you may want to suggest it.

Affective skills focus on managing the feelings provoked by the event and maintaining a reasonable balance. Venting feelings by talking, crying, or even screaming allows for emotional discharge of anger, despair, and frustration. The ability to identify and discuss one's feelings is an adaptive skill. To be able to tolerate ambiguity and maintain some hope is very helpful during a crisis period.

Spiritual skills help the individual find meaning in and understand the personal significance of an unexpected event. Finding meaning is an ongoing issue during and after the crisis period. The result of the search is dependent on the individual's spirituality or philosophy of life. Some

TABLE 9.1	Crisis Assessment

Individual Assessment

1. What is the most significant stress/problem occurring in your life right now?
2. For whom is this a problem? You? Family members? Employer? Community?
3. How long has this been a problem?
4. Is this a temporary or permanent problem?
5. What does this problem mean to you?
6. What are the factors that cause this problem to continue?
7. Have you had similar stresses/problems in the past?
8. What other stresses do you have in your life?
9. How are you managing your usual life roles (partner, parent, homemaker, worker, student, etc.)?
10. In what way has your life changed as a result of this problem?
11. Are you feeling like you want to harm yourself or others?
12. Describe how you have managed problems in the past.
13. What have you done to try and solve the problem so far?
14. What happened when you tried this?
15. Describe possible resources (e.g., family, friends, employer, teacher, financial, spiritual).
16. What are your expectations and hopes concerning this problem?
17. What is the most you hope for when this problem is resolved?
18. What is the least you will settle for to resolve this problem?
19. What part of the overall problem is most important to deal with first?

Family Assessment

1. How do you perceive the current problem?
2. In what way has the problem affected your roles in the family?
3. How has your lifestyle changed since this problem began?
4. Describe communication within the family before this current problem.
5. Describe communication within the family since the problem began.
6. How does the family typically manage problems?
7. What has the family done to try and solve the problem so far?
8. What happened when you tried this?
9. How well do you believe the family is coping at this time?
10. Describe possible resources (e.g., extended family, friends, financial).
11. What are your expectations and hopes concerning this problem?
12. Which part of the overall problem is most important to deal with first?

Community Assessment

1. What are the special demands of the client's community?
2. What are the living conditions of the neighborhood?
3. Are recreational centers available?
4. Are there affordable child care services available?
5. Is there a community mental health center?
6. What support groups are available in the community?
7. What are the possible funding resources?

people may find this by living for causes beyond themselves. Others believe in divine purpose, in which they find a great source of consolation.

Cognitive skills help the individual in coping temporarily and in long-term resolution of the crisis. Denial may be temporarily effective. To prevent feeling overwhelmed, individuals may deny the unexpected event or its possible consequences. Another cognitive skill is the ability to redefine the unexpected event. In this instance, the person accepts the basic reality of the event but reshapes the situation into something favorable. For example, the individual might focus on the potential positive outcomes or compare herself or himself with those less fortunate. The goal of adaptive cognitive skills is to maintain a satisfactory self-image and a sense of competence and mastery.

Psychosocial skills enable a person in crisis to maintain relationships with family and friends throughout and after the crisis period. The person must be open to accepting the comfort and support offered by others. Family and friends may be sources of information that will enable the person to make wise decisions. Not to be overlooked are community resources such as hotlines, mental health centers, support groups, and self-help groups.

In addition to behavioral, affective, spiritual, cognitive, and psychosocial skills, other factors influence the outcome of unexpected events. Demographic and personal factors influence how a person defines and resolves these crises. These factors include age, gender, ethnicity, economic resources, spiritual resources, and past experiences. Factors specific to the event also influence the outcome. Tasks and coping skills vary among biological, psychological, environmental, and social crisis events. The more control a person has over these factors, the more adaptive she or he is likely to be. Successful resolution of crisis leads to growth and an increased ability to cope in the future. Failure to resolve the issues contributes to decreased adaptation and potential problems in the future.

COGNITIVE–BEHAVIORAL THERAPY

Cognitive–behavioral therapy is a combination therapy. The *behavioral* aspect helps people identify habitual reactions to troublesome situations. It also teaches people how to relax and calm their bodies. The *cognitive* aspect focuses on distorted thinking patterns that cause unpleasant feelings or symptoms of mental disorders. The role of the therapist is that of a coach or tutor and there is shared responsibility to work as a team to explore problems. The goal of cognitive–behavioral therapy is accurate and rational thinking based on logic and available facts.

When participating in cognitive–behavioral therapy, clients initially identify the most troubling problems in their lives. The therapist then helps them problem solve in the following way:

- What happens? What do you *think* when this happens? What do you *feel*? What do you *do*?
- When does this happen? Where? With whom? What are the consequences?
- Why do you think this happens to you?
- How does this relate to your ideas about how things are or ought to be in your world?
- How often do you expect similar problems to happen to you in the future?
- How can you change this situation or learn to accept it?

Cognitive–behavioral therapists utilize various techniques. One is *cognitive modification* of negative automatic thoughts or maladaptive schemas. Every person has automatic thoughts, some of which are helpful and some of which are negative. An example is that a person's teenage daughter is 1 hour late for her curfew and has not called. The person's automatic thought might be: "She must have been in an accident and can't call," "She cares so little for me that she can't call even though she knows how I worry," "She is just trying to push my buttons and rebel against the rules," or "She is usually very responsible so I am certain that she will be home soon and will be able to tell me what happened."

Automatic thoughts that have a theme are called schemas. They are basic assumptions or beliefs about oneself and the world. Examples of maladaptive schemas are "Nobody in my life has ever respected me," "I am not lovable," or "My mother was right—I really am stupid." Cognitive–behavioral therapists help clients identify these patterns of irrational thinking and find ways to replace them with more logical and fact-based patterns of thinking.

Relaxation training is one of the behavioral techniques used in this type of therapy. It is difficult to think clearly

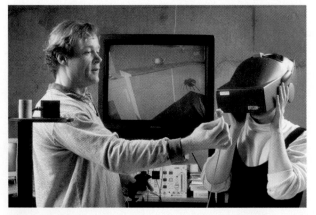

PHOTO 9.2 ■ Some cognitive behavior therapists are experimenting with using virtual reality for exposure therapy.

SOURCE: University of Washington HIT Lab/Mary Levin. Used with permission.

when one is anxious, angry, or resentful. *Behavioral activation* involves strategies that get clients actively involved in their treatment. For example, a person with depression may develop lists of pleasurable activities, schedule some of these, actually participate in the activity, and then evaluate the impact of the activity on thoughts and feelings.

Most often people go through daily routines with little awareness or attention. People read while they eat, exercise while watching television, or cook while talking to their children, and the nuances of these experiences are lost. This situation might be called living mindlessly by ignoring present moments. *Mindfulness,* another technique, is the opposite of living on "automatic pilot." It is the art of conscious living through focusing full attention on the activity at hand. While it may be simple to practice mindfulness, it is not necessarily easy. Habitual unawareness is persistent, and mindfulness requires effort and discipline. Cognitive–behavioral therapists believe that the way for people to start changing their minds is not to force it but to watch it. Through the process of mindfulness, people can learn to identify destructive thought patterns, simply label them, and watch them pass by whenever they appear in their minds. As people learn how their brains "tell stories," they can begin to change their negative automatic thoughts and schemas.

Cognitive–behavioral group therapy is often the treatment of choice for clients experiencing depression. The group setting allows people the opportunity to practice new ways of interacting with others while receiving immediate feedback (Chen, Lu, Chang, Chu, & Chou, 2006).

A somewhat similar therapy is the BE SMART trauma reframing program for clients who have experienced trauma and abuse. It is based on the theory that trauma alters the way in which the brain processes information and feelings. Those changes that facilitated survival during the traumatic period of time are no longer effective in the posttraumatic period of time. BE SMART focuses on four domains of wellness: health, attitudes and behavior, environment, interpersonal relationships, and spirituality. The goal is that clients develop sound health practices, nondestructive behaviors, positive attitudes, safe relationships, and a beneficial sense of spirituality (Moller & Rice, 2006).

BEHAVIORAL THERAPY

Behavioral therapy is based on the principle that all behavior has specific consequences. Behavior is changed by conditioning—a process of reinforcement, punishment, and extinction. Consequences that lead to an increase in a particular behavior are referred to as *reinforcement*. Positive reinforcement is providing a reward for the desired behavior, such as an allowance for completing household responsibilities. Negative reinforcement is removing a negative stimulus to increase the chances that the desired behavior will occur. An example of negative reinforcement is ignoring a child who holds his breath in the midst of a temper tantrum in an effort to frighten the parents. Consequences that lead to a decrease in undesirable behavior are referred to as *punishment.* Positive punishment is the addition of a negative consequence if the undesirable behavior occurs; for example, the child who does not complete her schoolwork gets a demerit and has to stay after school. Negative punishment is the removal of a positive reward if the undesirable behavior occurs; for example, the child who does not complete her schoolwork is unable to attend the next field trip with her class. *Extinction* refers to the progressive weakening of an undesirable behavior through repeated nonreinforcement of the behavior.

Most behavioral therapists believe that reinforcement procedures are more desirable than punishment procedures. There is no doubt that punishment is effective and is sometimes necessary when the behavior is dangerous. But behavior changed through reinforcement is a more desirable clinical outcome than behavior changed through punishment.

Contingency contracts are basically "if-then" rules. If the client performs a targeted response, such as self-care activities, social responsiveness, or group participation, then the client receives desired reinforcers. Contingency contracts are only as effective as the rewards chosen. These may be food treats, activities, or privileges. What works for one person may not be a reward for another person. When a client is first learning the targeted behavior, rewards are given immediately, along with verbal praise and specific feedback. An example is, "Good job. You put the dishes away in the cabinet. Here is the reward we talked about."

Token economies are formalized programs of contingency contracts. They are established for all members of a group. There are three parts to token economies:

1. Identifying behaviors that everyone in the group is expected to demonstrate
2. Specifying token continuances for doing these behaviors, (e.g., if you do your morning hygiene activities, you will receive 10 tokens). Inappropriate behaviors are also identified for which tokens may be lost.
3. Establishing rules for redeeming tokens: types of activities or privileges that may be swapped for tokens; how many tokens each one costs, and when and where tokens are swapped.

As with many of the other therapies, nurses are in an ideal position to evaluate client response to treatment. Because they spend a great deal of time with clients, nurses can see developing patterns of behavioral change.

PLAY THERAPY

Play therapy is the purposeful use of play to provide information for assessment and subsequent interventions. Play therapy is especially helpful for children younger than 12 years because their developmental level makes them less able to verbalize thoughts and feelings. The nurse must establish objectives for the use of play, as well as consider the age and needs of the child. Play therapy may be a one-to-one session or it may be used with a group of children. The limits, discussed prior to the session, are that children are not allowed to hurt themselves or others, and they must not destroy property. Within those limits, children are allowed to express any feelings and act out any of their experiences.

A typical play-therapy room is equipped with a variety of toys and objects, including dolls of various sizes, shapes, and colors; a doll house; puppets; stuffed animals; clay; a sandbox; a sink for water play; toy cars and trucks; toy airplanes; blocks; soft balls; punching toys; soft foam bats; and magic markers or crayons. As you observe and interact with the children, you learn about family dynamics, conflicts, and traumas, as well as positive experiences and people in the children's lives. Play therapy allows the nurse to develop a sense of how each child perceives and experiences the world.

The overall goals of play therapy are to:

- Establish rapport with children.
- Reveal the feelings that children are unable to verbalize.
- Enable children to act out feelings of anxiety or tension in a constructive manner.
- Understand children's relationships and interactions with significant others in their lives.
- Teach children adaptive socialization skills.

Sand play is often used with children. It is a nondirective form of play therapy in which the child is allowed to "play out" emotions or distressful situations in a sand box or sand tray. You can be more directive and ask children to create a picture of anything they would like to and to put some toy animals or people in the scene. You then ask the children to tell you about the picture, what is happening in the picture, how the people/animals feel, and what they would say if they could talk. You may wish to take a photograph of the creation for future reference. Children need to be told that other children use the sand to express their feelings and so, when they return, they will have a fresh box to express themselves. Otherwise, they will expect you to keep their "scene" exactly as they left it.

ART THERAPY

Art therapy—the use of painting, drawing, sculpting, or other media—is a way for children and adults to express what is contained in the unconscious. You may ask the children to draw or paint a picture themselves or to tell you

how to draw something. You may ask them to draw their family, draw themselves, draw feelings, draw what happened, draw a hero or an imaginary helper, or draw a nightmare. Art allows questions to be raised naturally. As clients are engaged in creative art, you should observe them. Are the clients timid? Worried about making mistakes? Bold? Haphazard? Anxious or relaxed? Is the style small and neat or messy and careless? Art therapy provides information on how people perceive themselves and others and how they interact with significant others in their lives.

INDIVIDUAL PSYCHOTHERAPY

Individual psychotherapy is a reciprocal agreement between client and therapist to enter into a therapeutic relationship. It is performed by a variety of health care professionals such as APNs, psychiatrists, psychologists, and psychiatric social workers. The goals of psychotherapy are to help clients:

- Clarify perceptions
- Identify feelings
- Make connections among thoughts, feelings, and events
- Gain insight
- Problem solve
- Modify problematic behavior

The process can also help clients develop better coping strategies such as stress reduction and crisis management. For some clients, it is an opportunity to feel supported in their struggle to overcome symptoms or interpersonal problems. Some individual therapies deal with specific issues, such as sex therapy or eating disorders. Certain therapies are short-term, such as crisis intervention, whereas other therapies may be longer in duration.

Part of individual therapy is the telling of one's story, through talking or journaling. When people tell their story, they are able to re-experience the associated emotions from a more objective perspective. In considering the telling of one's story from a *neurobiological* basis, it is believed that connections between the limbic system (emotional center) and the frontal cortex (thinking center) allow us to conceptualize and manage our emotions.

Student nurses will be doing individual counseling in their one-to-one relationships with clients. The details of the phases, goals, and process of this professional relationship are covered in chapter 1 ∞.

FAMILY THERAPY

Family therapy is a specialized area of study, and becoming a family therapist requires extensive preparation. In **family therapy**, the family system is treated as a unit and the focus

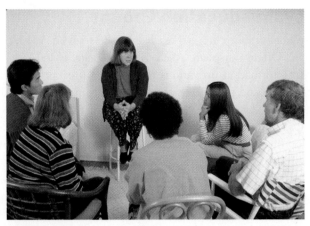

PHOTO 9.3 ■ Group therapy gives clients the opportunity to meet with and learn from other people who have similar problems.

SOURCE: Mary Kate Denny/PhotoEdit, Inc. Used with permission.

is on family dynamics. The goal is to help families cope, improve their communication and interpersonal skills, establish boundaries, and moderate family cohesion and flexibility. Families strive to maintain balance and harmony. When change affects this balanced state, families must use their internal and external resources to adapt. Competent families seem to adapt more efficiently than dysfunctional families. Change is so frightening or alien to some families that they invest their energies in maintaining the status quo. The result is that they seem more interested in enabling the illness of one of its members than in supporting changes that will improve health.

One of the problems with family therapy is that the Euro-American, middle-class, heterosexual family ideal has been used as the yardstick for determining "normal family function." This traditional stance has ignored families from other cultures, social classes, or family structures—all of whom may have very different values. Currently, family therapists are committing to not "pathologize" that which is different. Using multicultural theory, they take a more investigative approach and help family members define their unique culture and values.

Family therapy is recommended when the nurse or family determines that the family system is impaired because of the presence of a psychosocial problem or mental disorder in one or more family members. Schools, courts, or health care providers may identify impairment of family functioning. All family members must feel that they are part of the problem-solving and decision-making processes and that their personal welfare is always considered. Some advanced practice nurses are providing home-based family therapy. This allows the nurse-therapist to observe the family in the natural setting of the home. Comfort with one's environment encourages family member participation. In addition, the therapist becomes a guest; thus, a measure of control remains with the family.

Direct observation illuminates family dynamics rather quickly and can effectively guide nursing interventions (Falloon, 2002).

Family therapy is often the preferred approach when a child or adolescent is the identified client. Family therapists help family members look at a number of issues. They assess the family hierarchy, which defines power relationships among the members. They identify subsystems—groups of people within the family who join together to perform various functions—such as the parental or sibling subsystem. Therapists identify and discuss boundaries, which define the degree of emotional closeness among family members and subsystems.

The overall goals of family therapy are to:

■ Develop better parenting and nurturing skills
■ Reinstate generational boundaries in the family hierarchy
■ Improve family communication
■ Teach the family how to problem solve

Although most nurses are not family therapists, this is not to say that nurses in the mental health care system will not intervene with families at all. It is very likely that nurses in both the inpatient and outpatient settings will have a great deal of contact with the families of their clients. Family members are usually not in formal family therapy and have contact only with the nurse who assumes the responsibility of working with the family and client.

When nurses work with families informally, they assess for a number of factors, including:

■ Relationships between individual members of the family
■ Roles assumed by various members of the family
■ Family communication patterns
■ Achievement of the developmental tasks of the family
■ Normal coping strategies used by the family
■ Past and current efforts to cope with identified problems
■ Family support systems
■ Sociocultural norms and values of the family
■ Personal goals for each family member

Disagreements and conflicts in family relationships are normal. The problem is not that people disagree, but that they do not know how to resolve their differences. Teaching families general principles for resolving conflict is a helpful nursing intervention. Box 9.3 lists eight steps to resolve family disagreements. See chapter 2 ∞ for more in-depth information about families.

| BOX 9.3 | Eight Steps to Resolve Family Disagreements |

1. *Stay calm.* When people are calm, they think much more clearly. Calmness is difficult to maintain when people call each other names, become sarcastic, or drag up past injustices. Do not try to solve problems when members are very angry.
2. *Express commitment to the relationship.* Arguments often leave people feeling like enemies rather than members of a caring family unit. It is important to defuse that by saying, "I love you. Let's work together to work this problem out."
3. *Identify areas of agreement or success.* Teach people to look for similarities in their viewpoint or find positive characteristics in the other person. Family members often get stuck on arguing about one small point and overlook that they agree on many other points.
4. *Identify the specific problem.* It is difficult to resolve problems when arguments keep escalating with the addition of more and more problems.
5. *Express the desired outcome.* Family members should clearly state what they want to happen so that everybody is clear about each other's goals.
6. *Listen carefully to the other person's concerns.* Each person needs to hear what the other is saying. If necessary, have them repeat the essence of what they heard to show that they understand. Problems cannot be solved if individuals are planning what they are going to say next, rather than listening carefully to what is being said to them.
7. *Seek solutions that benefit the relationship.* Teach family members to brainstorm possible solutions and how to look for ways to compromise and meet everyone's needs.
8. *Assess the outcome.* Teach family members to analyze the solution before it is implemented. Has everyone felt respected and heard? Is everyone at least partially satisfied with the solution? If so, the conflict has probably been resolved successfully.

GROUPS

There are different kinds of groups with a variety of purposes. In your professional career, you most likely will have the opportunity to lead and participate in many different kinds of groups.

Task Groups

Task groups are designed to carry out a particular type of task and are product oriented. It is called a task group because its purpose is very specific. This kind of group usually meets once or just a few times and ends when the task is completed. The emphasis is on problem solving and decision making. Staff meetings, case conferences, and planning sessions are examples of task groups. Client task groups might plan and prepare a community meal or draw up a list of responsibilities and privileges for the clinical setting. The nurse's role in the task group is to keep the group on task and to facilitate appropriate interaction.

Psychoeducation Groups

Psychoeducation groups teach members about a specific topic. Often, nurses are asked to provide clients and families with information on various topics. The nurse provides information and then elicits reactions and comments from the members. Knowledge about the disorder and treatment helps family members provide for the needs of the client, develop their own coping strategies, and develop a collaborative relationship with professionals and other families.

Psychoeducation includes information about the etiology, treatment, and prognosis of the mental disorder. Clients and families are taught stressors associated with relapse, how to set realistic expectations, stress management, communication skills, and problem-solving skills. When families' educational needs are met, they have an increased ability to cope, understand, and deal with their loved one's illness. (See chapter 7 ∞ for more information on psychoeducation.)

Group Therapy

Therapeutic groups provide support to the members as they work through their problems. **Group therapy** is a beneficial experience in which the group members and group therapist help people with psychological, cognitive, behavioral, or spiritual dysfunctions through a process of change. Groups can be held in an inpatient unit, an outpatient clinic, a community mental health center, or a variety of other settings.

Ballinger and Yalom (1995) identified mechanisms of change within a group and called them *curative factors* of group therapy. These factors provide a rationale for a variety of group interventions. Table 9.2 ■ describes the curative factors.

Ballinger and Yalom (1995) also identified two concepts basic to group therapy: the group as a social microcosm and the here-and-now quality. *Social microcosm* refers to the concept that group members eventually behave in the therapy group in the same way they behave with their families

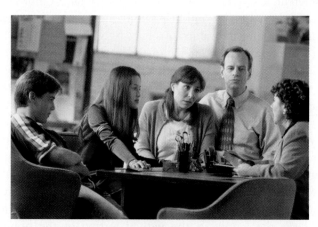

PHOTO 9.4 ■ Family therapy includes at least two or perhaps more or all family members in treatment. Family therapists strive to improve mental health by altering family relationships.

SOURCE: Bruce Ayres/Getty Images, Inc.—Stone Allstock. Used with permission.

TABLE 9.2	Curative Factors of Group Therapy

Factor	Description
Instillation of hope	As clients observe other members farther along in the therapeutic process, they begin to feel a sense of hope for themselves.
Universality	Through interaction with other group members, clients realize they are not alone in their problems or pain.
Imparting of information	Teaching and suggestions usually come from the group leader but may also be generated by the group members.
Altruism	Through the group process, clients recognize that they have something to give to the other group members.
Corrective recapitulation of the primary family group	Many clients have a history of dysfunctional family relationships. The therapy group is often like a family, and clients can learn more functional patterns of communication, interaction, and behavior.
Development of socializing techniques	Development of social skills takes place in groups. Group members give feedback about maladaptive social behavior. Clients learn more appropriate ways of socializing with others.
Imitative behavior	Clients often model their behavior after the leader or other group members. This trial process enables them to discover what behaviors work well for them as individuals.
Interpersonal learning	Through the group process, clients learn the positive benefits of good interpersonal relationships. Emotional healing takes place through this process.
Existential factors	The group provides opportunities for clients to explore the meaning of their life and their place in the world.
Catharsis	Clients learn how to express their own feelings in a goal-directed way, speak openly about what is bothering them, and express strong feelings about other members in a responsible way.
Group cohesiveness	Cohesiveness occurs when members feel a sense of belonging.

SOURCE: From THEORY AND PRACTICE OF GROUP PSYCHOTHERAPY by PSYCHOTHERAPY by IRVIN YALOM (Copyright notice exactly as it appears in the book). Reprinted by permission of BASIC Books a member of Perseus Books Group. Adapted with permission from Ballinger, B., & Yalom, I. D. (1995). *The theory and practice of group psychotherapy* (4th ed.). New York: Basic Books.

and friends. The group becomes a living example of how each member relates to others outside the group. The therapist's task is to help members recognize dysfunctional ways of relating to others. As group members interact with one another and discuss this process, individuals engage in self-reflection, leading to affective, behavioral, cognitive, and spiritual changes. The *here-and-now concept* refers to the present moment of group experience. Although past and future have some importance, changes can be made only in the present time. People who get stuck in the past ruminate over what was and what might have been. Others spend a great deal of time worrying about the future. The therapist's task is to keep the focus in the present time by discussing what happens and why it happens.

Nurses function as group therapists in many different settings, establishing the type of group that is appropriate for the desired outcomes. A single nurse may lead groups, or two cotherapists may share the leadership. Initially, the members are strangers, and the leader, as the unifying force, helps the members relate to one another. Some of the important tasks of the group leader include (Ballinger & Yalom, 1995):

1. Encouraging members to remain in the group
2. Helping the group develop a sense of cohesiveness
3. Establishing a code of behavior and norms with the group

Throughout the therapeutic process, the nurse leader assumes two basic roles (Ballinger & Yalom, 1995):

1. *Technical expert:* Using a variety of nondirective or directive approaches, the leader moves the group in a desirable direction. The leader may give explicit directions for conduct or imply suggestions.
2. *Model-setting participant:* The leader shapes behavior by the example set in personal behavior within the group. The leader molds the group in a health-oriented direction by encouraging adaptive behavior. Through encouraging frank expression of feelings, the leader sets a model in which responsibility and restraint temper honesty with concern for others' feelings and defenses. By modeling the leader's responses, the group members work toward improving interpersonal skills.

Group therapy can be effective with *children* and *adolescents.* In working with young children, the size of the group is usually limited to five people. Age and attention span determine the duration of the group session. Group therapy with children is usually activity oriented, for example, daily goal setting, art projects, music or movement therapy, and play therapy.

Because adolescents can reason and talk about their behavior, thoughts, and feelings, group therapy is a verbal process, rather than an activity process, used with children. Peers, as a source of support, feedback, and information, are very important in teenagers' lives. Group therapy with adolescents is often more productive than individual sessions.

There is often a parallel group for the *parents* of children and adolescents so that the entire family can receive treatment simultaneously. Such a group enables the parents to support each other, learn growth and developmental stages, gain an awareness of their contribution to family dynamics, increase parenting skills, and explore their own needs and problems.

Support Groups

Nurses frequently refer clients and their families to support groups, which are very important for mental health clients. In this type of group, members share thoughts and feelings and help one another examine issues and concerns. The characteristics of support groups include the following:

- Clients define own needs.
- Members have equal power.
- Groups may or may not be autonomous from mental health professionals.
- Attendance is voluntary.
- Groups may be responsive to a special population, such as a bilingual population, those with eating disorders, those experiencing domestic violence, or those defined by racial, gender, or sexual identity.

Support groups function to educate community members, to help family and friends support the individual, and to act as a crisis support, a source of referrals, and an advocate to help people get their needs met through the health care system. Because people with severe mental illness often have a very restricted social network or are even socially isolated, the interpersonal contact of support groups is vitally important. These groups contribute to an increased self-esteem, a sense of identity, increased dignity, and improved self-responsibility.

Twelve-Step Programs

In the United States, an estimated 3.5 million people attend 12-step programs annually. **Twelve-step programs** are fundamentally a spiritual plan for recovery. The first one, Alcoholics Anonymous (AA), originated in Akron, Ohio, in 1935; the first edition of the "Big Book" was published in

1939 and continues today as the principal guideline for AA. Today, worldwide AA membership is estimated at 2 million scattered across 100 countries. Other 12-step programs emerged in the 1950s and 1960s, including Al-Anon, Narcotics Anonymous, Cocaine Anonymous, Adult Children of Alcoholics, Emotions Anonymous, Gamblers Anonymous, Overeaters Anonymous, and Sex Addicts Anonymous.

The 12-step program consists of prescribed beliefs, values, and behaviors. The sequential plan for recovery is stated in 12 steps, as described in Box 9.4. Step work is considered to be a lifelong process and is usually accomplished with the aid of a sponsor. Twelve-step fellowship includes the activities of the organization, such as helping others, building relationships among members, and the sharing of joys and hardships.

The only requirement for membership is the sincere desire to change the target behavior. Any interested person can attend open meetings. Closed meetings are reserved only for the members. Some 12-step groups cater to demographic

BOX 9.4	The 12 Steps of Alcoholics Anonymous

We

1. Admitted we were powerless over alcohol, that our lives had become unmanageable.
2. Came to believe that a Power greater than ourselves could restore us to sanity.
3. Made a decision to turn our will and our lives over to the care of God as we understood Him.
4. Made a searching and fearless moral inventory of ourselves.
5. Admitted to God, to ourselves, and to another human being the exact nature of our wrongs.
6. Were entirely ready to have God remove all these defects of character.
7. Humbly asked Him to remove our shortcomings.
8. Made a list of all persons we had harmed and became willing to make amends to them all.
9. Made direct amends to such people wherever possible, except when to do so would injure them or others.
10. Continued to take personal inventory and when we were wrong promptly admitted it.
11. Sought through prayer and meditation to improve our conscious contact with God as we understood Him, praying only for knowledge of His will for us and the power to carry that out.
12. Having had a spiritual awakening as the result of these steps, we tried to carry this message to alcoholics and to practice these principles in all our affairs.

SOURCE: The Twelve Steps are reprinted with permission of Alcoholics Anonymous World Services, Inc. (A.A.W.S.). Permission to reprint the Twelve Steps does not mean that A.A.W.S. has reviewed or approves the contents of this publication, or that A.A.W.S. necessarily agrees with the views expressed herein. A.A. is a program of recovery from alcoholism only—use of the Twelve Steps in connection with programs and activities which are patterned after A.A., but which address other problems, or in any other non-A.A. context, does not imply otherwise.

subsets such as women, men, adolescents, gays or lesbians, nurses, and so on. There are four common meeting formats:

1. *Open discussion:* Individuals are asked to share thoughts and feelings regarding a general topic introduced at the beginning of the meeting.
2. *Speaker meetings:* One to three members talk for the entire meeting, usually about what life was like before membership, what happened to facilitate membership, and what life is like now as the result of membership.
3. *Big Book or 12-by-12 meetings:* Often called step meetings, the primary focus is on the meaning and practice of the 12 steps.
4. *Birthday meetings:* Once a month, members recognize specified periods of continuous abstinence. Thirty-, 60-, and 90-day intervals are recognized, as well as 6-, 9-, and 12-month birthdays. Thereafter, birthdays are celebrated annually.

TECHNOLOGY AND THERAPIES

Online support groups are becoming more popular. Some support groups offer a variety of services such as chat rooms, reference materials, "ask an expert," and assessment services and referrals. Other online support groups limit their offerings to online support for people with similar concerns. The advantages of online support groups include 24-hour-a-day service from anywhere in the world; a high level of anonymity, which protects confidentiality; and a reasonable cost. While more women participate in face-to-face support groups, equal numbers of men and women participate in online support groups. A disadvantage for those who are socially isolated is the lack of face-to-face human interaction. Since nonverbal communication is extremely important in communicating with others, the lack of these cues makes the nuances of communication more difficult to understand (Houston, Cooper, & Ford, 2002).

Computer programs for cognitive–behavioral therapy have been developed in an effort to make therapy available to more people. These programs utilize a multimedia format to teach the basic concepts and have a variety of interactive exercises designed to help people build these skills. The multimedia format makes the program accessible for people who do not have computer or keyboard skills. A study comparing the computer-assisted form with standard cognitive–behavioral therapy found that they were equally effective. That being the case, computer-assisted therapy could reduce costs and improve access to care (Pull, 2006).

Recent advances in telecommunications have led to increasing availability of inexpensive, user-friendly equipment. With this, *telepsychiatry* is becoming a more common way to provide treatment for mental disorders from a distance. In a randomized, controlled trial, 119 individuals experiencing depression were assigned to either telepsychiatry or in-person treatment. Both forms of treatment lasted 6 months and consisted of medications, psychoeducation, and brief supportive counseling. Researchers found no significant differences between the two groups in terms of symptom improvement, remission, treatment adherence, or client satisfaction (Ruskin et al., 2004).

BIOLOGICAL THERAPIES

Electroconvulsive Therapy

Electroconvulsive therapy (ECT) produces a deliberate, artificially induced grand mal seizure of the brain lasting about a minute. No one is sure exactly why ECT works and what the seizure does to the brain. It is thought that the treatment enhances dopamine (DA) sensitivity, reduces uptake of serotonin (5-HT), increases the amount of gamma-aminobutyric acid (GABA), and activates the systems in the brain that use norepinephrine (NE). ECT also increases slow-wave activity, reduces regional cerebral blood flow and glucose metabolism, and increases the blood–brain permeability. It is also thought to reduce brain activity in the prefrontal cortex (Sanacora et al., 2003).

ECT may lead to shorter and less costly inpatient care. Even though it is a safe and effective treatment, the use of ECT varies widely and depends on geographic location; some areas in the United States do not use the treatment at all. In addition, socioeconomically disadvantaged clients do not have equal access to ECT. Groups associated with a decreased probability of receiving ECT include African Americans, Latinos, those who live in a poor area, those on Medicaid, and those who lack health insurance. ECT is rarely available in state and county hospitals (Breakey & Dunn, 2004).

The most common indications for ECT are major depressive disorder and bipolar I disorder, depressed. It is indicated for clients in the following situations:

- Failure to respond to medications
- Severe symptoms, such as severe psychosis or dangerously suicidal or homicidal behaviors
- Adverse reactions to psychotropic medications
- Medical conditions, such as heart disease or glaucoma, that could be worsened by psychotropic medications
- Previous successful response to ECT
- Client preference

ECT is sometimes used in the treatment of people with schizophrenia. It is primarily used in clients experiencing

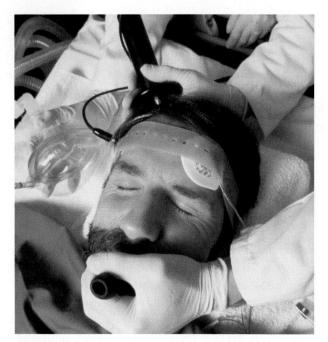

PHOTO 9.5 ◼ A physician prepares a client for unilateral electro-convulsive therapy (ECT).

SOURCE: W&D McIntyre/Photo Researchers, Inc. Used with permission.

catatonia, those who have predominant affective symptoms, those who have had a previous successful response to ECT, and those who do not respond to medications. Because of concurrent medical conditions, poor tolerance of psychotropic medications, and marked disability with depression, ECT is often the treatment of choice in older clients. Even the oldest clients, and younger clients, tolerate ECT. Several studies have shown that ECT is a safe and effective treatment for adolescents with catatonic or psychotic symptoms of depression. ECT is safe in all trimesters of pregnancy and may be less harmful to the fetus than psychotropic medications (American Psychiatric Association, 2001).

ECT is usually given as a series of 6 to 12 treatments administered three times a week. Before a client is given ECT, a complete history is taken, along with physical and neurological examinations. There are several *contraindications* for ECT: brain tumor, recent cerebrovascular accident (CVA) or brain attack, subdural hematoma, recent myocardial infarction (MI), congestive heart failure, angina pectoris, retinal detachment, acute or chronic respiratory disease, and current use of cocaine or heavy use of alcohol.

The client should ingest nothing by mouth for at least 8 hours prior to the treatment. Thirty minutes prior to the treatment, the client is given 1 mg atropine sulfate intramuscularly (IM) to control secretions and to prevent bradycardia, which sometimes occurs with ECT. A short-acting barbiturate is administered intravenously as a general anesthetic. Succinylcholine chloride (Anectine) is injected to induce muscle relaxation and prevent the full-body muscular response to the grand mal seizure. The client is preoxygenated with 95% to 100% oxygen before treatment, and oxygen is provided until the client awakens. Electrodes are placed either on one side of the temples or on both sides, through which a very small current of electricity is delivered. Side effects are more severe or persistent with the use of bilateral placement as opposed to nondominate unilateral electrode placement. The client usually awakens 10 to 15 minutes after the procedure. Upon awakening, clients may experience a headache, some muscle aches, confusion, and disorientation, which usually disappear within an hour (Table 9.3 ◼ describes nursing care for clients receiving ECT).

Memory is often affected by ECT—both memory of past events and newly learned information. More recent memories are more easily disrupted because they have not yet been stored in final long-term memory form. People often experience retrograde amnesia for the weeks or months closest to ECT treatment. Within 6 to 9 months, the ability to learn new material returns to normal. As many as half the people receiving ECT may experience persistent memory loss (Rose, Fleischmann, Wykes, Leese, & Bindman, 2003; Stern & Sacheim, 2004).

Transcranial Magnetic Stimulation

Repetitive transcranial magnetic stimulation (rTMS) is a fairly new biological treatment. It is based on the principle of mutual induction, that is, that electrical energy can be converted into magnetic fields and magnetic fields can be converted into electrical energy. rTMS is the use of a magnetic field that passes through the skull, which causes cells in the cerebral cortex to fire. rTMS shows promise as a noninvasive tool in improving mental disorders. One study

TABLE 9.3	Nursing Care for Clients Receiving ECT

Nursing Diagnosis	Interventions
Deficient Knowledge	Teach client and family about treatment and side effects. Allow client and family time to verbalize their understanding of the procedure. Document teaching.
Anxiety	Assure client that no pain will be experienced. Stay with client before and after treatment.
Altered Thought Processes	Reassure client that memory deficits and confusion are reversible. Reorient client as needed.

found that participants with schizophrenia had an improvement in negative and depressive symptoms offset by a trend for worsening positive symptoms. In a review of the literature, ECT was superior to rTMS for clients with psychosis, but among nonpsychotic clients, both treatments had similar success rates at 60% and 64%. Another study found that smokers experienced fewer cravings when treated with rTMS. rTMS can also speed the response to antidepressant medications. rTMS is being evaluated for treatment response in Tourette syndrome, hallucinations, anxiety disorders, and posttraumatic stress disorder (Hoffman & Cavus, 2002; Johann et al., 2003; Rossini et al., 2005).

With rTMS, the client sits in a lounge chair and a small, powerful, coiled electromagnet is placed on the scalp. The client usually wears ear protection because of the noise of the machine. Forty stimulations are given in 2 seconds and this is repeated 20 times. As there is no pain or discomfort, no anesthesia is necessary. Five treatments are given over 2 to 4 weeks. The most dangerous side effect is the induction of epileptic seizures. There are no other known lasting side effects in adults.

rTMS is *contraindicated* in clients with increased intracranial pressure, brain tumors, recent CVA or brain attack, meningitis, encephalitis, severe head trauma, untreated epilepsy, and current use of cocaine or heavy alcohol use.

Magnetic Seizure Therapy

Magnetic seizure therapy (MST) is the use of very-high-frequency rTMS to induce a controlled seizure in selected areas of the brain. It is administered three times a week under general anesthesia, similar to the process for ECT. The client is given earplugs to diminish the loud vibrations from the machine. MST is a substitute for ECT (Howland, 2005).

Vagus Nerve Stimulation

Vagus nerve stimulation (VNS) involves the surgical implant of a small generator, much like a pacemaker. This generator provides intermittent stimulation to the left vagus nerve. Side effects include mild to moderate hoarseness, cough, neck pain, and shortness of breath, which tend to decrease over time. Unlike antidepressant medications, there is no weight gain, sleep disturbance, or sexual dysfunction. VNS has been used to treat refractory epilepsy and has both behavioral and anticonvulsant effects. In the psychiatric field it is used for treatment-resistant depression, with a 40% rate of effectiveness (Carpenter et al., 2006; Howland, 2005).

Deep Brain Stimulation

Deep brain stimulation (DBS) involves the surgical implant of electrodes in deep subcortical nuclei. These electrodes provide intermittent stimulation. Currently, DBS is approved for unremitting tremors and for Parkinson disease. It is being researched for effectiveness in obsessive–compulsive disorder. Potential side effects include bleeding, seizures, infections, and paresthesia (Howland, 2005).

Psychosurgery

Neurosurgical treatment of mental disorders has a history dating back to antiquity. The twentieth century saw a great abuse of this intervention by performing frontal lobotomies for aggression and abnormal behavior. Tragically, this resulted in people who lost their personality and in many cases could not even do self-care. Due to this abuse, current procedures are under strict control by independent review panels. At the present time, **psychosurgery** is considered a last-ditch option for people whose conditions have not responded to other treatments. As few as 1% of clients may be candidates for surgical treatment, particularly people with severe and unremitting obsessive–compulsive disorder, depression, and Tourette syndrome. Methods include surgical incisions or a radiation treatment called a *Gamma Knife*. Some physicians implant tiny electrodes in the brain, which is gaining favor because it is reversible. The risks of psychosurgery have lessened in recent years due to enhanced radiological imaging, better surgical techniques, and a rapidly expanding knowledge of the brain's structure and function (Anandan, Wigg, Thomas, & Coffey, 2004; Mashour, Walker, & Martuza, 2005; Ruck et al., 2003).

Psychosurgery is a controversial issue in the medical community. Although some physicians see the benefit in very specific cases, others say that there is never any excuse to mutilate the brain to control someone's emotions or behavior.

Light Therapy

Light therapy, or phototherapy, is often the treatment of choice for seasonal affective disorder (SAD), which appears to be directly related to the amount of light a person is exposed to. Light has an inhibiting effect on the production of melatonin, a hormone that affects mood, sensations of fatigue, and sleepiness. It may also be effective for depression during pregnancy and postpartum (Oren et al., 2002).

Clients are exposed to very bright (10,000 lux) full-spectrum fluorescent lamps for 30 minutes for a minimum of 5 days. Light therapy is done in the home, and clients often read or watch TV during the painless treatment. It is thought that the bright light suppresses the production of melatonin and normalizes the disturbance in circadian rhythms. Light therapy may also be used prophylactically with clients susceptible to SAD or postpartum depression (Golden et al., 2005).

Temporary eye or vision problems and headaches are experienced by about 20% of clients receiving light therapy.

To prevent insomnia, the treatment is done in the morning or by 5:00 p.m. at the latest.

Sleep Deprivation

A biological treatment for depression is sleep deprivation. This may be total, for 36 hours, or partial, with the person being awakened after 1:30 a.m. and kept awake until the next evening. During this time, clients may be alone, in a group, or participating in activities. Some improve steadily after only one night of sleep deprivation. Others respond better if the deprivation is conducted once a week for several weeks. Others quickly return to their baseline level of depression. The way by which sleep deprivation acts as an antidepressant is still unknown (Voderholzer et al., 2004).

Gene Therapy

With the discovery of the human genome, there has been increasing interest in gene therapy. The goal of **gene therapy** is to transfer genes that will have a therapeutic effect on cellular function. In the area of neuroscience, research is being conducted with the slow neurodegenerative diseases and acute injury to the brain. In contrast to these situations, the biology of psychiatric disorder is much more complicated than ischemia, seizures, or a concussion. It is unlikely that gene therapy will be clinically useful in psychiatry for some time to come (Sapolsky, 2003).

Seclusion and Restraint

Seclusion is the removal of a client from the general milieu into a single room, with or without a locked door. Restraint is physical restriction of movement; the most common form is to restrain arms and legs (four-point) or arms, legs, and waist (five-point) on a specially designed bed. Human restraint is the use of physical force to restrict freedom of movement. The use of involuntary seclusion or mechanical or human restraints is justified only as an emergency safety measure to imminent danger to oneself or others and only after less restrictive methods have been deemed inadequate to prevent injury. Seclusion and restraints are not treatment interventions but security measures, and these are extreme measures that are very controversial in mental health care.

Tragically, seclusion and restraint have sometimes been imposed for *staff convenience* to control individual behavior without having to use adequate staffing or clinical interventions. They also have been used for *coercion* to force a client to comply with the staff's wishes. And they have been used as *retaliation* to punish or penalize clients. None of these are legitimate reasons to impose seclusion or restraints.

Studies show that seclusion and restraint lead to feelings of fear, anger, anxiety, humiliation, depression, and helplessness. Clients perceive this as punishment, a form of torture, and of little therapeutic value. To some clients, these experiences are as devastating as physical abuse or rape. In these situations, nurses become perpetrators and are consequently feared by clients (Bower, McCullough, & Timmons, 2003).

In addition to negative feelings, clients in seclusion and restraints experience problems with sensory deprivation similar to prison inmates in solitary confinement. Problems include a hypersensitivity to external stimuli and hallucinations. A tragic consequence of restraints is accidental death from asphyxiation, strangulation, or cardiac arrest.

Many states have strict guidelines for the use of seclusion and restraints, and many hospitals have instituted "no-seclusion" policies. The Health Care Financing Administration (HCFA), which finances and regulates Medicare and Medicaid, and the Joint Commission on Accreditation of Healthcare Organizations (JCAHO) have revised their standards regarding seclusion and restraint. The changes are geared toward staff education and changes in the milieu, with the goal of preventing the need for these aversive measures. Both agencies require that there exists a high risk of harm to others, with seclusion and restraint being a last-resort, emergency measure (Guido, 2006).

Research shows that seclusion and restraints are related to milieu factors such as overcrowding, high noise level, staffing shortage, and an authoritarian attitude of the staff. Progressive institutions have made changes in the milieu to prevent or deescalate agitation and violence in clients. These changes include (Guido, 2006; Schreiner, Crafton, & Sevin, 2004):

- High staff–client ratios
- Rules and regulations that are less rigid
- Decreased noise related to decreased overcrowding
- Improved recreational activities and facilities
- One-to-one care during a psychological crisis
- Staff education regarding alternative interventions
- Medications
- Behavioral system to reward positive behavior

Chapter 6 ∞ covers triggers to aggression, assessment, prevention, and nonviolent interventions using interpersonal skills, nonverbal communication skills, and verbal communication skills.

COMPLEMENTARY/ALTERNATIVE THERAPIES

Complementary/alternative therapies is an umbrella term for hundreds of therapies drawn from all over the world. Many forms have been handed down over thousands of years, both orally and as written records. These are based on the medical systems of ancient peoples, including Egyptians, Chinese, Asian Indians, Greeks, and Native Peoples. Others, such as osteopathy and chiropractic therapy, evolved in the United States over the past two centuries. Still others, such as some of the mind–body and bioelectromagnetic approaches, are on the frontier of scientific knowledge and understanding.

Contemporary nursing is advancing beyond the Western biomedical model to incorporate many healing tools used by our Asian, Latino, Native People, African, and European ancestors. The health care field is rapidly rediscovering that these ancient principles and practices have significant therapeutic value. Clients do not wish to abandon conventional medicine, but they do want to have a range of options available to them, including herbs, nutrition, manual healing methods, mind–body techniques, and spiritual approaches. Some healing practices, such as exercise, nutrition, meditation, and massage, promote health, manage stress, and prevent disease. Others, such as herbs or homeopathic remedies, address specific illnesses. Many other healing practices do both.

Studies show that 36% of adult Americans use alternative treatments in a given year. When prayer specifically for health reasons is included as a treatment, the number rises to 62%. Among people with mental disorders, the use is even more common. Around 43% of individuals with anxiety attacks and 41% of adults with severe depression utilize alternative therapies. Most of them also continue to use conventional health care (Barnes, Powell-Griner, McFann, & Nahin, 2004; Kessler, Walters, & Forthofer, 2001).

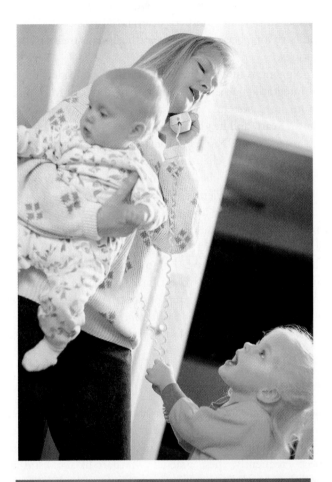

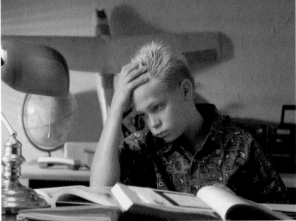

PHOTO 9.6 ■ People who exercise experience less depression and anxiety. Exercise also has a positive effect on self-concept, mastery, self-sufficiency, body image, and cognitive processing.

SOURCE: Dennis MacDonald/PhotoEdit, Inc. Used with permission.

PHOTO 9.7 ■ Stress is a part of everyday life. Stress cannot be avoided, but some ways of coping with life's challenges are more effective than others.

SOURCE: Chris Lowe/Photolibrary.com; Superstock, Inc. Used with permission.

Ethnocentrism, the assumption that one's own cultural or ethnic group is superior to others, has often prevented Western health care practitioners from learning "new" ways to promote health and prevent chronic illness. With client demand for a broader range of options, the health care field must be open to the idea that other cultures and countries have valid ways of preventing and curing disease that could be good for Western societies. Although the information may be new to contemporary Western medicine, many of these traditions are hundreds or even thousands of years old and have long been part of the medical mainstream in other cultures.

Nursing is in a unique position to take a leadership role in integrating alternative healing methods into Western health care systems. Nurses have historically used their hands, heart, and head in more natural and traditional healing interactions. Nurses, by virtue of their education and relationships with clients, can help clients assert their right to choose their own healing journey and the quality of their life and death experiences (Fontaine, 2005).

This section of the chapter provides an extremely brief definition of the more common forms of alternative therapies. Chapters 11 through 17 ∞ present more information on alternative therapies for the specific mental disorders. If you wish to explore alternative practices in more depth, from a nursing perspective, an excellent reference is *Complementary & Alternative Therapies for Nursing Practice,* second edition, by the author of this text, Karen Lee Fontaine.

Acupuncture

Acupuncture, acupressure, Jin Shin Jyutsu, Jin Shin Do, and reflexology are different forms of the same practice of stimulating points on the body to balance the body's life energy. Frequently, these practices are part of a holistic approach to wellness and are combined with diet, herbs, mind–body techniques, and spiritual therapies.

When the flow of energy becomes blocked or congested, people experience discomfort or pain on a physical level, may feel frustrated or irritable on an emotional level, and may experience a sense of vulnerability or lack of purpose in life on a spiritual level. The goal of care is to recognize and manage the disruption before illness or disease occurs. Pressure-point practitioners bring balance to the body's energies, which promotes optimal health and well-being, and facilitates a person's healing capacity.

Animal-Assisted Therapy

Animal-assisted therapy is the use of specifically selected animals as a treatment method in health and human service settings. Accredited professionals guide the human–animal interaction toward specific, individualized therapeutic goals. A variety of goals can be addressed: cognitive goals such as improved memory or verbal expression; emotional goals such as increased self-esteem and motivation; social goals such as building rapport and improved socialization skills; and physical goals such as balance and mobility.

For many people, interacting with a pet is less stressful than interacting with other people. In comparison with people, animals are nonjudgmental and accepting. This unconditional support system can be accessed at any time of day or night when one lives with a pet. Loneliness, lack of companionship, and lack of social support are major risk factors for depression and suicide that can be offset by the presence of a loved pet. Animals also facilitate socializing within the neighborhood by getting owners out of the house and providing a topic of conversation. Even sitting and looking at fish in an aquarium relaxes and relieves anxiety for many people. Children with short attention spans are able to sustain attention longer when interacting with animals.

Aromatherapy

Aromatherapy is the therapeutic use of essential oils in which the odor or fragrance plays an important part. It is an offshoot of herbal medicine, with the basis of action the same as that of modern pharmacology. The chemicals found in the essential oils are absorbed into the body, resulting in physiological or psychological benefit. Essential oils are extracted from plants and are massaged into the skin, inhaled, placed in baths, used as compresses, or mixed into ointments. Different oils may calm, stimulate, improve sleep, change eating habits, or boost the immune system. Some oils cause the brain to release enkephalins that decrease the perception of pain and increase the sense of well-being (LaTorre, 2003). Oils used in the mental health field include:

- *Anxiety*: Basil, bergamot, chamomile, green apple, lemon balm, neroli, and orange
- *Depression*: Bergamot, geranium, jasmine, lemon balm, rose, and ylang ylang
- *Insomnia*: Chamomile, clary sage, lavender, marjoram, neroli, and vetiver
- *Memory/mental function*: Basil, black pepper, coriander, ginger, rosemary, thyme
- *Alertness*: Peppermint

Essential oils are potent and can irritate the skin, so they should be diluted with a carrier oil before being used on the skin. Carrier oils contain vitamins, proteins, and minerals that provide added nutrients to the body. Carrier oils include apricot kernel oil, sunflower oil, soy oil, sweet almond oil, grape seed oil, sesame oil, avocado oil, jojoba, and wheat germ oil.

Ayurveda

The Indian system of medicine, *Ayurveda*, is at least 2,500 years old. Illness is viewed as a state of imbalance among the body's systems. Ayurveda emphasizes the interdependence of the health of the individual and the quality of societal life. Mentally healthy people have good memory, comprehension, intelligence, and reasoning ability. Emotionally healthy people experience evenly balanced emotional states and a sense of well-being or happiness. Physically healthy people have abundant energy with proper functioning of the senses, digestion, and elimination. From a spiritual perspective, healthy people have a sense of aliveness and richness of life, are developing in the direction of their full potential, and are in good relationships with themselves, other people, and the larger cosmos.

Nutritional counseling, massage, natural medicines, meditations, yoga, and other methods are used to treat many disorders. This ancient system has adapted to modern science and technology, including biomedical science and quantum physics.

Traditional Chinese Medicine

Traditional Chinese medicine (TCM) has developed over 3,000 years and seeks to balance the flow of *qi*, the energy or life force of a person. In TCM the mind, body, spirit, and emotions are never separated. Thus, the heart is not just a blood pump; it also influences one's capacity for joy, one's sense of purpose in life, and one's connectedness with others. The kidneys filter fluids, but they also manage one's capacity for fear, one's will and motivation, and one's faith in life. The lungs breathe in air and breathe out waste products, but they also regulate one's capacity to grieve, as well as one's acknowledgment of self and others. The liver cleanses the body, and it also influences one's feeling of anger and that of vision and creativity. The stomach has a part in digestion of food and influences one's ability to be thoughtful, kind, and nurturing as well. These are just a few of the mind–body connections that TCM practitioners recognize.

Practitioners are trained to use a variety of ancient and modern therapeutic methods, including acupuncture, herbal medicine, massage, heat therapy, Qigong, t'ai chi, and nutritional and lifestyle counseling.

Chiropractic

Chiropractic is the third largest independent health profession in the Western world after conventional medicine and dentistry. It is based on the premise that the spine is literally the backbone of human health. Misalignments of the vertebrae or loss of mobility in the facet joints caused by poor posture or trauma result in pressure on the spinal cord, which may lead to diminished function and illness. Three primary clinical goals guide chiropractic intervention: reduce or elim-

inate pain; correct the spinal dysfunction; and preventative maintenance to ensure the problem does not recur.

Curanderismo

Curanderismo is a cultural healing tradition found in Latin America and among many Latinos in the United States. Although it is a traditional healing system, it utilizes Western biomedical beliefs, treatments, and practices. Three levels of care are practiced among *curanderos* and *curanderas*: the material level, the spiritual level, and the mental level. Healers have the gift for working at only one of these levels. Healers working at the mental level have the ability to transmit, channel, and focus mental vibrations in a way that directly affects a person's mental or physical condition. When working with mental conditions, healers send vibration into the person's mind to manipulate energies and modify behavior.

Herbal Medicine

Herbal medicine is used by 80% of the world's population. Even though only a tiny fraction of plants have been studied for medicinal benefits, plant-derived products are used regularly by conventional health care providers. Around 25% of all prescription drugs sold in the United States are derived from plants. Because herbs are marketed as "natural" or promoted as foods, clients may assume incorrectly that herbs are safe and without side effects. Remember that natural remedies should be approached with respect and teach clients that, although herbs are generally much safer than prescription drugs, if abused or overused they can cause harm. Herbs used in the mental health field include:

- *Anxiety*: Chamomile and kava
- *Depression*: St. John's wort and SAMe
- *Mood swings*: Ginseng
- *Insomnia*: Catnip, hops, lemon balm, melatonin, passion flower, or valerian
- *Memory*: Ginkgo
- *Alcohol or drug withdrawal*: Chamomile, evening primrose oil, ginseng, and valerian

Herbs are drugs and you must treat them with respect. The majority of herbal medicines present no danger. Some can, however, cause serious side effects if taken in excess or, for some, if taken over a prolonged period of time. For example, kava may cause liver damage at high doses. Herbs can also interact with drugs and caution should be used when combining herbs with prescription and over-the-counter (OTC) medications. For example, St. John's wort should not be combined with antidepressants as their effects may increase. St. John's wort reduces the effectiveness of birth control pills, HIV treatment medications, and the asthma medication theophylline. Kava should not be mixed with antianxiety medication and some antihypertensives. It is important that people investigate herb–drug interactions before using herbs as an alternative therapy.

Homeopathy

Practitioners use infinitesimal doses of natural substances, called *remedies*. If taken in large amounts, these natural compounds will produce symptoms of the disease. In the doses used by homeopaths, however, these remedies stimulate a person's self-healing capacity. Homeopaths also believe that it is necessary to have adequate nutrition, exercise, rest, good hygiene, and a healthy environment to adapt to and maintain homeostasis. In other words, health is the ability of people to adapt their equilibrium in response to internal and external change. Remedies that are used in the mental health field include pulsatilla (windflower) for insomnia and for people who are highly emotional, weepy, impressionable, easily influenced, fearful of abandonment, and worried about what others think of them; and ignatia (St. Ignatius bean) and arsenicum album (arsenic) for anxiety.

Hypnotherapy and Guided Imagery

Hypnosis and guided imagery are states of attentive and focused concentration during which people are highly responsive to suggestion. Therapists help people learn methods to take advantage of the mind–body–spirit connection through the medium of relaxation and imagination. Hypnosis and imagery cannot make people do anything against their will. These therapies can be used to help people gain self-control, improve self-esteem, and become more autonomous. People who are imprisoned by negative beliefs see themselves as hopeless, helpless victims. With hypnosis or guided imagery, they can learn how to substitute positive, empowering messages. These procedures are unsuitable for people with active psychosis or somatic delusions. It is generally considered that these individuals are often bombarded with too many images already and are unable to differentiate between voluntary and involuntary images.

Kinesiology/Applied Kinesiology

Applied kinesiology is both a diagnostic method and a treatment method using energy and lymphatic, neurovascular, and muscle systems. Well-being and health are determined by the nature of the flow of energy within and without the body. Disease and pain occur when energy is blocked, fixed, or unbalanced. When someone's thoughts and emotions are misaligned with the energy necessary to meet a life challenge, an energy imbalance results. It is believed that people are responsible for their own health and that they can take simple steps to improve and maintain their level of wellness.

Massage Therapy

Massage therapy, the scientific manipulation of the soft tissues of the body, is a healing art, an act of physical caring, and a way of communicating without words. The goal of massage therapy is to achieve or increase health and well-being and to help people heal themselves. On the mental level, massage therapy induces a relaxed state of alertness; reduces mental stress, thus clearing the mind; and increases one's capacity for clearer thinking. On the emotional level, massage therapy satisfies the need for caring and nurturing touch, increases feelings of well-being, decreases mild depression, enhances self-image, reduces levels of anxiety, and increases awareness of the mind–body connection.

Massage has been used with severely ill individuals as an adjunct to conventional psychiatric interventions. Clients are given an *executive massage*, done with the client fully dressed and seated on a massage chair. The head, neck, back, arms, and legs are massaged for 10 to 20 minutes per session. Hilliard's study (1995) found that massage was an effective stress reducer for inpatient and outpatient clients who sought safe touch and relaxation, resulting in a sense of emotional well-being. Massage is also effective in decreasing agitation in persons with Alzheimer's disease.

Meditation

Meditation is a general term for a wide range of practices that involve relaxing the body and easing the mind. Meditation is a process that anyone can use to calm down, cope with stress, and, for those with spiritual inclinations, feel as one with God or the universe. Meditation can be practiced individually or in groups and is easy to learn. It requires no change in belief system and is compatible with most religious practices. People who meditate say that they have clearer minds and sharper thoughts. The brain seems to clear itself so that new ideas and beliefs become available. This clearer mind may be accompanied by a cognitive restructuring in which people interpret life events in a more positive, more realistic fashion. Meditation's residual effects—improved stress-coping abilities—are a protection against daily stress and anxiety.

Native American Healing

Spirituality and medicine are inseparable in Native American tradition. Medicine women and men see themselves as channels through which the Great Power helps others achieve well-being in mind, body, and spirit. The only healer is the One who created all things. Medicine people consider that they have certain knowledge to put things together to help the sick person heal and that knowledge has to be dispensed in a certain way, often through ritual or ceremony. The healer enters into the healing relationship with love and compassion. The two individuals experience a joining or merging as this process unfolds. This merger symbolizes the cementing together of people and the Divine Spirit.

Health is viewed as a balance or harmony of mind and body. The goal is to be in harmony with all things, which means first being in harmony with oneself. It is believed that most illness begins in the head and people must get rid of ideas that predispose illness. If the mind is negative, the body will be drained, making it more vulnerable. When people open up to the universe, learn what is good for them, and find ways to be happier, they can begin to work toward a longer and healthier life.

Naturopathy

Naturopathy is a primary health care system emphasizing the curative power of nature, working to restore and support the body's healing ability using nutrition, herbs, homeopathic remedies, and Chinese medicine. It involves a 4-year course of study beyond the bachelor's degree, much like conventional medical school.

Prayer

Prayer is most often defined simply as a form of communication and fellowship with the Deity or Creator. The universality of prayer is evidenced in all cultures that have some form of prayer. Prayer has been, and continues to be, used in times of difficulty and illness, even in the most secular societies. Nine of 10 Americans believe in prayer; 72% to 82% have prayed for personal healing; and 87% have prayed for the healing of others (Taylor, 2003).

Life-affirming beliefs and philosophies nourish people. They meditate and say prayers that elicit physiological calm and a sense of peacefulness, both of which contribute to longer survival.

Reiki

Reiki is an ancient Tibetan healing system that uses light hand placements to channel healing energies to the client. It is commonly used to treat distress and acute and chronic health problems, and to achieve spiritual focus.

Spiritual/Shamanic Healing

A shaman is a woman or man who enters an altered state of consciousness, at will, to contact and utilize another type of reality to acquire knowledge and power and to help other people. Shamans use ancient techniques to achieve and maintain well-being and healing for themselves and members of their communities, serving as a link between the world of matter and spirit. Shamanism is not a belief system. Rather, it covers ancient, indigenous, and holistic healing practices worldwide.

T'ai Chi

T'ai chi and *Qigong* are Chinese practices consisting of breathing and mental exercises combined with body movements. They are easy and nontiring exercises that contain sets of moves designed to gather *qi*, or energy. Most people spend 30 minutes a day doing the exercises and another 30 minutes in meditation. Practitioners discover how to generate more energy and conserve what they have in order to maintain health or treat illness. The benefits of t'ai chi are seen in conditions such as hypertension, osteoporosis, and arthritis. T'ai chi can decrease stress and fatigue, improve mood, and increase energy. It is especially helpful in improving balance in older adults, which decreases the risk for falls (Fontaine, 2005).

Therapeutic Touch

Popularized by nursing professor Dolores Krieger in the 1970s, Therapeutic Touch is practiced by registered nurses and others to relieve pain and stress. It is believed that people must, and do, heal themselves. Healing environments are created when nurses enter into caring moments with clients in which the nurse becomes a resource for clients to self-heal. The nurse assesses where the person's energy field is weak or congested and then uses her or his hands to direct energy into the field to balance it. Indications include irritability and anxiety; lethargy, fatigue, and depression; premenstrual syndrome; nausea and vomiting, chemotherapy and radiation sickness; wound and bone healing; acute

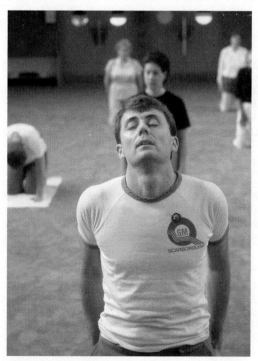

PHOTO 9.8 ■ Yoga is one form of relaxation training.
SOURCE: Stu Rosner/Stock Boston.

Using Research Evidence | Helping Clients With Medications

Kozuki, Y., Poupore, E., & Schepp, K. (2005). **Visual feedback therapy to enhance medication adherence in psychosis.** *Archives of Psychiatric Nursing, 19,* 70–80.

What is the study about?

For persons living with psychotic disorders, a serious problem is that many fail to adhere to their medication plans. A meta-analysis reports a medication adherence rate of approximately 58%. Therefore, the purposes of this study were primarily to test feasibility of a specific protocol for persons with psychotic disorders, test effectiveness of visual feedback therapy (VFT), and examine how well an electronic monitoring (EM) system tracks patterns of continuous medication adherence for a 3-month period.

How was the study done?

This was a quantitative quasi-experimental pilot study using participants recruited from both inpatient psychiatric units and a community mental health center (outpatients). This study was approved by an institutional review board, and the researchers recruited a total of 23 consenting participants, all living with DSM-IV diagnoses of psychotic disorder(s). Of these 23 participants, 9 were female and the remaining were male; all were taking at least one psychotropic drug; 16 were living with schizophrenia, 2 with schizoaffective disorder, and the remaining 5 with mood disorders with psychotic episodes. Eight participants were living at an inpatient psychiatric unit and the rest were enlisted from a community mental health center.

Medication adherence rates were measured for each prescribed medication by a separate EM device: a medication bottle cap with a computer processor in it allowed for recording the frequency and times of day when the bottle was opened. These stored data were downloaded to a computer with a special software package for analysis. To verify these EM records, participants were asked to self-report daily on their medication adherence, and a pharmacist followed up by counting pills. For the intervention and measurements, all participants met with one or two intervention clinicians weekly for the first month, and then once at months 2 and 3. Intervention meetings lasted from 30 to 60 minutes. There were three interventions: visual feedback of medication-taking patterns presented on a computer screen and recorded continuously by the EM device; attentive listening by the intervention clinician (who listened to concerns but did not discuss treatment); and teaching about medication and symptom-management strategies. The Positive and Negative Syndrome Scale (PANSS) was administered at baseline and at 1, 2, and 3 months into the study. The PANSS measured how psychiatric symptoms fluctuated in intensity so that that fluctuation could be associated with adherence to medication plan. In addition, the participants were given the Scale to Assess Unawareness of Mental Disorders to assess their insights about mental illness and the importance of adhering to medication plans.

What were the results of the study?

Final EM records showed that clients had taken 83.3% of prescribed medications, 64.2% at the correct time. The rate of adherence to medication plans did not change significantly over the 3-month study. Of the outpatients, 60% maintained or increased their adherence rates. However, of the total partici-

pants, half decreased adherence rates within 2 weeks. The EM device also allowed for assessment of behavioral patterns of adherence. The patterns included: 1) missing doses, 2) irregularity seen in more-than-once-per-day regimen, 3) complete irregularity, 4) complete cessation, 5) treatment effects, and 6) correlations between adherence rates and psychiatric symptoms.

Most clients missed doses. A pattern of irregularity emerged: doses prescribed more than once a day were taken irregularly, and the irregular patterns appeared at both morning and night doses. *Complete irregularity* meant that no regular pattern could be discerned; these clients missed doses as well. In the pattern of *complete cessation*, no patterns preceded cessation, nor did participants resume the medication. A *treatment-effects pattern* was discerned in some participants: they took medications irregularly at first, then more regularly, and they gradually missed fewer doses. Data analysis revealed that the average compliance rate based on participants' self-report was 74.3%; however, the EM device identified that the average compliance rate was 83.3%, indicating that these clients underestimated their adherence rates. Verification by counting pills showed that the EM had an error rate below 5%; thus EM was more reliable than self-report. For the outpatient group, adherence rate at 2 weeks into the study was 84.6%; after 1 month 83.3%, after 2 months 80.8%, and after 3 months 68.85%. For the inpatient group, adherence rates changed as follows: after 2 weeks 91.2%; after 1 month 80.9%, after 2 months 78.9%, and after 3 months 73.8%. Researchers concluded that clients whose adherence rates are low need more intensive intervention. Data from the PANSS and SUMD showed that, in most participants, nonadherence or underadherence to psychotropic medications worsened psychiatric symptoms at several weeks and months later. Further, adherence rates correlated with two factors: insight into having a mental illness with psychotic episodes and insight into the illness's social consequences. The weekly visual feedback at 1, 2, and 3 months did not statistically increase the number of participants who improved their adherence.

What additional questions might I have?

How would the results of the study differ with a larger sample size or use of a control group? What other strategies might be helpful in assisting persons living with psychosis to take their medications as prescribed?

How can I use this study?

Nurses need to be ever-vigilant regarding medication adherence in clients living with psychosis, especially those with multiple medications and varied dosing schedules. In persons living with serious psychosis, opening medication containers at specified times might not be practical. The behavioral patterns identified in this study indicate that medication adherence needs to be addressed in a manner that produces improved compliance. Using an EM system to provide visual feedback may be effective for persons living with psychotic disorders; although, in this study, the treatment did not reach statistical significance, it may be clinically significant and warrant further investigation. In addition, nurses who monitor adherence should know that clients' self-reports can be erroneous.

SOURCE: Contributed by Dolores Huffman, PhD, RN, Associate Professor of Nursing, Purdue University Calumet, Hammond, Indiana.

musculoskeletal problems such as sprains and muscle spasms; and fibromyalgia syndrome. Therapeutic Touch produces a sense of well-being and relaxation for both the nurse and the client (Denison, 2004; Moore, 2005).

Yoga

Yoga has been practiced for thousands of years in India, where it is a way of life that includes ethical models for behavior and mental and physical exercises aimed at producing spiritual enlightenment. It is a method for life that can complement and enhance any system of religion, or it can be practiced completely apart from religion. The Western approach to yoga tends to be more fitness oriented with the goal of managing stress, learning to relax, and increasing vitality and well-being. A typical yoga session lasts 20 minutes to an hour. Some people spend 30 minutes doing the poses and another 30 minutes doing breathing practices and meditations. Others spend the majority of the time doing poses and end with a short meditation or relaxation procedure. Even for those who are stiff and out of shape, sick, or weak, sets of easy exercises can help to loosen the joints and stimulate circulation. If practiced regularly, these simple exercises alone make a great difference in people's health and well-being.

Nursing and alternative therapies share the focus on what is unique about the individual and her or his role in healing. The individual is always at the center of treatment interventions, with the emphasis on growth toward health. Health promotion is a lifelong process that focuses on optimal development of one's physical, emotional, mental, and spiritual selves.

Focus Your Study

OBJECTIVES	KEY CONCEPTS
1. Differentiate between the professional roles that exist in mental health settings.	■ At the basic level of practice, nurses provide primary mental health services to individuals, families, groups, and communities. This practice includes health promotion, intake screening and evaluation, case management, milieu therapy, promotion of self-care activities, psychobiological interventions, health teaching, counseling, crisis care, and psychiatric rehabilitation. ■ Advanced practice nurses provide psychotherapy and consultation, design and implement research activities, and have prescriptive authority. They are accountable for using evidence-based practice research and implementing the results in direct client care. ■ Psychiatric consultation liaison nurses provide mental health care in nonpsychiatric settings. They bridge the gap between mental health and medical–surgical nursing care by providing crisis intervention. ■ Nurse informaticists integrate nursing, computer, and information sciences to develop, customize, or update computer information and clinical documentation systems. ■ Psychiatrists are physicians who admit clients to the inpatient setting. They are responsible for diagnosing mental disorders and prescribing treatment. ■ Psychologists and psychiatric social workers conduct individual, couple, family, and group therapy. ■ Occupational therapists provide activities that help clients improve activities of daily living.
2. Describe characteristics of milieu therapy.	■ Clear communication ■ Safe environment ■ Activity schedule with therapeutic goals ■ Support network

3. Outline psychosocial nursing interventions.	■ Social skills training includes:
	  • Activities of daily living (ADLs) and instrumental activities of daily living (IADLs)
	  • Vocational skills
	  • Leisure-time skills
	  • Communication skills
	  • Conflict management skills

(continued)

(continued)

3. Outline psychosocial nursing interventions.

■ Self-esteem interventions:
  • Acknowledge strengths.
  • Accept compliments—do not accept put-downs.
  • Set achievable realistic goals and work to accomplish them.
  • Reward yourself for your successes.
  • Take up a new hobby or interest, join a new group, or try volunteering.
  • Counteract negative thoughts with positive thoughts.
■ Remotivation therapy:
  • Based on client autonomy and the concept of acceptance
  • Outcomes include increased interactions with others, improved self-care, active involvement in treatment decisions, improved self-esteem, and increased feelings of belonging to a group
■ Reminiscence therapy:
  • Older adults are encouraged to remember the past through the process of life review.
  • Outcomes are improved self-esteem, increased self-awareness, and an improved sense of identity in the face of cognitive disorders.

4. Describe the key points in assessment and intervention in crisis situations.

■ The primary goal of crisis intervention is to resolve the immediate problem, regain emotional equilibrium, and adapt and return to the precrisis level of functioning.
■ Crisis intervention skills include:
  • Problem solving
  • Management of emotions
  • Ability to redefine the unexpected event
  • Maintaining interpersonal relationships

5. Compare and contrast different forms of psychological and biological therapies.

■ Cognitive–behavioral therapy involves clients learning how to relax and calm their bodies and changing negative automatic thoughts or maladaptive schemas.
■ Behavioral therapy utilizes contingency contracts and token economies to increase positive behaviors.
■ Play therapy is used with children younger than 12 years to establish rapport, reveal feelings that children are unable to verbalize, enable children to act out anxiety or tension in a constructive manner, understand children's relationships with significant others, and to teach children adaptive socialization skills.
■ The goals of individual psychotherapy are to help clients clarify perceptions, identify feelings, make connections among thoughts, feelings, and events, gain insight, problem solve, and modify problematic behavior.
■ The goals of family therapy include helping families cope, improve their communication and interpersonal skills, establish boundaries, and moderate family cohesion and flexibility. All family members must feel that they are part of the problem-solving and decision-making processes and that their personal welfare is always considered.
■ There are many types of groups in the mental health setting. These are task groups, psychoeducation groups, group therapy, support groups, and 12-step programs.
■ Electroconvulsive therapy (ECT) involves the application of a very small current of electricity through electrodes placed on the temples. ECT is used for people with depression, for older clients, for pregnant clients, and for some people with schizophrenia.

6. Describe the different roles nurses play in group settings.

■ The nurse's role in a task group is to keep the group on task and to facilitate appropriate interaction.
■ In psychoeducation groups, nurses provide information to clients and families and elicit reactions and comments from the group members.
■ In group therapy, the nurse:
  • Encourages members to remain in the group
  • Helps the group develop a sense of cohesiveness
  • Establishes a code of behavior and norms with the group
  • Acts as a technical expert
  • Models appropriate, adaptive behavior

7. Discuss the use of alternative therapies in mental health settings.

- Repetitive transcranial magnetic stimulation (rTMS) is a noninvasive tool using magnetic fields. rTMS is used with clients who have a nonpsychotic mental illness and sometimes for people who are trying to quit smoking.
- Magnetic seizure therapy (MST) uses a very high frequency rTMS to induce a therapeutic seizure, similar to the process for ECT.
- Vagus nerve stimulation (VNS) involves the surgical implant of a small generator which provides intermittent stimulation to the left vagus nerve. It is used for treatment-resistant depression.
- Light therapy, used for seasonal affective disorder, involves 30 minutes a day of exposure to full-spectrum fluorescent lamps.

Explore MediaLink

For review questions, case studies, and other resources for this chapter see the Pearson Health MediaLink CD-ROM that accompanies this book and the Companion Website.

CD-ROM
- Audio Glossary
- NCLEX-RN® Review Questions

Companion Website www.prenhall.com/fontaine
- Audio Glossary
- NCLEX-RN® Review Questions
- Case Study
  - Crisis Intervention
- Care Plan
  - Depression Intervention
- Critical Thinking
  - Milieu Therapy
- Medialink Application
  - The Illness Management and Recovery Program
- MediaLinks
  - Books for Clients and Families
  - Community Resources

NCLEX-RN®Review Questions

9-1. Which of the following roles is not within the scope of practice for an advanced practice mental health nurse?
   1. Performing physiological and psychological assessments of clients
   2. Prescribing psychotropic medications
   3. Administering and interpreting psychological tests
   4. Providing psychotherapy to individuals, groups, and families

9-2. In managing the therapeutic milieu, the nurse is responsible for which of the following activities?
   1. Taking clients on excursions to go bowling or swimming to develop healthy leisure activities and social skills
   2. Providing classes on activities of daily living and social skills to improve healthy lifestyles and communication skills
   3. Providing assistance with placement after discharge and community resources
   4. Providing classes on resume writing and job interview skills to prepare for future employment opportunities

9-3. Which one of the following clients would receive the most benefit from social skills training?
   1. A 20-year-old college student who is afraid to speak in front of large groups
   2. A 41-year-old mother of two teenage children recently divorced and entering the dating scene
   3. A 35-year-old homeless man who has a history of chronic paranoid schizophrenia
   4. A 29-year-old waitress who works two jobs and is planning to go back to nursing school

9-4. A 17-year-old high school senior is referred to the outpatient mental health clinic after learning that she is 5 months pregnant. Despite her decision to keep the baby after it is born, she wants to start college next fall. Her parents have offered no financial or emotional support and her boyfriend broke up with her after learning of her pregnancy. Which of the following actions should the nurse take to help the client deal with this crisis?
   1. Call the client's parents and suggest they attend a family therapy session.

2. Give the client information about homes for unwed mothers and adoption agencies.

3. Explore with the client different options available to her and the possible consequence of each.

4. Encourage the client to attend classes to get her GED after the baby is born.

9-5. The nurse is applying principles of cognitive–behavioral therapy (CBT) in the treatment of a client with depression. Which of the following interventions is an example of CBT?

1. Rewarding the client with five tokens for attending group therapy

2. Encouraging the client to identify destructive thoughts and practice mindfulness

3. Fostering hope in the client by encouraging a focus on abilities rather than problems

4. Encouraging the client to review the past and focus on strengths and accomplishments

9-6. The nurse is leading a medication education group for clients who are taking an antidepressant medication. Which of the following goals is appropriate for this type of group?

1. Clients will identify common side effects of selective serotonin reuptake inhibitors.

2. Clients will recognize the common side effects of St. John's wort and SAMe.

3. Clients will understand the 12 steps of recovery from drug addiction.

4. Clients will identify one advantage and one disadvantage of electroconvulsive therapy.

9-7. The client has been nonresponsive to antidepressant medication and the treatment team has recommended transcranial magnetic stimulation (TMS). An hour after the psychiatrist explained the procedure the client asks, "What exactly does this procedure involve?" Which of the following explanations is correct?

1. "You will have tiny little electromagnets placed in your brain under a local anesthetic that will give off alternating electrical impulses. You will need to stay in the hospital overnight and go home the next day."

2. "After you are given a general anesthetic, the doctor will place an electrode on your temple and you will be given enough electrical current to cause a seizure. You will have 6 to 12 treatments, approximately 3 treatments per week."

3. "You will sit in a lounge chair and a small electromagnet will be placed on your scalp. There will be loud noises for approximately 1 minute so you'll need to wear earplugs. You will have 5 treatments over 2 to 4 weeks."

4. "After you are given a general anesthetic, you will have electrodes surgically implanted in your brain that will give off alternating electrical impulses that will feel like tingling sensations."

See Appendix D for answers.

References

American Nurses Association. (2001). *Scope and standards of nursing informatics practice*. Washington, DC: American Nurses Publishing.

American Psychiatric Association. (2001). Practice of electroconvulsive therapy: Recommendations for treatment, training, and privileging. *A task force report of the American Psychiatric Association* (2nd ed.). Washington, DC: Author.

American Psychiatric Nurses Association. (2005). Psychiatric–mental health nursing practice, APNA position papers. Retrieved August 20, 2005, from www.apna.org/resources/positionpapers/psychiatric

Anandan, S., Wigg, C. L., Thomas, C. R., & Coffey, B. (2004). Psychosurgery for self-injurious behavior in Tourette's disorder. *Journal of Child & Adolescent Psychopharmacology, 14*(4), 531–538.

Ball, J. W., & Bindler, R. C. (2006). *Child health nursing*. Upper Saddle River, NJ: Prentice Hall.

Ballinger, B., & Yalom, I. D. (1995). *The theory and practice of group psychotherapy* (4th ed.). New York: Basic Books.

Barnes, P., Powell-Griner, E., McFann, K., & Nahin, R. (2004). Complementary and alternative medicine use among adults: United States, 2002. *CDC Advance Data Report #343*. Washington, DC: U.S. Department of Health and Human Services.

Bierma, J. R. (2005a). Evidence-based remotivation. In J. A. Dyer & M. L. Stotts (Eds.), *Handbook of remotivation therapy* (pp. 43–54). New York: Haworth Clinical Practice Press.

Bierma, J. R. (2005b). The role of remotivation in abuse prevention, treatment and relapse prevention. In J. A. Dyer, & M. L. Stotts (Eds.), *Handbook of remotivation therapy* (pp. 147–156). New York: Haworth Clinical Practice Press.

Bower, F. L., McCullough, C. S., & Timmons, M. E. (2003). A synthesis of what we know about the use of physical restraints and seclusion with patients in psychiatric and acute care settings: 2003 update. *The Online Journal of Knowledge Synthesis for Nursing, 10*(1).

Breakey, W. R., & Dunn, G. J. (2004). Racial disparity in the use of ECT for affective disorders. *American Journal of Psychiatry, 161*(9), 1635–1641.

Carpenter, L. L., Friehs, G. M., Tyrka, A. R., Rasmussen, S., Price, L. H., & Greenberg, B. D. (2006). Vagus nerve stimulation and deep brain stimulation for treatment resistant depression. *Medicine and Health, Rhode Island, 89*(4), 140–141.

Chen, T. H., Lu, R. B., Chang, A. J., Chu, D. M., & Chou, K. R. (2006). The evaluation of cognitive–behavioral group therapy on patient depression and self-esteem. *Archives of Psychiatric Nursing, 20*(1), 3–11.

Cummings, J., & Cummings, E. (1962). *Ego and milieu*. New York: Atherton Press.

Denison, B. (2004). Touch the pain away: New research on Therapeutic Touch and persons with fibromyalgia syndrome. *Holistic Nursing Practice, 18*(3), 142–151.

Falloon, I. R. H. (2002). Cognitive–behavioral family and educational interventions for schizophrenic disorders. In S. G. Hofmann & M. C. Tompson (Eds.), *Treating chronic and severe mental disorders*. New York: Guilford Press.

Fisher, J. E. (2005). Mental health nurse practitioners in Australia. *International Journal of Mental Health Nursing, 14*(4), 222–229.

Fontaine, K. L. (2005). *Complementary & alternative therapies for nursing practice* (2nd ed.). Upper Saddle River, NJ: Prentice Hall.

Golden, R. N., Gaynes, B. N., Ekstrom, R. D., Hamer, R. M., Jacobsen, F. M., Suppes, T., et al. (2005). The efficacy of light therapy in the treatment of mood disorders. *American Journal of Psychiatry, 162*(4), 565–662.

Guido, G.W. (2006). *Legal and ethical issues in nursing*. Upper Saddle River, NJ: Prentice Hall.

Heitkemper, M. M., & Bond, E. F. (2004). Clinical nurse specialists: State of the profession and challenges ahead. *Clinical Nurse Specialist, 18*(3), 135–140.

Herlihy-Chevalier, B. (2005). What is remotivation therapy? In J. A. Dyer & M. L. Stotts (Eds.), *Handbook of remotivation therapy* (pp. 13–17). New York: Haworth Clinical Practice Press.

Hilliard, D. (1995). Massage for the seriously mentally ill. *Journal of Psychosocial Nursing, 33*(7), 29–30.

Hoffman, R. E., & Cavus, I. (2002). Slow transcranial magnetic stimulation, long-term depotentiation, and brain hyperexcitability disorders. *American Journal of Psychiatry, 159*(7), 1093–1102.

Houston, T. K., Cooper, L. A., & Ford, D. E. (2002). Internet support groups for depression. *American Journal of Psychiatry, 159*(12), 2062–2068.

Howland, R. H. (2005). Therapeutic brain stimulation for mental disorders. *Journal of Psychosocial Nursing, 43*(2), 16–19.

Hsieh, H. F., & Wang, J. J. (2003). Effect of reminiscence therapy on depression in older adults: A systematic review. *International Journal of Nursing Studies, 40*(4), 335–345.

Johann, M., Wiegand, R., Kharraz, A., Bobbe, G., Sommer, G., Hajak, G., et al. (2003). Transcranial magnetic stimulation for nicotine dependence. *Psychiatrische Praxis, Supplement 2,* 129–131.

Kessler, R. C., Walters, E. E., & Forthofer, M. S. (2001). The use of complementary and alternative therapies to treat anxiety and depression in the United States. *American Journal of Psychiatry, 158*(2), 289–294.

Kozuki, Y., Poupore, E., & Schepp, K. (2005). Visual feedback therapy to enhance medication adherence in psychosis. *Archives of Psychiatric Nursing, 19,* 70–80.

Kraft, A. (1966). The therapeutic community. In S. Arieti (Ed.), *American handbook of psychiatry* (Vol. 2). New York: Basic Books.

LaTorre, M. A. (2003). Aromatherapy and the use of scents in psychotherapy. *Perspectives in Psychiatric Care, 39*(1), 35–37.

Mashour, G. A., Walker, E. E., & Martuza, R. I. (2005). Psychosurgery: Past, present, and future. *Brain Research. Brain Research Reviews, 48*(3), 409–419.

McCabe, S. (2002). The nature of psychiatric nursing: The intersection of paradigm, evolution, and history. *Archives of Psychiatric Nursing, 16*(2), 51–60.

McDevitt, J., Snyder, M., Miller, A., & Wilbur, J. (2006). Perceptions of barriers and benefits to physical activity among outpatients in psychiatric rehabilitation. *Journal of Nursing Scholarship, 38*(1), 50–55.

Milstein, G. (2003). Clergy and psychiatrists: Opportunities for expert dialogue. *Psychiatric Times, 20*(3), 36–39.

Minarik, P. A., & Neese, J. B. (2002). Essential educational content for advanced practice in psychiatric consultation liaison nursing. *Archives of Psychiatric Nursing, 16*(1), 3–15.

Moller, M. D., & Rice, M. J. (2006). The BE SMART trauma reframing psychoeducation program. *Archives of Psychiatric Nursing, 20*(1), 21–31.

Moore, T. (2005). Best practice guidelines: An invitation to reflect on Therapeutic Touch practice. *Journal of Nursing Care Quality, 20*(1), 90–94.

Oren, D. A., Wisner, K. L., Spinelli, M., Epperson, C. N., Peindl, K. S., Terman, J. S., et al. (2002). An open trial of morning light therapy for treatment of antepartum depression. *American Journal of Psychiatry, 159*(4), 666–669.

Peplau, H. (1952). *Interpersonal relations in nursing.* New York: Putman.

Pull, C. B. (2006). Self-help Internet interventions for mental disorders. *Current Opinion in Psychiatry, 19*(1), 50–53.

Rose, D., Fleischmann, P., Wykes, T., Leese, M., & Bindman, J. (2003). Patients' perspectives on electroconvulsive therapy. *British Medical Journal, 326*(7403), 163.

Rossini, D., Magri, L., Lucca, A., Giodani, S., Smeraldi, E., & Zanardi, R. (2005). Does rTMS hasten the response to escitalopram, sertraline, or venlafaxine in patients with major depressive disorder? *Journal of Clinical Psychiatry, 66*(12), 1569–1575.

Ruck, C., Andrewitch, S., Flyckt, K., Edman, G., Nyman, H., Meyerson, B. A., et al. (2003). Capsulotomy for refractory anxiety disorders. *American Journal of Psychiatry I, 160*(3), 513–521.

Ruskin, P. E., Silver-Aylaian, M., Kling, M. A., Reed, S. A., Bradham, D. D., Hebel, J. R., et al. (2004). Treatment outcomes in depression: Comparison of remote treatment through telepsychiatry to in-person treatment. *American Journal of Psychiatry, 161*(8), 1471–1476.

Sanacora, G., Mason, G. F., Rothman, D. L., Hyder, F., Ciarcia, J. J., Ostroff, R. B., et al. (2003). Increased cortical GABA concentrations in depressed patients receiving ECT. *American Journal of Psychiatry, 160*(3), 577–579.

Sapolsky, R. M. (2003). Gene therapy for psychiatric disorders. *American Journal of Psychiatry, 160*(2), 208–220.

Schreiner, G. M., Crafton, C. G., & Sevin, J. A. (2004). Decreasing the use of mechanical restraints and locked seclusion. *Administration and Policy in Mental Health, 31*(6), 449–463.

Sensmeier, J., West, L., & Horowitz, J. K. (2004). Survey reveals role, compensation or nurse informaticists. *Computers, Informatics, Nursing, 22*(3), 178–182.

Sharrock, J., Grigg, M., Happell, B., Keeble-Devlin, B., & Jennings, S. (2006). The mental health nurse: A valuable addition to the consultation-liaison team. *International Journal of Mental Health Nursing, 15*(1), 35–43.

Stern, Y., & Sacheim, H. A. (2004). Neuropsychiatric aspects of memory and amnesia. In S. C. Yudofsky & R. E. Hales (Eds.), *Essentials of neuropsychiatry and clinical neurosciences* (pp. 201–238). Washington, DC: American Psychiatric Publishing.

Taylor, E. J. (2003). Prayer's clinical issues and implications. *Holistic Nursing Practice, 17*(4), 179–188.

Ussher, M., Sampuran, A. K., Doshi, R., West, R., & Drummond, D. C. (2004). Acute effect of a brief bout of exercise on alcohol urges. *Addiction, 99*(12), 1542–1547.

Voderholzer, U., Hohagen, F., Klein, T., Jungnickel, J., Kirschaum, C., Berger, M., et al. (2004). Impact of sleep deprivation and subsequent recovery sleep on cortisol in unmedicated depressed patients. *American Journal of Psychiatry, 161*(8), 1404–1410.

Wang, P. S., Lane, M., Olfson, M., Pincus, H. A., Wells, K. B., & Kessler, R. C. (2005). Twelve-month use of mental health services in the United States. *Archives of General Psychiatry, 62*(6), 590–592.

Woods, B., Spector, A., Jones, C., Orrell, M., & Davies, S. (2005). Reminiscence therapy for dementia. *The Cochrane Database of Systematic Reviews 2005, 2,* Art. No.: CD001120.pub2.DOI:10.1002/14651858.CD001120.pub2.

Wortans, J., Happell, B., & Johnstone, H. (2006). The role of the nurse practitioner in psychiatric/mental health nursing. *Journal of Psychiatric and Mental Health Nursing, 13*(1), 78–84.

Chapter 10

Illness Management: Medications

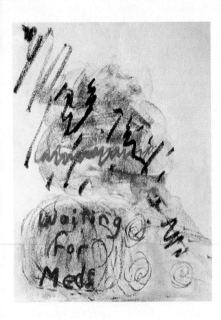

❝*Major source of irritability*❞

—Brian, Age 19

OBJECTIVES

After reading this chapter, you will be able to:

1. Outline the physiological and therapeutic effects of common psychotropic medications.

2. Outline frequently occurring side effects of common psychotropic medications.

3. Discuss toxicity and overdose with common psychotropic medications.

4. Discuss the use of psychotropic medications in special populations.

5. Develop medication teaching plans for a person with mental illness and her/his family.

MediaLink www.prenhall.com/fontaine

Go to the Pearson Health MediaLink CD-ROM and the Companion Website at www.prenhall.com/fontaine for interactive resources for this chapter.

More psychotropic medications are available these days than ever before. The good news is that there are more options and more people have found medications that work better and help them lead more fulfilling lives. However, more choices can complicate things. The challenge is to find the most effective medications and use them in ways that maximize client quality of life.

INTRODUCTORY CONCEPTS

Pharmacokinetics

The way the body handles medications, or what the body does to medications, is referred to as **pharmacokinetics**. This includes the absorption, distribution, metabolism, and excretion of medications. These processes determine the concentration of medications in the blood. *Absorption* refers to the way in which the medication passes from dose form to available molecules. The fastest rate of absorption is intravenous (IV), followed by intramuscular (IM), subcutaneous (SC), and oral. *Distribution* is the process by which the medication is transported to various sites in the body. Many psychiatric medications bind with transport proteins and only the unbound medications are active and capable of crossing the blood–brain barrier. Changes in the concentration of medication-binding proteins are very important to the effectiveness of medications.

The primary site of *metabolism* is the liver. Metabolism is critical to therapeutic blood levels and is affected by environmental and genetic factors. Environmental factors include stress, social support, personality styles, compliance, and prescribing patterns, all of which may influence the way individuals respond to medications. Genetic differences in the medication-metabolizing enzymes are responsible for ethnic variations in therapeutic response (Ruiz, 2000). Age and functional status of the liver also impact metabolism.

The *CYP* enzyme system (cytochrome P450) is the main pathway of medication metabolism. The three CYP enzymes of interest in psychiatry are *CYP2D6* (the enzyme that metabolizes most of the antipsychotic and antidepressant medications), *CYP2C19* (the enzyme that metabolizes benzodiazepines and some antidepressants), and *CYP3A4* (the enzyme that metabolizes mood stabilizers, benzodiazepines, calcium channel blockers, and antidepressants). There are significant genetic variations or mutations that inactivate, impair, or accelerate the function of these enzymes. The interaction of genetics and ethnicity is discussed later in this chapter. Other factors that affect the function of these enzymes include toxins, other medications, sex hormones, tobacco, alcohol, and caffeine. Depending on enzyme activity, some people are slow metabolizers of medications and have higher levels of medication in their blood, more severe side effects, and a potential for toxicity. Those who are superextensive metabolizers have very low medication levels in the blood with typical doses and may even be thought to be noncompliant with their medications. The nurse has a role in monitoring effectiveness of medications. It is important that the nurse consider the role of environmental factors, genetic factors, health status, and age in assessing objective and subjective responses (Ruiz, 2000).

Excretion of most medications is through the kidney, although some medications are secreted through bile, feces, skin evaporation, or lungs. The *half-life* of a medication is the time required for half of the medication to be eliminated. This is an important consideration in determining the proper amount and frequency of dose of the medication to be administered. The estimated half-life of medications is based on normal liver and kidney function. Medications with a short half-life are given in more frequent doses than are those with a long half-life.

Potency refers to the strength of a medication. It is the power to produce the desired effects per milligram of the medication. Medications that are low potency need higher doses to create the desired effect. High-potency medications have lower dosage levels and thus the dosage range provides information regarding potency.

Pharmacodynamics

Pharmacodynamics refers to medication action at the cellular level, or what the medication does to the body. Psychotropic medications act on cell receptors and turn postsynaptic cellular functions on or off. Medications act as either agonists or antagonists. As discussed in chapter 6 ∞, an agonist stimulates receptor actions and antagonists prevent cellular response.

Pharmacogenomics

The International HapMap Project is a multicountry effort to identify genes that affect health, disease, and individual responses to medications and environmental factors. It is hoped that this will enable the customization of medications to maximize effectiveness and minimize side effects, referred to as **pharmacogenomics**. Rather than the current trial-and-error method of figuring out which medications work best for a client, primary care providers will be able to examine each person's genomic information when making that determination. In addition, genome-based research will be critically important in the development of new medications for mental illness.

Discontinuation Syndrome

Most psychotropic medications should be discontinued over a period of weeks. When people abruptly stop taking these medications, they are likely to experience **discontinuation**

syndrome. They may experience flulike symptoms, gastrointestinal problems, headaches, fatigue, anxiety, insomnia, or restlessness. This may occur within hours after the last dose. While this is not a dangerous situation, it is uncomfortable and easily prevented (van Geffen, Hugtenburg, Heerdink, van Hulten, & Egberts, 2006).

Smoking, Alcohol, Hydration, and Nutrition

It is important to assess clients for any usual habits that may influence the effectiveness of their medications. *Smoking* has a direct impact on liver enzymes, blood flow, and nicotine receptors in the central nervous system. Smoking increases the rate of metabolism of antidepressants and antianxiety agents, contributing to a need for higher doses. The combination of nicotine and antipsychotics puts the individual at higher risk for tardive dyskinesia. Nicotine decreases the therapeutic effect of propranolol (Inderal). Cocaine causes vasoconstriction, which is further enhanced by the use of nicotine (Turkoski, Lance, & Bonfiglio, 2004).

Excessive *alcohol* affects liver and kidney function, affecting metabolism and excretion of medications. Alcohol also has an additive effect with medications that depress the central nervous system.

Poor *hydration* lessens blood flow to the kidney, decreasing the excretion rate. Poor *nutrition* may result in less protein available for binding medications. A recent discovery finds that *grapefruit* may cause potentially serious interactions when taken with a number of medications. A compound specific to grapefruit has the ability to block CYP3A4, which metabolizes medications, resulting in increased blood levels of medications such as nefazodone (Serzone) and alprazolam (Xanax) and the calcium channel blockers used to stabilize mood.

Disease states can change all aspects of pharmacokinetics. For example, cirrhosis impairs enzyme metabolism of medications, as does abnormal thyroid function. Circulatory problems affect absorption, distribution, and excretion, and kidney disease decreases excretion of medications (Turkoski et al., 2004).

Off-label Use

Many medications on the market have not been officially approved by the Food and Drug Administration (FDA) for a variety of disorders. For example, some antidepressants (FDA approved for depression) are used to treat some of the anxiety disorders (off-label use). For some medications, the off-label use is supported by data from studies, whereas in other situations off-label use is supported by anecdotal reports. As more is learned about neuropsychiatry, there will be a better understanding of how a variety of medications are effective in a number of disorders.

PSYCHOTROPIC MEDICATIONS

Psychotropic medications affect cognitive function, emotions, and behavior. They are categorized into classes: antipsychotic, antidepressant, mood-stabilizing, antianxiety, and stimulant medications. They may be used alone (monotherapy) or in combination with one another (polytherapy). The increased frequency of comorbid disorders, more severe symptoms, and availability of a growing number of medications have contributed to a steady increase in the use of polytherapy. Polytherapy is a controversial issue at the present time. Those who prescribe a combination of psychotropic medications believe that they are better tolerated and safer when used in combination, especially for clients with chronic or severe disease. Those who are opposed to polytherapy believe that there are increased side effects with often no apparent gain in clinical benefit. Current studies address safety concerns but do not address efficacy concerns (Centorrino et al., 2005; Janssen, Weinmann, Berger, & Gaebel, 2004; Preskorn, 2006).

ANTIPSYCHOTIC MEDICATIONS

Physiological Effects

Symptoms of severe mental illness are classified as positive and negative. To make sense of this, it is important to understand that positive does not mean good and negative does not mean bad. Rather, positive symptoms are added behaviors not normally seen in mentally healthy adults, such as hallucinations, delusions, or loose associations. Positive symptoms are thought to result from an excess of dopamine (DA) or from hypersensitive DA receptors and are usually responsive to medication. Negative symptoms are the absence of behaviors normally seen in mentally healthy adults, such as social withdrawal, minimal self-care, concrete thinking, and flat affect. (See chapter 14 ∞ for further description of positive and negative symptoms in schizophrenia.) Until recently, negative symptoms have been less responsive to treatment with antipsychotic medications. First-generation antipsychotic medications act by blocking the overreactive DA receptors or by decreasing the amount of available DA. The second-generation medications also block serotonin (5-HT) receptors (Love & Conley, 2004).

Therapeutic Effects

The therapeutic purpose of antipsychotic medications is to decrease as many of the psychotic symptoms as possible. This action allows clients to assume more control over their lives. With reduced symptoms, they can participate more effectively in other forms of treatment.

Initially, clients take or receive their medication in divided doses, two to four times a day, which decreases the occurrence of side effects. It may take 2 to 4 weeks before the client shows a significant response to the medication. Many clients, however, show a significant degree of improvement in the first few days. Once the client's symptoms are under control, the dosage may be changed to once a day. Once maintenance on a particular medication is established, the client is kept on the lowest possible dosage (Kapur et al., 2005).

First-Generation Antipsychotics

It may take 2 to 4 weeks to see clinical improvement from first-generation antipsychotic medications. Although there is no evidence to suggest the superiority of any one first-generation antipsychotic agent, some people respond better to one medication than another. Choosing which medication to use with individual clients also depends on its side effects. For example, one client may respond well to haloperidol (Haldol) but have dangerous episodes of hypotension, while another client may do well with haloperidol with little or no side effects. Approximately 15% to 25% of clients with schiz-

ophrenia experience little clinical improvement with antipsychotic medication. Treatment-resistant schizophrenia remains highly symptomatic and requires extensive periods of hospitalization. Half the people will experience one or more side effects and, in response, many will discontinue their medication (Schooler et al., 2005). See Table 10.1 ■ for a list of first-generation antipsychotics.

Second-Generation Antipsychotics

In September 2005 the first results from the Clinical Antipsychotic Trials of Intervention Effectiveness (CATIE) surprised both health care providers and clients. Prior to this study it was thought that second-generation medications were more effective, had fewer side effects, and were thought to be the medication of choice for clients experiencing their first episode of schizophrenia. The CATIE study compared perphenazine (Trilafon), a first-generation antipsychotic, with olanzapine (Zyprexa), quetiapine (Seroquel), risperidone (Risperdal), and ziprasidone (Geodon)—all second-generation antipsychotics. Of the medications used, olanzapine appeared to work best in terms of controlling symptoms; however, it also produced the highest rate

TABLE 10.1	Antipsychotic Medications		
Class	**Generic Name**	**Trade Name**	**Adult Dosage (mg/day)**
Second-generation antipsychotics	Aripiprazole	Abilify	10–25
	Clozapine	Clozaril	300–900
	Olanzapine	Zyprexa	5–20
	Olanzapine/fluoxetine	Symbyax	6/25–12/50
	Quetiapine	Seroquel	150–750
	Risperidone	Risperdal	4–16
	Sertindole	Serlect	12–24
	Ziprasidone	Geodon	40–160
Phenothiazines	Acetophenazine	Tindal	40–120
	Chlorpromazine	Thorazine	30–800
	Fluphenazine	Prolixin, Permitil	1–40
	Mesoridazine	Serentil	75–300
	Perphenazine	Trilafon	8–64
	Thioridazine	Mellaril	150–800
	Trifluoperazine	Stelazine, Suprazine	15–20
	Triflupromazine	Vesprin	60–150
Thioxanthenes	Chlorprothixene	Taractan	75–600
	Thiothixene	Navane	6–120
Butyrophenones	Haloperidol	Haldol	1–50
Dibenzoxazepine	Loxapine	Loxitane	10–160
Dihydroindolone	Molindone	Moban	15–225
	Diphenylbatylperidine Pimozide	Orap	1–10

of side effects. In spite of the side effect profile, fewer participants stopped or switched their medications because they thought the better control of symptoms was more important than the weight gain (Lieberman et al., 2005).

Clients in their first episode of schizophrenia are more responsive to the therapeutic effects of medications and are more susceptible to side effects compared to later stages of the disorder. Most clients in their first episode respond equally well to first- or second-generation antipsychotics (Lieberman et al., 2005). Doses should be 50% lower than in people who have chronic schizophrenia.

The determination of which medication to use is often made on the basis of an individuals side effect profile, which is determined by medication history. If an individual has a history of EPS side effects, she or he would most likely be prescribed a second-generation antipsychotic. If an individual is prone to weight gain and high blood lipid levels, she or he would most likely be prescribed a first-generation antipsychotic.

Risperidone (Risperdal) and olanzapine (Zyprexa) are effective for persons with oppositional defiant disorder, conduct disorder, and rage disorder, though these are off-label uses. The FDA has approved olanzapine (Zyprexa) and aripiprazole (Abilify) for the short-term treatment of acute manic episodes associated with bipolar disorder.

Ziprasidone (Geodon) and aripiprazole (Abilify) are second-generation antipsychotics for which an oral and a rapid-acting intramuscular form have been developed. The IM form is used for the control and short-term management of clients who are acutely psychotic and agitated. Effect is apparent within 1 hour after injection without being profoundly sedating. Ziprasidone is also effective for decreasing the anger associated with bipolar disorder. It may be used to treat social withdrawal for persons with autistic disorder or Asperger syndrome. Olanzapine and fluoxetine (Symbax) is a combination antipsychotic/antidepressant medication for the treatment of depressive episodes associated with bipolar disorder. (See Table 10.1 for a list of second-generation antipsychotics.)

Side Effects
First-Generation Antipsychotics

First-generation antipsychotic medications provide relief from the symptoms of severe mental illness for many people, but side effects are common. Some are bothersome (e.g., dry mouth), some affect movement (e.g., akathisia), some are disfiguring (e.g., tardive dyskinesia), some are frightening (e.g., dystonia), and others are dangerous (e.g., neuroleptic malignant syndrome). These adverse effects interfere with function, reduce the quality of life, and contribute to clients' stopping their medication. The most common side effects of first-generation antipsychotic medications include anti-

cholinergic effects, photosensitivity, weight gain, sexual difficulties, and extrapyramidal side effects.

Anticholinergic side effects occur when the medication blocks the acetylcholine receptors, resulting in the inhibition of the transmission of parasympathetic nerve impulses. These side effects are more bothersome than anything else and include dry mouth, blurry vision, trouble urinating, constipation, memory difficulties, and confusion.

Photosensitivity is the increased sensitivity of the skin to sunlight. Relatively brief exposure to sunlight may cause edema, rashes, or severe burns. Instruct clients to wear protective clothing and use high-potency sunscreen to avoid this complication.

The amount of *weight gain* varies by medication because of how the various neurotransmitters differ in degree of action. The degree of weight gain also increases with length of time of administration. It is believed that the weight gain is associated with a medication-induced rise in the level of leptin, a hormone involved in weight regulation. Weight gain may cause clients to discontinue their medications, which may predispose them to relapse. The medications with the highest weight gain are thioridazine (Mellaril) and chlorpromazine (Thorazine).

Interference with *sexual function* is very common. Some side effects are direct; that is, they are the result of chemical action of the medication. These include decreased sex drive, erection difficulties, ejaculation irregularities, and decreased ability to achieve orgasm. Indirect sexual side effects are related to other side effects such as anticholinergic effects, sedation, changes in energy, weight gain, or body image. Therefore, individuals may avoid sexual interaction because of fatigue, dry mucous membranes, indigestion, dizziness, tremors, or self-image. Sexual side effects are one of the most important factors influencing medication compliance. It is important that nurses integrate sexual health questions in their ongoing assessment of clients (Higgins, Barker, & Begley, 2005).

Smooth body movements and body posture depend on a critical ratio of DA to acetylcholine (ACh) in the brain. When medications block DA receptors, they lower this ratio, and **extrapyramidal side effects (EPSs)** occur in about 35% of clients. EPSs include akinesia, akathisia, parkinsonism, dystonia, oculogyric crisis, and tardive dyskinesia. **Akinesia** is muscular weakness or a partial loss of muscular movement. **Akathisia** is the inability to sit or stand still, along with an intense feeling of anxiety. This side effect usually begins within the first 60 days of treatment and persists as long as the client is taking medication. It is extremely distressing to people and is a frequent cause of medication nonadherence. Akathisia is less responsive to treatment than parkinsonism and dystonia. Medications to counteract akathisia are propranolol (Inderal), diphenhydramine (Benadryl), and benztropine (Cogentin) (Janno, Holi, Tuisku, & Wahlbeck, 2004).

Parkinsonism is evidenced in clients' stooped posture and shuffling gait. Their faces resemble masks, and they may drool. They experience tremors and pill-rolling motions of the thumb and fingers at rest. This reaction is likely to begin within the first 30 days of treatment and occurs throughout the use of the medication.

Dystonia has an abrupt onset, with frightening muscle spasms in the head and neck. *Oculogyric crisis* and *laryngospasm* are terms used to describe acute dystonic reactions in specific body regions. In oculogyric crisis, the person's eyes roll up and sideways and are held in a fixed position for minutes or several hours. In laryngospasm, there is a spasmodic closure of the larynx. These reactions usually occur within the first 5 days of therapy or when dose is significantly increased. Episodes are more likely to occur during the afternoon and evening than during the night and morning. Treatment is IM benztropine (Cogentin) or IM diphenhydramine (Benadryl).

Tardive dyskinesia, a form of EPS, occurs in 20% to 46% of clients who take first-generation antipsychotic medications for more than 2 years. Females and older people are at higher risk for tardive dyskinesia. The symptoms of strange face and body movement make it very difficult for others to interact with them. Symptoms include frowning, blinking, grimacing, puckering, blowing, smacking, licking, chewing, tongue protrusion, and spastic facial distortions. Abnormal movements of the arms and legs include rapid, purposeless, irregular movements; tremors; and foot tapping. Body symptoms include dramatic movements of the neck and shoulders and rocking, twisting pelvic gyrations, and thrusts. If severe, other people may be so distracted by the abnormal body movements that interactions become almost impossible. Because tardive dyskinesia is often irreversible, the goal is prevention. If symptoms begin to appear, the medication is reduced or the person is switched to a newer antipsychotic medication (Janno et al., 2004).

Neuroleptic malignant syndrome (NMS) is a potentially fatal side effect related to sympathetic nervous system hyperactivity. It affects 1% to 2% of clients who take first-generation antipsychotic medication. The risk is higher when clients are taking two or more of these medications or suffering from organic brain disease. Symptoms of NMS develop suddenly and include muscle rigidity and respiratory problems. Hyperpyrexia ranges from 101°F to 107°F (38°C to 41.6°C). During the next 2 to 3 days, tachycardia, hypertension, respiratory problems, diaphoresis, urinary incontinence, confusion, and/or delirium develops. The mortality rate with NMS is 14% to 30%; it is estimated that 1,000 to 4,000 people die every year. There is no specific treatment for NMS other than discontinuation of the medication and supportive measures in the intensive care setting. Bromocriptine (Parlodel) may be of some help in halting the DA blockage. Muscle relaxants such as dantrolene (Dantrium) may lessen the rigidity (Gill, Singh, & Nugent, 2003).

Recently, concerns have been raised about antipsychotic medications associated with *QT prolongation* in cardiac conduction. QT prolongation may be associated with palpitations, dizziness, and lightheadedness. In some cases, it may progress to ventricular fibrillation and sudden death. Females are at higher risk because they have normally longer QT intervals. Risk for the elderly is higher due to an increased risk for coronary disease and the use of multiple medications. The antipsychotics with the most risk include thioridazine (Mellaril) and mesoridazine (Serentil). Ziprasidone (Geodon) prolongs the QT interval, but there is no evidence that this leads to sudden death (Turkoski et al., 2004).

Because of the side effects, many people do not like the way their bodies feel when taking first-generation antipsychotic medication. Identifying and managing side effects may help people stay on the medication and maintain a higher level of functioning, thus avoiding acute hospitalization. Some people will stop taking their medication and relapse, while others relapse first and, as a result of their symptoms, stop taking their medication.

Second-Generation Antipsychotics

Among the second-generation antipsychotics, clozapine (Clozaril) has the most significant side effect in that agranulocytosis develops in about 0.5% of those taking this medication. This carries a 40% fatality rate, usually from an overwhelming infection. Monitoring white blood counts (WBCs) weekly for the first 6 months, then every other week for a year, and then once a month is required to administer this medication safely. It is desirable that the WBCs stay above 3,500 cells/cm (Reuters Health Information, 2003).

Because there is less DA receptor action, second-generation antipsychotic agents have fewer EPSs, making them more tolerable to clients. Other side effects of these antipsychotic medications include sedation, hypersalivation, nervousness, headache, and dizziness. Neuroleptic malignant syndrome is less likely but is a possibility.

Weight gain is more of a problem with second-generation medications than with the first-generation antipsychotic agents. Medications that cause the most weight gain are clozapine (Clozaril) and olanzapine (Zyprexa). Sertindole (Serlect), quetiapine (Seroquel), and risperidone (Risperdal) cause a moderate weight gain while ziprasidone (Geodon) and aripiprazole (Abilify) cause little or no weight gain. Between 50% and 80% of clients gain weight, ranging from a few pounds to more than 20% of their baseline weight. As weight increases, so does the risk for coronary heart disease, osteoarthritis, hypertension, and gallbladder disease. Medication-induced weight gain prompts some people to discontinue their medications. Treating the obesity problem with sibutramine (Meridia), an FDA-approved appetite suppressant, along with behavior modification, has resulted in weight loss for clients. Amantadine (Symmetrel), used for the treatment of EPSs, shows some promise in stabilizing the weight gain associated with antipsychotics (Graham, Gu, Lieberman, Harp, & Perkins, 2005: Henderson et al., 2005).

Metabolic syndrome related to second-generation antipsychotics include (Citrome, Blonde, & Damatarca, 2005):

- Abdominal obesity defined as waist measurement in men greater than 40 in. (102 cm) and greater than 35 in. (88 cm) in women
- Triglyceride level of 150 mg/dL or greater
- High-density lipoprotein (HDL) cholesterol level less than 40 mg/dL for men and less than 50 mg/dL for women
- Blood pressure of 130/85 mm Hg or higher
- Fasting glucose of 100 mg/dL or higher

Obesity is the risk factor for the development of *type 2 diabetes* or worsening of preexisting diabetes and an increase in triglyceride and cholesterol levels. Those medications with the highest weight gain have the highest metabolic side effects. All of these side effects are associated with higher morbidity and mortality because of cardiovascular disease. An infrequent, but very serious, side effect is *diabetic ketoacidosis*. This is a medical emergency that involves the rapid onset of symptoms and alteration in cognition and level of consciousness.

Clients taking second-generation antipsychotics should undergo baseline screening and ongoing monitoring. This includes a personal and family history of obesity, diabetes, hypertension, and any cardiovascular diseases. Body mass index should be calculated at baseline and monthly until week 12, and every 3 months thereafter. An increase in 5% or more from baseline weight should be an indication to consider changing to a different medication. Fasting plasma glucose and fasting lipid profile should be done at baseline, after 12 weeks, and then annually (Rettenbacher, 2005).

Another rare but significant side effect is *priapism*. Priapism is a prolonged and painful penile erection not associated with sexual arousal. It is a urologic emergency that necessitates prompt intervention to prevent permanent damage to the penis. The agents most likely to be associated with priapism are clozapine (Clozaril), risperidone (Risperdal), and olanzapine (Zyprexa) (Reeves & Mack, 2002).

Toxicity and Overdose

The primary symptom of overdose is central nervous system (CNS) depression, which may extend to the point of coma. Other symptoms include agitation and restlessness, seizures, fever, EPSs, arrhythmias, and hypotension. Caring for a client who has overdosed includes monitoring vital signs, especially cardiac function; maintaining a patent airway; and gastric lavage. Antiparkinsonian medications may be given for EPSs. Diazepam (Valium) may be given for seizures.

Administration

Administration of antipsychotic medications is oral, in liquid or pill form, or by injection. Long-acting injectable medications such as fluphenazine (Prolixin Decanoate), haloperidol (Haldol Decanoate), and risperidone (Risperdal), are often used to treat clients with schizophrenia. These medications are administered IM once every 2 to 6 weeks, a helpful regimen for clients who have difficulty remembering to take medications daily.

ADJUNCTIVE MEDICATIONS FOR EPS

A number of medications may be used to lessen the EPS effects of first-generation antipsychotics. Some reduce ACh, thereby restoring the DA:ACh ratio (see Table 10.2 ■ for a list of these medications). Amantadine (Symmetrel) is an antiviral medication that also works as an antidyskinetic by stimulating the release of DA.

Anticholinergic agents should be used with caution in people who have difficulty urinating or an enlarged prostate; glaucoma; myasthenia gravis; or cardiovascular, kidney, or liver disease. Side effects include blurry vision, dizziness, orthostatic hypotension, and drowsiness. Clients may find sunglasses are necessary if their eyes become more sensitive to light. Decreased sweating may result in a rise in body temperature. Symptoms of overdose include unsteadiness; seizures; severe drowsiness; severe dryness of the mouth, nose, and throat; tachycardia; shortness of breath; hallucinations; and coma.

ANTIDEPRESSANT MEDICATIONS

Physiological Effects

The neurotransmitters involved in depression are DA, 5-HT, norepinephrine (NE), and ACh. It is believed that during a depressive episode, there is a functional deficiency of these neurotransmitters or hyposensitive receptors. Antidepressant medications increase the amount of available neurotransmitters by inhibiting neurotransmitter reuptake, by inhibiting monoamine oxidase (MAO), by blocking certain receptors, or by modulating the effect of neurotransmitters.

TABLE 10.2	Adjunctive Medications for EPSs		
Class	**Generic Name**	**Trade Name**	**Adult Dosage (mg/day)**
Anticholinergic	Amantadine	Symmetrel	100–300
	Benztropine	Cogentin	1–6
	Biperiden	Akineton	2–8
	Diphenhydramine	Benadryl	50–300
	Ethopropazine	Parsidol	50–200
	Orphenadrine	Disipal, Norflex	50–300
	Procyclidine	Kemadrin	5–30
	Trihexyphenidyl	Artane	6–10
Specialized agents	Bromocriptine	Parlodel	5–50
	Dantrolene	Dantrium	60–600
	Propranolol	Inderal	30–120
	Pindolol	Visken	10–60

Therapeutic Effects

Antidepressant medications can be classified as older generation agents—the tricyclics, tetracyclics, and MAO inhibitors (MAOIs)—and the new-generation agents—the selective dopamine–norepinephrine reuptake inhibitors (DNRIs), selective serotonin reuptake inhibitors (SSRIs), the serotonin–norepinephrine reuptake inhibitors (SNRIs), the serotonin modulators, and the norepinephrine–serotonin modulators. The new-generation medications have dramatically changed the treatment of depression, with more effective action and fewer side effects.

Because depression is heterogeneous in terms of which neurotransmitters are depleted, different people respond differently to various antidepressants. At times, a period of trial and error is necessary to determine which medication is most effective. The therapeutic purpose of antidepressants is to decrease as many depressive symptoms as possible, thereby enabling clients to participate more effectively in other forms of treatment. Maintenance continues until clients are free of symptoms for 4 months to 1 year. Then the medications are slowly discontinued.

Antidepressants do not cause dependence, tolerance, addiction, or withdrawal. It takes an average of 10 to 14 days for the beginning effect of most antidepressants, and the full effect may not be apparent for 2 to 4 weeks. Some of the newer antidepressants such as duloxetine (Cymbalta) may show an effect as soon as 1 week. Approximately 30% of clients do not respond after a trial of 4 to 6 weeks. At that point, the health care provider may try a different antidepressant or augment with other medications.

Selegiline (Eldepryl), a patch-delivered MAOI, shows dramatic improvement within 1 week. The quick results are seen because patches send medications on a direct route to the blood and the brain, while pills are diluted as they pass through the liver. (See Table 10.3 ■ for a list of antidepressant medications.)

Suicide rates related to depression have dropped in association with increased use of SSRIs and new-generation non-SSRIs, according to the results of an analysis of a U.S. Centers for Disease Control and Prevention (CDC) national study. There was no decrease in the suicide rates for people who were prescribed tricyclic antidepressants. It has been found, however, that some clients have an increase in suicidal behavior when taking newer generation antidepressants (Gibbons, Hur, Bhaumik, & Mann, 2005).

A significant number of clients improve when 600 mg of lithium is added to the antidepressant treatment. Other clients improve when triiodothyronine (T_3) is administered daily. For clients who are delusional or severely agitated, antipsychotic medication may be indicated.

Bupropion (Zyban) is used in smoking cessation programs. It is thought that DA counters the craving associated with nicotine withdrawal. Fluoxetine (Sarafem) is the same medication as Prozac and has been FDA approved for the treatment of premenstrual dysphoric disorder. Studies show that women's moods improved and they had fewer physical complaints. Sertraline (Zoloft) is the first medication to receive FDA approval for the treatment of posttraumatic stress disorder. It is also used for panic disorder and obsessive–compulsive disorder.

Side Effects

Anticholinergic side effects occur when the medication blocks the ACh receptors, resulting in the inhibition of the transmission of parasympathetic nerve impulses. These side

TABLE 10.3	Antidepressant Medications		
Class	**Generic Name**	**Trade Name**	**Adult Dosage (mg/day)**
Dopamine–norepinephrine reuptake inhibitor (DNRI)	Bupropion	Wellbutrin, Zyban Wellbutrin XL	100–450
Selective serotonin reuptake inhibitor (SSRI)	Citalopram	Celexa	20–60
	Escitalopram	Lexapro	10–20
	Fluoxetine	Prozac, Sarafem	20–80
	Fluvoxamine	Luvox	50–300
	Paroxetine	Paxil, Paxil CR	20–50
	Sertraline	Zoloft	50–200
Serotonin–norepinephrine inhibitor (SNRI)	Venlafaxine	Effexor, Effexor XR	75–225
Serotonin modulators	Trazodone	Desyrel	50–400
Norepinephrine–serotonin modulator	Mirtazapine	Remeron	15–45
	Duloxetine	Cymbalta	40–60
Tricyclic	Amitriptyline	Elavil, Endep	50–300
	Clomipramine	Anafranil	75–250
	Desipramine	Norpramin, Pertofrane	50–300
	Doxepin	Adapin, Sinequan	50–300
	Imipramine	Tofranil	50–300
	Nortriptyline	Aventyl, Pamelor	40–150
	Protriptyline	Vivactil	10–60
	Trimipramine	Surmontil	50–300
Tetracyclic	Amoxapine	Asendin	75–300
	Maprotiline	Ludiomil	50–225
MAOI	Isocarboxazid	Marplan	20–60
	Phenelzine	Nardil	45–90
	Tranylcypromine	Parnate	30–90
	Selegiline	Eldepryl	Patch 20

effects are more bothersome than dangerous and include dry mouth, blurry vision, trouble urinating, constipation, memory difficulties, and confusion. The SSRIs, SDNIs, SNRIs, and the modulators have fewer anticholinergic effects. There are additional problems with the anticholinergic properties of these medications for the older person. If the client has dentures, an extremely dry mouth can lead to gingival erosion. If the older male client has prostatic enlargement, the anticholinergic effect of urinary retention can cause very serious problems. Anticholinergic properties can also intensify unsuspected glaucoma, resulting in increased intraocular pressure. Antidepressant medications may also cause orthostatic hypotension, resulting in a higher risk for dizzy spells and falls. Relatively brief exposure to sunlight may cause edema, rashes, or severe burns. Clients need to be cautioned to wear protective clothing and use high-potency sunscreen to avoid this side effect.

Some of the most common, troublesome, and most frequently overlooked side effects are *sexual difficulties.* Bupropion (Wellbutrin) is the medication of choice in terms of sexual side effects as it causes virtually no sexual problems. For people taking SSRIs, the rate of sexual dysfunction ranges from 58% to 73%. Men and women may experience desire disorders. Women may have orgasmic problems and decreased lubrication. Men may have difficulty with erections, inhibited ejaculation, and decreased ejaculatory volume. Sexual problems may be a major factor, leading to noncompliance with antidepressant medication. Making decisions about medication choice or change often leaves the client facing important quality-of-life issues. If the medication is effective but has sexual side effects, should the client risk changing medications? Is the client's partner more disturbed than the client about the sexual side effects? SSRIs have been used to treat rapid ejaculation, but the value may be complicated by decreased desire. Men who experience erectile difficulties may find that sildenafil (Viagra) helps them stay on the antidepressant medication (Seagraves & Balon, 2003).

Weight gain is a significant problem with these medications and can contribute to poor body image and avoidance of sexual activity. Fluoxetine (Prozac) is associated with modest weight loss during treatment. Medications with the least weight gain (0 to 10 lb) are desipramine (Norpramin) and nortriptyline (Pamelor). Those with the greatest weight gain (5 to 40 lb) include amitriptyline (Elavil), doxepin (Adapin and Sinequan), and clomipramine (Anafranil).

MAOIs decrease the amount of monoamine oxidase in the liver, which breaks down the essential amino acids tyramine and tryptophan. If a person eats food rich in these substances while taking an MAOI, he or she risks a *hypertensive crisis.* The first sign of a hypertensive crisis is a sudden and severe headache, followed by neck stiffness, nausea, vomiting, sweating, and tachycardia. Death can result from circulatory collapse or intracranial bleeding. Due to these interactions, MAOIs are used in treatment-resistant depression only. Box 10.1 lists the foods and medications clients must avoid while taking an MAOI. Because of the unique properties of selegiline (Eldepryl), food interactions are not a problem and there are no dietary restrictions. Individuals may experience some skin irritation from the patch.

The SSRIs and SNRIs increase the availability of 5-HT, which relieves depression but can also cause the hyperserotonergic state known as the **serotonin syndrome (SS)**. This syndrome is more likely to occur when these agents are used in combination with MAOIs, lithium, St. John's wort, and triptans—the class of medications used to treat migraines. Serotonin syndrome develops very quickly and is characterized by:

- Mental changes such as agitation, confusion, or hypomania
- Altered muscle tone such as hyperreflexia, rigidity, twitching, or tremor
- Autonomic changes such as hyper- or hypotension, tachycardia, or diaphoresis
- CNS changes such as discoordination, coma, or seizures
- Hyperthermia with temperatures as high as 101°F to 107°F (30°C to 41.6°C)

Treatment of SS is supportive, which includes controlling hyperthermia with antipyretics and cooling devices. Muscle rigidity and twitching can be treated with clonazepam (Klonopin), benztropine (Cogentin), and lorazepam (Ativan). Anticonvulsants are used for seizures secondary to serotonin syndrome (Turkoski et al., 2004).

Toxicity and Overdose

Symptoms of toxicity include confusion, disturbed concentration, agitation, irritability, hallucinations, seizures, dilated pupils, delirium, hypotension or hypertension, hyperactive reflexes, tachycardia, arrhythmia, respiratory depression, coma, kidney failure, and cardiac arrest. Caring for a client who has overdosed includes monitoring vital signs, especially cardiac function, and maintaining a patent airway. Vomiting is induced if the client is alert, while gastric lavage is initiated for the client who is stuporous. Following this procedure, activated charcoal may be administered to minimize absorption. Physostigmine (Antilirium) 1 to 3 mg may be given IV to counteract the toxic effects. Diazepam (Valium) may be administered for seizures and vasopressors or lidocaine for cardiovascular effects (Turkoski et al., 2004).

If MAOIs and other antidepressants are administered together, serious reactions may occur. Symptoms include hyperthermia, severe agitation, delirium, and coma. Between 2 and 5 weeks should elapse between the use of MAOIs and other antidepressants.

Administration

Administration of antidepressant medications is primarily oral. It usually takes 2 to 4 weeks to reach therapeutic levels, at which point the client is able to notice a reduction in symptoms. Other people may actually see changes in energy and mood before the client experiences an improvement. It is important to educate clients about this fact so that they do not become frustrated and stop taking the medication before it becomes effective.

BOX 10.1	Foods to Avoid With MAOIs

Absolutely Restricted

- Aged cheeses
- Aged and cured meats
- Dried or pickled fish
- Liver
- Flavor cubes or meat extracts
- Bananas
- Broad bean pods
- Sauerkraut
- Soy sauce and other soy condiments
- Draft beer
- Vitamins with Brewer's yeast

Consume in Moderation

- Red or white wine (no more than two 4-oz glasses per day)
- Bottled or canned beer, including nonalcoholic (no more than two 12-oz servings per day)
- Chocolate
- Yogurt (4 ounces per day)

SOURCE: Adapted with permission from Roach, S. S., & Scherer, J. C. (2000). *Clinical pharmacology* (6th ed.). Philadelphia, PA: Lippincott Williams & Wilkins.

Selegiline (Eldepryl) is the only antidepressant in a skin patch. It is not known whether all antidepressants can be administered through a patch-delivery system. Individuals who are stabilized on 20 mg daily of fluoxetine (Prozac) may consider Prozac Weekly, the first once-a-week medication for depression.

MOOD-STABILIZING MEDICATIONS

Physiological Effects

The mood stabilizers include a small group of diverse medications that are useful in stabilizing clients' affect. The FDA does not officially recognize the term *mood stabilizers*. Most professionals consider a medication to be a mood stabilizer if it is effective in:

- Treating manic symptoms
- Treating acute depressive symptoms
- Preventing manic symptoms
- Preventing depressive symptoms

Lithium is the best known and most often prescribed mood stabilizer. In recent years, several anticonvulsant medications have been added to this category: carbamazepine (Tegretol), valproate (Depakene and Depakon), divalproex (Depakote), and clonazepam (Klonopin). Calcium channel blockers (verapamil [Calan and Isoptin]) are increasingly being used with success in manic disorders either alone or in combination with other mood stabilizers. Antihypertensives (clonidine [Catapres] and guanfacine [Tenex]) help in controlling rage attacks. Table 10.4 ■ lists the mood-stabilizing medications.

Lithium

Lithium potentiates the therapeutic effects of antidepressants. In the body, lithium substitutes for sodium, calcium, potassium, and magnesium. Clients experiencing an acute manic episode have been found to have increased levels of intracellular calcium, which decrease when lithium is administered. It also interacts with DA, NE, and 5-HT. Lithium affects a complex biological system called the phosphatidyl inositol cycle inside many cells. This cycle is referred to as a *second messenger* system that relays and amplifies signals. It is thought that this system may be overactive in mania and depression, and lithium serves to inhibit the activity of this pathway. Approxi-

TABLE 10.4	Mood-Stabilizing Medications		
Class	**Generic Name**	**Trade Name**	**Adult Dosage (mg/day)**
Antimanic	Lithium carbonate	Eskalith, Lithane, Lithobid	900–2,400; acute
			300–1,200; maintenance
	Lithium citrate	Cibalith-S	900–2,400; acute
			300–1,200; maintenance
Anticonvulsants			
	Carbamazepine	Tegretol	200–1,400
	Clonazepam	Klonopin	1.5–20
	Gabapentin	Neurontin	900–1,800
	Lamotrigine	Lamictal	100–500
	Levetiracetam	Keppra	
	Tiagabine	Gabitril	32
	Topiramate	Topamax	100–400
	Valproate/divalproex	Depakene, Depacon, Depakote	750–1,000
	Zonisamide	Zonegran	
Calcium Channel Blockers			
	Isradipine	DynaCirc	5
	Nimodipine	Nimotop	90–360
	Verapamil	Calan, Isoptin	120–480
Antihypertensives			
	Clonidine	Catapres	0.1–0.6
	Guanfacine	Tenex	1–3

mately 70% to 80% of clients experiencing mania respond to lithium treatment. This medication should never be abruptly discontinued. To prevent clinical relapse, lithium is gradually tapered off over a minimum of 14 days (Geddes, Burgess, Hawton, Jamison, & Goodwin, 2004; Gill et al., 2003).

Anticonvulsants/Calcium Channel Blockers/Antihypertensives

It is thought that carbamazepine (Tegretol) reduces the rate of impulse transmission and that divalproex (Depakote) increases levels of the inhibitory neurotransmitter gamma-aminobutyric acid (GABA). Increasing GABA activity seems to have an antimanic, antipanic, and antianxiety effect. Manic episodes may be triggered by persistent low-level stimulation of the brain. The anticonvulsants may be effective in that they block this persistent stimulation. Calcium channel blockers have been found to be effective in the treatment of bipolar disorder and seem to work best in people who also respond to lithium. Two antihypertensives, clonidine (Catapres) and guanfacine (Tenex), have been found to stabilize mood in some individuals. The molecular action is unclear but it is thought that clonidine binds to the hypothalamic receptors, thus affecting the hypothalamus–pituitary–adrenal axis (Papolos & Papolos, 2002).

Therapeutic Effects

For clients with problems such as bipolar disorder, major depression, schizoaffective disorder, treatment-resistant schizophrenia, alcohol and opiate withdrawal, rage outbursts, and other problems concerning the regulation of mood, mood-stabilizing medications are helpful.

The antimanic effectiveness of lithium is 70% to 80%; some people are resistant to it and others cannot tolerate the side effects. Because it takes 1 to 3 weeks to control symptoms, antipsychotic medications or benzodiazepines are given initially for relief that is more immediate. Lithium reduces the frequency, duration, and intensity of manic and depressive episodes and is the medication of choice for long-term treatment of bipolar disorder. Individuals who are considered to be "rapid cyclers" (those who have four or more bipolar cycles in a 1-year period) may not do as well with lithium as they do with other mood stabilizers.

Divalproex (Depakote) has a 57% response rate. It may improve a person's response to lithium. Divalproex may be especially useful in rapid-cycling bipolar disorder and in treating the mood disorders associated with organic syndromes. Clonazepam (Klonopin) is a benzodiazepine that is also an anticonvulsant. Its use is typically in addition to lithium, the combination of which lengthens the periods of remission. It has a more rapid onset than the other anticonvulsants, which may take 2 to 3 weeks to be effective.

Carbamazepine (Tegretol) has a favorable response rate in about 60% of clients and is most often used with persons who are unable to take lithium. If given in combination, it may also increase the effectiveness of lithium. Carbamazepine also has antiaggressive properties, which makes it useful for people with frequent rage attacks.

Gabapentin (Neurontin), lamotrigine (Lamictal), topiramate (Topamax), tiagabine (Gabitril), and zonisamide (Zonegran) are anticonvulsant medications that are often effective for controlling rapid-cycling bipolar disorder and for some people with social phobia. Gabapentin and lamotrigine should not be given to children under the age of 16.

Calcium channel blockers are involved in cellular electrical activity and neurotransmitter release as well as regulation of circadian rhythms. This group of medications, which includes verapamil (Calan and Isoptin), nimodipine (Nimotop), and isradipine (DynaCirc), has recently been established as mood stabilizers. It is unlikely that you will see nimodipine prescribed because it is extremely expensive and must be taken three to four times a day, 1 to 2 hours before or after meals.

Clonidine (Catapres) and guanfacine (Tenex) are antihypertensive agents that are helpful for rage attacks, tic disorders, attention deficit/hyperactivity disorder, and pervasive developmental disorders. They are also used for opioid and alcohol withdrawal syndromes (Seagraves & Balon, 2003).

Side Effects

Lithium is nonsedating and nonaddictive. The early side effects of lithium often disappear after 4 weeks. These side effects include lack of spontaneity, memory problems, difficulty concentrating, nausea, vomiting, diarrhea, a metallic taste in the mouth, and hand tremors. Weight gain and a worsening of acne often persist throughout treatment.

The side effects of carbamazepine (Tegretol) are primarily related to the CNS and include drowsiness, dizziness, blurred or double vision, ataxia (unsteady or staggered gait), and nystagmus (involuntary rolling of the eyes). They often disappear over time and are less likely to occur when dose is gradually increased. Women taking oral contraceptives should understand that carbamazepine interferes with the contraceptive ability of the pills and they may experience breakthrough bleeding and false-positive pregnancy tests.

Likewise, the side effects of divalproex (Depakote) tend to occur early in treatment and include sedation, tremor, ataxia, and gastrointestinal effects. Weight gain tends to persist throughout treatment, and clients may stop taking their medication as a result. Low doses of topiramate (Topamax) may counteract the extreme hunger associated with divalproex.

Lamotrigine (Lamictal), topiramate (Topamax), tiagabine (Gabitril), and gabapentin (Neurontin) have few side effects except for some fatigue, dizziness, ataxia, and tremor. They cause no weight gain, and topiramate and lamotrigine actually cause weight loss.

Lamotrigine may cause a rash within the first 8 weeks of treatment. If this occurs, the primary health care provider must be notified immediately since the rash may be associated with a life-threatening syndrome known as **Stevens–Johnson syndrome**. This is a severe and sometimes fatal allergic reaction that attacks the skin, mucous membranes, lungs, and kidneys. Stevens–Johnson syndrome can be caused by sulfa medications, penicillin, phenytoin (Dilantin), and lamotrigine, especially when lamotrigine is combined with divalproex (Depakote) (Lacro, 2004; Nasrallah & Kuo, 2003).

Anticonvulsant hypersensitivity syndrome (AHS) is a rare, but potentially fatal, syndrome that can begin anytime within the first 12 weeks of starting anticonvulsants. AHS is characterized by fever, rash, and involvement of internal organs. Treatment includes symptomatic therapy and discontinuation of the medication (Gogtay, Bavdekar, & Kshirsagar, 2005).

The most common side effects of calcium channel blockers are due to excessive vasodilation and include dizziness, hypotension, headaches, facial flushing, and nausea. Clients must be cautioned not to eat grapefruit or drink its juice because it inhibits an enzyme in the intestines that breaks down calcium channel blockers and can lead to toxic levels in the blood.

Children and adults who are taking clonidine (Catapres) or guanfacine (Tenex) should never stop the medication abruptly. A gradual weaning over 2 to 4 days is necessary to prevent rebound high blood pressure. Side effects of the antihypertensives include agitation, depression, dizziness, drowsiness, orthostatic hypotension, decreased sex drive, and difficulty with erections. Blood pressure should be monitored frequently.

Toxicity and Overdose

There is a fine line between therapeutic levels and toxic levels of lithium. The kidneys excrete both lithium and sodium. If there is a low sodium level in the body, lithium will be retained in its place, which could result in toxicity. Therefore, a normal sodium balance is needed to ensure a therapeutic lithium level. Lithium can rapidly rise to toxic levels whenever there is a severe loss of fluids, such as that caused by fevers, vomiting and diarrhea, or excessive sweating. Other causes of toxicity include excessive intake (deliberate or accidental) and reduced excretion of lithium (resulting from kidney disease and low salt intake).

At the beginning of lithium treatment, blood levels are monitored at least three times a week. Blood must be drawn about 12 hours after the last lithium dose and before the person takes the next dose. Because the initial side effects

---

BOX 10.2	Signs of Lithium Toxicity

Mild (serum level about 1.5 mEq/L)

- Slight apathy, lethargy, drowsiness
- Decreased concentration
- Mild muscular weakness, slight muscle twitching
- Coarse hand tremors
- Mild ataxia

Moderate (serum level about 1.5–2.5 mEq/L)

- Severe diarrhea
- Nausea and vomiting
- Mild to moderate ataxia
- Moderate apathy, lethargy, drowsiness
- Slurred speech
- Tinnitus (ringing in the ears)
- Blurred vision
- Irregular tremor
- Muscle weakness

Severe (serum level above 2.5 mEq/L)

- Nystagmus
- Dysarthria (speech difficulty due to impairment of the tongue)
- Deep tendon hyperreflexia
- Visual or tactile hallucinations
- Oliguria or anuria
- Confusion
- Seizures
- Coma or death

---

are similar to signs of toxicity, it is impossible to know clinically what is happening in the body. After the side effects disappear and the medication has stabilized in the body, blood levels typically are obtained every 3 to 4 months. If symptoms occur during this maintenance period, it is certain that they are signs of toxicity. Box 10.2 lists the signs of lithium toxicity. Caring for a client who is toxic includes monitoring vital signs, maintaining a patent airway, and administering intravenous fluids (adding NaCl if hyponatremic). Severe toxicity is treated with hemodialysis.

Symptoms of toxicity with carbamazepine (Tegretol) include seizures, hypotension, arrhythmia, respiratory depression, and coma. Divalproex (Depakote) overdose can cause severe coma and death. There is no specific treatment other than monitoring vital signs, maintaining a patent airway, and decreasing absorption by the use of activated charcoal. Naloxone (Narcan) may be used to reverse the coma.

Symptoms of toxicity with clonidine (Catapres) and guanfacine (Tenex) include hypotension, bradycardia, lethargy, irritability, weakness, and hypoventilation.

Administration

The administration of lithium is oral, in capsule or liquid form. There is some speculation that the liquid form is absorbed more quickly and is therefore more beneficial when initiating the medication. Some capsules are in slow-release or controlled-release forms. Lithium is usually administered in divided doses, and the ultimate dose is determined by the reduction of symptoms and blood lithium levels.

Carbamazepine (Tegretol) and divalproex (Depakote) both are available in tablet and liquid forms. They are given in divided dosages, beginning with low dosage and a gradual increase. The ultimate dose is determined by the reduction of symptoms, blood levels, and side effects. Calcium channel blockers are increased gradually over several days, during which clients are monitored for hypotension and bradycardia.

Clonidine (Catapres) given orally is likely to cause significant drowsiness. A steady dose via a patch is less likely to be a problem. For those who experience skin sensitivity to the patch or want to swim, clonidine cream (0.1 mg/0.1 mL) is available. To avoid another person receiving the medication, the client should be the one to rub the cream into the skin.

ANTIANXIETY MEDICATIONS

Physiological Effects

Benzodiazepines

Benzodiazepine antianxiety medications act on the limbic system and the reticular activating system (RAS). They produce a calming effect by potentiating the effects of GABA, one of the inhibitory neurotransmitters. CNS depression can range from mild sedation to coma. Other physiological effects include skeletal muscle relaxation and anticonvulsant properties.

Azaspirones

Azaspirone antianxiety medications do not bind at GABA receptors but rather balance 5-HT activity by stimulating the 5-HT receptors. These medications do not tranquilize and sedate and may have mild antidepressant effects. Typically, it takes 1 to 2 weeks for the level of anxiety to decrease.

Therapeutic Effects

Although antianxiety medications will not eliminate all symptoms of anxiety, they will decrease the level of anxiety, enabling clients to function more effectively. These medications are used for anxiety symptoms, anxiety disorders, acute alcohol withdrawal, and convulsive disorders.

Individual benzodiazepines differ in potency, speed in crossing the blood–brain barrier, and degree of receptor binding. High-potency and short-acting benzodiazepines include alprazolam (Xanax), lorazepam (Ativan), halazepam (Paxipam), and oxazepam (Serax). Low-potency and long-acting benzodiazepines include cloazepate (Tranxene), diazepam (Valium), and chlordiazepoxide (Librium). (Table 10.5 ■ lists the various antianxiety medications.)

Side Effects

Benzodiazepines

Side effects of benzodiazepines are primarily related to the general sedative effects and include drowsiness, fatigue, dizziness, and psychomotor impairment. Sedation usually disappears within 1 to 2 weeks of treatment. These medications potentiate the effects of alcohol on the CNS, leading to severe CNS depression. Consuming alcohol while taking benzodiazepines can lead to fatal consequences. When administered

TABLE 10.5	Antianxiety Medications		
Class	**Generic Name**	**Trade Name**	**Adult Dosage (mg/day)**
Benzodiazepines	Alprazolam	Xanax	0.75–4.0
	Chlordiazepoxide	Librium	15–100
	Clonazepam	Klonopin	5–20
	Clorazepate	Tranxene	15–60
	Diazepam	Valium	6–40
	Halazepam	Paxipam	60–160
	Hydroxyzine	Atarax, Vistaril	200–400
	Lorazepam	Ativan	4–12
	Oxazepam	Serax	30–120
	Prazepam	Centrax	10–60
Azaspirones	Buspirone	BuSpar	15–60
Metathizanone	Chlormezanone	Trancopal	300–800

IV, there is a potential for cardiovascular collapse and respiratory depression. There is a potential for addiction and abuse in vulnerable client populations. Benzodiazepines may improve sexual aversion, vaginismus, and rapid ejaculation.

Azaspirones

BuSpar (buspirone) has no potential for dependence and does not potentiate the effects of alcohol on the CNS. It is the medication of choice for clients prone to substance abuse or for those who require long-term treatment with antianxiety medications. Side effects include drowsiness, dizziness, headache, and nervousness. This medication does not negatively affect sex drive or arousal; in fact, sexual desire is often enhanced. It may improve delayed ejaculation and may worsen rapid ejaculation (Seagraves & Balon, 2003).

Toxicity and Overdose

Symptoms of toxicity include euphoria, relaxation, slurred speech, disorientation, unsteady gait, and impaired judgment. Symptoms of overdose include respiratory depression, cold and clammy skin, hypotension, weak and rapid pulse, dilated pupils, and coma. Caring for a client who has overdosed includes monitoring vital signs, especially of cardiac function, and maintaining a patent airway. If the client is alert, vomiting is induced, while gastric lavage is initiated for a stuporous client. Following this procedure, activated charcoal may be administered to minimize absorption. Forced diuresis may increase elimination of the medication.

Flumazenil (Romazicon) is the antidote for overdose and can reverse sedation, respiratory depression, and coma within 2 minutes. Doses may need to be repeated. The initial dose is 0.2 mg IV, followed by 0.3 mg 1 minute later and then as necessary to counteract the overdose symptoms (Turkoski et al., 2004).

Administration

All the antianxiety medications may be taken orally. Antacids interfere with the absorption of these medications and should not be taken until several hours later. Hydroxyzine (Atarax and Vistaril) may also be administered IM. Chlordiazepoxide (Librium), diazepam (Valium), and lorazepam (Ativan) may be administered IM and IV.

Two medications, alprazolam (Niravam) and clonazepam (Klonopin), are available in an orally dissolving form. Clients who wish to take their medication discreetly and without the necessity for water may prefer these wafers of medication.

Benzodiazepines should not be discontinued abruptly after 3 to 4 months of therapy because of the risk for severe withdrawal symptoms, which include seizures, abdominal and other muscular cramps, vomiting, and insomnia. These medications must be gradually reduced very carefully.

CENTRAL NERVOUS SYSTEM STIMULANTS

In the next few years, we are likely to see the development of CNS stimulants referred to as "smart medications." Modafinil (Provigil), the medication used to treat narcolepsy, is one of the medications that promises improved concentration and mental acuity. Other medications that enhance thinking are methylphenidate (Ritalin) and donepezil (Aricept). As the baby-boomer generation ages, interest in these types of medications is increasing.

CNS stimulants are used in the management of attention deficit/hyperactivity disorder (ADHD) and Tourette disorder (see Table 10.6 ■ for these medications). These medications increase the ability to focus attention by blocking out irrelevant thoughts and impulses. CNS stimulants lead to significant improvement in 70% to 75% of cases. The use of CNS stimulants can be compared to the use of glasses for those who are nearsighted (myopic). Glasses allow the child to see the board in the front of the classroom, and CNS stimulants focus attention. One would never say to a myopic child, "You don't need your glasses. Just concentrate and you can read the material on the board." And yet, children with ADHD are often told to "just concentrate" and do the work. For most of these children, it is impossible without medication. See Box 10.3 for therapeutic effects of CNS stimulants.

There is an "anti-Ritalin" group of individuals who are totally against the use of medication for children with ADHD. One of their concerns is that children treated with ADHD medications are more likely to smoke, drink, or take illicit medications as teenagers or adults. There were earlier concerns that long-term stimulant use in children might alter the way the brain reacts to these and other medications, serving as a "gateway" for later tendency to abuse medications. This was based on research in the early 1990s on rats. Those researchers, however, were using doses far in excess of what would ever be used in humans. A study by Barkley, Fischer, Smallish, and Fletcher (2003) followed 147 children with ADHD for 13 years into adulthood. The study found that stimulant-treated children had no greater risk of ever trying drugs by their teens or any significantly greater use of drugs by young adulthood. Wilens, Faraone, Biederman, and Gunawardene (2003) examined six previous studies tracking nearly 1,000 clients with ADHD into adolescence and adulthood, finding that those taking stimulants had a lower rate of later substance abuse than children who were not treated with medication.

The advantage of methylphenidate (Ritalin) and dextroamphetamine (Dexedrine) is that effectiveness is almost immediate, whereas the same effect with pemoline (Cylert) may take 6 to 8 weeks. Clients are cautioned not to eat or drink citrus products within 1 hour of taking dextroam-

TABLE 10.6	Medications to Treat ADHD and Tourette Disorder	
Generic Name	**Trade Name**	**Dosage**
CNS Stimulants		
Dextroamphetamine	Dexedrine	5–15 mg every 4–6 hours
	Adderall	5–30 mg every 4–6 hours
Dexmethylphenidate	Focalin	2.5–10
Methylphenidate	Ritalin, Ritalin SR, Concerta	0.3–0.8 mg/kg BID or TID
	Metadate CD	
Modafinil	Provigil	200–400 mg once a day
Pemoline	Cylert	maximum dose 112.5 mg once a day
Nonstimulant		
Atomoxetine	Strattera	40–100
Mood Stabilizers/Antihypertensives		
Clonidine	Catapres	0.1–0.6 mg per day
		Available in patch
Guanfacine	Tenex	1–3 mg per day
Antidepressants		
Bupropion	Wellbutrin	100–450 mg per day
Antidyskinetic		
Pergolide	Permax	50–500 g per day
Antispastic		
Tizanidine	Zanaflex	8 mg every 6–8 hours

BOX 10.3	Therapeutic Effects of CNS Stimulants

Increases

- Attention
- Accuracy
- Concentration
- Coordination
- Learning
- Memory
- On-task behavior

Decreases

- Aggression
- Daydreaming
- Defiance
- Distractability
- Destructiveness
- Hyperactivity
- Lying
- Oppositional defiant disorder

phetamine because citrus interferes with absorption of the medication. Individuals taking CNS stimulants should avoid caffeine and products with ephedrine (e.g., cough medicine) as these will increase the sense of jitteriness. Common side effects include pallor, a pinched facial expression, dark hollows under the eyes, anorexia, insomnia, headache, and dryness of the mouth.

Atomoxetine (Strattera) is the first nonstimulant medication for ADHD. It inhibits the presynaptic norepinephrine transporter similar to antidepressants. A FDA black box warning has been added to atomoxetine for children and adolescents since there is an increased risk of suicidal behavior with this medication. Dextroamphetamine (Adderall XR) is no longer available because of safety concerns. There have been a number of sudden unexplained deaths with the extended release form of this medication.

Of special concern are preschoolers with ADHD. One group found that 28 preschoolers taking dextroamphetamine in a placebo-controlled study showed a significant improvement in 82% of the sample. No doubt there will be further studies on this population (Short, Manos, Findling, & Schubel, 2004).

ANTICRAVING MEDICATIONS

Medications in the treatment of addictions reduce medication craving and help prevent relapse. Except for a few older medications, this is a new and growing area. In some cases,

BOX 10.4   Medications Used to Prevent Relapse

Opiates

- Methadone
- Buprenorphine (Dilaudid)
- Naltrexone (ReVia)
- Acamprosate (Campral)
- Clonidine (Catapres)

Alcohol

- Ondansetron (Zofan)
- Acamprosate (Campral)
- Topiramate (Topamax)
- Disulfiram (Antabuse)

Cocaine

- Disulfiram (Antabuse)
- Topiramate (Topamax)
- Modafinil (Provigil)
- Propranolol (Inderal)
- Baclofen (Lioresal)
- Gabapentin (Neurontin)

Nicotine

- Nicotine replacement
- Bupropion (Wellbutrin/Zyban)

clients are given a medication similar to the medication of dependence to block withdrawal symptoms. The medication dose is then gradually reduced. An example is treating nicotine withdrawal with a nicotine patch. In other cases, the medication blocks the brain pathways involved in producing the withdrawal symptoms. An example is the use of clonidine (Catapres) for opiate withdrawal. Box 10.4 lists the medications used to prevent relapse of addictive disorders. More detailed information about these medications is found in chapter 15 ∞.

SPECIAL POPULATIONS AND PSYCHOPHARMACOLOGICAL TREATMENT

Certain groups of clients present a challenge to nurses when psychotropic medications are part of their treatment. These groups include older adults, pregnant women, children, medically complex clients, those with severe and persistent mental illness, and culturally diverse clients.

Older Adults

The physiological changes of aging affect the use of psychotropic medications. Absorption of medication is influenced by a decrease in gastric emptying time, a reduction in blood flow to the gastrointestinal (GI) system, and a decrease in GI motility. Once through the GI system, most psychotropic medications bind to albumin. Albumin levels de-

crease with aging, and there is more free-floating medication in the bloodstream, thereby contributing to increased sedation in older adults. At the same time, adipose tissue increases by 10% to 50% over the age of 65. Medications such as the long-acting benzodiazepines, which are stored in adipose tissue, are thus available for longer periods of time. Changes in liver metabolism contribute to slower metabolism of medications, which prolongs elimination and leads to increased toxicity. The renal filtration rate may decrease by 50% by age 70, which also contributes to increased toxicity. Aging reduces the amount of NE, 5-HT, DA, ACh, and GABA in the CNS, leading to increased receptor sensitivity. The result is a change in responsiveness to medications (Turkoski et al., 2004).

Older adults are more sensitive than younger adults to the side effects of antipsychotic medications. This is important information since 25% to 45% of geriatric nursing home residents are given these medications. Increased sedation may lead to confusion and agitation. Orthostatic hypotension increases the risk of falls and fractures. Older people are likely to have more severe EPSs, especially a higher risk of tardive dyskinesia. All second-generation antipsychotics now carry a black box warning that they are not to be used for older adults with dementia since they have an increased chance of death. Individuals with significant behavioral problems may be given first-generation antipsychotics. Older adults are also more sensitive to antidepressant side effects. The anticholinergic effects may increase symptoms of prostatic hypertrophy, blurred vision, and constipation. The anticholinergic properties of these medications may lead to short-term memory problems, disorientation, and impaired cognition. These side effects may be mistaken for organic brain disease (pseudodementia).

The second-generation of antidepressants, the SSRIs and SNRIs, are especially useful for treating depression in older people. The response time between initiation of the medication and relief of depressive symptoms is much shorter than with tricyclic antidepressants. The most commonly used are fluoxetine (Prozac) for people experiencing psychomotor retardation, and sertraline (Zoloft) for those experiencing anxiety.

Because the production of MAO increases with age, MAOIs may be more effective for older clients. Another benefit to older people is the absence of anticholinergic side effects. There is, however, a higher risk for hypotension, which may be a contributing factor in falls. The disadvantage of this group of medications is the strict dietary limitations. The nutritional options of many older clients are limited because of their finances; they may find it difficult to follow the severely restricted diet. Because of the unique properties of selegiline (Eldepryl), food interactions are not a problem and there are no dietary restrictions, and this MAOI may be helpful for older adults. Individuals may experience some skin irritation from the patch.

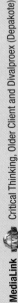

5. Develop medication teaching plans for a person with mental illness and her/his family.

→

- Prescribed medication: Include the purpose of medication, how to take, potential side effects, and when to call the doctor. Combine verbal and written instructions or use pictures for those unable to read English.
- Medication management: Adults have the right to refuse medications; clients and nurses mutually agree on goals and outcomes of medication; if client stops taking medication, determine the reasons; encourage clients to research further information for self-education about their medications.
- Weight management: It is better to prevent weight gain than try to lose excess weight; identify changes that need to be made; increase physical activity; and utilize community support groups.
- Temperature regulation: Provide information about side effect of heatstroke; teach need to maintain adequate fluid intake; utilize cooling centers.
- Family support: Supportive families can help with symptom monitoring, decision making regarding medications, and avoiding relapse.

Explore MediaLink

For review questions, case studies, and other resources for this chapter see the Pearson Health MediaLink CD-ROM that accompanies this book and the Companion Website.

CD-ROM
- Audio Glossary
- NCLEX-RN® Review Questions
- Animations/Videos
  - Liver Enzyme (Cytochrome P450) Inhibition and Activation
  - Diazepam (Valium)
  - Methylphenidate (Ritalin)
  - Fluoxetine (Prozac)

Companion Website www.prenhall.com/fontaine
- Audio Glossary
- NCLEX-RN® Review Questions
- Case Study
  - Family Teaching: Medications and the Client With Bipolar Disorder
- Care Plan
  - The Client With Lithium Toxicity
- Critical Thinking
  - Family Teaching: The Older Client on Divalproex (Depakote)
- MediaLink Application
  - Weight Gain and Antipsychotic Medications
- MediaLinks
  - Books for Clients and Families; Community Resources

NCLEX-RN® Review Questions

10-1. A client has been on antipsychotic medication for 20 years with little control of schizophrenic symptoms. The client was recently switched to clozapine (Clozaril). Which of the following behaviors would indicate a positive therapeutic response to this medication? (Select all that apply.)
1. A decrease in blood pressure
2. An increase in weight
3. A decrease in white blood cells
4. An increase in motivation
5. A decrease in hallucinations

10-2. A client is taking thioridazine (Mellaril) and is exhibiting restlessness, muscle rigidity, involuntary movements, and drooling. Which of the following medications would be most helpful in treating these side effects?
1. Fluoxetine (Prozac)
2. Lorazepam (Ativan)
3. Benztropine (Cogentin)
4. Olanzapine (Zyprexa)

10-3. A recent lab report on a client taking olanzapine (Zyprexa) reveals a triglyceride level of 300 mg/dL, high-density lipoprotein (HDL) cholesterol level of 30 mg/dL,

and a fasting blood glucose level of 215 mg/dL. In addition, the client has an abdominal girth of 41 inches. Which of the following syndromes does the client exhibit?
1. Serotonin syndrome
2. Metabolic syndrome
3. Parkinson syndrome
4. Cushing syndrome

10-4. A 29-year-old female client is worried that she may be pregnant. She has been taking lithium for the past year and is concerned about the effects of lithium on her unborn child. Which of the following statements is true?
1. Lithium interferes with oral contraceptives and may cause a false-positive pregnancy test.
2. Lithium does not cross the placental barrier and poses no risk to the fetus.
3. Lithium should be avoided during the latter part of the first trimester if possible.
4. Lithium should not be taken during pregnancy.

10-5. A client with bipolar disorder has been taking lithium for the past 2 years. Recently, the client has been experiencing a recurrence of manic symptoms approximately once a month. The psychiatrist has added clonazepam

(Klonopin) to help manage the client's mood swings. Which of the following statements should the nurse include in medication teaching?

1. "This medication will help to steady your moods by reducing the overstimulation of chemical messengers in your brain."

2. "This medication should not be taken with foods that contain tyramine such as aged cheese."

3. "This medication should not be taken with any other medication."

4. "This medication may cause a severe rash and should be reported to your physician immediately."

See Appendix D for answers.

References

Barkley, R. A., Fischer, M., Smallish, L., & Fletcher, K. (2003). Does the treatment of attention-deficit/hyperactivity disorder with stimulants contribute to drug use/abuse? *Pediatrics, 111*(1), 97–109.

Centorrino, F., Goren, J. L., Hennen, J., Salvatore, P., Kelleher, J. P., & Baldessarini, R. J. (2005). Multiple versus single antipsychotic agents for hospitalized psychiatric patients. *American Journal of Psychiatry, 161*(4), 700–706.

Citrome, L., Blonde, L., & Damatarca, C. (2005). Metabolic issues in patients with severe mental illness. *Southern Medical Journal, 98*(7), 714–720.

Crane, K., Kirby, B., & Kooperman, D. (1996). Patient compliance for psychotropic medications. *Journal of Psychosocial Nursing, 34*(1), 8–15.

dosReis, S., Zito, J. M., Safer, D. J., Gardner, J. F., Puccia, K. B., & Owens, P. L. (2005). Multiple psychotropic medication use for youths. *Journal of Child and Adolescent Psychopharmacology, 15*(1), 68–77.

Geddes, J. R., Burgess, S., Hawton, K., Jamison, K., & Goodwin, G. M. (2004). Long-term lithium therapy for bipolar disorder. *American Journal of Psychiatry, 161*(2), 217–222.

Gibbons, R. D., Hur, K., Bhaumik, D. K., & Mann, J. J. (2005). The relationship between antidepressant medication use and rate of suicide. *Archives of General Psychiatry, 62*(2), 165–172.

Gill, J., Singh, H., & Nugent, K. (2003). Acute lithium intoxication and neuroleptic malignant syndrome. *Pharmacotherapy, 23*(6), 811–815.

Gogtay, N. J., Bavdekar, S. B., & Kshirsagar, N. A. (2005). Anticonvulsant hypersensitivity syndrome. *Expert Opinion on Drug Safety, 4*(3), 571–581.

Graham, K. A., Gu, H., Lieberman, J. A., Harp, J. B., & Perkins, D. O. (2005). Double-blind, placebo-controlled investigation of amantadine for weight loss in subjects who gained weight with olanzapine. *American Journal of Psychiatry, 162*(9), 1744–1746.

Henderson, D. C., Copeland, P. M., Daley, T. B., Borba, C. P., Nguyen, D. D., Louie, P. M., et al. (2005). A double-blind, placebo-controlled trial of sibutramine for olanzapine-associated weight gain. *American Journal of Psychiatry, 162*(5), 954–962.

Higgins, A., Barker, P., & Begley, C. M. (2005). Neuroleptic medication and sexuality: The forgotten aspect of education and care. *Journal of Psychiatric and Mental Health Nursing, 12*(4), 439–446.

Janno, S., Holi, M., Tuisku, K., & Wahlbeck, K. (2004). Prevalence of neuroleptic-induced movement disorders in chronic schizophrenia inpatients. *American Journal of Psychiatry, 161*(1), 160–163.

Janssen, B., Weinmann, S., Berger, M., & Gaebel, W. (2004). Validation of polypharmacy process measures in inpatient schizophrenia care. *Schizophrenia Bulletin, 30*(4), 1023–1033.

Kallen, B. (2004). Neonate characteristics after maternal use of antidepressants in late pregnancy. *Archive of Pediatrics and Adolescent Medicine, 158*(4), 312–316.

Kapur, S., Arenovich, T., Agid, O., Zipursky, R., Lindborg, S., & Jones, B. (2005). Evidence for onset of antipsychotic effects within the first 24 hours of treatment. *American Journal of Psychiatry, 162*(5), 939–946.

Koren, G., Cohn, R., Chitayat, D., Kapur, B., Remington, G., Reid, D. M., et al. (2002). Use of atypical antipsychotics during pregnancy and the risk of neural tube defects in infants. *American Journal of Psychiatry, 159*(1), 136–137.

Kozuki, Y., Poupore, E., & Schepp, K. (2005). Visual feedback therapy to enhance medication adherence in psychosis. *Archives of Psychiatric Nursing, 19*(2), 70–80.

Lacro, J. (2004). Medication adherence. *Medscape Psychiatry & Mental Health, 9*(1), 1–4.

Lieberman, J. A., Stroup, T. S., McEvoy, J. P., Swartz, M. S., Rosenheck, R. A., Perkins, D. O., et al. (2005). Effectiveness of antipsychotic drugs in patients with chronic schizophrenia. *New England Journal of Medicine, 353*(12), 1209–1223.

Lin, K. M., & Smith, M. W. (2000). Psychopharmacotherapy in context of culture and ethnicity. In P. Ruiz (Ed.), *Ethnicity and psychopharmacology* (pp. 1–36). Washington, DC: American Psychiatric Press.

Love, R. C., & Conley, R. J. (2004). Long-acting risperidone injection. *American Journal of Health-System Pharmacy, 61*(17), 1792–1800.

Mahone, I. H. (2004). Medication decision-making by persons with serious mental illness. *Archives of Psychiatric Nursing, 18*(4), 126–134.

Munoz, C., & Hilgenberg, C. (2005). Ethnopharmacology. *American Journal of Nursing, 105*(8), 41–49.

Nasrallah, H. A., & Kuo, I. (2003). Side effects in the treatment of bipolar affective disorder. *Medscape Psychiatry & Mental Health, 8*(2), 1–4.

Nulman, I., Rovet, J., Stewart, D. E., Wolpin, J., Pace-Asciak, P., Shuhaiber S., et al. (2002). Child development following exposure to tricyclic antidepressants of fluoxetine throughout fetal life. *American Journal of Psychiatry, 159*(11), 1889–1895.

Papolos, D., & Papolos, J. (2002). *The bipolar child.* New York: Broadway Books.

Pomerantz, J. M. (2004). Controversy over suicide risk in children and adolescents taking antidepressants. *Drug Benefit Trends, 16*(10), 526–528.

Preskorn, S. H. (2006). Pharmacogenomics, informatics, and individual drug therapy in psychiatry. *Journal of Psychopharmacology, 20*(4 Suppl), 85–94.

Reeves, R. R., & Mack, J. E. (2002). Priapism associated with two atypical antipsychotic agents. *Pharmacotherapy, 22*(8), 1070–1073.

Rettenbacher, M. A. (2005). Disturbances of glucose and lipid metabolism during treatment with new generation antipsychotics. *Current Opinion in Psychiatry, 18*(2), 175–179.

Reuters Health Information. (2003). FDA advisors back reduced monitoring for patients on clozapine. *Reuters Health Information.* Retrieved June 30, 2003, from www.medscape.com/viewarticle/457338_print.

Ruiz, P. (2000). Foreword. In P. Ruiz (Ed.), *Ethnicity and psychopharmacology* (pp. xv–xx). Washington, DC: American Psychiatric Press.

Schooler, N., Rabinowitz, J., Davidson, M., Emsley, R., Harvey, P. D., Kopala, L., et al. (2005). Risperidone and haloperidol in first-episode psychosis. *American Journal of Psychiatry, 162*(5), 947–953.

Seagraves, R. T., & Balon, R. (2003). *Sexual pharmacology: Fast facts.* New York: WW Norton.

Seeman, M. V. (2004). Gender differences in the prescribing of antipsychotic drugs. *American Journal of Psychiatry, 161*(8), 1324–1333.

Short, E. J., Manos, M. J., Findling, R. L., & Schubel, E. A. (2004). A prospective study of stimulant response in preschool children. *Journal of the American Academy of Child and Adolescent Psychiatry, 43*(3), 251–259.

Trzepacz, P. T., & Kennedy, R. E. (2005). Delirium and posttraumatic amnesia. In J. M. Silver, T. W. McAllister, & S. C. Yudofsky (Eds.), *Textbook of traumatic brain injury* (pp. 175–200). Washington, DC: American Psychiatric Press.

Turkoski, B. B., Lance, B. R., & Bonfiglio, M. F. (2004). *Drug information handbook for advanced practice nursing* (4th ed.). Hudson, OH: Lexi-Comp.

van Geffen, E. C., Hugtenburg, J. G., Heerdink, E. R., van Hulten, R. P., & Egberts, A. C. (2006). Discontinuation symptoms in users of selective serotonin reuptake inhibitors in clinical practice. *European Journal of Clinical Pharmacology, 61*(4), 303–307.

Wilens, T. E., Faraone, S. V., Biederman, J., & Gunawardene, S. (2003). Does stimulant therapy of attention-deficit/hyperactivity disorder beget later substance abuse? A meta-analytic review of the literature. *Pediatrics, 111*(1), 179–185.

Unit 3

Mental Disorders

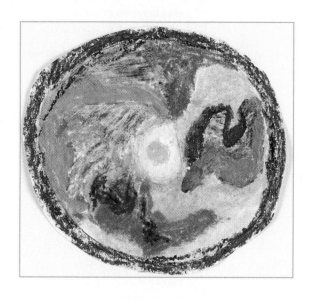

66 *This is where I see myself now. A face with no identity surrounded by a head of darkness, consumed by a fire turning my soul into ashes.* 99

—Brenda, Age 25

Chapter **11**

Anxiety, Dissociative, and Somatoform Disorders

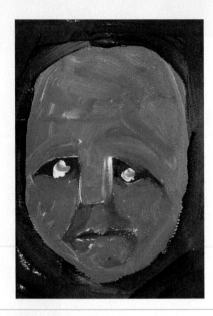

> *Anxiety/Depression*
>
> *dying inside*
> *invisible to others*
>
> *reaching out*
> *with arms not there*
>
> *trying to find hope*
> *in a dim light dying*
>
> *hope in anything*
> *to keep breathing*
>
> —Heather, Age 30

OBJECTIVES

After reading this chapter, you will be able to:

1. Compare and contrast the different theories regarding the etiology of anxiety, dissociative, and somatoform disorders.

2. Discuss the psychopharmacological treatment of the symptoms of a person with an anxiety, dissociative, or somatoform disorder.

3. Outline different treatment options for anxiety, dissociative, and somatoform disorders.

4. Outline the assessment process for a client with an anxiety, dissociative, or somatoform disorder.

5. Use the nursing process to develop a comprehensive plan of care for a client with an anxiety, dissociative, or somatoform disorder.

6. Develop illness management teaching plans for a person with an anxiety, dissociative, or somatoform disorder and her/his family.

7. Discuss the key points in effectively communicating with a person with an anxiety, dissociative, or somatoform disorder.

MediaLink www.prenhall.com/fontaine

Go to the Pearson Health MediaLink CD-ROM and the Companion Website at www.prenhall.com/fontaine for interactive resources for this chapter.

The ROAD to Critical Thinking   A Client Experiencing Anxiety Disorder

Travel this ROAD to understand Steve and his condition.

Read about Steve below and throughout this chapter.

Observe Steve on the CD-ROM accompanying this book.

Assess Steve by answering the questions at the end of this chapter.

Develop a Care Plan on the CD-ROM to address Steve's condition.

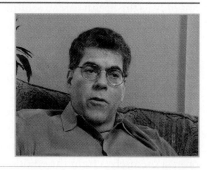

Steve

Steve is 54 years old and has had social phobia most of his life. School was traumatic for Steve, who coped by either acting as the class clown or by trying to be invisible. As an adult, he self-medicated with alcohol to cope with parties and other social gatherings. He perceives that others are watching him and find him ignorant or stupid.

You will meet Steve on the video clip on your CD-ROM and throughout this chapter. At the end of the chapter, you will find critical thinking questions relating to assessment and development of a plan of care for Steve.

Social phobias are fears of most social situations and affect more than 13% of the population. There are two peaks of incidence—at 11 to 15 years of age and at 18–25 years of age—with an unremitting course. Social phobias are characterized by the fear of situations in which an individual dreads humiliation or embarrassment when under the scrutiny of others. Unlike shyness, social phobias make victims actually sick with fear. Social phobias may take many forms, such as fear of meeting new people, attending social gatherings, talking to people in authority, stage fright, public speaking, using public bathrooms, eating in public, and being observed at work. Many people with social phobia fear and avoid a variety of situations, resulting in negative social, vocational, and financial consequences and functional impairment. Despite the availability of effective treatment for social phobias, most adults in the United States do not receive mental health care for their symptoms. They are often ashamed of their symptoms and fear what professionals may think or say about them (Bruce et al., 2005).

Anxiety is an uncomfortable feeling that occurs in response to the fear of being hurt or losing something valued. Some

Steve:

" When I'm at a party, I feel my heart racing. I feel there's a kind of hollowness inside my body. I sweat and I stammer. I start a conversation and usually for the first minute or two I'm on target where I say something that's amusing. Humor for me is a sort of social grease. But then there's a kind of halting pause after that because I don't quite know what to do. I'm really worried that someone's going to ask me a question that's going to reveal how ignorant I am on that topic. The biggest fear is that I'm going to appear as ignorant. "

professionals distinguish between fear and anxiety. When making this distinction, fear is a feeling that arises from a concrete, real danger, whereas anxiety is a feeling that arises from an ambiguous, unspecific cause or is disproportionate to the danger.

Anxiety is a common human emotion. It is a biologically mediated response to stress and change. Anxiety helps us mobilize the protective resources necessary for adaptation. When a person's anxiety loses its link with precipitating circumstances or becomes excessive or maladaptive, that person is said to be experiencing an anxiety disorder.

Since September 11, 2001, many Americans have experienced an unfamiliar level of anxiety related to the terrorist acts on the World Trade Center and the Pentagon. For the first time in our lives, we feel vulnerable in our homes, in our cities, and in our country. We were forced to forsake the illusion that we were untouchable. As we gave up our expectation of security, we moved into a time of uncertainty and, for many, a time of diffuse anxiety. Many of those directly affected by the attacks—survivors, rescuers, health care professionals, and the family members of each of these—experienced acute stress disorder and some developed posttraumatic stress disorder. Both of these disorders are presented in this chapter.

In terms of the "normal" or nonviolent world, you, like other people, probably are anxious about certain aspects of your life. When you began the study of nursing, you were introduced to a new and foreign subculture: health care professionals and institutions. Your first few days in the clinical setting were probably highly anxious times, as you were uncertain about your skills and insecure in your role as a nursing student. As your skills increased and your professional role became more comfortable, your level of anxiety decreased. Now, you begin your experience in mental health nursing, your anxiety again increases as you struggle with new skills and new professional roles. You are probably skeptical of your ability to intervene with clients and are uncertain about what is expected of you. Some of you must adapt not only to the health care subculture, but also to a different, larger culture because of geographical relocation or becoming part of a more culturally diverse group of people. Because too much anxiety interferes with learning, for both you and the clients, effective coping behaviors are necessary for optimal education.

In addition to understanding the meaning of anxiety, it is important to know its process and characteristics, as well as defenses against it. Consciously and unconsciously, people try to protect themselves from the emotional pain of anxiety. Conscious attempts at protection are referred to as **coping behaviors**, which may be effective. *Ineffective coping behaviors* can include such things as becoming involved in physical fights, abusing substances, social withdrawal, or addictive behaviors.

People often effectively use physical activity—walking, jogging, competitive sports, swimming, strenuous housecleaning—to counteract the tension associated with anxiety. *Effective cognitive coping behavior* includes realistically reviewing strengths and limitations, determining short- and long-term goals (both individual and family), and formulating a plan to confront the anxiety-producing situation. Useful affective coping behavior may include expressing emotions (laughter, words, tears) or seeking support from family, friends, or professionals. Stress-reduction techniques may also be used, such as meditation, progressive relaxation, visualization, and biofeedback. Effective coping mechanisms contribute to a person's sense of competence and self-esteem.

Unconscious attempts to manage anxiety are referred to as **defense mechanisms**. They often prevent a person from being sensitive to anxiety and, therefore, interfere with self-awareness. When they allow for gratification in acceptable ways, defense mechanisms may be adaptive; however, when the anxiety is not reduced to manageable levels, the defenses become maladaptive. (See chapter 1 ∞ for examples of defense mechanisms.)

The consistent use of certain defenses leads to the development of *personality traits* and characteristic behaviors. How a person manages anxiety and which defense mechanisms are used are more behaviorally formative than the source of the anxiety. Consider the basic human need to be loved and cared for by another person. The anxiety produced by fear of the loss of love may result in a variety of behaviors. One person may be driven to constantly look for love and affirmation by engaging in frequent one-night sexual encounters. Another person may seek out and develop a warm, intimate relationship. A third person may be so frightened of not finding love and so fearful of rejection that he or she avoids relationships to decrease the anxiety. The management of defenses can become so time consuming that little energy remains for other aspects of living.

It is estimated that 27 million adults suffer from anxiety disorders at some point, making these disorders the single largest mental health problem in the United States, with the exception of substance use disorders. Anxiety disorders are twice as common in women as in men. With the exception of panic disorder without agoraphobia, these disorders are chronic and have low rates of recovery and high rates of recurrence. In addition, individuals with one anxiety disorder often develop an additional anxiety disorder. Only 25% of sufferers receive psychiatric intervention; the remaining 75% use other health care services or go untreated. Without relief, anxiety disorders can dramatically reduce productivity and significantly diminish quality of life (Bruce et al., 2005; Gelernter, Page, Stein, & Woods, 2004).

Sometimes it is difficult to distinguish among the various anxiety disorders and the difference between anxiety disorders and depression is not always clear. It is thought that the neurobiological disruptions overlap for both disorder categories. Indeed, antidepressant medications are the pharmacological treatment of choice for anxiety disorders (Pennington, 2002).

Clients with varying levels of anxiety are found in all types of clinical facilities, from community clinics to medical–surgical settings to intensive care units. In a person with the added stress of a sudden or long-term physical illness, an anxiety disorder may be especially pronounced. The disorders associated with anxiety are thyroid problems, congestive heart failure, cardiac arrhythmias, chronic obstructive pulmonary disease, pneumonia, hyperventilation, neoplasms, pulmonary embolism, and hyperadrenalism.

Included with the anxiety disorders in this chapter are the dissociative disorders, somatoform disorders, factitious disorder, and malingering. These disorders are presented in the same chapter because anxiety is the underlying theme in each. The DSM-IV-TR feature lists the categories and different types of disorders presented.

KNOWLEDGE BASE

This section describes the various categories of disorders that develop in response to anxiety. At times, it may be difficult to determine which disorder the person is experiencing because the symptoms often cut across the various disorders. This should not be a great problem for nurses since their focus, as nurses, is on client responses to illness.

Anxiety Disorders

Generalized Anxiety Disorder

Generalized anxiety disorder (GAD) is a chronic disorder characterized by persistent anxiety, without phobias or panic attacks. Affecting 4% to 7% of the population, it usually begins in childhood or adolescence but may begin in one's 20s.

TABLE 11.1	Physiological Characteristics According to Levels of Anxiety

Anxiety Level	Physiological Response
Mild	Slightly elevated heart rate and blood pressure
	Feels safe and comfortable
	Perceptual field increased
	Ability to learn increased
Moderate	Occasional shortness of breath
	Mild gastric symptoms such as "butterflies" in the stomach
	Facial twitches, trembling lips
	Selective inattention
	Narrowing of the perceptual field
Severe	Frequent shortness of breath
	Increased heart rate, possible premature contractions
	Elevated blood pressure
	Dry mouth, upset stomach, anorexia, diarrhea, or constipation
	Body trembling, fearful facial expression, tense muscles, restlessness, exaggerated startle response, inability to relax, difficulty falling asleep
	Extremely narrowed perceptual field
	Difficulty problem solving or organizing
Panic	Shortness of breath, choking or smothering sensation, sweating
	Hypotension, dizziness, chest pain or pressure, palpitations, chills or hot flashes
	Nausea
	Agitation, poor motor coordination, involuntary movements, entire body trembling, facial expression of terror
	Feeling of losing control, fear of dying
	Completely disrupted perceptual field

It can be triggered by stress or come out of nowhere. Most sufferers worry excessively about everyday concerns, such as whether the boss thinks they are doing a good job or how they are going to pay the bills. In more severe cases, a victim may become preoccupied with catastrophic thoughts and visions. Other symptoms include overall fatigue, muscular tension, restlessness, irritability, difficulty concentrating, and sleep disturbance. Table 11.1 ■ lists the physiological characteristics according to levels of anxiety. Unremitting stress and tension can suppress the immune system, which makes a person more susceptible to disease (Kessler, Walters, & Wittchen, 2004).

Panic Disorder

Panic attack is the highest level of anxiety, characterized by disorganized thinking, feelings of terror and helplessness, and nonpurposeful behavior. It may occur in several anxiety disorders. During this intense experience, people believe they are about to die, lose control, or "go crazy." See Table 11.1 for symptoms of the panic level of anxiety. Some studies suggest that occasional panic attacks occur in 35% of the U.S. population. These episodes are usually associated with public speaking, interpersonal conflict, examinations,

or other situations of high stress (American Psychiatric Association [APA], 2000).

Panic disorder, which affects more than 1.5 million Americans, is diagnosed when there are recurrent panic attacks. It usually develops between the ages of 15 and 24 years; one third to one half of individuals also have agoraphobia. Those with agoraphobia tend to have a poor outcome in terms of daily functioning. Nearly 18% of postmenopausal women experience panic attacks, and the occurrence of the attacks seems to be tied to stressful life events and comorbid medical illness. Typically, the onset of panic attacks is sudden and unexpected, with intense symptoms lasting from a few minutes to an hour. The episodes involve intense fear and a premonition of doom, which is accompanied by a variety of symptoms, as listed in Table 11.1. Although panic attacks are an essential feature of panic disorder, other psychiatric symptoms include widespread catastrophic thinking, phobialike avoidance, anxiety, depression, and obsession (Bruce et al., 2005; Smoller et al., 2003).

The frequency of panic attacks varies widely among persons with panic disorder, as do symptom clusters. Some people experience primarily respiratory symptoms, some primarily experience cardiovascular symptoms, and others are more overwhelmed by cognitive symptoms. Many people

MediaLink

Critical Thinking, Panic Attack

TABLE 11.2	Psychiatric Rating Scale: Levels of Severity for Panic Disorders

Level	Description
6	At least one panic episode per day
5	At least one panic episode per week but less than one per day
4	Persistent fear of panic
3	Limited-symptom panic
2	Sometimes feels on the verge of an attack but is able to control it
1	None of the above

SOURCE: Adapted with permission from Yonkers, K. A., Zlotnick, C., Allsworth, J., Warshaw, M., Shea, T., & Keller, M. B. (1998). Is the course of panic disorder the same in women and men? *American Journal of Psychiatry, 155*(5), 596–602. Reprinted with permission from *American Journal of Psychiatry,* Copyright © (1998).

with panic disorder believe they are suffering from heart or lung disease, which may lead to avoidance of exercise due to their fear that it could precipitate a heart attack (Cloos, 2005).

A rating scale for the severity of the symptoms provides direction for the multidisciplinary team in helping people with panic disorders improve their quality of life (see Table 11.2 ■).

Dowoyne has been experiencing panic attacks for the past 6 months. He feels very stressed at work because his new boss is "riding everyone." The same boss recently fired Dowoyne's girlfriend. He describes his panic attacks as a combination of dizziness, trembling, sweating, gasping for breath, and severe pounding of his heart. When the panic subsides, he feels exhausted, as if he has survived a traumatic experience. It has become very stressful for him to commute to work on the train because he fears having an attack in front of everyone. Dowoyne is seriously considering changing jobs so he won't have to take the train.

A variation of panic disorder is *nocturnal panic.* Panic attacks awaken the person and usually occur within 1 to 4 hours after falling asleep, usually during non-REM sleep. No one knows the cause of nocturnal panic, although some believe it may be related to sleep apnea. Panic is further discussed later in the chapter along with agoraphobia, since the two disorders often occur together.

Phobic Disorders

Phobic disorders are behavioral patterns that develop as a defense against anxiety. They progress as a way of objectifying underlying anxiety, displacing it to something concrete that can then be identified and avoided. Other features common to these disorders include fear of losing control, fear of appearing inadequate, defense against threats to self-esteem, and perfectionist standards of behavior.

Almost all people try to avoid physical dangers. If this avoidance is generalized to situations other than realistic danger, it is called a *phobia.* It is estimated that 20% to 45% of the general population have some mild form of phobic behavior. However, actual phobic disorders occur in only 5% to 15% of the

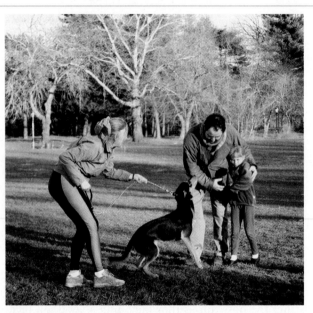

PHOTO 11.1 ■ People with specific phobias experience high levels of anxiety when confronted with the feared situation or object.
SOURCE: Innervisions. Used with permission.

population (Pennington, 2002). There are many phobic disorders, and they all have four features in common:

1. Unreasonable behavioral response
2. Persistent fears
3. Avoidance behavior
4. Disabling behavior

Although the feared object or situation may not be symbolic of the underlying anxiety, the *primary* fear in all phobic disorders is the fear of losing control.

Ever since they were married, Mike has been emotionally abusive to Velda, telling her what a worthless wife, a terrible housekeeper, and an unimaginative lover she is. Velda has now developed a phobic fear of dirt, germs, and contamination. This phobia so dominates her life that whenever Mike comes home, she immediately scrubs the floor where he has walked because "you can't tell where he has been or what dirt or germs he is bringing in on his shoes." Because the anxiety caused by Mike's abuse and his threats to abandon her were too painful to confront, repression forced her fears out of conscious awareness. Because repression is never successful by itself, the anxiety became displaced from her inadequacies in the relationship and transferred representatively to dirt, germs, and contamination. Constant cleaning then became symbolic of her fears and threatened self-esteem, over which she had more control than her husband's behavior.

A *specific phobia* is a fear of only one object or situation; it can arise after a single unpleasant experience. The most common phobias are of "old" dangers, such as closed spaces, heights, snakes, and spiders. Very seldom are people phobic about current dangers, such as guns, knives, and speeding cars. Phobias usually begin early in life and are experienced as often by men as by women. People with specific phobias experience *anticipatory anxiety,* that is, they become anxious even thinking about the feared object or situation. A specific phobia is not disabling unless the feared object or situation cannot be avoided.

Ever since a rattlesnake bit Carlos 5 years ago, he has developed a specific phobia of snakes. Normally, his phobia causes no disability because he lives in a large urban area. However, the phobia has prevented him from participating in certain leisure activities such as hiking and camping.

Janelle has a specific phobia of being in an elevator with other people. Her phobia is mildly disabling; she must use the stairs almost all the time. Her vocational opportunities are somewhat limited because she is unable to work on the upper floors of a high-rise office building.

For social phobias, please see the ROAD feature at the beginning of this chapter.

Agoraphobia, the most common and serious phobic disorder, is a fear of being away from home and of being alone in public places when assistance might be needed and where escape might be difficult. A person with agoraphobia will avoid groups of people, whether on busy streets or in crowded stores, on public transportation or at town beaches, at concerts or in movie theaters. Places where the person might become trapped, such as in tunnels or on elevators, are also sometimes avoided.

Agoraphobia is often triggered by severe stress. Moving, changing jobs, relationship problems, or the death of a loved one may precipitate it. The two peak times for the onset are between the ages of 15 and 20 years and then again between the ages of 30 and 40 years. Some people may experience a brief period of agoraphobia, which then disappears, never to recur. If it persists for more than a year, the disorder tends to be chronic, with periods of partial remission and relapse (Paris, 1999).

People who suffer from disabling agoraphobia are excessively dependent because their avoidance behavior dominates all activities. They may even be so panic-stricken outside the home that they become housebound (see Table 11.3 ■).

Edith, who lives in a large urban area, developed agoraphobia 10 years ago during a time of severe marital distress. In the beginning, she merely avoided large crowds of people. She then began to fear leaving her neighborhood. Five years ago, she became housebound and experienced panic attacks if she attempted to leave her home. Two years ago, her phobia progressed to the point that she cannot leave her living room couch. She now needs a great deal of assistance in the activities of daily living. Her husband and a cleaning woman provide for her basic needs. She is alert and continues to manage all the household finances and any other activities that can be accomplished from her couch.

Obsessive–Compulsive Disorder

Obsessions are unwanted, repetitive thoughts that lead to feelings of fear, anxiety, or guilt, such as the thought of killing someone or of being contaminated with germs. **Compulsions** are behaviors (e.g., frequent hand washing) or thoughts (e.g., silently counting) used to decrease the fear or guilt associated with obsessions.

TABLE 11.3	Psychiatric Rating Scale: Levels of Severity for Agoraphobia
Level	**Description**
6	Severe avoidance resulting in near or total restriction to home or inability to leave home unaccompanied
5	Avoidance resulting in constricted lifestyle or fear endured with great anxiety (e.g., able to leave house alone but unable to go more than a few miles unaccompanied)
4	Some avoidance and relatively normal lifestyle (e.g., travels unaccompanied when necessary, such as to work or to shop, but otherwise avoids traveling alone)
3	Moderate anxiety when in a phobic situation but no avoidance
2	Slight anxiety in a phobic situation (or anticipation of the situation) but no avoidance
1	None of the above

SOURCE: Adapted with permission from Yonkers, K. A., Zlotnick, C., Allsworth, J., Warshaw, M., Shea, T., & Keller, M. B. (1998). Is the course of panic disorder the same in women and men? *American Journal of Psychiatry, 155*(5), 596–602. *Reprinted with permission from American Journal of Psychiatry,* Copyright © 1998.

Almost all people have experienced a mild form of obsessive–compulsive behavior known as *folie du doute*, consisting of thoughts of uncertainty and *compulsions to check* a previous behavior. Some common forms are setting the alarm clock and checking it before being able to sleep, turning off an appliance and then returning to make sure it is off, and locking the door and then checking to be sure it is locked. People are bothered by uncertainty and have such thoughts as "Are you sure you locked the door?" There is a feeling of subjective compulsion: "You better check to make sure you locked the door." But there is often a resistance to the compulsion: "You don't have to check the door because you know you locked it." The obsessive thoughts continue and anxiety increases until the compulsive behavior is performed.

Jeanine's mother always worried that the house would be set on fire if she forgot to unplug the iron. Now an adult, Jeanine always checks three times that she unplugged the iron before she leaves the laundry room. Her obsessive thoughts focus on the house burning down with her two children in it. Returning to check the iron reduces her fear to manageable levels. If she resists the urge to perform the compulsion, her anxiety mounts until she is forced to check the iron.

When obsessive–compulsive thoughts and behaviors dominate a person's life, the person is described as having **obsessive–compulsive disorder (OCD)**. OCD affects approximately 3% of the U.S. population. Males usually develop this disorder at a younger age (6 to 15 years) than females (20 to 29 years). In one half to two thirds of cases, onset is abrupt following a significant life event. In the other one half to one third of cases onset is gradual (Landsman, Rupertus, & Pedrick, 2005; Szeszko et al., 2004).

The degree of interference in the lives of OCD sufferers can range from slight to incapacitating. Often, there is significant interference with home, school, work, and interpersonal functioning. Once begun, OCD usually runs a lifelong course, waxing and waning in severity, but seldom stopping spontaneously. About 10% of people with OCD are disabled by this illness. Rapoport (1989) describes the severity in terms of time involved in the compulsive behavior:

- *Mild:* Less than 1 hour a day
- *Moderate:* 1 to 3 hours a day
- *Severe:* 3 to 8 hours a day
- *Extreme:* Nearly constant

People with OCD often display *consuming*, and at times bizarre, *behavior*. People with OCD describe their behavior as being forced from within. They say, "I have to. I don't want to, but I have to." Of women with OCD, 90% are compulsive cleaners who have an unreasonable fear of contamination and avoid contact with anything thought to be unclean. They may spend many hours each day washing themselves and cleaning their environment. Cleaning rituals and avoidance of contamination decrease their anxiety and reestablish some sense of safety and control. With increased public awareness of AIDS, one third of people with OCD now cite the fear of AIDS to explain their washing behavior.

Jay feels a drop in his eye as he looks up while passing a building and cannot dismiss the thought that someone with AIDS has spit out of a window. To reassure himself, he proceeds to knock on the door of every office on that side of the building, asking whether anyone there has spit out the window.

Men with OCD are more likely to experience *compulsive checking* behavior, which is often associated with "magical" thinking. They hope to prevent an imagined future disaster by compulsive checking, even though they may recognize it to be irrational.

Other examples of obsessive behavior are arranging and rearranging objects, counting, hoarding, seeking order and precision, and repeating activities such as going in and out of a doorway. The *ritualistic behavior* may become so severe that the person may not be able to work or socialize. Professional help may not be sought until the individual is unable to meet basic needs or the family can no longer tolerate the symptoms (Clark, 2003).

About 10% to 20% of individuals with OCD have **hoarding compulsions**, defined as the acquisition of and inability to discard worthless items. The obsessional fears underlying this behavior are of losing important items that might be needed at a later time, extreme beliefs about the importance of possessions, or an excessive emotional attachment to possessions. People are unable to decide what to keep and what to discard, so they save everything, including newspapers, magazines, old clothing, junk mail, and so on. Living spaces become so cluttered that there may only be paths through the rooms. Since the disorder is egosyntonic, the behavior can be especially troublesome for family members. As living space rapidly decreases, family members are forced to modify their daily activities. Some families acquire additional storage facilities, but these too are soon overrun with clutter. Family members are ashamed of the clutter but have little control over it. Embarrassment over the appearance of the home leads to social isolation of the family. Hoarders often have little insight into their symptoms, making them less likely to seek treatment and more likely to divorce or never marry (Saxena et al., 2004).

Two years after Betty moved in, her two-bedroom condominium was so cluttered with junk mail, newspapers, unfinished craft projects, old clothes, and broken gadgets that the only spot to sit was on one side of the bed. When Betty finally asked a friend for help, he spent 14 hours throwing out her junk—which she reclaimed from the dumpster as soon as he left. She feared that something dreadful would happen if she threw those things away.

BOX 11.1 — Types of Obsessions and Compulsions

Aggressive, Sexual, and Religious Obsessions With Checking Compulsions

- Checking, such as doors, locks, appliances, written work
- Frequent confession (of anything)
- The need to ask others repeatedly for reassurance

Symmetry Obsessions With Ordering, Arranging, and Repeating Compulsions

- The need to have objects in fixed and symmetrical positions
- Repeating movements, such as going in and out of doorways, getting in and out of chairs, touching objects
- Counting or spelling silently or out loud

Contamination Obsessions With Washing and Cleaning Compulsions

- Grooming, such as washing hands, showering, bathing, brushing teeth
- Cleaning personal space

Hoarding, Saving, and Collecting Symptoms

- Compulsive acquisition of items
- Difficulty discarding items
- Extreme clutter

The most common *preoccupations* involve dirt; safety; and violent, sexual, or blasphemous thoughts. There may be magical thinking, false beliefs, superstitions, or religious ideation, the content of which is culturally determined. They say, "No matter how hard I try, I cannot get these thoughts out of my mind." See Box 11.1 for types of obsessions and compulsions.

Ramona has persistent thoughts such as: What if the smell of gasoline gets in my lungs? What if I breathe it in when I am pumping gas and get lung cancer? What if my cat licks the gasoline off my hands? What if she gets sick? What if she dies? What if I spread it to my mom? What if I die?

Some people believe that OCD is really a spectrum disorder, that is, not one disorder but several that exhibit repetitive, unwanted behavior. Spectrum disorders include compulsive shopping; compulsive gambling; other compulsions related to television, computers, and pornography; substance abuse; nail biting; hair pulling; autism; anorexia and bulimia; somatization disorders; paraphilias; stuttering; and tic disorders. People with these disorders exhibit intrusive obsessive thoughts and repetitive behaviors. Other features they share include family history, course of illness, neurobiological alterations, and response to behavioral treatment and medications (Clark, 2003).

Posttraumatic Stress Disorder

People exposed to extremely dangerous and life-threatening situations may develop **posttraumatic stress disorder**

(PTSD). Only a minority of people exposed to extreme stress develop PTSD. Those more vulnerable to the disorder include people with low social support systems, preexisting mental disorders, childhood physical or sexual abuse, childhood separation from parents, and family instability. Additional high-risk factors include physical injury during the event, situations that are more malicious and grotesque, and active involvement versus witnessing the trauma (King, Vogt, & King, 2004).

Symptoms of PTSD usually begin within the first 3 months after the trauma, although there may be a delay of months or in some cases years before symptoms appear. Any time a trauma occurs, the potential to develop PTSD exists. In severe trauma, a person confronts extreme helplessness and terror in the face of possible annihilation. Ordinary coping behaviors are ineffective, action is of no avail, and the person can neither resist nor escape. Some people describe the traumatic events as happening in slow motion, some say the situation seems unreal, like a dream, and some actually feel disconnected from their bodies. This is referred to as *peritraumatic dissociation,* which temporarily protects them from feeling intense fear or pain (Brewin, 2003).

For example, rape, child sexual abuse, and battering involve the use of force by the perpetrator. Whether it is a sudden shock or a repetitive torment, the stress of the assault is inescapable and the result is often PTSD. Disaster workers are also at risk for PTSD, thought to be related to exposure to violent death, severely mutilated bodies, the impact of life-threatening situations, and physically demanding activities.

It is important to understand that people with PTSD are normal people who have experienced abnormal events, such as terrorist attacks, physical or sexual assault, motor vehicle accidents, hostage situations, natural disasters, and military combat. Chapters 22, 23, 24, and 25 ∞ discuss domestic violence, sexual violence, community violence, and terrorism and natural disasters, respectively.

People with PTSD often exhibit a *hyperalertness* resulting from their need to constantly search the environment for danger. Increasing anxiety can cause unpredictably *aggressive* or *bizarre behavior.* PTSD sufferers may resort to abusing drugs or alcohol in an effort to decrease this anticipatory anxiety. They may also behave as if the original trauma were actually recurring. Thus, they may try to defend themselves against a past enemy who is perceived to be in the present. Triggering events create a continuous cycle of reminders. Examples are the anniversary of the crime or event; holidays and family events, especially if a perpetrator is involved; tastes, touches, and smells; and media coverage, such as articles, talk shows, and movies. Many people with PTSD develop a phobic avoidance of the triggers that remind them of the original trauma. *Avoidance* may become so all-encompassing that the person develops a socially isolated lifestyle.

> Holly was robbed and beaten at gunpoint on a Sunday evening as she put her car in her garage. A few days later, she tried to return to work. "I tried to walk to the corner to take the bus and was terrified to walk just half a block for fear I would be assaulted again. When I came home from work, I was terrified again to walk the half block and I cried all the way home. I was afraid to come out of the house after that and would ask family and friends to come and get me when I had to go somewhere. I felt like a prisoner."

Guilt is common with PTSD. When a traumatic event entails the death of others, the guilt stems from the fact that the person survived when others did not. If the person is a war veteran, she or he may feel guilty about the acts she or he was forced to commit to survive combat.

In addition to anxiety, tension, irritability, aggression, and guilt, there can be a *numbing* of other *emotions*. Often, people with PTSD discover they can no longer appreciate previously enjoyed activities. Feeling detached from others, they are unable to be intimate or tender. Obviously, this difficulty contributes to relationship problems.

A sudden, life-threatening trauma often causes people to reevaluate themselves and their experiences. In the face of imminent death, the fantasy of personal immortality is exploded. Confrontation with severe injury or death results in long-lasting changes in a person's thinking patterns.

Memory may be affected by trauma. Memory of the traumatic event may be erased by amnesia, which may vary from a few minutes, to months, to years. Some individuals may have intermittent memories about the trauma that range from quick flashes to entire recollections of the event. Although this experience is distressing, it may be tolerable if the memories are infrequent. Some people, in contrast to amnesia, experience memories that return in the form of unpredictable and uncontrollable *flashbacks*. These memories can be so intrusive and persistent that people become obsessed with them. In a sense, victims of trauma live with ghosts and are haunted by their past. Recurring nightmares, in which the person reexperiences the event, are also common. A person may become preoccupied with thoughts of the trauma recurring. All these cognitive changes contribute to the development of an external locus of control, and PTSD sufferers feel themselves to be at the mercy of the environment.

> Jeanmarc, 35 years old, has a home decorating business. Three months ago he was stabbed in the back by a client while working in her home. The attack was unprovoked, and Jeanmarc did not attempt to defend himself for fear of hurting the woman and thus ending up in prison. His attacker lives in his neighborhood and is now out on bail. He states that since the incident he has been preoccupied with death. His sleep has deteriorated to 2 to 3 hours a night, and he has terrible nightmares. Other symptoms include decreased appetite, a 20-pound weight loss, decreased concentration, listlessness, decreased sex drive, headaches, and diarrhea. Prior to the event, he lived by himself in an apartment. Since the attack, he has moved in with his sis-

> ter and her three children. His relationships with both his sister and his girlfriend are strained due to his recurrent symptoms.

Another cognitive characteristic that may accompany PTSD is *self-devaluation*. For some, the sense of self is shattered, while for others it is not allowed to develop at all. Repetitive childhood trauma interferes with the developmental organization of the personality. Being treated like an object results in feelings of dehumanization. A rape survivor may be influenced by cultural myths and begin to believe she was responsible for the act of violence committed against her. Survivors of disasters often feel guilty, believing that other, more capable people deserve to live more than they do. Upon returning from Vietnam, many veterans were assailed by society's reproach and indifference. This devaluation became a part of the self-image of many veterans. Studies on Vietnam veterans show that 15% of all male veterans suffer from PTSD many years after the war experience. The same longterm effect is also true for nurses who served in Vietnam. About 8.5% suffered from and continue to suffer from PTSD. Soldiers and nurses who have survived serving in Afghanistan and Iraq are returning home with PTSD (Finke, 2003; Perkonigg et al., 2005).

Acute Stress Disorder

Many people who experience or witness an extreme traumatic stressor develop **acute stress disorder**. During or shortly after the trauma, these individuals may feel numb and emotionally nonresponsive, have a decreased awareness of their environment, and may experience amnesia for part, or all, of the event. Like PTSD sufferers, they often experience recurrent images and flashbacks, which contribute to the avoidance of stimuli that remind them of the trauma. These events cause significant distress and impair activities of daily living. Acute stress disorder begins within a month of the traumatic event, lasts at least 2 days, and goes away within 4 weeks. If symptoms persist beyond 4 weeks, the person is given the diagnosis of PTSD.

Dissociative Disorders

Dissociation is defined in the *Diagnostic and Statistical Manual of Mental Disorders* (4th ed., Text Revision) (DSM-IV-TR) (APA, 2000) as a disruption in the usually integrated functions of consciousness, memory, identity, and perception of the environment. Dissociative symptoms exist along a continuum ranging from common experiences such as daydreaming and lapses in attention to a pathological failure to integrate thoughts, feelings, and actions.

Dissociative disorders are characterized by an alteration in conscious awareness of behavior, affect, thoughts and memories, and identity, particularly in the consistency of personality. The alteration in identity may be identity loss or the presence of more than one identity. Regardless of the type of dissociative

DSM-IV-TR   Diagnostic Criteria for Anxiety Disorders

Diagnostic Criteria for Panic Disorder Without Agoraphobia and Panic Disorder With Agoraphobia

A. Both 1 and 2:
1. Recurrent unexpected Panic Attacks
2. At least one of the attacks has been followed by 1 month (or more) of one (or more) of the following:
   a. Persistent concern about having additional attacks
   b. Worry about the implications of the attack or its consequences (e.g., losing control, having a heart attack, "going crazy")
   c. A significant change in behavior related to the attacks

B. The presence of Agoraphobia (for 300.21 Panic Disorder With Agoraphobia)
OR
The absence of Agoraphobia (for 300.01 Panic Disorder Without Agoraphobia)

C. The Panic Attacks are not due to the direct physiological effects of a substance (e.g., a drug of abuse, a medication) or a general medical condition (e.g., hyperthyroidism).

D. The Panic Attacks are not better accounted for by another mental disorder, such as Social Phobia (e.g., occurring on exposure to feared social situations), Specific Phobia (e.g., on exposure to a specific phobic situation), Obsessive–Compulsive Disorder (e.g., on exposure to dirt in someone with an obsession about contamination), Posttraumatic Stress Disorder (e.g., in response to stimuli associated with a severe stressor), or Separation Anxiety Disorder (e.g., in response to being away from home or close relatives).

Diagnostic Criteria for Obsessive–Compulsive Disorder

A. Either obsessions or compulsions:

Obsessions as defined by 1, 2, 3, and 4:
1. Recurrent and persistent thoughts, impulses, or images that are experienced, at some time during the disturbance, as intrusive and inappropriate and that cause marked anxiety or distress
2. The thoughts, impulses, or images are not simply excessive worries about real-life problems

3. The person attempts to ignore or suppress such thoughts, impulses, or images, or to neutralize them with some other thought or action
4. The person recognizes that the obsessional thoughts, impulses, or images are a product of his or her own mind (not imposed from without as in thought insertion)

Compulsions as defined by 1 and 2:
1. Repetitive behaviors (e.g., hand washing, ordering, checking) or mental acts (e.g., praying, counting, repeating words silently) that the person feels driven to perform in response to an obsession, or according to rules that must be applied rigidly
2. The behaviors or mental acts are aimed at preventing or reducing distress or preventing some dreaded event or situation; however, these behaviors or mental acts either are not connected in a realistic way with what they are designed to neutralize or prevent or are clearly excessive

B. At some point during the course of the disorder, the person has recognized that the obsessions or compulsions are excessive or unreasonable. Note: This does not apply to children.

C. The obsessions or compulsions cause marked distress, are time consuming (take more than 1 hour a day); or significantly interfere with the person's normal routine, occupational (or academic) functioning, or usual social activities or relationships.

D. If another Axis I disorder is present, the content of the obsessions or compulsions is not restricted to it (e.g., preoccupation with food in the presence of an Eating Disorder; hair pulling in the presence of Trichotillomania; concern with appearance in the presence of Body Dysmorphic Disorder; preoccupation with drugs in the presence of a Substance Use Disorder; preoccupation with having a serious illness in the presence of Hypochondriasis; preoccupation with sexual urges or fantasies in the presence of a Paraphilia; or guilty ruminations in the presence of Major Depressive Disorder).

E. The disturbance is not due to the direct physiological effects of a substance (e.g., a drug of abuse, a medication) or a general medical condition.

Specify if:
With Poor Insight: if, for most of the time during the current episode, the person does not recognize that the obsessions and compulsions are excessive or unreasonable

Diagnostic Criteria for Anxiety Disorders

Diagnostic Criteria for Posttraumatic Stress Disorder

A. The person has been exposed to a traumatic event in which both the following were present:
1. The person experienced, witnessed, or was confronted with an event or events that involved actual or threatened death or serious injury, or a threat to the physical integrity of self or others
2. The person's response involved intense fear, helplessness, or horror. Note: In children, this may be expressed instead by disorganized or agitated behavior.

B. The traumatic event is persistently re-experienced in one (or more) of the following ways:
1. Recurrent and intrusive distressing recollections of the event, including images, thoughts, or perceptions. Note: In young children, repetitive play may occur in which themes or aspects of the trauma are expressed.
2. Recurrent distressing dreams of the event. Note: In children, there may be frightening dreams without recognizable content.
3. Acting or feeling as if the traumatic event were recurring (includes a sense of reliving the experience, illusions, hallucinations, and dissociative flashback episodes, including those that occur on awakening or when intoxicated). Note: In young children, trauma-specific reenactment may occur.
4. Intense psychological distress at exposure to internal or external cues that symbolize or resemble an aspect of the traumatic event

continued

DSM-IV-TR Diagnostic Criteria for Anxiety Disorders—(continued)

5. Physiological reactivity on exposure to internal or external cues that symbolize or resemble an aspect of the traumatic event

C. Persistent avoidance of stimuli associated with the trauma and numbing of general responsiveness (not present before the trauma), as indicated by three (or more) of the following:
1. Efforts to avoid thoughts, feelings, or conversations associated with the trauma
2. Efforts to avoid activities, places, or people that arouse recollections of the trauma
3. Inability to recall an important aspect of the trauma
4. Markedly diminished interest or participation in significant activities

5. Feeling of detachment or estrangement from others
6. Restricted range of affect (e.g., unable to have loving feelings)
7. Sense of a foreshortened future (e.g., does not expect to have a career, marriage, children, or a normal life span)

D. Persistent symptoms of increased arousal (not present before the trauma), as indicated by two (or more) of the following:
1. Difficulty falling or staying asleep
2. Irritability or outbursts of anger
3. Difficulty concentrating
4. Hypervigilance
5. Exaggerated startle response

E. Duration of the disturbance (symptoms in Criteria B, C, and D) is more than 1 month.

F. The disturbance causes clinically significant distress or impairment in social, occupational, or other important areas of functioning.

Specify if:
Acute: if duration of symptoms is less than 3 months
Chronic: if duration of symptoms is 3 months or more

Specify if:
With Delayed Onset: if onset of symptoms is at least 6 months after the stressor.

SOURCE: American Psychiatric Association. (2000). *Diagnostic and statistical manual of mental disorders* (4th ed., Text Revision) (pp. 440–441, 462, 463, 467–468). Washington, DC: Author. Reprinted with permission.

---

disorder, all sufferers at times demonstrate behavior different from their usual behavior. Dissociative disorders are often precipitated by a traumatic event, such as a disaster, rape, or war (Simeon, Guralnik, Knutelska, & Schmeidler, 2002).

Dissociative Amnesia **Dissociative amnesia**, memory loss not caused by an organic problem, is usually related to an acute, precipitating, traumatic event. The most common type is *localized amnesia*, in which memory loss occurs for a specific time related to the trauma. *Selective amnesia* is localized for a specific time, with partial memory of events during that time. The least common types of psychogenic amnesia are *generalized amnesia*, a complete loss of memory of one's past, and *continuous amnesia*, in which memory loss begins at a particular point in time and continues to the present.

Yuki's firstborn child died of sudden infant death syndrome 3 months ago. Although she remembers arriving in the emergency department with her baby, she continues to have no memory of finding him in his crib, calling the paramedics, or hearing the doctor telling her that her baby was dead.

Dissociative Fugue **Dissociative fugue** is a rare dissociative disorder in which people, while either maintaining their identity or adopting a new identity, wander or take unexpected trips. The disorder is often precipitated by subacute, chronic stress. The episode may last several hours or several days. During the fugue state, these people may appear either normal or disoriented and confused; they usually behave in ways inconsistent with their usual personality and values. The fugue state often ends abruptly, and there is either partial or complete amnesia for that period. Dissociative amnesia and dissociative fugue both are most commonly seen during war and in the aftermath of disasters.

Depersonalization Disorder **Depersonalization disorder** is characterized by persistent or recurrent feelings of being detached from one's body or thoughts. People describe feeling like robots, being an outside observer of their bodies or thoughts, or feeling like they are living in a dream. They remain oriented to reality in that they know they are not really robots or living in a dream. The incidence and prevalence of this disorder are unknown as it is one of the least studied dissociative conditions. It is thought to result from emotional abuse in childhood; the more severe the abuse, the more severe the symptoms. Depersonalization disorder usually begins in adolescence and is often not responsive to therapy or medication (Michal et al., 2005).

Dissociative Identity Disorder **Dissociative identity disorder (DID)**, formerly multiple-personality disorder, is the most severe form of dissociative disorders. This diagnosis is given when at least two personalities exist in the same person. Each personality, or *alter*, is integrated and complex; that is, each has its own memory, value structure, behavioral pattern, and primary affective expression. The host personality, which is the original personality, has at best only a partial awareness of the alters. People with DID suffer from an alteration in conscious awareness of their total being.

Efrain has been working for several years with Judith in outpatient therapy. Over a period of time he has been introduced to the following personalities within her "family" system:

Judith—35 years old, married, one son; very traditional, good housekeeper, attends church regularly, dresses in a careful and "proper" manner; good at art, draws with right hand. Role in the "family" is to be responsible.

Little Judy—5 years old; gentle, shy, playful; likes to draw "pretty" pictures, draws with her left hand. Role in the "family" is to serve as a distraction when there is too much pain and fear.

Mary—14 years old; assertive and outgoing; does not attend church, does not like housework, prefers to wear blue jeans and T-shirts; very knowledgeable about drugs; assumes large gaps of missing time related to drug use. Role in the "family" is the "party animal," able to have fun and play with peers.

Sue—15 years old; has a chip-on-the-shoulder, I-don't-care attitude; out only at night; sees self as totally separate from the "family"; plans to use men as she has been used. Role in the "family" is to try to understand sexuality, express anger for entire family.

Gail—powerful and wise; knows all the personalities and is known by all the others; position of trust in the "family"; role is as a spiritual guide to everyone. Sometimes Judith finds herself at one of Mary's parties, wearing blue jeans and a sweatshirt. At times Mary finds herself sitting in church wearing a dress; both Judith and Mary are horrified by these experiences.

Recent reports agree that the origin of DID is severe, sadistic, often sexual, child abuse. The abusive incidents are repeated over time and inconsistently alternate with expressions of care and concern from the abuser. Another factor may be the secrecy and denial associated with this form of abuse. Subjectively, the child lives in a fragmented reality, and social support is limited because traumatization occurs through exactly the persons on whom the child is dependent.

In DID, the defense mechanisms of *repression* and *dissociation* are used to manage the anxiety, rage, and helplessness the child experiences in response to severe abuse. The only way for these people to survive the pain of the trauma is to eliminate it from conscious awareness. Dissociation is accomplished by self-hypnosis, which correlates with the onset of the abuse. This soon becomes the dominant method of managing severe stress, and people with DID are able to quickly and spontaneously enter hypnotic trances. What is a life-saving process in childhood becomes a self-destructive tool in adulthood.

Somatoform Disorders

The **somatoform disorders**—somatization, conversion, pain disorder, hypochondriasis, and body dysmorphic disorder—all involve physical symptoms for which no underlying organic basis exists. Common to all these disorders is dysfunction of physical self-awareness. Somatoform disorder sufferers are *obsessively interested in bodily processes* and diseases. Almost all their attention is focused on the discomfort they are experiencing. So obsessed are they with their bodies that they are constantly aware of very small physical changes and discomforts that would go unnoticed by others. In hypochondriasis, these changes are regarded as concrete evidence of an active disease process. They are highly resistant to reassurance from health care providers. Information, education, and explanation only temporarily lessen their disease fears.

Conversion disorders are rare, but the other somatoform disorders are frequently seen in community settings, health care offices, and acute care units. These three disorders account for a large portion of the medical expense in the United States. It is estimated that 4% to 18% of all physician visits are made by the "worried well." People with these disorders truly suffer; they must not be discounted as malingerers or manipulators. The nurse can often provide a long-term caring relationship, which may be the most important intervention in preventing needless tests, medications, and surgeries. When people with somatoform disorders feel that no one is listening to or caring for them, they often go from one health care professional to another, duplicating tests and medical interventions. By being knowledgeable and sensitive, the nurse can protect these clients by keeping them within one health care system.

Somatization Disorder People diagnosed with a **somatization disorder** have multiple physical complaints involving a variety of body systems. This is a chronic disorder that usually begins in the teenage years and is identified more often in women than in men. Men may express symptoms of the disorder less dramatically, or perhaps physicians have been less likely to perceive men as having multiple unexplained somatic symptoms.

In the past year, Dorothy has been seen by eight health care providers, including her family physician, a cardiologist, an internist, an orthopedist, a chiropractor, a proctologist, and a cancer diagnostician. After extensive and repeated testing, no evidence of organic disease was found. Dorothy continues to complain about the incompetence of these people and is in the process of finding new health care providers.

Conversion Disorder A **conversion disorder**, characterized by the presence of deficits in voluntary motor or sensory functions, can appear at any age but typically begins and ends abruptly. It is usually precipitated by a severe trauma such as war or childhood abuse. Sensory symptoms range from paresthesia and anesthesia to blindness and deafness. Motor symptoms range from gait disturbances to seizures to paralysis.

Some people with conversion disorders exhibit *la belle indifference*, a relative lack of concern for their physical symptoms. People showing a sudden onset of symptoms, even severe ones like paralysis or blindness, sometimes seem nonchalant about their condition. This reaction usually occurs in people who do not want to be noticed by others. But others with conversion disorders may be very verbal about their distress over the sudden appearance of symptoms. This reaction is more likely to occur in people with a high need for attention and sympathy.

Pain Disorder Pain that cannot be explained organically is the primary symptom of a **pain disorder**. Unconscious conflict and anxiety are believed to be the basis for the pain. The pain may severely disrupt the person's life, and inadvertent substance abuse may occur.

MediaLink

MediaLink Application, Somatoform Disorders

Hypochondriasis People with **hypochondriasis** believe they have a serious disease involving one body system, despite all medical evidence to the contrary, or they are terrified of contracting certain diseases. These people are extremely sensitive to internal sensations, which they misinterpret as evidence of disease. This disorder usually begins in midlife or late in life and affects women and men equally.

Ray is convinced that he has AIDS in spite of all negative diagnostic test results. He is not reassured by the fact that he is at low risk because of having been in a monogamous relationship for 20 years, having never used intravenous drugs, and having never had a blood transfusion. He is hyperalert to all slight variations in bodily function and regards these normal variations as evidence of AIDS.

Body Dysmorphic Disorder **Body dysmorphic disorder** is a serious long-term, and often disabling, condition. The prevalence is not well known because it is believed that people underreport their symptoms because of shame. Body dysmorphic disorder is a preoccupation with an imagined or slight defect in physical appearance. The most common concerns involve the face—facial skin, nose, and hair. As with those suffering from eating disorders, there is a lot of concern with bodily appearance. The disorder is probably related to OCD in that their thoughts are intrusive and they compulsively check their body appearance. They may avoid social and work activities because of embarrassment, leading to social isolation. They experience feelings of low self-esteem, shame, and worthlessness, which may lead to suicidal thoughts and attempts (Carroll, Scahill & Phillips, 2002).

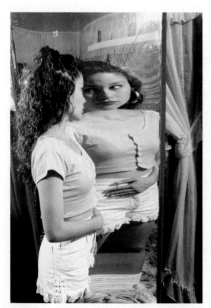

PHOTO 11.2 ■ Body dysmorphic disorder is characterized by a preoccupation with some imagined defect in appearance.
SOURCE: Tony Freeman/PhotoEdit, Inc.

Factitious Disorder

Individuals are diagnosed with **factitious disorder** when they intentionally simulate or produce physical or psychological symptoms in order to assume the sick role. *Subjective* complaints may concern feeling unwell or the presence of pain. They may ingest psychoactive substances to produce symptoms such as restlessness, insomnia, or hallucinations. Examples of falsified *objective* signs are hematuria (by ingesting anticoagulants), fever (manipulating a thermometer), self-inflicted conditions (injecting toxic substances such as poisons or own urine or feces; creating bruises, lesions, or other injuries consistent with illness), or an exaggeration of a preexisting condition (feigning a hypoglycemic attack with a history of diabetes). They may present with predominantly physical complaints, predominantly psychological complaints, or with combined complaints. The most severe and chronic form of this disorder is referred to as *Munchausen syndrome*. (See chapter 22 ∞ for Munchausen syndrome by proxy as a form of child abuse.)

People with factitious disorder usually present in a dramatic manner but are extremely vague and inconsistent during the medical history. When extensive workups demonstrate no underlying disease, they may complain of other problems and new symptoms. The only motivation for the behavior is to assume the sick role and gain attention. Factitious disorder usually consists of intermittent episodes with an onset in early adulthood (APA, 2000).

Malingering

Malingering is similar to factitious disorder in that the individual intentionally produces false physical or psychological symptoms. Unlike factitious disorder, the motivation in malingering is external incentives such as getting sick leave from work, obtaining financial compensation, evading criminal prosecution, or obtaining drugs.

Comorbid Disorders

There is a high correlation between anxiety disorders and *substance abuse.* As many as 50% to 60% of those who abuse substances also have one of the anxiety disorders. Typically, severe anxiety precedes the onset of the substance abuse, although for some the abuse precedes the anxiety. People with anxiety disorders often self-medicate to feel better because they believe that alcohol decreases anxiety. In fact, alcohol actually increases anxiety. The combination of increased anxiety, addiction, and continued self-medication contributes to an ever increasing self-destructive cycle (Sukhodolsky et al., 2005).

Frequently, *depression* follows the onset of an anxiety disorder. It is thought that depression and anxiety disorders share a common biological predisposition, which may be activated by stress. Comorbidity between anxiety disorders and major depression is associated with more impairment than either anxiety or depression alone and predicts poorer outcomes. The depression may be a response to feelings of loss of control, hopelessness, helplessness, decreased self-esteem, and severe restrictions on lifestyle. Suicide can be a lethal complication. People with panic attacks and PTSD have high rates of suicidality (Ghaemi, 2004; Leonard, Brann, & Tiller, 2005).

Children with anxiety disorders often struggle with depression, attention deficit disorders, oppositional behaviors, and peer deficits. An anxious child is less likely to have friends or even to develop relationships with peers. It is possible that feeling anxious and alone leads to depression. Some behaviors of anxious children, such as fidgeting and distractibility, are also criteria for attention deficit disorder. Anxious children often exhibit oppositional behavior such as tantrums, refusal to do things, and arguing with authority. See chapter 17 ∞ for more information on these spectrum disorders.

Some medical conditions are associated with high levels of anxiety. Restless leg syndrome is a common cause of insomnia and anxiety. Other conditions include multiple sclerosis, brain attack, and early Alzheimer disease. PANDAS (pediatric autoimmune neuropsychiatric disorder) associated with streptococcal infections can cause OCD. See chapter 20 ∞ for further information on PANDAS.

OCD may also be related to autoimmune diseases such as rheumatic fever and lupus as well as brain tumors and head trauma (Landsman et al., 2005; Stein & Hugo, 2004).

Etiologies

No single theory can adequately explain the cause and maintenance of any of the anxiety disorders. They are best understood as a complex interaction of neurobiological and environmental factors.

Genetics

Based on studies of twins, the heritability for anxiety disorders is 30% to 40%. These genetic influences appear to be general rather than disorder-specific; that is, people inherit a general predisposition toward anxiety. Anxious behaviors are often identified at an early age. Mothers of clinically diagnosed anxious children report that these children cried more and had difficulty sleeping during the first year of life and experienced more fears than other children during the second

year of life. Shyness and social phobia seem to be related to a gene involved with the serotonin transporter system (Arbelle et al., 2003; Hudson & Rapee, 2004).

Social phobia clusters in families and has a significant genetic component estimated at 51%. The more severe the disorder, the stronger the genetic influence. The norepinephrine (NE) transporter gene on chromosome 16 is the most likely candidate. The NE transporter takes NE and dopamine back into the presynaptic neurons, ending that particular neurotransmission. Studies of twins suggest that there is a significant heritable component in panic disorder and generalized anxiety disorder, with the concordance rate of 35% for monozygotic twins and only 6% to 12% for dizygotic twins (Gelernter et al., 2004).

Research in OCD focuses on a number of vulnerability genes. In OCD, children and adults experience identical symptoms, whereas in most of the other mental disorders, children's symptoms are different from those of adults. In addition, 50% of adults with OCD state that their symptoms began when they were children; whereas only 5% of adults with other mental disorders state that their symptoms began in childhood. Of OCD sufferers, 20% have a first-degree relative with the same problem. It is unlikely that the behavior is learned within the family, given the high level of secrecy. In addition, children and parents may have very different rituals; for example, the parent may engage in checking rituals, whereas the child may engage in washing rituals. Compulsive hoarding has a more distinctive pattern of genetic influence than the other forms of OCD, which may explain the poorer prognosis with hoarding symptoms. Body dysmorphic disorder may be related to OCD. Four percent of first-degree relatives of people with OCD experience body dysmorphic disorder, compared with only 1% of the control group's first-degree relatives (Carroll et al., 2002; Saxena et al., 2004).

Neurobiology

Some believe anxious individuals have an overly responsive autonomic nervous system related to a *dysfunction of serotonin* (5-HT), *NE, dopamine* (DA), and *GABA* (gamma aminobutyric acid) neurotransmission. A hyperactive autonomic nervous system may be responsible for the characteristics of high levels of anxiety such as impulsiveness, agitation, restlessness, sleep and cognitive disturbances, and aggression. People with panic disorder and PTSD suffer from an *abnormally sensitive fear network* that includes the amygdala, hippocampus, and other brain stem areas. The oversensitivity means that the brain is instantly hyperaroused by fearful stimuli, with the cortex so overwhelmed that it is unable to focus (Olszewski & Varrasse, 2005; Warden & Labbate, 2005).

There appear to be biological changes in PTSD that illustrate the influence of psychological events on neurobiology. When high levels of adrenaline and other stress hormones are circulating, *memory traces* are deeply imprinted. These are then reactivated as if the traumatic event were actually occurring. Each time the traumatic experience is recalled, the amygdala releases more stress hormones and intensifies the stressful memories even more. Traumatic nightmares can occur in stages of sleep in which people do not ordinarily dream. Thus, traumatic memories appear to be based in altered neurophysiological organization. People with PTSD tend to have low levels of the stress hormone cortisol but have an overabundance of epinephrine and NE, which could be why they continue to feel anxious after the trauma. In addition, they tend to have higher than normal levels of corticotropin-releasing factor (CRF), which switches on the stress response and may explain why people with PTSD startle so easily (Lanius et al., 2004).

Panic attacks often occur in areas such as restaurants, elevators, cars, and planes, where there is an *increased concentration* of people and *carbon dioxide* (CO_2). Fresh air has a CO_2 level of 300 parts per million (ppm). In cars, the CO_2 level reaches 750 ppm, and in elevators and planes it reaches as high as 900 ppm. As CO_2 increases in the brain, neurons in the brain stem activate and send signals to the locus coeruleus, which increases the release of NE, leading to the fight-or-flight response. Stimulants that alter NE transmission (including caffeine, cocaine, and amphetamines) can precipitate panic attacks. It is believed that some biological vulnerability is present, which—when combined with certain psychological, social, and environmental events—leads to the development of panic disorder (Kent et al., 2001).

Positron-emission tomography (PET) and magnetic resonance imaging (MRI) provide evidence of neurologic deficit in many individuals with OCD. The abnormality apparently lies in a pathway that links the orbitofrontal cortex with the basal ganglia. Heightened activity in the cortex may reflect obsessional thinking, while compulsions may originate in the basal ganglia where body movements are planned and executed. Individuals with OCD have impairment in executive functioning located in the frontal lobes. They are unable to process all the features of a situation and therefore are unable to set goals and plan strategies. This dysfunction contributes to automatic, repetitive behaviors (Clark, 2003; Mataix-Cols, Rosario-Campos, & Leckman, 2005).

Little is known about the biology of depersonalization disorder. PET demonstrates higher than normal glucose metabolism in portions of the *sensory cortex* in the temporal, parietal, and occipital lobes. Normally, it is in these areas where visual and somatosensory information is integrated to provide an intact, well-integrated body image (Simeon et al., 2000).

Intrapersonal Factors

Intrapersonal theorists view anxiety disorders as a reaction to anticipated future danger based on past experiences such as separation, loss of love, and guilt. The resulting anxiety is pushed out of conscious awareness by the use of *defense mechanisms*, such as repression, projection, displacement, or symbolization. As stress increases, the defenses become increasingly inefficient, symptoms develop, and the person engages in repeated self-defeating behavior.

In dissociative disorders, stressful life events are disowned and kept out of conscious awareness by *amnesia*. For example, a young girl who is abused physically and sexually by her father remains dependent on her family system. The perpetrator is a trusted parent, and the other parent is incapable of protecting or rescuing her from the situation. The trauma of abuse leaves the child terrified, depressed, angry, and filled with shame and guilt. Dissociating the abuse and denying the events enable the child to remain in the family with the least amount of pain.

People suffering from anxiety disorders often have an *external locus of control*. They regard life events as out of their control, occurring by luck, chance, or fate. When stressful events occur, they attribute the feeling of anxiety not to themselves, but to external sources, which then can be phobically avoided.

Adaptation to stress and anxiety depends to some extent on *personality traits*, which determine how one views stress and determines the coping activities that follow. For example, individuals with negative expectations may have less successful coping strategies when confronted with high levels of anxiety. Other people fear anxiety-related sensations and believe that these sensations have harmful consequences. For example, a person may fear that the sensation of palpitations indicates a heart attack. According to *expectancy theory*, such a person may become anxious whenever this symptom is experienced and may tend to avoid activities or places that are believed to bring it on.

The tendency to react to stressful situations with somatic complaints may be part of an *avoidant coping style*. The original source of anxiety is unrecognized, and the discomfort is experienced as physical symptoms or disorders. Somatoform disorders may also be unconscious expressions of anger in those unable to communicate such feelings directly. Because physical distress provides an acceptable excuse for avoiding certain activities and situations, people may unconsciously use physical limitations to *rationalize* their inadequacies.

Interpersonal Factors

Interpersonal theorists believe people with anxiety disorders become anxious when they sense or fear disapproval from significant others. They may feel trapped in unpleasant circumstances, believing they are unable to leave the situation. Fearing abandonment, they are unable to behave assertively during conflict. Thus, the anxiety experienced during *interpersonal conflict* is displaced onto the immediate surroundings, thereby allowing them to deny the interpersonal problem. Obsessive–compulsive or phobic behavior protects the self and the relationship during interactions with significant others.

Interpersonal theories focus on the *secondary gains* for people suffering from somatoform disorders. For those with a high degree of dependency, physical symptoms may receive a great deal of attention and support from significant others. The sympathy and nurturing these people receive may be a major factor in maintaining the disorders. The attention from others may be viewed as seeking reassurance of care and love or, since sick or weak people are often in a position of power, as an unconscious attempt to gain power and control.

Cognitive Theory

Cognitive theorists believe symptoms develop from ideas and thoughts. On the basis of limited events, people with anxiety disorders magnify the significance of the past and overgeneralize the future. They become preoccupied with impending disaster and self-defeating statements. These *cognitive expectations* then determine reactions to, and behavior in, various situations (Pennington, 2002).

Cognitive theory explains phobic disorders in a three-part sequence:

1. Phobic people have negative thoughts that increase anxiety and actually precede the feeling of fear in the phobic situation. Phobic people think irrationally and have unrealistic expectations about what might occur if they encounter the phobic situation.
2. These anticipatory thoughts and feelings enhance the physiological arousal level even before the person encounters the phobic situation.
3. The physiological arousal level is misinterpreted. Although thought to be caused by an external object or situation, the arousal is caused by the negative thoughts and *irrational expectations*. This mislabeling of feelings causes phobic people to displace the feelings onto objects or situations that can be avoided.

Learning Theory

Phobias may be *learned* from significant others. If a child observes a parent experiencing anxiety in certain situations, the child may learn that anxiety is the appropriate response. For example, if the mother has a phobic avoidance of elevators, the child soon learns to fear entering an elevator. A child can also learn parental fears through information given by the parent. A father may talk about the dangers of going outside when it is dark, and the child may develop agoraphobia during the nighttime.

People who develop dissociative disorders often consider themselves passive and helpless. They are fearful of others' anger and aggressive behavior. Unable to behave assertively or aggressively, they learn to cope by escaping or avoiding the anxiety-producing situations. Thus, they learn to avoid pain through *amnesia* or developing dissociative identities.

Behavioral Theory

Closely related to learning theory is the behavioral theory of how phobic disorders develop. Behavioral theorists believe phobias are *conditioned, learned responses.* Classic conditioning occurs when a stimulus results in anxiety or pain. The person then develops a fear of that particular stimulus. An example is a person who fears all dogs after being bitten by one dog. The learning component of behavioral theory states that the avoidance of the phobic object or situation is reinforced negatively by a decrease in anxiety. Because the person experiences less anxiety when avoiding the object or situation, avoidance becomes a habitual response.

Behavioral theorists view OCD as learned responses to anticipatory anxiety. It is thought that people with OCD always expect bad things to happen and worry constantly. The compulsive behaviors and thoughts are maladaptive attempts to reduce anxiety.

According to behavioral theory, the somatoform disorders are learned somatic responses. It is thought that these individuals are unable to deal directly with stress and habitually respond to stress with physical sensations or symptoms.

Gender-Bias Factors

Gender-bias theory is used to explain the disproportionate number of women who experience agoraphobia. These theorists believe women have been reinforced to behave *dependently, passively,* and *submissively.* This behavior often results in adult women who are unable to assume responsibility for themselves and who view themselves as incompetent and helpless. Often, the symptoms are reinforced by family members who also have been socialized to expect women to be helpless and dependent. Thus, the pattern of withdrawal can continue until the woman is completely homebound.

In the general population in North America, women and men both are exposed to multiple traumas. Women are more often exposed to indirect, sexual, and domestic violence whereas men are more often exposed to direct threats and military and civilian violence. Although the trauma to women could be considered less severe direct trauma, women are more likely than men to develop PTSD. This trend, however, reverses when veterans are studied. In Vietnam veterans, twice as many men than women developed PTSD. With more women being exposed to combat experiences in current wars, it is anticipated that the numbers will be fairly equal (Punamaki, Komproe, Qouta, Elmasri, & de Jong, 2005).

Psychopharmacological Interventions

Medications are often used on a short-term basis to help people manage anxiety disorders (see Table 11.4 ■). Antidepressants are the mainstay for pharmacological treatment of

TABLE 11.4	Medications Commonly Used to Treat Anxiety Disorders

Generic Name	Trade Name	Disorders
Antianxiety Agents		
buspirone	BuSpar	GAD, panic disorder, agoraphobia, PTSD
alprazolam	Xanax	PTSD
Tricyclic Antidepressants		
imipramine	Tofranil	GAD, agoraphobia
Selective Serotonin Reuptake Inhibitors (SSRIs)		
citalopram	Celexa	Panic disorder, OCD, GAD, body dysmorphic
escitalopram	Lexapro	disorder, social phobia, PTSD
fluoxetine	Prozac	
fluvoxamine	Luvox	
paroxetine	Paxil	
sertraline	Zoloft	
Serotonin-Norepinephrine Inhibitors (SNRIs)		
venlafaxine	Effexor	Anxiety associated with depression, GAD
duloxetine	Cymbalta	
Monoamine Oxidase Inhibitors (MAOIs)		
phenelzine	Nardil	Social phobia, agoraphobia
beta-Blockers		
atenolol	Tenormin	Social phobia (given before the event), PTSD
propranolol	Inderal	
Anticonvulsants		
levetiracetam	Keppra	Social anxiety disorder
Antihypertensives		
prazosin	Minipress	PTSD
Antibiotics		
cycloserine	Seromycin	Phobias

anxiety disorders. They are effective for a wide range of symptoms and have minimal abuse potential.

In GAD, the therapeutic goal in using antianxiety agents is to limit unpleasant symptoms to help the person return to a high level of functioning. Venlafaxine (Effexor) and escitalopram (Lexapro), selective norepinephrine reuptake inhibitor (SNRI) antidepressants, have Food and Drug Administration (FDA) approval for use in GAD. For clients who do not respond to the SNRIs, the addition of olanzapine (Zyprexa), an antipsychotic, may be helpful. Another medication choice is the nonbenzodiazepine antianxiety agent buspirone (BuSpar),

which is more effective than the benzodiazepines in managing GAD. Buspirone blocks 5-HT receptors and causes minimal sedation. This medication is better than the benzodiazepines for the addiction-prone and self-medicating–prone person because dosage increases result in a general sense of feeling ill. In addition, buspirone reacts only minimally with alcohol because it interacts very little with other central nervous system (CNS) depressants. However, clients should be cautioned not to expect an immediate effect.

Because anxiety may be related to a dysregulation of 5-HT and NE, tricyclic antidepressants have been used in the medical treatment of GAD. Imipramine (Tofranil) is the most effective medication in this group.

Selective serotonin reuptake inhibitors (SSRIs) are rapidly becoming the first-line medication treatment for panic disorder. The goal of treatment is to reduce the intensity and frequency of panic attacks, decrease anticipatory anxiety, and treat the associated depression. Typically, it takes 4 weeks before a therapeutic response occurs, but some people will not experience a full response for 8 to 12 weeks. Combining an antidepressant with an antianxiety agent (benzodiazepines) provides for rapid stabilization of panic symptoms (Pollack, 2005).

Social phobias severe enough to interfere with social and occupational functioning may be treated with paroxetine (Paxil), an FDA-approved antidepressant for social phobias. Paroxetine does not eliminate the anxiety but controls it enough that other interventions are more effective. Levetiracetam (Keppra), an anticonvulsant, is also effective for social phobias (Simon et al., 2004).

Social phobias severe enough to interfere with occupational functioning may be treated with a beta-blocker, either propranolol (Inderal) or atenolol (Tenormin). Beta-blockers are particularly effective in situations in which cardiovascular symptoms of anxiety are disruptive to the individual. Because they do not cross the blood–brain barrier, beta-blockers have no effect on neurotransmission, nor do they produce loss of fine motor control.

Cycloserine (Seromycin) is an antibiotic used in the treatment of tuberculosis. It has also been shown to reduce fear in people who suffer from specific phobias. It is used in combination with behavioral exposure therapy (Ressler et al., 2004).

The following SSRIs are often effective in the treatment of OCD: fluoxetine (Prozac), sertraline (Zoloft), fluvoxamine (Luvox), citalopram (Celexa), and paroxetine (Paxil). Of people suffering from OCD, 70% to 80% respond to these medications. The drug riluzole (Rilutek), used to treat amyotrophic lateral sclerosis, may help individuals who do not respond to SSRIs. Antipsychotic medications such as risperidone (Risperdal) and quetiapine (Seroquel) may also be helpful for people who do not respond to SSRIs. Compulsive hoarding syndrome usually does not respond to SSRIs or any other medications (Carroll et al., 2002; Coric et al., 2005).

Probably the most useful drugs for people with PTSD are antidepressants, which not only relieve depression, but also improve sleep and suppress intrusive thoughts, jumpiness, and explosive anger. Sertraline (Zoloft) and paroxetine (Paxil) are the only FDA-approved drugs for PTSD. The beta-blockers propranolol (Inderal) and atenolol (Tenormin) may reduce the restlessness and anxiety by depressing the sympathetic nervous system. Propranolol interferes with the amygdala's receptors, which "turns down" the intensity of the traumatic memory. Prazosin (Minipress), an antihypertensive, seems to counteract the excessive brain activity in PTSD.

Sertraline (Zoloft) and paroxetine (Paxil) are being used in the treatment of pediatric OCD. They are effective and generally well-tolerated. Children and adolescents must be assessed carefully for suicidal thoughts when taking antidepressants. Benzodiazepines are known to cause cognitive and psychomotor impairments in elderly individuals, which contribute to falls and fractures. For this reason, benzodiazepines are not recommended. Citalopram (Celexa) is the drug of choice for older individuals with anxiety disorders (Geller et al., 2004). See chapter 10 ∞ for more in-depth information on these medications.

Multidisciplinary Interventions

Medications play an important role in medical interventions, but intrapersonal and interpersonal aspects must also be treated. Clients and their families must cope with various aspects of anxiety, learn to take control of their lives, and manage family stress. All are accomplished through a blending of techniques and the use of individual, family, and group psychotherapy.

Cognitive–behavioral therapy is considered the best psychotherapy for anxiety disorders. The cognitive part of this therapy includes education about symptoms of the disorder, as well as the rationale for asking clients to recall their feared experiences. Therapists help clients examine and change distorted thinking and faulty beliefs. The next step is *exposure and response prevention*. Clients are exposed, in reality or in their mind, to feared situations or objects for about 30 minutes. This is followed by instructions to try to refrain from or delay their usual phobic or ritualistic response for 2 more hours. The therapist is present the entire time and coaches the client using relaxation techniques, distraction, conversation, and encouragement. Cognitive–behavioral therapy is not effective for people with hoarding symptoms but is effective for other symptoms of OCD. It is also effective for children and adolescents experiencing anxiety disorders.

Florean has a strong fear of contamination. Whenever she touches any surface that she thinks might be contaminated, she washes her hands for 5 minutes. With the help of her therapist, Florean has planned a program in which she will touch a wastebasket several times and stop herself from washing her hands until 1 minute has passed. The goal is to refrain from hand washing for longer and longer periods of time. After that goal has been reached, Florean will work on reducing the length of time she spends washing her hands until the behavior is largely under her control.

Individual psychotherapy and hypnosis are used to uncover the abuse and trauma of DID. Nonverbal therapies, such as play therapy, art therapy, occupational therapy, and journal writing, are also extensively used. One goal is to help the client discover that the various personalities are real and distinct but are not separate individuals. The client learns that all the personalities belong to each other and that they are all parts of the same person and same body. Hypnosis helps the personalities come to know each other, communicate with each other, and share skills.

Individuals with body dysmorphic disorder may seek cosmetic surgery to decrease anxiety related to their bodies. It appears, however, that surgical and dermatologic treatments do not ease the distress about the body parts (Carroll et al., 2002).

Repetitive transcranial magnetic stimulation (rTMS) over the right frontal cortex may improve the symptoms of PTSD. This treatment is usually given in 10 daily sessions. The main side effect is headache but is generally well tolerated (Cohen et al., 2004).

Severe OCD that does not respond to treatment causes tremendous suffering in those affected and in their families. Of this group of nonresponders, 35% to 70% respond to deep brain stimulation. This involves the implantation of electrodes in specific brain areas that are then connected to pulse generators placed in the chest, much like pacemakers. It is not intended to cause significant damage to brain tissue and the stimulation can be modified or ended (Greenberg et al., 2003).

Alternative Therapies

Several *herbs* are used for the treatment of anxiety disorders. Chamomile can be infused by pouring hot water over the herb, steeped for 3 to 5 minutes, and strained before drinking. Honey or lemon may be added to taste. Chamomile can also be purchased as a tincture for a dosage of 1 teaspoon three times a day. Chamomile, a member of the ragweed family, should not be used by people who have ragweed allergy (Fontaine, 2005).

Kava, a South Pacific herb, contains alpha-pyrones, a recently discovered class of potent skeletal muscle relaxants. It is unknown whether kava affects the GABA (benzodiazepine) receptors. Kava should not be taken with St. John's wort, antianxiety medications, antidepressants, or with alcohol because its effects may be increased. Reports of liver damage have led many countries to remove kava from their shelves. Currently, in the United States, the FDA recommends caution in the use of kava (Basch & Ulbricht, 2005).

Many people find lavender relaxing and some find it helpful in reducing anxiety. Lavender may be made into a tea, inhaled, added to bath water, or used with massage oil. Likewise, passion flower has a long history for use in agitation or anxiety.

Essential oils influence health on physical, mental, and emotional levels. The basis of action is thought to be the same as modern pharmacology, using smaller doses. The purity and authenticity of essential oils is critical to their effective-ness. Oils that are diluted, adulterated, or synthetic should not be used for aromatherapy. Essential oils are potent and can irritate the skin, so they should be diluted with a carrier oil before being used on the skin. Oils used to decrease anxiety include chamomile, green apple, lemon balm, neroli, and orange. Oils to improve sleep include chamomile, clary sage, lavender, marjoram, neroli, and vetiver.

Homeopathic remedies are believed to stimulate a person's self-healing capacity. Pulsatilla (windflower) is helpful for people who are highly emotional, weepy, fearful of abandonment, and worried about what others think of them. Ignatia (St. Ignatius bean) is helpful for those experiencing anxiety.

Massage has been used with people having anxiety disorders as an adjunct to conventional psychiatric interventions. Clients are given an "executive massage," which is a massage done with the client fully dressed and seated on a massage chair. The head, neck, back, arms, and legs are massaged for 10 to 20 minutes per session.

Therapeutic Touch (TT) works in conjunction with other medical or therapeutic techniques to alleviate anxiety and irritability. It also significantly reduces "state anxiety" in some clients and reduces stress in children and adults. TT also reduces anxiety levels for people who are hospitalized for medical–surgical problems (Newshan & Schuller-Civitella, 2003).

Yoga is tailored to the individual and can be done with great benefit at the beginner level as well as at the most advanced level. Attention is paid to how the body feels and what it is doing. Every movement is made gently and slowly. Every yoga session ends with a few minutes of complete relaxation. The psychiatric benefits of yoga include increasing brain endorphins, enkephalins, and serotonin; promoting relaxation; and managing stress. In PTSD due to sexual and physical abuse, yoga postures should be used with extreme caution because they may stimulate flashbacks to the traumatic situation.

If practiced regularly, even 15 minutes twice a day, *meditation* produces widespread positive effects on physical and psychological functioning. The autonomic nervous system responds with a decrease in heart rate, lower blood pressure, decreased respiratory rate and oxygen consumption, and a lower arousal threshold. All of this is helpful in reducing levels of general anxiety and worry. There are as many ways to meditate as there are people. When people say they have tried meditation and cannot do it, they just have not found the right practice for them. There is a variety of ways that one can meditate, including sitting, through repetitive prayers, swimming or running, walking, or through yoga or t'ai chi. Encourage clients to explore a variety of techniques and develop the habit of meditation on a daily basis.

Nursing Process

CLIENTS WITH ANXIETY, DISSOCIATIVE, AND SOMATOFORM DISORDERS

ASSESSMENT

Assess clients using the knowledge base provided in this chapter. Because of the shame and secrecy surrounding anxiety disorders, clients may not reveal symptoms unless the nurse asks direct, specific questions. An organized scheme of focused assessment ensures that all areas—behavioral, affective, cognitive, and social characteristics—are assessed. As always, assessment questions must be modified to the individual's cognitive, developmental, educational, and language abilities. See the Focused Nursing Assessment feature for assessment questions.

Nurses will see the majority of clients suffering from anxiety disorders in community settings, clinics, physician of-

fices, emergency rooms, and medical–surgical units. Because these clients often have complicated and detailed medical histories, careful physical assessment is necessary. Remember that, at any given time, a client with an anxiety disorder may develop an organic illness. Continual physical assessment, therefore, is a necessary component of nursing care.

Children can be assessed through verbal interaction, nonverbal observations, and parental or teacher reports. Young children may not have the language skills to describe their thoughts and feelings, but they are often able to communicate through play, sand trays, and art. Nonverbal assessments should be consistent with the child's developmental level.

Assessment: Behavior

The dominant behavioral characteristic of people with phobic disorders is *avoidance*. Fearing loss of control, they avoid the phobic object or situation that increases their level of anxiety.

Focused Nursing Assessment	**Clients With Anxiety Disorders**		
Behavior Assessment	**Affective Assessment**	**Cognitive Assessment**	**Social Assessment**
Obsessive–Compulsive Disorder			
What kinds of objects or situations do you feel a need to check or recheck frequently?	Describe how you experience the feeling of anxiety.	Describe the qualities you like about yourself. Describe the qualities you do not like about yourself.	In what way do habits or thoughts get in the way of work? Social life? Personal life?
How much time during a day do you spend on checking activities?	What happens to you when you feel out of control in situations?	What are your thoughts about your compulsive behavior?	Describe situations in which you feel close to and warm with your family members.
Describe any movements you are forced to repeat.	Describe your relationships with significant others.	Would you like to decrease the need for your compulsive behavior?	In what ways do you feel dependent on your family?
What kinds of things do you count, silently or out loud?	How do these others relate to you?	How much time a day do you spend doubting what you have done?	
	What are your greatest fears in life?		
Phobic Disorders			
What situations or objects do you try to avoid in life?	What are your greatest fears in life?	Do you dislike being controlled by your fears?	Who is able to support you in avoiding your feared situations or objects?
Describe what you do to avoid these situations or objects.	Do you fear others laughing at you? Being humiliated? Being abandoned by others? Being alone in an unfamiliar situation?	What does the future look like for you?	Describe how family living patterns have changed around your fears.
To what degree do these fears interfere with your daily routines?	What feelings do you experience when you are confronted with the situation or object that you fear?	Describe the qualities you like about yourself. Describe the qualities you do not like about yourself.	Under what circumstances are you able to socialize with friends?
Are your social or work activities limited to a prescribed geographic area?	What else happens to you at this time?	How much support do you need from others to cope with life?	
How often and in what circumstances are you able to leave home?	To what degree do you fear having future panic attacks?	How helpless and dependent on others do you feel?	

continued

Focused Nursing Assessment   Clients With Anxiety Disorders—*continued*

Behavior Assessment	Affective Assessment	Cognitive Assessment	Social Assessment
Posttraumatic Stress Disorder			
Under what circumstances do you experience outbursts of aggressive behavior?	How much time during a day do you feel tense or irritable?	Describe difficulties you have had with concentration.	In what ways do your family members and friends tell you that you are distant or cold in your relationships with them?
In what ways have you been reexperiencing the original trauma?	Have you been experiencing panic attacks?	Describe difficulties you have had with your memory.	Describe your communication patterns with family members and friends.
In what ways do you attempt to avoid situations or activities that may remind you of the original trauma?	Describe the guilt you have been experiencing in relation to the original trauma.	How often, in a day, do you have recurrent thoughts about the original trauma? Do you feel you have control over these thoughts?	Describe what happens when you lose control of your anger.
How frequently do you participate in social activities?	What types of activities do you enjoy doing?	Describe any nightmares you have.	How is violence handled within your family system?
Have you had any employment difficulties since the original trauma?	What are sources of pleasure for you in your life?	Describe the qualities you like about yourself.	Are you experiencing relationship difficulties?
	Describe relationships in which you feel emotionally close to other people.	Describe the qualities you do not like about yourself.	
Dissociative Identity Disorder*			
Does the client have widely varying behavior patterns, such as at times being submissive and quiet and at other times loud and outspoken?	Does the client experience anxiety about "lost" time?	Describe the frequency of amnesic periods.	Do family members describe the client as having different personalities?
Does the client have different styles of dressing that correspond to a change in behavior?	In what ways is the client passive and submissive?	Under what circumstances does this amnesia seem to appear?	How has the family tried to manage the situation thus far?
Are vocational or leisure skills inconsistent; that is, are these skills apparent at some times and not at other times?	In what ways is the client angry and aggressive?	Are there times when the client can remember specific events and other times when there is amnesia for the same events?	Is there a known history of child abuse for the client?
			Describe the client's relationship to his or her parents as a child.
Somatoform Disorders			
What OTC medications are you currently taking? How effective are they?	In what situations do you experience feelings of anger?	How often, in a day, are you aware of your physical symptoms?	How is your family managing with your illness?
What prescription medications are you currently taking? How effective are they?	In what situations do you experience feelings of anxiety?	How aware are you of bodily sensations?	Who is supportive to you in this illness?
What medications have you taken in the past? What results were obtained with them?	In what way do you share your feelings with others?	Do you believe you have a serious illness? Has this illness been confirmed by a health care provider?	Who cares for you when you are unable to care for yourself?
Who have you consulted professionally for your illness in the past 5 years? What diagnostic procedures have been performed? What surgeries have you had in your lifetime?	How do you respond when others become angry with you?	Describe your level of concern for your physical health.	How has your illness affected the family's financial situation?

*Since the client is unaware of changes in personalities, the assessment data are based on your observations and family reporting.

They dread the next encounter and develop elaborate strategies intended to avoid it. If the person demonstrates minor rechecking or ritualistic behavior, avoidance may take on an obsessive–compulsive aspect. Even when they know their fears are irrational, they still try to avoid the object or situation. If they cannot avoid the object or situation easily, the behavior may interfere with overall functioning and even lifestyle.

Typically, clients experiencing somatoform disorders purchase many over-the-counter (OTC) medications to reduce their symptoms or pain. Inadvertent *drug abuse* may result when medications are prescribed for long periods by a variety of physicians. Dependence on pain relievers or antianxiety agents is a common complication of these disorders.

These clients frequently discuss their symptoms and disease processes. Many adapt their behavior patterns and lifestyle to the disorder. Adaptation can range from a minor restriction of activities to the role of a complete invalid.

Assessment: Affect

People experiencing anxiety disorders worry a great deal. Their worries are focused on negative future events that may or may not occur. They also cannot tolerate uncertainty so they avoid ambiguous situations.

For people suffering from phobic disorders, *fear* predominates. Mainly, there is fear of the object or situation. There are also fears of exposure, which could result in being laughed at and humiliated, and of being abandoned during a phobic episode.

When confronted with the feared object or situation, phobic people feel panic, which may include a feeling of impending doom. Panic in itself is often accompanied by additional fears, such as fear of losing control, causing a scene, collapsing, having a heart attack, dying, losing one's memory, and going crazy. Having once experienced an unexpected attack of panic, individuals begin to fear that the attack will happen again. Because these attacks are so terrifying, the fear of another attack becomes the major stress in their lives. This *fear of fear*, which is extreme anticipatory anxiety, may become the dominant affective experience, particularly for people with agoraphobia.

People with OCD often experience a great deal of *shame* about their uncontrollable and irrational behavior, and they may try to hide it. They may be consumed with fears of being discovered. OCD sufferers respond to anxiety by feeling tense, inadequate, and ineffective. To alleviate the anxiety, *control* is all-important. They fear that if they do not act on their compulsion, something terrible will happen. Thus, in most cases, compulsions serve to temporarily reduce anxiety. But the behavior itself can create further anxiety. The affective distress may range from mild anxiety to almost constant anxiety about thoughts and behaviors. Obsessive–compulsive people often

experience *hopelessness* that their situation will never improve. They may also develop phobias when faced with situations in which they can no longer maintain control.

People suffering from PTSD experience *chronic tension*. They are often irritable and feel edgy, jittery, tense, and restless. They commonly experience labile affective responses to the environment. Anxiety is frequent and ranges from moderate to severe (panic).

The primary gain in somatoform disorders is the *reduction of conflict and anxiety*. People with these disorders are usually unable to express anger directly out of fear of abandonment and loss of love. They actively avoid situations in which others will become angry with them. As a result, there is an unconscious use of physical symptoms to manage the anxiety caused by conflicting issues.

When they fail to get relief from the physical symptoms, these clients experience more anxiety. It may be manifested by obsessions about the physical illness, depression, or phobic avoidance of activities associated with the spread of disease.

Assessment: Cognition

The symptoms of people with phobic disorders are *egodystonic*. Although sufferers recognize that their responses are unreasonable and their thoughts are irrational, they are unable to explain them or rid themselves of them. They are consumed with thoughts of anticipatory anxiety and have negative expectations of the future. Phobic people develop low self-esteem and describe themselves as inadequate and as failures. They believe they are in great need of support and encouragement from others. They begin to define themselves as helpless and dependent and often despair of ever getting better. They may even begin to believe they are mentally ill and fear ending up in an institution for the rest of their lives.

In an attempt to localize anxiety, phobic people often use *defenses* that allow them to remain relatively free of anxiety as long as the feared object or situation is avoided. Defenses—such as repression, displacement, symbolization, and avoidance—can also keep the original source of anxiety out of conscious awareness. In agoraphobia, however, defense mechanisms are not adequate to keep anxiety out of conscious awareness. People with agoraphobia live in terror of future panic attacks, and anticipatory anxiety is a constant state.

Steve:

" My biggest fear is that I'm going to appear ignorant. And it's so counter to who I am, but it still is this distortion of thought. It's a cognitive distortion. Call it what you will, but it's a cognitive distortion that I am going to come across as stupid. "

Traditionally, it has been thought that OCD is ego-dystonic because many sufferers feel tormented by their symptoms. These people recognize the senselessness of much of their behavior and want to resist it. The drive to engage in the behavior is overpowering, however, and they often feel extreme distress about their actions. A smaller number have limited recognition of their behavior, and a few are unable to see their behavior as senseless. Those who hoard typically have little or no insight into their disorder, making hoarding ego-syntonic.

OCD sufferers are consumed with constant *doubts*, leading to difficulty with concentration and mental exhaustion. They doubt everything related to their particular compulsion and cannot be reassured by what they see, feel, smell, touch, or taste. Their OCD symptoms make them very slow in solving problems but do not interfere with accuracy in problem solving.

Yvette is a 27-year-old mechanical engineer. Her obsessive–compulsive behavior has been increasing during the past 5 years, and she is in danger of losing her job because of decreased productivity. She checks and rechecks every project she is assigned to the degree that she is unable to complete any project. She is able to identify when a project is complete, but her fear of making a mistake drives her to continue to recheck her work and avoid handing it in to her supervisor. She recognizes that her behavior is unrealistic and will likely result in the loss of her job.

Denial is the major defense mechanism in clients with somatoform disorders. Initially, these clients deny the source of anxiety and conflict, and the energy is transformed into physical complaints. Along with physical symptoms is a denial that there could be any psychological component to the physical symptoms. If confronted with the possibility of a psychological cause, clients often change health care providers in an effort to maintain their system of denial. Rarely will they follow through on referrals for psychotherapy.

Assessment: Interpersonal Relationships

The impact of agoraphobia on the family system is usually severe and may cause considerable disruption to family patterns of behavior. People with agoraphobia are often unable to leave home, which means they cannot be employed outside the home, cannot go out with friends, and cannot attend their children's school or sports activities. Thus, though appearing weak, they actually have a great deal of power to control family and friends through their dependency and helplessness.

Unconscious advantages from, or rewards for, being ill are referred to as **secondary gains**. The secondary gains of agoraphobia are the relinquishing of responsibilities, the satisfying of dependency needs that cannot be met directly, and the power to control others. Weakness as a form of control cannot work without another's cooperation. The secondary gains for the partner may be in fulfilling nurturing needs or being the main support of the family.

OCD is a devastating illness that alters the lives of clients and their family members. OCD symptoms are all-encompassing and involve family members and the home itself. Relationships are often strained and at times destroyed. Compulsive behavior may be so bizarre at times that family members go to great extremes so outsiders do not see the behaviors. They may even invent excuses for the public absence of their loved one (Stengler-Wenzke, Trosbach, Dietrich, & Angermeyer, 2004).

Family members may believe that if they "help" their loved one with the compulsions, the person will eventually be able to get the behaviors under control. But OCD symptoms progress over time and consume more of the entire family's life. Family members find themselves manipulated into enabling behavior to keep the peace and often end up bitter and resentful.

Family members of people with PTSD have a great deal of anxiety. One of the defenses for coping with the traumatic event is the numbing of emotions, or emotional anesthesia. Because of the PTSD sufferer's feelings of detachment, alienation, and doubts about ability to trust and love, interpersonal relationships are strained to the limit. Loss of the ability to communicate feelings makes relationship problems inevitable. Outbursts of anger and aggression further alienate family and friends.

The media are a contributing factor in somatoform disorders. Magazines, radio, and television bombard us with advertisements for "cures" for every imaginable physical problem. In addition, there has recently been an emphasis on staying healthy—an emphasis that, at times, seems like a morbid preoccupation with death. Another form of the somatoform disorders is an obsessive, unrealistic fear of contracting HIV, the virus that causes AIDS. Individuals at low risk for AIDS and who have a somatoform disorder are terrified they may have AIDS. With such intense media attention, it is hardly surprising that people become obsessed with bodily processes.

Any one of the somatoform disorders may completely disrupt a person's life. Sufferers may need to change their vocation to one more adaptable to their physical symptoms. Others may be unable to work in any capacity, either inside or outside the home. The chronic nature of these disorders often places a severe financial and emotional strain on the family. Physician, diagnostic, and hospital expenses may place the family in debt. The emotional drain on client and family leads to increased stress and interpersonal conflict, especially when there is no physical improvement. This increased level of conflict contributes to the continuation of the disorder, and a vicious cycle is established.

Assessment: Cultural Influences

While anxiety may be a universal emotion, the context in which it is experienced, the meaning it is given, and the responses to it are strongly influenced by cultural beliefs and practices. Cross-cultural studies have found significant differences in the expression of anxiety. These include differences in the type of specific fears as well as the associated

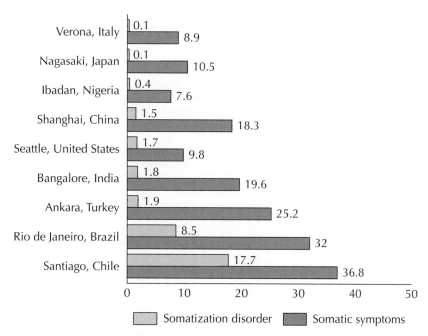

Figure 11.1 ■ Prevalence of somatization disorder and somatic symptoms in different countries. Somatization is *not* more common in nonindustrialized countries, contrary to common assumptions. (*Note*: Somatization disorder was based on ICD-10 diagnosis; somatic symptoms included a minimum of four for men and six for women.)

SOURCE: Reprinted with permission; rights held by APA. Gureje, O., Simon, G. E., Usrun, T. B., & Goldberg, D. P. (1997). Somatization in cross-cultural perspective: A World Health Organization study in primary care. *American Journal of Psychiatry, 154,* 989–995.

behavioral, affective, and cognitive characteristics. Some cultures do not use the word "anxiety" but rather they discuss "nervousness" or "tension." In some cultures, anxiety is expressed predominantly through somatic (physical) symptoms. A physical problem may be seen as a more legitimate reason to get help and gain support from family members and friends. Figure 11.1 ■ describes the prevalence of somatization disorder and somatic symptoms in various cultures.

In some cultures, panic attacks are believed to be caused by evil spirits. Individuals whose culture teaches fear of spirits, ghosts, and witches would not be diagnosed as having a phobia. Those who are socialized not to give offense to others in social situations would also not be diagnosed as having a social phobia. Chapter 4 ∞ describes culture-bound syndromes related to anxiety.

People from countries with a history of wars and social unrest may have a high rate of PTSD. Most of the symptoms of PTSD are not culture bound but are similar cross-culturally. Fear may prevent these individuals from divulging their experiences of torture and trauma until the therapeutic relationship is well established.

Assessment: Age-Specific Characteristics
Children

It is common for children to experience anxiety. This experience is usually temporary and requires no professional intervention. Infants fear loud and sudden noises, loss of support,

and heights. Very young children fear strangers, being left alone, and the dark; preschoolers fear separation from caregivers, imaginary creatures, animals, and the dark. Anxiety about physical safety and storms are common among young school-age children. During the middle-school years, the focus of anxiety changes to academic, social, and health-related issues. This focus continues into adolescence. Table 11.5 ■ provides a description of anxiety disorders in children and adolescents.

Developmentally appropriate fears and anxieties must be distinguished from those that are inappropriate or pathological. Anxiety disorders are the most prevalent form of mental disorders in children. Some anxiety disorders are specified as Axis I disorders and as other disorders of infancy, childhood, or adolescence. Other anxiety disorders of children and adolescents are described under the adult disorders. Estimates for the presence of any anxiety disorder are 6% to 18%. Anxiety disorders are three to four times higher in children who also suffer from depression and two to three times higher in children with oppositional or conduct disorders. Preadolescent girls and boys experience the same rate of anxiety disorders. This changes, however, in puberty when rates of anxiety in girls are higher than those in boys.

Characteristics of anxiety in children and adolescents include fears, worries, uneasiness, apprehension, restlessness, decreased concentration, self-doubt, decreased school performance, dizziness, lightheadedness, shortness of breath, nausea and vomiting, headaches, and stomachaches. Between 10% and 30% of schoolchildren experience anxiety severe enough

TABLE 11.5	Anxiety Disorders in Children and Adolescents	
Disorder	**Age**	**Description**
Obsessive—compulsive disorder (OCD)	As young as 2 years; mean age 10 years	Most common behaviors are washing and cleaning, followed by checking, counting, repeating, touching and straightening, and hoarding. Fears include contamination, harm to self, and harm to familiar person. Many are embarrassed and secretive, and the disorder is often unrecognized.
Posttraumatic stress disorder (PTSD)	Related to traumatic event	Traumatic events prior to age 11 are three times more likely to result in PTSD. Younger children may repeatedly act out specific themes of the trauma. Some engage in high motor activity in an effort to keep minds off recurring thoughts.
General anxiety disorder (GAD)	5–17 years	Formerly referred to as overanxious disorder of childhood. Affects about 3–15% of children and adolescents. Variety of worries such as future events, performance, personal safety, and the social environment. Often have somatic complaints. Self-conscious and excessive need for reassurance from others. Perfectionistic, eager to please, hypermature.
Specific phobia	Childhood, adolescence	Common phobia include heights, small animals, doctors, dentists, darkness, noises, and thunder and lightning. Behaviors include screaming, crying or running to loved one for safety. There is a common belief that confrontation with phobic stiumulus will result in personal harm.
Social phobia	As young as 8 years; early to midadolescence	Persistent fear of one or more situations such as formal speaking, eating in front of others, using public restrooms, speaking to authority figures. Fear is of criticism or failure. Sixty percent of distressing events occur at school.

SOURCES: American Psychiatric Association. (2000). *Diagnostic and statistical manual of mental disorders* (4th ed., Text Revision). Washington, DC: Author; and Malcarne, V. L., & Handsdottir, I. (2001). Vulnerability to anxiety disorders in children and adolescence. In R. E. Ingram & J. M. Price (Eds.), *Vulnerability to psychopathology* (pp. 271–303). New York: Guilford Press.

to impair academic achievement. Highly anxious adolescents engage in more problem behavior, are more disliked by peers, have poorer self-concepts, and have lower school achievement than less anxious teens. Individuals who experience anxiety disorders in childhood or adolescence are at a significantly higher risk for a recurrent anxiety disorder in young adulthood. It must also be noted that many anxious children do not develop anxiety disorders as adults (Albano & Hack, 2004).

Steve:

❝ I would describe my high school years as an incredibly alien experience. I felt terribly alienated. Going to school every day was an effort. It was a terrible effort. When I think back on it, it's kind of upsetting. I remember getting a call some years ago from a guy who was an alumnus at the high school. He wanted to know if I wanted to come for a high school reunion. And I said, 'Why would I want to relive one of the most painful periods of my life?' And it was absolutely one of the most painful periods of my life. ❞

Separation Anxiety Disorder A mild form of separation anxiety is fairly common in young children. Most children fear losing their parents. **Separation anxiety disorder** may develop at any age, although it is more common in children than in adolescents, and onset can be as early as age 2 to 3 years, with the peak onset between 7 and 9 years. The child may follow the parent around the house, needing to be close at all times. Their worries may focus on separation themes such as being kidnapped or killed or the parents being killed. The school-age child may refuse to go to school, although not all refusals are due to separation anxiety. Physiological manifestations include nausea, vomiting, stomachache, and sore throat. Older children may have palpitations, respiratory distress, and dizziness (Albano & Hack, 2004).

Separation anxiety disorder may have either an acute or an insidious onset. Many children recover without any further problems, while others may have periodic exacerbations. Some may have symptoms into adulthood, especially when attachments are threatened or disrupted.

Selective Mutism **Selective mutism**, a form of social phobia, is the steady failure to speak in specific social situations in which speaking is expected. Onset is usually between 3

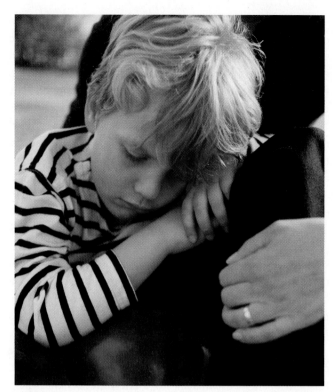

PHOTO 11.3 ■ Some children are overly dependent on parents.
SOURCE: Mel Curtis/Getty Images, Inc.—PhotoDisc, Inc. Used with permission.

and 6 years of age and occurs more frequently among girls. The extent to which the child speaks varies greatly. Some children speak loudly and freely at home but never say a word at school. Some speak to strangers in public, while others do not. Some are unable to speak to others face to face but may be able to speak to these same individuals on the phone. As is obvious, this disability interferes with education and social relationships. The majority of the children "outgrow" the disorder, although it may persist for several years (APA, 2000).

Reactive Attachment Disorder **Reactive attachment disorder** is associated with grossly pathological care, resulting from parental inexperience, extreme poverty, or prolonged institutionalization of the child. Not all children in these circumstances develop this disorder. The primary characteristic of this disorder is developmentally inappropriate social interactions. There are two subtypes: inhibited and disinhibited. Children suffering from the inhibited subtype do not initiate social contact nor do they appropriately interact with others. Those with the disinhibited subtype have few social boundaries and become quickly attached to multiple individuals. The course of the disorder appears to be related to the severity and duration of the pathological care as well as the effectiveness of a corrective supportive environment (APA, 2000).

Generalized Anxiety Disorder In children and adolescents with generalized anxiety disorder (GAD), anxieties often concern school performance, athletic performance, and catas-

trophes such as war, massive bombings, earthquakes, tornadoes, or hurricanes. They typically seek approval and frequent reassurance from adults. They may obsessively redo school work out of an excessively high standard of achievement that is usually unrealistic or unnecessary. Since they also worry about social relationships, it is difficult at times to distinguish between GAD and social phobia (Albano & Hack, 2004).

Panic Disorder Panic disorder occurs in children and, more commonly, adolescents. It often is preceded by or is comorbid with separation anxiety disorder. Panic disorder is often accompanied by a variety of specific phobias including fear of the dark, monsters, kidnappers, bugs, small animals, heights, and open or closed-in spaces. These specific phobias may be common triggers for panic and are responsible for many of the avoidance behaviors seen in children and adolescents with panic disorder.

Social Phobia Behavioral inhibition refers to the tendency among some young children to respond to unfamiliar people and situations with wariness and avoidance. This is considered to be an early temperamental precursor of later anxiety disorders. Children with behavioral inhibition are shy and fearful as toddlers; shy with strangers and timid in unfamiliar situations as preschoolers; and cautious, quiet, and introverted at school age. Those diagnosed with **social phobia** may fail to achieve in school, refuse to go to school, or avoid age-appropriate social activities. The terms *school phobia* and *school refusal* are often used to refer to children with social phobia.

Obsessive–Compulsive Disorder There are two peak ages of onset for obsessive–compulsive disorder (OCD), with one peak around age 10 and another during young adulthood. It is unknown whether these are different subtypes of the disorder. Juvenile-onset OCD has a stronger family genetic transmission; affects boys more than girls; has a higher incidence of attention deficit hyperactivity disorder (ADHD), tics and other neurological symptoms, and attention deficit; and is less responsive to treatment. As with adults, OCD is characterized by repetitive, ritualistic behaviors and thoughts. Children with OCD may be misdiagnosed with learning disabilities when the compelling need to count or check interferes with homework and testing (Piacentini, Bergman, Keller, & McCracken, 2003).

Posttraumatic Stress Disorder Children who experience natural disasters, war, unexpected personal tragedies, and ongoing interpersonal violence are at risk for development of posttraumatic stress disorder (PTSD). Urban children and adolescents experience a distressingly high rate of trauma. Forty percent of urban adolescents report having experienced or witnessed frightening violent events. About 25% of these individuals develop PTSD. Children who were in automobile accidents are also at risk for PTSD. PTSD can last for months or years, creating peer and school difficulties (Gill, 2002). See chapters 24 and 25 ∞ for a complete discussion of community violence, terrorism, and natural disasters.

Older Adults

Anxiety symptoms and disorders are among the most common psychiatric illnesses experienced by older adults. Panic attacks and phobic disorder often begin earlier in life and continue in older years, especially when those affected have received no treatment. People who develop late-onset panic attacks, after age 55, have less avoidance behavior than those who have early onset panic attacks. Panic attacks are common among postmenopausal women and seem to be associated with stressful life events and comorbid medical disorders (Smoller et al., 2003).

Anxiety can manifest in various ways, including somatic complaints, rigid patterns of behavior, fatigue, hostility, and confusion. Sleep disturbances are common in persons with anxiety. Many have difficulty getting to sleep and staying asleep and have poor quality of sleep.

Anxiety is often associated with medical illness. The symptoms of cardiovascular disease, such as angina pectoris and myocardial infarction, may simulate panic attacks. Medications such as cold and allergy drugs, amphetamines, bronchodilators, and some calcium channel blockers may produce anxietylike symptoms. Akathisia, a side effect of antipsychotic agents, is often indistinguishable from anxiety. Alcohol withdrawal and sedative/hypnotic withdrawal produce high levels of anxiety. There is a high prevalence of anxiety disorders in persons with Parkinson disease. In addition, the medications used to treat Parkinson disease may themselves cause anxiety. See chapter 20 ∞ for further information on Parkinson disease. People suffering from dementing disorders often experience concomitant anxiety. See chapter 19 ∞ for in-depth information on dementia.

Assessment: Physical

Healthy people can usually adapt to anxiety for brief periods of time. However, when the cause is unknown, the intensity is severe, or the duration is chronic, normal physiological mechanisms no longer function efficiently. Refer to Table 11.1 for the physical characteristics of anxiety.

In *mild anxiety*, people experience an agreeable, perhaps even a pleasant, increase in tension. Mild anxiety helps people deal constructively with stress. This level of anxiety also motivates learning and produces creativity.

In *moderate anxiety*, a person remains alert but the perceptual field narrows. The focus is on the immediate concerns while blocking out extraneous sensory stimuli—a process called *selective inattention*. Individuals may also experience a twitch in the eyelid, trembling lips, and mild gastric symptoms.

As anxiety increases to the *severe* level, the survival response of fight or flight begins. Starting in the cerebral cortex, this response is mediated through the body's nervous system and endocrine system. The sympathetic nervous system and the response of the adrenal glands lead to changes throughout the body. Heart rate increases and blood pressure rises to send more blood to the muscles. There may be frequent episodes of shortness of breath. The pupils dilate, the person may sweat, and the hands may feel cold and clammy. Some body trembling, a fearful facial expression, tense muscles, restlessness, and an exaggerated startle response may all be noticeable. There is an increased blood glucose level due to increased glycogenolysis. The moderately anxious person may verbalize subjective experiences such as a dry mouth, upset stomach, anorexia, tension headache, stiff neck, fatigue, inability to relax, and difficulty falling asleep. There may also be urinary urgency and frequency as well as diarrhea or constipation. Sexual dysfunction may include painful intercourse, erectile disorder, orgasmic difficulties, lack of satisfaction, or a decrease in sexual desire.

When anxiety continues to the *panic level*, the body becomes so stressed it can neither adapt effectively nor organize for fight or flight. At this level of anxiety, the person is helpless to care for or defend the self. As blood returns to the major organs from the muscles, the person may become pale. Hypotension, which causes the person to feel faint, may also occur. Other signs are a quavering voice, agitation, poor motor coordination, involuntary movements, and body trembling. The facial expression is one of terror, with dilated pupils. A person feeling panic may complain of dizziness, lightheadedness, a sense of unreality, and, at times, nausea. Some of the most frightening symptoms of the panic level of anxiety are chest pain or pressure, palpitations, shortness of breath, a choking or smothering sensation, and fear of imminent death. Each person tends to experience the physiological sensations in a pattern that repeats itself with every episode of anxiety. Some people are primarily aware of internal organ reactions, whereas others primarily exhibit symptoms of muscular tension. Still others experience both visceral and muscular responses.

The physical assessment must differentiate anxiety responses from various organic conditions that have similar symptoms. Medical conditions that may cause *secondary anxiety* or produce symptoms mimicking panic include hypoglycemia, hyperthyroidism, hypoparathyroidism, Cushing syndrome, pheochromocytoma, pernicious anemia, hypoxia, hyperventilation, audiovestibular system disturbance, paroxysmal atrial tachycardia, and withdrawal from alcohol or benzodiazepines. Similar symptoms may also occur during withdrawal from barbiturates and antianxiety medications and with the use of cocaine. High levels of caffeine, amphetamines, theophyllines, beta agonists, steroids, and decongestants may also be initially confused with anxiety disorders. Anxiety will frequently be seen as another symptom in people who have been diagnosed with schizophrenia, a mood disorder, or an eating disorder.

People with panic disorder, including agoraphobia, have a higher incidence of mitral valve prolapse (MVP) than the general population. The exact relationship between MVP and panic is unclear. The symptoms of MVP—particularly tachycardia, palpitations, and shortness of breath—are similar to the symptoms of panic levels of anxiety. People predisposed to panic attacks often interpret the sensations of MVP as increased anxiety. The interpretation or expectation then evokes panic.

Individuals with panic disorder frequently have significantly higher cholesterol levels than control groups do. It is thought that chronic anxiety, like stress, increases blood cholesterol (McLaughlin, Geissler, & Wan, 2003).

People with somatization disorders have multiple physical symptoms involving a variety of body systems. These symptoms may be vague and undefined, and they do not follow a particular disease pattern.

Pain is the primary symptom in pain disorder. The pain is severe and prolonged and usually does not follow the nerve-conduction pathways of the body.

Conversion disorder symptoms can occur in any of the sensory or motor systems of the body. The person may become suddenly blind or deaf. Loss of speech may range from persistent laryngitis to total muteness. Body parts may tingle or feel numb. Motor symptoms range from spasms or tics to paralysis of hands, arms, or legs.

In hypochondriasis, symptoms may be limited to one or several body systems. The most frequent symptoms appear in the head and neck. These include dizziness, loss of hearing, hearing one's own heartbeat, a lump in the throat, and chronic coughing. Symptoms in the abdomen and chest are common, including indigestion, bowel disorders, palpitations, skipped or rapid heartbeats, and pain in the left side of the chest. Some people may also have skin discomfort, insomnia, and sexual problems.

DIAGNOSIS

The next step in the nursing process is to analyze and synthesize the assessment data to form nursing diagnoses. The nurse must consider the client's level of anxiety as well as the behavioral, affective, cognitive, and physical responses to the anxiety. Other considerations are the client's self-evaluation, degree of insight, positive coping behavior, defense mechanisms, and the family/friendship systems.

The following are those diagnoses most commonly identified for clients with anxiety disorders (North American Nursing Diagnoses Association, 2007):

- Anxiety, Mild, related to threat to self-concept due to fear of being out of control
- Ineffective Breathing Pattern related to choking or smothering sensations, shortness of breath, and hyperventilation associated with the panic level of anxiety
- Sensory-Perceptual Alteration related to decreased perceptual field nursing panic level of anxiety
- Alteration in Thought Processes related to difficulty in concentrating and concrete thinking during panic level of anxiety
- Fear related to confrontation with feared object or situation
- Ineffective Individual Coping related to being consumed with obsessive and/or compulsive behavior
- Interrupted Family Process related to detachment and inability to express feelings, or to struggle for power and control or excessive dependency needs or repeated accommodating behaviors
- Social Isolation related to fear of leaving neighborhood or home or to physical symptoms and disability
- Spiritual Distress related to a view of the world and people as threatening after a severe traumatic event
- Disturbed Body Image related to preoccupation with imagined or slight defects in physical appearance
- Powerlessness related to a lifestyle of helplessness
- Posttrauma Syndrome related to traumatic experiences thought to be life-threatening
- Impaired Skin Integrity related to compulsive washing and cleaning

OUTCOME IDENTIFICATION AND GOALS

Based on the assessment data, select outcomes appropriate to the nursing diagnoses. Examples of broad outcomes are:

- Reduce high levels of anxiety.
- Improve quality of life.

Once the nurse has established outcomes, the nurse and the client mutually identify goals for change. Client goals are specific behavioral prescriptions that the nurse, the client, and significant others identify as realistic and attainable. The following are examples of goals that may be pertinent to those with anxiety disorders:

- Verbalize feeling less anxiety.
- Experience fewer episodes of panic.
- Verbalize less shame about the disorder.
- Develop effective coping behaviors.
- Utilize support systems when anxious.
- Describe a state of spiritual well-being.

In the section on implementation, goals are specified for each client issue or problem.

PLANNING

Once the nursing diagnoses, outcome criteria, and goals have been identified, the plan of care is developed to assist clients toward a higher level of functioning and an enriched quality of life. Priorities of care for clients with anxiety, somatoform, and dissociative disorder are as follows:

- Panic attack
- Altered thought process
- Comorbid physical problems
- Ability to function in daily life
- Social and family relationships

IMPLEMENTATION

Nursing diagnoses give direction for the development of goals and outcome criteria, which help focus nursing care. If possible, involve the client in developing the plan of care. If the client wants something different from what the nurse expects, the nursing care plan will not be appropriate; in fact, the client will likely sabotage it. The overall goal is to help the client improve the response to anxiety and develop more constructive behavior to manage anxiety.

The purpose of crisis intervention following traumatic events is to reduce the panic response, prevent PTSD, and maintain function and quality of life. Details on the implementation of crisis intervention and critical incident stress debriefing are found in chapters 24 and 25 ∞.

Complementary/Alternative Therapies

How to Help Clients Decrease Anxiety

The next time you feel anxious, try this procedure to decrease your anxiety:

1. Hold the frontal eminences on your forehead either with the first two fingers of your hands—the right and the left at the same time—or place the palm of your hand flat on your forehead.
2. While applying light pressure, in your mind go over exactly what you are thinking and how you are feeling. Continue holding these points and going over what is bothering you for a few minutes or until you feel the anxiety becoming less strong.
3. Let go with your hands and look around you. Mentally review the issue again. If anxiety is still there or has changed to other stressful feelings (frustration or anger, for example), go back and begin the process again. After a few more minutes, release the pressure and check your feelings about the situation again.

Hopefully your mind feels clearer and the anxiety no longer has the same stressful effect.

SOURCE: Fontaine, K. L. (2005). *Complementary & alternative therapies for nursing* (2nd ed.). Upper Saddle River, NJ: Prentice Hall.

Clinical Interactions   A Client With Obsessive–Compulsive Disorder

Detra, age 23, lives with her parents and has recently become obsessed with thoughts of her parents' deaths. She has developed several compulsions to manage the associated anxiety. When walking outside, she must never step on a crack in the sidewalk, and she silently repeats to herself over and over again: "Step on a crack, break your mother's back." She also fears that if she does not keep the house clean enough, her parents will get sick and die. She usually spends at least 8 hours a day cleaning their two-bedroom apartment. She insists that the windows and doors remain closed to prevent contamination and allows no one into the apartment other than immediate family members. Lately, she has begun to use a magnifying glass to see whether she has missed cleaning any fingerprints off the tables and chairs. In the interaction, you will see evidence of:

- Ego-dystonic feelings about the obsession
- A desire to resist the obsession
- Shame about the uncontrollable behavior
- Temporary relief of anxiety by compulsive behavior

NURSE: "It sounds like you have a lot of worries."

DETRA: **"Yeah."**

NURSE: "Your mother said you worry about the family a lot. Is that true?"

DETRA: **"Yeah."**

NURSE: "Are you worried about your parents right now?"

DETRA: **"No, not if I don't think about it."**

NURSE: "Well, when you're worried about your parents, does anything help?"

DETRA: **"Yeah." [Pauses, looks embarrassed.] "It's really stupid. I clean the apartment over and over all day long."**

NURSE: "You are constantly cleaning. Does that help?"

DETRA: **"Sort of, but it's stupid."**

NURSE: "What do you mean 'stupid'?"

DETRA: **"Just stupid. I wish I could quit thinking about it."**

NURSE: "Do you have other worries you wish you could quit thinking about?"

DETRA: **"Yeah."**

NURSE: "Tell me about one of your other worries that you think is kind of stupid."

DETRA: **"I worry about dirt and germs coming in through the windows and doors."**

NURSE: "Do you do anything when you have these worries?"

DETRA: **"I go around the apartment and keep checking that all the windows and doors are sealed. I search to see if there is any way germs can get in."**

NURSE: "When you check the windows and doors, that helps your worry about germs?"

DETRA: **"Yeah. That's stupid, isn't it?"**

NURSE: "Well, it sounds like you have a problem, but I don't think you're stupid."

NURSING CARE PLAN for Clients With Anxiety, Dissociative, and Somatoform Disorders

Managing Panic

Nursing Diagnosis: Client at risk for anxiety, panic level

Outcomes: Clients will decrease physiological arousal and verbalize feeling safe.

Psychiatric service animals are trained to "alert" the person that a specific event is going to occur in the near future and are able to notify the human partner of this impending event. They may also be trained to "respond," that is, to act in a predetermined manner when a specific event occurs. These animals alert or respond to human partners experiencing panic attacks, social phobias, agoraphobia, PTSD, stress disorder, dissociative amnesia, and depersonalization disorder. Training service animals is an expensive and time-consuming project. The benefit, of course, is that people can lead more independent and fulfilling lives (Gonser, 2000).

Clients who are in a panic state of anxiety respond best to a calm, direct approach. Stay with clients to promote safety and reduce fear.

Intervention	Rationale	Goals
Reassure client you will stay and the panic attack will subside.	This will decrease fears of being abandoned in a frightening situation.	Verbalizes less fear
Speak slowly, in a gentle voice and use short, simple sentences such as "Sit down," or "I will help."	Highly anxious people have great difficulty focusing or concentrating.	Responds to simple directions
Loosen any tight clothing.	This will ease the sensation of choking.	Clothing nonrestrictive
Instruct and demonstrate deep, slow breathing.	This will decrease hyperventilation.	Breathing is deeper and slower.
Direct client to imagine inhaling and exhaling through the soles of the feet.	During a panic attack, people feel disconnected from the environment, and this imagery helps them feel grounded and therefore safer.	Verbalizes a feeling of connection to the surroundings
Decrease environmental stimuli and interactions with other people.	This minimizes the communicable elements of anxiety to and from others in the environment.	Levels of anxiety decrease

Reducing Anxiety/Fear

Nursing Diagnosis: Client at risk for fear

Outcomes: Clients will identify sources of anxiety/fear, utilize coping behaviors, and experience anxiety at a manageable level.

Help clients label the feeling as anxiety because accurate identification is the first step in the problem-solving process. Ask clients to identify one anxiety-producing situation, which is a more manageable place to begin than with multiple fears. Ask clients to identify their negative anticipatory thoughts that may be the basis for feeling anxious. Help them analyze the fear of losing control and make the connection between this fear and increased anxiety. Have clients review how anxiety has been handled in the past and the effectiveness of these past coping behaviors. Help clients select and practice alternative behaviors such as relaxation, stress management, or biofeedback.

Intervention	Rationale	Goals
Teach how to monitor their physiological level of arousal.	This allows the client to implement coping strategies before anxiety escalates to an intolerable level.	Describes symptoms associated with the various levels of anxiety
Teach use of abdominal breathing at the first sign of anxiety. Have them practice this during nonanxiety states. Suggest the purchase of relaxation tapes.	The techniques should become familiar responses. Tapes reinforce this learning.	Utilizes deep breathing to control escalating anxiety
For clients who have phobias, help them express the fears that interfere with their lives. Use a nonjudgmental approach.	They are often afraid of the response of others to their fears.	Expresses fears clearly

continued

NURSING CARE PLAN for a Client With Anxiety, Dissociative, and Somatoform Disorders

Reducing Anxiety/Fear   *continued*
Nursing Diagnosis: Client at risk for fear

Intervention	Rationale	Goals
Encourage client to search for, confront, and relieve the source of the original anxiety that has become a phobia.	Insight into the development of the phobia may provide some control over the response.	Verbalizes an understanding of the development of the phobia
Ask client to picture the phobic response step by step, then picture coping effectively. Encourage the use of relaxation techniques during this process.	Visualization helps client move in the direction of expectations. Visualizing effective coping reinforces self-image as a person capable of dealing with fear. Relaxation techniques reduce physical sensations that provoke anxiety.	Modifies or eliminates phobic response
Limit the amount of time clients with somatization disorder talk about their physical complaints.	Repeatedly speaking about their problems reinforces the disorder.	Decreases the amount of time talking about physical problems
Encourage clients to recognize and identify their fears.	Discussing fears directly rather than to "somatize" feelings will decrease need for the symptom.	Discusses fears; verbalizes a decrease in somatic symptoms
Avoid implying that physical symptoms are imaginary.	Anxiety will increase if client does not feel believed.	Verbalizes a feeling of acceptance
Teach distraction techniques that can control moderate levels of anxiety (e.g., listening to music, reading a book, talking to a close friend, playing a game, counting backward by threes, counting the number of items on a shelf, or vigorous physical activity).	Distraction techniques allow person to remain in control during episodes of moderate anxiety.	Utilizes distraction techniques
Teach the use of positive imagery such as sitting quietly on a beach, being held by a trusted person, playing with a pet.	Positive imagery allows focus away from anxiety-producing stimulus and onto a positive image that feels safe.	Utilizes positive imagery
Teach journal keeping—making entries one or several times a day. Encourage them to identify events preceding, during, and after anxiety. Write down coping strategies that are effective.	Journal keeping is a useful way to keep track of thoughts, feelings, and memories. Self-monitoring increases self-control. The client can refer back to journal to review coping strategies in future times of anxiety.	Keeps journal
Encourage journal keeping for clients with DID. In some instances, journal keeping groups help clients talk about their self-discovery through writing.	Journal keeping is less threatening than sharing details verbally with staff. Because several of the personalities often write, the journal becomes one way the personalities can communicate and cooperate with one another.	Verbalizes that journal keeping is an effective coping behavior
Teach calming techniques such as muscle relaxation. Help them focus on relaxing specific muscle groups: while taking a deep breath through the nose, inhaling to the count of 5 and exhaling to the count of 5. Practice 2 times a day for 20 minutes.	Calming techniques provide clients with a skill response so they can experience anxiety without feeling overwhelmed.	Uses calming techniques to limit anxiety levels
Teach them positive affirmations such as "I am calm and happy," "My breathing is slow and even," "I am very relaxed."	Affirmations quiet the mind and set the expectation for remaining calm.	Practices positive affirmations several times a day

NURSING CARE PLAN for a Client With Anxiety, Dissociative, and Somatoform Disorders

Managing Worry

Nursing Diagnosis: Client at risk for anxiety

Outcomes: Clients will decrease the amount of time spent ruminating over worries; verbalize more accurate predictions of future events.

People with anxiety disorders often feel overwhelmed with worries. They tend to live in a largely negative world of their own making. Many believe that worry gives them some control over outcomes; that is, worry can prevent bad things from happening.

Clients who worry a great deal can be taught to control their worrying thoughts. The process begins with identifying the thoughts, which are often so automatic that clients are no longer aware of them. They can then choose to counter the thoughts or challenge the thoughts. Countering the thoughts involves distraction, which prevents the buildup of anxiety.

Intervention	Rationale	Goals
Ask clients: ■ Is the event (what is being worried about) highly unlikely or highly implausible? ■ Is this a current problem or a possible problem? ■ Is there an action that can be taken?	This process helps clients distinguish between productive and unproductive worrying.	Decreases unproductive worrying
Point out that time spent worrying often has no impact on actual outcomes.	This counters the belief that worry will prevent bad things from happening.	Verbalizes less worry
Identify situations that trigger worries such as interpersonal conflict or uncertainty at work.	This helps clients make the connection between these events and the onset of worry.	Identifies personal triggers to worry

Stabilizing Mood

Nursing Diagnosis: Client at risk for ineffective coping

Outcomes: Clients will express feelings appropriately and verbalize increasing stability of mood.

Clients need reassurance and encouragement during times of stress. Assist clients in distinguishing between feelings such as anxiety, frustration, guilt, and hostility.

Intervention	Rationale	Goals
Discuss appropriate ways to express negative feelings.	This provides more effective options for managing feelings.	Identifies ways to effectively express feelings
Teach that suppressing feelings requires energy.	This constant drain on energy is depleting.	Expresses feelings rather than suppressing them
Identify safe physical outlets for negative feelings such as exercise, working out in a gym, or pounding clay.	These activities help limit explosive anger.	Utilizes physical activities to manage negative feelings.

Managing Cognitive Problems

Nursing Diagnosis: Client at risk for disturbed thought processes

Outcomes: Clients will decrease cognitive distortions and decrease ruminations or obsessions.

Cognitive intervention techniques concentrate on teaching people to change the maladaptive beliefs, self-statements, and phobic imagery that contribute to anxiety disorders. A technique used with anxious children is to separate the fearful part of the child from the calm and nonanxious part of the child. Because anxious children have become accustomed to viewing themselves as constantly fearful, they ignore the times that they are successful and brave. You can provide opportunities for success. Praise and reinforce their behavior whenever possible. Focusing on positive characteristics and behaviors is often more helpful than focusing on problems. Ask children to create a list of all their strengths; for example: I am honest, I am a good friend, I can throw a ball, I can skip rope, I am a good brother, and so on. You can discuss this list and discover ways to use these characteristics in a positive manner.

continued

NURSING CARE PLAN for a Client With Anxiety, Dissociative, and Somatoform Disorders

Managing Cognitive Problems   *continued*
Nursing Diagnosis: Client at risk for disturbed thought processes

Intervention	Rationale	Goals
Teach clients to think certain thoughts before acting, such as "I will get on the elevator and go to the second floor successfully."	Negative self-statements reinforce phobias.	Replaces negative expectations with positive expectations
Teach them to challenge negative thoughts that are not facts and to identify what part of the thought is unrealistic or improbable; for example, "Yesterday was terrible, today is likely to be awful too" can be changed to "Yesterday was terrible; no, parts of it were good and although parts were uncomfortable, I coped." Another example is "My son is late—he's had an accident," which can be changed to "My son is late; maybe he got held up in traffic."	Identifying when thoughts are unrealistic, exaggerated, and catastrophic is the first step in learning cognitive restructuring.	Decreases the number of cognitive distortions
In working with clients with PTSD, explore how they interpreted the trauma. Ask what it means to them that the event happened. Ask them to write a detailed account of the event.	Emotions are more the result of beliefs and interpretations than of the events themselves.	Verbalizes the meaning of the trauma
Ask clients to write a detailed account of the traumatic event.	This reinforces reality versus cognitive distortions.	Writes a detailed account
Teach clients to ask themselves: ■ How well do my beliefs fit the facts? ■ Do other beliefs fit the facts better?	This process challenges their negative beliefs.	Verbalizes beliefs more consistent with the reality of the traumatic event

Managing Flashbacks

Clients who are experiencing a flashback respond best to a calm, direct approach. You intervene in the same way as someone who is in a panic state of anxiety. In addition, reorient them to the present environment as they are experiencing the old traumatic environment. As clients gain experience in relaxation techniques, guided imagery, and other comfort measures they will be able to calm themselves during flashbacks.

The desired outcome is that the client will utilize self-calming techniques.

EVALUATION

To complete the nursing process, the nurse evaluates client responses in terms of outcomes the nurse and the client estab-

lished. It is seldom an all-or-nothing phenomenon, but rather an ongoing process of movement toward the goals of better health and improved quality of life. If there is little movement toward achieving the outcome, the nurse must determine the problem. Considerations are:

■ Assessment data were incomplete or inaccurate.

■ The diagnosis was inappropriate to the situation.

■ Outcomes were not realistic.

■ Client disagreed with the outcomes.

■ Interventions were not appropriate.

When the problem is identified, changes can be made in the nursing process, and the nurse, the client, and the family can move forward.

Using Research Evidence   Self-care: Anxiety

Kemppainen, J. K., Holzemer, W. L., Nokes, K., Eller, L. S., Corless, I. B., Bunch, E. H., Kirksy, K. M., Goodroad, B. K., Portillo, C. J., & Chou, F-Y. (2003). Self-care management of anxiety and fear in HIV disease. *Journal of the Association of Nurses in AIDS Care, 14,* 21–29.

What is the study about?

Persons living with HIV disease have an increased incidence of mood and anxiety disorders. The purpose of this study was to describe self-care practices they use to manage the symptom cluster of fear and anxiety.

How was the study done?

This was a quantitative study using the critical-incident technique. Data for this study were obtained from a convenience sample of 73 participants from a larger national study on self-care for symptoms in HIV disease. The sample included 49 men and 24 women with a mean age of 41.8 years and an average time since diagnosis of 4.9 years. Most data were obtained through interview, and the rest through Web-based questionnaires. First, participants were asked to describe their most troublesome symptoms and to identify the symptoms' causes. Then they were asked to identify self-care behaviors they used to ease the symptom, and finally to identify sources of information about self-care. The interviews lasted about 20 minutes and were transcribed verbatim. Reponses from the participants were documented on specially designed critical-incident forms. Using Ethnograph® software, researchers transcribed the data verbatim and analyzed it by grouping data into major behavioral categories. Then the same data were independently re-sorted by two HIV/AIDS advanced practice nurse experts. Using these nurse experts' results, a third sort was done.

What were the results of the study?

The most frequently perceived causes of anxiety and fear were thoughts of death and the future. All 73 participants described a total of 212 incidents of anxiety and/or fear, which elicited self-care behaviors that the researchers placed into seven mutually exclusive categories: 1) using activities for distraction, 2) talking to others, 3) using complementary/alternative therapies, 4) taking medications, 5) using self-talk, 6) using substances, and 7) using avoidance behaviors.

Activities for distraction were usually solitary and included physical exercise, card games, watching television, or housework. When participants talked to others, they sought out supportive family, friends, providers, and others living with HIV. Complementary/alternative therapies were most often praying and increasing spirituality, followed by relaxation and meditation. The fourth category was use of prescribed antianxiety drugs to relieve feelings of anxiety and fear. Self-talk was described as "thinking about something else," "talking myself through it," and "telling myself to take positive action." In the sixth category, using substances, participants described the use of street drugs as a self-care management technique. The last identified self-care behavior was using avoidance behaviors such as withdrawal, crying and screaming, and overeating. As for sources of self-care advice, notably, these participants rarely, if ever, appealed to health care providers.

What additional questions might I have?

What is the relationship between self-care practices and stages of HIV? What therapeutic interventions are most effective in helping persons living with anxiety and fear related to a diagnosis of HIV? What are the dynamics that cause persons with HIV not to use health care providers to manage their anxieties and fears? Would vastly different results emerge if data were gathered from more than a one-time self-report or Web questionnaire?

How can I use this study?

Nurses need to be aware of the importance of self-care management techniques used by persons living with HIV, and incorporate these strategies in the plan of care. Nurses should continuously assess for symptoms and signs of anxiety, and realize that levels of anxiety can change quickly with the situation. Nurses need to develop strong therapeutic relationships with persons living with HIV, who may then feel more comfortable discussing their fears and anxieties. Nurses can promote positive coping; they may bring up the subject of self-management to encourage persons with HIV to take an active part in both recognizing their fears and anxieties and coping with them positively. In addition, coping can involve an open discussion between nurse and client about advance directives or other end-of-life concerns.

SOURCE: Contributed by Dolores Huffman, PhD, RN, Associate Professor of Nursing, Purdue University Calumet, Hammond, Illinois.

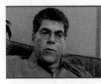

ROAD Assessment: Critical Thinking Questions

1. Steve identified several manifestations of anxiety during his interview. Identify at least four of his reported symptoms and indicate whether the symptom is physical or cognitive. Also, for each symptom of anxiety you record, indicate a nursing intervention you could implement. Support your answers in detail.

2. Steve talked about his high school years as being painful. Why would the high school environment be especially difficult for someone with anxiety disorder? Why would someone with Steve's symptoms experience feelings of alienation in the high school setting?

3. During his marriage, Steve reported that he found relief for his anxiety when he drank alcohol.
   a. Discuss the factors that you think influenced his perception of anxiety relief.

   b. What would have been the critical nursing medication assessment for any antianxiety medications Steve was prescribed during this time?

5. View the last video again. What was the coping technique Steve reported using when he encountered anxiety while talking to groups of people? Discuss whether you think this technique was or was not helpful for Steve. In further discussion with Steve about this technique, what questions or interventions would you implement to assist him in making it more effective?

ROAD: DEVELOP A CARE PLAN

Go to the CD-ROM to Develop a care plan based on your assessment of Steve. Identify nursing diagnoses, outcomes, goals, and interventions.

SOURCE: Contributed by Susan Siwinski-Hebel, RN, MSN

Focus Your Study

OBJECTIVES

1. Compare and contrast the different theories regarding the etiology of anxiety, dissociative, and somatoform disorders.

KEY CONCEPTS

- Genetics:
  - Heritability for anxiety disorders is 30% to 40%.
- Neurobiology:
  - Anxious individuals have an overly responsive autonomic nervous system related to dysfunctions of 5-HT, NE, DA, and GABA.
  - Those who are fearful have an abnormally sensitive fear network.
  - Those with OCD have an abnormality in the pathway linking the orbitofrontal cortex with the basal ganglia.
- Intrapersonal factors:
  - Reaction to anticipated future danger based on past experiences
  - Anxiety is pushed out of conscious awareness by use of defense mechanisms.
  - Other factors include external locus of control and an avoidant coping style.
- Interpersonal factors:
  - Interpersonal conflict results in anxiety, which is displaced onto the immediate surroundings.
  - Secondary gains reinforce the anxiety disorders.
- Cognitive theory:
  - Magnify the significance of the past, overgeneralize to the future, and develop negative cognitive expectations.
- Learning theory:
  - Learn to cope by escaping or avoiding anxiety-producing situations.
- Behavioral theory:
  - Learned responses to anticipatory anxiety
- Gender-bias factors:
  - Traditionally, women have been reinforced to behave dependently, passively, and submissively.

2. Discuss the psychopharmacological treatment of the symptoms of a person with an anxiety, dissociative, or somatoform disorder.

- GAD:
  - Venlafaxine (Effexor)
  - Escitalopram (Lexapro)
  - Olanzapine (Zyprexa)
  - Buspirone (BuSpar)
  - Imipramine (Tofranil)
- Panic disorder:
  - Selective serotonin reuptake inhibitors
- Social phobias:
  - Paroxetine (Paxil)
  - Levetiracetam (Keppra)
  - Propranolol (Inderal)
  - Atenolol (Tenormin)
- Specific phobias:
  - Cycloserine (Seromycin)
- OCD:
  - Fluoxetine (Prozac)
  - Sertraline (Zoloft)
  - Fluvoxamine (Luvox)
  - Citalopram (Celexa)
  - Paroxetine (Paxil)
  - Riluzole (Rilutek)
  - Risperidone (Risperdal)
  - Quetiapine (Seroquel)
- PTSD:
  - Sertraline (Zoloft)
  - Paroxetine (Paxil)
  - Propranolol (Inderal)
  - Atenolol (Tenormin)

3. Outline different treatment options for anxiety, dissociative, and somatoform disorders.

- Cognitive–behavioral therapy
- Repetitive transcranial magnetic stimulation (rTMS)
- Deep brain stimulation
- Herbs, essential oils, homeopathic remedies, massage, Therapeutic Touch, yoga, meditation

4. Outline the assessment process for a client with an anxiety, dissociative, or somatoform disorder.

- Assessment of behavior:
  - Avoidance
  - Use of OTC medications to self-medicate
  - Change in lifestyle to adapt to the disorder
- Assessment of affect:
  - Intense worry or fear
  - Shame
  - Chronic tension
- Assessment of cognition:
  - Ego-dystonic
  - Constant doubts
- Assessment of interpersonal relationships:
  - Family often distressed
  - Secondary gains of disorder
- Assessment of children:
  - Anxiety disorders specific to children include separation anxiety disorder, selective mutism, and reactive attachment disorder.

5. Use the nursing process to develop a comprehensive plan of care for a client with an anxiety, dissociative, or somatoform disorder.

→

- Managing anxiety, fear, panic, and flashbacks:
  - Use problem-solving process when anxiety is at a low level.
  - Teach the use of coping strategies or distraction techniques before anxiety escalates.
  - Advise client to use journal keeping to keep track of effective coping strategies.
  - Use a calm, direct approach with short simple sentences when anxiety is very high.
  - Advise client to loosen tight clothing and direct slow, deep breathing.
- Enhancing relaxation response:
  - Teach and practice muscle relaxation and deep breathing.
  - Identify other calming techniques specific to the individual such as guided imagery, exercise, or talking to friends.
- Managing helplessness:
  - Support defenses until they can gain control over their lives.
  - Identify secondary gains that maintain the disorder.
  - Problem solve ways to meet these needs in a more adaptive fashion.
- Managing cognitive problems:
  - Teach and practice thought stopping and guided self-dialogue.
  - Teach how to challenge unrealistic or catastrophic thoughts.
  - Provide opportunities for success in coping with anxiety-producing situations.
- Reducing compulsive behavior:
  - Explore the relationship between obsessive behavior and anxiety reduction.
  - Help clients problem solve ways to modify their routines to accommodate harmless rituals.
  - Help clients and families improve the safety in the home for those who are hoarders.
- Enhancing spirituality:
  - Encourage the search for meaning in the trauma.
  - Identify spiritual support systems.
  - Encourage meditation or prayer, which evokes the relaxation response.
- Improving socialization:
  - Provide assertiveness training.
  - Practice communication and social skills.
- Promoting nutrition:
  - Avoid substances that increase anxiety such as caffeine, chocolate, and alcohol.
  - Diets should include L-tryptophan, niacin, vitamin B_6, vitamin B_1, vitamin C, calcium, and magnesium.
- Promote exercise:
  - Help clients choose an exercise routine and design a progress graph to monitor their involvement.
- Improving sleep:
  - Establish a consistent sleep schedule.
  - Increase physical activity during the day, use relaxation techniques or guided imagery, avoid caffeine and alcohol, and take a warm bath or a warm drink just before bedtime.

6. Develop illness management teaching plans for a person with an anxiety, dissociative, or somatoform disorder and her/his family.

→

- Plan ways to directly meet the needs evidenced by the secondary gains of the anxiety disorders.
- Describe ways in which family members find themselves manipulated into enabling behaviors.
- Plan constructive ways to respond to outbursts of anger and aggression that alienate family and friends.
- Provide social skills training to improve the ability to negotiate stressful interpersonal situations.
- Improving family process:
  - Help define and clarify relationships.
  - Identify secondary gains of all family members.
  - Teach "I" language to express thoughts and feelings.
  - Help family formulate behavioral contracts regarding how they want to change and how their loved one wants to change.
  - Help the family develop behavioral contracts.

7. Discuss the key points in effectively communicating with a person with an anxiety, dissociative, or somatoform disorder.

→

- Ask direct, specific questions when seeking information about the disorder.
- Modify questions to the individual's cognitive, developmental, educational, and language abilities.
- Use play, sand trays, and art to help young children communicate.
- Use a calm, direct approach with short simple sentences when anxiety is very high.

Explore MediaLink

For review questions, case studies, and other resources for this chapter see the Pearson Health MediaLink CD-ROM that accompanies this book and the Companion Website.

 CD-ROM

- Audio Glossary
- NCLEX-RN® Review Questions
- ROAD Care Plan: *Steve*
- Animations/Videos
  - Panic Disorder–Parts 1, 2, and 3
  - Dissociative Disorders–Parts 1, 2, and 3
  - Obsessive-Compulsive Disorders–Parts 1, 2, and 3

 Companion Website www.prenhall.com/fontaine

- Audio Glossary
- NCLEX-RN® Review Questions
- Case Study
  - Anxiety
- Care Plan
  - Obsessive–Compulsive Behavior
- Critical Thinking
  - Panic Attack
- MediaLink Application
  - Somatoform Disorders
- MediaLinks
  - Books for Clients and Families
  - Community Resources

NCLEX RN® Review Questions

11-1. The nurse in the emergency department (ED) is caring for a client who suffers recurrent panic attacks. The client states, "I want to know what causes these panic attacks so I can do something to keep it from happening again." Which of the following responses by the nurse is correct?
  1. "No one really knows what causes panic attacks."
  2. "One current theory is that panic attacks are caused by high levels of carbon dioxide."
  3. "Panic attacks are caused by low levels of epinephrine."
  4. "Some people believe that panic attacks are caused by an abnormal pathway in the brain."

11-2. Which of the following medications would be used to treat a client who is experiencing ritualistic behavior that interferes with job performance and activities of daily living?
  1. Fluphenazine (Prolixin)
  2. Fluoxetine (Prozac)
  3. Lorazepam (Ativan)
  4. Carbemazepine (Tegretol)

11-3. A treatment plan is developed for a client diagnosed with dissociative identity disorder (DID). The nurse should object if which of the following was included in the plan for this client?
  1. Encourage the client to explore feelings of anger and helplessness.
  2. Encourage the client to keep a journal.
  3. Teach the client self-hypnosis.
  4. Teach the client to visualize lying in a meadow under the warm sun.

11-4. A client presents to the emergency department (ED) with a history of chest pain, nausea, and dizziness. These symptoms decreased after talking with the health care

provider. Vital signs were T-98.8, P-120, R-20, and BP 140/82. An electrocardiogram (ECG) revealed normal sinus rhythm with a rate of 120/minute. The client was recently fired and is worried about paying his bills. The client was driving to file for bankruptcy when the symptoms occurred. After assessing the client, the nurse would decide that which of the following nursing diagnoses is most important for this client?
  1. Ineffective Coping related to recent life changes
  2. Hopelessness related to loss of job and inability to pay bills
  3. Panic and Anxiety related to loss of job and financial changes
  4. Ineffective Denial related to worrying about paying bills

11-5. The nurse is leading a group for clients who have returned from fighting in Iraq. Which of the following client statements indicates the need for further interventions?
  1. "I slept 7 hours last night and didn't wake up once."
  2. "I know I'm not in danger now, but certain sounds make me remember the war."
  3. "I need to forget the war and get used to my life at home again."
  4. "I am writing down my thoughts about my experiences in Iraq."

11-6. A nurse is teaching clients about various techniques for stress management. Which of the following client statements indicates the correct use of a stress management technique?
  1. "Writing my feelings down every day helps me focus more attention on my anxiety."
  2. "Exercising my leg muscles makes them ache and keeps me awake at night."

3. "Breathing in and out through my nose several times helps me feel energized."
4. "Imagining myself on a beach and listening to the waves makes me fall asleep at night."

11-7. The client is a 25-year-old pregnant mother of two children under the age of 6. She is a very protective mother and will not allow her children to play outdoors for fear of tick bites. She is worn out from cleaning the house from top to bottom every day. She asks the nurse how she can stop worrying so much. What is the most appropriate response for the nurse?

1. "Allow your children to play outside after you spray them with an insect repellent."
2. "Why do you worry about the children getting tick bites?"
3. "Tell me your concerns about the children playing in your backyard."
4. "Have you sprayed your backyard for ticks?"

See Appendix D for answers.

References

Albano, A. M., & Hack, S. (2004). Children and adolescents. In R. G. Heimberg, C. L. Turk, & D. S. Mennin (Eds.), *Generalized anxiety disorder* (pp. 383–408). New York: Guilford Press.

American Psychiatric Association. (2000). *Diagnostic and statistical manual of mental disorders* (4th ed., Text revision). Washington, DC: Author.

Arbelle, S., Benjamin, J., Golin, M., Kremer, I., Belmaker, R. H., & Ebstein, R. P. (2003). Relation of shyness in grade school children to the genotype for the long form of the serotonin transporter promoter region polymorphism. *American Journal of Psychiatry, 160*(4), 671–676.

Basch, E. M., & Ulbricht, C. E. (2005). *Natural standard. Herb & supplement handbook.* St. Louis, MO: Elsevier/Mosby.

Brewin, C. R. (2003). *Posttraumatic stress disorder.* New Haven, CT: Yale University Press.

Bruce, S. E., Yonkers, K. A., Otto, M. W., Eisen, J. L., Weisberg, R. B., Pagano, M., et al. (2005). Influence of psychiatric comorbidity on recovery and recurrence in generalized anxiety disorder, social phobia, and panic disorder. *American Journal of Psychiatry, 162*(6), 1179–1187.

Carroll, D. H., Scahill, L., & Phillips, K. A. (2002). Current concepts in body dysmorphic disorder. *Archives of Psychiatric Nursing, 16*(2), 72–79.

Clark, D. A. (2003). *Cognitive-behavioral therapy for OCD.* New York: Guilford Press.

Cloos, J. M. (2005). The treatment of panic disorder. *Current Opinions in Psychiatry, 18*(1), 45–50.

Cohen, J., Kaplan, Z., Kotler, M., Kouperman, I., Moisa, R., & Grisaru, N. (2004). Repetitive transcranial magnetic stimulation of the right dorsolateral prefrontal cortex in posttraumatic stress disorder. *American Journal of Psychiatry, 61*(3), 515–524.

Coric, V., Taskiran, S., Pittenger, C., Wasylink, S., Mathalon, D. H., Valentine, G., et al. (2005). Riluzole augmentation in treatment-resistant obsessive–compulsive disorder. *Biological Psychiatry, 58*(5), 424–428.

Finke, L. M. (2003). Conspiracy of silence. *Reflections on Nursing Leadership, 1*(3), 17–18.

Fontaine, K. L. (2005). *Complementary and alternative therapies for nursing practice* (2nd ed.). Upper Saddle River, NJ: Prentice Hall.

Gelernter, J., Page, G. P., Stein, M. B., & Woods, S. W. (2004). Genome-wide linkage scan for loci predisposing to social phobia. *American Journal of Psychiatry, 161*(1), 59–66.

Geller, D. A., Wagner, K. D., Emslie, G., Murphy, T., Carpenter, D. J., Wetherhold, E., et al. (2004). Paroxetine treatment in children and adolescents with obsessive–compulsive disorder. *Journal of the American Academy of Child and Adolescent Psychiatry, 43*(11), 1387–1396.

Ghaemi, S. N. (2004). Anxiety and bipolar disorder. *Medscape Primary Care, 6*(2), 1–4.

Gill, A. C. (2002). Risk factors for pediatric post-traumatic stress disorder after traumatic injury. *Archives of Psychiatric Nursing, 16*(4), 168–175.

Gonser, R. (2000). Prescription protocols for psychiatric service animals. Presentation on October 28, 2000, at the American Psychiatric Nurses' Association annual conference. Retrieved November 4, 2003, from http://www.petsandpeople.org

Greenberg, B. D., Price, L. H., Rauch, S. L., Friehs, G., Noren, G., Malone, D., et al. (2003). Neurosurgery for intractable obsessive–compulsive disorder and depression. *Neurosurgical Clinical of North America, 14*(2), 199–212.

Hudson, J. L., & Rapee, R. M. (2004). From anxious temperment to disorder. In R. G. Heimberb, C. L. Turk, & D. S. Mennin (Eds.), *Generalized anxiety disorder* (pp. 51–74). New York: Guilford Press.

Kemppainen, J. K., Holzemer, W. L., Nokes, K., Eller, L. S., Corless, I. B., Bunch, E. H., Kirksy, K. M., Goodroad, B. K., Portillo, C. J., & Chou, F. Y. (2003). Self-care management of anxiety and fear in HIV disease. *Journal of the Association of Nurses in AIDS Care, 14,* 21–29.

Kent, J. M., Papp, L. A., Martinez, J. M., Browne, S. T., Coplan, J. D., Klein, D., et al. (2001). Specificity of panic response to CO_2 inhalation in panic disorder. *American Journal of Psychiatry, 158*(1), 58–67.

Kessler, R. C., Walters, E. E., & Wittchen, H. U. (2004). Epidemiology. In R. G. Heimberg, C. L. Turk, & D. S. Mennin (Eds.), *Generalized anxiety disorder* (pp. 29–50). New York: Guilford Press.

King, D. W., Vogt, D. S., & King, L. A. (2004). Risk and resilience factors in the etiology of chronic posttraumatic stress disorder. In B. T. Litz (Ed.), *Early intervention for trauma and traumatic loss* (pp. 34–64). New York: Guilford Press.

Landsman, K. J., Rupertus, K. M., & Pedrick, C. (2005). *Loving someone with OCD.* Oakland, CA: New Harbinger.

Lanius, R. A., Williamson, P. C., Densmore, M., Boksman, K., Neufeld, R. W., Gati, J. S., et al. (2004). The nature of traumatic memories. *American Journal of Psychiatry, 161*(1), 36–44.

Leonard, D., Brann, S., & Tiller, J. (2005). Dissociative disorders. *The Australian and New Zealand Journal of Psychiatry, 39*(10), 940–946.

Mataix-Cols, D., Rosario-Campos, M. C., & Leckman, J. F. (2005). A multidimensional model of obsessive–compulsive disorder. *American Journal of Psychiatry, 162*(2), 228–238.

McLaughlin, R., Geissler, E. C., & Wan, G. J. (2003). Comorbidities and associated treatment charges in patients with anxiety disorder. *Pharmacotherapy, 23*(10), 1251–1256.

Michal, M., Kaufhold, J., Grabhorn, R., Krakow, K., Overbeck, G., & Heidenreich, T. (2005). Depersonalization and social anxiety. *Journal of Nervous and Mental Disease, 193*(9), 629–632.

Newshan, G., & Schuller-Civitella, D. (2003). Large clinical study shows value of Therapeutic Touch program. *Holistic Nursing Practice, 17*(4), 21–29.

North American Nursing Diagnoses Association. (2007). *Nursing Diagnoses Definitions and Classification 2005–2006.* Philadelphia, PA: Author.

Olszewski, T. M., & Varrasse, J. F. (2005). The neurobiology of PTSD. *Journal of Psychosocial Nursing, 43*(6), 41–47.

Paris, J. (1999). *Nature and nurture in psychiatry.* Washington, DC: American Psychiatric Press.

Pennington, B. F. (2002). *The development of psychopathology.* New York: Guilford Press.

Perkonigg, A., Pfister, H., Stein, M. B., Hofler, M., Lieb, R., Maercker, A., et al. (2005). Longitudinal course of posttraumatic stress disorder and posttraumatic stress disorder symptoms in a community sample of adolescents and young adults. *American Journal of Psychiatry, 162*(7), 1320–1327.

Piacentini, J., Bergman, R. L., Keller, M., & McCracken, J. (2003). Functional impairment in children and adolescents with obsessive–compulsive disorder. *Journal of Child and Adolescent Psychopharmacology, 13*(2), 61–69.

Pollack, M. H. (2005). The pharmacotherapy of panic disorder. *Journal of Clinical Psychiatry,* (66 Suppl 4), 23–27.

Punamaki, R. L., Komproe, I. H., Qouta, S., Elmasri, M., & de Jong, J. T. V. M. (2005). The role of peritraumatic dissociation and gender in the association between trauma and mental health in a Palestinian community sample. *American Journal of Psychiatry, 162*(3), 545–551.

Rapoport, J. L. (1989). *The boy who couldn't stop washing.* Washington, DC: Dutton.

Ressler, K. J., Rothbaum, B. O., Tannenbaum, L., Anderson, P., Graap, K., Zimand, E., et al. (2004). Cognitive enhancers as adjuncts to psychotherapy. *Archives of General Psychiatry, 61*(11), 1136–1144.

Saxena, S., Brody, A. L., Maidment, K. M., Smith, E. C., Zohrabi, N., Katz, E., et al. (2004). Cerebral glucose metabolism in obsessive–compulsive hoarding. *American Journal of Psychiatry, 61*(6), 1038–1048.

Simeon, D., Guralnik, D., Hazlett, E. A., Spiegel-Cohen, J., Hollander, E., & Buchsbaum, M. S. (2000). Feeling unreal: A PET study of depersonalization disorder. *American Journal of Psychiatry, 157*(11), 1782–1788.

Simeon, D., Guralnik, O., Knutelska, M., & Schmeidler, J. (2002). Personality factors associated with dissociation. *American Journal of Psychiatry, 159*(3), 489–491.

Simon, N. M., Worthington, J. J., Doyle, A. C., Hoge, E. A., Kinrys, G., Fischmann, D., et al. (2004). An open-label study of levetiracetam for the treatment of social anxiety disorder. *Journal of Clinical Psychiatry, 65*(9), 1219–1222.

Smoller, J. W., Pollack, M. H., Wassertheil-Smoller, S., Barton, B., Hendrix, S. L., Jackson, R. D., et al. (2003). Prevalence and correlates of panic attacks in postmenopausal women. *Archives of Internal Medicine, 163*(17), 2041–2050.

Stein, D. J., & Hugo, F. J. (2004). Neuropsychiatric aspects of anxiety disorders. In S. C. Yudofsky & R. E. Hales (Eds.), *Essentials of neuropsychiatry and clinical neurosciences* (pp. 519–533). Washington, DC: American Psychiatric Publishing.

Stengler-Wenzke, K., Trosbach, J., Dietrich, S., & Angermeyer, M. C. (2004). Experience of stigmatization by relatives of patients with obsessive–compulsive disorder. *Archives of Psychiatric Nursing, 18*(3), 88–96.

Sukhodolsky, D. G., Rosario-Campos, M. C., Katsovich, L., Pauls, D. L., Peterson, B. S., King, R. A., et al. (2005). Adaptive, emotional, and family functioning of children with obsessive–compulsive disorder and comorbid attention deficit hyperactivity disorder. *American Journal of Psychiatry, 162*(6), 1125–1132.

Szeszko, P. R., MacMillan, S., McMeniman, M., Chen, S., Baribault, K., Lim, K. O., et al. (2004). Brain structural abnormalities in psychotropic drug-naïve pediatric patients with obsessive–compulsive disorder. *American Journal of Psychiatry, 161*(6), 1049–1056.

Warden, D. L., & Labbate, L. A. (2005). Posttraumatic stress disorder and other anxiety disorders. In J. M. Silver, T. W. McAllister, & S. C. Yudofsky (Eds.), *Textbook of traumatic brain injury* (pp. 231–243). Washington, DC: American Psychiatric Press.

Chapter **12**

Eating Disorders

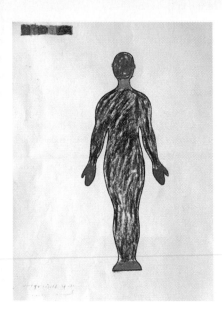

> **❝** *I felt fine doing this. I am very uncomfortable with my body and always have been. I hate pretty much everything about myself.* **❞**
>
> —Jeanne, Age 30

Color scale 1–5 represents confortablity with self.
Brown # 5 = most uncomfortable.

OBJECTIVES

1. Compare and contrast the different theories regarding the etiology of eating disorders.

2. Describe the treatment options for a client with an eating disorder.

3. Outline the assessment process for a client with an eating disorder.

4. Use the nursing process to develop a safe, comprehensive plan of care for a client with an eating disorder.

5. Develop illness management teaching plans for a person with an eating disorder and her/his family.

6. Discuss the key points in effectively communicating with a person with an eating disorder.

MediaLink www.prenhall.com/fontaine

Go to the Pearson Health MediaLink CD-ROM and the Companion Website at www.prenhall.com/fontaine for interactive resources for this chapter.

The ROAD to Critical Thinking | A Client Experiencing Eating Disorder

Travel this ROAD to understand Jessica and her condition.

Read about Jessica below and throughout this chapter.

Observe Jessica on the CD-ROM accompanying this book.

Assess Jessica by answering the questions at the end of this chapter.

Develop a Care Plan on the CD-ROM to address Jessica's condition.

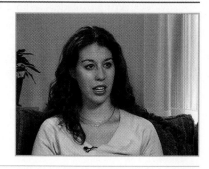

Jessica

The onset of Jessica's eating disorder coincided with her entry into a theater school in New York City. Her pattern was one of anorexia, purging, and compulsive exercise. Competing with other talented people led to her believing that her talents were negligible and that she was an insignificant person. Feeling out of control in many aspects of her life, she focused her attention on eating and her body. Rather quickly, she developed anorexia.

Determining the incidence of anorexia and bulimia is difficult because of the variety of definitions. The frequency of these disorders has been increasing, but the increase may be partly due to increased reporting. Ninety percent of women and 25% of men diet at some time in their lives. More than half of teenage girls and one third of teenage boys use unhealthy weight control behaviors such as skipping meals, fasting, vomiting, using laxatives, and smoking cigarettes. Clinical eating disorders are estimated to affect 8% to 20%

of the population. They are more commonly seen among females; estimates of the male–female ratio range from 1:6 to 1:10, although 19% to 30% of younger people with anorexia are male. The estimate may be low since primary health care providers are less likely to diagnose an eating disorder in a male than in a female. The disorders usually develop during adolescence: age 13 to 17 for anorexia and age 17 to 23 for bulimia. The age of onset has been dropping in recent years, and we now see children as young as age 7 with anorexia. Anywhere from 30% to 70% of people with anorexia develop chronic symptoms (Neumark-Sztainer, 2005; Tozzi et al., 2005).

You meet Jessica on the video clip on your CD-ROM and throughout this chapter. At the end of the chapter you will find critical thinking questions relating to assessment and development of a plan of care for Jessica.

ANOREXIA NERVOSA AND BULIMIA NERVOSA

Anorexia nervosa and bulimia nervosa are not single diseases but syndromes with multiple predisposing factors and a variety of characteristics. Although the most obvious symptom is the eating problem, these disorders are not simply a matter of eating too much or too little. It is because of the complex interaction of biological, psychological, developmental, familial, and sociocultural factors that certain people develop eating disorders.

There is no clear-cut distinction between the two disorders, and they have many features in common. The traditional division of anorexia and bulimia is still appropriate until more is known about eating disorders. Body weight may be a significant distinguishing characteristic; people with anorexia are severely underweight and people with bulimia are at normal or near-normal weight. About 30% of people with bulimia have a history of anorexia. As many as 62% of people with anorexia exhibit bulimic behaviors. Conversion from anorexia to bulimia may be a way of moving from a "visible" to an "invisible" eating disorder to deceive family, friends, and health care providers. Thus, the two disorders can occur

in the same person, or the person can go from one disorder to the other. There are far more similarities than differences between anorexia and bulimia (Finfgeld, 2002; Tozzi et al., 2005). However, to help you understand the differences, the disorders have been separated in this chapter (see the DSM-IV-TR Classifications feature).

People with **anorexia nervosa** lose weight by dramatically decreasing their food intake and sharply increasing their amount of physical exercise. Individuals with **bulimia nervosa** develop cycles of binge eating followed by purging. The severity of the disorder is determined by the frequency of the binge–purge cycles.

KNOWLEDGE BASE

Eating disorders are more common among competitive athletes than the general age-matched population. Female athletes are especially at risk in sports that emphasize a thin body such as gymnastics, ballet, figure skating, and distance running. Males in sports such as bodybuilding and wrestling are also at greater risk. Parents and coaches may support problematic eating behavior in a misguided effort to increase their competitive edge. Other groups at risk include dancers and models.

MediaLink Care Plan, Client with Bulimia: Binge Eating and Purging

Nurses will encounter people with eating disorders in a number of clinical settings. In schools, camps, community health care settings, pediatric units, medical–surgical units, and intensive care units, nurses must be aware of the characteristics of eating disorders so they can provide prompt attention to those in need. Eating disorders have generally been considered to have one of the highest mortality rates of all the mental disorders. They have a suicide rate that is much higher than the rate in the general population. Therefore, it is extremely risky to underestimate the seriousness of eating disorders (Keel et al., 2003; McIntosh et al., 2005).

Purging Disorder

Purging disorder is a separate clinical disorder from bulimia. People with purging disorder do not binge eat but do purge frequently. Screening tests may miss this group of individuals because they are of normal weight and respond negatively to the binge-eating questions. Given that purging itself has serious medical consequences, it is important to identify these clients (Keel, Haedt, & Edler, 2005).

Binge Eating Disorder

The bulimic pattern is different from **binge eating disorder**, which is often associated with obesity. This is a proposed new category that needs further study before inclusion into the *Diagnostic and Statistical Manual of Mental Disorders* (4th ed., text revision) (DSM-IV-TR) (APA, 2000). The prevalence in the general population is 1% to 3% and as high as 25% in those people seeking help for weight loss (Pull, 2004).

Obese individuals who overeat tend to follow one of two patterns, neither of which includes purging the body after excessive food intake. The first pattern is overeating and feeling out of control in response to a number of feelings such as anxiety or depression. The diagnosis of binge eating disorder is given when binging occurs at least twice a week for 6 months. Some binge in response to losing control over a weight-loss diet. Although these people lose weight in weight-control programs, they regain it after going off the diet. People with this eating pattern say that their eating or weight interferes with their relationships and their self-esteem. Women are more likely to have this eating pattern than men. There is evidence that several drugs are effective for this disorder including sibutramine (Meridia), an appetite suppressant; citalopram (Celexa), a selective serotonin reuptake inhibitor (SSRI) antidepressant; and topiramate (Topamax), an anticonvulsant and mood stabilizer (Appolinario et al., 2003; Neumark-Sztainer, 2005; Pull, 2004).

The second pattern is overeating because of the enjoyment of food. Seldom attempting to diet, these people have no sense of loss of control. They are more accepting of their body size and understand it to be the result of their enjoyment of eating.

Nocturnal Sleep-related Eating Disorder

Nocturnal sleep-related eating disorder is a newly recognized form of binge eating. It is characterized by sleepwalking and sleep eating. Safety becomes a problem when individuals actually prepare meals while asleep, resulting in burns or even a fire. Some sufferers discover bruises and lacerations from bumping into walls or furniture while sleepwalking. Upon awakening, the individual may have no recall or may have vague recall of the nighttime behavior. This eating disorder is found in those individuals of normal weight and those who are overweight. Some may also experience a daytime eating disorder such as anorexia or bulimia (Pull, 2004).

Obesity

Obesity is the most common form of malnourishment in the United States. Using the body mass index, it is estimated that 59 million adults in the United States are obese and 9 million youth are obese. The prevalence of obesity has increased in all age, gender, and ethnic/racial groups during the past three decades. Since the mental health of obese people is comparable to that of the general population, obesity is not considered a mental disorder. The only similarity between obesity and anorexia and bulimia is dissatisfaction with body size and shape. Therefore, a brief overview is presented here; consult other resources, books, and journals for a more comprehensive description (Eissa & Gunner, 2004; Long & Stevens, 2004).

Obesity is thought to result from a variety of combinations of psychosocial and physiological factors. There is no universal cause and therefore no single treatment approach. There are many ways of becoming and staying obese.

A variety of psychosocial factors may contribute to the development and maintenance of obesity. Eating habits are primarily learned *patterns of behavior* in response to hunger (a physiological sensation) and appetite (social and psychological cues). Some people manage negative feelings—such as anxiety, anger, and loneliness—by overeating. Others may view eating as a reward. These patterns may have been learned in childhood if parents used food as a way to decrease stress or reward good behavior. Because social events are frequently associated with food, some people make a connection between pleasure and eating—a connection that may predispose them to overeating. Increased caloric and fat intake and decreased physical activity also contribute to the rise in obesity.

Many researchers believe *physiological factors* are more significant than psychosocial factors. More than 200 genes have been identified that contribute to appetite, hunger, satiety, metabolism, fat storage, and activity tendencies. Recently, a gene for obesity, *ob,* and its protein product, leptin, were discovered. Leptin is produced in fat cells and travels to the

| **DSM-IV-TR** | **Diagnostic Criteria for Eating Disorders** |

ANOREXIA NERVOSA

A. Refusal to maintain body weight at or above a minimally normal weight for age and height (e.g., weight loss leading to maintenance of body weight less than 85% of that expected; or failure to make expected weight gain during period of growth, leading to body weight less than 85% of that expected).

B. Intense fear of gaining weight or becoming fat, even though underweight.

C. Disturbance in the way in which one's body image or shape is experienced, undue influence of body weight or shape on self-evaluation, or denial of the seriousness of the current low body weight.

D. In postmenarcheal females, amenorrhea, i.e., the absence of at least three consecutive menstrual cycles. (A woman is considered to have amenorrhea if her periods occur only following hormone, e.g., estrogen, administration.)

RESTRICTING TYPE

During the current episode of Anorexia Nervosa, the person has not regularly engaged in binge-eating or purging behavior (i.e., self-induced vomiting or the misuse of laxatives, diuretics, or enemas).

BINGE-EATING/PURGING TYPE

During the current episode of Anorexia Nervosa, the person has regularly engaged in binge-eating or purging behavior (i.e., self-induced vomiting or the misuse of laxatives, diuretics, or enemas).

BULIMIA NERVOSA

A. Recurrent episodes of binge eating. An episode of binge eating is characterized by both of the following:
1. Eating, in a discrete period of time (e.g., within any 2-hour period), an amount of food that is definitely larger than most people would eat during a similar period of time and under similar circumstances.
2. A sense of lack of control over eating during the episode (e.g., a feeling that one cannot stop eating or control what or how much one is eating).

B. Recurrent inappropriate compensatory behavior in order to prevent weight gain, such as self-induced vomiting; misuse of laxatives, diuretics, enemas, or other medications; fasting; or excessive exercise.

C. The binge eating and inappropriate compensatory behaviors both occur, on average, at least twice a week for 3 months.

D. Self-evaluation is unduly influenced by body shape and weight.

E. The disturbance does not occur exclusively during episodes of Anorexia Nervosa.

PURGING TYPE

During the current episode of Bulimia Nervosa, the person has regularly engaged in self-induced vomiting or the misuse of laxatives, diuretics, or enemas.

NONPURGING TYPE

During the current episode of Bulimia Nervosa, the person has used other inappropriate compensatory behaviors, such as fasting or excessive exercise, but has not regularly engaged in self-induced vomiting or the misuse of laxatives, diuretics, or enemas.

RESEARCH CRITERIA FOR BINGE-EATING DISORDER

A. Recurrent episodes of binge eating. An episode of binge eating is characterized by both of the following:
1. Eating, in a discrete period of time (e.g., within any 2-hour period), an amount of food that is definitely larger than most people would eat in a similar period of time under similar circumstances
2. A sense of lack of control over eating during the episode (e.g., a feeling that one cannot stop eating or control what or how much one is eating)

B. The binge-eating episodes are associated with three (or more) of the following:
1. Eating much more rapidly than normal
2. Eating until feeling uncomfortably full
3. Eating large amounts of food when not feeling physically hungry
4. Eating alone because of being embarrassed by how much one is eating
5. Feeling disgusted with oneself, depressed, or very guilty after overeating

C. Marked distress regarding binge eating is present.

D. The binge eating occurs, on average, at least 2 days a week for 6 months. Note: The method of determining frequency differs from that used for Bulimia Nervosa; future research should address whether the preferred method of setting a frequency threshold is counting the number of days on which binges occur or counting the number of episodes of binge eating.

E. The binge eating is not associated with the regular use of inappropriate compensatory behaviors (e.g., purging, fasting, excessive exercise) and does not occur exclusively during the course of Anorexia Nervosa or Bulimia Nervosa.

brain, where it decreases appetite and increases metabolic rate. A hormone produced in the stomach called *ghrelin* boosts appetite. A competing hormone, *obestatin,* suppresses the appetite. Adoption, twin, and family studies note that obesity has a strong inheritable component: 30% to 80% of variability in body weight or fat mass is genetically determined (Devlin, Yanovski, & Wilson, 2000).

In obese and nonobese people, the amount of *body fat* seems to be precisely regulated and maintained. This explains the difficulty most people have in changing the amount of their body fat. There is frequently no clear difference between the amount of food eaten by obese people and by nonobese people. The belief that all obese people overeat is inaccurate and underlies many of our culture's negative stereotypes about obesity.

Weight gain is among the most problematic *side effects* of psychotropic medications and is one of the most frequent reasons individuals stop taking their medications. Weight gain is a side effect for all the antipsychotic agents, lithium and other mood stabilizers, and many of the antidepressants.

Some people are blatantly hostile toward overweight people. It is no longer acceptable to stigmatize people on the basis of race or ethnic origin and therefore obesity remains one of the last socially acceptable forms of *prejudice*. Because of the high level of prejudice against obese people in America, the social consequences of being overweight can be severe. Obese individuals may suffer from job discrimination because employers assume they are less healthy, less diligent, and less intelligent than their thinner peers. In stores, obese customers may be treated with less respect and less consideration. When obese people eat in public, they are often given disapproving looks and comments from thinner people. Frequent exposure to such treatment increases feelings of hurt and failure. Being bombarded with anti-fat values further increases the obese person's level of self-disgust. Health care professionals add to this discrimination by viewing obesity not only as a health hazard, but also as an indication of emotional disturbance. In fact, it is the internalization of the culture's hatred and rejection, rather than body weight and size, which contributes to psychological problems.

People who are 35% or more above ideal body weight are at high risk for developing a number of *medical conditions*. These include diabetes mellitus, hypertension, cardiovascular disease, hyperlipidemia, gallbladder disease, arthritis, polycystic ovary syndrome, sleep apnea, and complications of pregnancy. The risk of death is higher for women than men and higher for the young than the old (Eissa & Gunner, 2004).

Obesity is among the easiest of medical conditions to recognize and the most difficult to treat. A wide variety of treatment approaches have been tried. In all the approaches, there is a general tendency to regain lost weight. At this point, preventing obesity is more effective than treating it.

Prader–Willi Syndrome

Prader–Willi syndrome (PWS) is a congenital disorder of the 15th chromosome. Estimated prevalence is 1 in 10,000 to 15,000 live births. PWS not only causes an unrelenting feeling of hunger, but also low muscle tone, short stature, incomplete sexual development, mild to severe mental retardation, and behavioral problems. By age 2 or 3 years, the child's appetite becomes insatiable and there is a rapid and excessive weight gain. The physiologically driven eating behavior is not under the individual's cognitive control. The person cannot decide "not to eat." Compounding the excessive appetite is decreased calorie utilization in those with PWS due to low muscle mass and inactivity. Their calorie needs are about 60% of other persons. Access to food must be rigidly enforced if they are not to become morbidly obese. Restricting food intake must extend from the home and into school, work, and community settings. Hoarding food and stealing money to buy food are very common problems for this group of individuals. Morbid obesity may lead to serious medical consequences, including cardiovascular diseases, diabetes mellitus, sleep disturbances, and respiratory compromise. These are the most common causes of premature death among those suffering from PWS (Nolan, 2003).

Behavioral problems can lead to curtailed psychosocial development and poor social functioning. Symptoms may include temper tantrums, oppositional behavior and stubbornness, labile emotions, and obsessive thinking or compulsive behaviors, such as skin picking. Some individuals compulsively engage in rectal digging, which often causes embarrassment to them and their families. Rectal digging has potential risks, ranging from fecal contamination to rectal bleeding and sphincter problems. Treatment of PWS is growth hormone that increases muscle tone and enhances growth. For those who are depressed or anxious, antidepressants are often prescribed (Nolan, 2003).

Comorbid Disorders

For those with anorexia or bulimia, the most frequently observed disorder is *depression*. In some cases, this may be the result of abnormal eating and weight loss. In other cases, the depression is the primary disorder to which the eating disorder is a response. And for other people, the depression and eating disorder both are primary disorders.

There is a high prevalence of several *anxiety disorders* associated with eating disorders. *Social phobias* may occur in people with eating disorders, possibly in response to others' awareness of their abnormal eating behaviors. *Obsessive–compulsive symptoms* are common, especially among people with anorexia. Obsessive–compulsive symptoms often continue even after weight is restored in anorexia. *Panic attacks* are likely when anorexic people are prohibited from exercising their usual behavior patterns. It is unclear whether these are primary disorders or are secondary to the eating disorders (Kaye, Bulik, Thornton, Barbarich, & Masters, 2004).

People with eating disorders often *abuse substances*. In some, this may be an effort to self-medicate the symptoms of anxiety or depression. Others may abuse substances, such as cocaine, to decrease their appetite. Eating disorders share many features with problem drinking. Both begin with a decrease in anxiety in response to the behavior (drinking or not eating). Eventually both groups of people lose control over the behavior and continue on a path of self-destruction. There is a compulsive need to engage in the behavior, with considerable distress if the behavior is disrupted. Denial is the central defense mechanism of both disorders, and both have a long-term course with frequent relapses (Anderson, Martens, & Cimini, 2005; Finfgeld, 2002).

Etiologies

The causes of eating disorders are multiple in individuals and across a variety of people. Fatness and thinness are outcomes of biological, psychological, and social processes. The balance between energy intake and expenditure determines weight, and this balance is the product of many influences. Although family and culture may provide a trigger, it seems increasingly likely that hormones and brain chemicals prime a certain group of people to push themselves to starvation. Having a knowledge base about the major theories will help the nurse understand individual clients from a composite perspective.

Genetics

Family risk studies show that relatives of clients with eating disorders are five to ten times more likely to develop an eating disorder. It appears that in anorexia, the more severe the disorder, the more likely a strong genetic predisposition. Twin studies for anorexia show that the concordance rate for monozygotic twins is 55% to 71% and for dizygotic twins it is 0% to 32%. These data suggest that there may be a *genetic predisposition* to anorexia. Concordance rates for bulimia range from 23% to 83% for monozygotic twins and 0% to 27% for dizygotic twins (Slof-O't Landt et al., 2005).

Genetic research focuses on behavioral, neurobiological, and temperamental variables that may represent core features of these disorders. These features include perfectionism, orderliness, low tolerance for new situations, low self-esteem, and overall high anxiety. Even if an individual has a high genetic risk, however, he or she might develop an eating disorder even if he or she did not live in a culture that stresses dieting and thinness (Bulik, 2005).

Neurobiology

Recent studies indicate that *neurotransmitter dysregulation* may be involved in eating disorders, particularly serotonin (5-HT). Being full of food to the point of satisfaction is referred to as *satiety*. Normally, a low level of 5-HT decreases a person's satiety and thereby increases food intake. In contrast, a high level of 5-HT increases satiety and thereby decreases food intake. Carbohydrates (CHOs) are involved in the synthesis of 5-HT by increasing tryptophan, the precursor of 5-HT. The neurotransmitter hypothesis of bulimia is that the recurrent binge episodes may result from a deficiency in 5-HT and low satiety levels. Since people with bulimia tend to binge on high-CHO foods, this may be a reflection of the body's adaptive attempt to increase 5-HT levels. The neurotransmitter hypothesis of anorexia is that decreased food intake is related to excess 5-HT and increased satiety (Romano, Halmi, Sarkar, Koke, & Lee, 2002).

The level of spontaneous physical activity appears to be related to energy expenditure and thus to body weight.

Orexin neurons in the lateral hypothalamus appear to integrate this activity with feeding behavior (Kotz, 2006).

Other neurotransmitters affect eating behavior. Norepinephrine (NE) and neuropeptide Y (NPY) increase eating behavior while dopamine (DA) suppresses food intake. DA agonists such as amphetamines and cocaine are appetite suppressants (Frank et al., 2005).

Endogenous opioids, such as endorphins, are associated with food intake and mood. Opioids increase food intake and enhance positive mood states; therefore, insufficient levels cause decreased food intake and depressed mood. It has been found that underweight people have significantly lower levels of endorphins compared to healthy volunteers. When the person's weight is returned to normal levels, the endorphin level is also within normal limits.

Neuroimaging studies have shown a low level of functioning in the frontal lobes, parietal lobes, and the anterior cingulate of individuals with anorexia and bulimia. When these individuals viewed high-calorie foods, they experienced abnormally increased activity in those same brain regions (Uher et al., 2004).

Intrapersonal Factors

Intrapersonal theorists believe that people at higher risk for eating disorders have low self-esteem, experience significant adolescent turmoil, and have difficulty with identity formation. Personality characteristics of people with anorexia are perfectionism, low tolerance for new situations, low self-esteem, and difficulty achieving the maturational tasks of adolescence. People with bulimia are described in terms of perfectionism, affective instability, and poor impulse control. Feelings of incompetence and fear of losing control contribute to a tenuous self-definition, which is masked by the eating disorder (Stein & Corte, 2003).

Impulsive personality traits are characteristic of many people suffering from bulimia. The loss of control and the inability to stop binging once started is the typical bulimic pattern. This impulsivity resembles other addictive disorders.

Cognitive Theory

Cognitive theorists believe that cognitive distortions and dysfunctional thoughts such as dichotomous thinking and catastrophizing (exaggerating failures in one's life) contribute to disordered eating patterns. The extreme belief is: "It is absolutely essential that I be thin." This belief leads to dieting, avoidant behavior, and increased isolation, which in turn cause a lack of responsiveness to alternative cognitive input. Given the cultural emphasis on thinness, there is a sense of gratification, self-control, mastery, and approval of or concern from others.

Behavioral Theory

Behavioral theorists are concerned with what the disordered behavior accomplishes rather than why the behavior occurs. Eating disorders are considered phobias. In this context, anxiety increases with eating and decreases with fasting or purging. Anxiety reduction is the reinforcer for anorexia and bulimia both.

Family Factors

Most family theorists believe family issues are not specific to eating disorders. The family is viewed more as an enabler of the disorder than as a primary causative factor. Some people with eating disorders are survivors of childhood or adolescent sexual abuse, which may or may not have occurred within the family or extended family system. (Sexual abuse is discussed further in chapter 23 ∞.)

As the result of anorexia, some families become enmeshed; that is, the boundaries between the members are weak, interactions are intense, dependency on one another is high, and autonomy is minimal. Everybody is involved in each member's concerns, and there is minimal privacy. The enmeshed family system becomes overprotective of the child, and the entire family system becomes preoccupied with food, eating, and rituals involving meals. In contrast, current research indicates that families of people with bulimia are less enmeshed than those of anorexic people. Family members tend to be isolated from one another, and eating behavior may be an attempt to decrease feelings of loneliness and boredom.

Many families of individuals with eating disorders have difficulty with conflict resolution. An ethical or religious value against disagreements within the family supports the avoidance of conflict. When problems are denied for the sake of family harmony, they cannot be resolved, and growth of the family system is inhibited. The anorexic child may protect and maintain the family unit. In some family systems, the parents avoid conflict with each other by uniting in a common concern for the child's welfare. In other family systems, the issues of marital conflict are converted into disagreements over how the anorexic child should be managed. In both systems, the marital problems are camouflaged to prevent the disruption of the family unit. (See chapter 2 ∞ for more details on family dynamics.)

Many families of clients with eating disorders are achievement and performance oriented, with high ambition for the success of all members. In these families, body shape is related to success, and priorities are established for physical appearance and fitness. The family's focus on professional achievement as well as on food, diet, exercise, and weight control may become obsessional.

Gender-Bias Factors

From the gender-bias perspective, eating disorders arise out of a conflict between female development and traditional developmental theories. Western culture has viewed male development as the norm, and autonomy as the opposite of dependency. For women, the opposite of dependency is isolation. Conflict arises when women believe they must become autonomous and minimize relationships to be recognized as mature adults. For some, this conflict is acted out in self-destructive eating behavior.

Cultural stereotypes contribute to women's preoccupation with their bodies. Attractiveness is determined by how closely a woman's appearance matches the cultural ideal of thinness. Thus, identity and self-esteem are dependent on physical appearance. Being disgusted with one's flesh is the same as having an adversarial relationship with the body—a relationship that often results in eating disorders.

Psychopharmacological Interventions

Medications, primarily antidepressants, are used to reduce the frequency of disturbed eating behaviors such as binge eating and vomiting. In addition, medications are used to ease symptoms that may accompany eating disorders such as depression, anxiety, obsessions, or impulse control problems.

For people with anorexia, drug trials have been disappointing, although there is some interest in exploring the use of second-generation antipsychotic medication. Fluoxetine (Prozac), an SSRI, is effective for clients with bulimia when given at the higher dose of 50 to 60 mg per day. Typically, the medication is continued until 6 months following the disappearance of symptoms. In the past, tricyclic antidepressants have been used but the dropout rate is higher than with the SSRIs (Bacaltchuk & Hay, 2003).

Multidisciplinary Interventions

The current therapeutic approach for eating disorders relies on a combination of psychological, behavioral, and nutritional techniques often provided in an intensive outpatient setting and, less often, in an inpatient setting. If the anorexic client is evaluated as highly endangered, as assessed by weight, current rate of weight loss, nutritional status, organ functioning, and cardiac health, she or he may be admitted to an acute care medical facility. Bulimic clients may also be hospitalized for uncontrolled vomiting, hematemesis, hypothermia, substance abuse, or suicide risk. Medical treatment may include a feeding schedule, potassium supplements, and bed rest. Tube feeding and parenteral nutrition are avoided unless absolutely necessary because they do not help clients assume responsibility for their own health.

Psychological treatment may include individual therapy, group work, family therapy, cognitive therapy, and systematic desensitization. The majority of centers that treat clients with eating disorders also use cognitive behavior therapy, which is based on the belief that the symptoms of anorexia, such as food restriction and avoidance, become habit patterns independent of the initial "reasons" for giving up food. Techniques include challenging dysfunctional thoughts, thought restructuring, self-monitoring homework, prescription of normal eating, and a negotiated weight range goal (McIntosh et al., 2005).

When people have incorporated their eating disorder into their identities, therapy can be a threat. Unlike many clients with other mental disorders who wish to be free of their symptoms, people with eating disorders are often very reluctant to give up the drive for thinness or low weight. They may also believe that there is a positive stigma to having an eating disorder—such as being a member of the "eating disorder club." Their lives can become filled with support groups, and they continually discuss their obsessions regarding food, weight, and shape. Groups of people with eating disorders can become competitive: Who is the thinnest? Who ate the least? Who exercised the most? Understanding the function that the eating disorder serves in terms of creating an identity is essential in treatment planning.

Alternative Therapies

Clients with eating disorders should take vitamin and mineral complexes. They are usually taken in very high doses because they are passed through the gastrointestinal tract rapidly and are poorly assimilated. The multivitamin complex should contain:

- Natural beta-carotene 25,000 IU daily
- Vitamin A 10,000 IU daily
- Vitamin D 400 IU daily
- Calcium 1,500 mg daily
- Copper 3 mg daily
- Magnesium 1,000 mg daily
- Potassium 99 mg daily
- Selenium 200 mcg daily
- Zinc 80 mg daily

Clients who are vomiting or using laxatives should take acidophilus, which replaces the "friendly" bacteria lost through purging. Acidophilus should be taken on an empty stomach so that it passes quickly to the small intestine. The following herbs may be used as appetite stimulants: ginger root, ginseng, gotu kola, and peppermint. Clients should not use ginseng if they are hypertensive.

Animal studies of repetitive transcranial magnetic stimulation (rTMS) have shown promise in changing eating behaviors. Further studies are being done to translate this finding with human subjects (Tsai, 2005). Further information on rTMS is found in chapter 9 ∞ .

Nursing Process

CLIENTS WITH EATING DISORDERS

ASSESSMENT

Clients with bulimia may welcome the opportunity to talk about their disorder with a caring, nonjudgmental nurse. Moreover, learning that they are not alone in having bulimia may relieve some of their anxiety and distress. Clients with anorexia, on the other hand, may not be as willing to talk about their disorder. Client denial of problems or illness may interfere with the nurse's ability to obtain an accurate nursing assessment. A supportive and caring approach is necessary to establish rapport with these clients.

In general, nursing assessment includes a detailed analysis of eating patterns and weight fluctuations, methods of weight control, food avoided and the reasons they are avoided, and the occurrence and frequency of binge eating and purging. In addition, the nurse should explore the individual's and family's beliefs about nutrition and attitudes toward eating, exercise, and appearance. Side effects of steroid abuse may include several psychiatric symptoms such as hallucinations, manic symptoms, and depression. Other mental disorders that must be taken into consideration include depression, anxiety disorders, and substance abuse. If left untreated, these comorbid conditions can significantly reduce treatment effectiveness.

Nurses who work with adolescent and young adult athletes, particularly those athletes participating in the at-risk sports, must be alert to early symptoms of eating disorders. Simple screening questions about weight, possible dissatisfaction with appearance, exercise routine, and nutritional intake on the day before evaluation may help identify a person who is developing an eating disorder.

Assessment: Behavior

Anorexia

Rigidity and overcontrol are the hallmarks of anorexia. To control themselves and their environment, these individuals develop rigid rules. Such rigidity often develops into *obsessive rituals,* particularly concerning eating and exercise. Cutting all food into a predetermined size or number of pieces, chewing all food a certain number of times, allowing only certain combinations of food in a meal, accomplishing a fixed number of

Focused Nursing Assessment   Clients With Eating Disorders

Behavior Assessment	Affective Assessment	Cognitive Assessment
What type of eating patterns do you have? Do you have rules for eating, such as places to eat? Combination of foods? Number of pieces of food? Number of times to chew food? What time of day do you usually binge? Where do you do this? How often? How long does it last? Foods that trigger a binge? Favorite foods to eat on a binge? After binge eating, how do you rid your body of the food? Vomit? Laxatives? Diuretics? How much time do you spend exercising each day? How does the use of alcohol or drugs help you cope with your problems?	Describe any of the following fears: gaining weight, being fat, rejection by others, losing control over eating. What kinds of situations make you feel guilty? Ashamed? Anxious? Frustrated? Helpless? What are your feelings when you eat more than your diet allows?	Do you believe your eating pattern is in any way unusual? Do you have any desire to alter your eating behavior? Describe your body to me. Describe what an attractive person looks like. What would your life be like if you were as thin as you wished? What will happen if you gain weight?

exercise routines, and having an inflexible pattern of exercises are rituals common to anorexic people. These rules and rituals help keep anxiety beyond conscious awareness. If the rituals are disrupted, the anxiety becomes intolerable. Paradoxically, all these efforts to stay in control lead to out-of-control behaviors (Tozzi et al., 2005).

Many people with anorexia are hyperactive and discover that *overexercise* is a way to increase their weight loss. Solitary running tends to be the exercise of choice and there are often obsessional qualities to it. For example, they feel that before they can eat, they have to earn calories by exercising. Conversely, if they overeat, they feel they have to punish themselves with excessive exercise. Excessive exercise signifies the

Jessica:

" I would go to the gym no matter what. For me the gym was never something that was enjoyable. It was something I did to negate the calories that I'd eaten during the day. It was a really long period of exercise done after hours of dance classes. I hated running but I would run for an hour on the treadmill and then I would lift weights for another half hour. It was very punishing exercise on my body. It was just sort of another form of purging for me. "

triumph of will over the body and is a possible indication of poor prognosis in recovery (Neumark-Sztainer, 2005).

Anorexic young women have a desperate need to please others. Their self-worth depends on responses from others, rather than on their own self-approval. Thus, their behavior is often *overcompliant*; they always try to meet the expectations of others in order to be accepted. They may overachieve in academic and extracurricular activities, but these accomplishments are usually an attempt to please parents rather than a source of self-satisfaction.

People with anorexia often feel hopeless, helpless, and ineffective. Because of being overcompliant with their parents, they believe they have always been controlled by others. Their *refusal to eat* may be an attempt to assert themselves and gain some control within the family. As weight is lost, they are rewarded with praise, admiration, and envy from their peers, which reinforces the restricted eating pattern.

Phobias in people with anorexia are common. Initially, the fear is of weight gain, but it develops into a *secondary food phobia*. The mechanism of phobic avoidance in anorexic people is different from that in others. In nonanorexic people, the phobia has an external stimulus, such as an animal or an object, a place, or a situation. Avoidance prevents the escalation of anxiety, but the person receives no pleasure in the

Social Assessment	Physiological Assessment
How often do you socialize with friends? What activities do you do together?	*Weight* What is your present weight? What is the most you have ever weighed? What is the least you have ever weighed?
How close are the members of your family?	
What are the family rules about disagreements?	*Endocrine* Are you having menstrual periods? Describe your usual cycle to me.
Describe your family's standards for physical fitness and appearance.	
How do other members of the family control their weight?	*Cardiovascular* Do you get dizzy when you stand up from a lying position? Have you experienced any heart palpitations? Irregular heartbeat? Are you having any problems with your ankles and feet swelling? Your fingers?
	Gastrointestinal Have you had an increase in the number of dental caries? Have you lost any teeth? Do you have frequent sore throats? Do you experience heartburn? Do you have problems with constipation?
	Neurological Have you experienced any seizures or convulsions?

process. In people with anorexia, the phobia has an internal stimulus: the fear of being fat. Avoidance of food provides a feeling of control and a sense of pleasure when weight is lost.

The onset of Ann's anorexia was in the 6th grade. The disorder has gradually become more severe until now, at age 16, she is in very serious condition. She changes the food she eats every month and describes a sense of pride in her self-control. For example: in November she ate 10 pieces of lettuce at 5 P.M. and at 7 P.M.; in December she ate 1/2 cup of low fat macaroni and cheese at 5 P.M.; and in January she ate 1/2 cup of cereal with 1/2 cup of water at 5 P.M. and 2 teaspoons of ice cream at 7 P.M. Ann is 5 feet 6 inches tall and her current weight is 72 pounds (32.7 kg).

Bulimia

Impulsivity and affective dysregulation are hallmarks of bulimia. Because they have difficulty with self-directedness, individuals are unable to regulate their behavior and affect. This impulsivity contributes to additional problems of substance abuse, self-injury behavior, and impulse control disorders.

Individuals with bulimia often learn this maladaptive pattern of weight control from peers who have used purging as a method of losing weight. This sort of bulimia may go undetected for years because often there is no significant weight loss. For males and females both, the behavior rapidly becomes impulsive and compulsive, and the frequency and severity of the eating disorder tend to increase.

There is a *cyclic behavioral pattern* in bulimia. It begins with skipping meals sporadically and overstrict *dieting* or fasting. In an effort to refrain from eating, the person may use amphetamines, which can lead to extreme hunger, fatigue, and low blood glucose levels. The next part of the cycle is a period of *binge eating*, in which the person ingests huge amounts of food (about 3,500 kcal) within a short time (about 1 hour). Binges can last up to 8 hours, with consumption of 12,000 kcal. Binge eating usually occurs when the person is alone and at home, and is most frequent during the evening. The cycle may occur once or twice a month for some and as often as five or ten times a day for others. The binge part of the cycle may be triggered by the ingestion of certain foods, but this is not consistent for everyone. Although eating binges may involve any kind of food, they usually consist of junk foods, fast foods, and high-calorie foods.

The final part of the cycle is *purging* the body of the ingested food. After excessive eating, people with bulimia force themselves to vomit. They often abuse laxatives and diuretics to purge their bodies of the food. Some use as many as 50 to 100 laxatives per day. In rare cases, they

Jessica:

" I was essentially abusing diet pills and laxatives. I was not using them in the prescribed amounts and was taking them for incorrect uses, especially the laxatives. And I was on diet pills all the time. So, of course that produced other effects like shakiness and heart palpitations and weakness, especially when I was combining that with exercise. When I first started using diet pills the weight dropped off pretty quickly. And then they sort of became a security blanket. They were something I needed to affirm the fact that I was doing enough to control my body. "

may resort to syrup of ipecac to induce vomiting. Purging becomes a purification rite and a means of regaining self-control. Some describe it as feeling "completely fresh and clean again."

After the purging, the cycle begins all over again, with a return to strict dieting or fasting. Some people with bulimia eat highly nutritious meals when not binging/purging to repair harm done to the body.

Binge eating and purging begin as a way to eat and stay slim. Before long, the behavior becomes a response to stress and a way to cope with negative feelings such as anger, anxiety, and depression. For some, it is poor impulse control, and for others it is an expression of rebellion against family members.

People with bulimia may engage in *sporadic excessive exercise,* but they usually do not develop compulsive exercise routines. They are more likely to abuse street drugs to decrease their appetite and alcohol to reduce their anxiety. Since their binges are often expensive, costing as much as $100 per day, they may resort to *stealing* food or money to buy the food. The binge–purge cycle can become so consuming that activities and relationships are disrupted. To keep the secret, the person often resorts to excuses and lies.

Assessment: Affect

Anorexia

People with anorexia are often beset by *fears;* some fear maturing and assuming adult responsibilities. Because of their need to please others with high levels of achievement, some fear they are not doing well enough. Almost all have an extreme terror of weight gain and fat. A paradoxical response occurs when this fear actually increases as body weight decreases. If weight gain (real or imagined) occurs, anxiety surfaces to the conscious level and is perceived as a threat to the entire being. People with anorexia also fear a loss of control. Although this fear is usually related to losing control over eating, it may extend to other physiological processes such as sleeping, urination, and bowel functioning. The steady loss of weight becomes symbolic of mastery over self and environment. However, if they lose control and eat more than they believe to be appropriate, they experience severe guilt.

Bulimia

Because of their need for acceptance and approval, people with bulimia repress feelings of frustration and anger toward others. *Repressing feelings* and avoiding conflict protect them from rejection. As the ability to identify feelings decreases, they often confuse negative emotions with sensations of being hungry. Food then becomes a source of comfort and a way to defend against anger and frustration. Life is often viewed as tragic and *hopeless.* Talents and interests are abandoned and their lives are devoid of fun, humor, or genuine self-pleasure.

Like people with anorexia, people with bulimia experience multiple *fears.* They fear a loss of control, not only over their eating but also over their emotions. They are extremely fearful of weight gain and, with real or perceived changes in their weight, they feel panic. Motivating much of their behavior is fear of rejection.

The binge–purge cycle can be understood from the affective perspective as well as the behavioral perspective. *Anxiety* increases to a high level, at which point the person engages in binge eating to decrease the anxiety. Afterward, the person experiences *guilt* and self-disgust because of the loss of control. Guilt and disgust increase the anxiety, and purging, through vomiting and other methods, is then used to decrease this anxiety. Because this behavior is an indirect and ineffective way to manage anxiety, the levels rebuild, and the cycle starts anew. Some are able to talk about their feelings of helplessness, hopelessness, and worthlessness, while others do not seem to have the language to talk about their feelings.

Jessica:

" I think my depression was related to these perfectionistic ideals that I had set up for myself. If I didn't live up to perfect, I wasn't worth anything. I had no coping mechanisms, no ways of expressing my feelings. When I was feeling angry or anxious, or when I was feeling lonely or upset or sad, or whatever it was, I didn't have any way of either talking about those emotions or dealing with them in other ways. How I coped with my feelings was my eating disorder. "

Assessment: Cognition

Anorexia

The desire to be thin and the behavioral control over eating are ego-syntonic in the anorexic client. **Ego-syntonic behavior** is behavior that agrees with one's thoughts, desires, and values. Anorexic people regard their obsession with food and eating as conventional behavior. The major defense mechanism for defining the behavior in an ego-syntonic manner is *denial:* denial of sensations of hunger, denial of physical exhaustion, and denial of any disorder or illness.

People with anorexia experience **cognitive distortions** similar to those experienced by people with mental disorders. These cognitive distortions are considered errors in thinking that continue even when there is obvious contradictory evidence. Cognitive distortions involve food, body image, loss of control, and achievement. One type of distortion is **selective abstraction**, or focusing on certain information while ignoring contradictory information. Another distortion is **overgeneralization**, in which the person takes information or an impression from one event and attaches it to a wide variety of situations. Using such words as *always, never, everybody,* and *nobody* indicates that the client is overgeneralizing. Anorexic people also have a tendency toward **magnification**, attributing a high level of importance to unpleasant occurrences. Through **personalization**, or **ideas of reference**, they believe that what occurs in the environment is related to them, even when no obvious relationship exists. There is also a tendency for **superstitious thinking**, in which the person believes that some unrelated action would magically influence a course of events. A further distortion is **dichotomous thinking**, an all-or-none type of reasoning that interferes with people's realistic perceptions of themselves. Dichotomous thinking involves opposite and mutually exclusive categories such as eating or not eating, all good or all bad, and celibacy or promiscuity. See Table 12.1■ for examples of cognitive distortions.

Rachael, 18, has been diagnosed with anorexia. She does not believe that her 5 foot 9 inch frame is underweight at 102 pounds (46.3 kg). Rachael believes she will look better when she reaches 85 pounds (38.6 kg). She says that when she goes to college, she wants to be active in student government and that fat people are never elected. Her superstitious thinking relates to white clothing, which she feels decreases her hunger.

Body image is an integration of people's perceptions, thoughts, and feelings about their own body. *Perceptions* involve how big or small they estimate their body to be. *Thoughts* include an evaluation of body attractiveness, and *feelings* are the emotional association with their body shape and size. Body image is a psychological phenomenon but it is significantly affected by social factors. See Figure 12.1■ for ideal body image. By age 13, 53% of girls in the United States are unhappy with their bodies and consider themselves to be fat. By age 18, that number jumps up to 78%. As men's bodies become more exposed by the media, men are becoming more dissatisfied with their bodies. In one study of 548 men, 43% reported that they were dissatisfied with their overall appearance, 63% were dissatisfied with their abdomen, and 52% were unhappy with their weight. Body image disorders are more prevalent in North American, European, and Australian men than in men in non-Western cultures. This difference may reflect a greater decline in traditional male roles in the West, leading to greater emphasis on the body as a measure of masculinity. Researchers have discovered that men are just as unhappy as women about their bodies (Keel, 2005; Yang, Gray, & Pope, 2005).

People suffering from anorexia experience *a severely distorted body image* that often reaches delusional proportions. Incapable of seeing that their bodies are emaciated, they continue to perceive themselves as fat. Some perceive their total body as obese, whereas others focus on a particular part of the body as fat, such as their hips, stomach, thighs, or face. While others see these people as starving and disappearing, they view themselves as strong and in the process of creating a whole new person.

Jessica:

❝No matter how thin I got, I was never going to be perfect enough. I was never going to be thin enough. I looked in the mirror and I saw something completely different than reality. And even as the numbers on the scale went down, the image in the mirror got bigger. I just was very, very out of touch with what my real appearance was.❞

Anorexic individuals believe they are in charge of their lives and in complete control. They believe their peers are jealous of their willpower and thinness, which gives them an additional sense of power. The disorder becomes an issue of *autonomy* because no one can make them eat or make them gain weight. They think of food not as a necessity for survival

TABLE 12.1	Examples of Cognitive Distortions
Distortion	**Example**
Selective abstraction	"I'm still too fat—look at how big my hands and feet are."
Overgeneralization	"You don't see fat people on television. Therefore, you have to be thin to be successful at anything in life."
Magnification	"If I gain 2 pounds, I know everyone will notice it."
Personalization	"Jim and Bob were talking and laughing together today. I'm sure they were talking about how fat I am."
Superstitious thinking	"If I wear all white, I'll lose weight faster." "Sitting still will cause my weight to go up rapidly."
Dichotomous thinking	"If I gain even 1 pound, that means I am totally out of control and I might as well gain 50 pounds." "If I eat one thing, I will just keep eating until I weigh 300 pounds." "If I'm not thin, I'm fat."

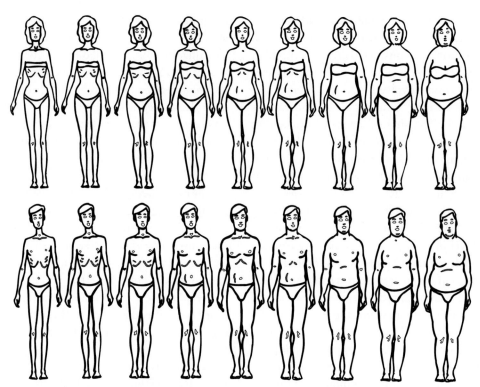

Figure 12.1 ■ Ideal body image—Which image do you think is ideal for your sex? And which comes closest to your body? This task is commonly used to assess whether a person has a positive or a negative body image.

SOURCE: Kassin, S. (2001). *Psychology* (3rd ed.). Upper Saddle River, NJ: Prentice Hall.

but as something that threatens survival. Cognitively, fat represents need and loss of control; thinness represents strength and control. These people are frequently secretive about their behavior. The secrecy is not viewed as manipulative but rather protective. From their point of view, anorexia is the solution, not the problem.

Anorexia contributes to distorted perceptions of internal physical sensations, a distortion referred to as **alexithymia**. Hunger is not recognized as hunger. When they eat a small amount of food, they often complain of feeling too full. There is also a decreased internal perception of fatigue, so they often push their bodies to physical extremes. Even after long and strenuous exercise, they seem unaware of any sensations of fatigue.

Young people with anorexia are overly concerned with how others view them. Many are convinced that other people have more insight into who they are than they do themselves. This *self-deprecation* and fear of self-definition contribute to beliefs and fears of being controlled by others. Feeling they have no power in their interpersonal relationships, they attempt to please and placate significant others whom they perceive to be more powerful.

People with anorexia develop *perfectionistic standards* for their behavior and moralistic guidelines about all aspects of life. Their decision-making ability is hampered by their need to make absolutely correct decisions. They are in such dread of losing control that they impose extremes of discipline on themselves. During the times clients are able to maintain control, their perfectionist behavior and dichotomous thinking

lead them to believe they are better than other people. However, these standards of behavior become self-defeating when clients fail to achieve them consistently. Another part of perfectionism is the ability to exceed other's expectations. Clients develop an identity as a person who can survive and flourish with little food.

> Kunjali, a 35-year-old woman, developed anorexia at age 12. She claims that life without an eating disorder would be a life without an identity. She believes she has not been "successful" as an anorexic because she has never reached an extremely low weight. She believes that truly successful anorexics die of starvation and that somehow they should be respected for their accomplishment. She believes that she has "failed" as an anorexic.

While it is unclear whether anorexia is a type of obsessive–compulsive disorder (OCD), anorexic people typically exhibit *obsessive–compulsive symptoms*. They spend a great deal of time obsessing about their weight and their bodies. They are preoccupied with thinking about food. Often, they develop complex rituals around food preparation, even though they refuse to eat the final product. Even after long-term weight recovery, their obsessions and compulsions continue (Bulik et al., 2003).

Bulimia

In contrast to people with anorexia, bulimic individuals are troubled by their behavioral characteristics. They experience ego-dystonic behavior, behavior that does not conform to the person's thoughts, wishes, and values. Another facet of ego-dystonic symptoms is that one feels the symptoms are beyond personal control. The person feels compelled to binge, purge, and fast; feels helpless to stop the behavior; and feels full of self-disgust for continuing the pattern.

Although bulimic people are not pleased with their body shape and size, they usually do not experience the delusional distortions of anorexic people. There is a direct correlation between the frequency and severity of the disorder and the degree of perceived distortion of body size. Many were overweight before the disorder, so there is an *obsessional concern* about not regaining the lost weight. It is difficult for them to think of anything other than food. Since they eat in response to hunger, appetite, and thoughts of food, the obsessions also involve getting rid of the food ingested to counteract the caloric effects of binge eating.

People with bulimia also experience the *cognitive distortions* discussed for anorexic people. They tend to relate their problems to weight or overeating. Their fantasy is that if they could only be thin and not overeat, all other problems would be solved. Another example of this all-or-none thinking is the belief that one bite will automatically lead to binge eating. The person may say, "As long as I have eaten one cookie, I have failed, so I might as well eat the entire package."

Bulimic people are *perfectionistic* in their personal standards of behavior. Even with their typically high level of professional achievement, they are extremely self-critical and often feel incompetent and inadequate. They set unrealistic standards of weight control and feel like failures when unable to maintain these standards. The thought of failure is a contributing factor to the binge phase of the cycle. Following the purge phase, they promise themselves to be more steadfast and disciplined with their diet. Because these resolutions are unrealistic, they set themselves up for another failure. Characteristics of people with anorexia and bulimia are listed in Table 12.2 ■.

Bill, who suffers from bulimia, states: "If I see another guy my age at the gym with perfectly defined abs, it really ruins my day."

TABLE 12.2	Characteristics of Eating Disorders

Characteristic	People With Anorexia	People With Bulimia
Self-evaluation	Are dependent on response from others; are self-depreciating	Are self-critical; view themselves as incompetent
Decision making	Need to make perfect decisions	Need to make perfect decisions
Rituals	Are obsessive in eating and exercise	Perpetuate the binge/purge/fast cycle
Sense of control	Create a sense of control and achievement by refusing to eat	Set unrealistic standards for own behavior; feel out of control
Phobia	Initially fear weight gain; develop food phobia	None specific
Exercise	Have obsessive routines	Exercise sporadically
Fears	Fear not being perfect, weight gain, fat, loss of control	Fear loss of control, weight gain, rejection
Guilt	Experience guilt when they eat more than they believe appropriate	Experience guilt when they binge eat and purge
Defense mechanisms	Deny hunger, exhaustion, disease	Do not deny hunger
Insight into illness	Are ego-syntonic; do not believe they have a disorder; see anorexia as the solution, not the problem	Are ego-dystonic; are disgusted with self but helpless to change
Cognitive distortions	Practice selective abstraction, overgeneralization, magnification, personalization, dichotomous thinking	Practice selective abstraction, overgeneralization, magnification, personalization, dichotomous thinking
Body image	Experience delusional distortion	See themselves as slightly larger
Relationships	Attempt to please and placate others	Experience conflicts between dependency and autonomy
Social isolation	Tend to isolate themselves to protect against rejection; tend to be more introverted	Need privacy for binge eating and purging; tend to be extroverted
Weight loss	Experience 25–50% weight loss	Maintain normal weight or experience slight weight loss
Death	Results usually from starvation, when body proteins are depleted to half the normal levels	Often results from hypokalemia, a deficiency of potassium (leading cause), and suicide (second most frequent cause)

Assessment: Interpersonal Relationships

Women's bodies, much more so than men's, have always been perceived as unfinished and in need of revamping to make them conform to the cultural standards of beauty. From Chinese women binding their feet in the 12th and 13th centuries, to corsets in the 19th century, to binding breasts in the early 20th century, to today's lean, physically fit, and surgically altered body, women have tried to change their bodies to "look good."

In American society, *female attractiveness* is strongly equated with thinness. Models, actresses, and the media glamorize extreme thinness, which is then equated with success and happiness. This cultural obsession for an extremely thin female body has led to widespread prejudice against overweight people. This prejudice has a significant impact on overall self-esteem and self-acceptance. Self-worth is enhanced for those who are judged attractive and diminished for those deemed unattractive (Stein & Corte, 2003). Box 12.1 lists the cultural values that are extremely harmful to all women, whether overweight, normal weight, or underweight.

Magazines marketed for adolescent women often present diet and weight control as the solutions for adolescent crises and contain 90% more articles and advertisements promoting dieting than do magazines read by young men. Frequent exposure to articles about dieting is significantly associated with lower self-esteem, depressed mood, and lower levels of body satisfaction. Thus, the body becomes the central focus of existence, and self-esteem becomes dependent on the ability to control weight and food intake. This *preoccupation with body image* continues throughout women's lives. In fact, dieting and concerns about weight have become so perva-

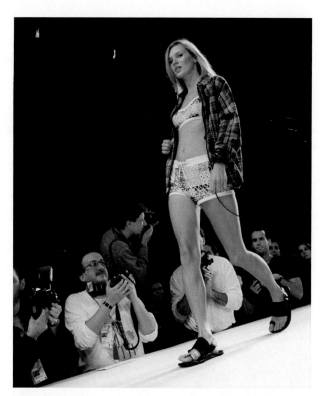

PHOTO 12.1A ■ Images of women in advertising and popular media often equate thinness with beauty, success, and happiness.
SOURCE: Ron Frehm/AP Wide World Photos. Used with permission.

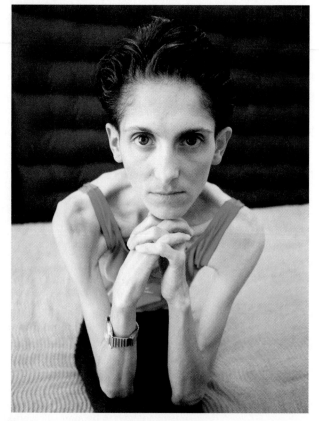

PHOTO 12.1B ■ Caraline, 28 years old, told a reporter, "I'm not telling you how much I weigh because I'm ashamed I don't weigh less." She later died of complications due to anorexia nervosa.
SOURCE: Express Newspapers/Getty Images/Time Lite Pictures. Used with permission.

BOX 12.1	Cultural Values Harmful to All Women

Thinness equals power and control, and fat equals helplessness and lack of self-control. Those who are fat are viewed as helpless people who are weak-willed, nonachieving, and out of control. What often goes unrecognized, however, is the fact that it's the compulsion for thinness that is out of control.

Thinness equals beauty, and fat equals ugliness. Thinness is the most important aspect of physical attractiveness, and fat women are considered to be sexually unattractive.

Thinness equals happiness, and fat equals unhappiness. The main determining factor of joy in life becomes tied to body size and shape. A slim body is seen as the only way to achieve a happy life.

Thinness equals goodness, and fat equals immorality. The message is that those who diet and are thin are good, whereas those who eat normally are fat and bad. Because fat is considered a moral issue, discrimination is accepted as an appropriate response.

Thinness equals fitness, and fat equals laziness. The fitness movement has perpetuated the glorification of thinness as the cultural ideal. Those people who are overweight or even normal weight are considered lazy and have only themselves to blame for their body size.

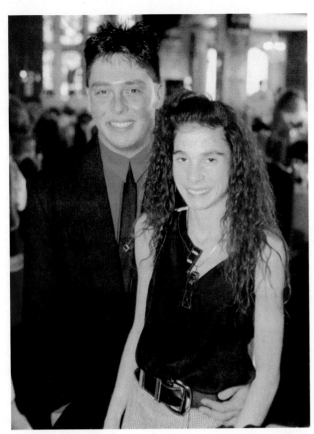

PHOTO 12.1C ■ Olympic-class gymnast, Christy Heinrich, with her boyfriend in 1993. After a 3-year struggle with anorexia nervosa, she died of multiple organ failure in 1994. She weighed less than 50 pounds at the time.

SOURCE: AP Wide World Photos. Used with permission

sive that they are now the norm for American women (Utter, Neumark-Sztainer, Wall, & Story, 2003).

Fear of fat is a constant companion. Young girls are often rewarded for their attempts at weight control. Peers, family members, coaches, dance teachers, and others may actively support the attainment or maintenance of low body weight. Those who go on to develop eating disorders may have internalized an exaggerated version of the cultural ideal, the basis of which is that women define their value and worth in terms of being attractive to and obtaining love from men. No wonder eating disorders occur, when women have grown up in a culture that is fat phobic, where they may have been ridiculed for being overweight or may have participated in ridiculing others. Discovering that thin girls frequently have more friends, go on more dates, and receive higher grades in school, they believe they can win approval, parental love, and social recognition by a frantic pursuit of thinness.

Young women with anorexia usually find that severe dieting does not produce the reward of being sought after by young men. In response to this real or perceived rejection, they feel even more unattractive and undesirable. To protect themselves, they begin to lose interest in social activities and *withdraw* from their peers. Dating is minimal or nonexistent,

and they purport to have no interest in sexual activities. High scholastic achievement may be an attempt to compensate for the lack of peer relationships (Ghizzani & Montomoli, 2000).

The ideal of *male attractiveness* in American society has been changing and has contributed to an increase in eating disorders among men. Magazines targeted for a predominantly male audience tend to focus on body building, weight lifting, or muscle toning. The "ideal" male body is one with well-developed muscles on the chest, arms, and shoulders with a slim waist and hips. This ideal is becoming more and more difficult for the average boy or man to attain. Little boys are being taught to value their self-esteem on being strong and athletic. Their action toys have washboard abdominal muscles, and their heroes are members of World Wrestling Entertainment (WWE). Men with eating disorders have an overwhelming fear of fatness and a desire to maintain a masculine appearance or shape. It is not uncommon to see males with eating disorders use anabolic steroids to improve muscle tone and build strength (Keel, 2005).

Research has shown that a disproportionately high number of men with eating disorders are gay or bisexual. Much like expectations for women, within the gay male culture there are strong pressures on men to be physically attractive, thin, and youthful looking, especially among gay men whose social life is centered on the "gay scene"—clubbing, drinking, and the like. Less likely to be satisfied with their body weight and shape, gay men have an increased risk for developing anorexia or bulimia (Keel, 2005).

People with bulimia experience shame and guilt about their behavior and may *withdraw socially* to hide it. They also need privacy for binge eating and purging, which contributes further to their isolation. The more isolated they become, the more the behavior tends to escalate as food is used to fill the void and provide a source of comfort. Generally, they do not become as socially isolated as those do with anorexia. Although they are sexually active, they have difficulty enjoying sex because of fears relating to loss of control. Feeling inadequate and incompetent, they may fear the intimacy of a long-term relationship.

Assessment: Cultural Influences

There is considerable evidence that eating disorders occur predominantly in industrialized, developed countries and that they occur less often in traditional societies. For example, Native Canadians (Ojibway-Cree) tend to show a preference for heavier body types than the Euro-Canadian population does. The incidence is changing, however, as cultures around the world become more Westernized. In a sense, anorexia and bulimia could be considered to be culture-reactive syndromes in the Western world (Keel, Leon, & Fulkerson, 2001).

A surprising influence in a girl's vulnerability may be her ethnic background. Recent studies have found, for instance, that African American women's perceptions of beauty are less media driven than those of Euro-American women. Dieting is less rampant, as are unhealthy weight management practices, and African American teens may be more accepting of the way they look. African American women and men are more positive about higher weights in women than are Euro-American women and men. African American women who are obese have a more positive body image than their Euro-American counterparts. In the Caribbean island of Curacao the incidence of anorexia among the majority Black population is zero, whereas the incidence among the minority mixed and White population is similar to that in the United States (Hoek et al., 2005; Striegel-Moore et al., 2003).

Typically, Asian American and Latino women were less likely to describe themselves as fat, were less dissatisfied with their body size, and were less likely to diet. Recent research, however, indicates that a cultural shift is occurring. Asian American and Latino women are becoming less satisfied with their bodies, and cultural media are presenting thin ideal body sizes for women, similar to those presented in the Anglo media.

Women in other cultures experience behaviors and symptoms that superficially appear to be similar but may not be identical in the causes or meanings of the disorder. Arab women in Qatar experience a culture-bound syndrome characterized by nausea, poor appetite, breathing difficulty, palpitations, faintness, and fatigue. The majority of these victims is either unmarried or has fertility problems. The disorder is rooted in the cultural belief that the value of women is based on their husbands and the children they have. As women become more educated and are exposed to Western media, they discover the different female–male relationships of more developed nations. Therefore, they find themselves caught between traditional cultural values and new values and role expectations (Keel, 2005).

Assessment: Physical

The nurse must be on the alert for medical emergencies such as acute cardiac failure, acute gastric dilatation or rupture, esophageal bleeding or rupture, and massive peripheral edema. Ongoing physical assessment is a critical need when working with clients with eating disorders.

There are many physiological effects of starvation and purging. *Electrolyte imbalance* may cause muscle weakness, seizures, arrhythmias, and even death; hypokalemia is the most critical electrolyte abnormality. Hypokalemia develops in several ways. With vomiting, there is some loss of potassium. Perhaps more important is metabolic alkalosis, which results from the loss of stomach acid through vomiting. This, in turn, causes a shift of potassium from the extracellular space into the cells, thereby lowering the serum potassium level. In addition, laxative abuse causes loss of potassium through the lower gastrointestinal system (Finfgeld, 2002).

Decreased blood volume results in lowered blood pressure and in postural hypotension. Lessened sympathetic nervous system activity is reflected in symptoms such as hypotension, bradycardia, and hypothermia. Elevated blood urea nitrogen (BUN) indicates decreased blood flow to the kidneys, which predisposes these individuals to edema. Cardiovascular changes include a decrease in cardiac chamber dimensions and thinning of the heart muscle wall. With underoxygenation of the heart muscle and bradycardia, cardiac output is decreased (Takimoto et al., 2004).

Gastrointestinal complications such as constipation, cathartic colon, and laxative dependence may develop. When food is in short supply, gastric emptying slows to improve the efficiency of nutrient absorption. This also delays the expenditure of energy required for digestion, absorption, and storage. Frequent vomiting can lead to esophagitis, with scarring and stricture. Changes in the epithelial lining of the esophagus have the potential to advance to cancer. If perforation or rupture of the esophagus occurs, there is a 20% mortality rate, even with immediate treatment. Gastric rupture, fortunately a fairly rare occurrence, carries a mortality rate of 85%. Repeated vomiting decreases tooth enamel, causing dental caries and tooth loss. There may be a chronic sore throat, and salivary glands are usually swollen and tender. Some people with bulimia may demonstrate **Russell's sign**, a callus on the back of the hand, formed by repeated trauma from the teeth when forcing vomiting.

Amenorrhea is common in females with anorexia, and irregular menses is frequently associated with bulimia. Although the exact mechanism is unclear, menstrual problems are thought to be related to the degree of stress the person is experiencing, the percentage of body fat lost, and altered hypothalamic function. There are also abnormalities in the secretion of luteinizing hormone and follicle-stimulating hormone, resulting in low estrogen and progesterone levels. In women who conceive, there is an increased risk for preterm delivery and fetuses that are small for gestational age (Sollid, Wisborg, Hjort, & Secher, 2004).

With low estrogen levels, these young women are at higher risk for osteopenia, leading to *osteoporosis*. This is a serious medical complication with no effective treatment. In a similar fashion, testosterone levels drop in male sufferers. In an adaptive effort to limit energy expenditure and conserve protein, thyroid hormone levels drop. People with anorexia develop *lanugo hair* on their body, reflecting their state of starvation. Lanugo is the soft, downy hair covering a fetus beginning in the 5th month of gestation and which is almost entirely shed by the 9th month.

People with anorexia usually experience a *weight loss* of 25%, but a loss as high as 50% is possible. People with bulimia do not reach such low levels of weight and may remain at normal weight. Since a large food intake speeds up the gastric emptying rate, a significant number of calories are absorbed before the purging begins.

BOX 12.2	Physical Complications of Anorexia

Organ System	Signs and Symptoms
Whole body	Weakness; malnutrition; low weight; low body fat
Central nervous system	Apathy; poor concentration; cognitive impairment; depression; irritable mood; enlarged ventricles, sleep disorders
Cardiovascular system	Palpitations; irregular pulse; dizziness; hypotension; shortness of breath; chest pain; peripheral vasoconstriction with cold extremities; decrease in cardiac chamber dimensions; thinning of heart muscle walls; refeeding edema; sudden cardiac death
Skeletal	Bone pain with exercise; arrested skeletal growth; osteoporosis
Muscular	Weakness; muscle wasting
Reproductive	Loss of menses or primary amenorrhea; arrested sexual development; decreased sex drive; pregnancy and neonatal complications
Endocrine, metabolic	Low body temperature; fatigue; electrolyte abnormalities; low thyroid levels; elevated serum cortisol; dehydration
Hematological	Anemia; neutropenia; low erythrocyte sedimentation rate; thrombocytopenia
Gastrointestinal	Abdominal pain; distention and bloating with meals; delayed gastric emptying; constipation; abnormal bowel sounds; hypokalemic ileus; refeeding pancreatitis
Urinary	Low glomerular filtration rate; elevated BUN; pitting edema; kidney failure
Skin	Hair loss; presence of lanugo hair on body; dry skin, brittle hair/nails; petechiae

SOURCE: American Psychiatric Association. (2000). *Practice guideline for the treatment of patients with eating disorders* (2nd ed.). Washington, DC: Author; Levenkron, S. (2000). *Anatomy of anorexia.* New York: Norton; and White, J. H. (2000). Symptom development in bulimia nervosa: A comparison of women with and without a history of anorexia nervosa. *Archives of Psychiatric Nursing, 14*(2): 81–92. Used with permission.

BOX 12.3	Physical Complications of Bulimia

Organ System	Signs and Symptoms
Whole body	Weakness; malnutrition; average body weight
Central nervous system	Irritability; depression; sleep disorders
Cardiovascular system	Palpitations; arrhythmias; hypotension; sudden cardiac death
Reproductive	Fertility problems; irregular menses
Endocrine, metabolic	Hypokalemia; hypochloremic alkalosis (vomiting); hypomagnesemia and hypophosphatemia (laxative abuse)
Gastrointestinal	Abdominal pain; gastritis; esophagitis; perforation of the esophagus; increased rate of pancreatitis; constipation; bowel irregularities; cathartic colon; hypokalemic ileus
Oropharyngeal	Dental decay; chronic sore throat; swollen salivary glands
Skin	Scarring on back of hand (Russell's sign); finger calluses/abrasions

SOURCE: American Psychiatric Association. (2000). *Practice guideline for the treatment of patients with eating disorders* (2nd ed.). Washington, DC: Author; Boskind-White, M., & White, W. C. (2000). *Bulimia/anorexia* (3rd ed.). New York: Norton; and White, J. H. (2000). Symptom development in bulimia nervosa: A comparison of women with and without a history of anorexia nervosa. *Archives of Psychiatric Nursing, 14*(2): 81–92. Used with permission.

The physiological effects of malnutrition and vomiting are widespread throughout the body. In some cases, death occurs as a result of these disruptions. See Boxes 12.2 and 12.3 for an overview of the physical complications of eating disorders.

DIAGNOSIS

After analyzing and synthesizing the client assessment data, the nurse develops nursing diagnoses. The client's level of malnourishment must be identified because, in some cases,

death could be imminent. It is generally agreed that nutritional rehabilitation and weight restoration are the first steps in the recovery process. The client's binge eating or purging patterns must be identified, as well as her or his fears, cognitive distortions, and relationships with family and friends.

The following are those diagnoses most commonly identified for clients with eating disorders (North American Nursing Diagnosis Association, 2007):

- Imbalanced Nutrition: Less Than Body Requirements related to reduced intake

- Imbalanced Nutrition: More Than Body Requirements related to binge eating episodes
- Imbalanced Nutrition: Less Than Body Requirements related to purging
- Deficient Knowledge about nutritional value of foods
- Body Image Disturbance related to delusional perception of body
- Disturbed Thought Process related to cognitive distortions such as dichotomous thinking, overgeneralization, personalization, obsessions, and superstitious thinking
- Anxiety related to fears of gaining weight and losing control
- Chronic Low Self-Esteem related to striving to please others to obtain acceptance
- Powerlessness related to having no control over bulimic pattern
- Potential for Injury related to excessive exercise
- Impaired Social Interaction related to withdrawal from peer group and fears of rejection
- Altered Family Processes related to enabling disorder eating or enmeshed family system

The nursing process in relation to the many physical complications from eating disorders is beyond the scope of this text. Refer to a medical–surgical textbook for this information.

OUTCOME IDENTIFICATION AND GOALS

Based on the assessment data, the nurse selects outcomes appropriate to the nursing diagnoses. Broad outcomes include:

- Weight stabilizes within normal parameters
- Abnormal eating patterns decrease or cease
- Verbalizes an improved quality of life

Once the nurse has established outcomes, the nurse and the client mutually identify goals for change. Client goals are specific behavioral prescriptions that the nurse, the client, and significant others identify as realistic and attainable. The following are examples of goals appropriate to people with eating disorders:

- Verbalizes increased satisfaction with self
- Demonstrates more flexible daily routines
- Exercises appropriately
- Decreases frequency of binge eating and purging
- Verbalizes fewer fears
- Achieves target weight

- Identifies secondary gains
- Verbalizes fewer cognitive distortions
- Family problem-solves together

PLANNING

Once the nursing diagnoses, outcome criteria, and goals have been identified, the nurse develops the plan of care to assist clients toward a higher level of functioning and an enriched quality of life.

Priorities of care for clients with eating disorder are as follows:

- Critical physical alterations
- Imbalanced nutrition
- Excessive exercise
- Delusional body image
- Impaired cognitions

IMPLEMENTATION

In response to the unrelenting demand of the cultural ideal, fat has become a "weightism" issue. It is time for nursing to challenge the cultural ideal and respond appropriately to people suffering from eating disorders. Nurses must become leaders in fostering a humane approach to body size.

Because nurses are products of their culture, they have probably internalized the prejudice against fat. Before intervening with clients, nurses must rethink their values and rid themselves of unrealistic ideals. When working with overweight clients, nurses must understand that these clients do not necessarily have more emotional problems than people of normal weight. Their emotional problems are most likely a result of prejudice and stigma and the cultural pressure to lose weight. Decreasing the stigma as well as the internalized disgust will greatly benefit overweight clients. Nurses must be careful not to perpetuate the misconception that losing weight will solve all other problems in life. A thin body is neither a magical cure nor a guarantee for living happily ever after.

The nurse can actively challenge idealized cultural values by eliminating all negative references to overweight people in verbal and written communications. Support people of average weight and express concern for people who are severely underweight. Speak up about the potential life-threatening aspects of dieting behavior. Help expand the standard of feminine beauty. Nurses can teach their daughters how to defend against cultural pressures for weight loss and how to love, respect, and celebrate their bodies. Nurses can teach their sons that women are not ornaments or sex objects, teach them to respect and appreciate women who have many qualities and many sizes and shapes. Finally, nurses must help all

NURSING CARE PLAN for a Client With an Eating Disorder

Promoting Food Intake
Nursing Diagnosis: Client at risk for imbalanced nutrition, less than body requirements

Outcomes: Clients will increase food intake to meet body requirements.

Dangerously underweight clients may need *nasogastric refeeding* in an inpatient setting. This intervention has a history of controversy on clinical and ethical grounds. Those who are opposed to it believe that forced feeding may place people with anorexia at greater risk for relapse or for developing bulimia. No research studies support this view. The current trend is oral refeeding with supplemental nighttime nasogastric refeeding for those who are seriously ill. The nighttime supplement provides a gradual increase in calories over 24 hours. Since it is administered slowly, it should not cause distention and pain. Daytime oral intake continues to be encouraged and monitored. These nighttime feedings are stopped when the target weight has been achieved (Robb et al., 2002).

Intervention	Rationale	Goal
Negotiate a reasonable contract for meals with client.	Contract usually begins with 1,000 to 1,500 kcal per day; gradually increased.	Contracts for amount of daily intake
Begin diet low in fats and milk products.	Starvation has led to insufficient bowel enzymes for digestion of these foods.	Digests food with minimal difficulty
Spread calories across 6 meals a day; no longer than 2 to 3 hours between periods of eating.	Decrease the sensation of bloating.	Reports few sensations of bloating
Encourage client to plan meals.	Active involvement with meal planning will increase client's feeling of control.	Plans balanced meals according to contract
Encourage client to keep a food diary to record all food ingested, as well as thoughts and feelings associated with eating or not eating.	Patterns can be analyzed by client and staff and plan of care altered as necessary.	Keeps daily food diary; maintains normal eating pattern
Teach nutritional information about calories, food values, and balanced diets.	Accurate information will dispel magical beliefs about food.	Verbalizes accurate knowledge of nutrition
Encourage supplementation with vitamins and minerals, especially calcium.	Most diets do not provide adequate daily requirements.	Uses supplements
Assess clients for literacy; provide dietary information in written handouts in preferred language.	Verbal information should be reinforced with written information.	Uses written information

Binge Eating
Nursing Diagnosis: Client at risk for imbalanced nutrition, more than body requirements

Outcome: Client will decrease binge eating.

There are a number of ways you can assist people to gain control over their binge eating.

Intervention	Rationale	Goal
Help client differentiate between emotions and sensations of hunger.	Misinterpretation of emotions contributes to binge eating.	Differentiates emotions from hunger
Help client identify particular foods that trigger binge eating.	Identification of trigger foods will help client gain control of binges.	Identifies trigger foods
Help client assess situations that precede binging.	Insight into high-risk situations will help client gain control on binges.	Identifies stressful situations
Encourage delay in responding to urge to binge by trying alternative behaviors such as talking to a teacher or counselor, calling a friend, or using relaxation techniques.	The delay interrupts the habitual cycle of behavior.	Delays urge to binge

continued

NURSING CARE PLAN for a Client With an Eating Disorder

Binge Eating   *continued*

Nursing Diagnosis: Client at risk for imbalanced nutrition, more than body requirements

Intervention	Rationale	Goal
Help client solve ways to avoid privacy at usual times of binges.	Most binging occurs in isolation. Being with others will decrease opportunities to binge.	Formulates plan to avoid privacy
Help client identify other positive behaviors (e.g., avoiding fast-food restaurants, formulating a list of "safe" foods, shopping for food with a friend).	These activities will inhibit the binging behavior.	Implements plan to decrease binge eating
Teach clients to eat three to six meals a day and avoid periods of fasting.	Fasting increases the risk of binge-eating episodes.	Eats three to six meals a day
Teach client to include a carbohydrate at each meal.	Carbohydrate deprivation may trigger binge eating.	Eats appropriate amounts of carbohydrates

Purging

Nursing Diagnosis: Client at risk for ineffective coping

Outcome: Client will discontinue purging activities.

The following are strategies to manage purging behavior.

Intervention	Rationale	Goal
Discuss how purging is used to cope with negative feelings.	Insight into purging behavior as a way to decrease anxiety, guilt, and self-disgust will help client manage the dynamics of the behavior.	Associates purging with ineffective management of feelings
Point out that purging began as a method of control and that now the purging is out of control.	Insight into the paradox of the behavior will assist clients in finding alternative methods of control.	Formulates alternative plan to gain control
If client continues to vomit, restrict bathroom use for 1–2 hours after meals unless accompanied by a staff member.	Staff needs to set limits on purging behavior until client is able to establish own limits.	Does not vomit after meals
Encourage clients to talk to staff when they feel urge to vomit.	Talking about feelings will increase clients' ability to control impulsive behavior.	Utilizes resources to resist urge to vomit

Fear and Anxiety

Nursing Diagnosis: Client at risk for fear

Outcomes: The client will verbalize fewer fears and lowered levels of anxiety.

People with anorexia or bulimia have multiple anxieties and fears, most of which get translated into fears of weight gain and loss of control. Clients with eating disorders often believe that weight loss will bring happiness and freedom from becoming fat. As they lose more and more weight, however, they tend to become more and more terrified of weight gain.

Intervention	Rationale	Goal
Discuss fears of weight gain and loss of control; help them identify underlying fears, such as fear of rejection, that have been transformed into a fear of gaining weight.	Fears must be openly discussed before they can be managed.	Discusses fears
Discuss how obsessions with food and weight are used to protect oneself.	Obsessions decrease anxiety and contribute to avoidance of negative feelings and problems.	Identifies purpose of obsessions

NURSING CARE PLAN for a Client With an Eating Disorder

Fear and Anxiety   *continued*

Nursing Diagnosis: Client at risk for fear

Intervention	Rationale	Goal
Discuss how feelings are confused with sensations of hunger.	The binge eater uses food as a source of comfort and as a way to defend against anxiety.	Differentiates emotions from hunger
Help clients identify feelings experienced when they lose control over rigid diet.	It is important to attach the feelings of shame and guilt to the rigid diet standards rather than to personal inadequacy.	Relates guilt and shame to rigid standards
Discuss how weight loss is symbolic of self-control and mastery of self and the environment.	Insight into symbolic meaning of the behavior assists clients in establishing more adaptive behavior.	Identifies need for self-control
Discuss measures other than weight loss to exert control.	Active involvement in the problem-solving process increases clients' use of more adaptive behavior.	Implements alternative control measures
Teach alternative methods to manage fears (e.g., relaxation techniques, self-hypnosis, assertiveness training).	Healthful techniques to decrease anxiety and fears will decrease need to use food in an unhealthy manner.	Implements alternative measures to manage feelings
Use term "weight restoration"; provide repeated assurance that they will not be allowed to become fat.	The term "weight gain" often creates an instant phobic response; reassurance is needed as you ask them to do the very thing of which they are the most frightened.	Responds positively to term "weight restoration"

Secondary Gains

Nursing Diagnosis: Client at risk for ineffective coping

Outcomes: With the help of others, clients will identify the unconscious benefits of their disorder and develop ways to meet these secondary gains in more constructive ways.

Intervention	Rationale	Goal
Have client list pros and cons of eating disorder.	Often they have been warned of the dangers but have never identified benefits. Treatment will not be successful if they do not compensate for loss of benefits.	Formulates list
Help clients identify secondary gains that are the ultimate, unconscious purpose the disorder serves, e.g.: ■ Ideal body will protect from all future pain. ■ Gain a sense of control. ■ Individuate from parents. ■ Compete with siblings for attention. ■ Response to depression. ■ Regress to a younger and safer time in life.	Accurate identification will lead to effective interventions.	Identifies secondary gains
Help clients problem solve ways to meet these needs in constructive and healthy ways, e.g., if there is a need to be in control, point out that the binge–purge cycle is now out of control.	As clients develop insight into the paradox of the behavior, they can begin to explore alternative behaviors for maintaining control.	Utilizes problem-solving process
Help them identify pleasurable and leisure activities as well as vocational interests.	Increases ability to define and control themselves while decreasing feelings of powerlessness.	Verbalizes improved self-esteem and decreased dependency on others

continued

NURSING CARE PLAN for a Client With an Eating Disorder

Cognitive Distortions

Nursing Diagnosis: Client at risk for disturbed thought processes

Outcomes: Client will verbalize a logical and realistic thinking process.

Several interventions are effective for clients who believe that achieving an ideal body will solve all problems in life. When clients say that people will only love them if they are thin, they are experiencing the cognitive distortion of *overgeneralization*. You can challenge this belief by asking clients to make observations. Ask them whether there is anyone in their lives whom they love who is not thin. Ask them to go to the mall and look at couples of all sizes. Do they notice that average size and overweight people seem to be in happy relationships? As this process continues, clients may come to believe that others will love them no matter what they weigh.

Intervention	Rationale	Goal
Point out the process of overgeneralization in developing the belief that all life's problems will be solved if enough weight is lost.	The loss of weight is symbolic of other problems; interpersonal problems must be separated from physical problems.	Reduces use of overgeneralization
Confront all-or-none thinking patterns such as food is either good or bad or the choice is to eat nothing or eat everything.	Decreasing dichotomous thinking increases realistic perceptions; in reality, no food is necessarily good or bad.	Verbalizes less dichotomous thinking
Discuss how perfectionism influences perception of reality.	Clients need to understand relationship between need for perfectionism and cognitive distortion.	Identifies perfectionistic thinking
Discuss unrealistic goals and promises to self.	Rigid goals and promises contribute to superstitious thinking.	Identifies rigidity of goals
Help formulate realistic goals.	Realistic goals help clients remain in control and decrease feelings of helplessness.	Establishes reasonable goals

Improving Body Image

Nursing Diagnosis: Client at risk for disturbed body image

Outcomes: Clients will verbalize realistic perception of own bodies and identify cultural stereotypes that influence perceptions.

Body image is an important part of self-concept. Clients with anorexia have a distorted and even delusional body image. To facilitate movement from a negative and distorted body image to a realistic perception, have clients keep a body image diary. In this diary they record situations that provoke concerns over their appearance, their body image beliefs, and the effect of these on their mood and behavior. Cognitive interventions involve the identification of multiple automatic thoughts linking body image to self-worth. They may have thoughts such as: "What I look like affects my worth in the world. What I look like is unacceptable." As they learn to identify their maladaptive thoughts, they can begin to reframe those thoughts by saying positive affirmations aloud. Encourage clients to develop a list of these affirmations in a variety of areas such as school, leisure, achievements, interactions with others, and roles. Affirmations are always said in the present tense and as if they are occurring. Examples are "I am a good student"; "I am a good friend"; "My body is healthy"; "I like my body"; "Food is good for me"; "I enjoy doing things with my friends." Discuss with clients the interaction of sociocultural factors and body image. Topics include the pressures for women to be thin, the consequences of evaluating oneself largely in terms of weight, and how the female body is used in advertising and in the media. Explain media images do not represent people as they actually look because the photos are touched up. Explore how thinness of models is at a level that is impossible for many women to achieve by healthy means.

Help clients appraise messages about body image as information they will evaluate in relation to their own experiences, goals, and values. If the media messages are incongruent with the self, suggest that they simply ignore these messages. As they learn to do this they generate their own criteria regarding body image. It is important that clients see themselves as *being in control* rather than as passive sex objects valued mainly for appearance. See the Complementary/Alternative Therapies feature on teaching clients how to alter negative cognitions.

NURSING CARE PLAN for a Client With an Eating Disorder

Improving Body Image   *continued*
Nursing Diagnosis: Client at risk for disturbed body image

Intervention	Rationale	Goal
Discuss with clients how they perceive their bodies.	Gain an understanding of the particular distortions of each client.	Verbalizes perceptual distortions
Do not argue with body perceptions.	Arguments increase clients' need to defend the delusion.	
Point out your perception and objective data about their bodies.	Introduction of reality may assist clients in focusing on a more realistic body image and decrease self-criticism.	Listens to nurse's perceptions
Discuss clients' perceptions of other people's bodies.	Ability to accurately perceive other's bodies assist clients in becoming more realistic about own body.	Verbalizes realistic perception of own and others' bodies

Managing Family Dynamics
Nursing Diagnosis: Client at risk for interrupted family processes

Outcomes: Family will assist client toward autonomy.

For young clients with a short duration of anorexia, the initial phase of family therapy is the phase of refeeding. Family members are considered part of the treatment team rather than as clients. To reinforce generational boundaries, siblings are encouraged to be supportive of the client and parents are encouraged to form a united front. Families are counseled to determine and implement their individualized refeeding plan. If there is any teasing, criticism, or social comparisons about weight occurring in the family, these behaviors must be stopped if the client is to improve (le Grange, 1999).

Once the client begins refeeding and is willing to work toward the target weight, other family issues will be introduced in therapy. Refeeding continues to be monitored during this phase. Interventions may include discussions on family cohesion, the degree of emotional bonding that occurs within a family. At one end of the continuum of cohesion is the family system that is disengaged; that is, the family members are isolated and alienated from one another. At the other end of the continuum is the enmeshed family system in which the members are immersed in and absorbed by one another. Eating disorders often lead to an enmeshed family system as everyone becomes concerned and involved with the eating behavior of one family member. The family may also develop rigid rules for and expectations of the identified client. Since the most adaptive family systems function between the two extremes of disengaged and enmeshed, families may need help problem solving to achieve a healthy balance. Increasing the autonomy of young people may decrease the use of food as passive–aggressive adolescent rebellion and increase feelings of self-control.

Once the client has achieved and maintained a healthy weight, the termination process begins. The focus shifts from the eating disorder to healthy family interactions. The family must let the client take responsibility for her or his own eating behavior. Normal developmental stages and individuation from parents are discussed in preparation for the adolescent's departure from home and family (Keel, 2005).

Intervention	Rationale	Goal
Discuss inappropriate dependency on family.	Extreme dependency inhibits normal separation and autonomy of adolescents and young adults.	Identifies examples of inappropriate dependency
Problem solve ways to increase independence appropriate to client's developmental stage.	Increasing autonomy decreases use of food as a method of passive–aggressive rebellion.	Implements plan to increase independence from family unit
Problem solve ways to obtain appropriate privacy within the family.	Decreasing family's overinvolvement in client's life increase feelings of self-control.	Implements plan to increase privacy within family unit

Complementary/Alternative Therapies

How to Help Clients Alter Negative Cognitions

Often, we endure such runs of negative thoughts that we are unaware of the process until we have been "beating ourselves up" for 10 to 15 minutes. To become more aware of this habitual process and to counter with positive thoughts, try this procedure:

■ When you become aware of your thoughts, tap your left finger on a firm surface for every negative thought. When your finger becomes quite sore, you will have another level of awareness of your negativity.

■ Negative thoughts can be countered with positive ones. When you catch yourself thinking and feeling a negative thought, such as how fat your body is or how inadequate you are, STOP.

■ Look for and substitute a positive thought or feeling in the place of the one you removed, such as how lovely your hair looks or how well you have succeeded at something.

■ Now listen to yourself saying the positive phrase out loud.

■ Continue in this way, adding other phrases and wishes for yourself.

SOURCE: Fontaine, K. L. (2000). *Healing practices: Alternative therapies for nursing.* Upper Saddle River, NJ: Prentice Hall.

clients view themselves as competent people who have many talents and traits—creativity, humor, empathy, warmth, and wisdom. Everyone must work together to eliminate the deprecation of women and instead celebrate womanhood.

Inpatient care is the most expensive treatment and the least desirable form of treatment for clients with eating disorders. It is, however, necessary when clients are in life-threatening circumstances related to starvation, are at risk for suicide, or are experiencing extreme social isolation. Most clients will be seen in an outpatient setting. There are day programs, evening programs, intensive group therapy, and intensive individual therapy. In day and evening treatment programs, clients are in a controlled environment for one or two meals and snacks during the treatment time. As clients are more able to modify their behaviors, they may move to weekly, biweekly, and monthly outpatient sessions.

It is a challenge to develop a therapeutic alliance with eating-disordered clients. They often resist interventions and are angry about being in treatment. Use a kind, firm, and consistent approach and work toward a collaborative relationship. It is sometimes difficult to maintain the balance between setting clear limits on behaviors and helping these clients grow in autonomy. The ultimate goal is to have them take responsibility for their own behavior.

Moderating Excessive Exercise Pattern

Physical activity should be adapted to the client's food intake and with consideration of bone mineral density and cardiac function. For the severely underweight person, exercise should be restricted and always carefully supervised. Help clients problem solve an appropriate exercise pattern. The focus is on helping clients assume responsibility for themselves as they move from the destructive use of exercise to healthy exercise. The desired outcomes are that the client will not exercise to extreme physical limits and will implement a safe and realistic exercise routine.

Managing Impulsivity

Clients with eating disorders often go through their daily routines with little awareness or attention. They read while they eat and exercise while they watch TV. When feelings arise, they often respond with an impulsive action. Help them identify feelings and problem solve wise choices. Help them plan safe ways of coping with painful emotions without resorting to impulsive and often self-destructive behaviors.

Some clients find that meditation helps them decrease their impulsive behavior. Meditation is a general term for a wide range of practices that involve relaxing the body and stilling the mind, such as prayer, yoga, or t'ai chi. It is a process that anyone can use to calm down, cope with stress, and for those with spiritual inclinations, feel as one with God or the universe. Meditation can be practiced individually or in groups and is easy to learn. It requires no change in belief system and is compatible with most religious practices. The desired outcome is that the client will verbalize consequences of impulsive behavior and implant plan to think before acting.

Refining Self-definition

Discuss the belief that other people have more insight into who they are than they do themselves. This belief contributes to an ever-changing self-definition depending on who is in the immediate moment. Explain that, as children, we form a self-concept from repeated interactions with significant others in our lives. As we mature, our self-definition becomes more internalized and less subject to random changes. Rather than reacting to others' input, encourage them to explore how they feel and what they believe. The desired outcome is that the client will verbalize a decreasing need to placate and please others, an identity based on self-definition, increased self-confidence, and increased life satisfaction.

Ask clients to write down 10 traits that describe the kind of person they *actually* are (intelligent? kind? honest? friendly? interesting? strong?). Next ask them to list the 10 traits that describe the kind of person they *ought* to be, in terms of their sense of responsibility and duty. Finally, have them make a list of 10 traits that describe the *ideal* of what they would like to be, based on their hopes and dreams. The more similar these three lists, the less distressed people are. Major differences between the actual and the "ought-selves" contribute to feelings of guilt, shame, and fear. Major differences between the actual and ideal selves contribute to disappointment, frustration, and sadness. This exercise is a good starting point in developing a stable self-definition.

Encourage clients to pursue their own interests and not what others tell them to do. Ask them to identify pleasurable activities and ones that give a sense of satisfaction. Point out behaviors that are part of their self-definition. As they are able to identify their personal values and goals, their lives will have more of a sense of direction. Over time they will develop an identity that is self-initiated and self-regulated.

EVALUATION

To complete the nursing process, the nurse evaluates client and family responses in terms of established outcomes. It is seldom an all-or-nothing phenomenon, but rather an ongoing process of movement toward the goal of better health and improved quality of life.

Recovery from eating disorders is a long process. Individuals with anorexia are ambivalent about treatment and often terminate treatment early. Symptoms correlated with early termination include higher levels of weight concerns, greater maturity fears, and impulsivity. For those who continue treatment, about 40% recover, and the rest experience a chronic course, some with fewer symptoms and some with the same symptoms. Similarly, 50% of people with bulimia recover. The time to recovery ranges from 3 years to 11 or more years (Finfgeld, 2002; Woodside, Carter, & Blackmore, 2004).

Clinical Interactions | A Client With Anorexia

Lorna, 23 years old, entered the eating disorders unit at the urging of her husband and physician. Lorna and her husband would like to start a family, and she has been told that her eating disorder (anorexia) would be very dangerous to a fetus. She weighed 95 pounds (43 kg) when she was admitted, and now, 3 weeks later, weighs 102 pounds (46 kg). In the interaction, you will see evidence of:

- Denial
- Distorted body image
- Obsessions
- Fear of gaining weight

NURSE: *"You said that you still have difficulty believing you have a problem."*

LORNA: ***"Well, my doctor says I do, but it's just hard for me to see it."***

NURSE: *"What do you see?"*

LORNA: ***"I see a lot of fat."***

NURSE: *"You see a lot of fat—on yourself? You mean, you look in the mirror and see yourself as fat?"*

LORNA: ***"Yes. That's all I can see."***

[Period of silence]

LORNA: ***"All I think about is food. My mind is like a computer—it just keeps going on thinking about food."***

NURSE: *"Do you feel trapped?"*

LORNA: ***"Very trapped. It's like a habit. I just can't stop it. And now, here on the unit, we spend so much time talking about food and weight and everything. I think you are all as obsessed as I am."***

NURSE: *"Do you think the staff is as out of control as you feel you are? That might be a scary thought."*

LORNA: ***"No, not really. I'm just so frustrated. Getting on the scale every few days is frightening. Seeing the numbers going up—I just want to stop it. I want to lose weight—go back to where I was. Yet I want a future, too. I want to have a baby, and part of me knows that I have to get healthier before I can get pregnant. So it's an immense conflict every single day."***

NURSE: *"As painful as the conflict sounds, I also see some progress in you. When you first came to the unit, you believed there was nothing dangerous with your lack of eating. Now it sounds like you understand that your eating disorder is a real problem, especially in terms of becoming a mother."*

LORNA: ***"Yeah, I know. My husband's being very supportive. I just wish I didn't have to gain this weight in order to become pregnant."***

Using Research Evidence | Discharge Readiness: Anorexia

Turrell, S. L., Davis., R., Grahan, H., & Weiss, I. (2005). Adolescents with anorexia nervosa: Multiple perspectives of discharge readiness. *Journal of Child and Adolescent Psychiatric Nursing, 18*(3), 116–126.

What is the study about?

The purpose of this study was to survey discharge criteria for Canadian adolescents with anorexia nervosa, as verbalized by nurses, clients, and parents during a first hospitalization for this disorder.

How was the study done?

This was a qualitative pilot study of a nonrandomized sample of registered nurses (RNs) (n=14), adolescent clients with a diagnosis of anorexia nervosa (n=14), and these adolescents' parents (n=14) at the Hospital for Sick Children in Toronto, Canada. The mean age of the adolescents was 14.6 years; the mean period since diagnosis was 9.9 months. Following the first weekend pass, the adolescent completed an open-ended questionnaire. Adolescents were asked, "As a teenager who has been hospitalized with anorexia nervosa, what conditions should exist for you to feel ready for discharge, to continue your recovery at home?" A parallel version of the questionnaire was given to the parents and the RNs. Of the parents, 12 were married and 2 were separated, 12 were mothers and 2 were fathers of the adolescent participants. The RN group had a mean age of 41.5 years and had worked with adolescents with the diagnosis of anorexia nervosa for a mean of 17.9 years. Completed questionnaires were given to three independent reviewers for the purpose of content analysis of the responses. Reviewers did not know identities of the respondents. Reviewers were to sort responses according to "broad thematic similarity."

What were the results of the study?

Researchers found six themes. As theme 1, all three groups identified *medical stability* as necessary for discharge. All groups required that the "heart is good and your vital signs are stable."

For all groups, theme 2 was *education,* but groups differed as to who needed it. RNs requested that adolescents have a "clear understanding of the outpatient process, goals, and expectations prior to discharge." They expected that adolescents would know how to manage meals at home. Parents needed their child living with anorexia nervosa to be educated, but did not express a need for their own education.

For all groups, theme 3 was *psychological changes,* which also focused on the client. Adolescents made statements such as "I have to be able to eat without supervision" and "I have to be more assertive and speak up for myself." Parents identified psychological changes for the adolescent to make: for example, better coping skills to deal with anxiety, an increased understanding of body image, and less distortion. Many parents indicated that they desired to have a "guarantee of compliance

from their adolescent prior to discharge" regarding adhering to the meal plan. Parents did not indicate any psychological changes that *they* needed to make prior to adolescent discharge. However, RNs believed that discharge called for psychological changes by both the adolescent clients and their parents. This theme was summed up in statements such as "family needs to know how to help kids with eating problems, to supervise meals, and to understand their child will not be cured right away."

Theme 4 was *planning for resources in the community*. Adolescent clients requested "individual counseling near our home." Parents requested "coordination of follow-up with local family doctor, including a list of recommendations." RNs expressed a desire "for planned community involvement, such as social activities, after school groups, and peer support network."

Theme 5, unique to adolescent participants, was *support*. Adolescents wrote statements such as "make sure you have a trustworthy person for all meals and snacks, someone who can help you get through this."

Theme 6, unique to the RNs, was *parents as members of the treatment team*. RNs believed that parents "must agree about the severity of illness and treatment plan."

What additional questions might I have?

Would the themes have remained the same with a larger participant group at various stages of recovery or discharge status? How would discharge criteria change in adolescent participants with multiple hospitalizations for anorexia nervosa? Why did parents perceive no need to be educated? Would the themes have differed if more fathers were involved in the study? Did the setting of the study in a country with national health insurance influence the outcome since length of hospital admission was not a financial issue?

How can I use this study?

Nurses have an important role in educating both the adolescent living with anorexia nervosa and the family. Adolescents living with anorexia nervosa and parents need to be informed regarding the disease process, plans, and expectations through a working team relationship with the health care staff. After discharge, nurses need to work closely with families and support both the adolescent and the parents. Nurses must know community resources that can help the adolescent living with anorexia nervosa to feel supported, and nurses should advocate for additional support groups and after-school groups if needed. Nurses should model good communication skills with adolescents and their families, demonstrating how to set limits and to avoid talking about food and appearance in a demeaning manner.

SOURCE: Contributed by Dolores Huffman, PhD, RN, Associate Professor of Nursing, Purdue University Calumet, Hammond, Indiana.

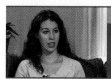

ROAD Assessment: Critical Thinking Questions

Go to the CD-ROM to assess Jessica by answering the following critical thinking questions based on what you have **R**ead about Jessica and **O**bserved on the videos.

1. Jessica's eating disorder began at the age of 19 years, 6 months after she started her freshman year. She struggled through the Christmas holiday and noted that the severity of the eating disorder seemed to peak around Easter. Fixed cognitive distortions, maladaptive defense and coping mechanisms, along with specific eating and exercise rituals were predominant ways of functioning in her daily life. Listen to section A on your student ROAD CD-ROM for chapter 12. Considering the above information, what additional mental disorder is Jessica at risk for developing? Be sure to explain your rationale and identify the specific data that correlate with the areas of mental functioning that require further assessment. (*Hint*—also refer to chapter 8 from the textbook for additional information that will help you in formulating your answers.)

2. People diagnosed with eating disorders will have differing degrees of self-perception and acceptance of the behaviors that are manifested during their illness. Listen to section B of your student ROAD CD-ROM for chapter 12. What chapter-specific term would you use to describe Jessica's self-appraisal of her behavior and why? Provide a rationale for your answer.

3. Developing a knowledge base and assessment skills in mental health nursing requires one to expand his or her awareness and recognition of the similarities between disorders and reoccurring patterns of behavior and thought. As in other mental disorders, people with eating disorders will utilize maladaptive defense mechanisms and also develop altered thought processes that present as cognitive distortions. Listen to the three interview segments from section C of your student ROAD CD-ROM for chapter 12. Identify the cognitive distortion and/or the defense mechanism Jessica is verbalizing and the rationale for selecting your answer(s). (*Hint*— refer to chapter 1 from the textbook for additional information that will help you in formulating your answers.)

4. Consider that Jessica is a client recently admitted to your unit. During your nursing assessment she verbalizes the information found in section D of your student ROAD CD-ROM for chapter 12.
   a. Identify what specific issue(s) need further evaluation, especially those that pertain to improving family functioning. Provide the rationale for your answer. (*Hint*—also refer to chapter 3 from the textbook for additional information that will help you in formulating your answers.)
   b. Identify a communication technique and an example of the phrasing you would use to implement your nursing communication. Provide the rationale for your answer. (*Hint* – also refer to chapter 2 from the textbook for additional information that will help you in formulating your answers.)

ROAD: DEVELOP A CARE PLAN

 Go to the CD-ROM to Develop a care plan based on your assessment of Steve. Identify nursing diagnoses, outcomes, goals, and interventions.

SOURCE: Contributed by Susan Siwinski-Hebel, RN, MSN.

Focus Your Study

OBJECTIVES

1. Compare and contrast the different theories regarding the etiology of eating disorders.

2. Describe the treatment options for a client with an eating disorder.

3. Outline the assessment process for a client with an eating disorder.

KEY CONCEPTS

- Genetics:
  - There is a genetic predisposition for anorexia.
  - The variables being studied include a genetic predisposition to perfectionism, orderliness, low tolerance for new situations, low self-esteem, and overall high anxiety.
- Neurobiology:
  - Those with bulimia have a deficiency of 5-HT and low satiety levels while those with anorexia have an excess of 5-HT and increased satiety.
  - Insufficient levels of endogenous opioids are associated with decreased food intake.
  - Dysfunction may occur in the frontal lobes, the parietal lobes, and the anterior cingulate.
- Interpersonal factors:
  - People with anorexia are described as perfectionists who have low tolerance for new situations, low self-esteem, and difficulty achieving the maturational tasks of adolescence.
  - People with bulimia have an unstable affect, feelings of incompetence, fear of losing control, and poor impulse control.
- Cognitive theory:
  - Dysfunctional thoughts such as dichotomous thinking and catastrophizing contribute to disordered eating patterns.
- Behavioral theory:
  - Eating disorders are considered phobias.
- Family factors:
  - Family is more of an enabler than a causative factor.
  - Some families are enmeshed, some have difficulty with conflict resolution, and many are focused on high achievement and performance.

- Medications:
  - Fluoxetine (Prozac) 50–60 mg per day for persons with bulimia
  - Acute, inpatient care may be necessary for those with anorexia whose weight, nutritional status, organ functioning, and cardiac health may be significantly compromised. Treatment may include a feeding schedule, potassium supplements, and bed rest.
  - Psychological treatment may include individual therapy, group work, family therapy, cognitive therapy, and systematic desensitization. Cognitive–behavioral therapy is the treatment of choice.

- Anorexia:
  - Rigidity and overcontrol as reflected by obsessive rituals and overexercise.
  - Overcompliant.
  - Food phobia, terror of weight gain and body fat, fear loss of control.
  - Ego-syntonic.
  - Cognitive distortions include selective abstraction, overgeneralization, magnification, ideas of reference, superstitious thinking, dichotomous thinking, and delusional body image.
  - Amenorrhea, osteoporosis, weight loss of 25% to 50%, cardiovascular problems, anemia, bloating with meals, death from starvation.
- Bulimia:
  - Impulsive and affect instability contributing to substance abuse, self-injury, and impulse control disorders.
  - Cyclic pattern of dieting, binge eating, and purging; engage in sporadic excessive exercise.
  - Repress feelings, view life as hopeless, fear weight gain and loss of control.
  - Ego-dystonic.
  - Similar cognitive distortions as in anorexia; perfectionistic.
  - Electrolyte imbalance, gastrointestinal complications, cardiovascular problems, death from hypokalemia or suicide.

4. Use the nursing process to develop a safe, comprehensive plan of care for a client with an eating disorder.

- Setting target weight:
  - 90% of average weight with a range of 4–6 pounds.
- Promoting food intake:
  - Contract for amount of calories spread over six meals a day.
  - Food diary to record food eaten and feelings associated with eating or not eating.
  - Teach a balanced diet.
- Discouraging binge eating:
  - Discuss differences between emotions and sensations of hunger.
  - Food diary to identify triggers to binge eating, the consequences, alternative coping behaviors, and ways to decrease opportunities to binge.
- Discouraging purging:
  - Discuss how purging is used to manage negative feelings.
  - Limit use of the bathroom for 2 hours after eating.
  - Provide support before, during, and after meals.
- Modifying the exercise routine:
  - Adapt physical activity to food intake, bone mineral density, and cardiac function.
- Decreasing impulsivity:
  - Help clients connect emotions with impulsive action.
  - Implement meditation practices or relaxation techniques.
- Coping with fears:
  - Identify underlying fears that have been transformed into a fear of gaining weight; model ways to share feelings with others.
  - Discuss how obsessions with food and weight are used to decrease anxiety, shame, and guilt; discuss how disordered eating is no longer under their control.
- Identifying secondary gains:
  - Ask clients to write out pros and cons of their eating disorder; help clients identify secondary gains the disorder serves.
  - Problem solve constructive ways to meet these needs; identify pleasurable activities.
- Rectifying cognitive distortions:
  - When distortions occur, point them out to clients; discuss how these distortions are not reality.
- Improving body image:
  - Keep a body image diary recording concerns over appearance, beliefs about the body, and the effect of these thoughts on mood and behavior.
  - Discuss the impact of media on their body image.
  - Help them use positive affirmations to counter negative beliefs.
- Facilitating self-definition:
  - Ask clients to identify positive traits; encourage them to pursue their own interests, goals, and activities.

5. Develop illness management teaching plans for a person with an eating disorder and her/his family.

- Managing family dynamics:
  - Family members are part of the treatment team; assess family for enmeshment or disengagement.
  - Formulate a refeeding plan.
  - Help family be supportive while letting the client take responsibility for own eating behavior.
- Educating:
  - Teach about the potential complications if the eating disorder is left untreated.
  - Teach the problem-solving process.
  - Refer to self-help groups.

6. Discuss the key points in effectively communicating with a person with an eating disorder.

- Use a caring, nonjudgmental approach to establish rapport and encourage talking about the disorder.
- Use a kind, firm, and consistent approach and work toward a collaborative relationship.
- Be alert for clients responding in an overcompliant manner in an attempt to win your approval.
- Discuss multiple fears and phobias.
- Discuss feelings of frustration and anger. Model how these feelings can be expressed appropriately.
- When cognitive distortions occur, gently point them out to the client.
- Discuss body image and cultural expectations.
- Discuss how perfectionistic standards interfere with decision making and self-image.

Explore MediaLink

For review questions, case studies, and other resources for this chapter see the Pearson Health MediaLink CD-ROM that accompanies this book and the Companion Website.

CD-ROM
- Audio Glossary
- NCLEX-RN® Review Questions
- ROAD to Critical Thinking: Jessica
- Animations/Videos
  - Anorexia Nervosa—Parts 1 and 2
  - Bulimia Nervosa—Parts 1 and 2

Companion Website www.prenhall.com/fontaine
- Audio Glossary
- NCLEX-RN® Review Questions
- Case Study
  - Anorexia Nervosa: A Case for the School Nurse
- Care Plan
  - Client With Bulimia: Binge Eating and Purging
- Critical Thinking
  - Anorexia Nervosa: The Client With a Feeding Tube
- MediaLink Application
  - Prader-Willi Syndrome
- MediaLinks
  - Books for Clients and Families; Community Resources

NCLEX-RN® Review Questions

12-1. A client with bulimia asks the nurse, "I wish I knew more about what causes bulimia. I read on the Internet that some people with bulimia have trouble knowing when they're full and that's why they keep bingeing." Which of the following responses by the nurse would be most appropriate?
1. "That's right. Some people with bulimia have a low level of serotonin, the neurotransmitter that lets you know when you're full."
2. "That's right. A high level of serotonin in some people prevents them from knowing when they are full to the point of satisfaction."
3. "You can't really believe everything you read on the Internet. Bulimia is caused by anxiety so bingeing on comfort foods is a learned behavioral response."
4. "The Internet is not really a good source for medical information. Bulimia has a strong genetic correlation and in your case it may have been inherited."

12-2. A high school wrestler fasts before every wrestling meet and then binges immediately after the meet. On the way to each meet, he walks rapidly up and down the bus aisle and spits repeatedly into a cup. Which of the following is the best intervention for this client?
1. Discuss secondary gains that are unconsciously driving the client's behavior.
2. Teach the client's mother about nutritional requirements of teenage boys.
3. Ask the health care provider for medication to treat the eating disorder.
4. Call the high school principal to report the wrestling coach for not stopping this behavior.

12-3. A female Asian American client who has a BMI of 25 kg/m² is referred to the outpatient clinic by her primary care provider to be assessed and treated for an eating disorder. Which of the following signs and symptoms would the nurse recognize as supporting the diagnosis of bulimia? (Select all that apply.)

1. The client has become socially withdrawn and never eats out with friends.
2. The client has a serum potassium level of 5.7 mEq/L.
3. The client has a callous on the back of her hand.
4. The client has an obsession with fad diets in order to lose weight.
5. The client expresses a fear of her inability to maintain her normal body weight.

12-4. A 30-year-old female client has been admitted to the intensive care unit (ICU) with metabolic alkalosis. She was diagnosed with anorexia nervosa 10 years ago and says that she is "too fat" even though she weighs 70 pounds and is 5 feet 4 inches. Her primary nursing diagnosis is Imbalanced Nutrition: Less Than Body Requirements related to reduced food intake and self-induced vomiting. Which of the following nursing diagnoses is the greatest priority immediately after she is medically stable in the ICU?
1. Hopelessness related to lack of control over environment
2. Potential for Injury related to excessive exercise
3. Body Image Disturbance related to delusional perception of body
4. Risk for Suicide related to self-neglect and starvation

12-5. A nurse is teaching clients with anorexia nervosa methods of normalizing eating behaviors. Which of the following statements by a client indicates to the nurse that the client needs further teaching?
1. "I will eat six small meals a day, 2 to 3 hours apart."
2. "I will eat a diet high in protein, fiber, and fat."
3. "I will record all food eaten including thoughts associated with foods."
4. "I will write a contract to plan balanced, nutritious meals."

12-6. Which of the following statements made by a client with anorexia require the nurse's counsel to address the client's distorted cognitive views?
1. "If I stick to my diet and eat the right foods I will be able to live a normal life."

2. "If I follow a nutritional diet and watch my tendency to over-exercise I will feel better."

3. "If I continue my therapy and deal with my anxiety in a healthy manner I will get better."

4. "If I exercise less and eat a little more every day I will be able to reach my target weight."

See Appendix D for answers.

References

American Psychiatric Association. (2000). *Diagnostic and statistical manual of mental disorders* (4th ed., Text revision). Washington, DC: Author.

Anderson, D. A., Martens, M. P., & Cimini, M. D. (2005). Do female college students who purge report greater alcohol use and negative alcohol-related consequences? *International Journal of Eating Disorders, 37*(1), 65–68.

Appolinario, J. C., Bacaltchuk, J., Sichieri, R., Claudino, A. M., Godoy-Matos, A., Morgan, C., et al. (2003). A randomized, double-blind, placebo-controlled study of sibutramine in the treatment of binge-eating disorder. *Archives of General Psychiatry, 60*(11), 1109–1116.

Bacaltchuk, J., & Hay, P. (2003). Antidepressants versus placebo for people with bulimia nervosa. *Cochrane Database of Systematic Reviews* (4): CD003391.

Bulik, C. M. (2005). Exploring the gene-environment nexus in eating disorders. *Journal of Psychiatry & Neuroscience, 30*(5), 335–339.

Bulik, C. M., Tozzi, F., Anderson, C., Mazzeo, S. E., Aggen, S., & Sullivan, P. F. (2003). The relation between eating disorders and components of perfectionism. *American Journal of Psychiatry, 160*(2), 366–368.

Devlin, M. J., Yanovski, S. Z., & Wilson, G. T. (2000). Obesity: What mental health professionals need to know. *American Journal of Psychiatry, 157*(6), 854–866.

Eissa, M. A .H., & Gunner, K. B. (2004). Evaluation and management of obesity in children and adolescents. *Journal of Pediatric Health Care, 18*(1), 35–38.

Finfgeld, D. L. (2002). Anorexia nervosa: Analysis of long-term outcomes and clinical implications. *Archives of Psychiatric Nursing, 16*(4), 176–186.

Frank, G. K., Bailer, U. F., Henry, S. E., Drevets, W., Meltzer, C. C., Price, J. C., et al. (2005). Increased dopamine D2/D3 receptor binding after recovery from anorexia nervosa. *Biological Psychiatry, 58*(11):908–12. Published ahead of print June 29, 2005.

Ghizzani, A., & Montomoli, M. (2000). Anorexia nervosa and sexuality in women. *Journal of Sex Education and Therapy, 25*(1), 80–88.

Hoek, H. W., van Harten, P. N., Hermans, K. M. E., Katzman, M. A., Matroos, G. E., & Susser, E. S. (2005). The incidence of anorexia nervosa on Curacao. *American Journal of Psychiatry, 162*(4), 748–752.

Kaye, W. H., Bulik, C. M., Thornton, L., Barbarich, N., & Masters, K. (2004). Comorbidity of anxiety disorders with anorexia and bulimia nervosa. *American Journal of Psychiatry, 161*(12), 2215–2221.

Keel, P. K. (2005). *Eating disorders.* Upper Saddle River, NJ: Prentice Hall.

Keel, P. K., Haedt, A., & Edler, C. (2005). Purging disorder. *International Journal of Eating Disorders, 38*(3), 191–199.

Keel, P. K., Dorer, D. J., Eddy, K. T., Franko, D., Charatan, D. L., & Herzog, D. B. (2003). Predictors of mortality in eating disorders. *Archives of General Psychiatry, 60*(2), 179–183.

Keel, P. K., Leon, G. R., & Fulkerson, J. A. (2001). Vulnerability to eating disorders in childhood and adolescence. In R. E. Ingram & J. M. Price (Eds.), *Vulnerability to psychopathology* (pp. 389–411). New York: Guilford Press.

Kotz, C. M. (2006). Integration of feeding and spontaneous physical activity. *Physiology & Behavior, 88*(3), 294–301.

Long, J. D., & Stevens, K. R. (2004). Using technology to promote self-efficacy for healthy eating in adolescents. *Journal of Nursing Scholarship, 36*(2), 134–139.

McIntosh, V. V. W., Jordan, J., Carter, F. A., Luty, S. E., McKenzie, J. M., Bulik, C. M., et al. (2005). Three psychotherapies for anorexia nervosa. *American Journal of Psychiatry, 162*(4), 741–747.

Neumark-Sztainer, D. (2005). *"I'm, like, SO fat!"* New York: Guilford Press.

Nolan, M. E. (2003). Anticipatory guidance for parents of Prader-Willi children. *Pediatric Nursing, 29*(6), 427–430.

North American Nursing Diagnosis Association. (2007). *Nursing Diagnoses Definitions and Classification 2005-2006.* Philadelphia, PA: Author.

Pull, C. B. (2004). Binge eating disorder. *Current Opinions in Psychiatry, 17*(1), 43–48.

Robb, A. S., Silber, R. J., Orrell-Valente, J. K., Valadez-Meltzer, A., Ellis, N., Dadson, M. J., et al. (2002). Supplemental nocturnal nasogastric refeeding for better short-term outcome in hospitalized adolescent girls with anorexia nervosa. *American Journal of Psychiatry, 159*(8), 1347–1353.

Romano, S. J., Halmi, K. A., Sarkar, N. P., Koke, S. C., & Lee, J. S. (2002). A placebo-controlled study of fluoxetine in continued treatment of bulimia nervosa after successful acute fluoxetine treatment. *American Journal of Psychiatry, 159*(1), 96–102.

Slof-O't Landt, M. C., van Furth, E. F., Meulenbelt, I., Slagboom, P. E., Bartels, M., Boomsma, D. I., et al. (2005). Eating disorders: From twin studies to candidate genes and beyond. *Twin Research and Human Genetics, 8*(5), 467–482.

Sollid, C. P., Wisborg, K., Hjort, J., & Secher, N. T. (2004). Eating disorder that was diagnosed before pregnancy and pregnancy outcome. *American Journal of Obstetrics and Gynecology, 190*(1), 206–210.

Stein, K. F., & Corte, C. (2003). Reconceptualizing causative factors and intervention strategies in the eating disorders: A shift from body image to self-concept impairments. *Archives of Psychiatric Nursing, 17*(2), 57–66.

Striegel-Moore, R. H., Dohm, F. A., Kraemer, H. C., Taylor, C. B., Daniels, S., Crawford. P. B., et al. (2003). Eating disorders in White and Black women. *American Journal of Psychiatry, 160*(7), 1326–1331.

Takimoto, Y., Yoshiuchi, K., Kumano, H., Yamanaka, G., Sasaki, T., Suematsu, H., et al. (2004). QT interval and QT dispersion in eating disorders. *Psychotherapy and Psychosomatics, 73*(5), 324–328.

Tozzi, F., Thornton, L. M., Klump, K. L., Fichter, M. M., Halmi, K. A., Kaplan, A. S., et al. (2005). Symptom fluctuation in eating disorders. *American Journal of Psychiatry, 162*(4), 732–740.

Tsai, S. J. (2005). Repetitive transcranial magnetic stiumulation. *Medical Hypotheses, 65*(6), 1176–1178.

Turrell, S. L., Davis. R., Grahan, H., & Weiss, I. (2005). Adolescents with anorexia nervosa: Multiple perspectives of discharge readiness. *Journal of Child and Adolescent Psychiatric Nursing, 18*(3), 116–126.

Uher, R., Murphy, T., Brammer, M. J., Dalgleish, T., Phillips, M. L., Ng, V. W., et al. (2004). Medial prefrontal cortex activity associated with symptom provocation in eating disorders. *American Journal of Psychiatry, 161*(7), 1238–1246.

Utter, J., Neumark-Sztainer, D., Wall, M., & Story, M. (2003). Reading magazine articles about dieting and associated weight control behaviors among adolescents. *Journal of Adolescent Health, 32*(1), 78–82.

Woodside, D. B., Carter, J. C., & Blackmore, E. (2004). Predictors of premature termination of inpatient treatment for anorexia nervosa. *American Journal of Psychiatry, 161*(12), 2277–2281.

Yang, C. F. J., Gray, P., & Pope, H. G. (2005). Male body image in Taiwan versus the West. *American Journal of Psychiatry, 162*(2), 263–269.

Chapter 13

Mood Disorders

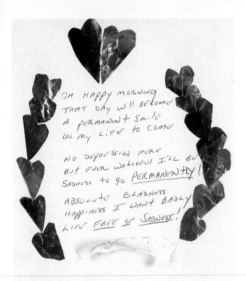

> **❝** *Oh happy morning*
> *That day will become*
> *A permanent smile*
> *On my life to come.*
>
> *No depression here*
> *But ever watchful I'll be*
> *Sadness to go PERMANENTLY!*
>
> *Absolute gladness*
> *Happiness I want badly*
> *Life FREE OF SADNESS!* **❞**
>
> —Rosalie, Age 57

OBJECTIVES

After reading this chapter, you will be able to:

1. Compare and contrast the different theories regarding the etiology of mood disorders.
2. Discuss the psychopharmacological treatment of the symptoms of mood disorders.
3. Outline the different treatment options for a person with a mood disorder.
4. Outline the assessment process for a client with a mood disorder.
5. Use the nursing process to develop a comprehensive plan of care for a client with a mood disorder.
6. Develop illness management teaching plans for a client with a mood disorder and her/his family.
7. Discuss the key points in effectively communicating with a person with a mood disorder.

MediaLink 🌐💿 www.prenhall.com/fontaine

Go to the Pearson Health MediaLink CD-ROM and the Companion Website at www.prenhall.com/fontaine for interactive resources for this chapter.

The ROAD to Critical Thinking   A Client Experiencing Bipolar Disorder

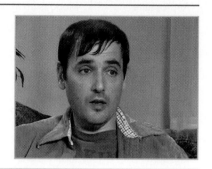

Travel this ROAD to understand Josh and his condition.
Read about Josh below and throughout this chapter.
Observe Josh on the CD-ROM accompanying this book.
Assess Josh by answering the questions at the end of this chapter.
Develop a Care Plan on the CD-ROM to address Josh's condition.

Josh

Josh's bipolar disorder began when he was in the 8th grade. Beginning then, and for some years after, Josh would self-medicate with alcohol and marijuana to shut out his thoughts and shut off his internal dialogue. When not taking his medications, Josh experiences paranoid delusions and hallucinations, not unusual for people with bipolar disorder. He recognizes that his mental illness has interfered with his ability to have a career or a family. During manic episodes, families may be subjected to bizarre, hostile, and even destructive behavior. Bipolar disorder can devastate individual and family life and often leads to a downward spiral in interpersonal, economic, and occupational functioning.

Approximately 60% of people with bipolar disorder also have a substance abuse diagnosis—the highest rate of all people with major psychiatric illness. Josh's substance abuse began as an attempt to self-medicate his bothersome symptoms. No doubt, his use of substances was also the natural result of his impulsive, expansive lifestyle and poor judgment during manic episodes. Substance abuse worsens the course of bipolar disorder.

Emotions are feeling responses to a wide variety of emotional stimuli. Positive emotions such as joy stimulate you to remain in the situation while negative emotions such as fear stimulate you to avoid or withdraw from the situation. **Mood** is defined as a sustained emotional state and how you subjectively feel. The way in which you communicate your mood to others is called affect. **Affect** is the immediate and observable emotional expression of mood, which you communicate verbally and nonverbally. *Verbal cues* we may use to describe our emotional state are words such as elation, happiness, pleasure, frustration, anger, or hostility. *Nonverbal cues* to emotions include facial expressions such as smiling, frowning, and looking blank; motor activities such as making hands into fists and pacing; and physiological responses such as profuse sweating and increased respirations. We may choose not to communicate verbally to another person, but it is almost impossible to prevent nonverbal expression of our feelings.

A variety of descriptors of affect are used to facilitate communication among health care professionals. Table 13.1 ■ gives definitions of affect descriptors and behavioral examples. Emotions, mood, and affect can be pictured along a continuum ranging from depression through normal to mania. The normal range of mood is stable and appropriate to the situation. Emotions, mood, and affect become dysfunctional when they occur in inappropriate situations or when the response is out of proportion to the stimulus. People diagnosed with mood disorders experience disrupting disturbances at varying points along the continuum.

KNOWLEDGE BASE

The mood spectrum disorders are characterized by changes in feelings ranging from severe depression to inordinate elation. They are best understood as syndromes with a core cluster of symptoms. We are beginning to understand that there are many different subtypes of mood disorders, each with different patterns and probably a different prognosis. These subtypes of depressive and bipolar disorders are just now becoming clear.

Types of Disorders

Major depressive disorder (MDD, also called **unipolar disorder**) is made when, along with a loss of interest in life, a person experiences a depressed mood that moves from mild to severe, with the severe phase lasting at least 2 weeks. MDD often has a chronic course with lengthy episodes or incomplete remission between episodes

Dysthymic disorder is a chronic disorder in which periods of depressed mood are interspersed with normal mood. With this disorder, people experience a depressed mood for most of the day more days than not for at least 2 years. Symptoms in dysthymic disorder tend to be less severe than those in MDD, and there are fewer physiological symptoms (disturbed sleep, altered appetite, and weight loss or gain). Most people with dysthymic disorder also experience one or more episodes of MDD. When this occurs it is referred to as **double depression**. Individuals

TABLE 13.1	Descriptors of Affect	
Affect	**Definition**	**Behavioral Example**
Appropriate	Mood is congruent with the immediate situation.	Juan cries when learning of the death of his father.
Inappropriate	Mood is not related to the immediate situation.	When Sue's husband tells her about his terrible pain, Sue begins to laugh out loud.
Stable	Mood is resistant to sudden changes when there is no provocation in the environment.	During a party, Dan smiles and laughs at the appropriate social interchanges.
Labile	Mood shifts suddenly in a way that cannot be understood in the context of the situation.	During a friendly game of checkers, Dorothy, who has been laughing, suddenly knocks the board off the table in anger. She then begins to laugh and wants to continue the game.
Elevated	Mood is one of euphoria not necessarily related to the immediate situation.	Sean bounces around the dayroom, laughing, singing, and telling other clients how wonderful everything is.
Depressed	Mood is one of despondency not necessarily related to the immediate situation.	Leo sits slumped in a chair with a sad facial expression, teary eyes, and minimal body movement.
Overreactive	Mood is appropriate to the situation but out of proportion to the immediate situation.	Karen screams and curses when her child spills a glass of milk on the kitchen floor.
Blunted	Mood is a dulled response to the immediate situation.	When Tom learns of his full-tuition scholarship, he responds with only a small smile.
Flat	There are no visible cues to the person's mood.	When Juanita is told about her best friend's death, she says "Oh" and does not give any indication of an emotional response.

with double depression have more severe symptoms and higher rates of suicide than clients with MDD (Klein, Shankman, Lewinsohn, Rohde, & Seeley, 2004).

The medical diagnosis of **bipolar disorder** is given when a person's mood alternates between the extremes of depression and elation (mania), with interspersing periods of normal mood. *Bipolar I disorder* is characterized by the occurrence of one or more manic episodes and one or more depressive episodes. *Bipolar II disorder* is characterized by one or more hypomanic episodes (less severe) and one or more depressive episodes. There is evidence that some individuals experience a unipolar mania with no depressive episodes. Data suggests that unipolar disorder and bipolar disorder are not two separate disorders but rather the same disorder with fluctuations in mood (Cassano et al., 2004; Schneck et al., 2004; Solomon et al., 2003).

Bipolar disorder is further classified as:

- *Mixed:* The person has rapidly alternating moods.
- *Manic:* The person is presently in the manic phase.
- *Depressed:* The person is in the depressed phase but has a history of manic episodes.

Rapid cycling describes the course for some people of bipolar disorder. It is defined as four or more episodes of illness within a 12-month period. A person with rapid cycling could be diagnosed as bipolar I, II, or mixed, manic, or depressed.

Rapid cycling occurs in 10% to 20% of persons with bipolar disorder, with 70% to 90% of rapid cyclers being women. This form of the disorder tends to be more resistant to treatment than the non–rapid-cycling course (Schneck et al., 2004)

Cyclothymic disorder is characterized by a mood range from moderate depression to hypomania, which may or may not include periods of normal mood, lasting at least 2 years. Clients with cyclothymic disorder do not experience the severe symptoms that qualify for a diagnosis of MDD or bipolar disorder. Figure 13.1 ■ illustrates our current understanding of mood disorders.

Schizoaffective disorder is diagnosed when clients have symptoms that appear to be a mixture of schizophrenia and the mood disorders. The person with schizoaffective disorder experiences one or more of the following symptoms: delusions, hallucinations, disorganized speech, disorganized behavior, or negative symptoms (see chapter 14 ∞ for more detailed discussion of these symptoms). In addition, the person experiences symptoms of the mood disorders: major depressive symptoms, manic symptoms, or mixed symptoms. Clients often have difficulty maintaining job or school functioning, experience problems with self-care, are socially isolated, and often suffer from suicidal ideation. The age of onset is typically late adolescence or early adulthood.

See the DSM-IV-TR feature for the diagnostic criteria for major depression and manic episodes.

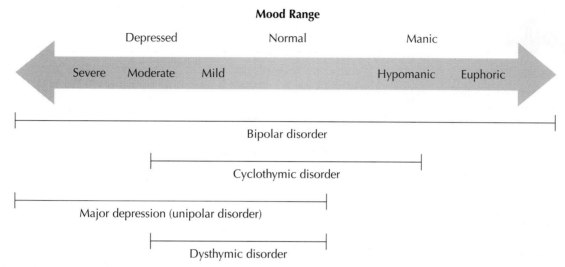

Figure 13.1 ■ Mood disorders and ranges.

Pregnancy and Postpartum

Although 10% to 15% of *pregnant women* meet criteria for depression, they often remain undiagnosed because the symptoms of depression are similar to the somatic changes of pregnancy. The prevalence of depression among pregnant adolescents is almost twice as high as among adult pregnant women and is more severe between the second and third trimesters. Untreated maternal mood disorders are associated with poor prenatal care, preterm delivery, small infant size, postpartum depression/mania, and maternal suicide (Suppaseemanont, 2006; Yonkers et al., 2004).

Mood disorders in women after delivering a child are fairly common. During pregnancy, levels of estrogens, glucocorticoids, and amino acids increase by as much as 200 times only to drop sharply within 24 hours after delivery. This results in a hypoactive hypothalamic–pituitary axis that may last for months. Symptoms can be described along a continuum from postpartum blues to postpartum depression to the rare form, postpartum psychosis. These disorders may be complicated by postpartum panic disorder and postpartum obsessive–compulsive disorder (Bailara et al., 2005).

Postpartum blues begin within the first 10 days postpartum and last a few days to 2 weeks with symptoms disappearing spontaneously. The mood may be unstable, accompanied by sadness, weepiness, irritability, anxiety, and fatigue. As many as 80% of new mothers may experience these symptoms, which are thought to be caused by hormonal fluctuations. Most of these women have not had previous emotional problems (Ugarriza, 2004).

Postpartum depression is estimated to occur in 13% of new mothers, often beginning within 3 months of delivery but may strike at any time during the first year after having a child. Women who give birth to multiple children and/or to preterm children are at higher risk for postpartum depression. Symptoms include insomnia, loss of energy, inability to concentrate, anxiety, mood swings, periods of crying, and feelings of despair as they ruminate over perceived inadequacies as a mother. If depression is untreated, it will affect the ability to parent and to cope with stressful situations. These symptoms are more intense and longer lasting than those in postpartum blues. Any symptoms lasting longer than 2 weeks qualify as postpartum depression. Contributing factors are hormonal changes, family history of depression, feeling overwhelmed by parenting tasks, changes in family dynamics, and inadequate support. Those who develop postpartum depression are at an increased risk for depression after subsequent pregnancies (Beck, 2003; Ugarriza, 2004; Wisner et al., 2004).

In some cases *postpartum panic disorder* accompanies postpartum depression. Symptoms include shortness of breath, heart palpitations, dizziness, and chest pain. *Postpartum obsessive–compulsive disorder* consists of persistent thoughts of hurting or killing the child and an inability to stop or ignore these thoughts (Ugarriza, 2004).

One to two women in 1,000, with no history of a mood disorder, experiences a *postpartum psychosis*—a medical emergency. The incidence of relapse for women who have a diagnosed bipolar disorder is 25% to 40% during postpartum or 260 women per 1,000 deliveries. The symptoms usually occur between the first 2 to 6 weeks after delivery but may occur as early as 48 hours postpartum. Symptoms develop rapidly and include insomnia, hallucinations, agitation, and bizarre feelings or behavior. An inordinate concern with the baby's health, guilt about lack of love, and delusions about the infant's being dead or defective also may be present. The mother may deny having given birth or hear voices that command her to hurt the baby. In extreme cases, the mother may even kill the child and/or herself. Unlike other types of psychoses, the woman with postpartum psychosis may alternate

DSM-IV-TR Diagnostic Criteria for Depressive Disorders

Major Depressive Episode

A. Five (or more) of the following symptoms have been present during the same 2-week period and represent a change from previous functioning; at least one of the symptoms is either (1) depressed mood or (2) loss of interest or pleasure. Note: Do not include symptoms that are clearly due to a general medical condition, or mood-incongruent delusions or hallucinations.

1. Depressed mood most of the day, nearly every day, as indicated by either subjective report (e.g., feels sad or empty) or observation made by others (e.g., appears tearful). Note: In children and adolescents, can be irritable mood.
2. Markedly diminished interest or pleasure in all, or almost all, activities most of the day, nearly every day (as indicated by either subjective account or observation made by others).
3. Significant weight loss when not dieting or weight gain (e.g., a change of more than 5% of body weight in a month), or decrease or increase in appetite nearly every day. Note: In children, consider failure to make expected weight gains.
4. Insomnia or hypersomnia nearly every day.
5. Psychomotor agitation or retardation nearly every day (observable by others, not merely subjective feelings of restlessness or being slowed down).
6. Fatigue or loss of energy nearly every day.
7. Feelings of worthlessness or excessive or inappropriate guilt (which may be delusional) nearly every day (not merely self-reproach or guilt about being sick).
8. Diminished ability to think or concentrate, or indecisiveness, nearly every day (either by subjective account or as observed by others).
9. Recurrent thoughts of death (not just fear of dying), recurrent suicidal ideation without a specific

plan, or a suicide attempt or a specific plan for committing suicide.

B. The symptoms do not meet criteria for a Mixed Episode.

C. The symptoms cause clinically significant distress or impairment in social, occupational, or other important areas of functioning.

D. The symptoms are not due to the direct physiological effects of a substance (e.g., a drug of abuse, a medication) or a general medical condition (e.g., hypothyroidism).

E. The symptoms are not better accounted for by bereavement, i.e., after the loss of a loved one, the symptoms persist for longer than 2 months or are characterized by marked functional impairment, morbid preoccupation with worthlessness, suicidal ideation, psychotic symptoms, or psychomotor retardation.

Major Depressive Disorder, Single Episode

A. Presence of a single Major Depressive Episode

B. The Major Depressive Episode is not better accounted for by Schizoaffective Disorder and is not superimposed on Schizophrenia, Schizophreniform Disorder, Delusional Disorder, or Psychotic Disorder Not Otherwise Specified.

C. There has never been a Manic Episode, a Mixed Episode, or a Hypomanic Episode. Note: This exclusion does not apply if all of the manic-like, mixed-like, or hypomanic-like episodes are substance or treatment induced or are due to the direct physiological effects of a general medical condition.

Major Depressive Disorder, Recurrent

A. Presence of two or more Major Depressive Episodes.
Note: To be considered separate episodes, there must be an interval of at least 2 consecutive months in which criteria are not met for a Major Depressive Episode.

B. The Major Depressive Episodes are not better accounted for by Schizoaffective Disorder and are not superimposed on Schizophrenia, Schizophreniform Disorder, Delusional Disorder, or Psychotic Disorder Not Otherwise Specified.

C. There has never been a Manic Episode, a Mixed Episode, or a Hypomanic Episode. Note: This exclusion does not apply if all of the manic-like, mixed-like, or hypomanic-like episodes are substance or treatment induced or are due to the direct physiological effects of a general medical condition.

Dysthymic Disorder

A. Depressed mood for most of the day, for more days than not, as indicated either by subjective account or observation by others, for at least 2 years. Note: In children and adolescents, mood can be irritable and duration must be at least 1 year.

B. Presence, while depressed, of two (or more) of the following:
1. Poor appetite or overeating
2. Insomnia or hypersomnia
3. Low energy or fatigue
4. Low self-esteem
5. Poor concentration or difficulty making decisions
6. Feelings of hopelessness

C. During the 2-year period (1 year for children or adolescents) of the disturbance, the person has never been without the symptoms in Criteria A and B for more than 2 months at a time.

D. No Major Depressive Episode has been present during the first 2 years of the disturbance (1 year for children and adolescents); i.e., the disturbance is not better accounted for by chronic Major Depressive Disorder, or Major Depressive Disorder, in Partial Remission. Note: There may have been a previous Major Depressive Episode provided there was a full remission (no significant signs or symptoms for 2 months) before development of the Dysthymic Disorder. In addition, after the initial 2 years (1 year in children or

---

DSM-IV-TR | **Diagnostic Criteria for Depressive Disorders** *continued*

adolescents) of Dysthymic Disorder, there may be superimposed episodes of Major Depressive Disorder, in which case both diagnoses may be given when the criteria are met for a Major Depressive Episode.

E. There has never been a Manic Episode, a Mixed Episode, or a Hypomanic Episode, and criteria have never been met for Cyclothymic Disorder.

F. The disturbance does not occur exclusively during the course of a chronic Psychotic Disorder, such as Schizophrenia or Delusional Disorder.

G. The symptoms are not due to the direct physiological effects of a substance (e.g., a drug of abuse, a medication) or a general medical condition (e.g., hypothyroidism).

H. The symptoms cause clinically significant distress or impairment in social,

occupational, or other important areas of functioning.

Seasonal Pattern Specifier
Specify if:
With Seasonal Pattern (can be applied to the pattern of Major Depressive Episodes in Bipolar I Disorder, Bipolar II Disorder, or Major Depressive Disorder, Recurrent)

A. There has been a regular temporal relationship between the onset of Major Depressive Episodes in Bipolar I or Bipolar II Disorder or Major Depressive Disorder, Recurrent, and a particular time of the year (e.g., regular appearance of the Major Depressive Episode in the fall or winter).
Note: Do not include cases in which there is an obvious effect of seasonal-related psychosocial stressors (e.g., regularly being unemployed every winter).

B. Full remissions (or a change from depression to mania or hypomania) also occur at a characteristic time of the year (e.g., depression disappears in the spring).

C. In the last 2 years, two Major Depressive Episodes have occurred that demonstrate the temporal seasonal relationships defined in Criteria A and B, and no nonseasonal Major Depressive Episodes have occurred during that same period.

D. Seasonal Major Depressive Episodes (as described above) substantially outnumber the nonseasonal Major Depressive Episodes that may have occurred over the individual's lifetime.

SOURCE: Reprinted with permission from the Diagnostic and statistical manual of mental disorders, 4th ed., Text Revision (pp. 375, 376, 380–381, 427). Copyright 2000 American Psychiatric Association.

---

between lucid states and a "zombie-like" psychotic state (Spinelli, 2004; Ugarriza, 2004).

Lavonne, a 22-year-old nurse, has been admitted to the acute care unit for postpartum psychosis. Her father has bipolar disorder and is an alcoholic, her mother is depressed, and her grandmother committed suicide. She was treated 9 years ago for depression. She stopped taking her Prozac 4 years ago and her depression resurfaced a few months before this pregnancy (her first). She and her fiancé moved to this area 10 months ago and she has made few friends during that time. Prior to the birth she learned her fiancé's divorce was never finalized and she is not certain if he lied to her or was "conned by his ex-wife." After her delivery 2 weeks ago, she started having irrational thoughts and saw visions of her baby boy being hurt by her with a knife. She then began to see very graphic, violent images of her son's butchered body. She feels guilty that she is a bad mother since she is having these thoughts. She feels sad, depressed, and hopeless with intermittent suicidal thoughts.

Fathers also need to adjust during pregnancy and after childbirth, and there is evidence that some men experience depressive symptoms following the birth of their children. Mothers and fathers show that they have similar levels of parenting-related stress and anxiety. Factors increasing the risk for depression include inexperience with childcare, unemployment, relationship conflict with partner, and less emotional and social support from family and friends.

Onset and Course of Disorders

The World Health Organization estimates that by the year 2020, major depressive disorder will be the second most important cause worldwide of disability (behind heart disease). At any given time, 20 million people worldwide suffer from depression. It is thought that 5% to 12% of men and 10% to 25% of women will suffer a major depression in their lifetime (Arnault, Sakamoto & Moriwaki, 2005; Draucker, 2005; Valdivia & Rossy, 2004).

Men and women are equally at risk for bipolar disorder, which affects 1.5% of people in the United States. The disorder most commonly begins during adolescence but has often been under-recognized and misdiagnosed in this age group. It is difficult to predict the course of the disorder; some may have only one episode every 10 years, while others may have several episodes a year (Bellivier et al., 2003).

Mood disorders tend to be chronic in nature. As many as 85% of people who have one major depressive episode will experience another episode and 35% experience residual symptoms between acute episodes. Relapse rates for bipolar disorder range from 44% in 1 year to 73% to 89% over 4 to 5 years. Between 30% to 60% of individuals with bipolar disorder do not fully recover between episodes. In addition, bipolar disorder has the highest suicide risk of all psychiatric disorders (Steinhauer, 2003; Tohen et al., 2005; Valdivia &

Rossy, 2004). Descriptions of the course of these disorders include (Tohen et al., 2003):

- *Recovery:* Return to or exceed pre-illness levels of functioning
- *Remission:* Sustained recovery of at least 8 weeks
- *Switching:* A new illness phase (manic or depressed) without recovery
- *Relapse:* Return of disorder soon after recovery
- *Recurrence:* A later recurrence after recovery

The high rate of mood disorders makes these disorders a major concern for nurses. Mood-disordered clients are found in the community and in all types of clinical settings and are not restricted to psychiatric settings. It is vital that the nurse be alert to cues because one of the tragic results in untreated depression is suicide.

Comorbid Disorders

Severe depression and *anxiety disorders* frequently occur at the same time. Studies indicate that as many as 40% of those suffering from agoraphobia, 50% of those experiencing panic attacks, 44% of those with obsessive–compulsive disorder, and 17% of those with generalized anxiety disorder are also clinically depressed. An estimated 85% of adults with depression experience significant symptoms of anxiety. Individuals with bipolar disorder are more likely to have concomitant panic disorder and generalized anxiety disorder than the general population. Major depression increases the risk of developing posttraumatic stress disorder. People with both mood and anxiety disorders have fewer personal and social resources and demonstrate poorer overall functioning (Ghaemi, 2004; Oquendo et al., 2005; Steinhauer, 2003).

The rate of comorbidity between mood disorders and *substance-related disorders* is high. In some cases, the primary diagnosis is a mood disorder, with substance abuse being an attempt to self-medicate. In other situations, the substance-related disorder is the primary diagnosis. An example is the person who becomes depressed during withdrawal from amphetamines or cocaine. A third possibility is that the person has both disorders as primary diagnoses. Research reports that major depression tends to come before alcohol problems in women, while the opposite is true for men. Unfortunately, the use of alcohol to relieve depression can also aggravate depression by causing other problems for the drinker and also by intensifying the level of depression. Thirty-two percent of all depressed adolescents have a comorbid substance abuse disorder. As stated earlier, people with bipolar disorder have the highest rate of comorbid substance abuse disorder of all the major psychiatric illnesses. Treatment for both mood and substance abuse disorders should be concurrent (Baethge et al., 2005; Davis et al., 2005; Wilens et al., 2004).

Josh:

❝ I was so nervous that I couldn't feel anything. I shut down, basically. And that was the only way for me to deal with my illness. That's why I loved marijuana. I wouldn't get high, I'd just get stoned. I'd turn into a piece of stone and a grin. That's why I was doing drugs, because it helped me shut off this dialogue I had within myself and these thoughts. ❞

People with bipolar disorder have a 30% rate of comorbid pathological gambling. Of those hospitalized for pathological gambling, 38% have been diagnosed with hypomania and 24% with bipolar disorder. The pleasure-seeking behavior and poor judgment of bipolar disorder contribute to this comorbidity (Hollander, Pallanti, Allen, Sood, & Rossi, 2005).

Secondary causes of depression may be related to a variety of medications and medical conditions. Medications implicated in secondary depression include antianxiety agents, antihypertensives, corticosteroids, estrogen/progesterone, and chemotherapeutic agents. Metabolic disorders that may cause depression include hyperthyroidism, hypothyroidism, adrenal diseases, parathyroid disorders, and vitamin B_{12} deficiency. Neurological disruptions include brain tumors or acute traumatic brain injury (especially in the frontal or basal ganglia areas), Huntington disease, multiple sclerosis, Alzheimer disease, AIDS dementia, migraine, and carbon monoxide exposure. People who have Parkinson disease have a 30% to 50% chance of also having a major depression. Often the mood disorder precedes the motor changes. Of people who have a cerebral vascular accident, 20% to 50% experience depression at a more severe level than people who become depressed after other medical diagnoses such as chronic pain syndromes, sleep apnea, cancer, and heart disease (Mayberg, Keightley, Mahurin, & Brannan, 2004; Valdivia & Rossy, 2004). See chapter 20 ∞ for more detailed information on the psychiatric implications of medical disorders.

It is vital that the nurse is alert to cues for self-harm, since as many as 15% of people with major depressive disorder and 10% to 20% of people with bipolar disorder go on to commit suicide. Suicidal behavior and suicide prevention is covered in chapter 21 ∞.

Etiologies

Multiple theories have been developed to explain the cause of mood disorders. Depression, like schizophrenia, is considered a spectrum disorder. At one end of the spectrum is an incapacitating illness such as a double depression or bipolar disorder with psychosis. At the other end is a depressive personality characterized only by a pessimistic outlook on life or mood swings that are mild in nature. Most cases fall somewhere in between these two extremes.

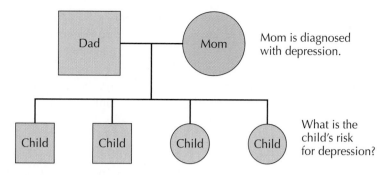

Figure 13.2 ■ Top-down sampling.

In understanding people with mood disorders, the nurse must look at how factors interacted within the person's past and how they interact in present circumstances. A person may have a genetic predisposition to abnormalities in neurotransmission. The abnormalities may occur only if certain psychological mechanisms are present, and these mechanisms may operate only if particular social interactions occur. Many factors in both the individual and the environment increase or decrease the risk of mood disorders. Different forms of the illness may have different risk factors. In some forms, predisposition may have a stronger role, and in other forms, stressors may have a stronger role. It is likely that mood disorders represent a common final pathway of multiple underlying factors. By applying genetic, neurobiological, intrapersonal, learning, cognitive, social, and gender bias theories, the nurse can approach the client from a holistic perspective.

Genetics

Some evidence suggests that people who experience mood disorders have a genetic predisposition to these disorders. It is not yet clear what is inherited, neurobiological vulnerability, cognitive vulnerability, or social vulnerability. The inheritability of major depression is 40% to 50%. The more severe the depression, the stronger the genetic link. The general population rate of recurrent unipolar depression is 8%. Children of depressed parents (top-down sampling as shown in Figure 13.2 ■) have twice the risk or about 16% over a lifetime. If both parents have depression, the risk rises to

75%. First-degree relatives of depressed children (bottom-up sampling as depicted in Figure 13.3 ■) also have a twofold greater risk of depression. Studies of the incidence in twins show that in 60% of monozygotic twins, both twins developed a unipolar depression, compared with only 12% of dizygotic twins (Faraone, Glatt, Su, & Tsuang, 2004).

Bipolar disorder has the greatest inheritability, where about 85% of the risk appears to be inherited. Early onset of the disorder may be the result of a particularly strong genetic effect. Studies of the incidence in twins demonstrate that in 50% to 80% of monozygotic twins, both twins developed bipolar disorder, compared with only 17% to 24% of dizygotic twins (Badner, 2003; Fisfalen et al., 2005).

Studies suggest that a complex mode of inheritance exists, rather than a single dominant gene. It is probably the individual mix of these multiple genes that determines differences such as age of onset, symptoms, severity, and course of the mood disorders.

Neurobiology

The *prefrontal cortex* has been the subject of increasing attention in research on mood disorders. Studies of depressed people have shown lower than normal activity, low glucose metabolism, and decreased blood flow in the anterior cingulate cortex. These abnormalities may be associated with abnormal processing of emotion. Neuroimaging findings in bipolar disorder include ventricular enlargement and smaller volumes in the posterior hippocampus, left amygdala, and temporal lobe. The amygdala plays a role in keeping social

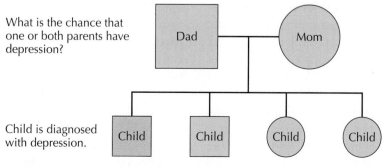

Figure 13.3 ■ Bottom-up sampling.

and emotional behavior within bounds, both of which are impaired in manic episodes (Caetano et al., 2006; Frazier et al., 2005; Neumeister, Charney, & Drevets, 2005).

The *neurotransmission hypothesis* is specifically concerned with the levels of serotonin (5-HT), dopamine (DA), norepinephrine (NE), and acetylcholine (ACh) in the central nervous system. It is believed that there is a functional deficiency of these neurotransmitters during a depressive episode and a functional excess during a manic episode (Meyer et al., 2003).

Most likely there are different combinations of problems with the neurotransmitter systems. Both DA and the balance between DA and ACh are responsible for difficulties with motivation. ACh is implicated in the sleep disturbances of both bipolar and unipolar disorders. NE is important in motor arousal, movement, energy, concentration, and motivation. The principal neurotransmitter for mood states is 5-HT, which is associated with anxiety and aggression, especially self-destructive behavior. A newly found protein named p11 appears to regulate how brain cells respond to 5-HT by increasing the number of receptors. Compared to people who are not depressed, people who are depressed have lower levels of p11. In addition, endogenous opioids are necessary to moderate sad moods. The interactions between these different neurotransmitters explain how clinical features tend to vary from client to client (Svenningsson et al., 2006).

One way this imbalance may occur is through the action of the enzyme *monoamine oxidase (MAO)*, which is responsible for deactivating neurotransmitters after they have been released from the receptor sites. If there is an excess of MAO, neurotransmitter levels will be low, resulting in decreased impulse transmission. If there is insufficient MAO to deactivate the neurotransmitters, they will accumulate at the synapse and increase the transmission of impulses.

This hypothesis may be one explanation for the higher incidence of depression in women and older people. Throughout life, women and older adults have consistently higher levels of MAO than do men and younger people. The result may be a functional decrease in the necessary neurotransmitters.

Another part of the hypothesis concerns the *sensitivity of the receptors* to the neurotransmitters. During depression, the receptors may be subsensitive, so that fewer impulses are transmitted. During the manic state, receptors may be supersensitive, resulting in an increase in the transmission of impulses.

Although peripheral *thyroid hormone levels* may be normal, 35% of people with depression experience central nervous system (CNS) thyroid dysfunction, which has a major effect on serotonin (5-HT), dopamine (DA), and gamma-aminobutyric acid (GABA). It is believed that people who are depressed have a lower level of transthyretin, a protein important for transporting thyroid hormones in the brain. Current or past hypothyroidism may be associated with rapid-cycling bipolar disorder (Mayberg et al., 2004).

Continuing research into the relationship between *stress* and mood disorders indicates that the limbic system of the brain is the major site of stress adaptation. With stress, neurotransmitter production in the limbic system increases. When the stress becomes chronic or recurrent, the body can no longer adapt as efficiently, and a shortage of neurotransmitters results. During manic episodes, there appears to be a defective feedback mechanism in the limbic system. Even after the stressful event has been resolved, the limbic system continues to produce excessive neurotransmitters; the increased transmission of impulses continues. Different areas of the limbic system play a major role in the regulation of emotions such as fear, rage, excitement, and euphoria. The signs and symptoms of limbic dysfunction correlate to the characteristics seen in the mood disorders.

Another hypothesis involves **biological rhythms**. In some individuals, internal desynchronization may result in depression. The tendency toward internal desynchronization is probably inherited, but stresses, lifestyle, and normal aging also influence it. It is unclear, however, whether changes in circadian rhythms cause mood disturbances or whether changes in mood alter circadian rhythms. (See chapter 1 ∞ for a more detailed discussion of circadian rhythms.)

The **sleep–wake cycle** has an important role in mood disorders. In 50% to 75% of adults and 90% of old age people with depression there is an earlier onset of REM sleep and alternations in brain activity during REM sleep. For those with bipolar disorder, lack of sleep can trigger a manic episode (Rao, 2003).

Some forms of mood disorders are related to the time of year and the amount of available sunlight. In **seasonal affective disorder (SAD)**, depression occurs annually during fall and winter, and normal mood or hypomania occurs in spring and summer. The depressive state appears to be directly related to the amount of light because symptoms disappear if the person is exposed to more sunlight. Light has an inhibiting effect on the production of melatonin, a hormone that affects mood, sensations of fatigue, and sleepiness. Seasonal light changes are not the only trigger. A change of living quarters, such as a move into a darker basement apartment or into a windowless office, can trigger the disorder in some people (Wehr et al., 2001).

The majority of SAD sufferers are women with a family history of mood disorders. Unlike major depression, in which symptoms for children and adults differ, children and adults with SAD exhibit similar symptoms: fatigue, decreased activity, irritability, sadness, crying, worrying, and decreased concentration. A symptom seen more frequently in SAD, compared to the other mood disorders, is increased appetite, carbohydrate craving, and weight gain.

Intrapersonal Factors

Intrapersonal theory focuses on the theme of loss, either real or symbolic. The loss may be of another person, a relationship, an object, self-esteem, or security. When grief concerning the loss is unrecognized or unresolved, depression may result. A normal feeling accompanying all losses is anger, a compensatory response to feelings of powerlessness. People who have been taught it is inappropriate to experience and express anger learn to repress it. The result is that anger is turned inward and against the self. Some theorists believe the repressed anger and aggression against the self are the cause of depressive episodes. Other theorists believe the cause of depression is an inability to achieve desired goals, the loss of these goals, and a feeling of lack of control in life.

People who are unusually sensitive to loss or abandonment issues are said to have dependent traits. People who are unusually sensitive to failure to achieve their goals are said to have self-critical traits. Both of these cognitive–personality features increase the likelihood that environmental stressors will lead to depression.

Learning Theory

Learning theory states that people learn to be depressed in response to an external locus of control, as they perceive themselves lacking control over their life experiences. Throughout life, depressed people experience little success in achieving gratification, and little positive reinforcement for their attempts to cope with negative incidents. These repeated failures teach them that what they do has no effect on the final outcome. The more that stressful life events occur, the more their sense of helplessness is reinforced. When people reach the point of believing they have no control, they no longer have the will or energy to cope with life, and a depressive state results.

Cognitive Theory

The cognitive schemas influence the way people with mood disorders experience themselves and others. Those who are depressed focus on negative messages in the environment and ignore positive experiences. These negative schemas contribute to a view of the self as incompetent, unworthy, and unlikable. All present experiences are viewed as negative, and there is no hope for the future. In the manic phase, people focus on positive messages in the environment and ignore negative experiences. These positive schemas contribute to a grandiose view of themselves. Everything that occurs is seen as positive, and the future holds no limits. When people get caught up in this process, a number of cognitive distortions may occur. See Table 1.6 in chapter 1 ∞ for examples of cognitive distortions.

Sociocultural Factors

A variety of sociocultural conditions may contribute to a person's depressive feelings of powerlessness, hopelessness, and low self-esteem. Racism, classism, sexism, ageism, and homophobia are predominant sociocultural characteristics in the United States. Whatever way *minorities* are defined, they experience

discrimination psychologically, educationally, vocationally, and economically. When one is the subject of cultural stereotypes in comments or jokes, it is difficult not to feel inadequate and shameful. When education has been substandard, one cannot expect to be successful without remedial work. When promotions are based on race, gender, age, or sexual orientation, it is difficult to feel hopeful about advancing in one's career. It is also difficult to combat the helplessness felt when one's financial compensation is clearly inadequate for the job being done.

There is a much higher rate of depression among *women* than among men. One of the contributing factors in Western society may be the stress of being a single parent. With the high divorce rate, there are increasing numbers of single parents, 85% of whom are women. These women must deal with financial hardships, parenting problems, loneliness, and lack of a supportive adult relationship. A major predisposing factor for depression in women is having three or more children under the age of 14 living at home. When the children grow up and leave, the rate of depression decreases. This is contrary to the theory that depression results from the empty-nest syndrome. It appears that being responsible for children is a source of stress that contributes to depression (Peden, Rayens, Hall, & Grant, 2005; Peden, Rayens, Hall, & Grant, 2004).

Another sociocultural factor that may contribute to depression is the occurrence of *stressful life events*. Some events cause expansion of the family system: marriage, births, adoptions, and other people moving into the home. Other events cause a reduction of the family system: children leaving, marital separations, divorce, and death. Some life events involve a threat, as in job problems, difficulties with the police, and illness. Others can be emotionally exhausting, such as holidays, changing residences, and arguing with family and friends. Many people who experience major stressful events do not become depressed. However, for those who are vulnerable to depression, stressors may play a significant role in the exacerbation and course of the disorder.

A number of factors influence the degree of stress that accompanies significant life events. Figure 13.4 ■ illustrates the relationship between life events and depression. The presence of a social support network can decrease the impact an event may have on a person. People who have developed adaptive coping patterns such as problem solving, direct communication, and use of resources are more likely to maintain their normal mood. Those who feel out of control, are unable to problem solve, and ignore available resources are more apt to feel depressed. Thus, an individual's perception and interpretation of significant events may contribute to depression.

Childhood sexual abuse is a significant risk factor for depression, both during childhood, and as an adult. Although the depressive episodes do not seem to be more severe, the onset is often earlier and the survivors are more likely to self-mutilate and attempt suicide (Gladstone et al., 2004). See chapter 23 ∞ for more detailed information on childhood sexual abuse.

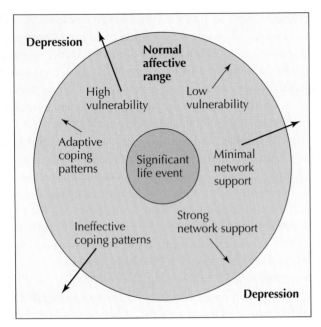

Figure 13.4 ■ The relationship between life events and depression.

Gender-Bias Theory

In the definition of mental health there has, in the past, been a double standard for women and men. A healthy woman has been described as acquiescent, subdued, dependent, and emotionally expressive. A healthy man, on the other hand, has been described as logical, rational, independent, aggressive, and unemotional. These stereotypes have had unfortunate consequences for both women and men. There is, however, movement toward an androgynous definition of mental health. This perspective stresses positive human qualities such as assertiveness, self-reliance, sensitivity to others, intimacy, and open communication—qualities that legitimately belong in the repertoire of both women and men.

Throughout the world, *women* experience more depression than do men. Certainly, there are cross-cultural similarities in the way women are socialized and in the inferior status that they experience in many societies. Psychosocial stressors, including multiple work and family responsibilities, poverty, sexual and physical abuse, gender discrimination, lack of social supports, and traumatic life experiences, may contribute to women's increased vulnerability to depression. In the United States and Canada, African American women are at higher risk for depression than Euro-American women are. Research suggests that additional risk factors include minority status, socioeconomic stress, and multiple roles (Schreiber, Stern, & Wilson, 2000).

Gender socialization differences may be a factor in the higher rate of depression in women. It starts early, when many girls are encouraged to play with dolls and help take care of other children in the family. Girls are taught to be "nice," nonargumentative, and docile. They become more concerned than boys about fitting in and backing down in the face of conflict. Gradually, they begin to question the worth of their abilities and opinions, which decreases self-esteem. Boys are socialized to be individualistic, to speak up, to raise their hands more in class. Gradually they begin to see themselves as autonomous individuals with good self-esteem (Brommelhoff, Conway, Merikangas, & Levy, 2004).

Rigid expectations about gender roles continue to linger and contribute to higher rates of depression among women. Women who are full-time homemakers may develop no identity other than that of wife and mother. The tremendous duties of managing a household are often invisible to others and lack prestige. Positive feedback or positive reinforcement such as compliments, a paycheck, and retirement benefits are uncommon. And the position is continuous, 24 hours a day. Since one lives in the workplace, there is no stimulation from a change in the environment. Indeed, being a full-time homemaker is one of the most isolating professions in society today.

Women who are employed outside the home, in both professional and blue-collar positions, are less depressed than those who remain at home. This is true even for women who must assume the responsibility for two full-time jobs with minimal or no support from other family members. Employed women must often accept lower pay, inferior jobs, and fewer opportunities for career advancement. The legal system has been slow to redress employment discrimination, which increases women's frustration, anger, and distress. Thoughts of the future focus on the helplessness of their situations and contribute to depression.

Gender bias theory can also be applied to the situation in which some older adults find themselves. In a society that places a premium on youth, older people feel useless, unimportant, incapable, and at times even repulsive. Role changes and losses may threaten their self-esteem. With aging, physiological changes may lead to a self-perception of being unfit, which then extends to further thoughts of being ineffectual and inferior. All these changes may contribute to despair about one's entire life and a sense of hopelessness about the limited future. Considering these effects, it is not surprising to find a higher rate of depression among older people. See Table 13.2 ■ for an overview of the etiologies of mood disorders, with specific relevance to women and older adults.

Psychopharmacological Interventions

Antidepressant medications are often prescribed for clients with mood disorders. Because depressions are heterogeneous in terms of which neurotransmitters are depleted, different people respond differently to various antidepressants. At times, a period of trial and error is necessary to determine which medication is the most effective. Approximately 30%

TABLE 13.2	Causative Theories of Mood Disorders	
Theory	**Main Points**	**Relevance to Women and Older Adults**
Genetic	Increased sensitivity to chemical changes related to stress	
Neurobiologic	Impaired neurotransmission; limbic dysfunction	Higher levels of MAO in CNS in women and older people
Biologic rhythms	Internal desynchronization of circadian rhythms	
Sunlight	Decreased exposure to sunlight increases production of melatonin	Older people do not go outside as much during the winter months
Intrapersonal	Loss of person, object, self-esteem; hostility turned against the self; goals unachieved	Women are more dependent on others for self-esteem; older people suffer multiple losses
Learning	Lack of control over experiences; learned helplessness; failure to adapt	Expectation of women's dependency reinforces helplessness; older people have increased stress with decreased resources, which contributes to loss of control
Cognitive	Negative view of self, the present, and the future; focus on negative messages; cognitive errors	
Feminist	Internalization of cultural norms of behavior; rigid gender-role and age expectations	Women's identity may be limited to homemaker role; employment positions less prestigious; may hold two full-time jobs. Older people suffer from the cultural value on youth; many role changes and losses

of clients do not respond to their antidepressant after a trial of 4 to 6 weeks. At that point, the primary care provider may try a different antidepressant or augment with other medications such as antipsychotics or mood stabilizers. Maintenance continues until clients are free of symptoms for 4 months to 1 year, then the drugs are slowly discontinued. See chapter 10 ∞ for a detailed discussion of these medications (Quitkin et al., 2005; Trivedi et al., 2006).

People with bipolar disorder who are in the depressive phase and prescribed *only* an antidepressant are at high risk for switching to a manic episode. For that reason, mood stabilizers are always prescribed at the same time (Brown, 2004).

To date, no psychotropic medication has been approved by the FDA for use during *pregnancy*. Tricyclic antidepressants and SSRIs have not generally been associated with a high risk of major birth defects. On the other hand, abrupt discontinuation of maintenance medications including antipsychotics, antidepressants, and mood stabilizers has been associated with a high, early relapse risk. The practice of abrupt discontinuation of these medications to minimize potential birth defects can place a woman and her fetus at risk due to impulsive or self-injurious behavior, substance abuse, or inattention to prenatal care. Untreated mood disorders during pregnancy have been associated with premature delivery, low birth weight, and lower Apgar ratings of the infant. Lamotrigine (Lamictal) appears to be safer than the other anticonvulsants. Lithium doses should be decreased at the onset of labor to avoid maternal toxicity at delivery. Divalproex

(Depakote) should be switched to another mood stabilizer before conception as there is a higher than average risk for neural tube defects. Carbamazepine (Tegretol) should be used during pregnancy only if there are no other options, as this medication is associated with craniofacial defects and developmental delay (Yonkers et al., 2004).

Women who are *breast-feeding* and need antidepressant medication can usually take the SSRIs and anticonvulsants safely, although the infant should be monitored periodically. Taking medication immediately after breast-feeding minimizes the amount present in milk and maximizes clearance before the next feeding. Dosage should be as low as possible while still being clinically effective (Gjerdingen, 2003; Yonkers et al., 2004).

Women with *postpartum depression* have a risk of recurrence of 25% with future pregnancies. It is suggested that at-risk women be treated with antidepressants after birth for as long as 26 weeks.

Medication is considered for *children* and *adolescents* in the following situations:

- Severe symptoms that prevent effective psychotherapy
- Psychosis
- Chronic or recurrent episodes

Antidepressants now come with Food and Drug Administration (FDA) warning labels that describe a link between the drugs and increased suicidal thought and behavior in children and youth especially during the first several months of administration. In contrast, many mental health professionals are worried that not medicating seriously ill children can also lead to an increase in suicidal behavior. In addition, the consequences of not treating with medications may, in itself, be detrimental to neurodevelopment in children with mood disorders (Pruett & Luby, 2004).

The mood stabilizers lamotrigine (Lamictal) and gabapentin (Neurontin) should never be used in clients younger than 16 due to the risk of developing Stevens-Johnson syndrome (see chapter 10 ∞).

The clinical response to antidepressant medications in *older depressed clients* is often delayed. The average time to easing of symptoms is 12 to 13 weeks. Studies show that while only 30% of older adults responded by week 6 of treatment, the number jumped to 55% at week 12. This suggests that longer treatment periods may be important to evaluate the effectiveness in older adults (Bondareff et al., 2000).

Multidisciplinary Interventions

Electroconvulsive therapy (ECT) may be useful for a variety of clients. ECT is a safer alternative for highly suicidal clients, those who suffer from psychotic depression, and those who are medically deteriorated. In addition, it is a safe alternative for children and adolescents. ECT is safe in all trimesters of pregnancy and may be less harmful to the fetus than psychotropic medications. Clients who do not respond to medications or cannot tolerate the side effects often respond positively to ECT. Because of concurrent medication conditions, poor tolerance of the side effects of psychotropic medications, and marked disability with depression, ECT is often the treatment of choice in older clients (Valdivia & Rossy, 2004). See chapter 9 ∞ for more detailed information on ECT.

Another medical treatment for depression is *sleep deprivation*. Sleep deprivation is the only known intervention in depression that has proven benefits within 24 hours. It is beneficial for individuals ranging in age from adolescence through late life. It is believed that DA and 5-HT activity is altered in response to sleep deprivation. The deprivation may be total, for 36 hours, or partial, with the person being awakened after 1:30 A.M. and kept awake until the next evening. During this time, clients may be alone, in a group, or participating in activities. Some improve steadily after only one night of sleep deprivation. Sleep deprivation is inappropriate for people with rapid cycling bipolar disorder. For reasons that are unknown, these individuals have very delicate "internal clock" mechanisms, and disruption of these mechanisms by losing even a single night's sleep often results in a manic episode

Phototherapy is often the treatment of choice for clients of any age who are experiencing SAD. Clients are exposed to very bright full-spectrum fluorescent lamps for 30 minutes a day. Clinical improvement is typically seen within 3 to 5 days.

Phototherapy may be used prophylactically with clients susceptible to SAD. It is thought that the bright light suppresses the production of melatonin and normalizes the disturbance in circadian rhythms. See chapter 9 ∞ for more information on phototherapy.

When one family member suffers from a mood disorder, there is frequently a detrimental effect on all family members. Families need information and support during this time, and *family therapy* is often very beneficial. Roles and relationships must be redefined during acute episodes and clients and families may need help with this process. If family interactions are dysfunctional, therapists may be able to assist in the development of healthier and more adaptive coping behaviors. Most family members want to be involved in treatment and believe that it is difficult to support the person with a mood disorder if they are excluded from the therapeutic process. Chapter 2 ∞ covers family issues, and chapter 9 ∞ covers family therapy in more detail.

Alternative Therapies

Depression, fatigue, insomnia, and anxiety are among the most commonly reported reasons for the use of alternative therapies in community surveys. The following are some alternative therapies used for mood disorders.

Transcranial Magnetic Stimulation

Repetitive transcranial magnetic stimulation (rTMS) is the use of a magnetic field that passes through the skull, which causes cells in the cerebral cortex to fire. rTMS in depression is the most-studied clinical application in psychiatry. The target area is the left prefrontal cortex, which is the brain area thought to be disrupted in depression. The opposite lobe, the right prefrontal cortex, has therapeutic effects in manic episodes. rTMS has a rapid onset of action of 1 to 2 weeks, which is faster than most psychotropic medications. ECT and rTMS have the same effectiveness in depression without psychosis, while depression with psychosis is best treated with ECT. There are several ongoing studies using oscillating magnetic fields similar to those used in functional magnetic resonance imaging (fMRI) especially with people having bipolar disorder See chapter 9 ∞ for more detailed information on rTMS (Brown, 2004; Rohan et al., 2004).

Vagus Nerve Stimulation

Vagus nerve stimulation (VNS) has been used successfully with hard-to-treat seizure disorders and has FDA approval for this use. Noticing an improvement in subjects' moods, researchers are now studying VNS for people suffering from treatment resistant depression. A cookie-size generator is surgically implanted in the chest under the skin that conveys electrical impulses via a connecting wire to the vagus nerve.

The nerve is a leading provider of information from the heart and other organs to the brain; it also affects areas of the brain involved with mood. It provides continuous therapy for 8 to 12 years, which is the life of the implant's battery. VNS is most effective in people who have low to moderate, but not severe, resistance to antidepressants (Brown, 2004).

Exercise

There have been numerous studies on the effect of exercise on depression. Short periods of vigorous aerobic exercise or longer periods of nonaerobic exercise, for at least several weeks, is most helpful in mild to moderate depression. Exercise raises levels of endorphins, which enhance one's feelings of well-being. Exercise also increases levels of DA, 5-HT, and NE, which are related to feelings of reward, motivation, and attention.

Yoga has been found to improve wellness and prevent disorders such as depression. The gentle nature of the exercises allows its use in almost any condition. People who practice yoga on a regular basis report improved life satisfaction, alertness, enthusiasm, and mental and physical energy, all of which are the opposite of the symptoms of depression (Kabat-Zinn, 2003).

St. John's Wort

St. John's wort (hypericum perforatum) has been the most widely publicized alternative treatment for *mild to moderate depression*. The side effects of St. John's wort in higher doses are similar to that of SSRIs. The dosage is 300 to 600 mg/day of 0.3% hypericin, the active component in St. John's wort. It should *not* be combined with prescription antidepressants. It may also interfere with the action of anticonvulsants. There is insufficient data to recommend this herb for children. St. John's wort has been found to reduce the effectiveness of birth control pills, HIV treatment medications, and the asthma medication theophylline (Basch & Ulbricht, 2005).

SAMe

A nutritional supplement called SAMe (pronounced "sammy") has been used by more than 1 million people in Europe, primarily for depression and arthritis. SAMe (S-adenosylmethionine), a compound made by every cell in the body, helps produce DA, 5-HT, and NE. Numerous trials have found SAMe to be effective in depression, postpartum depression, and postmenopausal depression. It may, however, worsen bipolar depression. Its rapid onset (10 to 12 days), low side effects (no weight gain or sexual dysfunction), and ability to boost antioxidants give it many advantages in the treatment of depression. The dose is 800 to 1,600 mg/day and is best taken 30 minutes before meals. It has been successfully used as augmentation of all categories of antidepressants without adverse effects and there is no evidence that it interacts with other medications. Side effects are generally mild and temporary such as headaches, loose bowels, anxiety, and insomnia. Like tricyclic antidepressants, SAMe should be used with caution in people who have a history of cardiac arrhythmia. Infants normally have a three to four times naturally higher level of SAMe than do adults. Given this knowledge, the amount of SAMe passing to infants through breast milk may be inconsequential (Goren, Stoll, Damico, Sarmiento, & Cohen, 2004).

Vitamin B

Vitamin B is necessary for the production of DA, 5-HT, and NE as well as for the natural synthesis of SAMe. One study found that individuals with a significant vitamin B deficiency were at twice the risk of depression than those who had normal levels. Depression itself could cause low levels through decreased appetite and resulting decreased food intake. In addition, many of the tricyclic antidepressants deplete the body of vitamin B (Hvas, Juul, Bech, & Nexo, 2004).

Tyrosine

Tyrosine, an amino acid, is the precursor for DA and NE and, as such, acts as a mood elevator. Supplemental tyrosine has been used in depression, stress reduction, anxiety, and chronic fatigue. People taking MAO inhibitors should not take any supplements containing tyrosine, as it may lead to a hypertensive crisis. Tyrosine combined with vitamin B_6 and vitamin C will provide better absorption.

Melatonin

Insomnia is a frequent complaint among people suffering from depression. Melatonin, a hormone secreted by the pineal gland, plays a critical role in the regulation of the day–night cycle. Studies have shown that melatonin is effective in inducing sleep and has no notable side effects. Slow-release melatonin combined with standard antidepressant treatment often improves the sleep pattern in depressed individuals.

DHEA

Dehydroepiandrosterone (DHEA) is a corticosteroid produced primarily in the adrenal glands. In addition to serving as a precursor to testosterone and estrogen, DHEA may be involved in regulating mood and one's sense of well-being. The method of action is unclear but it may stimulate GABA receptors or increase 5-HT levels. It has been used alone or as an adjunct to antidepressants. Since there is little known about long-term risks, it is probably best used under medical supervision. The usual dose is up to 90 mg/day (Basch & Ulbricht, 2005).

Omega-3 Fatty Acids

A number of studies have been done on the effects of omega-3 fatty acids from concentrated fish oils on mood disorders. Omega-3 fatty acids are thought to act on cells similar to lithium, block calcium channels as do the other mood stabilizers, and help regulate 5-HT. It appears to be antidepressant, antimanic, and a mood stabilizer. Research shows significantly low levels of omega-3 fatty acids in depression and the lower the levels, the more severe the depression. The recommended dose is 5 grams per day, which is usually 7 or 8 capsules. The maximum dose is 15 grams daily. Taking the capsules at night and with orange juice cuts down on the fishy aftertaste (Basch & Ulbricht, 2005).

Aromatherapy

Olfactory receptors are the only sensory pathways that open directly to the brain. Nerve cells relay this information directly to the limbic system, influencing emotions and behavior. Inhaling essential oils through the use of a diffuser or using essential oils in massage may be beneficial in relieving depressive symptoms. The following oils are the most helpful: bergamot, geranium, jasmine, lemon balm, rose, and ylang-ylang.

Acupuncture

Acupuncture is helpful in relieving feelings of depression and anxiety, most likely related to the rise in endorphin levels as a result of the treatment. Adding electrostimulation to acupuncture needles usually increases the effectiveness of the treatment. After only a single session, many people report a sense of well-being. Two rigorous studies found acupuncture to be as effective as tricyclic antidepressants. It is unclear how helpful acupuncture is for bipolar disorder. Client response appears to be quite variable at the present time (Larzelere & Wiseman, 2002).

Animal-Assisted Therapy

Companionship with animals is associated with people experiencing less depression and loneliness. Animals provide meaningful and substantial comfort for many individuals. Studies show elderly women (who are at higher risk for depression) who live alone to be in better emotional health if they lived with an animal. They were less lonely, more optimistic, and more interested in the future than those women who lived alone without a pet (Hart, 2000).

Music Therapy

Music is often used in healing from the ancient sounds of the drum, rattle, bone flute, and other primitive instruments to the current use of music as a prescription for health. In a study of 54 people who were clinically depressed and on medication, there was meaningful clinical improvement following 2 weeks of music therapy (Hsu & Lai, 2004).

Nursing Process

A CLIENT WITH MOOD DISORDER

ASSESSMENT

Assessing clients with mood disorders is often done in segments of 15 to 20 minutes each. Those who are depressed do not have the energy to talk for longer periods, and those who are in a manic phase are unable to concentrate and sit still for longer periods. The nurse must exercise a great deal of patience when assessing these clients. Clients who are depressed may take a long time to answer questions, and the nurse may need to repeat them. If family members are present, discourage them from answering questions for the client who is responding slowly. Clients in a manic phase with flight of ideas must frequently be refocused on the topic at hand. Their elevated mood may interfere with their ability to give accurate information. The nurse may wish to use the Beck Depression Inventory (Table 13.3 ■). This is a self-rating scale that measures levels of depression.

People with mood disorders display a variety of characteristics involving changes in behavior, affect, cognition, and physiology. Somewhat similar changes occur for people ex-periencing grief. Table 13.4 ■ differentiates between depression and grief during the assessment process.

Assessment: Behavior

One of the changes in people with mood disorders is their level of *desire to participate in activities*. As people participate less, they begin to regard themselves as incompetent and inadequate. Severe depression results in an inability to do anything, even the simplest activities of daily living (ADLs). If the nurse suggests that clients attempt ADLs, they will often respond with something like, "It's pointless to even try because I can't do it."

In the early stages of an elevated mood (hypomania), people with bipolar disorder increase their work productivity. This leads to positive feedback from employers and family members, which contributes to increased self-esteem around the issues of competency and power. When they reach the manic end of the continuum, however, their productivity decreases because of a short attention span. People in a manic phase are interested in every available activity and are supremely confident of being able to accomplish them all perfectly. *Poor judgment* can result in reckless driving, spending sprees, and foolish business investments. Many clients have poor impulse control and have episodes of spending enormous amounts of money.

TABLE 13.3	Beck Depression Inventory

The Beck Depression Inventory is a self-rating scale that measures depression. The patient can complete the questionnaire in about 10 minutes. The total score provides an estimate of the degree of severity of the depressed mood. Add the raw scores. The mean scores can be interpreted as follows.

Total Score	Levels of Depression
1–10	Normal ups and downs
11–16	Mild mood disturbance
17–20	Borderline clinical depression
21–30	Moderate depression
31–40	Severe depression
Over 40	Extreme depression

(A persistent score of 17 or above indicates professional treatment might be necessary)

1. 0 I do not feel sad.
   1 I feel sad.
   2 I am sad all the time and I can't snap out of it.
   3 I am so sad or unhappy that I can't stand it.

2. 0 I am not particularly discouraged about the future.
   1 I feel discouraged about the future.
   2 I feel I have nothing to look forward to.
   3 I feel that the future is hopeless and that things cannot improve.

3. 0 I do not feel like a failure.
   1 I feel I have failed more than the average person.
   2 As I look back on my life, all I can see is a lot of failures.
   3 I feel I am a complete failure as a person.

4. 0 I get as much satisfaction out of things as I used to.
   1 I don't enjoy things the way I used to.
   2 I don't get real satisfaction out of anything anymore.
   3 I am dissatisfied or bored with everything.

5. 0 I don't feel particularly guilty.
   1 I feel guilty a good part of the time.
   2 I feel quite guilty most of the time.
   3 I feel guilty all of the time.

6. 0 I don't feel I am being punished.
   1 I feel I may be punished.
   2 I expect to be punished.
   3 I feel I am being punished.

7. 0 I don't feel disappointed in myself.
   1 I am disappointed in myself.
   2 I am disgusted with myself.
   3 I hate myself.

8. 0 I don't feel I am worse than anybody else.
   1 I am critical of myself for any weaknesses or mistakes.
   2 I blame myself all the time for my faults.
   3 I blame myself for everything bad that happens.

9. 0 I don't have any thoughts of killing myself.
   1 I have thoughts of killing myself, but I would not carry them out.
   2 I would like to kill myself.
   3 I would kill myself if I had the chance.

10. 0 I don't cry any more than usual.
    1 I cry more now than usual.
    2 I cry all the time now.
    3 I used to be able to cry, but now I can't even though I want to.

continued

TABLE 13.3	Beck Depression Inventory *continued*

11. 0   I am no more irritated by things than I ever am.
   1   I am slightly more irritated now than usual.
   2   I am quite annoyed or irritated a good deal of the time.
   3   I feel irritated all the time now.

12. 0   I have not lost interest in other people.
   1   I am less interested in other people than I used to be.
   2   I have lost most of any interest in other people.
   3   I have lost all of my interest in other people.

13. 0   I make decisions about as well as I ever could.
   1   I put off making decisions more than I used to.
   2   I have greater difficulty in making decisions than before.
   3   I can't make decisions at all anymore.

14. 0   I don't feel that I look any worse than I used to.
   1   I am worried that I am looking old or unattractive.
   2   I feel that there are permanent changes in my appearance that make me look unattractive.
   3   I believe that I look ugly.

15. 0   I can work about as well as before.
   1   I take an extra effort to get started doing something.
   2   I have to push myself very hard to do anything.
   3   I can't do any work at all.

16. 0   I can sleep as well as usual.
   1   I don't sleep as well as I used to.
   2   I wake up 1–2 hours earlier than I used to and cannot get back to sleep.
   3   I wake up several hours earlier than I used to and cannot get back to sleep.

17. 0   I don't get more tired than usual.
   1   I get tired more easily than I used to.
   2   I get tired from doing almost anything.
   3   I am too tired to do anything.

18. 0   My appetite is no worse than usual.
   1   My appetite is not as good as it used to be.
   2   My appetite is much worse now.
   3   I have no appetite at all anymore.

19. 0   I haven't lost much weight, if any, lately.
   1   I have lost more than 5 pounds.
   2   I have lost more than 10 pounds.
   3   I have lost more than 15 pounds.

20. 0   I am no more worried about my health than usual.
   1   I am worried about physical problems such as aches and pains, or upset stomach, or constipation.
   2   I am very worried about physical problems and it's hard to think of much else.
   3   I am so worried about my physical problems that I cannot think about anything else.

21. 0   I have not noticed any recent change in my interest in sex.
   1   I am less interested in sex than I used to be.
   2   I am much less interested in sex now.
   3   I have lost interest in sex completely.

SOURCE: Reprinted with permission from Beck, A. T., Ward, C. H., Mendelson, M., Mock, J., & Erbaugh, J. (1961). Inventory for measuring depression. *Archives of General Psychiatry, 4,* 561–571.

TABLE 13.4	Differences Between Depression and Grief	
Trait	**Depression**	**Grief**
Trigger	Specific trigger not necessary	Trigger usually loss or multiple losses
Active/passive	Passive behavior tends to keep them "stuck" in sadness	Actively feel their emotional pain and emptiness
Emotions	Generalized feeling of helplessness, hopelessness	Experience a range of emotions that are usually intense
Ability to laugh	Likely to be humorless and incapable of being happy or even temporarily cheered up; likely to resist support	Sometimes will be able to laugh and enjoy humor; more likely to accept support
Activities	Lack of interest in previously enjoyed activities	Can be persuaded to participate in activities, especially as they begin to heal
Self-esteem	Low self-esteem, low self-confidence; feels like a failure	Self-esteem usually remains intact; does not feel like a failure unless it relates directly to the loss
Feeling of failure	May dwell on past failures; catastrophize	Any self-blame or guilt relates directly to the loss; feelings resolve as they progress toward healing.

Josh:

"When I was off my meds I couldn't function at work. I was delusional, I was argumentative, I was hysterically laughing. There's a point, though, when you get off the meds where you're hyper and you're high and you're manic and you can do anything, or at least you think you can. Sometimes I'll be really high and manic and I'll get so much done. I'll clean, I'll cook, I'll organize my papers. I'm up to 2:00 or 3:00 in the morning organizing my papers and making labels for things. But then the reverse happens and I come down. For every high there's a low. You're really low—can't get out of bed, don't shower, don't shave. I just feel terrible about the world."

Interaction with others is altered in people with a mood disorder. In the beginning of a depressive episode, people may avoid social activities that are not highly interesting and stimulating. As the depression deepens, the tendency is to withdraw from most social interactions because they require too much effort. Depressed people say they feel lonely but also say they feel incapable of halting the process of withdrawal and isolation. Family and friends often respond with criticism and anger, further contributing to isolation. In depression, people may experience more conflict than usual. Difficulty communicating often leads to disputes and hostility within the family.

During manic episodes, people are unusually talkative and gregarious. Unable to control the impulse to interact with everyone in the environment, they are oblivious to the social convention of not interrupting a private discussion. They may share intimate details of their lives with anyone who will listen. When their mood returns to its normal range, they are often embarrassed about what they have said to others.

A change in *affiliation needs* also occurs in the mood disorders. During a depressive episode, normally self-sufficient people experience a significant increase in dependency. If others reject their demands, they view this as validation of being unlovable. If, on the other hand, intense assistance is given to them, their dependency needs are reinforced, which contributes to a lack of self-confidence. In severe depression, they want total care and attention.

Those experiencing a shift in mood toward elation show a decreased need for affiliation. They view themselves as independent and completely self-sufficient. They also believe themselves to be indispensable to others.

Assessment: Affect

During depression, the mood begins with an intermittent sense of sadness. It begins with statements such as "I feel down in the dumps." As depression deepens, people become more gloomy and dejected and describe their lives as having no joy. In severe levels of depression, their misery is constant with no hope for improvement.

Ghada describes her changes in this way: "I worry about what's going to happen to me. I mean, I didn't have this numbness a month ago. I could be lying here dying and not even know it. I just don't have any feeling anymore."

On the manic end of the continuum, there is an *unstable mood* state. Beginning with cheerfulness, it escalates toward euphoria. The instability of mood is observed when, with minimal environmental stimulus, the person suddenly becomes irritable, argumentative, openly hostile, and even combative. As the stimulus is withdrawn, however, the person's mood rapidly returns to euphoric.

MediaLink   Critical Thinking, A Manic Episode

Guilt is another common affective experience on which depressed people focus. For some, the source of guilt is vague; for others, it is specific. Depressed people ruminate over incidents they feel guilty about, and it is difficult to change their focus of attention.

Mark says: "I yelled at my mom the night before she died. Now I can't say I'm sorry. If I killed myself, I would be able to tell her I'm sorry." This theme is continually repeated throughout the day.

During a manic episode, people are unable to experience any sense of guilt. Confronted with behavior that has hurt another person, they respond with indifference, laughter, or anger. The ability to experience guilt returns when their affect returns to a normal level.

Crying spells may occur during a depressive state. In mild and moderate depressions, people have an increased tendency to cry in situations that would not normally provoke tears. In a severe depression, people may not even have the energy to cry. During the manic state, sudden and unpredictable crying spells may occur. These may last only 20 to 30 seconds before a rapid return to a euphoric mood.

People's feelings of *gratification* are altered in mood disorders and their participation in normally pleasurable activities decreases. In severe depression, people become **anhedonic**, that is, incapable of experiencing pleasure.

People who are manic, on the other hand, try to participate in every available pleasurable activity. There is a constant need for fun, excitement, and stimulation. They become involved in activities without considering any possible negative outcomes. For instance, because of their certainty that every investment will be a wonderful success, they are open to abuse in business ventures. They often go on buying sprees without concern for the consequences of incurring great debt.

Accompanying a depressive state is a loss of *emotional attachment*. It begins with decreased affection for family members and friends, along with dissatisfaction with these relationships. As the depression deepens they may become indifferent to their loved ones.

People in the manic state form intense emotional attachments very rapidly. They feel affectionate toward everyone in the environment and may "fall in love" in a matter of minutes and with a number of people. During a manic state, a person may think nothing of having simultaneous sexual relationships. Accompanying this is a preoccupation with sex, which others may find offensive.

Juanita, a nurse, is doing a nursing history admission on Sid, a 73-year-old man with bipolar disorder, manic phase. He is sexually preoccupied throughout the interview. When asked what his major strengths are, he replies, "Making love." When asked how he handles stress at home, the response is, "Making it with as many girls as I can."

Assessment: Perception

Psychotic features, including delusions and hallucinations, are common in mood disorders. About 75% of people with mania and 14% of people with MDD have psychosis. Symptoms typically reflect the extreme mood state at the time (i.e., grandiosity during mania and worthlessness during depression). Less than 40% of these individuals attain functional recovery as measured by independent living, occupational stability, and interpersonal relations (Cassano et al., 2004).

Sherry describes her hallucinations this way: "I'm hearing voices telling me to kill myself. I hear them all the time. I feel like I'm going crazy. The voices are getting clearer. They tell me to kill myself and I'll be at peace. They say, 'Kill yourself and your problems will be solved'."

Assessment: Cognition

A person's thoughts about personal worth and value contribute to an overall sense of *self-esteem*. In mild depression, people overreact to mistakes they may make and reproach themselves for minor errors. As the depression worsens, however, people focus much of their attention on past, present, and future failures. A good deal of their thinking is self-deprecatory and self-

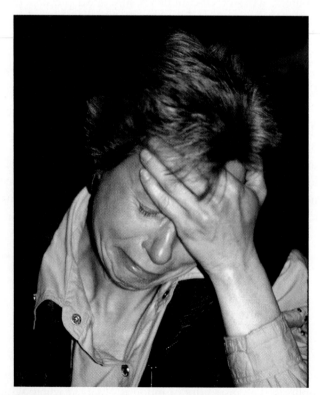

PHOTO 13.1 ■ The quality of a depressed mood is often different from the sadness that might arise from an event such as the loss of a loved one. Some depressed people say that they feel like they are drowning or suffocating.

SOURCE: Vincent DeWitt/Stock Boston. Used with permission.

accusatory. This magnification of failures is called **catastrophizing**. These negative thoughts then make clients feel more helpless, powerless, and depressed.

People on the manic end of the continuum have an exaggerated self-concept. They have *grandiose beliefs* about their physical and intellectual talents. In any undertaking, there is a supreme sense of self-confidence.

Josh:

❝ When I stopped taking my meds, I had racing thoughts, I talked very quickly and had grandiose ideas. I wanted to win the Nobel Prize and I wanted to cure cancer. I wanted to win the Boston Marathon. I weighed 205 pounds. I wanted to win the Boston Marathon? Sure, Josh, whatever you say. ❞

People's *expectations* are altered during mood disorders. In depression they exaggerate the importance of negative information and minimize positive information resulting in the cognitive distortion of selective abstraction. In severe depression, the present and future are viewed as completely *hopeless*. Even simple goals are viewed as unachievable. They see no reason to make an effort, since life is not worth living and they might as well be dead. The inability to cope is evidence of an *external locus of control*. In contrast, people in a manic state have inordinate expectations of themselves, others, and the future. They feel all powerful and in total control.

Dee: "I don't want to lose my husband. He's my soul mate."
Nurse: "Are you afraid he will leave you?"
Dee: "God, yes. Here I am in the loony bin. He's probably out having an affair. No, he's not. That's just me making things up. But don't you think he's going to leave me?"
Nurse: "Has he said anything about leaving you?"
Dee: "No, he's never said that. But he does things that make me think he'll leave."
Nurse: "Could you give me an example of the things he does?"
Dee: "Well, for one, he doesn't ever listen to me. I mean, really listen to me. He pretends to listen, but he's not."

People's *decision-making* ability deteriorates in mood disorders. In mild depression, people often seek advice and affirmation from others before making even simple decisions. As the depression deepens, there is a decreased ability to concentrate on a subject long enough to formulate a decision. A person might stand in front of the closet for 20 minutes, trying to decide what clothes to wear. Planning meals, shopping, or concentrating on homework may be very difficult. In severe depression, people are incapable of making decisions.

During manic episodes, people also have difficulty making decisions. Easily distracted by stimuli in the environment, they cannot concentrate long enough to go through the problem-solving process. Their short attention span causes them to make impulsive decisions.

Flow of thought is disrupted in people with mood disorders. In depression, there may be slowed speech, an inability to think of specific words, or an inability to complete sentences, referred to as *poverty of speech*. In severe depression, it may take the person several minutes to respond to a question and the person may even be mute.

During manic episodes, *flight of ideas* is often present. The flow of thought is fragmented by any external stimuli. Thoughts come so quickly that there is not enough time to completely express one idea before another is stimulated. As the nurse listens, the nurse may be able to determine a theme or the underlying emotions.

Geoff describes the police bringing him to the hospital in this way: "My neighbor and I rigged this up. We called about six police guys that we knew and an ambulance and set it up. We wanted to teach the kids about law and order. Everything is closed on holidays. No doctors, no pharmacies, no police. It's hard to get hold of anyone. No pharmacies are open. If you need something, you're in trouble. I don't like the medical profession, especially doctors. No, especially psychiatrists. They don't do anything. They give you medicine. You can fix yourself up. I know everything there is to know about medicine in the pharmacy. I don't need a doctor to tell me."

Yuki: "I'm a 55-year-old woman and my mother just needs to understand that. Not that I would do anything. Honor thy mother and father and all that. My dad was artsy but not my mom. She doesn't believe me but my demons are real."
Nurse: "Tell me more about those demons."
Yuki: "It's a long story about life and work and the world is such a terrible place. You can't even turn on the TV anymore. My son is named Sam. He's a night owl. He's a good boy. He just needs to find himself. That's how it is sometimes. Looking and finding. I found this t-shirt at K-Mart."

Thoughts about *body image* are also distorted in those clients with mood disorders. In a mild or moderate depression, distortion begins as an obsessional concern over physical appearance, with a focus on the disliked body parts. As the depression worsens, people believe they are unattractive and may actually erroneously perceive their body as being disfigured or deformed.

People in a manic state have exaggerated self-esteem, which may contribute to believing they look like well-known people or famous beauties. If others challenge this perception, they often respond with a great deal of anger.

Sue is 25 years old and comes in to the clinic complaining of racing thoughts, decreased concentration, inability to keep a job, not sleeping, and lots of energy. She tells an elaborate life story: She states she was a prostitute for 4–5 months but that she only did it for her boyfriend who was very controlling. She also states that she ran an escort service that she started as a teenager and that by the time she was 19 years old she had 3 million dollars, which she "blew."

Faulty perceptions of body image may escalate into *delusions*. Depressed people may experience *somatic delusions*, in which they believe themselves to be hopelessly ill or that part of the body has been infected or contaminated by outside agents. An example is the person who says, "I'm afraid I might have rabies because my friend spit in my throat. My sister has rabies because a wild rabid wolf pissed on her cocaine." Manic people may experience *delusions of grandeur* focusing on beliefs of being famous or *erotomanic delusions*, which are delusions of having personal relationships with prominent, well-known people. These delusions may include paranoid content.

John is sexually and religiously preoccupied. He often sings and shouts as he walks around the unit. He believes that he rose from the dead and that he came from heaven. He says that when he was in heaven he had sex with several people. He believes that he has special powers and can make any liquid into alcohol.

Loss of faith is a common experience during depressive episodes. People lose faith in their ability to ever again feel love for family members, in the possibility of their negative thoughts ever going away, and in their religion. Unable to find meaning in their illness, they feel a sense of injustice in life. This loss of faith contributes to an overwhelming sense of *spiritual distress*.

Assessment: Interpersonal Relationships

The impact of mood disorders on the *family* must not be underestimated. Many families report that for several of their extended family and friends, mental illness is still associated with moral weakness or failure. This results in being treated differently or stigmatized.

The family's frustration, confusion, and anger in response to the multiple changes in their loved ones are all understandable. Initially, family members may react with support and concern but in some families, when the depression does not improve, support changes to frustration and anger. A vicious cycle may be established. Increased conflict causes increased symptoms, further rejection, and deepening depression. Other families may become overly solicitous and assume total care of the depressed person. Total care may contribute to increased symptoms because the person feels helpless and indebted to the family.

Nearly every family who has a loved one with bipolar disorder perceives the illness as a moderate to severe *caregiver burden*. About 33% of people with bipolar I disorder are unable to live independently. During manic episodes, a person's family may be subjected to bizarre, hostile, and even destructive behavior. Family members often call the police to protect themselves and their property. Untreated bipolar disorder can devastate individual and family life and often leads to a downward spiral in interpersonal, economic, and occupational functioning (Hammen & Cohen, 2004).

After an acute illness episode, families often have problems in one or more of the following areas (Miklowitz, 2004):

- Disagreements over illness management such as medication compliance, sleep–wake routines, and/or substance abuse
- Establishing a routine for work, school, and social responsibilities
- Household management roles and financial responsibilities
- Interpersonal problems: parent/child—boundaries; couple—intimacy issues

There has been increasing awareness of the impact of *parental mood disorders* on children and adolescents. During an acute episode, youngsters must try to cope with parental behavior that is not easily understood. They may also experience repeated separations from the parent. Children of depressed parents experience greater social, education, behavioral, and vocational difficulties. Since both genetic and psychosocial influences are involved in the transmission of these disorders from parent to child, they are at higher risk for experiencing symptoms by the end of their adolescence.

Mood disorders are costly in terms of both direct medical costs and indirect costs, such as lost productivity caused by absenteeism and work impairment. The onset of mood disorders often occurs at what should be a productive time of life and the economic impact can be substantial. While some individuals are able to function well in high-level professions, others never work due to disability. The majority has difficulty sustaining jobs (Hammen & Cohen, 2004).

Josh:

"I began to really just be too bizarre for the world. People couldn't relate to me. I thought I could relate to them but they couldn't relate to me. I was too out there to have relationships with anybody. The only people who I could depend on were custodians of my life—my parents and an older brother who's a doctor. I just never fit in when I was sick. I couldn't find a niche...."

Mood disorders often disrupt a couple's *sex life*. Depressed people lose interest in sexual activity, both autoerotic and with their partner. The depressed person often decreases initiation of sexual activity but continues to give and receive pleasure in the usual pattern. With deepening depression, further change in sexual activity is common. Some people, needing comfort, seek out the partner more frequently. Others may change their patterns by increasing sexual behavior that takes less energy such as cuddling or oral sex. In severe depression, most people experience a complete *loss of sexual desire* and fulfillment. The person and the partner must understand that these changes are symptoms of the depression, not necessarily a reflection of the relationship.

During a manic state, there is an *exaggerated sexual desire,* which is often acted out with a variety of partners. People's ethical and moral restraints on sexual activity do not function during the elevated mood state. Seductive behavior, frequency of activity, and number of partners may all increase. Families are often angry and hurt, and this may be the particular behavior that forces treatment or hospitalization. At the height of manic episodes, a paradoxical decrease in sexual behavior may occur. Because they may be constantly trying to seduce everyone in the environment, there is no time for consummating any of the relationships. When mood levels return to normal, they often feel embarrassed and guilty about their behavior.

Assessment: Cultural Influences

Appropriate *expressions of mood* are largely culturally determined. For example, situations in which people are expected to experience sadness, anger, loneliness, frustration, joy, or happiness are defined by the culture. The culture also determines how people are to behave when experiencing a variety of feelings. For example, cultural expectations of grieving individuals may be self-control and a "stiff upper lip" or may be loud mourning and ripping of clothing. Extreme pleasure may be expressed with a nod and a smile or may be expressed with loud laughter and exuberant behavior.

The Western interpretation of feelings is that emotions are intrapersonal. In contrast, in Micronesia, emotions are considered to be not within a person but rather between people. In some Middle Eastern, African, Hispanic, and Chinese cultures, emotions are viewed and expressed in somatic (bodily) terms. The process by which psychological distress is experienced and communicated in the form of somatic symptoms is called **somatization**. Because these cultures are not subject to the mind–body dualism of Western thinking, psychological distress is viewed as arising from bodily imbalances (Chou, 2005).

Emotions of suffering and depression have dramatically *different meaning and forms* of expression in different cultures. Many Americans view suffering as unexpected or unacceptable and perceive depression as something to overcome through personal striving. Latin American cultures associate suffering with a deep sense of tragedy. Shi'ite Muslims view suffering within a religious context of martyrdom, while Buddhist cultures view suffering as a positive feature of life. Throughout the entire world, most cases of depression are experienced and expressed in bodily terms such as fatigue, headaches, heart distress, dizziness, and so on. It is only in Western cultures that depression is considered to be a mental disorder (Sethabouppha & Kane, 2005).

When nurses assess clients from cultures different from their own, it is important for nurses to understand that the expression of depression is culturally determined. Immigrants are at higher risk for depression as they cope with multiple stressors such as family at a long distance, un- or underemployment, discrimination, language problems, and a new environment. Immigrant children are at risk for depression as they are often expected to interpret the concerns of adult family members to outside authority figures, such as doctors, nurses, teachers, and government officials (Aroian & Norris, 2002; Heilemann, Coffey-Love, & Frutos, 2004).

African Americans and Latinos often look to family and their faith communities for help rather than seeking professional help. There is a strong fear of hospitalization and involuntary commitment, and both of those are more likely than for Euro-Americans. Children are less likely to receive outpatient treatment when compared to their Euro-American peers. Among the elderly, African Americans are less likely to receive treatment for depression (37%) compared to 24% of Hispanics, 22% of Euro-Americans, and 14% of Asians. African Americans and Latinos who experience mood disorders are often misdiagnosed as having schizophrenia. As a result of this misdiagnosis, they may receive antipsychotic medication and no antidepressants. Thus, appropriate treatment is delayed, resulting in poorer therapeutic response (Draucker, 2005; Strothers et al., 2005).

Assessment: Age-specific Characteristics

The incidence of depression in children is often underestimated. The cultural norm is that childhood is a carefree and happy time and that there is no reason for children to be depressed. The reality, however, is that at least 1% of *preschoolers,* 2% to 3% of *children,* and 6% to 8% of *adolescents* are depressed at any point in time. Furthermore, half of all adults with depression report onset before age 20. While the recovery rate from a single episode of major depression in young people is quite high, episodes are likely to recur (Dopheide, 2006).

In childhood, boys and girls appear to be at equal risk for depressive disorders; but during adolescence, girls are twice as likely as boys to develop depression. Children and adolescents who develop major depression are more likely to have a family history of the disorder than people with adult-onset depression. Between 20% and 40% of adolescents with major depression develop bipolar disorder within 5 years after the initial diagnosis. People with early-onset bipolar disorder (before the age of 21) are more likely to be male, have a more severe form of the disorder, and experience a more chronic course. The presence of substance abuse appears to lower the age at onset of bipolar disorder.

Depression is often manifested through negativism, acting-out behaviors, and/or unexplained physical complaints. Symptoms are often related to the developmental levels. See Box 13.1 for problem behaviors associated with depression at the various age levels. Depressive disorders can have far-reaching

BOX 13.1	Behaviors Associated With Depression

Infants

- When separated from parent, may have weepy and withdrawn behavior
- Frozen facial expression
- Weight loss
- Increased incidence of infections

1 to 3 Years

- Delays or regression in toileting, eating, sleeping, intellectual growth
- Increase in nightmares
- Loss of interest and pleasure in playing
- May appear sad or expressionless
- Apathetic or more clingy

3 to 5 Years

- Loss of interest in newly acquired skills
- Nightmares with themes of annihilation
- Decreased socialization
- Tantrums
- Nonspecific somatic complaints
- Enuresis, encopresis, anorexia, or binge eating may occur
- May also experience separation anxiety
- Frequent negative self-statements and thoughts or impulses of self-harm

6 to 12 Years

- Depressed mood, irritable, aggressive
- Academic difficulties, absence from school
- Social isolation
- Blames self for bad things
- Decreased concentration
- Eating and sleeping disturbances
- Severe self-criticism and guilt
- Suicidal ideation and plans

Adolescents

- Intense mood swings
- Academic difficulties
- Argumentative and/or assaultive
- Substance abuse
- Involvement with law enforcement
- Risk taking or antisocial behavior
- Hypersomnia
- Very low self-esteem

SOURCES: Adapted from: Luby, J. L., Mrakotky, C., Heffelfinger, A., Brown, K., Hesler, M., & Spitznagel, E. (2003). Modification of DSM-IV criteria for depressed preschool children. *American Journal of Psychiatry, 160*(6), 1169–1172; Luby, J. L., Mrakotsky, C., Heffelfinger, A., Brown, K., & Spitznagel, E. (2004). Characteristics of depressed preschoolers with and without anhedonia. *American Journal of Psychiatry, 161*(11), 1998–2004; and Reinherz, H. Z., Paradis, A. D., Giaconia, R. M., Stashwick, C. K., & Fitzmaurice, G. (2003). Childhood and adolescent predictors of major depression in the transition to adulthood. *American Journal of Psychiatry, 160*(12), 2141–2147.

effects on the functioning and adjustment of young people. Children and teens have school difficulties related to an inability to concentrate and their grades often worsen. Lack of energy and irritability may interfere with their participation in school and leisure activities, leading to disruption in peer relationships (Draucker, 2005).

Trevor, 12 years old, is referred to the clinic for treatment of depression. He states that he is irritable and doesn't enjoy anything. In 4th grade he received all As, in 5th all Bs, in 6th all Ds, and in his current year is getting all Fs. He says he is disappointed in himself. His classmates call him "fat and stupid" and tell him he should hang himself. He thinks about stabbing himself in the heart with a knife. Both his mother and brother are depressed and his mother has a history of suicide attempts.

The incidence of bipolar disorder in children and adolescents is probably underestimated when researchers use adult criteria. At least 1.2% of youth have bipolar I disorder, 0.1% to 0.6% have bipolar II disorder, and 0.3% have bipolar disorder not otherwise specified. In early-onset bipolar disorder, manic symptoms are similar to the externalizing symptoms associated with childhood disruptive disorders, especially attention deficit hyperactivity disorder and conduct disorder. (See chapter 17 ∞ for more in-depth information on bipolar disorder and disruptive disorders.) Instead of a euphoric mood, the most frequent mood disturbance is severe irritability, with accompanying hostile, violent, and long-lasting temper outbursts. They often engage in extreme risk-taking behaviors. Youth are more likely to be rapid cycling and may experience ultradian cycling. Adolescents also experience the classic symptoms of grandiosity, hypersexuality, increased energy, and decreased need for sleep. Early age onset predicts more psychotic symptoms, more mixed episodes, increased incidence of panic attacks, and decreased response to lithium (Badner, 2003; Youngstrom, Findling, & Feeny, 2004).

Depression is a common and troublesome mental disorder among *older adults,* who are at higher risk because of changes in self-concept and the multiple losses they have likely experienced. Many older people have an increase in stressful life events at the very time when they may have limited resources for managing such difficult circumstances. The more that stressful life events occur, the more their sense of helplessness becomes reinforced. If they reach the point of believing they have no control, they lose the will and the energy to cope with life, and depression frequently results.

Although depression is common, it may not be recognized and is frequently undertreated because health care professionals mistakenly view it as a "natural" part of aging. The consequences of this ageism include poor quality of life, cognitive impairment, nursing home placement, and increased risk of death by suicide. Of the older people living in the United States, about 10% to 20% are significantly depressed. For those living in residential care, the rate of depression is as high as 32% (Cole & Dendukuri, 2003; Rapp et al., 2005; Weeks, McGann, Michaels, & Penninx, 2003).

Some studies report that older adults experience symptoms of depression similar to those of younger adults. Other studies indicate that older people experience symptoms related to anxiety and somatic complaints rather than feelings of sadness. Older people with depression may exhibit signs of cognitive impairment leading to incorrect diagnoses of dementia. Symptoms include short-term memory problems, word-finding difficulty, confusion, and disorientation. Depression that simulates dementia is referred to as *pseudodementia*. This form of depression must be recognized and differentiated from irreversible dementia, and appropriate treatment measures must be implemented.

Bipolar disorder accounts for 5% to 19% of all mood disorders treated in the older population. Only a few of these individuals become ill for the first time after age 50. The cause of late-onset bipolar disorder is often a neurological disease. One common precipitant is a cerebrovascular accident in the right hemisphere affecting the limbic system. Other causes include hyperthyroidism; epilepsy; trauma; and degenerative, vascular, or neoplastic disease of the right hemisphere. Medications that produce manic symptoms include adrenal steroids, levodopa, antidepressants, bronchodilators, and decongestants (Russ, 2003).

Assessment: Physical

People experience many physiological symptoms during episodes of the mood disorders. A change in *appetite* is not unusual. Many people lose their desire for food when depressed, and statements such as "Nothing tastes good to me" are common. Others discover their appetites increase when they become depressed, and their eating patterns cause them to gain weight. Another pattern is for people to overeat and gain weight when mildly depressed and to lose their appetite and weight when severely depressed. Obesity may also be the result of side-effects of psychotrophic medications. People in a manic state may not obtain sufficient food and fluid because they cannot remain still long enough to eat a meal.

Sleep patterns are disrupted in people with mood disorders and sleep dysregulation may precede the onset of both major depression disorder and bipolar episode. During mild or moderate depression, people may sleep more than usual or they may awaken earlier than usual. In severe depression, people usually have difficulty falling asleep and may sleep for only a few hours a night. The person often awakens in the early morning and is unable to return to sleep (Fava, 2004).

During a manic episode, people experience a dramatic decrease in their amount of sleep. Although they may sleep only 1 or 2 hours a night, they are full of energy throughout the day. They have great difficulty taking naps or relaxing during the day to compensate for their lack of sleep.

Another change characteristic of mood disorders is in *motor activity.* Some people who are depressed experience extremely slowed motor activity. They walk slowly with a trudging gait. When speaking, they use a minimum of gestures to illustrate their thoughts. Others experience constant and nonpurposeful activity such as wringing the hands, picking at the skin, or agitated pacing.

In manic episodes, people experience hyperactivity without being aware of fatigue. They move constantly and have great difficulty remaining seated for more than a few minutes. When they are seated, constant swinging of the legs is typical. Dramatic arm and facial gestures accompany their speaking. Because they are unaware of fatigue, they are in danger of total physical exhaustion.

As many as one third of people in a manic episode develop *catatonia* exhibited as stereotypic motor excitement. The person exhibits behavior that is nonfunctional and repetitive such as rocking or picking at one's skin. The presence of catatonia predicts an increased severity of the disorder and a poorer outcome.

The vast majority of people who are depressed experience *somatic symptoms.* Complaints of headache, chest pain, back pain, joint pain, and fatigue are often heard. Women tend to report more somatic symptoms than men.

Bowel activity may be a problem in both unipolar and bipolar disorder. A marked decrease in food and fluid intake and decreased physical activity can result in constipation. Constipation in manic episodes is related to distractibility and therefore the ignoring of bodily signals or the inability to take the time to have a bowel movement.

There is a high rate of *nicotine dependence* (31% to 61%) among mood-disordered people compared to the rate for the general population (21% to 30%). Nicotine increases dopamine release in the reward center of the brain, which may be one of the few pleasurable experiences available to a depressed person. These individuals are able to describe the negative impact of smoking but consider that advantages of smoking outweigh the disadvantages. Smoking cessation programs have not been very effective for this group (Spring, Pingitore, & McChargue, 2003).

Physical appearance is often indicative of an altered mood state. Depressed people may wear the same clothes for days without laundering them. Personal hygiene may be poor because they do not have the energy to brush their teeth, shower, or wash their hair. During a manic state, people may change clothes as often as every hour. Separates, such as skirts, pants, and tops, may clash and seem to be chosen for their brightness rather than for their coordination. Personal hygiene may become a problem if distractibility interferes with normal ADLs. Women who wear makeup and jewelry have extravagant tastes during an elevated mood state. Their cosmetics tend to be very bright and may be carelessly applied.

Pam has been diagnosed as having a bipolar disorder, manic phase. Since admission 2 days ago, she has been averaging 2 hours of sleep a night. The rest of the nighttime hours are spent pacing hallways and talking to staff. She is in constant motion and brags about how energetic she is. Her clothing consists of startlingly bright miniskirts, low-cut sweaters, and high heels. Every few hours she reapplies her makeup to match each change of clothing.

Depression is also a risk factor of *osteoporosis* in both women and men and carries an increased risk of fractures. Loss of bone density may be the result of neuroendocrine alterations during depression (Gold & Charney, 2002).

For a review of the behavioral, affective, cognitive, sociocultural, and physiological characteristics of people with mood disorders, see Table 13.5 ■. See the Focused Nursing Assessment feature on pages 322–323 for examples of assessment questions you may ask. Given the potential for serious consequences of depression, it is imperative that health care professionals assess all new mothers and anyone else at risk for a mood disorder. A simple two-question assessment, developed by Whooley, Avins, Miranda, and Browner (1997), is very effective. The two questions are: 1) "Over the past 2 weeks, have you felt down, depressed, or hopeless?" and 2) "Over the past 2 weeks, have you felt lit-

TABLE 13.5	Characteristics of Mood Disorders	
Characteristic	**Depressed State**	**Manic State**
Behavioral		
Desire to participate in activities	Decreased to absent	Interested in all activities; increase in high-risk behaviors
Interaction with others	Limited; client withdraws	Talkative, gregarious
Affiliation needs	Increased dependency	Independent, self-sufficient
Affective		
Mood	Despair, desolation	Unstable: euphoric and irritable
Guilt	High level	Unable to experience guilt
Crying spells	Frequent crying to inability to cry	May have brief episodes
Gratification	Loss of interest in pleasurable activities	Constantly seeking fun and excitement
Emotional attachments	Indifference to others	Forms intense attachments rapidly
Cognitive		
Self-evaluation	Focuses on failures; sees self as incompetent; catastrophizes and personalizes	Grandiose beliefs about self
Expectations	Believes present and future hopeless; overgeneralizes one experience or fact	Inordinate positive expectations; unable to see potential negative outcomes
Self-criticism	Harshly critical of self; is a perfectionist; anticipates disapproval from others	Approves of own behavior; irate if criticized by others
Concentration	Decreased	Decreased
Decision-making ability	Decreased ability or inability to make decisions	Difficulty due to distractibility and impulsiveness
Flow of thought	Decrease in rate and number of thoughts	Flight of ideas; can't be interrupted
Body image	Believes self unattractive or ugly	Believes self unusually beautiful
Delusions	Somatic delusions	Delusions of grandeur
Hallucinations	Occur in 15% to 25% of cases	Occur in 15% to 25% of cases
Sociocultural		
Sexual desire	Loss of desire	Increase in activity and partners
Physiological		
Appetite	Increased or decreased in mild and moderate depression; decreased in severe depression	Difficulty eating due to inability to sit still
Amount of sleep	Increased or decreased in mild and moderate depression; decreased in severe depression	Sleeps only 1 or 2 hours a night
Activity level	Impaired motor activity; loss of energy	Hyperactivity; high energy
Bowel activity	Constipation	Constipation
Physical appearance	Unkempt; poor hygiene	Bright clothing; frequently changes clothing

tle interest or pleasure in doing things?" A positive response to either question indicates the nurse should complete a more in-depth assessment.

DIAGNOSIS

The next step in the nursing process is to analyze and synthesize the assessment data to form nursing diagnoses. You must consider the client's level of mood alteration as well as the behavioral, affective, cognitive, and physiological responses to their disorder. Another consideration is danger to self or others through suicide, homicide, or impulsive behavior. The following are those diagnoses most commonly identified for clients with eating disorders (North American Nursing Diagnosis Association, 2007).

- High Risk for Violence, Self-Directed related to a sense of hopelessness or to poor impulse control
- High Risk for Violence, Directed at Others, related to unrealistic thoughts of being inadequate as a parent, delusions, or command hallucinations
- Impaired Verbal Communication related to fragmented thought, flight of ideas, or slowed thought processes
- Decisional Conflict related to inability to utilize the problem-solving process
- Deficit in Diversional Activity related to lack of interest in any activities, inability to focus on an activity
- Altered Thought Process related to delusions, hallucinations, or cognitive distortions
- Self-esteem Disturbance related to inability to evaluate self objectively, catastrophizing, or grandiose beliefs about physical and intellectual characteristics
- Spiritual Distress related to lack of connection with others, hopeless view of the future, and no sense of purpose in life
- Caregiver Role Strain related to stigma, frustration, and increased conflict
- Altered Sexuality Patterns related to no desire for sex or to sexually acting-out behavior
- Deficient Knowledge related to disease process, treatment options, medications
- Sleep Pattern Disturbance related to insomnia or hyperactivity
- Imbalanced Nutrition, Less Than Body Requirements related to anorexia, hyperactivity
- Imbalanced Nutrition, More Than Body Requirements related to decreased activity, overeating in response to emotions
- Self-care Deficits, Bathing/Hygiene related to lack of motivation, decreased concentration

OUTCOME IDENTIFICATION AND GOALS

Once you have established diagnoses, you select outcomes appropriate to the nursing diagnoses. Broad outcomes include:

- Remains safe
- Engages in positive interpersonal relations
- Improves quality of life

Following this, the nurse and the client mutually identify goals for change. Client goals are specific behavioral measures that the nurse, the client, and significant others identify as realistic and attainable. The following are several examples of goals that may be pertinent to the client with a mood disorder:

- Verbalizes decreasing suicidal ideation
- Utilizes the problem-solving process
- Makes decisions that reflect good judgment
- Employs self-help strategies
- Mood stabilizes

PLANNING

Once the nursing diagnoses, outcome criteria, and goals have been identified, the nurse develops a plan of care to assist clients toward a higher level of functioning and improved mental health. Priorities of care for clients with mood disorders are as follows:

- Suicide
- Violence toward others
- Inadequate nutrition
- Altered thought processes
- Inability to problem solve or make decisions
- Impaired communication
- Self-care deficits

IMPLEMENTATION

For clients who are depressed, the focus of intervention is relief of symptoms and an improved quality of life. For clients who are in the midst of a manic episode, the focus of intervention is on symptom management and containment until the client recovers enough to participate in more structured nursing interventions.

Spiritual Distress

The desired outcome is that the client identifies meaning and purpose in life, verbalizes a connectedness to others, and utilizes religious resources if desired.

Focused Nursing Assessment | Clients With Mood Disorder

Behavior Assessment	Affective Assessment	Cognitive Assessment
How are you managing your work/household/school responsibilities?	How would you describe your overall mood?	What qualities do you like about yourself?
Has there been a change in your activity level?	Do you have mood swings?	What would you like to change about yourself?
Are you having difficulty doing basic activities of daily living?	What kinds of things make you feel guilty?	Give me an example of past success in your life.
What are your leisure activities?	How much time each day do you spend thinking about failure or guilt?	Overall, how would you evaluate your life in the past?
How much exercise are you getting?	How often do you cry?	What are your hopes for the future?
Do you enjoy doing things with other people?	What activities have given you pleasure in the past? In the present?	What does criticism or rejection by others mean to you?
	How have you used food, alcohol, or drugs to increase your pleasure?	Are you having difficulty concentrating?
		Does it seem as though your thoughts come slowly or quickly?
		Do you make decisions easily?

Remember that people are spiritual beings and be alert to spiritual concerns. Promote an atmosphere that accepts and encourages many forms of spiritual expression. Respecting people's beliefs and experiences also means that the nurse should not force spiritual issues on clients, push religion on them, or attempt to convert them to a particular faith.

In the midst of depression, many people experience spiritual distress related to a lack of purpose or joy in life and feeling disconnected with others. Be open to their expressions of loneliness, powerlessness, and loss of faith. Review their past joys and successes in life and help them identify "small" purposes of current life such as contributions to their family, value to friends, and goals for next day or week. Help them identify possible new functions or purposes in life to counteract the depressed feelings. Review with them the availability of supportive people, as those people will increase their sense of connectedness to others.

For clients who are religious, use religious resources to decrease distress. Facilitate their use of worship, meditation, or prayer. Remember that nurses are not meant to replace clergy. In the best of worlds, health care professionals and clergy work closely together to provide meaningful holistic care. For many people with mood disorders, religious beliefs improve self-esteem, life satisfaction, and the ability to cope.

Helplessness and Hopelessness

The desired outcome is that the client will identify personal strengths, verbalize an internal locus of control, act as a self-advocate, and develop advance directives.

Nursing interventions to counteract helplessness and hopelessness include exploring clients' previous achievements of success, encouraging them to identify their own strengths and abilities, and facilitating the evaluation of their own behavior. Help them identify ways in which they have control of their lives. The nurse can help them problem-solve situations in which they can become more autonomous, especially through vocational, social, and community activities.

Many people with mood disorders feel they have lost control over their own lives, rights, and responsibilities, and have lost the ability and right to effectively advocate for themselves. Nursing activities designed to help clients advocate for themselves give them hope and self-esteem. The nurse may assist clients in the following way:

- Encourage them to believe in themselves.
- Inform them of their rights.
- Help them clarify what they need and want by setting clear goals.
- Provide them with accurate information, preferably in writing.
- Help them strategize by using the problem-solving process.
- Facilitate their identification of resources such as friends, family, self-help groups, and advocacy organizations.
- Encourage them to identify the best person(s) to assist them with this problem.
- Foster effective communication so they can get their message across by suggestions such as: Be brief, stick to the point, don't get diverted, and state the concern and how things should be changed.

Social Assessment	Cultural Assessment	Physiological Assessment
Who lives in your household?	What is your ethnic identity?	How is your appetite?
With whom do you communicate most easily?	What is your religious affiliation?	How much weight have you gained or lost? In what period of time?
Who can you depend on in a crisis?	What do you believe is the source of your problems?	Are you having difficulty sleeping?
Who can depend on you in a crisis?	What home remedies or alternative therapies have you tried to make yourself better?	Do you tire easily or have a high level of energy?
What roles and responsibilities do you assume in your family?		Has your partner commented on a change in your level of sexual desire?
How do people seem to be treating you?		
What kinds of losses have you sustained during the past year?		

- Promote firmness and persistence so clients can get what they need for themselves.

Another activity to enhance clients' coping abilities is through the development of *advance directives*. While not legally binding in all states, these plans assist families and caregivers who must make decisions for clients when they are unable to make them for themselves. Advance directives are initiated by the client, formulated between acute episodes, and include:

- Symptoms that indicate the person is not able to make decisions at this time
- The names and phone numbers of at least three people, including health care professionals, and family members who should make decisions on their behalf
- A listing of medications, other treatments, and treatment facilities—ranked as preferred, acceptable, and unacceptable—including reasons

Clients are encouraged to develop their own mental health file containing information about their diagnoses, medications, self-help strategies, and resources. The advance directives should be kept in this file and a copy should be given to each specific supporter or health care professional.

Postpartum Depression

The desired outcome is that the client will verbalize an understanding of symptoms, utilize resources to cope with mood changes, and successfully parent the new infant.

It is important to teach all pregnant women the signs and symptoms of postpartum depression. With this information, women are likely to understand what is occurring and seek help at an earlier stage.

Group therapy for women experiencing postpartum "blues" or depression may be most helpful. Interacting with other women experiencing the same situation improves socialization and provides ideas for managing symptoms. They are able to support one another through the issues of feeling like a "bad" mother, finding parenthood to be more of a stress than a joy, and coping with family and friends who do not comprehend the disorder.

In some communities, women who have experienced postpartum depression have formed home management support groups. They organize and provide help in several forms: sessions with a psychotherapist, nutritionist, personal trainer, and professional childcare by mothers' helpers. A combination of these resources for 9 to 10 weeks helps mothers overcome the debilitating effects of postpartum depression and successfully parent their infants.

Disrupted Family Process

The desired outcome is that the client will utilize community resources, problem-solve resolution of conflict, and utilize effective communication skills.

Mood disorders affect not only the client but also family and friends. Nurses must consider all significant others to be recipients of their care. During acute episodes, clients may be very dependent and needy or may need firm direction and limit setting. Help caregivers acknowledge clients' dependency and assume appropriate responsibility. Provide information about clients' condition in accordance with client preferences, remembering the importance of confidentiality. Provide the family with a list of community resources and encourage them to participate in support groups.

MediaLink   Books for Clients and Families and Community Resources

NURSING CARE PLAN for a Client With Mood Disorder

Preventing self-harm

Nursing Diagnosis: Client at risk for self-directed violence

Outcomes: Client remains safe.

The first priority of care is client safety. Since as many as 20% of clients with mood disorders commit suicide, it is extremely important that you assess for suicide potential. Chapter 21 ∞ gives detailed information on assessment and interventions for clients who are suicidal.

Intervention	Rationale	Goal
When severely suicidal and not in the hospital, someone must remain with clients at all times until they can be moved to a safe environment.	Clients must be protected from self-destruction until safety can be guaranteed.	Does not act on suicidal plan
Teach family members: ■ People who talk about suicide are at high risk. ■ Suicide attempts may follow loss of an important person, position, or possession. ■ Attempts may increase as the depression is beginning to improve and there is more energy to act. ■ Getting one's "life in order" is a high-risk signal.	Family members should recognize risk factors that increase suicide risk.	Families verbalize an understanding of risk factors

Preventing Harm to Others

Nursing Diagnosis: Client at risk for other-directed violence

Outcomes: Client will not threaten others, and will control aggressive impulses.

Aggressive behavior may occur in a manic episode because of mood instability, command hallucinations, or impulse control problems. It is important that you continually assess for ongoing signs of escalation of aggressive behavior. If you assess accurately and respond early and appropriately, you may be able to halt the progression of aggressive behavior. Chapter 8 ∞ has detailed nursing interventions in regard to aggression.

Intervention	Rationale	Goal
Use a calm, professional, confident approach.	This often diffuses hostility.	Level of aggression lessens
Do not argue.	This avoids giving the person a reason to continue to be angry.	Level of aggression lessens
Give people limited choices on what they can do.	This supports the feeling that they have some control in the situation.	Makes appropriate choices
When clients are not angry, teach nonviolent coping strategies; role-play these behaviors.	This expands options in response to provocative situations.	Identifies and practices new ways of responding

Managing Impulsive Behavior

Nursing Diagnosis: Client at risk for ineffective coping

Outcomes: Client will stop and think before acting, and will get input from others before acting.

Cognitive disruptions for clients in the manic phase of bipolar disorder often result in impulsive behavior, which may or may not be dangerous to themselves or others. There are a number of actions you can take to assist clients in impulse control training. An example might be impulse buying. Clients may decide that every time they take out their wallet, they must "stop and think" if they really need the item they are about to purchase. They might choose to leave their credit cards and checkbooks at home, as well. If absolutely necessary, they may elect to have another person control access to credit cards, checkbooks, ATMs, and cash disbursements. The benefits from these decisions are financial stability and self-management.

NURSING CARE PLAN for a Client With Mood Disorder

Managing Impulsive Behavior   *continued*
Nursing Diagnosis: Client at risk for ineffective coping

Intervention	Rationale	Goal
Help clients identify situations that require thoughtful action.	This provides preparation for more thoughtful action.	Identifies personal situations
Teach them to cue themselves to "stop and think" before acting impulsively.	This slows down impulsive behavior.	Implements "stop and think" action
Help them identify other courses of action.	Identifying the potential benefits of alternative behavior may limit impulsive actions.	Lists other ways to respond
Have client identify two trusted people with whom they can discuss their plans. These people will provide feedback to clients.	If the plan is a reasonable one, two other people ought to be able to agree that it is reasonable; if plan is not reasonable, friends can provide feedback on potential negative consequences.	Identifies two friends and discusses plans with them

Stabilizing Mood
Nursing Diagnosis: Client at risk for ineffective coping

Outcome: Expression of mood will be within normal limits, and client will utilize a daily mood chart.

The way you interact, as a nurse, may decrease or increase mood instability. A calm, professional, confident approach is important when interacting with people experiencing labile affect. Instructions for mood charting and an example of a completed mood chart are available from the National Depressive and Manic Depressive Association at http://www.manicdepressive.org/moodinstruct.html. Mood charts for children may be found at http://www.bpkids.org/learning/mood.html.

Intervention	Rationale	Goal
Teach mood charting process including three categories of mood: ■ Depressed ■ Elevated ■ WNL (within normal limits)	This is a method to identify and control mood swings.	Implements mood charting
Each day clients enter their mood, any psychotic symptoms, significant events, and medications.	Over time, this chart is a record that can be used to better manage their disorder.	Maintains mood chart
Parents can help children complete the daily charting.	Young children need parental guidance.	Parents and children work together

Managing Hallucinations
Nursing Diagnosis: Client at risk for disturbed sensory perception

Outcomes: Client experiences hallucinations without major difficulties.

Hallucinations are frightening experiences, and most clients welcome opportunities to discuss them. It is critical that you monitor the hallucinations for content that is self-harmful, suicidal, or violent toward others. Encourage clients to express these feelings appropriately rather than act on the violent messages. Chapter 8 ∞ provides more detailed nursing interventions for clients who hallucinate.

Intervention	Rationale	Goal
Encourage clients to validate their perceptions with others.	Choosing a trusted person such as you or a family member will result in more success.	Identifies trusted people
If clients ask you to verify a hallucination, point out that you are not experiencing the same stimuli.	Arguments about the validity of the hallucination should be avoided.	Validates their perceptions with others

continued

NURSING CARE PLAN for a Client With Mood Disorder

Managing Hallucinations *continued*
Nursing Diagnosis: Client at risk for disturbed sensory perception

Intervention	Rationale	Goal
If hallucinations are interfering with conversation, try to refocus the client to the topic.	This may distract from the hallucination.	Participates in conversations
Involve clients in reality-based activities such as a game or preparing a meal.	This may distract from the hallucination.	Participates in activities
Focus on the underlying feelings or content themes rather than particulars about the hallucination, (e.g., "That sounds like a frightening experience" or "You seem worried about your mother").	Identification of feelings and themes may help clients focus on what they are trying to explain.	Acknowledges feelings and themes

Enhancing Self-esteem
Nursing Diagnosis: Client at risk for chronic low self-esteem

Outcome: Client verbalizes a realistic self-evaluation.

Clients in manic episodes often experience grandiose views of themselves. Do not argue about their delusions, as that would place them in the position of having to defend their belief. If they are excessively preoccupied, set limits on the amount of time they can discuss their beliefs, such as, "We will talk about how good you feel about yourself for 5 minutes and then we will talk about something else for 15 minutes." Ask clients to identify the significance of their culture, religion, race, gender, sexual orientation, and age on their self-esteem. When appropriate, discuss more positive values, which will lead to a higher self-esteem. For example, if the client has experienced discrimination related to lesbian identification, help her develop a list of positive aspects of her sexual orientation.

People suffering from depression often experience self-esteem disturbances related to criticism and negative self-evaluation. Attentive listening is critical since it communicates that you consider the client to be a person of value.

Intervention	Rationale	Goal
Set limits on time spent discussing past failures.	Rumination intensifies guilt and low self-esteem.	Spends less time discussing negative characteristics
Review past achievements and present successes; provide feedback whenever possible.	Reinforces strengths that they bring to a variety of situations.	Identifies own strengths and abilities; discusses current situations in which they are successful
Encourage behaviors that foster an internal locus of control.	Acknowledging control lessens feelings of helplessness.	Verbalizes an internal locus of control
Teach positive affirmations in a variety of areas such as work, school, leisure, achievements, interactions with others, etc. Examples are: ■ I am a good mother. ■ I like my job. ■ I am a good friend. ■ I am honest. ■ I am a good student.	This is a method of changing distorted negative cognitions.	Speaks affirmations aloud several times a day; verbalizes improved self-esteem
Assess negative thought patterns for logic and validity; ask clients if these are realistic evaluations.	Global statements about guilt and inadequacy contribute to a negative self-esteem. Cognitive distortions increase feelings of depression.	Verbalizes fewer feelings of inadequacy and guilt
Discuss perfectionism.	Unrealistic self demands increase associated guilt.	Verbalizes decreased need for perfectionism
Help clients formulate realistic self-standards.	Realistic standards are achievable and thereby increase self-esteem.	Identifies realistic self-evaluation criteria

NURSING CARE PLAN for a Client With Mood Disorder

Managing Cognitive Problems

Nursing Diagnosis: Client at risk for disturbed thought processes

Outcome: Client verbalizes fewer cognitive distortions.

Assess clients for altered thought processes such as overgeneralization, dichotomous thinking, catastrophizing, or personalization. See the Complementary/Alternative Therapies feature for teaching clients how to moderate their level of depression.

Intervention	Rationale	Goal
Help clients identify negative self-statements by asking: ■ What do you say about yourself? ■ Is that true? ■ Have these thoughts increased your depression?	Negative thoughts are so automatic, they occur outside of conscious awareness.	Identifies negative thinking as a symptom of the disorder rather than reality
Teach them to question if there are alternative explanations when they find themselves interpreting ambiguous situations in a negative way.	This increases awareness of typical thought processes.	Challenges negative patterns
Brainstorm alternative explanations.	With practice they may be able to keep a more open mind.	Verbalizes a more realistic perspective
When clients have negative predictions of the future, ask: ■ What is the worst that can happen? ■ What is the best that can happen? ■ What is the most likely to happen?	This challenges automatic negative thoughts.	Verbalizes more positive predictions of the future

Improving Socialization

Nursing Diagnosis: Client at risk for social isolation

Outcome: Client will socialize appropriately with others.

People who are depressed often say they have no energy or motivation to participate in social activities, which results in social isolation. The more alone and isolated people are, however, the more depressed they feel. When people connect to and interact with others, they feel less lonely and their mood often begins to lift.

Intervention	Rationale	Goal
Provide brief, frequent contacts.	Ability to concentrate is decreased in depression.	Increases attention span
You or family participate with clients during activities.	This fosters connection to others.	Verbalizes less loneliness
Provide feedback on efforts to socialize with others.	This reinforces positive changes.	Connects the frequency and intensity of social interaction to mood state
Help clients and families identify benefits of social interactions.	This reinforces positive changes.	Identifies personal changes
Encourage clients to make a list of things they enjoy doing such as going for a walk, listening to music, watching funny DVDs, or visiting with friends.	Part of self-management is making the time to include one or more of these activities on a regular basis.	Participates in selected social activities

continued

NURSING CARE PLAN for a Client With Mood Disorder

Improving Socialization

Nursing Diagnosis: Client at risk for impaired social interaction

Outcomes: Client will socialize appropriately with others.

In contrast to those who are depressed, people experiencing manic episodes are interested in every person and every activity, whether appropriate or not. Thus, they may be very intrusive in other people's conversations and create socially awkward situations. Social skills training is covered in more depth in chapter 9 ∞.

Peer counseling may be another activity to enhance clients' socialization. Peer counseling is a free, safe, and effective self-help tool that encourages expression of feelings. It puts clients in control of their own healing process. In a peer counseling session, two people agree to spend a certain amount of time together, dividing the time equally, paying attention to each other's issues, needs, and distresses. Judging, criticizing, and giving advice are not allowed.

Intervention	Rationale	Goal
Set limits on intrusive or interruptive behaviors.	This reduces chances of rejection from other people.	Modifies intrusive behavior
Keep activities simple and short and consistent with clients' physical, emotional, and social capabilities.	This ensures success in these endeavors.	Participates in activities
Engage clients in nonstimulating activities.	This avoids escalation of mood by competition or sensory stimulation.	Mood does not escalate

Enhancing Decision Making

Nursing Diagnosis: Client at risk for disturbed thought processes

Outcomes: Client will make logical decisions with minimal difficulty.

Nurses can enhance decision making by teaching clients to utilize the problem-solving process. This process is presented in more detail in chapter 7 ∞. Discourage clients from making important decisions when under severe stress or during the acute phase of their disorder.

Intervention	Rationale	Goal
Give limited choices, (e.g., "Would you like to take your shower before or after breakfast?").	Activity is directed while giving clients limited control until decision-making ability is improved.	Makes decisions within limited context
When clients talk about being overwhelmed by all the decisions that have to be made, have them identify only one decision to work toward.	Narrowing the focus to one decision decreases feelings of helplessness.	Focuses on one decision at a time
Explore previous methods of managing problems and the outcomes of these past attempts.	This increases awareness of what works and what doesn't work.	Explores past coping behaviors

Managing Low Activity Level

Nursing Diagnosis: Client at risk for activity intolerance

Outcome: Client will increase physical activity.

Exercise is the least expensive and most available antidepressant. It is nature's way of increasing neurotransmitters and endorphins, thus decreasing feelings of sadness and tension. A daily walk or some other kind of enjoyable exercise makes most people feel better. Clients who are depressed may tell you that they will exercise when they feel better. Teach them that, in contrast, they will feel better when they exercise. Finding an "exercise buddy" may facilitate this aspect of self-management.

NURSING CARE PLAN for a Client With Mood Disorder

Managing Low Activity Level *continued*
Nursing Diagnosis: Client at risk for activity intolerance

Intervention	Rationale	Goal
Ask clients what physical activities are most enjoyable.	Planning with client demonstrates respect for clients' ability to collaborate and control life.	Identifies acceptable exercises
Provide clients with materials to keep a record of activities and set realistic goals.	This allows client to assume responsibility for own behavior.	Keeps record of exercises
Encourage clients to evaluate mood on a scale from 1 to 10 before and after exercise.	This provides a subjective measurement of effects of exercise.	Verbalizes subjective effects of exercise

Managing High Activity Level
Nursing Diagnosis: Client at risk for fatigue

Outcome: Client's level of physical activity moderates.

Clients experiencing a manic episode may become exhausted when excessive levels of activity are combined with decreased awareness of fatigue. See the Complementary/Alternative Therapies feature for teaching clients how to slow down their behavior.

Intervention	Rationale	Goal
Teach clients to avoid stimulating places such as bars or busy shopping malls.	This prevents escalation of mood and activity level.	Verbalizes understanding of need for a quieter environment
Limit intake of caffeinated food and fluids.	This facilitates self-control.	Monitors food and fluids
Provide high-calorie foods that can be eaten while walking.	Intake must be sufficient to provide energy for high activity level; may be unable to sit down to eat a meal.	Intake appropriate to energy output
Set short rest periods such as 10 minutes every hour.	This prevents physical exhaustion.	Sits quietly for short periods of time
Avoid activities that need intense concentration such as complicated games or puzzles.	Attention span is too short for client to be successful at these activities.	Completes simple, short projects

Reinforcing Sexual Health
Nursing Diagnosis: Client at risk for sexual dysfunction

Outcome: Client returns to or develops satisfactory sexual experiences, discusses sexual concerns with partner, and decreases inappropriate sexual behavior.

Clients in a manic episode often exhibit an impulse increase in their sexual activity. Explain to family members that such behavior is a symptom of the manic state, is not within the client's control, and is not an indication of a change in ethics and values. As much as possible, clients should be protected from sexual acting out until they are able to assume control over this behavior. Set firm limits on inappropriate verbal and physical sexual behaviors. You may find that distracting clients to another activity is helpful.

Adult clients who are depressed often experience a diminished interest in sex. This stems from the inability to experience pleasure, lack of energy, and little interest in interacting with others.

Intervention	Rationale	Goal
Introduce the topic of sexuality with client and partner. You might say: "When people are depressed they often lose their interest in sexual intimacy. Is this a problem for the two of you?" or "Sometimes the medication you are taking causes sexual problems. Has this happened to you?"	This enables clients to share any concerns they may have.	Verbalizes concerns

continued

NURSING CARE PLAN for a Client With Mood Disorder

Reinforcing Sexual Health *continued*

Nursing Diagnosis: Client at risk for sexual dysfunction

Intervention	Rationale	Goal
If there are sexual problems, determine if these problems existed prior to the onset of depression.	Preexisting sexual problems may be unrelated to the mood disorder.	Identifies preexisting sexual problems
If sexual problems are the result of mood changes, explain that sexual desire usually returns as the depression recedes.	Understanding this as a symptom of depression will decrease feelings of hurt, inadequacy, and guilt.	Identifies lack of desire as symptom of disorder
If the sexual problem is related to medication side effects, a change in medication should be considered.	Some people stop taking their antidepressant medication because of sexual side effects.	Verbalizes reason for stopping medications
Stress importance of nonsexual expression of affection, such as hugging and holding each other.	Touch is a very important and reassuring form of communication.	Couple agrees on amount and type of nonsexual physical touch
If problems continue after the depression has lifted, suggest that the couple consider sex therapy.	Sexual problems may need the intervention of specialized sex therapists.	Follows up on referral

Educating

Nursing Diagnosis: Client at risk for deficient knowledge

Outcome: Client will be self-directed in managing the disorder.

People who are self-managers say that it is absolutely essential to learn everything they can about their particular diagnosis. Education is part of taking responsibility for wellness and facilitates appropriate decision-making. Clients are encouraged to become experts on their illness and work collaboratively with health care providers to manage their disorder. This educational process must be continuous to keep clients and families up-to-date with the latest findings about their disorder. Your role is not simply to hand out teaching sheets but to discuss, explain, and teach clients and their families. More detailed information on client and family teaching is found in chapter 7 ∞.

Intervention	Rationale	Goal
Identify barriers to learning such as a belief that they know everything or in total denial of having a disorder.	Barriers to learning must be identified and managed if your teaching is to be effective.	Improves readiness to learn
Provide information to clients and families: ■ Theories of mood disorders ■ Risk factors ■ Symptoms and course of disorder ■ Treatment options ■ Medications	Accurate information is basic to self-management.	Verbalizes an understanding of the disorder
Teach about early signs of relapse and risk factors: ■ Alcohol/drug use ■ Sleep deprivation ■ Family distress ■ Interpersonal conflict ■ Inconsistency with medications	Identification of signs of impending relapse can help ensure that treatment is begun as early as possible in the course of the relapse.	Verbalizes an understanding of relapse in the disorder
Teach about the protective factors in staying well: ■ Using mood charts ■ Maintaining consistent routines ■ Relying on social and family supports ■ Regular medication use ■ Psychosocial treatment programs	Incorporating protective factors may limit the incidence of relapse.	Incorporates protective factors

NURSING CARE PLAN for a Client With Mood Disorder

Maintaining Hygiene and Appearance

Nursing Diagnosis: Client at risk for self-care deficit: bathing/hygiene; dressing/grooming

Outcomes: Client will manage ADLs.

People who are depressed often have little motivation or energy to accomplish ADLs. Some merely need reminding while others may need step-by-step instruction.

Intervention	Rationale	Goal
If clients are unable to do basic hygiene, provide these measures.	Providing hygiene will prevent social embarrassment and improve self-esteem.	Is clean and neatly dressed each day
Assist in gathering hygienic articles and clean clothing appropriate to climate and situation.	Inability to make decisions may interfere with ADLs.	Accomplishes ADLs
Encourage clients to assume responsibility for own hygiene.	Self-directive behavior will increase self-esteem.	Initiates self-care measures
Provide positive feedback for assuming responsibility.	Positive feedback reinforces behavioral changes.	Maintains positive changes in behavior

Enhancing Sleep Patterns

Nursing Diagnosis: Client at risk for disturbed sleep pattern

Outcome: Client will attain normal sleep pattern: sleep 6 to 8 hours a night, report feeling rested, and establish consistent routines.

Since disrupted rhythms are a stimulus for a manic episode, regularity is of prime importance for people with bipolar disorder. They should have a job that never requires shift work or extended overtime, eat on a regular schedule, and maintain patterns of daily activities. They should avoid overscheduling stimulating activities in a short period of time. If they are unable to sleep, they should schedule rest periods throughout the day to avoid physical exhaustion. Changes in the daily schedule should be made gradually if at all possible. If the changes are predictable, such as adding a new baby to the family, preparations can be made over several weeks. If the changes are unexpected, clients will need to find ways to adapt and protect steady social rhythms.

People who are depressed or in a manic episode experience insomnia and frequent awakening. Working with the client, discover ways to improve sleep patterns.

Intervention	Rationale	Goal
Ask about past and present patterns. Keep a record of present pattern.	This establishes baseline data.	Identifies sleep patterns
Ask what measures to improve sleeping have been successful in the past.	Past measures may be adaptable to present setting.	Suggests measures to improve sleep
Discuss alternative methods to facilitate sleep: ■ Increase physical activity ■ Avoid exercise right before bedtime ■ Relaxation techniques ■ Avoid caffeine ■ Avoid emotional upsets prior to bedtime ■ Warm bath ■ Warm drink ■ Decrease amount of daytime napping	Natural sedative measures may improve sleeping pattern.	Initiates and evaluates measures that improve sleep; reports that sleep is more restful
Encourage reading, watching TV, or talking to someone when unable to sleep.	Nighttime may increase feelings of hopelessness and sleepless periods are often spent ruminating over problems. Redirection decreases excessive focus on problems.	Initiates positive activities when unable to sleep

Complementary/Alternative Therapies

How to Help Clients Moderate Level of Depression

This exercise is designed to empower yourself with your thoughts by transforming negative thoughts and events through imagery. Do this every day prior to bedtime.

1. Mentally go through your day and decide what you could have changed that would have brought better results.

2. Imagine that change occurring. For example, if you didn't enjoy lunch with your friends, imagine that you had a good time at lunch. If you are unhappy about something you said to a loved one, imagine saying something more caring.

3. As you progress in this exercise, pay attention to how your thoughts, feelings, and behaviors are becoming more positive and less depressing.

Complementary/Alternative Therapies

How to Help Clients Slow Down Behavior

This exercise is designed to decrease hyperactive behavior and induce a sense of peace and calm.

1. Gently close your eyes and focus all your attention on the flow of air as you breathe in and exhale.

2. After three to five breaths, imagine that you are breathing in peace and breathing out tension. Tell yourself that the clean, fresh air that you breathe in through your nose has the power to clear your mind of distracting thoughts. With every exhaled breath, you are releasing stress and tension.

3. Repeat this breathing cycle for 5 to 10 minutes.

Clinical Interactions   A Client With Bipolar Disorder

Ken, age 36, has been in a partial hospitalization program for the past 2 months. Both of his parents are deceased, and his two siblings are uninvolved with him. His mood ranges from euphoria to irritability. He believes he is very handsome, intelligent, and superior to other people. He is often preoccupied with sexual topics. The nurse is meeting Ken for the first time. In the interaction, you will see evidence of:

- Ken's grandiose beliefs about himself
- His flight of ideas
- His labile moods

KEN: "You would like to talk and help me?"

NURSE: *"I would like to get to know you first."*

KEN: "You will find me really interesting. I am rich."

NURSE: *"I would like to know a little bit about who you are, Ken."*

KEN: "I was a chosen child."

NURSE: *"Can you help me understand what that means, to be a chosen child?"*

KEN: "I was my parents' favorite child and they treated me special."

NURSE: *"What does 'special' mean to you?"*

KEN: "Love would come from my mother to me. Jesus is the love child. Did you know that?"

NURSE: *"Ken, let's concentrate on you and your family. You were telling me that your mother loved you very much."*

KEN: "Yes, she showed me how to love, but she died and left me. She went away. My father died later when I was 26."

NURSE: *"How did your parents' deaths affect you?"*

KEN: "I like women. There is no room for homosexuals. I'm a heterosexual."

NURSE: *"Ken, let's concentrate on the topic of you and your parents. How did you feel when your parents died?"*

KEN: "My father was a big man."

NURSE: *"Your father was a strong figure to you?"*

KEN: "Big man. He would slap my mother." [Acts out how his father would slap his mother; seems to be getting angry and aggressive.]

NURSE: *"Ken, did that anger you when your father hit your mother? Can you tell me about those times?"*

KEN: "My father would slap my mother and hit me here." [Jumps up and points to his backside and legs.]

NURSE: *"That must have been painful. How did you feel when that happened?"*

KEN: "He had to show me the way. Like God the Father."

NURSE: *"Ken, let's continue on with your childhood father."*

KEN: "I signed up for the army and went to Vietnam. I killed the evil people." [Angry tone and then starts laughing.]

NURSE: *"You sound angry about having killed but yet you laugh."*

KEN: "I had to kill those liars. My brother and sister were jealous."

NURSE: *"Ken, I don't understand. Slow down. Let's talk about the jealousy."*

KEN: "I was chosen. My mother loved me." [loudly] "I came home with shell shock. I have a tattoo on my nose and a fracture on my skull. I'm tired of talking. I'll see you later."

After the acute episode, families often have difficulties in one or more of the following areas:

- Disagreements over management of the disorder such as sleep–wake routines, medication inconsistencies, and alcohol/drug use

- Problems relating to the return to school or work, and the resumption of social responsibilities

- Disparity in household management rules and financial responsibilities

- Interpersonal problems such as intimacy issues for a couple and boundary issues for parent and child

When caring for families, observe interactional patterns and verbal communications. How do family members interact? Do they: speak for each other, cut each other off, listen to other viewpoints, blame each other, or use problem solving? Enhancing communication will decrease family stress, resolve conflict, and improve relationships. Have the family choose a nonthreatening event that happened within the past few days. Teach and model the following new ways of talking and listening to one another about this event:

- Express positive feelings about the event

- Utilize active listening, which includes eye contact, nodding head, asking clarifying questions

---

Using Research Evidence   Self-Care: Depression

Choenarom, C., Williams, R. A., & Hagerty, B. M. (2005). The role of sense of belonging and social support on stress and depression in individuals with depression. *Archives of Psychiatric Nursing, 19,* 18–29.

What is the study about?

Depression is a leading disability among Americans and is among the top five illnesses in every other country outside of Africa, where it ranks 11th. Therefore, the purpose of this study was to examine, in men and women both with and without a history of depression, how level of depression was related to perceived stress, and how that relationship might be mediated or moderated by three social factors: sense of belonging, social support, and spousal support. In addition, this study examined how well those three factors could predict severity of depression at four different times over a period of 9 months.

How was the study done?

This was a quantitative longitudinal, correlational, and comparative study using a convenience sample of clients diagnosed with major depressive disorder (MDD) as compared with a matching group of adults with no history of depression. Participants were matched for age, sex, and race/ethnic background. The researchers enrolled 90 participants: 63 females and 27 males. The mean age was 38.8; 89% were White and 11% identified themselves with other ethnic groups; 51 were diagnosed with MDD and 39 were in the comparison group. MDD diagnoses met DSM-IV criteria. The participants completed five self-report instruments: Beck Depression Inventory II (BDI-II), Perceived Stress Scale (PSS), Sense of Belonging Instrument (SOBI), Social Support Scale (SOCIAL-S), and Spousal Support (SPOUSE-S).

Candidates were initially screened by telephone for eligibility. Persons meeting eligibility criteria and consenting to participate were mailed a packet of the instruments at the start of the study and at 3, 6, and 9 months. Both the MDD and the comparison groups received the same instruments at the same intervals. Statistical analysis included t-tests and chi-squares to identify how or if the groups might differ demographically. Regression analysis was used to test whether the three social factors moderated or mediated depression/stress. Repeated measures of analysis of variance were used to determine the relationship between research variables over time.

What were the results of the study?

Demographic data analysis showed no differences between groups in their income or educational level. Group status was significantly associated with marital status: Married people were more likely to be in the comparison group, while the depressed group tended to be either single or divorced. The two groups differed significantly in their results on all of the five instruments. Thus, persons diagnosed with depression, but not currently experiencing a depressive episode, appear to have underlying psychological vulnerabilities that may differ from those of persons without such a diagnosis. In the comparison group, there were no significant correlations between PSS or BDI scores and the three social factors. This result suggests that the comparison group may have used different ways to manage stress so that stress did not influence depression. The findings also suggested that, for persons living with MDD, the effect of stress (any level of stress) on depression could be lessened by encouraging a sense of belonging and social support. Also among the MDD group, the experience of depression seemed to be lessened substantially by a sense of belonging. On the other hand, among these persons, the stress-and-depression interaction was not affected by spousal support.

What additional questions might I have?

Would the results be significantly different in a sample that was less homogenous in racial background? Could the research design have answered the study's questions by other methods than self-report questionnaires? What suggestions would help families and significant others give the person with MDD a sense of belonging?

How can I use this study?

Nurses need to be aware of the unique ways that persons living with depression experience it. Nurses should encourage initiatives that reappraise stress and foster a sense of belonging. For these clients, the plan of care should include careful assessment of social support, of spousal support if available, and of willingness to accept support.

SOURCE: Contributed by Dolores Huffman, PhD, RN, Associate Professor of Nursing, Purdue University Calumet, Hammond, Indiana.

■ Make a positive and specific request for change in others' behavior, (e.g. "I would really like it . . .").

■ Express any negative feelings about the event

Instruct the family to pick a time at home to practice these new skills. Encourage them to keep a journal about the process so it can be fine-tuned as they gain expertise in positive communication.

The goal is to help family members identify and change behaviors that maintain mood disorders. Because family therapy is a specialized area of nursing practice and requires additional education, the nurse should collaborate closely with colleagues who possess advanced practice skills. Managing family system problems with children who have mood disorders is covered in chapter 17 ∞.

EVALUATION

To complete the nursing process, you evaluate clients' responses in terms of the outcomes you and the client established. It is seldom an all-or-nothing phenomenon, but rather an ongoing process of movement toward the goal of better health and functioning. If there is little movement toward achieving the outcome, you must determine the problem. Considerations are:

■ Assessment data was incomplete or inaccurate.

■ The diagnosis was inappropriate to the situation.

■ Outcomes were not realistic.

■ Clients disagreed with the outcomes.

■ Interventions were not appropriate.

When the problem is identified, changes can be made in the nursing process, and the nurse, the client, and the family can move forward.

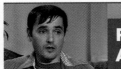

ROAD Assessment: Critical Thinking Questions

Go to the CD-ROM to assess Josh by answering the following critical thinking questions based on what you have **R**ead about Josh and **O**bserved on the videos.

1. You meet Josh during your psychiatric nursing clinical rotation at an outpatient partial hospitalization program. Based upon your observation of Josh's affect and his verbalizations, how would you document the affective and mood portion of his assessment?

2. Identify the prevailing issue(s) and Josh's symptoms of bipolar disorder present in the excerpt from your student ROAD CD-ROM segment B for chapter 13 Support your answer(s).

3. You are invited to join a therapy session between Josh and his therapist, from which a portion of the interaction is recorded on segment C of your student ROAD CD-ROM for chapter 13. Describe what you assess are, and have been, Josh's psychological issues.

4. After Josh's session has ended, his therapist asks if you would like to talk further. She reports that Josh has been more withdrawn during group sessions as well as voicing discouragement about his social life and himself during therapy sessions. She also states that he was recently started on an antidepressant medication. Later in the shift you are reviewing Josh's medication sheet and note the following prescriptions: Zoloft 50 mg

1 PO every A.M., Zyprexia 5 mg 1 PO bid, and acetaminophen 325 mg 1–2 PO every 4–6 hours prn. What is the specific data have you gathered (up until this point in question 3) which will cause you to discuss Josh's medication regimen with the unit RN? Provide a rationale for your answer.

5. Your next interaction with Josh takes place the following week. He tells you about how much he has been getting done. In a flurry of words, he recounts how during the past 5 days he has been writing a book on building a homemade weather radio. He states that with the low gas reserves in the United States the economy will surely collapse and people should have a way of being self-sufficient. His thoughts are that people won't be able to afford gas and if there were an energy emergency his radio may offer people a way to survive. He reports creating a 10-page outline and filling two binders with ideas and notes. Within the past 48 hours he tells you he hasn't slept so he could rearrange his office and organize his workspace. He has used colored signs to map out where each section of his book will be written. Based upon your knowledge of the characteristics of Josh's past illnesses, what areas of further assessment are indicated at this time?

ROAD: Develop a Care Plan

 Go to the CD-ROM to Develop a care plan based on your assessment of Josh. Identify nursing diagnoses, outcomes, goals, and interventions.

SOURCE: Contributed by Susan Siwinski-Hebel, RN, MSN

Focus Your Study

OBJECTIVES	KEY CONCEPTS

1. Compare and contrast the different theories regarding the etiology of mood disorders.

- Genetics:
  - There is a genetic predisposition to mood disorders with bipolar disorder having the greater inheritability.
- Neurobiology:
  - Decreased activity in the prefrontal cortex
  - Altered neurotransmission: 5-HT, DA NE, ACh
  - Altered receptor sensitivity
  - Disrupted biologic rhythms
  - Secondary to medications or medical conditions
- Intrapersonal theory:
  - Focus is on the theme of loss, grief, anger, and abandonment.
- Learning theory:
  - Repeated failures and an external locus of control contribute to depression.
- Cognitive theory:
  - Negative schemas contribute to a view of self as incompetent, unworthy, and unlikable.
- Sociocultural factors:
  - The experience of discrimination by cultural minorities may contribute to depression.
  - For those who are vulnerable to depression, stressors may play a significant role in the exacerbation and course of the disorder.
- Gender-bias theory:
  - Psychosocial stressors—including multiple work and family responsibilities, poverty, sexual and physical abuse, gender discrimination, lack of social supports, and traumatic life experiences—may contribute to women's increased vulnerability to depression.
  - In a society that places a premium on youth, older people feel useless, unimportant, incapable, and at times even repulsive.

2. Discuss the psychopharmacological treatment of the symptoms of mood disorders.

- Antidepressant medications are often prescribed for clients with mood disorders.
- About 30% of people do not respond to their antidepressant after 4 to 6 weeks. Mood stabilizers or antipsychotics may be added or a different antidepressant may be tried.
- For people with bipolar disorder, mood stabilizers are always prescribed at the same time as an antidepressant to lessen the risk of switching to a manic episode.
- Antidepressants now come with FDA warning labels that describe a link between the drugs and increased suicidal thought and behavior in children and youth, especially during the first several months of administration. In contrast, many mental health professionals are worried that not medicating seriously ill children can also lead to an increase in suicidal behavior.
- To date, no psychotropic medication has been approved by the FDA for use during pregnancy. Abrupt discontinuation of maintenance medications, including antipsychotics, antidepressants, and mood stabilizers, has been associated with a high, early relapse risk.
- Divalproex (Depakote) should be switched to another mood stabilizer before conception as there is a higher than average risk for neural tube defects. Carbamazepine (Tegretol) should be used during pregnancy only if there are no other options, as this medication is associated with craniofacial defects and developmental delay.
- Lamotrigine (Lamictal) appears to be safer than the other anticonvulsants. Lithium doses should be decreased at the onset of labor to avoid maternal toxicity at delivery.

continued

3. Outline the different treatment options for a person with a mood disorder.

- Electroconvulsive therapy (ECT) is a safe alternative for highly suicidal clients, those who suffer from psychotic depression, and those who are medically deteriorated. It is safe in all trimesters of pregnancy.
- Phototherapy is the treatment of choice for clients with SAD.
- Repetitive transcranial magnetic stimulation (rTMS) is helpful in depression without psychosis.
- Vagus nerve stimulation is being studied for people suffering from treatment-resistant depression.
- Alternative therapies for mood disorders include St. John's wort, SAMe, vitamin B, tyrosine, melatonin, DHEA, omega-3 fatty acids, aromatherapy, acupuncture, animal-assisted therapy, and music therapy.

4. Outline the assessment process for a client with a mood disorder.

- People with mood disorders display a variety of characteristics involving changes in behavior, affect, cognition, and physiology.
- Alterations in behavior include participation in activities, poor judgment, interaction with others, and affiliation needs.
- Alterations in affect include mood changes, instability of mood, guilt, anhedonia, and emotional attachment.
- Delusions and hallucinations may occur in mood disorders.
- Alterations in cognition include self-esteem, catastrophizing, locus of control, decision making, and flow of thought.

5. Use the nursing process to develop a comprehensive plan of care for a client with a mood disorder.

- Violence, self/other:
  - Ongoing suicide assessment
  - Watch for escalation of aggression
  - Behavioral contract
  - Talking down
  - Medications
- Impulsive behavior:
  - Impulse control training
  - Input from trusted others
- Mood instability:
  - Mood charting
  - Use to manage disorder
- Hallucinations:
  - Client validates perceptions
  - Identify triggers
  - Self-management techniques
- Self-esteem:
  - Set limits on ruminations or grandiosity
  - Identify strengths
  - Teach positive affirmations
  - Reality testing for irrational beliefs
- Cognitive distortions:
  - Identify patterns of dysfunctional thinking
  - Brainstorm alternative thoughts
- Social skill problems:
  - Brief, frequent contacts
  - Identify benefits of interactions
  - Set limits on intrusive behavior
  - Choose enjoyable activities
  - Peer counseling
- Helplessness/hopelessness:
  - Identify own strengths
  - Teach to advocate for self
  - Develop advance directives
- Decision-making difficulties:
  - Teach problem-solving process
- Decreased physical activity:
  - Select enjoyable form of exercise
  - Exercise with another person

- Increased physical activity:
  - Decrease environmental stimuli
  - Prevent exhaustion
- Spiritual distress:
  - Accept clients' belief system
  - Identify meaning and purpose in life
  - Refer to religious resource
- Low sex drive:
  - Teach couple that this is a symptom
  - Nonsexual expression of affection
- Inappropriate sexual behavior:
  - Teach couple that this is a symptom
  - Set limits to protect
  - Distracting activities
- Postpartum depression:
  - Teach symptoms
  - Group therapy
  - Support in home
- Hygiene:
  - Encourage ADLs
- Disrupted rhythms:
  - Reestablish normal sleep patterns
  - Establish consistent routines
- Gastrointestinal problems:
  - Six small meals
  - Finger foods
  - Increase tryptophan
  - Relieve constipation
- Weight gain:
  - Diet counseling
  - Exercise

---

6. Develop illness management teaching plans for a client with a mood disorder and her/his family.

- Discuss the impact of mood disorders on the family:
  - Stigma of mental illness
  - Frustration
  - Increased conflict
  - Anger
  - Disorder management
  - Caregiver burden
  - Financial difficulties
  - Sex problems
- Teach communication skills.
- Teach conflict management.
- Teach course of the disorder, including early signs of relapse.
- Teach self-management techniques.

---

7. Discuss the key points in effectively communicating with a person with a mood disorder.

- People who are depressed do not have the energy to talk for more than 15 to 20 minutes at a time. They may take a long time to answer questions and may need questions repeated.
- People in a manic phase are unable to concentrate or sit still for more than a few minutes during a conversation. If clients have flight of ideas, they should be refocused on the topic at hand.
- If you are unable to follow what clients are saying, try to identify underlying feelings and themes being expressed.

Explore MediaLink

For review questions, case studies, and other resources for this chapter see the Pearson Health MediaLink CD-ROM that accompanies this book and the Companion Website.

CD-ROM
- Audio Glossary
- NCLEX-RN® Review Questions
- ROAD to Critical Thinking: *Josh*
- Animations/Videos
  - Bipolar Disorder Interview–Parts 1, 2, and 3

Companion Website www.prenhall.com/fontaine
- Audio Glossary
- NCLEX-RN® Review Questions
- Case Study
  - Depressive Mood Disorder
- Care Plan
  - Assessing the Client With Mood Disorders
- Critical Thinking
  - A Manic Episode
- MediaLink Application
  - A Personal Account of Rapid-Cycling Bipolar Disorder
- MediaLinks
  - Books for Clients and Families
  - Community Resources

NCLEX-RN® Review Questions

13-1. The daughter of an 82-year-old depressed client asks the nurse why her mother has developed depression so late in life without a previous history of depression. Which of the following responses by the nurse is most appropriate?
1. "Women and older adults have higher levels of an enzyme called monoamine oxidase that results in slower signals in the brain, causing depression."
2. "Women and older adults have higher levels of a thyroid hormone which can lead to irritability, mood swings, and depression."
3. "Women and older adults have enlarged ventricles of the brain, which can lead to problems with emotional regulation and depression."
4. "Women and older adults have higher levels of chemical messengers in the brain that result in faster signals in the brain causing depression."

13-2. Which of the following outcomes indicates that a client taking lithium is responding effectively to therapy?
1. The client reports an increase in sexual desire.
2. The client verbalizes complete understanding of bipolar disorder.
3. The client completes a crossword puzzle in the daily newspaper.
4. The client reports feeling refreshed after sleeping for 3 hours.

13-3. A female client who has recently moved into a basement apartment asks the nurse what she can do to cope with her depressed mood, craving for carbohydrates, and increased appetite. Which of the following treatment modalities is most effective to recommend?
1. Phototherapy
2. Cognitive–behavioral therapy
3. Aromatherapy
4. Nutrition therapy

13-4. Which of the following symptoms can be assessed in clients with bipolar disorder during a hypomanic phase? (Select all that apply.)
1. Anhedonia
2. Guilt
3. Lack of sleep
4. Preoccupation with sex
5. Rapid speech

13-5. A 17-year-old client gave birth to her first child 2 months ago and tells the nurse in her obstetrician's office that she fears she's a terrible mother because she doesn't know what to do when her baby continues to cry after feeding and changing him. Which of the following nursing diagnoses is most appropriate for a single, new mother experiencing insomnia, lack of energy, poor concentration, and anxiety?
1. Disturbed Thought Processes related to hormonal changes
2. Risk for Self-mutilation related to feelings of guilt and shame
3. Disturbed Sensory Perceptions related to fear of parenting and anxiety
4. Ineffective Coping related to feeling overwhelmed by parenting tasks

13-6. A client with bipolar disorder has been experiencing more frequent mood swings even though his serum lithium level is 1.3 mEq/dL. Which of the following statements by the nurse would assist the client's understanding of bipolar disorder?
1. "The part of your brain that controls emotion becomes supersensitive to stress over time and it releases extra neurotransmitters, causing more rapid mood swings."
2. "Your body develops a tolerance to the medication after a few months and you need a higher dose to control the mood swings."

3. "Your sleep–wake cycle is disrupted by the medication causing you to sleep too much which, in turn, can trigger a manic episode."

4. "The shorter days in fall and winter mean you're not getting enough sunlight to produce melatonin, which affects your mood and circadian rhythm."

13-7. A client is admitted with a diagnosis of major depression. The client expresses feelings of worthlessness and a feeling of being abandoned by significant persons in her life.

Which of the following replies by the nurse conveys empathy to this client?

1. "Are you feeling like others have abandoned you?"

2. "I can understand what is going on with you."

3. "Can you tell me what you are thinking right now?"

4. "This must be a difficult time for you."

See Appendix D for answers.

References

American Psychiatric Association. (2000). *Diagnostic and statistical manual of mental disorders* (4th ed., Text revision). Washington, DC: Author.

Arnault, D. S., Sakamoto, S., & Moriwaki, A. (2005). The association between negative self-descriptions and depressive symptomology: Does culture make a difference? *Archives of Psychiatric Nursing, 19*(2), 93–100.

Aroian, K. J., & Norris, A. (2002). Assessing risk for depression among immigrants at two-year follow-up. *Archives of Psychiatric Nursing, 16*(6), 245–253.

Badner, J. A. (2003). The genetics of bipolar disorder. In B. Geller & M. P. Delbello (Eds.), *Bipolar disorder in childhood and early adolescence* (pp. 247–254). New York: Guilford Press.

Baethge, C., Baldessarini, R. J., Khalsa, H. K., Hennen, J., Salvatore, P., & Tohen, M. (2005). Substance abuse in first-episode bipolar I disorder. *American Journal of Psychiatry, 162*(5), 1008–1010.

Bailara, K. M., Henry, C., Lestage, J., Launay, J. M., Parrot, F., Swendsen, J., et al. (2005). Decreased brain tryptophan availability as a partial determinant of post-partum blues. *Psychoneuroendocrinology, 31*(3), 407–413

Basch, E. M., & Ulbricht, C. E. (2005). *Natural standard: Herb & supplement handbook.* St. Louis, MO: Elsevier Mosby.

Beck, C. T. (2003). Recognizing and screening for postpartum depression in mothers of NICU infants. *Advances in Neonatal Care, 3*(1), 37–46.

Bellivier, F., Golmard, J. L., Rietschel, M., Schulze, T. G., Malafosse, A., Preisig, M., et al. (2003). Age at onset in bipolar I affective disorder. *American Journal of Psychiatry, 160*(5), 999–1001.

Bondareff, W., Alpert, M., Friedhoff, A. J., Richter, E. M., Clary, C., & Batzar, E. (2000). Comparison of sertraline and nortriptyline in the treatment of major depressive disorder in late life. *American Journal of Psychiatry, 157*(5), 729–736.

Brommelhoff, J. A., Conway, K., Merikangas, K., & Levy, B. R. (2004). Higher rates of depression in women: Role of gender bias within the family. *Journal of Women' Health, 13*(1), 69–76.

Brown, A. B. (2004). New strategies for treatment-resistant depression. *National Alliance for Research on Schizophrenia and Depression Research Newsletter, 15*(4), 37–40.

Caetano, S. C., Kaur, S., Brambilla, P., Nicoletti, M., Hatch, J. P., Sassi, R. B., et al. (2006). Smaller cingulated volumes in unipolar depressed patients. *Biological Psychiatry, 59*(8), 702–706.

Cassano, G. B., Rucci, P., Frank, E., Fagiolini, A., Dell'Osso, L., Shear, M. K., et al. (2004). The mood spectrum in unipolar and bipolar disorder: Arguments for a unitary approach. *American Journal of Psychiatry, 161*(7), 1264–1269.

Choenarom, C., Williams, R. A., & Hagerty, B. M. (2005). The role of sense of belonging and social support on stress and depression in individuals with depression. *Archives of Psychiatric Nursing, 19,* 18–29.

Chou, J. C. Y. (2005). Eastern vs Western perspectives on depression. *Medscape Psychiatry & Mental Health, 10*(1), 1–4. Retrieved April 6, 2005, from http://www.medscape.com/viewarticle/501758

Cole, M. G., & Dendukuri, N. (2003). Risk factors for depression among elderly community subjects. *American Journal of Psychiatry, 160*(6), 1147–1156.

Davis, L. L., Rush, J. A., Wisniewski, S. R., Rice, L., Cassano, P., Jewell, M. E., et al. (2005). Substance use disorder comorbidity in major depressive disorder. *Comprehensive Psychiatry, 46*(2), 81–90.

Dopheide, J. A. (2006). Recognizing and treating depression in children and adolescents. *American Journal of Health-System Pharmacy, 63*(3), 233–243.

Draucker, C. B. (2005). Processes of mental health service use by adolescents with depression. *Journal of Nursing Scholarship, 37*(2), 155–162.

Faraone, S. V., Glatt, S. J., Su, J., & Tsuang, M. T. (2004). Three potential susceptibility loci shown by a genome-wide scan for regions influencing the age at onset of mania. *American Journal of Psychiatry, 161*(4), 625–630.

Fava, M. (2004). Daytime sleepiness and insomnia as correlates of depression. *Journal of Clinical Psychiatry,* Supplement 16, 27–32.

Fisfalen, M. E., Schulze, T. G., DePaulo, J. R., DeGroot, L. J., Badner, J. A., & McMahon, F. J. (2005). Familial variation in episode frequency in bipolar affective disorder. *American Journal of Psychiatry, 162*(7), 1266–1272.

Frazier, J. A., Chiu, S., Breeze, J. L., Makris, N., Lange, N., Kennedy, D. N., et al. (2005). Structural brain magnetic resonance imaging of limbic and thalamic volumes in pediatric bipolar disorder. *American Journal of Psychiatry, 162*(7), 1256–1265.

Ghaemi, S. N. (2004). Anxiety and bipolar disorder. *Medscape Primary Care, 6* (2), 1–4. Retrieved November 18, 2004, from http://www.medscape.com/viewarticle/492123

Gjerdingen, D. (2003). The effectiveness of various postpartum depression treatments and the impact of antidepressant drugs on nursing infants. *Journal of The American Board of Family Practice, 16*(5), 372–382.

Gladstone, G. L., Parker, G. B., Mitchell, P. B., Malhi, G. S., Wilhelm, K., & Marie-Paule, A., et al. (2004). Implications of childhood trauma for depressed women. *American Journal of Psychiatry, 161*(8), 1417–1425.

Gold, P. W., & Charney, D. S. (2002). Depression: A disease of the mind, brain, and body. *American Journal of Psychiatry, 159*(11), 1826–1827.

Goren, J. L., Stoll, A. L., Damico, K. E., Sarmiento, I. A., & Cohen, B. M. (2004). Bioavailability and lack of toxicity of s-adenosyl-l-methionine (SAMe) in humans. *Pharmacotherapy, 24*(11), 1501–1507.

Hammen, C., & Cohen, A. N. (2004). Psychosocial functioning. In S. L. Johnson & R. L. Leahy (Eds.), *Psychological treatment of bipolar disorder* (pp. 17–34). New York: Guilford Press.

Hart, L. A. (2000). Psychosocial benefits of animal companionship. In A. H. Fine (Ed.), *Handbook on animal-assisted therapy* (pp. 59–78). San Diego, CA: Academic Press.

Heilemann, M. V., Coffey-Love, M., & Frutos, L. (2004). Perceived reasons for depression among low income women of Mexican descent. *Archives of Psychiatric Nursing, 18*(5), 185–192.

Hollander, E., Pallanti, S., Allen, A., Sood, E., & Rossi, N. B. (2005). Does sustained-release lithium reduce impulsive gambling and affective instability versus placebo in pathological gamblers with bipolar spectrum disorders? *American Journal of Psychiatry, 162*(1), 137–145.

Hsu, W. C., & Lai, H. L. (2004). Effects of music on major depression in psychiatric inpatients. *Archives of Psychiatric Nursing, 18*(5), 193–199.

Hvas, A. M., Juul, S., Bech, P., & Nexo, E. (2004). Vitamin B6 level is associated with symptoms of depression. *Psychotherapy and Psychosomatics, 73*(6), 340–343.

Kabat-Zinn, J. (2003). Mindful yoga movement & meditation. *Yoga International, 70*, 86–93.

Klein, D. N., Shankman, S. A., Lewinsohn, P. M., Rohde, P., & Seeley, J. R. (2004). Family study of chronic depression in a community sample of young adults. *American Journal of Psychiatry, 161*(4), 646–653.

Larzelere, M. M., & Wiseman, P. (2002). Anxiety, depression, and insomnia. *Primary Care, 29*(2), 339–360.

Mayberg, H. S., Keightley, M., Mahurin, R. K., & Brannan, S. K. (2004). Neuropsychiatric aspects of mood and affective disorders. In S. C. Yudofsky & R. E. Hales (Eds.), *Essentials of neuropsychiatry and clinical neurosciences* (pp. 489–517). Washington, DC: American Psychiatric Publishing.

Meyer, J. H., McMain, S., Kennedy, S. H., Brown, G. M., DaSilva, J. N., Wilson, A. A., et al. (2003). Dysfunctional attitudes and 5-HT2 receptors during depression and self-harm. *American Journal of Psychiatry, 160*(1), 90–99.

Miklowitz, D. J. (2004). Family therapy. In S. L. Johnson & R. L. Leahy (Eds.), *Psychological treatment of bipolar disorder* (pp. 184–202). New York: Guilford Press.

Neumeister, A., Charney, D. S., & Drevets, W. C. (2005). Depression and the hippocampus. *American Journal of Psychiatry, 162*(6), 1057.

Oquendo, M., Brent, D. A., Birmaher, B., Greenhill, L., Kolko, D., Stanley, B., et al. (2005). Posttraumatic stress disorder comorbid with major depression. *American Journal of Psychiatry, 162*(3), 560–566.

Peden, A. R., Rayens, M. K., Hall, L. A., & Grant, E. (2005). Testing an intervention to reduce negative thinking, depressive symptoms, and chronic stressors in low-income single mothers. *Journal of Nursing Scholarship, 37*(3), 268–274.

Peden, A. R., Rayens, M. K., Hall, L. A., & Grant, E. (2004). Negative thinking and the mental health of low-income single mothers. *Journal of Nursing Scholarship, 36*(4), 337–344.

Pruett, J. R., & Luby, J. L. (2004). Recent advances in prepubertal mood disorders. *Current Opinions in Psychiatry, 17*(1), 31–36.

Quitkin, F. M., McGrath, P. J., Stewart, J. W., Deliyannides, D., Taylor, B. P., Davies, C. A., et al., (2005). *Journal of Clinical Psychiatry, 66*(6), 670–676.

Rao, U. (2003). Sleep and other biological rhythms. In B. Geller & M. P. Delbello (Eds.), *Bipolar disorder in childhood and early adolescence* (pp. 215–246). New York: Guilford Press.

Rapp, M. A., Dahlman, K., Sano, M., Grossman, H. T., Harutunian, V., & Gorman, J. M., et al. (2005). Neuropsychological differences between late-onset and recurrent geriatric major depression. *American Journal of Psychiatry, 162*(4), 691–698.

Rohan, M., Parow, A., Stoll, A. L., Demopulos, C., Friedman, S., Dager, S., et al. (2004). Title of article missing low-field magnetic stimulation in bioplar depression using an MRZ-based stimulator *American Journal of Psychiatry, 161*(1), 93–98.

Russ, N. (2003). Social support for the bipolar elderly. *Medscape Psychiatry & Mental Health, 8*(1), 1–3. Retrieved July 11, 2003, from http://www.medscape.com/viewarticle/457440

Schneck, C. D., Miklowitz, D. J., Calabrese, J. R., Allen, M. H., Thomas, M. R., Wisniewski, S. R., et al. (2004). Pheomenology of rapid-cycling bipolar disorder. *American Journal of Psychiatry, 161*(10), 1902–1908.

Schreiber, R., Stern, P. N., & Wilson, C. (2000). Being strong: How Black West-Indian Canadian women manage depression and its stigma. *Journal of Nursing Scholarship, 32*(1), 39–45.

Sethabouppha, H., & Kane, C. (2005). Caring for the seriously mentally ill in Thailand: Buddist family caregiving. *Archives of Psychiatric Nursing, 19*(2), 44–57.

Solomon, D. A., Leon, A. C., Endicott, J., Coryell, W. H., Mueller, T. I., Posternak, M. A., et al. (2003). Unipolar mania over the course of a 20-year follow-up study. *American Journal of Psychiatry, 160*(11), 2049–2051.

Spinelli, M. G. (2004). Maternal infanticide associated with mental illness. *American Journal of Psychiatry, 161*(9), 1548–1557.

Spring, B., Pingitore, R., & McChargue, D. E. (2003). Reward value of cigarette smoking for comparably heavy smoking schizophrenic, depressed, and nonpatient smokers. *American Journal of Psychiatry, 160*(2), 316–322.

Steinhauer, E. (2003). Current topic review: Psychosocial treatment of bipolar disorder. *Medscape Psychiatry & Mental Health, 8*(1), 1–3. Retrieved June 30, 2003, from http://www.medscape.com/viewarticle/457054

Strothers, H. S. 3rd, Rust, G., Minor, P., Fresh, E., Druss, B., & Satcher, D., et al. (2005). Racial disparities in depression care seen in elderly medicare patients. *Journal of the American Geriatric Society, 53*(3), 456–461.

Suppaseemanont, W. (2006). Depression in pregnancy. *The American Journal of Maternal Child Nursing, 31*(1), 10–15.

Svenningsson, P., Chergui, K., Rachleff, I., Flajolet, M., Zhang, X., Yacoubi, M. E., et al. (2006). Alterations in 5-HT1B receptor function by p11 in depression-like states. *Science, 6; 3*(5757), 77–80.

Tohen, M., Greil, W., Calabrese, J. R., Sachs, G. S., Yatham, L. N., Oerlinghausen, B. M., et al. (2005). Olanzapine versus lithium in the maintenance treatment of bipolar disorder. *American Journal of Psychiatry, 162*(7), 1281–1290.

Tohen, M., Zarate C. A., Hennen, J., Khalsa, H. K., Strakowski, S. M., Gebre-Medhin, P., et al. (2003). The McLean-Harvard first-episode mania study. *American Journal of Psychiatry, 160*(12), 2099–2107.

Trivedi, M. H., Fava, M., Wisniewski, S. R., Thase, M. E., Quitkin, F., Warden, D., et al. (2006). Medication augmentation after the failure of SSRIs for depression. *New England Journal of Medicine, 354*(12), 1243–1252.

Ugarriza, D. N. (2004). Group therapy and its barriers for women suffering from postpartum depression. *Archives of Psychiatric Nursing, 18*(2), 39–48.

Valdivia, I., & Rossy, N. (2004). Brief treatment strategies for major depressive disorder. *Topics in Advanced Practice Nursing eJournal, 4*(1), 1–12.

Weeks, S. K., McGann, R. E., Michaels, R. K., & Penninx, B. W. J. H. (2003). Comparing various short-form geriatric depression scales leads to the GDS-5/15. *Journal of Nursing Scholarship, 35*(2), 133–137.

Wehr, T. A., Duncan, W. C., Sher, L., Aeschback, D., Schwartz, P. J., Turner, E. H., et al. (2001). A circadian signal of change of season in patients with seasonal affective disorder. *Archives of General Psychiatry, 58*(12), 1108–1114.

Whooley, M. A., Avins, A. L., Miranda, J., & Browner, W. S. (1997). Case-finding instruments for depression: Two questions are as good as many. *Journal of General Internal Medicine, 12*(7), 439–445.

Wilens, T. E., Biederman, J., Kwon, A., Ditterline, J., Forkner, P., Moore, H., et al. (2004). Risk of substance use disorders in adolescents with bipolar disorder. *Journal of The American Academy of Child and Adolescent Psychiatry, 43*(11), 1380–1386.

Wisner, K. L., Perel, J. M., Peindl, K. S., Hanusa, B. H., Piontek, C. M., Findling, R. L., et al. (2004). Prevention of postpartum depression. *American Journal of Psychiatry, 161*(7), 1290–1292.

Yonkers, K. A., Wisner, K. L., Stowe, Z., Leibenluft, E., Cohen, L., Miller, L., et al. (2004). Management of bipolar disorder during pregnancy and the postpartum period. *American Journal of Psychiatry, 161*(4), 608–620.

Youngstrom, E. A., Findling, R. L., & Feeny, N. (2004). Assessment of bipolar spectrum disorders in children and adolescents. In S. L. Johnson & R. L. Leahy (Eds.), *Psychological treatment of bipolar disorder* (pp. 58–82). New York: Guilford Press.

Chapter **14**

Schizophrenic Disorders

❝ *The gold star (religious imagery) is bursting through the blackness of my life.* **❞**

—Carlos, Age 49

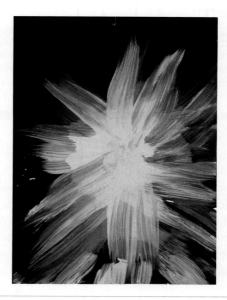

OBJECTIVES

After reading this chapter, you will be able to:

1. Discuss current thinking and research findings on the etiology of schizophrenia.

2. Compare assessment findings associated with the positive and negative characteristics of schizophrenic disorders.

3. Use the nursing process to develop a safe, comprehensive plan of care for a client with schizophrenia.

4. Develop illness management teaching plans for a person with schizophrenia and family.

5. Explain the different treatment options for a person with schizophrenia.

6. Discuss the key points in effectively communicating with a person with schizophrenia.

MediaLink www.prenhall.com/fontaine

Go to the Pearson Health MediaLink CD-ROM and the Companion Website at www.prenhall.com/fontaine for interactive resources for this chapter.

The ROAD to Critical Thinking

A Client Experiencing Paranoid Schizophrenia

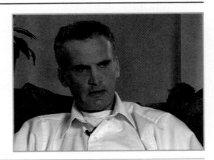

Travel this ROAD to understand Larry and his condition.

Read about Larry below and throughout this chapter.
Observe Larry on the CD-ROM accompanying this book.
Assess Larry by answering the questions at the end of this chapter.
Develop a Care Plan on the CD-ROM to address Larry's condition.

Larry

Larry has been diagnosed with paranoid schizophrenia. He had his "first difficulties" in seventh grade but was able to function fairly well until he went off to college. There, his symptoms became more severe, and, by his junior year, it was difficult for him to even make it to class. Currently, he volunteers as a clerk in a library.

Schizophrenia is a psychotic illness and onset is usually between late adolescence and early adulthood, as you see in Larry's experience. People with this disorder generally have problems with memory, attention, executive function, and affective symptoms, which often make activities of daily living difficult.

Schizophrenia is a disorder of the brain, like epilepsy or multiple sclerosis. It is diagnosed in about 1% of the U.S. population and is a devastating and often disabling disorder that affects not only the individual, but also family, friends, and the community as a whole. Although it is referred to as a single disease, it is more accurately a spectrum of disorders, characterized by a broad range of symptoms, physiologic malfunctions, etiologies, and prognoses. Included in the syndrome of schizophrenia are schizoid personality disorder, schizotypal personality disorder, paranoid personality disorder, schizoaffective disorder, schizophreniform disorder, delusional disorder, brief psychotic disorder, shared psychotic disorder, and schizophrenia. Relatives of people who have schizophrenia are often included in the spectrum since they are thought to have a genetic predisposition to schizophrenia but might not necessarily demonstrate full or any clinical manifestations of schizophrenia (Gottesman & Petronis, 2003; Seeman, 2004).

KNOWLEDGE BASE

Psychosis is a general term used to refer to the experience of pervasive mental changes, such as the inability to think clearly, perceive correctly, and manage intense emotions. Individuals with psychosis experience delusions (fixed, false beliefs) and hallucinations (abnormal sensory perceptions). Behavior and thinking both are disorganized. Psychosis can occur with any number of mental disorders representing the far end of the continuum of symptoms in each disorder.

In **schizoaffective disorder,** clients have symptoms that appear to be a mixture of schizophrenia and the mood disorders. The person experiences one or more of the following

psychotic symptoms: delusions, hallucinations, disorganized speech, disorganized behavior, or negative symptoms. In addition, the person experiences symptoms of the mood disorders, which may be major depressive symptoms, manic symptoms, or mixed symptoms. Schizoaffective disorder is most likely a distinct syndrome resulting from a high genetic liability to mood disorders and schizophrenia both. The age of onset, as with schizophrenia, is typically late adolescence or early adulthood. Like mood disorders, however, schizophrenia is much more common in women than in men. Women are also much more likely than men to have their diagnosis switched from schizophrenia to schizoaffective disorder. Clients with schizoaffective disorder often have difficulty maintaining job or school functioning, experience problems with self-care, are socially isolated, and often have suicidal ideation. The prognosis of schizoaffective disorder is somewhat better than for schizophrenia but significantly worse than the prognosis for mood disorders (Siever & Davis, 2004).

In **brief psychotic disorder**, there is a rapid onset of at least one of the following psychotic symptoms: delusions, hallucinations, disorganized speech, or disorganized and strange behavior. The episode lasts at least 1 day but less than 1 month, after which the person returns to the premorbid level of functioning. The symptoms of **schizophreniform disorder** are the same but last at least 1 month and less than 6 months. One third of those with schizophreniform disorder return to premorbid level of functioning, whereas two thirds progress to the diagnosis of schizophrenia or schizoaffective disorder. In a **shared psychotic disorder**, a person who is in a close relationship with another person who is delusional comes to share the delusional beliefs. This most commonly occurs between two people but may involve more individuals, such as when children adopt a parent's delusional beliefs (American Psychiatric Association [APA], 2000).

Cluster A personality disorders appear to be related to schizophrenia: *schizoid, schizotypal,* and *paranoid personality disorders.* Those with the personality disorders experienced disordered thinking and social withdrawal similar to those with schizophrenia but to a milder degree. Viewed on a continuum, schizophrenia is on the far end, with more severe symptoms, compared with the cluster A personality disorders (Keshavan et al., 2005). Personality disorders are covered in chapter 16 ∞.

Schizophrenia is a combination of disordered thinking, perceptual disturbances, behavioral abnormalities, affective disruptions, and impaired social competency. This means the person has difficulty thinking clearly, knowing what is real, managing feelings, making decisions, and relating to others. Typically, the person is fairly normal early in life, experiences subtle changes after puberty, and undergoes severe symptoms in the late teens to early adulthood. The early age of onset often shatters the lives of its victims and robs them of the opportunity for a productive adult life.

The onset and progression of schizophrenia are variable. It is believed that people with an abrupt onset of the illness have a different form of schizophrenia than those whose onset is more insidious. The majority develops the disorder in adolescence or young adulthood, with only 10% to 15% of cases first diagnosed in people older than 45. In some cases, the disorder progresses through relapse and remission; in other cases, it takes a long-term, stable course; while in some clients, a long-term, progressively deteriorating course evolves. Much too often, the illness results in lifelong problems coping with everyday living that reflect irreversible neurobiological deficits. Early diagnosis and treatment may reduce chronicity and improve the prognosis of people with schizophrenia. Women tend to have a later onset of illness, better treatment response, shorter and less frequent relapses, and an overall higher quality of life than their male counterparts (Seeman, 2004).

Larry:

❝ I had my first initial difficulties in seventh grade. It actually went unnoticed for many years. I was able to function in the academic community for many years. When I was in my senior year of high school, it manifested itself in a large way. They hospitalized me with an initial diagnosis of nervous breakdown. But then when I moved on to Tufts University, it blossomed into a real problem. I was able to complete my senior year of high school and I did spend two years at college—two very rough years at college. ❞

Individuals with schizophrenia have a 20% shorter life expectancy than the general population. Accidents, suicide, and homicide account for one third of these premature deaths. Two thirds die of coronary heart disease, hypertension, emphysema, or complications of type 2 diabetes mellitus. In part, this is attributable to a lifestyle with poor dietary habits, obesity, high rates of smoking, and the use of alcohol and street drugs. Side effects of antipsychotic medication include weight gain and metabolic syndrome (Ryan, Collins, & Thakore, 2003).

The classic subtypes described in the *Diagnostic and Statistical Manual of Mental Disorders* (4th ed., Text Revision) (DSM-IV-TR) (undifferentiated, catatonic, paranoid, disorganized, and residual) are difficult to apply and have many symptoms in common. Diagnoses are often changed from one category to another as symptoms fluctuate and, thus, the classification is unstable. See the DSM-IV-TR Criteria feature for the descriptions of the subtypes of schizophrenia. The classic subtypes have given way to new systems of classification. The most widely used system is one of positive symptoms, negative symptoms, and thought disorganization. This arrangement represents symptom types that are probably semi-independent of one another. To make sense of these groups, understand that positive does not mean good, and negative does not mean bad. Rather, **positive symptoms** are excessive or added behaviors that are not normally seen in mentally healthy adults. For example, healthy adults do not experience delusions; therefore, delusions are a positive symptom. Women are more likely to exhibit more positive than negative symptoms. Positive symptoms are most likely the result of physiological changes, including increased dopamine (DA) function in the subcortical areas of the brain and decreased glucose utilization in the brain. Medication is often successful in diminishing positive symptoms. Table 14.1 ■ lists the positive symptoms of schizophrenia.

Negative symptoms are the loss of normal function normally seen in mentally healthy adults. For example, healthy adults are able to complete activities of daily living (ADLs); therefore, an inability to care for oneself is a negative symptom of schizophrenia. Negative symptoms are related to decreased motivation and drive, the inability to express feelings, and the lack of spontaneity and curiosity. Negative symptoms are listed in Table 14.1. Men are more likely to exhibit prominent negative symptoms. Negative symptoms are most likely related to anatomical changes and decreased DA function in the prefrontal cortex. These symptoms are more treatment resistant.

Deficit schizophrenia is a distinct subtype of schizophrenia characterized by significant and persistent negative symptoms. Individuals with deficit schizophrenia often experience an insidious onset of schizophrenia, a progressive deteriorating course, poor social and occupational functioning, and resistance to antipsychotic medication. Evidence suggests that the deficit syndrome has important genetic or family environmental components (Galderisi et al., 2002).

DSM-IV-TR　Diagnostic Criteria for Schizophrenia Subtypes

Paranoid Type

A type of Schizophrenia in which the following criteria are met:

A. Preoccupation with one or more delusions or frequent auditory hallucinations.

B. None of the following is prominent: disorganized speech, disorganized or catatonic behavior, or flat or inappropriate affect.

Disorganized Type

A type of Schizophrenia in which the following criteria are met:

A. All of the following are prominent:
   1. Disorganized speech
   2. Disorganized behavior
   3. Flat or inappropriate affect

B. The criteria are not met for Catatonic Type.

Catatonic Type

A type of Schizophrenia in which the clinical picture is dominated by at least two of the following:

1. Motoric immobility as evidenced by catalepsy (including waxy flexibility) or stupor
2. Excessive motor activity (that is apparently purposeless and not influenced by external stimuli)
3. Extreme negativism (an apparently motiveless resistance to all instructions or maintenance of a rigid posture against attempts to be moved) or mutism
4. Peculiarities of voluntary movement as evidenced by posturing (voluntary assumption of inappropriate or bizarre postures), stereotyped movements, prominent mannerisms, or prominent grimacing
5. Echolalia or echopraxia

Undifferentiated Type

A type of Schizophrenia in which symptoms that meet Criterion A are present, but the criteria are not met for the Paranoid, Disorganized, or Catatonic Type.

Residual Type

A type of Schizophrenia in which the following criteria are met:

A. Absence of prominent delusions, hallucinations, disorganized speech, and grossly disorganized or catatonic behavior.

B. There is continuing evidence of the disturbance, as indicated by the presence of negative symptoms or two or more symptoms listed in Criterion A for Schizophrenia, present in an attenuated form (e.g., odd beliefs, unusual perceptual experiences).

SOURCE: Reprinted with permission from the Diagnostic and Statistical Manual of Mental Disorders, Fourth Edition, Text Revision, (Copyright 2000). American Psychiatric Association.

TABLE 14.1	Symptoms of Schizophrenia

Positive Symptoms	Negative Symptoms
Behavioral	
Hyperactivity	Decreased activity level
Bizarre behavior	Limited speech; conversation difficult
	Minimal self-care
Affective	
Inappropriate affect	Blunted or flat affect
Overreactive affect	Anhedonia
Hostility	
Perceptual	
Hallucinations	Inability to understand sensory information
Sensory overload	
Cognitive	
Delusions	Concrete thinking
Disorganized thinking	Attention impairment
Loose associations	Memory deficits
Suspiciousness	Impaired problem solving
	Lack of motivation
Social	
Aloof and stilted interactions	Social withdrawal, isolation
	Poor rapport with others
	Inadequate social and occupational skills

Comorbid Disorders

Many people with schizophrenia use *alcohol* or *drugs* to self-medicate and feel better. More than 50% of people with schizophrenia have problems with alcohol or drugs at some point during their illness. More than half are nicotine dependent. Prompt recognition and treatment of this *dual diagnosis* problem is essential for effective treatment. Substance-related disorders are discussed in chapter 15. ∞

Suicide accounts for the majority of premature deaths among people with schizophrenia. It is estimated that as many as half this population experience suicidal ideation, make suicide attempts, or both. Ten percent are successful suicides. Risk factors include young age, high socioeconomic status background, high IQ with a high level of preillness academic achievement, and a severe course of the disorder (Practice Guideline for the Treatment of Patients with Schizophrenia, 2004).

Comorbid *anxiety disorders*, especially social anxiety disorder, are present in more than half the people with schizophrenia. Because anxiety disorders are also disabling, the combination contributes to a more severe level of disability and decreased quality of life. Individuals with both disorders are less able to work, have poorer interpersonal relationships, and struggle more with ADLs (Pallanti, Quercioli, & Hollander, 2004).

Twenty-five percent of people with schizophrenia also experience obsessions and compulsions and, of this group, 26% could be diagnosed with *obsessive–compulsive disorder*. Typically, people are preoccupied with the content of their delusions and may ruminate for hours over their upsetting thoughts (Nechmad et al., 2003).

People with late-onset schizophrenia, diagnosed at age 50 or older, appear to be at high risk for Alzheimer's disease. In one study, half the subjects developed dementia between 1 and 5 years following a diagnosis of schizophrenia (Brodaty, Sachdev, Koschera, Monk, & Cullen, 2003).

Etiologies

The etiology of schizophrenia is unknown, but many studies support the view of environmental factors and genetic susceptibility as causes. In some individuals, a genetic defect may contribute to abnormal development of the brain or a neurochemical malfunction, whereas in other cases, factors such as nutrition, toxins, or trauma might interact in a genetically vulnerable person, resulting in schizophrenia. In still other cases, the cause may be completely environmental, such as viral infections or birth complications.

Genetics

It is well recognized that there is a genetic component in schizophrenia and it is thought that 85% of susceptibility to schizophrenia may be genetic. However, the amount of genetic vulnerability is not known because no single gene has been identified as a risk factor for schizophrenia. It is likely that a number of genes are involved and that different genes may be involved in different families. There may also be a different pattern of inheritance in early-onset versus late-onset schizophrenia. It is likely that the early-onset type has a higher genetic load for schizophrenia (Gochman et al., 2004).

A person has an 8% risk for schizophrenia if a sibling has the disorder, a 13% risk if one parent is affected, a 10% to 15% risk of sharing the disorder with a dizygotic twin, a 40% to 50% risk if both parents are affected, and a 50% risk if a monozygotic twin has schizophrenia. In addition, 21% of first-degree relatives of individuals with schizophrenia have schizotypal personality disorder or other traits in the schizophrenic spectrum (Tamminga, Thaker, & Medoff, 2004). Figure 14.1 ■ illustrates the average risk for development of schizophrenia.

In monozygotic twins, prenatal factors do not always affect each twin to the same extent. Because the hands are formed at the same time cells are migrating to the cerebral cortex during the second trimester of pregnancy, they have been a site for the

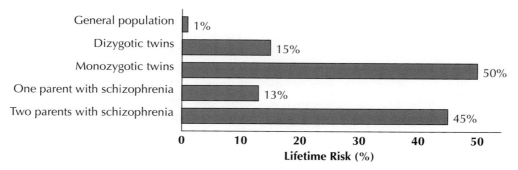

Figure 14.1 ■ Average risk for developing schizophrenia.

SOURCES: Gottesman, I. I, & Petronis, A. (2003). Schizophrenia genetics obscured by the realities of complex diseases. *NAMI Advocate, 1*(4), 31–32; Siever, L. J., & Davis, K. L. (2004). The pathophysiology of schizophrenia disorders: Perspectives from the spectrum. *American Journal of Psychiatry, 161*(3), 398–413; Tamminga, C. A., Thaker, G. K., & Medoff, D. R. (2004). Neuropsychiatric aspects of schizophrenia. In S. C. Yudofsky & R. E. Hales (Eds.), *Essentials of neuropsychiatry and clinical neurosciences* (pp. 457–487). Washington, DC: American Psychiatric Publishing.

indirect study of brain development. In studying sets of twins in which one has schizophrenia and the other does not, it was found that the affected twin had a number of small deformities in the hands and greater differences in fingerprints than the sibling. There was also a significant prenatal size difference between the twins during the second trimester. Conditions that could result in brain injury at this stage of development include anemia, anoxia, ischemia, maternal alcohol or drug abuse, toxin exposure, or viral infection (Tarrant & Jones, 2000).

Advanced paternal age may be a risk factor for schizophrenia and the other schizophrenia spectrum disorders. Compared with children of fathers younger than 25 years, the risk doubled for children of fathers in their 40s and tripled in children of men older than 50. The etiology is believed to involve mutations in the sperm (Sipos et al., 2005).

The more protective factors a person has, the less the chance of development of the disorder. Only a few people have such a strong genetic vulnerability that schizophrenia is almost inevitable. The majority of the population has little or no risk for schizophrenia. In between are the people who may develop the disorder if stressed enough but who could also survive and not experience schizophrenia if not sufficiently stressed.

Neurobiology

Neurodevelopment studies demonstrate evidence of abnormal brain development in persons with schizophrenia. The basic flaw seems to be that certain nerve cells migrate to the wrong areas when the brain is first taking shape, leaving small regions of the brain permanently out of place or miswired. In some cases, the neurons of the cortex may be deficient. From a developmental perspective it is not known whether these cells form normally and then fail to thrive or whether they are malformed from the beginning.

The question arises, if schizophrenia begins in utero, why does it not manifest for 20 years? Recent studies show that some people with schizophrenia may have early signs that are overlooked or misunderstood. For example, a child might sit up a month later than other children or speak 3 months later than other children. These signs may indicate a slight maturational lag in brain function that is later associated with schizophrenia. Later in childhood, there may be evidence of lagging development and cognitive perceptual abnormalities.

One factor related to the delay in the appearance of significant symptoms may be formation of the myelin sheath, which does not form on the outside of many brain cells until late adolescence. Between the ages of 16 and 22, there are also progressive changes in cortical interactions, especially between the left prefrontal and temporal regions. This failure of the cortex to reorganize during adolescence may be the final neurodevelopmental failure of schizophrenia.

Neurochemical factors likely involve DA, serotonin (5-HT), norepinephrine (NE), glutamate (glu), and gamma-aminobutyric acid (GABA) neurotransmission. At times, neurotransmitters work together (synergistically) to trigger the same biochemical reaction, while at other times they act as antagonists, with one inhibiting the action of another. Glu, involved in learning and memory, may be responsible for some of the cognitive symptoms of schizophrenia. Glu is necessary for the breakdown of DA and other transmitters, which affects the efficiency of prefrontal information processing. Glu receptors have a role in regulating the migration and pruning of neurons during brain development and, thus, may play a role in the structural abnormalities that have been seen in schizophrenia. Excessively high levels of NE are associated with positive symptoms, while paranoid symptoms have been related to increased DA activity. No single neurotransmitter is clearly responsible for schizophrenia. The important concept may be homeostasis: the absolute level of any neurotransmitter being much less important than its relative level with respect to all other transmitters. There may also be an undiscovered neurochemical factor. It will be a long time before this is understood clearly (Keltner, 2005; Yasuno et al., 2004).

A new area of research involves the *fat composition* of cell membranes. The neuronal membrane consists of two layers of fatty molecules, which determine the flexibility of the membrane. Soft and pliable membranes communicate more smoothly than stiff and rigid membranes. People with schizophrenia are depleted of both DHA (docosahexaenoic acid found in omega-3-type fish oil) and AA (arachidonic acid). These deficiencies may be related to the negative symptoms of schizophrenia.

On a larger scale, new brain imaging studies have revealed abnormalities of *brain structure* in schizophrenia. Although no single brain region has been found to be involved in the pathology of schizophrenia, the areas most noted for abnormalities include the prefrontal cortex, temporal lobes, hippocampus, limbic system, thalamus, and ventricles. The reason people with schizophrenia may not "look the same" clinically may be a function of individual deviations in brain structure. In some cases, tissue volume is decreased in specific areas; in others, cerebral blood flow is disrupted; in some clients, utilization of glucose and oxygen is decreased; and in still more, ventricular size is decreased. Individuals with childhood-onset schizophrenia demonstrate greater loss of cortical gray matter than those with later development of the disorder. The corpus callosum is defective in some people with schizophrenia. The resulting misconnection of the hemispheres may contribute to the affective symptoms and social isolation (Brambilla et al., 2005; Gogtay et al., 2004; Kim, Ha, & Kwon, 2004). See Box 14.1 for a list of brain abnormalities.

An example of one deviation is that decreased blood flow to the thalamus may affect the ability of the brain to filter sensory signals, causing a person to be flooded with sensory in-

BOX 14.1	Central Nervous System Abnormalities in Schizophrenia

Increased Ventricular Size

Decreased Volume

- Temporal lobes
- Hippocampus
- Prefrontal cortex
- Limbic system
- Thalamus

Decreased Cerebral Blood Flow

- Temporal lobes
- Basal ganglia
- Thalamus

Decreased Blood Glucose and Oxygen Utilization

- Frontal lobes
- Basal ganglia

Decreased Activity

- Prefrontal cortex

Decreased Nicotinic Receptors

- Hippocampus

formation (refer to Figure 14.2 ■). Changes in cerebral blood flow suggest abnormalities in the density, size, or configuration of blood vessels in a person with schizophrenia. Structural abnormalities are really only the result of some abnormal process and do not tell us much about the process.

For some people with schizophrenia, there is a deficiency of **nicotinic receptors** in the hippocampus, an area of the brain important in attention to new sensory stimuli and memory formation. Clients who smoke may be self-medicating with nicotine, which improves their attentiveness and ability to lay down memories. Nicotine may be especially reinforcing because it stimulates DA release in the nucleus accumbens and

the prefrontal cortex. DA deficiency and low activity in these regions are linked to the negative symptoms of schizophrenia. Only about 25% of the general U.S. population smokes, compared with 58% to 92% of people with schizophrenia. Nicotine addiction, therefore, is a serious problem for people with this disorder (Olincy et al., 2006).

Diathesis-Stress Model

The *diathesis-stress model* portrays the psychosis of schizophrenia as a final common result of neurodevelopmental, neurochemical, and structural abnormalities. This is a multiple-hit model in that there must be a genetic vulnerability and environmental risk factors, which are then combined with maturational changes or life events that trigger the onset of schizophrenia.

Studies suggest that environmental factors play a critical role in schizophrenia. Most of these factors occur early in development, particularly during pregnancy. Several maternal *infections* have been linked to schizophrenia. These infections include rubella, herpes simplex, polio, toxoplasmosis, varicella-zoster, and second-trimester influenza. When people are exposed to infectious agents, cytokines mediate the immune response. In maternal infections high levels of cytokines cause fetal brain damage (Bachmann, Schröder, Bottmer, Torrey & Yolken, 2005; Brown et al., 2004; Torrey & Yolken, 2003).

Obstetric complications are more frequent in people with schizophrenia and have been linked to earlier onset and greater severity of the disorder. There are three main categories of complications. The first is problems during pregnancy such as bleeding, preeclampsia, diabetes, and rhesus incompatibility. The second is problems with fetal growth and development, such as congenital malformations, small head circumference, and low birth weight. The third is complications during delivery, such as asphyxia, uterine atony, and emergency cesarean section. In addition, intrauterine exposure to famine is associated with an increased incidence of schizophrenia (Cannon, Jones, & Murray, 2002; St. Clair et al., 2005).

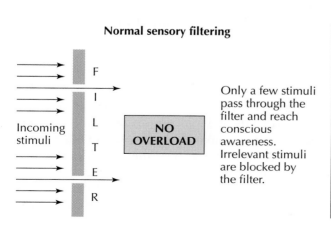

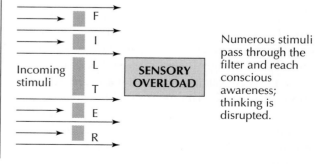

Figure 14.2 ■ Impaired sensory filtering in schizophrenia.

Psychopharmacological Interventions

During the first episode of schizophrenia, the majority of individuals respond quickly to relatively low doses of antipsychotic medication. Later episodes require higher doses, and 5% to 25% of people with schizophrenia become resistant to the effects of medications. In addition, side effects force other clients to decrease or stop their medication, which is a significant factor in relapse. The determination of which medication to use is often made on the basis of an individual side effect profile, which is determined by medication history. If an individual has a history of extrapyramidal symptoms side effects, she or he would most likely be prescribed a second-generation antipsychotic. If she or he is prone to weight gain and high blood lipid levels, she or he would most likely be prescribed a first-generation antipsychotic (Navon & Ozer, 2003). Chapter 10 ∞ discusses these medications in more detail.

When added to antipsychotic medications, *mood-stabilizing agents* such as lithium carbonate, Tegretol (carbamazepine), and Valproate (depakote) enhance the effectiveness of the response and improve negative symptoms specifically. They are also effective for people experiencing affective symptoms. *Benzodiazepines* may also be used as adjuncts to antipsychotic medications for agitation or catatonic symptoms. Studies have shown reductions in anxiety, agitation, and psychotic symptoms with the use of these agents.

The use of medications in older clients is problematic at times. These individuals are likely to have other medical illnesses and to be taking multiple medications. Because of their age, older clients are at increased risk for drug interactions and side effects. Low doses of the second-generation antipsychotics are the drugs of choice.

Multidisciplinary Interventions
Psychiatric Rehabilitation

The field of **psychiatric** (or **psychosocial**) **rehabilitation** grew out of a need to create opportunities for people with persistent psychiatric disability. The rehabilitation approach emphasizes the development of skills and support necessary for successful living, learning, and working in the community. This approach creates *collaborative partnerships* with all interested people—clients, families, friends, and mental health providers. It is assumed that the client will be "in charge" with regard to setting goals for where and how to live, work, learn, socialize, and enjoy recreation (see Box 14.2). Rehabilitation is a process, not a quick fix. It is also different than the traditional approach to long-term clients, which assumes that people with schizophrenia cannot make decisions and will continue to deteriorate in spite of interventions. It is now known that a substantial number of people with schizophrenia make good adjustments and lead satisfactory lives.

BOX 14.2	Beliefs and Values in Psychiatric Rehabilitation

Beliefs

- The most severely disabled psychiatric client has a potential for productivity.
- The opportunity to be gainfully employed is a generative force in human beings.
- Work can enhance self-esteem and reduce symptoms of mental illness.
- People require opportunities to be together socially.

Values

- Hope, optimism
- Wellness
- Choices
- Self-determination
- Individual responsibility
- Compassion

People who have severe and persistent mental illness differ little from the general population. They want work that is meaningful and self-enhancing and the opportunity to socialize with others. Psychiatric rehabilitation is anchored in the values of hope and optimism that people can grow, learn, and make changes in their lives. Other values include promotion of choices, self-determination, and individual responsibility. The essential element of self-help is *power*. People who are persistently ill need power and control in their relationships with professionals, in their own lives, and in the way resources are allocated. This allows them to take personal responsibility for where they are in their lives and where they are going (Lecomte, Wallace, Perreault, & Caron, 2005).

A nurse who functions as a resource for clients must not only be competent, but also be compassionate and caring. This includes searching for talents and skills in clients, even when these traits are obscured by multiple relapses and low self-esteem. The nurse's role is to teach skills, to coach skills as needed in a variety of social and work situations, and to identify supports in the community of choice. In this way, the nurse will promote independent living and successful coping for people with psychiatric disabilities.

Group Therapy

Group therapy is an effective psychosocial treatment method for persons with schizophrenia. It helps prevent the withdrawal and social isolation that may occur for people who are persistently ill. For those who live alone, the group may be their primary opportunity to relate to others. The group setting also provides an opportunity to discuss and help one another solve problems in everyday living, employment difficulties, or interpersonal conflicts. There are several types of group therapy. Some groups are highly structured, while others may be more spontaneous. Some may have a very narrow topic range, such as assertiveness training, while others may have a broader range, such as general problems living in the community. Groups focus on peer support, with an emphasis on development skills and changing behavior. Groups are also used for teaching and social support. See chapter 9 ∞ for more information on group therapy.

Assertive Community Treatment

People who are psychiatrically disabled are often ill prepared to find and maintain the multiple services needed to function in the community. One approach to help clients is the assertive community treatment (ACT) program. Clients are assigned to a specific multidisciplinary team that delivers all services when and where the client needs them. The main goal of the program is to prevent rehospitalization by providing comprehensive, integrated community services. The ACT program provides 24-hour coverage, including emergencies. Studies show that ACT reduces time spent in the hospital, improves housing stability, decreases the occurrence of symptoms, and improves quality of life (Marshall & Lockwood, 2000). Various other treatment settings within the community are discussed in chapter 3. ∞

Electroconvulsive Therapy

Electroconvulsive therapy (ECT) may be used in combination with second-generation antipsychotics for individuals with schizophrenia or schizoaffective disorder who have not responded to medication alone. Other candidates for ECT are

---

Using Research Evidence Schizophrenia and Physical Activity

Beebe, L. H. (2006). Describing the health parameters of outpatients with schizophrenia. *Applied Nursing Research, 19*, 43–47.

What is the study about?

Examine, among persons living with schizophrenia, physical health parameters and psychiatric symptoms as related to those three types of disease.

How was the study done?

- Quantitative descriptive pilot study of 11 veterans living with schizophrenia (9 men, 2 women) and receiving care from a veteran's outpatient facility in the Southeast.
- Sample included 9 Whites and 2 African Americans.
- Approved by an institutional review board.
- Investigated participant aerobic fitness, body mass index (BMI), body fat, severity of psychopathology, and perceptions of their own health.
- All participants medically approved to participate in a moderate exercise program; none reported a history of cardiovascular, neuromuscular, endocrine, or other disorders that would bar safe participation in the study.
- A trained research assistant unaware of treatment grouping obtained data over an 8-week period.
- All data obtained at same time of day to control for possible circadian variation and medication effects.
- Physical health measured by BMI, body fat percentages, and test of aerobic fitness: the 6-minute walking distance (6MWD).
- BMI calculated using height in meters and weight in kilograms.
- Body fat percentage assessed via three skinfold measures using calipers at three specific body sites.
- In 6MWD, participants walked around a path until signaled to stop; distance was measured to nearest foot.
- Severity of psychopathology measured by Positive and Negative Syndrome Scale (PANSS) and self-reported health perception by Duke Health Profile.

What were the results of the study?

- Subjects walked a distance ranging from 1,114 to 1,912 feet, with an average of 1,407 feet. Healthy men and women walk an average of 1,641 feet. BMIs ranged from 21.83 to 43.09, with an average of 31.58.

- 10 of 11 subjects exceeded the Centers for Disease Control (CDC) threshold for overweight (BMI between 25 and 29.9); 7 fell into the CDC category of obese (BMI>30).
- PANSS showed that the men were less ill on all scales than the women.
- White patients (n=9) had more negative symptoms and African American patients (n=2) more positive symptoms.
- Duke questionnaire revealed that none of the participants saw themselves as having a disability due to their diagnosis of schizophrenia, yet all had a history of inconsistent work patterns and 9 collected disability benefits from Veterans Affairs.
- Most common physical diagnoses were hypertension and peptic ulcer disease; the most commonly prescribed medications were antihypertensives.

What additional questions might I have?

- What results would be found from a larger sample?
- Since this was a pilot study, what follow-up studies might be planned to validate findings?
- How long had the participants been diagnosed with schizophrenia, and did length of diagnosis correlate with poorer physical health outcomes?
- What was the age range of the subjects; did younger patients experience fewer or milder physical health problems?

How can I use this study?

- Nurses caring for persons living with schizophrenia need to promote health by being attuned both to patients' mental and physical health.
- This kind of health promotion will involve addressing not only mental status but also physical fitness, good nutrition, and staying physically well.
- Nurses must monitor the physical health parameters of persons living with schizophrenia and make referrals as needed.
- All patients who receive medical clearance should be encouraged to participate in a physical fitness regimen.

SOURCE: Contributed by Dolores Huffman, PhD, RN, Associate Professor of Nursing, Purdue University Calumet, Hammond, Indiana.

people with unremitting depressive symptoms or severe suicidal ideation and behaviors (Practice Guideline, 2004).

Alternative Therapies

Transcranial Magnetic Stimulation

Transcranial magnetic stimulation (TMS) is the use of a magnetic field that passes through the skull, which causes cells in the cerebral cortex to fire. More studies have been conducted in the use of TMS for depression than for schizophrenia. Initial studies indicate that TMS of the left temporal-parietal area may decrease the frequency and duration of auditory hallucinations and may modulate other symptoms of schizophrenia (Saenger, 2004).

Omega-3 Fatty Acids

Individuals with a deficiency of omega-3 fatty acids will find the addition of fish oil helpful. It may not be that people with schizophrenia have a low intake, rather that they need more to overcome a metabolic disorder that uses up essential fatty acids at a faster rate. Initial studies suggest that omega-3 fatty acids reduce positive and negative symptoms and dyskinesia side effects. The recommended dosage is 5 g/day, usually seven or eight capsules. The maximum dosage is 15 g/day. Taking the capsules at night and with orange juice cuts down on the fishy aftertaste (Emsley, Myburgh, Oosthuizen, & van Rensburg, 2002).

Aromatherapy

Olfactory receptors are the only sensory pathways that open directly to the brain. Nerve cells relay this information directly to the limbic system, influencing emotions and behavior. Inhaling essential oils through the use of a diffuser or using essential oils in massage may be beneficial in inducing a sense of calmness. The following oils are the most helpful: basil, bergamot, chamomile, frankincense, juniper, lavender, lemon balm, and sandalwood. Coriander increases memory and mental function.

Acupuncture

The Chinese claim to have successfully treated schizophrenia with acupuncture. Research in Western medical practice is just beginning in this area. A 6-month study in Texas showed a decrease in the duration of hospital stays for acupuncture-treated individuals (Gerber, 2000).

Nursing Process

A CLIENT WITH SCHIZOPHRENIA

ASSESSMENT

The assessment of client responses to illness and functional status includes assessment of client reports, family or caregiver reports, and direct observation of performance. Clients who are not acutely ill are usually able to provide accurate information about their history with psychiatric disability and their current experiences.

If clients are acutely ill, it may be difficult to obtain information from them directly. This is especially true for those experiencing delusions and hallucinations. Family members, roommates, friends, group-home supervisors, or case managers may be the initial data sources when a client is admitted to the acute care setting. The Focused Nursing Assessment provides questions that can be used in the home, the residential or group-home setting, or the acute care setting.

Assessment: Behavior

Catatonia is a frequent psychomotor syndrome in people with schizophrenia. **Catatonic excitement** includes hyperactivity and bizarre behavior and is a positive symptom of the disorder. *Hyperactive behavior* most typically occurs during a period of relapse. Excitement may become so great that it threatens the person's safety or that of others. Behavior may also be unpredictable. Schizophrenia can cause people to engage in *bizarre behavior* such as repeating rhythmic gestures, doing ritualistic postures, or demonstrating freakish facial or body movements. Some people will imitate other people's movements (*echopraxia*) or words (*echolalia*) or may senselessly repeat the same word or phrase for hours or days. Another positive characteristic is a *decreased awareness of one's own behavior*. It is not unusual to hear clients describe their behavior as being under the influence of alien forces or of other people (Kruger, Bagby, Hoffler, & Braunig, 2003).

Catatonic inhibition involves decreased activity level, limited speech, minimal self-care, and, at times, a trancelike state. Catatonic inhibition is a negative symptom of schizophrenia. The *decreased activity level* includes a reduction of energy, initiative, and spontaneity. There is a loss of natural gracefulness in body movements that results in poor coordination: Activities may be carried out in a robotlike fashion. People with schizophrenia often have *limited speech*, referred to as *alogia*, which makes it difficult for them to carry on a continuous conversation or say anything new. They may say very little on their own initiative or in response to questions from others; some individuals with schizophrenia may be mute for several hours to several days. Some clients experience decreased responsiveness and appear to be in a *trancelike state*.

TABLE 14.2	Descriptors of Affect
Affect	**Example**
Appropriate	Juan cries when learning of the death of his father.
Inappropriate	When told it is time to turn off the TV and go to bed, Joe begins to laugh uproariously.
Stable	During a card game, Don smiles and laughs at the appropriate social interchanges.
Labile	During a friendly checkers game, Sean, who has been laughing, suddenly knocks the board off the table in anger. He then begins to laugh and wants to continue the game.
Elevated	Connor bounces around the cafeteria, laughing and singing and telling his classmates how wonderful everything is.
Depressed	Leo sits slumped in a chair with a sad facial expression, teary eyes, and minimal body movement.
Overreactive	Kathy screams and curses when her child spills a glass of milk on the floor.
Blunted	When Tom learns of his full-tuition scholarship, he responds with only a small smile.
Flat	When Juanita's mother tells her that her favorite dog has died, Juanita simply says, "Oh," and gives no indication of an emotional response.

Another difficulty for individuals and their significant others is a deterioration in appearance and manners. *Self-care* may become *minimal*; clients may need to be reminded to bathe, shave, brush their teeth, and change their clothes. Because of confusion and distraction, people with schizophrenia may not conform to social norms of dress and behavior.

Only a minority of people with schizophrenia demonstrate *violent behavior*. Risk factors include male sex; being poor, unskilled, or uneducated; a history of arrests; and a history of violent behavior. Some clients become violent when they act on the basis of their delusions and hallucinations. Comorbid alcohol and drug abuse increases the risk for violent behavior, as does severe akathisia (Practice Guideline, 2004).

Joran describes what led up to his admission to the acute care setting. "My girlfriend and I were at the bar and I was talking to a lady I knew and, when we got home, my girlfriend accused me of flirting. I told her I was just talking to the woman—someone I haven't seen in a long time. I told her I don't get jealous when I see her talking to men she knows. Then things went crazy and I pulled out my gun and threatened to kill her and myself."

Assessment: Affect

Positive affective characteristics include inappropriate affect, overreactive affect, and hostility. *Inappropriate affect* occurs when the person's emotional tone is not related to the immediate circumstances. An *overreactive affect* is appropriate to the situation but out of proportion to it.

Negative affective characteristics include blunted or flat affect and anhedonia. A *blunted affect* describes a dulled emotional response to a situation, and a *flat affect* describes the absence of visible cues to the person's feelings. Schizophrenia can make it difficult for people to identify and communicate feelings. Clients with schizophrenia show less emotion, laugh

less, and cry less. Do not confuse the inability to express emotions with the inability to experience emotions. Table 14.2 ■ gives examples of descriptors of affect.

Anhedonia, the inability to experience pleasure, causes many people with schizophrenia to feel emotionally barren. This may lead to eccentric social interaction and social withdrawal. Clients may not take much interest in the things around them, even things they used to find enjoyable. If the world feels "flat as cardboard," they may not feel that it is worth the effort to get out and do things.

People with schizophrenia have a normal ability to experience unpleasant emotions and often experience worries and fears. With little warning, some people with schizophrenia become *hostile* as anger turns into aggression with the intent to do harm.

Assessment: Perception

Positive perceptual characteristics include hallucinations and sensory overload. A **hallucination** is the occurrence of a sound, sight, touch, smell, or taste without an external stimulus to the corresponding sensory organ. Hallucinations are real to the person having them and may be triggered by anxiety or by functional changes in the central nervous system. The same brain area is activated when clients listen to audible speech as when they experience auditory hallucinations. In other words, the brain reacts as if unable to distinguish between its own internally generated speech and actual, audible speech.

The most common type of hallucination is an *auditory hallucination*, or the hearing of voices or unusual noises. The voice is often that of God, the devil, a neighbor, or a relative; the voice may say either bad or good things; and the voice seems to come from an external source. Auditory hallucinations occur in 50% to 80% of people with schizophrenia.

Focused Nursing Assessment | Clients With Schizophrenia

Behavior Assessment	Affective Assessment	Cognitive Assessment	Social Assessment
■ What are your responsibilities 　At home? 　At work? 　At school? ■ Signs of hyperactivity* ■ Evidence of decreased activity level* ■ Self-care activities* ■ Behaviors suggestive of hallucinations*	■ What kinds of activities/situations give you: 　Pleasure? 　Anxiety? 　Anger? 　Guilt? ■ Evidence of problems with affect:* 　Inappropriate 　Overreactive 　Blunted 　Flat ■ Signs of anhedonia* ■ Expressions of hostility*	■ Have you ever heard voices? ■ Are you hearing voices now? What do the voices say to you? What feelings are associated with the voices? ■ Have you ever seen things other people don't see? What things do you see? What feelings are associated with seeing things? ■ Do you believe that you are someone very important? ■ Do you feel anyone is trying to harm you? ■ Do you feel anyone is controlling you? ■ Do you think about religion a lot? ■ Do you believe that you are very guilty for something you have done? ■ Do you think anything abnormal is happening to your body? ■ Do you think people are talking about you often? ■ Do you believe others can hear your thoughts? ■ Do you believe others can put thoughts into your head? ■ Do you have thoughts of harming yourself? Harming others? ■ Have you ever thought you have special powers that other people do not have?	■ Are you employed? ■ What are your living arrangements?

*Observations by the nurse.

Larry:

66 I hear voices in my head and I have all kinds of companions, some fictional and some nonfictional. Some are from history and some are people I have invented. They speak to me about things, specifically about baseball. I love baseball. 99

The next most common type is a *visual hallucination*, which is usually nearby, clearly defined, and moving. Visual hallucinations are often accompanied by auditory hallucinations. *Tactile*, *olfactory*, and *gustatory hallucinations* are uncommon and are more likely to occur in people undergoing substance withdrawal or who are abusing drugs.

Hallucinations may considerably control the person's behavior. It is not unusual for people having auditory hallucinations to carry on a conversation with one of the voices. After a period of time, many people realize that if they admit they hear voices, they will be labeled as "sick" or "crazy." To avoid being labeled, people having auditory hallucinations may be very evasive about their hallucinations.

The body's sensory systems receive information from the environment and from the body through stimuli transmitted to the brain. Humans do not, however, consciously perceive much of this sensory information. Sensory information is processed in a series of relay stations within the brain where irrelevant stimuli are inhibited. This allows the brain to filter out unnecessary and distracting information—

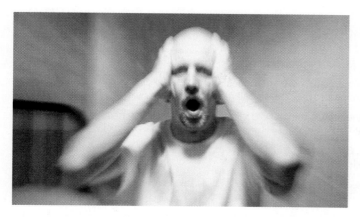

PHOTO 14.1 ■ Many symptoms of schizophrenia, including hallucinations and delusions, can be extremely distressing.

SOURCE: Carlton, Chuck/Photolibrary.com. Used with permission.

a process called **selective perception**—and focus on what is important at the given moment. Schizophrenia often disrupts the filtering process, causing *sensory overload*. When there are too many messages arriving at the cerebral cortex at the same time, thinking becomes disorganized and fragmented (see Figure 14.2).

The negative perceptual characteristic in schizophrenia is the inability to understand sensory information. People with schizophrenia sometimes have a hard time making sense of everyday sights, sounds, and feelings. Their *perception* of what is going on around them may be *distorted* so that ordinary things are distracting or frightening. They may be overly sensitive to background noises and colors and shapes.

Humans are highly evolved in face recognition. Survival demands that humans be able to distinguish between friend or foe, related from unrelated, and familiar from unfamiliar. People with schizophrenia often fail to recognize previously seen faces, which is likely related to dysfunction in the visual cortex. This may contribute to difficulties in social interactions (Onitsuka et al., 2005).

Assessment: Cognition

Schizophrenia impairs many cognitive functions, such as thought formation, memory, language, attention, and executive functions. This impairment interferes with daily functioning more than any other group of symptoms. Positive cognitive characteristics of schizophrenia are delusions, disorganized thinking, and loose associations.

Delusions are false beliefs that cannot be changed by logical reasoning or evidence. Clients attempt to make sense of delusions, even though they are the product of brain dysfunction in the context of who they are. Thus, people in an underdeveloped country might believe that evil shamans are after them, while in Canada they may believe that the Royal Canadian Mounted Police are following them.

When there is an extensively developed central delusional theme from which conclusions are deducted, the delusions are termed *systematized*. There are a number of delusional types: grandiosity (delusions of grandeur), persecution, control, somatic, religious, erotomanic, ideas of reference, thought broadcasting, thought withdrawal, and thought insertion (see Table 14.3 ■). It is believed that delusions represent dysfunctions in the information-processing circuits within and between the hemispheres of the brain. The severity of delusions can be a valuable indicator in monitoring the course of the illness.

Grandiosity, also known as *delusions of grandeur*, is an exaggerated sense of importance or self-worth. It is often accompanied by beliefs of magical thinking.

People with schizophrenia may experience *delusions of persecution*. They may believe someone is trying to harm them and, therefore, any personal failures in life are the fault of these harmful others.

Alegra has a right lower extremity cellulitis with gangrene. She believes her leg will heal on its own. Her family is going to court to get guardianship so they can sign for the amputation of Alegra's leg.

Alegra: "My sister told them where I live and now I can't go back to my own home because they're watching me all the time."

Nurse: "Who's watching you?"

Alegra: "The gangsters. That's why I'm here. The gang bangers were chasing me. I didn't think I was ever going to lose them."

Nurse: "They were chasing you because . . . ?"

Alegra: "This sore on my leg. Ever since I've had it they've been after me."

Nurse: "They chase you because of your sore?"

Alegra: "Yeah. They have been trying to get cocaine out of this thing (points to her wound) for weeks now. That's why I can't go home. They'll get me and get the cocaine out of my leg. They'll cut it off."

Delusions of control occur when the person believes that feelings, impulses, thoughts, or actions are not his/her own but are being imposed by some external force.

Samuel believes that a group of doctors is doing long-distance laser surgery on his back. He says his back twitches when the doctors do the surgery, and he can hear the voices of the doctors talking. "I have computer chips in my brain, and the computer sends out electrical impulses and tells me what to do. I really shouldn't be telling you this because now the security people are going to follow you."

Religious delusions involve false beliefs with religious or spiritual themes.

Pedro believes that he is Jesus, and his hand hurts where the nails had been placed. He wants to go to Washington, DC, and tell the president that he is God and can cure cancer. He states that he attempted suicide in the past but that "was a long time ago and I didn't know I was Jesus then."

TABLE 14.3	Examples of Delusions
Delusion	**Example**
Grandiosity	"Within 1 month I am going to be a billionaire and own 14 houses and 20 cars. I will be so rich and successful that Bill Gates and Alan Greenspan are going to call me for financial advice."
Persecution	"My neighborhood wants me dead or alive. They think I hold all of their secrets. They have tapped my phone and peek through my windows 24 hours a day."
Control	"My mother put a voodoo curse on me. She can control all of my thoughts and emotions through a remote-control car. I am completely under her spell."
Religious	"God told me that I am his Chosen One. I can perform miracles. I know this is real because my rosary beads revealed this to me."
Erotomanic	"I can have any guy I want. Matt Damon called me last night but I couldn't go out because I already had a date with Tom Cruise."
Sin and guilt	"I can't do anything right. I always mess everything up. I had so many friends from school, but now no one will come and see me because I am a failure."
Somatic	"I have a hammer in my heart. It pounds daggers in it all day long. Don't you hear it? Someday soon it is going to pound so hard that my heart will come flying out of my chest onto the floor."
Ideas of reference	"The headline of the *New York Times* told me that I have been assigned to stop crime. I am issuing a nationwide bulletin telling people to turn in their guns and knives. I take my assignments very seriously."
Thought broadcasting	"I don't have to tell you that. You already know because you can read my mind."
Thought withdrawal	"I'm trying to tell you something, but I keep losing it because someone keeps stealing my thoughts."
Thought insertion	"You think this is me talking, but it really isn't. My husband keeps putting these thoughts in my head."

People with *erotomanic delusions* believe that a person, usually someone famous and of higher status, is in love with them. Preoccupation with the "fantasy" lover may lead to stalking. Occasionally, the stalker turns violent, not because of hatred of the person, but because the object of their obsession cannot fulfill the romantic delusions.

Somatic delusions occur when people believe something abnormal and dangerous is happening to their bodies.

Rachel, looking at an orange she is holding, says: "I had a bowel movement yesterday. It looked like this. It was one of my ovaries, or it might have been a tumor."

Ideas of reference are remarks or actions by someone else that in no way refer to the person with schizophrenia but that are interpreted as related to her or him. *Thought broadcasting* occurs when people believe that others can hear their thoughts. *Thought withdrawal* is the belief that others are able to remove thoughts from one's mind. *Thought insertion* is the belief that others are able to put thoughts into one's mind.

Further information about delusions is found in chapter 8 ∞.

Disorganized thinking is another effect of schizophrenia. Adaptation to the environment and effective coping depend not only on learned responses, but also on the flexibility of the brain in organizing this incoming information. Schizophrenia is often referred to as a thought disorder, which is abnormal-ity in the form of thought, and it comes across to the the listener as disorganized speech. Because speech is a reflection of cognitive functioning, **loose association** is an indication of disorganized thinking. A person has a loose association when verbal ideas shift from one topic to another, there is no apparent relationship between thoughts, and the person speaking is unaware that the topics are unconnected. At times, a person with schizophrenia may change topic and direction so frequently that she or he is incoherent or impossible to understand (Bowie, Tsapelas, Friedman, Parrella, White, & Harvey, 2005).

Larry:

" The other major activity of mine is working at the library with a woman named Tuchman. You probably remember the name Tuchman, although this is no relationship whatsoever to the one I'm talking about—Barbara Tuchman, who was the daughter-in-law to Woodrow Wilson's secretary of state and who wrote the book, *The Guns of August*. That's a highly entertaining book, *The Guns of August*. "

The negative cognitive characteristics of schizophrenia are concrete thinking, attention impairment, memory deficits, impaired problem solving, lack of motivation, and lack of insight. These symptoms are most likely related to dysfunctions in the cerebral cortex.

Concrete thinking is characterized by a focus on facts and details and an inability to generalize or think abstractly. If one were to ask a client what brought her/him to the hospital, she or he would be likely to say, "A car."

Attention impairment interferes with the processing of information and the response to such information. A person with attention impairment has poor concentration and is easily distracted. Disturbances include responding to irrelevant external stimuli and difficulty completing tasks.

Recall from chapter 6 ∞ the two types of long-term memory: declarative and procedural. *Declarative memory* is memory related to people and facts, is consciously accessible, and can be verbally expressed. *Procedural memory* does not require conscious awareness and involves the memory of motor skills and procedures. *Memory deficits* in schizophrenia are one of the most severely impaired functions, which explains the day-to-day difficulties encountered by people with schizophrenia. The deficit is primarily in the area of declarative memory. The processes of responding emotionally, forming impressions about people, drawing inferences, and many other high-level cognitive functions are supported by declarative memory. Therefore, a person may display inappropriate behavior or make poor judgments when memory is impaired by schizophrenia (Kim et al., 2004).

Impaired problem solving may occur for a number of reasons. A person may be unaware that a problem exists, have impaired judgment, be unable to think logically, be unable to make a decision, or be unable to plan or follow through with a decision. Because one of the problems with schizophrenia is faulty information processing, a person with schizophrenia needs more time to think and problem solve.

Lack of motivation, referred to as *avolition*, is the inability to persist in goal-directed activities. Clients may have trouble starting projects or following through with things once begun. Their inability to persist at work or school activities gets them into significant employment or academic difficulties. At the extreme, these individuals may have to be reminded to do simple things such as taking a bath or changing clothes.

Poor insight, or lack of awareness of one's own mental illness, is more common in people with schizophrenia than in those with schizoaffective disorder or with major depressive disorder. Between 70% and 90% of clients have little awareness of their illness. Poor insight means that individuals have difficulty identifying their symptoms, which has implications when agreeing with treatment plans, recognizing early signs of relapse, and seeking treatment. Clients often believe that any difficulties they experience result from external causes. Insight often does not improve as the other symptoms improve (Flashman, 2004; Rickelman, 2004).

Assessment: Interpersonal Relationships

The primary positive social characteristic of schizophrenia is one of aloof and *stilted interactions* with others. People with schizophrenia may use outdated or very formal language and may have difficulty carrying on a conversation.

The negative social characteristics of schizophrenia are social withdrawal/isolation, poor rapport with others, and inadequate social and occupational skills.

Social withdrawal/isolation may result from paranoid delusions, severe difficulty participating in conversations, or an inability to experience feelings of friendship or intimacy. *Inadequate social skills* can interfere with the ability to develop rapport with others. These ineffective skills may drive away friends and family members who do not understand the behavior, further increasing the client's sense of isolation. People with schizophrenia may be socially incompetent, in part because they are unable to perceive the subtle cues critical to interpersonal interactions. In order to understand body cues during an interaction, one must be able to think abstractly. People with schizophrenia understand concrete cues better than abstract cues. For example, although a person with schizophrenia can identify and recall what someone said and did, she or he is less able to identify the emotional tone behind the words or comprehend the motivation for the interaction. Occupational skills may be problematic because of cognitive disruptions, behavioral abnormalities, inability to manage feelings, or inadequate social skills.

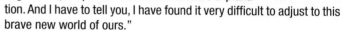

Larry:

Larry: "Having a mental illness still has very much stigma to it, despite all the modern world's explanation. And I have to tell you, I have found it very difficult to adjust to this brave new world of ours."

Nurse: "How do people react to you?"

Larry: "People don't react to me instantly because they don't know I'm sick. It'll take a little while for them to realize that I'm sick because obviously outwardly I don't display—I don't have a twitch, I don't have a physical twitch, I don't have a lame leg. I mean, these are things that people would notice immediately. But it does attach a certain social stigma to it once people have discovered that you are mentally ill."

Nurse: "What do they do?"

Larry: "They probably try to put a little bit of distance between themselves and me—physical and emotional distance."

Most people with schizophrenia experience *cycles of relapse and remission*. Families who have a loved one with a long-term medical illness, such as debilitating heart disease, usually receive social support and sympathy. But members of families with a loved one suffering from schizophrenia are often avoided. Many families are drained financially from the expense of long-term therapy, medications, and intermittent hospital stays. Mental health services are poorly covered in most medical insurance policies.

People with schizophrenia are not indifferent to their emotional and social environments. The *emotional climate of the family* has been shown to play a role in the relapse of the disorder. Clients who live in families that are highly critical, hostile, and overinvolved (referred to as *high expressed emotion*) have a significantly higher relapse rate than those who live in a supportive and caring family system. Families that are highly negative or excessively intrusive to the client can accelerate the time to relapse by causing physiological arousal and increased symptoms. On average, the relapse rate among clients who are not in family therapy is almost three times as high as those in family therapy (Jungbauer, Wittmund, Dietrich, & Angermeyer, 2003). Refer to chapter 2 ∞ , for more detailed information on family burden.

Approximately one third of the homeless population has a persistent mental illness; many have schizophrenia. The figures rise to 66% when chemical dependence is included in the estimate. In addition, all people, if left homeless for a sufficient period, will develop less effective coping skills and demonstrate some type of mental disorder (Bradford, Gaynes, Kim, Kaufman, & Weinberger, 2005; Philpot, 2005). Perhaps nothing is more upsetting than the sight of an individual who is homeless and clearly experiencing severe psychiatric problems. The image of a disheveled man angrily responding to voices only he can hear is an example of society's failure to address the problems of homelessness and mental illness. Homeless women with persistent mental illness represent one of the most vulnerable segments of society. They frequently face a choice between the dangers of life on the street and the hazards of overcrowded, unsafe, and poorly supervised shelters. Rape and physical battery are a daily risk for these women (Tucker, Wenzel, Straus, Ryan, & Golinelli, 2005).

Homeless people with persistent mental illness are often fearful and distrustful of the mental health system. The community health nurse must be prepared to work with homeless people in nonclinical settings, including on the streets, in shelters, on subways, in bus terminals, and in other public areas. The nurse will need a combination of patience, persistence, and understanding. Depending on the needs and wants of a particular person, providing food, clothing, or simply company can be essential in developing a therapeutic relationship (Dearing, 2004).

Assessment: Cultural Influences

A person's cultural and religious backgrounds must be considered when assessing individuals from cultures that are different from the nurse's. In some cultures, experiences labelled as delusional or hallucinatory are expected, normal experiences. Differences in styles of expression of feelings may be misunderstood and labeled as pathologic when in fact they are completely normal for that cultural group (APA, 2000).

Schizophrenia is recognized worldwide and affects about 1% of the population in different cultures. For unknown reasons, there are small areas of the population with increased incidence, such as second-generation African Caribbeans living in the United Kingdom. Unlike almost every other country in the world, in China the prevalence of schizophrenia is higher in women than in men. The symptoms of schizophrenia tend to be universal, but culture affects how the symptoms are interpreted (Phillips, Yang, Li, & Li, 2004).

Cultural factors affect the diagnosis of schizophrenia in the United States. Euro-Americans are more likely to receive a diagnosis of major depression and African Americans are more likely to receive a diagnosis of schizophrenia. Prescription practices may also vary with ethnicity. African Americans are less likely to be given a diagnosis of comorbid depression than Euro-Americans, leaving these clinically significant symptoms untreated. African Americans are more likely than Euro-Americans to receive psychotropic medications above recommended levels. In addition, African Americans are more likely to experience tardive dyskinesia than are Euro-Americans (Buchanan, Kreyenbuhl, Zito, & Lehman, 2002; Practice Guidelines, 2004; Wonodi, Adami, Cassady, Sherr, Avila, & Thaker, 2004).

Assessment: Age-specific Characteristics

Childhood schizophrenia is diagnosed when the onset of psychotic symptoms occurs before 12 years of age and before the completion of brain maturation. This form of schizophrenia is severe and may have a stronger genetic predisposition than other forms (Sporn et al., 2004).

Most children who develop schizophrenia seem healthy at birth and during the first years of life. Subtle behavioral and cognitive characteristics often precede the first psychotic episode. These signs include higher than expected rates of abnormal speech and motor abnormalities, such as clumsiness and abnormal movements. In addition, clients experience social withdrawal and isolation, decline in IQ over several years, and diminishing school performance. Prior to developing psychotic symptoms, there is a high rate of special education placement and failed grades (Sporn et al., 2004).

Symptoms in children are similar to those seen in adults, although the content of children's hallucinations and delusions comes from their experiences. For example, rather than believing that the FBI is following them, children may believe that a cartoon villain is out to get them.

The majority of *older adults* who have schizophrenia have had the disorder since youth. A number of older adults with schizophrenia show substantial improvement in symptoms, especially the positive symptoms, over the course of a lifetime.

Between 15% and 32% of people with schizophrenia have a late-onset type, which occurs after age 45 and affects more women than men. The clinical picture is somewhat different than in earlier-onset schizophrenia. People with the late-onset type have more delusions, which are often persecutory and bizarre. They are more likely to exhibit vivid hallucinations but have fewer cognitive disruptions and negative symptoms. It is thought that late-onset schizophrenia may be a less severe form of the disorder (Friedman et al., 2002).

Sensory impairment, such as hearing loss or cataracts, may increase the severity of the symptoms since environmental stimuli are often misinterpreted. In addition, people with hearing and vision loss tend to decrease social contacts and become socially isolated, which may increase suspicious thoughts.

Assessment: Physical

Velocardiofacial syndrome is a congenital defect related to chromosome 22. The predominant clinical signs include cleft palate, cardiac abnormalities, minor facial anomalies, and learning disabilities. Among adults with this syndrome, there is an increased incidence of schizophrenia and schizoaffective disorder. These anomalies develop during the first 16 weeks of gestation and coincide with early brain development. People with velocardiofacial syndrome demonstrate neuroanatomical abnormalities in the temporal lobe, as well as decreased total cerebral volume, both of which occur in people with schizophrenia (Moberg, Roalf, Gur, & Turetsky, 2004).

In comparison to men, women develop schizophrenia several years later and experience symptoms that are less severe. Research shows that *estrogens* protect against nerve cell loss and preserves connections between neurons. Estrogens also enhance the efficacy of antipsychotic medications. As estrogens decrease in the menopausal years, we find more women than men developing late-onset schizophrenia.

Rates of *cigarette smoking* (58% to 92%) are much higher for people with schizophrenia than for the general population (25%) and twice as high for those with other psychiatric diagnoses. There are three possible reasons for this heavy dependence on nicotine. First, clients may self-medicate with nicotine to improve cognition, lessen auditory hallucinations, and moderate the side effects of medications. Nicotine, like other drugs of addiction such as cocaine and amphetamines, appears to stimulate the reward center of the brain, through stimulation of nicotinic receptors, which increases DA synthesis and decreases DA metabolism. Thus, smoking may be a way to self-medicate a disturbance in the reward center. Second, smoking may be a risk factor for a person who has a genetic vulnerability to schizophrenia. This is supported by the data that those who start smoking at a young age have an earlier onset of schizophrenia. Third, genetic or environmental factors might work together, contributing to the co-occurrence of nicotine use and schizophrenia. Smoking places clients at greater psychiatric risk because components in cigarette smoke stimulate hepatic enzymes, increasing the rate of metabolism of psychotropic medications. Clients who smoke may need higher doses of their medication. Smoking also places clients at increased risk for cardiovascular and respiratory diseases (Compton, 2005).

Abnormalities in the ability to *identify smells* may be a marker of cerebral dysfunction in schizophrenia. Individuals have difficulty with odor detection, odor identification, and odor recognition memory. Research shows that people with schizophrenia are unable to identify when smells have a pleasing scent, just as they are unable to experience pleasure. The circuitry of the prefrontal brain regions used to assess emotional and olfactory pleasure appear to be dysfunctional (Turetsky, Moberg, Arnold, Doty, & Gur, 2003).

Schizophrenia is characterized by disturbed sleep patterns. In healthy adolescents, synaptic pruning occurs during delta- or slow-wave sleep patterns. An exaggeration of normal synaptic pruning processes is seen in adolescents with schizophrenia. This contributes to an impaired ability to process information and a decline in working memory (Keshavan, Cashmere, Miewald, & Yeragani, 2004).

Individuals with schizophrenia are at high risk for *polydipsia*, a condition in which a person ingests excessive amounts of liquids, 3 to 10 L. This can lead to hyponatremia, which may result in death. Symptoms include nausea and vomiting, diarrhea, headaches, delirium, ataxia, stupor, muscle tremors, seizures, and coma. Smoking makes the condition even more serious since nicotine causes the release of antidiuretic hormone (ADH), leading to increased water retention (Broome, 2004).

Clients taking antipsychotic medications should be assessed for *osteoporosis*. Antipsychotic medications act on the pituitary gland to increase prolactin. High levels of prolactin contribute to estrogen deficiency in women and testosterone deficiency in men, both of which reduce bone density. Other risk factors for people with schizophrenia include alcohol and drug abuse and heavy smoking (Hummer et al., 2005).

DIAGNOSIS

There are many potential nursing diagnoses for clients with schizophrenia. In synthesizing the assessment data, consider the following:

- How well clients are functioning in daily life
- What their skills and talents are
- How stable their affect is
- How well they are able to communicate
- How well they are getting along with others
- How well they function at work

The following is a list of the common diagnoses applicable to people with schizophrenia (North American Nursing Diagnosis Association, 2007).

- Risk for Violence, Self-Directed, related to command hallucinations
- Risk for Violence, Directed at Others, related to suspiciousness, fear, command hallucinations
- Altered Thought Process related to disruptions in cognitive processes such as delusions, loose association, concrete thinking
- Disturbed Sensory Perception, Auditory and Visual, related to disruptions in temporal lobe and occipital lobe causing hallucinations
- Impaired Verbal Communication related to cognitive disruptions
- Impaired Social Interaction related to withdrawal, preoccupation with symptoms, lack of a supportive network, negative reaction by others to client's social behavior
- Chronic Low Self-esteem related to feeling different from others; chronic nature of the disorder
- Anxiety related to environmental stimuli, reduced contact with reality
- Fatigue related to hyperactivity
- Noncompliance related to decreasing or stopping prescribed medication
- Self-care Deficit Bathing/Hygiene related to an inability to remember steps in self-care; low motivation
- Knowledge Deficit related to not understanding disease process
- Imbalanced Nutrition, More Than Body Requirements, related to side effects of antipsychotic medications
- Caregiver Role Strain related to fear of unknown, lack of social support, need to care for family member, inappropriate behavior on part of client
- Impaired Home Maintenance related to being homeless

OUTCOME IDENTIFICATION AND GOALS

Based on the assessment data, select outcomes appropriate to the nursing diagnoses. Three broad outcomes are:

- Reducing or eliminating symptoms
- Improving quality of life and adaptive functioning
- Enabling recovery by helping clients attain personal life goals

Once outcomes are established the nurse and the client mutually identify goals for change. Client goals are specific behavioral measures that the nurse, clients, and significant others identify as realistic and attainable. The following are examples of goals appropriate for people with schizophrenia:

- Communicates clearly
- Completes ADLs appropriately
- Exhibits increased attention span
- Makes appropriate decisions
- Displays affect appropriate to the situation
- Denies hallucinations
- Verbalizes logical thought processes
- Interacts well with others
- Develops occupational skills

PLANNING

Once the nursing diagnoses, outcome criteria, and goals have been identified, the plan of care is developed to assist clients toward a higher level of functioning and an enriched quality of life. Priorities of care for clients with schizophrenia are as follows:

- Prevention of violence
- Altered cognition
- Compromised social relationships

IMPLEMENTATION

Nurses have many opportunities to assist people with schizophrenia in a variety of settings, as previously described. These contacts may be long-term relationships or may be during crisis periods. Clients should be cared for in the least restrictive setting that is both safe and effective for treatment. Indications for hospitalization include the client's being a danger to self or others, the client's being unable to care for self and needing constant supervision, or a new onset of a psychotic episode.

It is important that clients identify their priority concerns for the plan of care to be effective. Change is more likely to happen when clients are invested in the treatment process. Families, significant others, or caregivers should be actively involved in the plan of care and be taught to implement many of these interventions.

The nature of the nurse–client relationship is one of the most effective nursing interventions. With rapport, communication, and trust, the nurse is able to help clients meet the outcome criteria they have identified. Review the material on communicating with clients in chapter 7 ∞. When the nurse listens to clients, accepts them for who they are, and understands their perspective, he/she is more likely to help empower them and thereby help them achieve their highest level of functioning.

NURSING CARE PLAN for a Client With Schizophrenia

Preventing Suicide

Nursing Diagnosis: Client at risk for self-directed violence

Outcomes: Client will remain safe.

An important priority of care is client safety. Command hallucinations may order clients to harm, mutilate, or kill themselves or others. Some clients have delusions so intensely for so long that suicide seems like the only way to escape the pain of being persecuted or controlled by outside forces. Living with such a complex, chronic illness induces feelings of hopelessness and depression, which in turn increases suicide risk. See chapter 21 ∞ for the specifics of caring for a suicidal client.

Intervention	Rationale	Goal
When severely suicidal and not hospitalized, clients must remain with someone at all times until they can be moved to a safe environment.	They must be protected from self-destruction until safety can be guaranteed.	Client does not act on suicidal plan.
Teach family members. ■ People who talk about suicide are at high risk. ■ Suicide attempts may follow loss of an important person, position, or possession. ■ Consider suicide risk at all stages of the illness.	Family members should recognize risk factors that increase suicide risk.	Families verbalize an understanding of risk factors.

Preventing Violence

Nursing Diagnosis: Client at risk for other or self-directed violence

Outcome: Clients' behavior remains nonaggressive.

Among the client population, African Americans are more likely to be perceived as being violent or dangerous than clients from other ethnic groups. This is true even when independent assessment of violent behavior showed they were significantly less likely to be violent. As a result of this racist misperception, African American clients receive more doses, more injections, and higher 24-hour doses of psychotropic drugs than do Euro-Americans (Lawson, 2000).

Some clients may be at risk for violence against others when they misperceive communication from others or when they perceive that they themselves are being threatened. See chapter 8 ∞ for further interventions with clients who are aggressive.

Intervention	Rationale	Goal
Encourage clients to talk out feelings rather than act out feelings.	This assists in maintaining control over behavior.	Clients should discuss feelings.
Help client identify triggers to aggression, such as noise, unfamiliar people, anxiety-provoking situations.	Elimination of potential triggers will help clients remain calm.	Client will identify triggers to aggression.
If behavior begins to escalate: ■ Remain calm ■ Use a low tone of voice ■ Give personal space ■ Avoid physical contact ■ Set limits on aggressive behavior	Remaining calm and focused will help client behavior de-escalate.	Client behavior de-escalates.
When working with clients who are suspicious: ■ Avoid startling ■ Give plenty of personal space ■ Never touch without specific permission ■ Avoid controversial issues such as politics, sex, and religion in conversation	Suspicious clients are always on the lookout for danger and function at a steady level of hyperalertness. If startled, they may strike out to protect themselves from perceived danger.	Client remains calm

continued

NURSING CARE PLAN for a Client With Schizophrenia

Preventing Violence   *continued*
Nursing Diagnosis: Client at risk for other or self-directed violence

Intervention	Rationale	Goal
When working with clients who are suspicious, avoid: ■ Talking softly with other staff ■ Laughing with other staff when client cannot hear what is being said	Because clients are hyperalert to everything in the environment, do not behave in ways that could be misinterpreted. The client may think, "They are talking about me" or "They are all laughing at me."	Client interprets interaction as nonthreatening

Coping With Hallucinations
Nursing Diagnosis: Client at risk for disturbed sensory perception

Outcome: Client develops effective coping strategies to manage hallucinations.

The experience of hallucinations can be especially troublesome for the person who does not have anyone to talk to about them. Discussion of hallucinations is important to the development of reality-testing skills. The person experiencing acute hallucinations has no voluntary control over the brain malfunction causing this symptom and needs immediate nursing interventions. See chapter 8 ∞ for more interventions for clients who are experiencing hallucinations.

Clients may wish to become involved in an international self-help movement called *voice hearer groups*. The goal of the group is to provide support and share practical ways to cope with problems related to experiencing hallucinations. For example, members in one group suggested using a cell phone (real or fake) to respond to the voices when out in public. Rather than being ridiculed for hallucinating, they blend in with others who are using cell phones. (Hagen & Mitchell, 2001).

Intervention	Rationale	Goal
Do not leave clients alone when they are hallucinating.	Inability to sort out reality may overwhelm the ability to cope.	Client remains calm.
Talk slightly louder using short, simple phrases and use client's name.	Focus the client's attention.	Client focuses attention.
Assess for clues that a person may be hallucinating: ■ Smiling or laughing inappropriately ■ Talking to someone whom the nurse cannot see ■ Slowed verbal responses	Continue with assessment.	Client responds to assessment questions.
Ask clients to describe what is happening. Assess for content of hallucinations. Help clients identify needs that may be reflected in the content of the hallucination, such as: ■ Power and control of decisions that affect daily life ■ Ability to express anger ■ Self-esteem issues	Safety may be a concern if command hallucinations are present. Presenting the nurse's perception of reality provides additional input to the sensory experience.	The client is able to identify needs and what is actually happening in the environment.
Ask which coping methods the client has used to manage hallucinations.	Support the client's positive efforts. They cannot turn off the voices but perhaps can influence the power or frequency of the voices.	The client identifies past successful coping methods.

NURSING CARE PLAN for a Client With Schizophrenia

Coping With Hallucinations   *continued*
Nursing Diagnosis: Client at risk for disturbed sensory perception

Intervention	Rationale	Goal
Identify ineffective coping behaviors, such as: ■ Eating more ■ Smoking more ■ Alcohol/drugs ■ Acting out against other people	More important than the presence of hallucinations is the ability or inability to effectively cope with the experience.	The client identifies ineffective behaviors.
Give suggestions such as: ■ Talk with family or friends ■ Participate in diversional activities ■ Exercise or sports ■ Listen to music ■ Relaxation techniques	More important than the presence of hallucinations is the ability or inability to effectively cope with the experience.	The client implements a plan of effective coping behaviors.
Encourage keeping a journal regarding hallucinations, triggers, and coping behaviors.	Keeping a journal helps the nurse see patterns and evaluate coping strategies.	The client keeps hallucination journal.

Managing Delusions
Nursing Diagnosis: Client at risk for disturbed thought processes

Outcome: Client develops effective coping strategies to manage delusions.

Persons experiencing delusions have difficulty processing language; therefore, nonverbal communication is critically important. Approach the person with calmness and empathy. It is normal to feel confused by a delusion. See chapter 8 ∞ for further information on working with clients who are delusional.

Intervention	Rationale	Goal
Carefully assess content of delusions without appearing to probe or be condescending.	Safety issues must be identified in case the client is a danger to self or others as directed by delusional thoughts.	The client remains safe and shares delusional thoughts.
Do not attempt to logically explain the delusion.	The person is unable to distinguish the delusion from reality.	The client verbalizes a sense of acceptance.
Assess the triggers, duration, frequency, and intensity of the delusion.	Delusions are often triggered by stress. Determine baseline patterns.	The client describes delusional process.
Respond to underlying feelings or themes of delusion.	Delusions are illogical to other individuals. Encourages discussion of fears, anxieties, or anger.	The client identifies feelings and themes underlying the delusion.
Engage the client in diversional activities.	Focus person away from the delusion.	The client participates in activities.

Promoting Effective Communication
Nursing Diagnosis: Client at risk for impaired communication

Outcome: Client will communicate clearly.

Sometimes clients are not able to hold thoughts together enough for you to comprehend what is being said. They may not remember how they started a sentence or where their thoughts were taking them (loose association). They are often more able to understand others than to make themselves understood.

continued

NURSING CARE PLAN for a Client With Schizophrenia

Promoting Effective Communication *continued*
Nursing Diagnosis: Client at risk for impaired communication

Intervention	Rationale	Goal
Interrupt politely but firmly, e.g., "I'm not understanding what you are saying. Could we try that again?"	Asking a question helps the client focus and communicate in a more direct manner.	The client repeats communication more clearly.
Listen for themes in the conversation.	Listening helps the nurse understand the client's current concerns.	The client validates identified themes.
Decrease environmental stimuli.	Sensory overload or the inability to screen unimportant stimuli interferes with listening and communicating.	The client remains focused on communication.
If the client is in large crowds or large family gatherings, encourage the client to talk with one person at a time.	Avoiding the noise and confusion will improve communication.	The client identifies environmental situations that improve communication.

Fostering Socialization
Nursing Diagnosis: Client at risk for impaired social interaction

Outcomes: Clients will identify specific social skill deficits; practice appropriate behaviors; utilize feedback from others to develop social skills; socialize with others on a regular basis; verbalize an improved quality of life.

Social difficulties frequently accompany schizophrenia, and social skills training is an appropriate nursing intervention. Because of the stigma attached to mental disorders and especially schizophrenia, clients have fewer opportunities to develop and practice social skills. This inexperience contributes to inappropriate responses when interacting with others. Poor social functioning has been found to be an important predictor of relapse and rehospitalization (Mueser et al., 2001). See chapter 9 ∞ for more information on social skills training. Chapter 3 ∞ describes a variety of vocational programs you may use as referral sources.

Intervention	Rationale	Goal
Design training strategies in organized sessions of practice of basic skills in a group format. Social communication skills: ■ Nonverbal behaviors (facial expressions, eye contact) ■ Paralanguage (voice loudness, sounds that are not words) ■ Initiating a conversation ■ Verbal content (appropriateness of what is said) ■ Avoiding topics inappropriate for casual conversation ■ Interactive balance (amount of time each person spends talking)	Reduce deficits. It is easier to learn social behavior in a social setting with peer modeling.	The client practices appropriate behaviors and improves level of social communication.
Use role-playing and social reinforcement to help clients learn behaviors step by step. Skills include: ■ How to interview for a job ■ How to set goals and develop motivation ■ Budgeting and money management ■ Self-advocacy ■ Structuring time ■ Managing conflict ■ Quality time spent with others	The ability to enjoy interpersonal relationships is a dimension of quality of life that is important to most people, including those with schizophrenia.	The client identifies specific deficits, socializes with others on a regular basis, verbalizes an improved quality of life.

NURSING CARE PLAN for a Client With Schizophrenia

Fostering Socialization   *continued*
Nursing Diagnosis: Client at risk for impaired social interaction

Intervention	Rationale	Goal
Practice until client masters the skill.	Mastery can result in improvement in social adjustment, leading to less withdrawal and isolation.	The client demonstrates improved social skills.
Vocational training programs.	For these programs to be successful, clients must be able to manage day-to-day living.	The client takes advantage of available vocational training programs.

Enhancing Self-Esteem
Nursing Diagnosis: Client at risk for low self-esteem

Outcome: Client will verbalize an improved self-esteem.

Many people with schizophrenia desperately desire to be "normal" and therefore suffer from low self-esteem. Self-esteem exercises can be implemented one-to-one and in group settings.

Intervention	Rationale	Goal
Encourage the keeping of a self-esteem journal in which clients can write their positive qualities.	Focusing on the positive is basic to improving self-esteem.	The client identifies his/her positive qualities.
In a group setting, ask clients to share their own positive qualities and to verbalize those of their peers.	Sharing this information provides an opportunity to learn how to give and receive positive feedback.	The client verbalizes increased comfort in giving and receiving positive feedback.
Encourage each client in the group to make a collage using magazines, scissors, glue, and blank paper. ■ Look for pictures that tell something about themselves and their interests. ■ Cut them out and glue them on the paper. ■ Take a turn in describing the significance of the collage to other group members. ■ Give feedback on the positive qualities each collage reveals.	Encourages creativity and provides a concrete way of talking about oneself.	The client participates in activity.
Give each group member two sheets of paper and crayons. ■ On one sheet of paper, ask them to draw the "real me." ■ On the other piece of paper, ask them to draw the "me others see." ■ Have each member present the "me others see." Client receives feedback from peers as to the accuracy of this perception. ■ The "real me" is presented and feedback is once again given.	This exercise focuses on the image a person presents to others and who we really are. This exercise is most successful with clients who have some ability to think abstractly.	The client participates in exercises.

continued

NURSING CARE PLAN for a Client With Schizophrenia

Monitoring Fatigue

Nursing Diagnosis: Client at risk for fatigue

Outcome: Client will limit excessive physical activity.

Some clients pace much of the day and are in danger of exhaustion and must be monitored for evidence of excess physical fatigue.

Intervention	Rationale	Goal
Provide firm direction to take short, frequent rest breaks; stay with the client for the designated rest time.	Limits must be set on hyperactivity to prevent fatigue.	The client rests for designated time periods.
Limit environmental stimuli.	Limiting stimuli facilitates relaxation.	The client slows physical activity.
Design calming and restful diversional activities.	Restful activities facilitate relaxation.	The client participates in activities.
Monitor food and fluid intake.	Monitoring prevents dehydration and ensures adequate energy resources.	The client balances intake with energy output.

Fostering Compliance with Medications

Nursing Diagnosis: Client at risk for noncompliance with medications.

Outcomes: Client will identify reason medication was stopped; verbalize benefits of taking medication; develop a method of self-administration of medications.

Some clients will be unhappy or frustrated with their medication. Discontinuation of medication is a significant factor in relapse. The first step in intervention is exploring the reasons people stop taking their medications. That understanding guides your interventions. For example, if clients stop taking their medication because they do not believe they have a mental illness, then teaching about the medication is not the appropriate first intervention. The appropriate intervention would be discussing their day-to-day lives in terms of level of functioning. The most common reasons for stopping medications include:

- Denial of the disorder and the desire to be normal
- Denial of the need for medication when they feel better
- Adverse side effects of medication
- Memory problems/forgetting to take medications
- Self-medicating with drugs and alcohol
- Lack of trust in health care providers
- No money to pay for medications
- If homeless, no place to store medications

Intervention	Rationale	Goal
Explore the pros and cons of continuing or discontinuing medication.	The client will understand the need for medication in the management of his/her disorder.	The client identifies pros and cons.
Explore how medication may be useful in helping the client progress toward personal goals.	A personal, vested interest in achieving goals may improve medication compliance.	The client verbalizes an understanding of how medication helps improve quality of life.
Provide guidance in the development of a routine for taking medication that fits into the client's daily habits, such as: - A weekly medication box with places for morning, noon, and evening medications - Using meal times as natural prompts - Putting a chart on the wall	Whatever system the client believes will help can usually be adapted for self-management.	The client develops a system that personally works.
Consider intramuscular antipsychotic medication if client is unable to manage medications.	Cognitive difficulties or homelessness makes daily medication management difficult for some clients.	The client keeps appointments at the medication clinic.

NURSING CARE PLAN for a Client With Schizophrenia

Facilitating Self-Care

Nursing Diagnosis: Client at risk for self-care deficit: Bathing/hygiene; dressing/grooming

Outcome: Client will manage self-care activities.

Some clients will need assistance with self-care because of a change in activity level, confusion, or a perceptual impairment.

Intervention	Rationale	Goal
Provide assistance: ■ List of step-by-step directions in bathroom and bedroom ■ "It's time for you to brush your teeth." ■ "Did you shower this morning?" ■ "Are your clothes appropriate for work."	Some clients need reminding or assistance with bathing, grooming, personal hygiene, and dressing.	The client is able to care for self with minimal assistance.
Provide social skills training as described in chapter 9 ∞ .	The client may need training in areas such as cleaning, cooking, shopping, or money management.	The client improves self-care.
As clients progress toward their goals, reward with greater responsibility and more privileges.	Although some clients may never live independently, they often can improve their quality of life through increased autonomy.	The client verbalizes an improved quality of life.

Reducing Relapse Episodes

Nursing Diagnosis: Client at risk for knowledge deficit: Relapse

Outcomes: Client will minimize chance for relapse; manage relapse at early stages; utilize protective factors to minimize chance of relapse; minimize risk factors for relapse; identify early signs of relapse.

Nursing theory believes that clients should be actively involved in the management of their illness. Thus, a psychoeducation program is an extremely important nursing intervention. The goal is to teach consumers about their illness and to cover the important behavioral, affective, cognitive, perceptual, and social problems they commonly experience.

Intervention	Rationale	Goal
Teach clients to identify risk factors: ■ Substance use ■ Sleep deprivation ■ Family distress ■ Interpersonal conflict ■ Inconsistency with medications	Knowledge improves ability to live with a chronic disorder.	The client minimizes risk factors for relapse.
Review early signs of relapse. The exact early warning signs vary from person to person but are repetitive for any one individual.	Because early intervention may prevent a relapse, this self-surveillance strategy allows people to influence the course of the disorder.	The client identifies personal early signs of relapse.
Teach clients protective strategies, such as: ■ Maintaining consistent day and night routines ■ Relying on social and family support systems ■ Participating in psychosocial treatment programs ■ Taking medication as prescribed	This self-surveillance strategy allows people to influence the course of the disorder.	The client uses protective strategies to minimize chance of relapse.

continued

NURSING CARE PLAN for a Client With Schizophrenia

Preventing Weight Gain

Nursing Diagnosis: Client at risk for imbalanced nutrition

Outcome: Client will maintain weight within normal limits.

The adverse effects of antipsychotic, antidepressant, and mood stabilizing medications include significant weight gain. This occurs even when clients do not increase their food intake.

Intervention	Rationale	Goal
Teach the client that weight gain is a common side effect of medications.	It is better to avoid weight gain than try to lose weight at a later time.	The client acknowledges the need to prevent weight gain.
Refer the client to a nutritional consultant.	Referral facilitates diet management.	The client follows recommended diet.
Encourage clients to identify physical activities they enjoy.	It is easier to establish a routine when preferred activities are included.	The client develops an exercise routine.
Teach that exercise not only helps people manage weight and reduces risk for cardiovascular problems, but also improves mood and psychosocial functioning (McDevitt, Wilbur, Kogan, & Briller, 2005).	Knowledge improves motivation to exercise on a regular basis.	The client continues exercise routine.

Promoting Employment

Nursing Diagnosis: Client at risk for powerlessness

Outcomes: Client will successfully manage employment; formulate a decisional balance sheet; discuss disadvantages of employment; formulate a plan of action.

The rates for employment for people with schizophrenia are very low. The reasons for this are high levels of negative symptoms, poor social skills, interpersonal stressors, lack of family support, relapses when medications are stopped, and inadequate job skills. In addition, those who are receiving federal benefits risk losing this financial assistance when they become employed. A way must be found to encourage employment while at the same time providing enough support to maintain community living and health care insurance. Details on supported employment are found in chapter 3 ∞.

Intervention	Rationale	Goal
Encourage clients to identify the benefits and disadvantages of finding employment.	Objectively listing benefits and disadvantages may clarify thinking about employment.	The client lists benefits and disadvantages.
Help clients make a decisional balance sheet based on this information.	If disadvantages outweigh advantages, clients will not be motivated to change.	The client makes decisional balance sheet.
Use reflective listening with an attitude of acceptance, not of confrontation.	Reflective listening helps clients clarify their reasoning.	The client reasons in a logical manner.
Discuss how remaining unemployed may block achievement of the client's important personal goals.	Personal goals are an important factor in motivation.	The client verbalizes increased motivation.
Express confidence that the client will be motivated when he/she is ready to change.	Motivation is an internal driving force for all people.	The client identifies readiness to change.
Refer the client to supported employment.	This may be the best route to improving vocational functioning (Corrigan, 2005).	Utilizes available resources.

Nicotine Addiction

People with schizophrenia have a very high rate of nicotine dependence and have been a very difficult group of individuals to involve in "quit smoking" programs. For many, the reward center in the brain functions below normal and nicotine stimulates this area. In fact, smoking may be one of the few dependable sources of pleasure for clients. Research has shown that clients know the disadvantages of smoking but they consider them outweighed by the advantages of smoking. Thus, it continues to be a challenge to motivate these individuals to quit smoking. Smoking cessation interventions should include both nicotine replacement therapies and behavioral approaches. The desired outcome is that the client quits smoking.

Need for Positive Reinforcement

Clients benefit from regular positive reinforcement and therefore it is important that you acknowledge the progress clients make and celebrate their successes. As they are able to accomplish more ADLs, increase interactions with others, cope with medication side effects, and live more independently, your support reinforces their personal gains (Dearing, 2004). The desired outcome is that the client will continue making positive behavioral changes.

Need for Family Education

Schizophrenia often strikes adolescents or young adults, leaving parents confused and frightened. Whether the child is living at home or away, employed or unemployed, parents report feeling a never-ending sense of responsibility for the child, which is at times overwhelming. Parents are likely to experience sorrow and grief as they begin to deal with the impact of their child's illness. Knowing that this is likely to occur, nurses can offer anticipatory guidance and interventions. Parents desire information and some level of involvement in their child's treatment plan. The question that health care professionals must answer is how to include the family within the context of client confidentiality. The desired outcome is that clients and families will verbalize an accurate understanding of the disorder; balance protective behaviors with encouraging independence; develop an advance directive; utilize effective communication skills; implement problem-solving process to manage family issues; negotiate individual roles and responsibilities within the family; and participate in family therapy.

Before intervening with the family, discover the answers to the following questions.

- How much does the family know about the illness?
- How do they react to symptoms?
- Is their reaction helpful or hurtful?
- How does the client respond to the family?
- Does the client understand the distress the family experiences?

Because so many people are afraid of and uninformed about schizophrenia, many families try to hide it from friends and deal with it on their own. The nurse must reach out to these families and offer them support and education. *Family education* often is conducted in a group setting, which enables families to begin to build a support network. The nurse must help them understand that they are not responsible for causing their loved one to develop schizophrenia and have no reason to feel guilty. They need to learn about the nature of schizophrenia and the variety of available treatment programs. Ask the client to teach the family what it is like to have schizophrenia. Similarly, the family members can share their observations and experiences.

Families need practical solutions on how to manage on a day-to-day basis. The nurse can assist families in achieving a *balance* between being protective and encouraging independence. For example, families should try to do things with the individuals rather than for them, so that clients are able to regain their sense of self-confidence. Increased family education often decreases caregiver burden and improves the quality of life for all family members (Czuchta & McCay, 2001). Box 14.3 provides an outline for family education.

Families may need help in *setting expectations and limits* on inappropriate behavior. The positive symptoms of schizophrenia can cause a great deal of family stress. That is also true of the negative symptoms, which are often misinterpreted as laziness or uncooperativeness. Families must understand that clients are not trying to be stubborn or difficult, but rather lack of insight accounts for some of the behaviors. Explain that just because clients can verbally describe problems, that does not mean that they can act on that knowledge. This information may help family members be more supportive.

Families can encourage their loved ones to stick with the treatment program, take their medications, and avoid alcohol and drugs. It is important to recognize *early signs of relapse*

MediaLink

Case Study, Family Teaching and the Client with Schizophrenia

---

BOX 14.3	Family Education

- Information about the disorder
- Managing symptoms
- Expectations during recovery
- Role of medications
- Handling crises
- Warning signs of suicide
- Early signs of relapse
- Housing and social resources
- Self-help groups

to prevent acute episodes and rehospitalization. Family members can ask clients with schizophrenia to agree that, if they notice warning signs of a relapse, it is okay for the family members to contact the physician so that the medication can be adjusted to stabilize the condition. All threats of suicide should be taken very seriously. Families should have an identified contact person they can call for help. If the situation becomes desperate, the family should call 911.

Clients are encouraged to develop an *advance directive* indicating permission for treatment in the case of future acute episodes. Advance directives assist the family and caregivers who must make decisions for clients when clients are unable to make the decision for themselves. Health care providers are given important information about the client's preferences for treatment. Family and friends experience less conflict and guilt during times of psychiatric crises. Chapter 5 ∞ describes what should be included in advance directives.

To prevent or delay relapse, it is critical to intervene with families who have high expressed emotion (EE), that is, those who are highly critical, hostile, and overinvolved. Clients who live in high EE situations have much higher relapse rates than those living in low EE environments. Teach family members to *moderate displays of all emotion* in an effort to provide a neutral emotional climate. They may need assistance in defining and reshaping appropriate boundaries.

Implementing effective communication styles is a way that families can decrease stress and improve family relationships. Choose a nonthreatening event and model new ways of talking and listening. Utilize role-playing and coach the family in these new skills. The four basic skills are (Miklowitz, 2004):

- *Expressing positive feelings.* When sharing feelings, family members are coached to use "I" language, such as "I feel really pleased when you get out of your bedroom in the morning."

- *Using active listening.* Family members are coached to ask clarifying questions of the speaker and use nonverbal attending behavior, such as eye contact and nodding of the head.

- *Making positive requests for change.* These requests should be specific and linked to a feeling, such as "I would really like it if you could help with the dishes after supper."

- *Expressing negative feelings.* Family members are reminded to use "I" language because "you" language leads to conflict. Rather than saying, "You are so lazy," it would be more effective to say, "I worry about you when it seems so difficult for you to participate in family activities."

Ask the family to pick a time and topic to practice these skills at home. The more they try the new skills, the more automatic they will become. Just as problem-solving skills are taught to individual clients, the *problem-solving process* is taught to families. A quick review of teaching the problem-solving process in chapter 7 ∞ follows:

- Identify and define the problem.
- List possible solutions.
- List advantages and disadvantages to each solution.
- Choose the best solution or combination of solutions.
- Develop an implementation plan.
- Evaluate the results of the action.

It is within the rights of a family to decide that a member who has an illness must get treatment for it. The family should also establish appropriate rules that must be followed. After an acute episode, the family may disagree over illness management around such issues as medication compliance, work/school activities, sleep–wake routines, or use of tobacco, alcohol, or drugs. Some families may disagree over role responsibilities and financial management. If the client is unwilling to comply with or modify behavior, the family may choose to look for alternative living arrangements. For more

Complementary/Alternative Therapies

How to Help Clients Improve Body Boundaries and Safe Touch

Massage is an effective method of reducing stress and tension that usually leads to a feeling of relaxation. Touch is a basic need, as necessary for growth and development as food, clothing, and shelter. Sometimes people are "touch starved" because they have few intimate relationships in their lives. This exercise is designed to help you nurture yourself through the sense of touch. It is also designed to help you improve your sense of the boundaries of your body.

1. Use olive oil or sesame oil for this exercise. If possible, warm a quarter cup of oil in the microwave for 10 to 15 seconds being careful not to overheat it.

2. Use one tablespoon of warm oil and rub it into your scalp. Use small, circular motions with the flat of your hand. Massage the forehead from side to side and gently massage your temples using circular motions. Gently rub the outside of the ears and the front and back of the neck.

3. Using more oil, massage your arms and hands.

4. Using more oil, massage your legs. Massage each toe with your fingertips. Vigorously massage the soles of your feet.

5. Sit quietly for a few seconds to relax and then shower or bathe as usual.

SOURCE: Adapted with permission from Chopra, D. (1991). *Perfect health*. New York: Harmony Books.

information, see the Community Resources and Books for Clients and Families features on your CD-ROM.

Clients who are discharged from an acute hospitalization episode with medication as the primary intervention have a 50% rehospitalization rate within 6 to 9 months. In contrast, clients discharged with medication and continuing family therapy only have a 2% to 10% rehospitalization rate. Family therapy moves beyond family education and helps people cope with the disorder of schizophrenia. Families learn how to manage conflict, avoid criticizing one another, decrease overprotective behaviors, and develop appropriate expectations of one another. Often, this is best accomplished with the help of a family therapist.

EVALUATION

Coping with schizophrenia is a lifelong process for most clients. Recovery rates from the first acute episode of schiz-

ophrenia are high, with almost 85% achieving remission. Remission is accomplished when symptoms no longer interfere with life. This is often referred to as the *stable phase*. The majority of clients alternate between acute psychotic episodes and stable phases. The current focus is on preventing relapse by maintaining medication and other treatment options. About 25% of individuals with schizophrenia are resistant to treatment and experience a "downward spiral" of functioning. They often become dependent on others for food, clothing, and housing. The negative symptoms and cognitive dysfunctions are more severe in this group. Recovery is a longer term phenomenon than remission and is characterized by few, if any, symptoms and an ability to function well in the community over a long period of time. Those who recover experience fewer cognitive and social problems during the acute phase of the illness (Andreasen, Carpenter, Kane, Lasser, Marder, & Weinberger, 2005; Scott, Kingdon, & Turkington, 2004).

Clinical Interactions | A Client With Schizophrenia

Sara is 41 years old and has suffered with schizophrenia for the past 15 years. She has a history of childhood sexual abuse. She has been able to live at home with her husband except for a few brief periods of hospitalization. Lately, her thinking has become more disorganized, and her therapist has recommended that she come to the day treatment program. The themes of the interaction below include raping and hurting little children and a desire to return to infancy, a period of time when she felt safe and cared for. In the interaction, you will see evidence of:

- Labile affect
- Loose associations
- Symbolism (attached at waist)
- Somatic delusions
- Grandiosity with magical powers

SARA: I killed a man when I was 6 years old, and he was raping and killing little babies. I killed him. Then my friends told me to run, so I ran. I got away with my underpants on. My twin brother died—he committed suicide. [crying]

NURSE: *Would you like to talk about this?*

SARA: Not right now. I loved my brother. [sobbing] I really miss him. You know I build houses.

NURSE: *You do?*

SARA: Yes, I start out 14 feet tall and when I'm done I've shrunk to 14 inches. [smiles and laughs]

NURSE: *You shrink?*

SARA: Yes. The aliens come and get me at night and tell me they'll make me safe and they make me into a baby and take care of me.

NURSE: *Do you feel safe as a baby?*

SARA: Yes; no one can hurt me then. They protect me. [smiling]

NURSE: *[Silence]*

SARA: My husband exhibits me, you know. [laughs]

NURSE: *Can you explain "exhibits"? I don't understand.*

SARA: He took movies of us having sex and set me down and showed them to me. He told me I had grown into a beautiful woman. He still loves me, you know, and I still love him even though I slapped him 3,600 times in the head.

NURSE: *How did you feel about his exhibiting you?*

SARA: It was okay because I really do love him. I was attached to my husband at the waist in the bedroom. [laughs] [Puts finger to ear and pauses]

NURSE: *Are you hearing voices?*

SARA: No. I have synthetic eardrums and I hear a buzz sometimes. Do you know I saved little boys from Alcatraz? I saved them to keep them safe. [laughs]

NURSE: *I didn't know that. What did you save them from?*

SARA: I saved them from the men raping them. They were raping and killing all those little boys. The president gave me permission to save as many as I could.

NURSE: *Is it a good feeling when you are able to help others?*

SARA: I build spaceships at night and escape to bars for smokes and men buy me whiskey.

NURSE: *Could we talk about one thing at a time? You are skipping to other subjects too quickly for me.*

SARA: Okay.

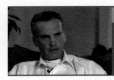

ROAD: Assessment   Critical Thinking Questions

Go to the CD-ROM to assess Larry by answering the following critical thinking questions based on what you have **R**ead about Larry and **O**bserved on the videos.

1. What conclusions do you draw about Larry's level of functioning prior to his developing symptoms of schizophrenia? Provide a rationale for your answer.

2. Review information about Belmont Hill School at http://www.belmont-hill.org/home/content.asp?id=1. What difficulties do you think Larry encountered during his academic years? How might his illness have influenced his social relationships? Support your answer with a rationale. (Hint: chapter 1 may help you in formulating an answer).

3. Within a case coordination meeting for Larry you learn that he has had long-term psychotropic treatment (antipsychotics). What characteristic(s) do you assess from segment B of your student ROAD CD-ROM that confirm(s) this information? Provide a rationale for your answer.

4. As Larry's treatment team focuses efforts on validating his diagnosis and specifying an appropriate plan of care, you have been asked to assess him for any characteristics that would correlate with acute positive or negative symptoms of his illness. Review segments A, B, and C of your student ROAD CD-ROM. Describe and support your assessment.

5. During an interaction with Larry, you gather data to formulate a neuropsychiatric assessment. What would be your assessment of his cognitive processes, specifically attention span and memory function, as displayed in segment C of your student ROAD CD-ROM?

6. In segment D of your student ROAD CD-ROM, Larry makes specific comments that have implications for his adjustment to his illness. What inferences do you make based on understanding the impact a diagnosis of schizophrenia can have on a person's ability to function? Provide rationale for your answer.

ROAD: Develop a Care Plan

 Go to the CD-ROM to Develop a care plan based on your assessment of Larry. Identify nursing diagnoses, outcomes, goals, and interventions.

SOURCE: Contributed by Susan Siwinski-Hebel, RN, MSN

Focus Your Study

OBJECTIVES	KEY CONCEPTS

1. Discuss current thinking and research findings on the etiology of schizophrenia.	■ Genetics
	  • Up to 85% of susceptibility may be genetic.
	  • Early-onset schizophrenia has a high genetic load.
	  • Protective factors may lessen the expression of genes.
	■ Neurobiology
	  • Abnormal brain development
	  • Abnormal levels of DA, 5-HT, NE, glu, and GABA
	  • Rigid cell membranes
	  • Decreased brain volume, disrupted cerebral blood flow, increased ventricular size
	■ Diathesis-Stress
	  • Genetic vulnerability combined with environmental risk factors and life events

2. Compare assessment findings associated with the positive and negative characteristics of schizophrenic disorders.

■ Positive symptoms
  • Hyperactivity
  • Bizarre behavior
  • Inappropriate or overreactive affect
  • Hostility
  • Hallucinations
  • Delusions
  • Disorganized thinking
  • Loose associations
  • Suspiciousness
  • Stilted interactions

■ Negative symptoms
  • Decreased activity level
  • Limited speech, conversation difficult
  • Minimal self-care
  • Blunted or flat affect
  • Anhedonia
  • Inability to understand sensory information
  • Concrete thinking
  • Attention impairment
  • Memory deficits
  • Impaired problem solving
  • Lack of motivation
  • Social withdrawal, isolation
  • Inadequate social and occupational skills

3. Use the nursing process to develop a safe, comprehensive plan of care for a client with schizophrenia.

■ Preventing suicide
  • Assess for command hallucinations and chronic delusions.
  • Review specific interventions in chapter 21 ∞.
■ Preventing violence
  • Identify triggering factors.
  • Remain calm, use low tone of voice, give personal space, avoid physical contact.
  • Review specific interventions in chapter 8 ∞.
■ Enhancing self-esteem
  • Ask client to list positive qualities and keep a self-esteem journal.
  • Provide positive reinforcement.
  • Provide a group format for giving and receiving positive feedback.
  • Institute self-esteem exercises.
■ Facilitating self-care
  • Make a list of step-by-step directions for hygiene and clothing.
  • Make a list of household tasks.
  • As clients progress toward their goal of independence, reward with more privileges and more responsibility.

4. Develop illness management teaching plans for a person with schizophrenia and his/her family.

■ Fostering compliance with medications
  • Explore reasons for stopping the medication.
  • Help clients understand the need for medication.
■ Promoting employment
  • Help clients identify the benefits and disadvantages of employment.
  • Identify personal goals.
  • Refer to Supported Employment—see chapter 3 ∞.
■ Facilitating self-care
  • Make a list of step-by-step directions for hygiene and clothing.
  • Make a list of household tasks.
  • As clients progress toward their goal of independence, reward with more privileges and more responsibility.
■ Teaching
  • Teach clients and families about the illness, the common problems, and ways to manage these problems.
  • Teach risk factors for relapse, early signs of relapse, and how to prevent relapse.
■ Involving family
  • Family education in group format is very helpful to build a support network and share coping strategies.
  • Help families find a balance between being protective and encouraging independence.
  • Help clients and families develop advance directives.
  • Help families who have high expressed emotion to moderate displays of emotion.
  • Teach effective family communication.
  • Teach family problem solving.

continued

5. Explain the different treatment options for a person with schizophrenia.

- Mediations
  - Antipsychotic medications
  - Medications to manage EPS
  - Mood-stabilizing medications
- Psychiatric rehabilitation
  - Development of social skills and supports necessary for successful living, learning, and working in the community
  - Collaborative partnerships with consumers, families, friends, and mental health providers
  - Emphasis on hope and optimism that people can grow, learn, and make changes in their lives
  - Stress values of choices, self-determination, and individual responsibility
- Assertive Community Treatment
  - Goal is to prevent rehospitalization through provision of comprehensive community services
- Electroconvulsive therapy
  - May be useful for individuals who have not responded to medication alone

6. Discuss the key points in effectively communicating with a person with schizophrenia.

- If you do not understand what the client is saying, help the person restate it.
- Listen for themes and feelings in communication.
- Decrease environmental stimuli and talk to one person at a time.
- Teach clients subtle cues that are critical to understanding communication from others.

Explore MediaLink

For review questions, case studies, and other resources for this chapter see the Pearson Health MediaLink CD-ROM that accompanies this book and the Companion Website.

CD-ROM
- Audio Glossary
- NCLEX-RN® Review Questions
- ROAD to Critical Thinking: *Larry*
- Animations/Videos
  - PET, SPECT of Schizophrenia
  - Tardive Dyskinesia: Mouth
  - Tardive Dyskinesia: Trunk
  - Tardive Dyskinesia: Ambulation
  - Extrapyramidal Signs: Akathisia
  - Extrapyramidal Signs: Akinesia and Pill Rolling
  - Extrapyramidal Signs: Bradykinesia–Shuffling Gait
  - Extrapyramidal Signs: Dystonia–Blepharospasm
  - Extrapyramidal Signs: Dystonia–Cervical Torticollis
  - Schizophrenia Interview–Part 1
  - Schizophrenia Interview–Part 2
  - Schizophrenia Interview–Part 3

Companion Website www.prenhall.com/fontaine
- Audio Glossary
- NCLEX-RN® Review Questions
- Case Study
  - Family Teaching and the Client With Schizophrenia
- Care Plan
  - The Client With Schizophrenia
- Critical Thinking
  - Positive and Negative Symptoms of Schizophrenia
- MediaLink Application
  - Schizophrenia
- MediaLinks
  - Books for Clients and Families
  - Community Resources

NCLEX-RN® Review Questions

14-1. A 45-year-old client with a diagnosis of paranoid schizophrenia, with auditory hallucinations, is in her third day on the unit and has refused all personal contact. She is sitting on her bed with her knees drawn to her chest and informs the staff nurse that she wants to call the FBI. The client states, "The FBI knows me and they will get me out of here." What would be the nurse's most appropriate therapeutic communication when talking to this client?
  1. Confront the client and explain that the FBI is not expecting a telephone call.

  2. End all conversations with this client until the client accepts reality.
  3. Confront the client with the reality and administer the client's PRN medication.
  4. Ask the client directly, "What do you want to talk to the FBI about?"

14-2. The therapeutic team has identified the need to formulate strategies for a client's inappropriate behavior and how to maintain a safe environment for the clients on the unit.

Of the following intervention strategies, which strategy must be initiated immediately?
1. Monitor the client's behavior
2. Identify the client's thought process that leads to this behavior
3. Help the client to identify why he demonstrates this behavior
4. Teach appropriate interpersonal skills to the client.

14-3. Select the response which accurately describes genetics and schizophrenia.
1. One single gene is responsible for producing schizophrenia.
2. There is strong evidence that environmental factors do not affect the risk of developing schizophrenia.
3. The chance of monozygotic (identical) twins both having schizophrenia is 100%, thus demonstrating the high level of genetic influence in schizophrenia.
4. A person has an 8% to 13% chance of being diagnosed with schizophrenia if a sibling or parent has the disorder.

14-4. Which of the following aspects of family communication patterns may be problematic for the client with schizophrenia? Select all that apply.

1. Family members appear to use language patterns that appear to be characteristic of the client's family only.
2. Family members appear to understand and respect individual boundaries.
3. Family members appear to be enmeshed or over-involved with each other.
4. Family members appear to be able to focus and discuss specific topics reasonably with each other.
5. Family members talk loudly at the same time and do not listen while others are talking.

14-5. An 18-year-old client is admitted with a diagnosis of paranoid-type schizophrenia. The student nurse asks the charge nurse about the approach to take with the client. The client has been exhibiting behavior of hostility and isolation. The best approach would be to:
1. Greet the client by gently touching her arm and telling her she can trust you.
2. Inform the client that she needs to receive care and you will assist her.
3. Respect the client's need for personal space and avoid physical contact with the client.
4. Tell the client that if she does not comply with the rules, you will inform the doctor.

See Appendix D for answers.

References

American Psychiatric Association. (2000). *Diagnostic and statistical manual of mental disorders* (4th ed., Text Revision). Washington, DC: Author.

Andreasen, N. C., Carpenter, W. T., Kane, J. M., Lasser, R. A., Marder, S. R., & Weinberger, D. R. (2005). Remission in schizophrenia. *American Journal of Psychiatry, 162*(3), 441–449.

Bachmann, S., Schröder, J., Bottmer, C., Torrey, E. F., & Yolken, R. H. (2005). Psychopathology in first-episode schizophrenia and antibodies to boxoplasma gondii. *Psychopathology, 38*(2), 87–90.

Bowie, C. R., Tsapelas, I., Friedman, J., Parrella, M., White, L., & Harvey, P. D. (2005). The longitudinal course of thought disorder in geriatric patients with chronic schizophrenia. *American Journal of Psychiatry, 162*(4), 793–795.

Bradford, D. W., Gaynes, B. N., Kim, M. M., Kaufman, J. S., & Weinberger, M. (2005). Can shelter-based interventions improve treatment engagement in homeless individuals with psychiatric and/or substance misuse disorders? *Medical Care, 43*(8), 763–768.

Brambilla, P., Cerini, R., Gasparini, A., Versace, A., Andreone, N., Vittorini, E., et al. (2005). Investigation of corpus callosum in schizophrenia with diffusion imaging. *Schizophrenia Research, 79*(2), 201–210.

Brodaty, H., Sachdev, P., Koschera, A., Monk, D., & Cullen, B. (2003). Long-term outcome of late-onset schizophrenia. *British Journal of Psychiatry, 183*(1), 213–219.

Broome, M. E. (2004). Polydipsia screening tool. *Archives of Psychiatric Nursing, 18*(2), 49–59.

Brown, A. S., Begg, M. D., Gravenstein, S., Schaefer, C. A., Wyatt, R. J., Bresnahan, M., et al. (2004). Serologic evidence of prenatal influenza in the etiology of schizophrenia. *Archives of General Psychiatry, 61*(8), 774–780.

Buchanan, R. W., Kreyenbuhl, J., Zito, J. M., & Lehman, A. (2002). Relationship of the use of adjunctive pharmacological agents to symptoms and level of function in schizophrenia. *American Journal of Psychiatry, 159*(6), 1035–1043.

Cannon, M., Jones, P. B., & Murray, R. M. (2002). Obstetric complications and schizophrenia: Historical and meta-analytic review. *American Journal of Psychiatry, 159*(7), 1080–1092.

Compton, M. T. (2005). Cigarette smoking in individuals with schizophrenia. *Medscape Psychiatry & Mental Health, 8*(2), 1–6.

Corrigan, P. W. (2005). Motivational interviewing of people with schizophrenia. *Medscape Psychiatry & Mental Health, 8*(2), 1–5. www.medscape.com/viewarticle/515818.

Czuchta, D. M., & McCay, E. (2001). Help-seeking for parents of individuals experiencing a first episode of schizophrenia. *Archives of Psychiatric Nursing, 15*(4), 159–170.

Dearing, K. S. (2004). Getting it, together: How the nurse patient relationship influences treatment compliance for patients with schizophrenia. *Archives of Psychiatric Nursing, 18*(5), 155–163.

Emsley, R., Myburgh, C., Oosthuizen, P., & van Rensburg, S. J. (2002). Randomized, placebo-controlled study of ethyl-eicosapentaenoic acid as supplemental treatment in schizophrenia. *American Journal of Psychiatry, 159*(9), 1596–1598.

Flashman, L. A. (2004). Disorders of insight, self-awareness, and attribution in schizophrenia. In B. D. Beitman & J. Nair (Eds.), *Self-awareness deficits in psychiatric patients* (pp. 129–158). New York: W.W. Norton & Company.

Friedman, J. I., Harvey, P. D., McGurk, S. R., White, L., Parrella, M., Raykov, T., et al. (2002). Correlates of change in function status of institutionalized geriatric schizophrenic patients. *American Journal of Psychiatry, 159*(8), 1388–1394.

Galderisi, S., Mau, M., Mucci, A., Cassano, G. B., Invernizzi, G., Rossi, A., et al. (2002). Historical, psychopathological, neurological, and neuropsychological aspects of deficit schizophrenia. *American Journal of Psychiatry, 159*(6), 983–990.

Gerber, R. (2000). *Vibrational medicine for the 21st century.* New York: Eagle Brook.

Gochman, P. A., Greenstein, D., Sporn, A., Gogtay, N., Nicolson, R., Keller, A., et al. (2004). Childhood onset schizophrenia: Familial neurocognitive measures. *Schizophrenia Research, 71*(1), 43–47.

Gogtay, N., Sporn, A., Clasen, L. S., Nugent, T. F. III, Greenstein, D., Nicolson, R., et al. (2004).

Comparison of progressive cortical gray matter loss in childhood-onset schizophrenia with that in childhood-atypical psychoses. *Archives of General Psychiatry, 61*(1), 17–22.

Gottesman, I. I., & Petronis, A. (2003). Schizophrenia genetics obscured by the realities of complex diseases. *NAMI Advocate, 1*(4), 31–32.

Hagen, B. F., & Mitchell, D. L. (2001). Might within the madness: Solution-focused therapy and thought-disordered clients. *Archives of Psychiatric Nursing, 15*(2), 86–93.

Hummer, M., Malik, P., Gasser, R. W., Hofer, A., Kemmler, G., Naveda, R. C. M., et al. (2005). Osteoporosis in patients with schizophrenia. *American Journal of Psychiatry, 162*(1), 162–167.

Jungbauer, J., Wittmund, B., Dietrich, S., & Angermeyer, M. C. (2003). Subjective burden over 12 months in parents of patients with schizophrenia. *Archives of Psychiatric Nursing, 17*(3), 126–134.

Kelly, C., & McCreadie, R. G. (1999). Smoking habits, current symptoms, and premorbid characteristics of schizophrenia patients in Nithsdale, Scotland. *American Journal of Psychiatry, 156*(11), 1751–1757.

Keltner, N. L. (2005). Genomic influences on schizophrenia-related neurotransmitter systems. *Journal of Nursing Scholarship, 37*(4), 322–328.

Keshavan, M. S., Cashmere, J. D., Miewald, J., & Yeragani, V. K. (2004). Decreased nonlinear complexity and chaos during sleep in first episode schizophrenia. *Schizophrenia Research, 71*(2), 263–272.

Keshavan, M. S., Duggal, H. S., Veeragandham, G., McLaughlin, N. M., Montrose, D. M., Haas, G. L., et al. (2005). Personality dimensions in first-episode psychosis. *American Journal of Psychiatry, 162*(1), 102–109.

Kim, M. S., Ha, T. H., & Kwon, J. S. (2004). Neurological abnormalities in schizophrenia and obsessive-compulsive disorder. *Current Opinions in Psychiatry, 17*(3), 215–220.

Kruger, S., Bagby, R. M., Hoffler, J., & Braunig, P. (2003). Factor analysis of the catatonia rating scale and catatonic symptom distribution across four diagnostic groups. *Comprehensive Psychiatry, 44*(6), 472–482.

Lawson, W. B. (2000). Issues in pharmacotherapy for African Americans. In P. Ruiz (Ed.), *Ethnicity and psychopharmacology* (pp. 37–53). Washington, DC: American Psychiatric Press.

Lecomte, T., Wallace, C. J., Perreault, M., & Caron, J. (2005). Consumers' goals in psychiatric rehabilitation and their concordance with existing services. *Psychiatric Services, 56*(2), 209–211.

Marshall, M., & Lockwood, A. (2000). Assertive community treatment for people with severe mental illness. *Cochrane Database Systematic Reviews, 2,* CD001089.

McDevitt, J., Wilbur, J., Kogan, J., & Briller, J. (2005). A walking program for outpatients in psychiatric rehabilitation. *Biological Research for Nursing, 7*(2), 87–97.

Miklowitz, D. J. (2004). Family therapy. In S. L. Johnson & R. L. Leahy (Eds.), *Psychological treatment of bipolar disorder* (pp. 184–202). New York: Guilford Press.

Moberg, P. J., Roalf, D. R., Gur, R. E., & Turetsky, B. I. (2004). Smaller nasal volumes as stigmata of aberrant neurodevelopment in schizophrenia. *American Journal of Psychiatry, 161*(12), 2314–2316.

Mueser, K. T., Bond, G. R., & Drake, R. E. (2001). Community-based treatment of schizophrenia and other severe mental disorders: Treatment outcomes. *Medscape Mental Health, 6*(1). www.medscape.com/ Medscape/psychiatry/journal/2001/v06.n01/.

Navon, L., & Ozer, N. (2003). Ordinary logic in unordinary lay theories: A key to understanding proneness to medication nonadherence in schizophrenia. *Archives of Psychiatric Nursing, 17*(3), 108–116.

Nechmad, A., Ratzoni, G., Poyurovsky, M., Meged, S., Avidan, G., Fuchs, C., et al. (2003). Obsessive-compulsive disorder in adolescent schizophrenia patients. *American Journal of Psychiatry, 160*(5), 1002–1004.

North American Nursing Diagnoses Association. (2007). Nursing Diagnoses Definitions and Classification 2005–2006. Philadelphia: Author.

Olincy, A., Harris, J. G., Johnson, L. L., Pender, V., Kongs, S., Allensworth, D., et al. (2006). Proof-of-concept trial of an alpha7 nicotinic agonist in schizophrenia. *Archives of General Psychiatry, 63*(6), 630–638.

Onitsuka, R., Nestor, P. G., Gurrera, R. J., Shenton, M. E., Kasai, K., Frumin, M., et al. (2005). Association between reduced extraversion and right posterior fusiform gyrus gray matter reduction in chronic schizophrenia. *American Journal of Psychiatry, 162*(3), 599–601.

Pallanti, S., Quercioli, L., & Hollander, E. (2004). Social anxiety in outpatients with schizophrenia. *American Journal of Psychiatry, 161*(1), 53–58.

Phillips, M. R., Yang, G., Li, S., & Li, Y. (2004). Suicide and the unique prevalence pattern of schizophrenia in mainland China. *Lancet, 364*(9439), 1016–1017.

Philpot, T. (2005). From hotel to home. *Nursing Standard, 19*(51), 22–23.

Practice Guideline for the Treatment of Patients with Schizophrenia (2nd ed.). (2004). Supplement to the *American Journal of Psychiatry, 161*(2), 1–56.

Rickelman, B. L. (2004). Anosognosia in individuals with schizophrenia: Toward recovery of insight. *Issues in Mental Health Nursing, 25*(3), 227–242.

Ryan, M. C. M., Collins, P., & Thakore, J. H. (2003). Impaired fasting glucose tolerance in first-episode, drug-naïve patients with schizophrenia. *American Journal of Psychiatry, 160*(2), 284–289.

Saenger, E. (2004). Treatment-resistant schizophrenia: An expert interview with Ralph Hoffman. *Medscape Psychiatry & Mental Health, 9*(2), 1–4. www.medscape.com/viewarticle/496285.

Scott, J., Kingdon, D., & Turkington, D. (2004). Cognitive-behavior therapy for schizophrenia. In J.

H. Wright (Ed.), *Cognitive-behavior therapy* (pp. 1–24). Washington, DC: American Psychiatric Press.

Seeman, M. V. (2004). Gender differences in the prescribing of antipsychotic drugs. *American Journal of Psychiatry, 161*(8), 1324–1333.

Siever, L. J., & Davis, K. L. (2004). The pathophysiology of schizophrenia disorders: Perspectives from the spectrum. *American Journal of Psychiatry, 161*(3), 398–413.

Sipos, A., Rasmussen, F., Harrison, G., Tynelius, P., Lewis, G., Leon, D. A., et al. (2005). Paternal age and schizophrenia: A population based cohort study. *British Medical Journal, 330*(7483), 147–148.

Sporn, A. L., Addington, A. M., Gogtay, N., Ordonez, A. E., Gornick, M., Clasen, L., et al. (2004). Pervasive developmental disorder and childhood-onset schizophrenia. *Biological Psychiatry, 55*(10), 989–994.

St. Clair, D., Xu, M., Wang, P., Yu, Y., Fang, Y., Zhang, F., et al. (2005). Rates of adult schizophrenia following prenatal exposure to the Chinese famine of 1959–1961. *JAMA, 294*(5), 557–562.

Tamminga, C. A., Thaker, G. K., & Medoff, D. R. (2004). Neuropsychiatric aspects of schizophrenia. In S. C. Yudofsky & R. E. Hales (Eds.), *Essentials of neuropsychiatry and clinical neurosciences* (pp. 457–487). Washington, DC: American Psychiatric Publishing.

Tarrant, C. J., & Jones, P. B. (2000). Biological markers as precursors to schizophrenia. In J. L. Rapoport (Ed.), *Childhood onset of "adult" psychopathology* (pp. 65–102). Washington, DC: American Psychiatric Press.

Torrey, E. F., & Yolken, R. H. (2003). Toxoplasma gondii and schizophrenia. *Emerging Infectious Diseases, 9*(11), 1375–1380.

Tsai, Y. F., & Ku, Y. C. (2005). Self-care symptom management strategies for auditory hallucinations among inpatients with schizophrenia at a veterans' hospital in Taiwan. *Archives of Psychiatric Nursing, 19*(4), 194–199.

Tucker, J. S., Wenzel, S. L., Straus, J. B., Ryan, G. W., & Golinelli, D. (2005). Experiencing interpersonal violence. *Violence Against Women, 11*(10), 1319–1340.

Turetsky, B. I., Moberg, P. J., Arnold, S. E., Doty, R. L., & Gur, R. E. (2003). Low olfactory bulb volume in first-degree relatives of patients with schizophrenia. *American Journal of Psychiatry, 160*(4), 703–708.

Wonodi, I., Adami, H. M., Cassady, S. L., Sherr, J. D., Avila, M. T., & Thaker, G. K. (2004). Ethnicity and the course of tardive dyskinesia in outpatients presenting to the motor disorders clinic at the Maryland psychiatric research center. *Journal of Clinical Psychopharmacology, 24*(6), 592–598.

Yasuno, F., Suhara, T., Okubo, Y., Sudo, Y., Inoue, M., Ichimiya, T., et al. (2004). Low dopamine D2 receptor biding in subregions of the thalamus in schizophrenia. *American Journal of Psychiatry, 161*(6), 1016–1022.

Chapter **15**

Substance-Related Disorders

"*Understand Me* **"**

—Brian, Age 19

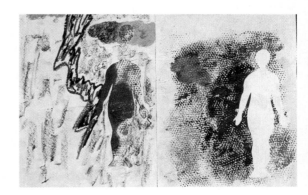

OBJECTIVES

After reading this chapter, you will be able to:

1. Outline information about the site of action, effects, complications, withdrawal, and overdose for commonly abused substances.

2. Compare and contrast the different theories regarding the etiology of substance-related disorders.

3. Discuss the psychopharmacological treatment of the symptoms of substance-related disorders.

4. Outline the different treatment options for a client with a substance-related disorder.

5. Outline the assessment process for a client with a substance-related disorder.

6. Describe the impact of a substance-related disorder on the functioning of family members.

7. Use the nursing process to develop a comprehensive plan of care for a client with a substance-related disorder.

MediaLink www.prenhall.com/fontaine

Go to the Pearson Health MediaLink CD-ROM and the Companion Website at www.prenhall.com/fontaine for interactive resources for this chapter.

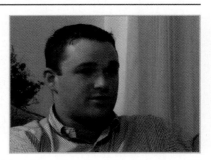

The ROAD to Critical Thinking

A Client Experiencing a Substance-Related Disorder

Travel this ROAD to understand Chris and his condition.

Read about Chris below and throughout this chapter.

Observe Chris on the CD-ROM accompanying this book.

Assess Chris by answering the questions at the end of this chapter.

Develop a Care Plan on the CD-ROM to address Chris's condition.

Chris

Chris, age 28, began stealing alcohol from his parents' liquor cabinet at age 12. Over the next several years he progressed to daily drinking but told himself he would never use drugs. In his junior year in high school he tried marijuana at a party one time and then a couple of weeks later he tried it again. Before long he was getting high a couple of times a day. He started using cocaine when he was 21 years old and by age 25 he was spending $1,000 a week on cocaine. At that point in time he decided he needed help and went into treatment.

Adolescents are quicker than adults to initiate and extend poly-drug abuses. Most adolescents abuse a wide number of substances, whereas adults tend to focus on one or two "drugs of choice." Males are more likely to abuse cocaine, majijuana, and opioids; females are more likely to abuse sedatives, antianxiety agents, and amphetamines (Compton, Thomas, Conway, & Colliver, 2005; O'Malley, 2005). For a list of the risk factors in teenagers, see Box 15.1.

You will meet Chris on the video clip on your disc and throughout this chapter. At the end of the chapter you will find critical thinking questions relating to assessment and development of a plan of care for Chris.

In our society, many people use substances recreationally to modify mood or behavior. There are, however, wide sociocultural variations in the acceptability of chemical use. Alcohol, caffeine, and tobacco are legal drugs, but the social acceptability of using them varies. Narcotics, sedatives, stimulants, and hallucinogens are often used illegally, and the general population considers recreational use to be socially unacceptable.

There are other forms of addiction, often referred to as *process addictions*, which are beyond the scope of this chapter. These process addictions include workaholism, gambling, shopping, spending and indebtedness, Internet, eating disorders, and sexual addiction. Process addictions involve compulsive behaviors that serve to reduce anxiety. Individuals who have reward deficiency syndrome (see chapter 6 ∞) are addicted to engaging in dangerous activities where there is a possibility of death. BASE jumpers are an example. The acronym refers to Buildings, Antennas, Spans (or bridges), and Earth (or cliffs), from which adherents leap. As they jump, their bodies start producing neurotransmitters, which provide the "high" to which they are addicted.

The *Diagnostic and Statistical Manual of Mental Disorders* (4th ed., Text Revision) (DSM-IV-TR) classifies the pathological use of chemicals as psychoactive substance-related disorders. The words *substance* and *chemical* are used interchangeably. **Substance abuse** is defined as recurrent use that results in a failure to manage work, school, or home roles; or use in hazardous situations such as driving a car; or use resulting in substance-related legal problems or related

BOX 15.1	Substance Dependence Risk Factors in Teenagers

- Peer pressure, group norms: prosubstance use
- A greater here-and-now orientation than adults; drugs provide immediate gratification
- Rebellion against authority
- Alienation from traditional social and religious values; drugs viewed as a way to individuate and disconnect
- Stressful situations, such as a dysfunctional family
- Insecurity and low self-esteem: powerful triggers for compensatory substance abuse

interpersonal problems. This diagnosis can be used only for someone who has never been diagnosed as dependent. **Substance dependence** occurs when the use of the drug is no longer under control and continues despite adverse effects. Substance-dependent individuals experience tolerance, with a need for increasing amounts of the drug, withdrawal symptoms, and increasingly higher doses. People who are dependent on drugs may spend a great deal of time obtaining drugs and limit their usual social, occupational, or recreational activities because of the substance use. As addiction continues, the need for the drug is so powerful that previously law-abiding people commit crimes and parents neglect children in the search for drugs (Hyman, 2005). This chapter focuses on substance dependence, which is the more severe form of the substance-related disorders. See the DSM-IV-TR diagnostic criteria box for a description of substance use disorders.

Substance **withdrawal** is physiological, behavioral, cognitive, and affective symptoms that occur after reduction or discontinuance of a drug that has been used heavily over a long period of time. When experiencing withdrawal, most individuals find themselves craving the drug, which they know would reduce the withdrawal symptoms. Withdrawal symptoms are specific for each drug (American Psychiatric Association, 2000).

Chemical dependence is a complex, chronic, progressive *disease* that can be fatal if left untreated. While it is true that a disease is not defined as a deficiency of willpower, this disease is composed of several biochemical processes that are subject to voluntary control. In addition, there are psychological, sociological, and spiritual aspects to chemical dependence.

A number of types of psychoactive substances are associated with chemical dependence. The days of the so-called "pure" drug addict or alcoholic are gone. Most people who are chemically dependent are poly-drug abusers. They may use amphetamines or cocaine to get high, and alcohol, diazepam (Valium), or marijuana to come down off the high. Some use sedatives to sleep and amphetamines to wake up. Whatever the pattern, clients must be treated for all secondary, as well as primary, addictions.

Substance use disorders in the United States cost over $414 billion a year, including the costs of treatment, related health problems, absenteeism, lost productivity, drug-related crime and incarceration, and education and prevention. Alcoholism (alcohol dependence) is a major health problem, one that is responsible for 100,000 deaths annually in the United States. Tobacco causes 431,000 deaths a year, while illicit drugs are related to 16,000 annual deaths. Studies indicate that alcohol and drugs are a factor in 50% of motor vehicle fatalities and 50% of all violent deaths from any cause. Between 40% and 60% of people seeking treatment are ordered to do so by the court system. The relapse rate for those who have been in treatment is 90% in the first year, with most occurring after 3 months of treatment (Murphy-Parker & Martinez, 2005; Nader & Czoty, 2005; Wright, 2003).

In general, women drink less heavily than men do. In the United States, 29% of males and 7% of females are diagnosed with alcoholism. The mean age of onset for males is 22 years, and for females it is 25 years. The illicit nature of drug use makes it nearly impossible to retrieve accurate information on the number of drug abusers in the United States. As much as 46% to 50% of all Americans 12 years of age and older have tried an illegal drug at least once during their lives. It is estimated that drug addiction is a problem for 9% to 20% of the U.S. population. The prevalence rate for alcohol or drug addiction in the medical population is 25% to 50%, and 50% to 75% in individuals with mental disorders (Miller & Adams, 2005).

In the 1960s, hallucinogens and amphetamines were the illegal drugs most commonly used. In the 1970s, heroin, marijuana, and sedatives were the most popular drugs. The 1980s was the decade of cocaine. Judging by the increase in cocaine-related visits to hospital emergency departments, we continue to have hard-core cocaine abuse problems in the United States. Eight million Americans use cocaine regularly, with 2.2 million considered dependent. Heroin has become a more popular drug with adolescents and young adults due to the change from injecting it to smoking it. Unfortunately, users mistakenly believe that smoking heroin is not addicting. Illicit use of prescription drugs has increased recently, especially among adolescents who mistakenly believe these

MediaLink

Care Plan, Risk for Relapse

DSM-IV-TR   Diagnostic Criteria for Substance Abuse Versus Substance Dependence

DIAGNOSTIC CRITERIA FOR SUBSTANCE ABUSE

A. A maladaptive pattern of substance use leading to clinically significant impairment or distress, as manifested by one (or more) of the following, occurring within a 12-month period:
   1. Recurrent substance use resulting in a failure to fulfill major role obligations at work, school, or home
   2. Recurrent substance use in situations in which it is physically hazardous
   3. Recurrent substance-related legal problems
   4. Continued substance use despite having persistent or recurrent social or interpersonal problems

caused or exacerbated by the effects of the substance

B. The symptoms have never met the criteria for substance dependence for this class of substance.

DIAGNOSTIC CRITERIA FOR SUBSTANCE DEPENDENCE

A. A maladaptive pattern of substance use, leading to clinically significant impairment or distress, as manifested by three (or more) of the following, occurring at any time in the same 12-month period:
   1. Tolerance
   2. Withdrawal
   3. The substance is often taken in larger amounts or over a longer period than was intended.

   4. There is a persistent desire or unsuccessful efforts to cut down or control substance use.
   5. A great deal of time is spent in activities necessary to obtain the substance.
   6. Important social, occupational, or recreational activities are given up or reduced.
   7. The substance use is continued despite knowledge of having a persistent or recurrent physical or psychological problem that is likely to have been caused or exacerbated by the substance.

SOURCE: Reprinted with permission from the American Psychiatric Association. (2000). *Diagnostic and statistical manual of mental disorders* (4th ed., Text Revision) (pp. 197–199). Washington, DC: Author.

DSM-IV-TR   **Diagnostic Criteria for Substance Intoxication and Withdrawal**

DIAGNOSTIC CRITERIA FOR SUBSTANCE INTOXICATION

A. The development of a reversible substance-specific syndrome due to recent ingestion of (or exposure to) a substance. Note: Different substances may produce similar or identical syndromes.

B. Clinically significant maladaptive behavioral or psychological changes that are due to the effect of the substance on the central nervous system (e.g., belligerence, mood lability, cognitive impairment, impaired judgment, impaired social or occupational functioning) and develop during or shortly after use of the substance.

C. The symptoms are not due to a general medical condition and are not better accounted for by another mental disorder.

DIAGNOSTIC CRITERIA FOR SUBSTANCE WITHDRAWAL

A. The development of a substance-specific syndrome due to the cessation of or reduction in substance use that has been heavy and prolonged.

B. The substance-specific syndrome causes clinically significant distress or impairment in social, occupational, or other important areas of functioning.

C. The symptoms are not due to a general medical condition and are not better accounted for by another mental disorder.

SOURCE: Reprinted with permission from the American Psychiatric Association. (2000). *Diagnostic and statistical manual of mental disorders* (4th ed., Text Revision) (pp. 201–202). Washington, DC: Author.

---

drugs are safer than illegal drugs. The rapidly escalating abuse of amphetamines, especially Ecstasy, is a significant problem at dance clubs and dance parties known as "raves." Young people take these "love drugs" for increased energy and sexual desire (Compton et al., 2005; O'Malley, 2005).

In the 1800s, alcohol, opiates, cocaine, and marijuana were part of many medications used to treat a variety of illnesses. The addictive potential of these chemicals were not known at the time. Those at highest risk for addiction were physicians, physicians' wives, housewives, and nurses. It was believed that for every male addict there were three female addicts. By the early 1900s, the process of addiction became clear but it was believed to be moral failing rather than a disease that could be treated. Addiction was criminalized with passage of the Harrison Narcotic Act of 1914, Prohibition, the Marijuana Tax Act of 1937, the Narcotic Control Act of 1956, the Controlled Substance Act of 1970, and the creation of the Drug Enforcement Agency in 1973.

In the early 20th century, nurses were identified as being at high risk for addiction due to high work loads and high stress levels. There were, however, no treatment options at the time. In the 1960s, nurses and physicians were identified as being at higher risk for narcotic addiction. Little was done about the problem of addiction and most instances were ignored. When nurses were identified as addicted or abusing alcohol or drugs, they were either fired or reported to state boards of nursing and disciplined by censure, suspension, or having their professional license revoked. In the 1970s research on **impaired nursing practice** began to appear and in 1982 the American Nurses Association (ANA) passed a resolution entitled "Action on Alcohol and Drug Misuse and Psychological Dysfunctions Among Nurses." The hope was to shift the focus from punishment to rehabilitation. In 2002, the ANA adopted an updated resolution entitled "The Profession's Response to the Problems of Addictions and Psy-

chiatric Disorders in Nursing," calling attention again to impaired nursing practice, stressing the need for peer assistance programs (Heise, 2003).

When nurses have an addiction, shame and guilt are magnified. After all, nurses are healers and nurturers. They are not expected to have their own problems, certainly not an addiction that could lead them to take drugs from clients or be less than 100% in control when they are at work. Early studies suggested that nurses are at higher risk for addiction than the general population. More recent studies contradict these findings and state that it is most likely that nurses are not at higher risk for substance abuse (Snow & Hughes, 2003).

Nurses now have access to peer assistance and statewide programs to seek treatment and save their licenses. Nurses with substance abuse problems are required to stop practicing and enter a 12-step treatment program for monitoring. Those who abuse alcohol are not allowed to perform client care or handle controlled substances for 6 months. For those who abuse substances other than alcohol, the ban is for 1 year (Fletcher, 2004; West, 2002). See Box 15.2 for signs of substance abuse among nurses.

BOX 15.2   **Signs of Substance Abuse Among Nurses**

- Frequent or unexplained disappearances from the unit
- Increasing difficulty meeting schedules or deadlines
- Sloppy or illogical charting
- Excessive number of mistakes
- Smell of alcohol on breath
- Labile emotions
- Diminished alertness
- Isolation from coworkers
- Frequent reports of medication spills or other waste
- Discrepancies in end-of-shift medication counts
- Increase in client complaints of unrelieved pain

KNOWLEDGE BASE

Comorbid Disorders/Dual Diagnosis of the Mentally III Chemical Abuser

Clients must be assessed for **dual diagnosis**, the presence of substance abuse as well as a mental disorder. A dual diagnosis indicates one of three things:

- Two disorders occur together, independent of each other.
- Substance abuse causes the other mental disorder.
- The person with the mental disorder uses substances in an effort to self-medicate and feel better.

Whatever the original cause of substance abuse, it usually complicates all other problems so much that it must be dealt with immediately. Substance abuse can precipitate psychiatric relapses and contribute to medication noncompliance, as well as relationship difficulties, financial mismanagement, disruptive behavior, and unstable housing. Therefore, people with dual diagnoses have a poorer prognosis than those with a single diagnosis (Havassy, Alvidrez, & Owen, 2004).

Individuals with a psychiatric disorder are at higher risk for having a substance abuse disorder. Of the general population, 13.8% abuse alcohol and drugs. The comorbidity of major depression with nicotine, alcohol, and drug abuse ranges from 32% to 54%. Sixty-one percent of people with bipolar disorder also experience substance abuse or dependence. Substance use disorders range from 22% to 43% in individuals with posttraumatic stress disorder. Rate of comorbid substance use disorders is 30% to 50% in adolescents with attention deficit hyperactivity disorder, oppositional defiant disorder, or conduct disorder. The rate of comorbid substance use disorders, excluding nicotine, is 50% in individuals with schizophrenia. The rate of nicotine dependence for those with schizophrenia is estimated at 70% to 90%. Smokers with mental disorders use nearly half of all cigarettes consumed in the United States (Brady & Sinha, 2005; Kessler, 2004; Ziedonis & Williams, 2003).

People with mental illnesses report that their reasons for using substances include attempting to improve unpleasant moods such as anxiety and depression, increasing social interactions, and increasing pleasure by feeling high. It is clear, however, that drugs and alcohol often increase psychiatric symptoms and are a factor in relapse of mental illness. Violence against others and violence against oneself also occur more frequently in substance-abusing persons with mental illness.

The following section begins with an overview of the commonly abused substances and provides specific information for each of the categories regarding site of action, effects, complications, withdrawal, and overdose. See Table 15.1 ■ for an overview of this information.

Alcohol

Types of alcohol include liquor, beer, and wine. Common street names for alcohol and mode of administration include:

- *Street names:* Booze, hooch, moonshine, sauce, brew
- *Mode of administration:* Oral

Site of Action

Alcohol acts as a central nervous system depressant in two ways. Alcohol potentiates gamma-aminobutyric acid (GABA) activity, a major inhibitory neurotransmitter. Alcohol decreases glutamate activity, a major excitatory neurotransmitter. In both cases, the outcome is depression of the central nervous system (CNS).

Effects

Alcohol is the most widely used drug in the United States and it is estimated that nearly 25% of all people admitted to a general hospital have alcohol problems. The *pattern of dependence* on alcohol varies from person to person. Some have a regular daily intake of large amounts of alcohol. Others restrict their use to drinking heavily on the weekends or days off from work. Some may abstain for long periods of time and then go on a drinking binge. The behavior may be inconsistent at the beginning of dependence. At times, people with alcohol dependence can drink with control, and at other times, they cannot control the drinking behavior. As the course of alcoholism continues, there may be behaviors such as starting the day off with a drink, sneaking drinks through the day, gulping alcoholic drinks, shifting from one alcoholic beverage to another, and hiding bottles at work and at home. They may give up hobbies and other interests in order to have more time to drink. It is not unusual for alcoholics to engage in what is known as *telephonitis*, making telephone calls to family and friends at inappropriate times, such as the middle of the night (Liska, 2004).

People with alcohol dependence can be separated into two groups. Those with type 1 alcoholism have a later onset, more psychological than physical dependence, and guilt related to their alcohol use. Those with type 2 alcoholism demonstrate problems with alcohol at an earlier age, compulsively seek alcohol, and are socially disruptive when drinking (Chai et al., 2005).

Ron describes his escalating substance abuse: "After my wife died from an asthma attack, I didn't care about anything. I tried to escape from it by drinking too much alcohol and using drugs because when I did that I didn't feel anything. It made me numb. But when I'm not using, I think about all my problems."

Mayfield, McCleod, and Hall (1974) developed the *CAGE Questionnaire*, which is simple and can be incorporated into

TABLE 15.1	Frequently Abused Substances			
Substance	**Psychological Effects**	**Physiological Effects**	**Overdose**	**Withdrawal**
Alcohol	Hostility, crying, shame, despair, blackouts, talkativeness	Slurred speech, lack of coordination, flushed face	Confusion, stupor, coma, possible death	6–8 hours after last drink: Irritability, tremors, elevated pulse and blood pressure 6–96 hours: Seizures, hallucinations 3–14 days: Alcohol withdrawal delirium
Sedatives	Sedation, euphoria, talkativeness, irritability, impaired attention and memory	Drowsiness, sleep, lowered pulse and blood pressure	CNS depression, respiratory arrest	Similar to alcohol withdrawal, seizures, anxiety, tremors, psychosis
Narcotics	Euphoria, sedation, attention and memory, motivation, apathy	Drowsiness, pinpoint pupils, pain motor retardation	Lowered respirations, pulse, and blood pressure; coma, death	Few hours to few days; craving, flulike symptoms, fearfulness
Cannabis	Pleasure, euphoria, slowed sense of time, altered perceptions	Dry mouth, fast pulse, appetite, fatigue, reddened eyes	Hallucinations	Craving, anxiety
Amphetamine	Elation, energy, anxiety, grandiosity, rapid speech, confusion	Elevated pulse and blood pressure, arrhythmias, visual disturbances, insomnia	Agitation, hallucinations, cardiovascular collapse, suicide	Sleep, fatigue, anhedonia, depression
Cocaine	Euphoria, energy, talkativeness, grandiosity, impaired judgment, paranoia, violence	Insomnia, anorexia, elevated pulse and blood pressure, runny nose, irritated nasal membrane	Delirium, hyperthermia, seizures, respiratory or cardiac arrest, cerebral hemorrhage	Severe craving, irritability
Hallucinogens	Euphoria, hallucinations, impulsiveness, paranoia, impaired judgment, body image changes	Intensified perceptions, sense of slowed time, elevated pulse and blood pressure, tremors, lack of coordination	Confusion, delirium, psychosis, accidents, suicide	No symptoms
Inhalants	Euphoria, uninhibited behavior, floating sensation, illusions, drowsiness, amnesia	Perceptual changes, hallucinations, eye irritation, sensitivity to light, nose/mouth irritation	Cardiac and respiratory arrest	No symptoms

any nursing assessment. Having one positive answer raises concern, and more than one positive answer is a strong indication of alcohol problems:

C Have you ever felt that you should **c**ut down on your drinking?

A Have people **a**nnoyed you by criticizing your drinking?

G Have you ever felt bad or **g**uilty about your drinking?

E Have you ever taken a drink in the morning as an "**e**ye-opener"?

Complications

Alcohol is a chemical irritant and has a direct toxic effect on many organ systems, as described in Table 15.2 ■.

Blackouts, a fairly early sign of alcoholism, are a form of amnesia about events that occurred during the drinking period. The alcoholic may carry out conversations and elaborate activities with no loss of consciousness, but have total amnesia about those activities the next day. This may be explained by the toxic effects of alcohol on glutamate transmission necessary for memory storage. A more advanced CNS problem is *Wernicke encephalopathy*, which is characterized by ataxia (lack of coordination), abnormal eye movements, and confusion. These symptoms result from long-term thiamine deficiency. About 80% of people with Wernicke encephalopathy also develop *Korsakoff syndrome*, characterized by intact intellectual functioning but an inability to retrieve long-term memory events or retain new

TABLE 15.2	Physiological Complications From Alcohol Dependence

Body Systems	Toxic Effects
Gastrointestinal	Esophageal reflux, esophagitis, esophageal varices, gastritis, decreased appetite, malabsorption, recurrent diarrhea, acute or chronic pancreatitis (75% of cases related to alcohol abuse)
Liver	Hepatomegaly, fatty liver, alcoholic hepatitis, cirrhosis, cancer. Elevated gamma-glutamyl transpeptidase (GGT) results
Cardiovascular	Hypertension, cardiomyopathy, arrhythmias, increased risk for stroke, coronary artery disease, sudden cardiac death
Respiratory	Pneumonia, bronchitis, tuberculosis
Hematologic	Bone marrow depression, anemia, leukopenia, blood clotting abnormalities
Neurologic	Seizures, peripheral neuropathy, optic neuropathy, Wernicke encephalopathy, Korsakoff syndrome, alcoholic dementia, impaired cognitive function, labile moods, sleep disturbances
Endocrine	Hyperglycemia, decreased thyroid function
Reproductive	Erectile problems, decreased testosterone, decreased sex drive, menstrual irregularities
Nutritional	Thiamine deficiency, folic acid deficiency, vitamin A deficiency, magnesium deficiency, zinc deficiency

SOURCE: American Psychological Association. (2000). *Diagnostic and statistical manual of mental disorders* (4th ed., Text Revision). Washington, DC: Author; Dunphy, L. M., & Winland-Brown, J. E. (2001). *The art and science of advanced practice nursing.* Philadelphia: Davis; and Naegle, M. A., & D'Avanzo, C. E. (2001). *Addictions and substance abuse: Strategies for advanced practice nursing.* Upper Saddle River, NJ: Prentice Hall.

information. **Confabulation**, making up information to fill memory blanks, develops in the person's attempt to protect self-esteem when confronted with memory loss. *Alcoholic dementia* is characterized by impaired abstract thinking and judgment, personality changes, and impaired memory. This is often seen in chronically heavy drinkers (Stern & Sacheim, 2004).

Withdrawal

Alcohol withdrawal syndrome (AWS) typically begins about 6 to 8 hours after the last drink. Early symptoms include irritability, anxiety, insomnia, tremors, sweating, and a mild tachycardia. In rare cases, the person may experience grand mal seizures or intermittent visual, tactile, or auditory hallucinations. Symptoms of withdrawal usually peak during the second day of abstinence and are likely to show significant improvement by the fourth or fifth day. For individuals who repeatedly withdraw from alcohol, symptoms become worse each time (Reoux & Ries, 2001).

Alcohol withdrawal delirium, formerly referred to as delirium tremens (DTs), usually occurs on days 2 and 3 but may appear as late as 14 days after the last drink. The person experiences confusion, disorientation, hallucinations, tachycardia, hypertension or hypotension, extreme tremors, agitation, diaphoresis, and fever. Death may result from cardiovascular collapse or hyperthermia. With improved diagnosis and medical treatment, the mortality rate has dropped from 20% to 1% (American Psychiatric Association, 2000).

Overdose

Signs of alcohol intoxication include nausea, vomiting, lack of coordination, slurred speech, staggering, disorientation, irritability, short attention span, loud and frequent talking, poor judgment, lack of inhibition, labile emotions, and, for some, violent behavior. Alcohol intoxication may result in accidents or falls that may cause contusions, sprains, and fractures and facial or head trauma. High blood alcohol levels may result in unconsciousness, coma, respiratory depression, and death. See Table 15.3 ■ for symptoms associated with blood alcohol levels. This becomes a *critical situation* in the emergency department and necessitates careful triage and monitoring to prevent death or permanent disability.

Sedatives/Hypnotics/Antianxiety Agents

Types of sedatives/hypnotics/antianxiety agents include barbiturates (Seconal, Nembutal, Amytal, Tuinal, phenobarbital, Quaaludes) and benzodiazepines (Valium, Librium, Xanax, Halcion, Ativan). Common street names for sedatives/hypnotics/antianxiety agents and mode of administration include:

- *Street names:* Downers, ludes, red devils, reds, blue angels, blues, yellow jackets, trenks, barbs, candy
- *Mode of administration:* Taken orally but can be used intravenously (IV)

| TABLE 15.3 | Blood Alcohol Levels and Symptoms |

Blood Alcohol Level (percentage of alcohol in blood)	Behavior
0.05	Changes in mood and normal behavior; loosening of judgment and restraint; person feels carefree
0.08–0.10	Voluntary motor action clumsy; legal level of intoxication
0.20	Brain motor area depression causes staggering; easily angered; shouting; weeping
0.30	Confusion; stupor
0.40	Coma
0.50	Death (usually due to medullar respiratory blocking effects)

Site of Action

They act by enhancing the action of GABA in the limbic system of the brain. They may cause significant CNS depression.

Effects

People using these drugs may experience drowsiness, sedated appearance, lack of coordination, euphoria, labile emotions, irritability, anxiety, impaired attention, and working memory loss. Clients taking therapeutic levels of benzodiazepines for a period of time develop physical dependence on the medication. This should be differentiated from intentional abuse of benzodiazepines. Intentional abusers usually have other substance abuse problems. They use benzodiazepines to augment the high received from another drug or to offset the adverse effects of other drugs (O'Brien, 2005a).

Complications

Two new designer drugs, Rohypnol (roofies, forget pills, R2) and GHB (G-riffic, Grievous Bodily Harm, Liquid G), have been called "date rape" drugs because they have been used to render rape victims unconscious. They also cause short-term memory loss, leading to horrifying stories of women whose only memory is of waking up naked with a stranger. Initially, they give a feeling of euphoria but combined with alcohol can lead to unconsciousness, coma, or, in some cases, death.

Withdrawal

Symptoms of withdrawal are similar to alcohol withdrawal: altered perceptions, hallucinations, depression, diaphoresis, marked agitation, tachycardia, anxiety, tremors, seizures, and delirium. If the individual has been taking high doses or has been taking these drugs for a long period of time, the withdrawal process should be medically supervised. Abrupt cessation can lead to serious problems, such as seizures and psychosis, and may even end in death. The medication is carefully titrated downward until the withdrawal process is completed.

Overdose

An overdose of sedative–hypnotics is very dangerous. Symptoms include weak and rapid pulse, shallow respirations, cold and clammy skin, and possible coma and death. When combined with alcohol, serious overdose can occur rapidly, with death from respiratory depression.

Opioids

There are almost a million long-term opiate users in the United States. Types of opioids include morphine, heroin, codeine, Vicodin, OxyContin, Dilaudid, Percodan, Demerol, methadone, Nubain, Darvon, Oxyfast, Percocet, Ultram, and Talwin. Common street names of opioids and modes of administration include:

- *Street names:* Smack, dope, H, horse, shit, Miss Emma, lords, D, dollies, china white, Captain Cody, oxy, big daddy, brown sugar, monkey, big O, black stuff
- *Modes of administration:* Oral, smoking, inhalation, injection, IV

Site of Action

Endorphins, enkephalins, and dynorphins are the naturally occurring substances that stimulate the opiate receptors in the brain, providing pain relief, pleasure, and motivation and regulating temperature, respiration, endocrine, and gastrointestinal activity. External opioids attach to those same opiate receptors.

Effects

When opioids are injected IV or inhaled, brain levels rise rapidly giving a brief, intense sensation called a rush or thrill. This is followed by a longer lasting period called a high, which includes a sense of calmness. The effects of opioids are a sedated appearance, motor retardation, slurred speech, impaired attention and memory, decreased awareness, and reduction of instinctual drives. Euphoria, pleasure, and relaxation also occur. Physically, opioids depress respiration, suppress coughs, and inhibit gastrointestinal motility. Cocaine and heroin may be used together as heroin maintains the euphoria after cocaine loses its effect. Continued use decreases the body's production of endorphin and enkephalin, resulting in a very low tolerance of pain and discomfort during withdrawal.

Christina describes the development of her substance dependence: "My husband and I had been out drinking. When we got home I decided to do the laundry. I slipped down the stairs and hit my tailbone on every stair. It hurt for 6 months. Then I was talking to my neighbor and she gave me some of her Vicodin. I didn't know what they were, I just called them "happy pills." I asked for more. She told me they were expensive so I bought them from her. When I needed more I went to the doctor to get a prescription. He didn't want to give them to me. I kept pushing him to give me the Vicodin. He finally gave me 90 pills plus three or four refills. Then I went to another doctor and got a prescription from him. Finally, I had to start getting them off the street. Right now I am taking 15 to 20 Vicodin a day and three Xanax to sleep."

Complications

Poisoning may be a problem because heroin is often "cut" with substances that may contain impurities to increase the quantity for sale. Because the potency of street heroin is unknown and because today's heroin is considerably more potent than it was 30 years ago, a number of overdose deaths occur every year. Since most users "shoot up" and share needles, they are at high risk for hepatitis, HIV infection, and AIDS. Other complications from heroin use include liver problems, malignant hypertension, strokes, and kidney failure, largely as the result of infections and impurities.

Withdrawal

Withdrawal symptoms usually begin within a few hours to a few days after the last dose. Symptoms are subjectively distressful and include craving, muscle aches, backaches, severe abdominal cramps and diarrhea, watery eyes, running nose, yawning, tremors, chills, sweating, and a crawling skin sensation. Symptoms peak in 2 to 3 days, and the discomfort may last as long as 2 weeks.

Overdose

Oxycodone (OxyContin) is a powerful and highly addictive time-released prescription pain medication. Some people in search of a rush chew or snort it, which can result in a dangerous or lethal drug overdose. Signs of opiate overdose include clammy skin, shallow respirations, pinpoint pupils (may be dilated with severe hypoxia), coma, and death from respiratory depression or sudden irreversible pulmonary edema. Naloxone (Narcan), a narcotic antagonist, 0.4 mg to 2 mg may be given IV to reverse respiratory depression and coma. The reversal is rapid but short-lived; thus, repeated treatments are needed every 2 to 3 minutes. The client must be contin-

ually assessed until the opioid is eliminated from the body. Furosemide (Lasix) may be helpful for pulmonary edema.

Cannabis

Types of cannabis include marijuana and hashish. The most common street names and modes of administration are:

- *Street names:* Grass, chronic, joint, pot, ganja, blang, reefer, weed, Mary Jane, Acapulco gold, Colombian, roach
- *Modes of administration:* It is smoked in cigarettes or pipes. Inhaling the smoke through a water-cooled apparatus called a *bong* lessens irritation and aids in deeper inhalation. Occasionally taken orally when mixed with food.

Site of Action

Delta-9-tetrahydrocannabinol (THC) is the psychoactive ingredient in cannabis. The content of THC ranges from 2% to 5% in marijuana, while hashish can contain up to 15% THC. THC acts on the cardiovascular and central nervous system. Recently, scientists have discovered a cannabis receptor in the brain. It is believed that we make our own endogenous cannabis in the form of anandamide, a derivative from arachidonic acid. Anandamide regulates memory, appetite, mood, learning, and motor coordination (Liska, 2004).

Effects

Cannabis is the most widely used illegal drug in the United States. Sixty million people have tried cannabis, and some 20 million use it regularly. Effects of cannabis include pleasure that may progress to euphoria, anxiety, apathy, detachment, passivity, enhanced appetite, slowed sense of time, altered perceptions, and sexual arousal.

Marijuana as a medical herb has been used for centuries, much longer than its use as a recreational drug. Marijuana appears to be a more potent antiemetic than prescription antiemetics. It is also useful in treating glaucoma, epilepsy, multiple sclerosis, hypertension, anorexia, and pain.

The debate regarding medical marijuana continues at the federal level, although several states have approved the use of marijuana for medical purposes. Americans who currently use marijuana medicinally do so illegally and without assurances of quality control. The National Institutes of Health and the Institute of Medicine have issued statements of support for medical marijuana. In 2006, the Food and Drug Administration (FDA) issued a statement that there were no scientific studies supporting the medical use of marijuana, ignoring the scientific studies that have been published in peer-reviewed medical journals. It appears politics, rather than science, influenced the FDA announcement (Carter & Mirken, 2006).

Complications

Since cannabis results in slowed response time and inattention, users should not drive motor vehicles for 12 hours after using the drug. Untoward effects include acute panic reactions, hostility, or vomiting. Cannabis is often used with other drugs, for example, to extend a heroin high or to lessen anxiety when snorting cocaine.

Embalming fluid is becoming an increasingly popular drug for users looking for a new and different high—one that often comes with violent and psychotic side effects. Users are buying marijuana cigarettes that have been soaked in the fluid and then dried. They are called by any number of names, including "wet," "fry," and "illy."

Withdrawal

Common withdrawal symptoms include irritability, anxiety, restlessness, sleep difficulties, and decreased appetite or weight loss.

Overdose

Overdose may result in a psychotic episode characterized by bizarre behavior, paranoia, and hallucinations. Cannabis is not lethal even at very high doses.

Cocaine

The most common street names for cocaine and modes of administration include:

- *Street names:* Coke, crack, blow, snow, C, powder, dust, flake, nose candy, rock
- *Modes of administration:* It is administered through smoking, inhalation, injection, and/or IV. When smoked, brain delivery rate is similar to IV.

Cocaine can be used in several ways. Snorting powdered cocaine into the nose, where it is absorbed through the mucous membrane, is a common method. There remains a persistent but erroneous belief that snorting cocaine is not addictive. It is addictive; it just takes longer. Snorting on a regular basis causes ulcerations of the nasal mucous membrane and may lead to perforation of the septum. The high is achieved about 2 to 3 minutes after use and may last as long as 20 to 30 minutes.

Smoking purified chips of cocaine, known as crack, has a higher potential for addiction and leads to more compulsive use than snorting does. It is the most efficient way to deliver cocaine, taking only 6 to 7 seconds for the drug to reach the brain. The high lasts only 2 to 5 minutes, and the crash is more severe than with snorting. Infants and children who live with crack abusers often test positive for cocaine, most likely from inhaling secondhand crack smoke.

Site of Action

The primary reason people use cocaine is to stimulate the CNS. It is believed that cocaine binds to the dopamine (DA) transporters, preventing them from picking up DA, resulting in an accumulation of DA and an out-of-control reward system. The cumulative effect is an intense feeling of euphoria. Persistent blockage of DA transporters may eventually lead to depletion of DA levels. Cocaine is the only drug laboratory animals prefer to food, water, and sex. Research animals allowed to self-administer cocaine with no limitations will often overdose and die (Liska, 2004).

Effects

Because of its action on the CNS, cocaine is a uniquely addicting drug. With its powerful rewarding properties, cocaine is even capable of making obsessive users of well-adjusted and mature individuals. **Positive reinforcement** occurs through the mood-altering effects of generalized euphoria, increased energy and mental alertness, a feeling of self-confidence, and increased sexual arousal. Tension, fatigue, and shyness disappear, and the person becomes more talkative and playful. Judgment may be impaired, and the person may become paranoid or even violent. The initial rush of euphoria lasts only 10 to 20 seconds followed by a less intense feeling of euphoria lasting 15 to 20 minutes.

Chris:

❝ I would smoke marijuana and drink. Then to stay awake, I resorted to cocaine, and that would just make me drink even more. At the end of my drugging career, I was snorting cocaine all day. At night I would consume a 12-pack [of beer] within 30 minutes or an hour in order to come down from the cocaine to get to bed. And that was a daily occurrence, every day. ❞

Following cocaine use, the intense pleasure is replaced by equally unpleasant feelings. This is referred to as a rebound dysphoria, or "crash." **Negative reinforcement** occurs when the person experiences the crash and takes more cocaine to overcome the dysphoria. Both positive and negative reinforcement sustain the use of cocaine. With increased use, there is a progressive tolerance of the positive effects while the negative effects steadily intensify. In other words, the highs are not as high and the lows are much lower.

Complications

Cocaine induces constriction of coronary and cerebral vessels, leading to cardiac and cerebral infarcts, with the risk being higher for those who smoke crack. Positron emission tomography (PET) studies in long-term cocaine users show decreased glucose utilization and generalized decreased blood flow in the frontal cortex (Gottschalk, Beauvais, Hart, & Kosten, 2001).

Complications from snorting cocaine may be loss of the sense of smell and necrosis leading to perforation of the nasal septum. Smoking cocaine can cause pulmonary damage and IV use may contribute to hepatitis. Since 27% to 75% of cocaine abusers also meet the criteria for alcohol abuse or dependence, there are added complications (Liska, 2004).

Crack cocaine can lead to marathon binge use, known as a *run*, lasting many hours or even days. A run can cost hundreds or thousands of dollars and leave the person in a state of total dysfunction.

Some people try speedballing, in which cocaine is mixed with heroin and injected intravenously. The high is reached in about 30 to 60 seconds. The appeal of a speedball is that the heroin decreases the unpleasant jitteriness and crash from cocaine. Speedballs are extremely dangerous. Heroin decreases the respiratory rate, as does cocaine in high enough doses. Heroin decreases the threshold for seizures, and cocaine is capable of inducing seizures. Because some users mistakenly believe that the effects cancel each other out, they overdose.

Space-basing is smoking crack cocaine that has been sprinkled with phencyclidine (PCP). This method may lead to intense panic and terror. People who have space-based sometimes become violent, and their behavior is uncontrollable.

Withdrawal

Symptoms of cocaine withdrawal include severe craving for cocaine and depression, which may be important triggers for relapse. Other symptoms include fatigue, irritability, vivid and unpleasant dreams, and insomnia or hypersomnia.

Overdose

Signs of cocaine intoxication include the feelings of euphoria, grandiosity, anger, combativeness, and impaired judgment. In addition, the person may experience tachycardia, elevated blood pressure, perspiration or chills, nausea and vomiting, seizures, respiratory depression, cardiac arrhythmias, hyperpyrexia, and death. Death can occur in as little as 2 to 3 minutes or up to 30 minutes after smoking crack (American Psychiatric Association, 2000).

Treatment of cocaine overdose may require ventilation of the client. Medications include lidocaine or propranolol IV for ventricular dysrhythmia, acetaminophen or dantrolene (Dantrium) for hyperthermia, propranolol or calcium channel blockers for tachycardia, hydralazine or nitroprusside for hypertension, and diazepam or phenobarbital for seizures.

Amphetamines

Types of amphetamines include benzedrine, methedrine, dexedrine, methamphetamine, and MDMA (methylenedioxymethamphetamine—a synthetic designed drug). Common street names of amphetamines and modes of administration include:

- *Street names:* Bennies, speed, dexies, hearts, uppers, pep pills, crystal, crank, meth, speed, ice, crystal, glass, Ecstasy, X, Adam, beans, E, Eve, lover's speed, peace
- *Modes of administration:* Oral, smoking, and IV

Site of Action

The stimulant effect on the neurotransmitters is similar to that of cocaine. It both blocks reuptake of DA and increases release of DA. The long-lasting effects on the brain are much greater than the changes found in people who abuse heroin, alcohol, or cocaine. One or two doses can cause permanent brain damage from vasoconstriction and neurotoxicity (Volkow et al., 2001).

Effects

In small amounts, amphetamines create a sense of mental alertness, euphoria, self-confidence, and increased sex drive. As use increases, people become hypervigilant, grandiose, agitated, and irritable, and experience intense sexual desire. Some individuals alternate between using amphetamines to "get going" and sedatives to "calm down."

Methamphetamine is cheap and easy to make in home labs using pseudoephedrine, the ingredient in many cold medicines. Ice, the smokable form of methamphetamine, is sometimes used as a substitute for cocaine because it is more easily available and less expensive. The effects of ice are similar to those of crack cocaine except that the euphoric state comes on a little slower and may last as long as 12 to 30 hours. People who use ice are more likely to become violent and unpredictable.

Instead of euphoria, MDMA users experience a warm state of empathy and good feelings for all those around them. This state of positive feelings has been described as a decrease in fear and aggression and an increase in connectedness.

Complications

Amphetamines greatly increase cardiac and respiratory rates and blood pressure. Long-term abuse frequently leads to paranoid, often violent, psychotic states accompanied by auditory and tactile hallucinations. Other complications include motor disturbances similar to Parkinson disease and poor memory performance, as well as tachycardia, arrhythmias, hypertension, altered respiration, headache, visual disturbances, and insomnia. Death may occur from cerebrovascular accident, cardiovascular collapse, or suicide (Liska, 2004).

Withdrawal

Withdrawal symptoms include exhaustion, fatigue, excessive need to sleep, unpleasant dreams, enhanced appetite, and depression. Drug craving may occur in some individuals. Depression may last for weeks and be accompanied by suicidal ideation.

Overdose

Amphetamine intoxication is often associated with impaired social or occupational functioning. Other symptoms include euphoria, hyperactivity, hypervigilance, interpersonal sensitivity, talkativeness, anxiety, anger, fighting, and impaired judgment. The person may experience tachycardia, arrhythmia, coronary artery spasms, myocardial infarction, hypertension, hyperthermia, and seizures. Medications include propranolol or calcium channel blockers for tachycardia, hydralazine or nitroprusside for hypertension, and diazepam (Valium) or phenobarbital for seizures. A protective environment may be necessary to prevent injury or suicide.

MDMA can cause death when combined with high levels of physical activity, such as at a rave. Death is usually the result of greatly increased body temperature, hypertension, muscle breakdown, and kidney failure.

Hallucinogens

Types of hallucinogens include lysergic acid diethylamide (LSD), mescaline, PCP, psilocybin, ketamine, and gamma-hydroxybutyrate (GHB). Common street names of hallucinogens and modes of administration include:

- *Street names:* Acid, cid, microdots, windowpane, barrel, blotter, sugar cubes, trips (LSD); mesque (mescaline); angel dust, crystal, hog, tranks, tea (PCP); magic mushrooms, shrooms (psilocybin); green mauve, L.A., special coke, Special K, bumps (ketamine); G, Liquid G (GHB)
- *Modes of administration:* Oral, smoking, inhalation, IV

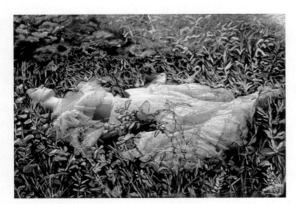

PHOTO 15.1 ■ Hallucinogenic drugs distort and intensify visual perceptions.

SOURCE: A. Rousseau/The Image Works. Used with permission.

Site of Action

These substances affect DA, serotonin (5-HT), norepinephrine (NE), and opioid receptors in the brain. The effects on the brain are somewhat unpredictable and may be influenced by the environment, the experience, and the expectations of the user (Liska, 2004).

Effects

People who take hallucinogens describe vivid visual images, altered perceptions, and a sensation of slowed time. They may also experience euphoria, anxiety, labile emotions, hostility, and depression. They may be impulsive or unable to perform simple tasks.

Hallucinogens are the only drugs that animals will not self-administer, indicating that they do not like the effects. The underlying reason is that the sensory, visual, and auditory misinterpretations have no beneficial effect for survival.

Complications

One of the dangers is a "bad trip," during which the person is in a psychotic state and terrified by perceptual changes. Flashbacks occur when the person is drug free but relives the experience of being on the drug. Hallucinogens can lead to violent and out-of-control behavior.

Herbal Ecstasy, also known as Cloud 9, X, and Ultimate Xphoria, is a legal (in many states) combination of herbs and other ingredients available cheaply at health food stores and truck stops as pills or tea. The main active ingredients are caffeine and ephedrine. Both of these drugs give a sense of euphoria and energy that lasts several hours. High doses can cause increased heart rate and blood pressure, heat stroke, stroke, and death. The FDA has issued warnings against the use of these drugs (Liska, 2004).

Withdrawal

Withdrawal is generally believed not to occur.

Overdose

Hallucinogen intoxication is evidenced by marked anxiety, ideas of reference, inattention, fear of losing one's mind, paranoia, and impaired judgment. Other changes include intensification of perceptions, depersonalization, illusions, hallucinations, dilated pupils, tachycardia, sweating, tremors, and incoordination. In most cases the person knows that the effects are substance induced. Cause of death may be due to accidents or suicide.

Inhalants

Types of inhalants include volatile solvents (gasoline, lighter fluid, paint thinner, spray paint, wax removers, hair spray, odorants, air fresheners, dry cleaning fluid, spot remover, analgesic sprays), propellant gases used in aerosols such as whipped cream dispensers, nitrates (amyl nitrite, butyl nitrite), and anesthetics (nitrous oxide). Common street names of inhalants and modes of administration include:

- *Street names:* Poppers, bombers, buzz bomb, snappers, rush, laughing gas
- *Modes of administration:* Fumes are inhaled directly from an open container or from a surface upon which the substance has been applied (sniffing), from a plastic bag (snorting, bagging), or from an inhalant-soaked rag next to or over the mouth or nose (huffing).

Site of Action

Substances displace oxygen and cause tachycardia and depression of the CNS.

Effects

Volatile substances produce a quick form of intoxication. with effects such as lightheadedness, tingling, euphoria, giddiness, impaired judgment, sense of well-being, sense of power, slurred speech, salivation, and loss of contact with reality. Other effects are sensations of floating and perceptual changes, including hallucinations.

Nitrates have been used by individuals to enhance sexual experience and pleasure. Nitrates may cause euphoria and alter perceptions. Nitrous oxide, often sold in large balloons from which the gas is released, induces a state of giggling and laughter.

Complications

Long-term use of inhalants can cause multiple organ damage. In the cardiovascular system, they can lead to myocarditis and fibrosis. Some cause direct pulmonary irritation with chemical pneumonitis. Toluene, the active substance in airplane glue, may cause chronic renal failure, peripheral neuropathy, and dementia. Contact dermatitis may be seen on the hands, nose, or around the mouth. Problems associated with nitrites include panic reactions, nausea, dizziness, and hypotension. Nitrous oxide can cause a paranoid psychosis with confusion. After several years of decline, the use of inhalants increased significantly from 2003 to 2004 (NIDA InfoFacts, 2005).

Withdrawal

There are no known withdrawal symptoms related to the use of inhalants.

Overdose

Anytime someone uses inhalants, she or he can die, even from the first experience. "Sudden sniffing death" is associated with arrhythmias, ventricular fibrillation, decreased cardiac output, respiratory depression, and accidents while intoxicated.

Anabolic Steroids

Types of anabolic steroids include Anadrol, Anavar, Dianobol, Durabolin, Equipose, Finajet, Halotestin, Maxibolin, Winstrol, Durabolin, and Depo-testosterone. Designer steroids often used by professional athletes include tetrahydrogestrinone (THG), Turinabol, Norbolethone, Sydnocarb, and Bromantan. Common street names of anabolic steroids and modes of administration include:

- *Street names:* Roids, Andro, juice
- *Modes of administration:* Anabolic steroids are administered by oral or IM injection. Users may "stack" steroids—mixing oral and injectable forms. Users often "pyramid"—set up 6- or 12-week cycles beginning with low doses, slowly increase the doses, midway start decreasing the doses, ending with zero use. This may be a continuous cycle, or the user may take a break from steroid use between cycles.

Site of Action

Anabolic steroids act on testosterone receptors concentrated in certain muscle groups, genitalia, hair follicles, and a few brain regions. Steroids increase calcium uptake in bones, increase protein synthesis, and alter the distribution of body fat (Liska, 2004).

Effects

Athletes and body builders use anabolic steroids to build body muscle mass and strength and improve physical appearance. Adolescent boys and girls may try steroids in an effort to look like body builders and supermodels. There is little evidence that steroids enhance athletic skill, although the ability to train longer and harder is enhanced. Some people report an increase in energy and may even experience a "high."

Complications

There is a potential for liver tumors, jaundice, kidney problems, fluid retention, hypertension, and cardiovascular problems. Other problems include headaches, nausea, vomiting, diarrhea, severe acne (especially on the face and back), halitosis, glucose intolerance, insomnia, and immune system compromise. A less well-known side effect is referred to as *roid rage*, with dramatic mood swings, maniclike episodes and a tendency toward aggressive behavior and violence. Women using anabolic steroids may increase muscle mass, develop a deeper voice, develop a larger clitoral size, experience breast atrophy, have absent menses, and be infertile. Steroids may cause a decreased sex drive, shrinking of the testicles, infertility, difficulty in urinating, and gynecomastia in males (Liska, 2004).

Withdrawal

There are no known withdrawal effects related to the use of anabolic steroids.

Overdose

Toxicity may be evidenced by abnormal liver, cardiac, and renal function tests.

Caffeine

Caffeine is ingested orally. Common street names for caffeine and modes of administration include:

- *Street names:* Java, Jo
- *Modes of administration:* Caffeine is administered through ingestion of liquids and food. Following are the average dosage amounts: brewed coffee, 125 mg/cup; instant coffee, 90 mg/cup; tea, 60 mg/cup; caffeinated soft drinks, 40 mg/cup. Chocolate and over-the-counter medications account for less than 10% of caffeine consumption by U.S. adults. Heavy use is daily or near-daily consumption of 625 mg or more of caffeine.

Site of Action

Absorption of caffeine occurs within minutes, and brain levels remain stable for at least 1 hour. Caffeine increases activity in the frontal lobe where working memory is centered and in the anterior cingulum, which controls attention. Caffeine is an adenosine receptor antagonist. Blockage of this receptor results in mental alertness, reduction in cerebral blood flow, and bronchodilation.

Effects

People use caffeine to decrease fatigue, increase alertness, and enhance a sense of well-being. People with asthma say that caffeine makes breathing easier. Caffeine is probably the most widely used drug in the world. Eighty percent of adults drink at least 3 cups of coffee a day.

Complications

The most well-known side effect is nervousness. For individuals who are susceptible to hypertension, caffeine may increase blood pressure. For those who are prone to anxiety, caffeine may increase levels of anxiety. Some people who consume large doses of caffeine experience gastroesophogeal reflux.

Withdrawal

Caffeine withdrawal, occurring within 24–48 hours, is marked by headaches, marked fatigue or drowsiness, anxiety or depression, irritability, muscle tension, and nausea or vomiting.

Overdose

Caffeine toxicity results in feeling ill, shaky, or jittery.

Nicotine

Types of nicotine include tobacco products: cigarettes, cigars, pipes, and chewing tobacco. Common street names of nicotine and modes of administration include:

- *Street names:* Smokes, fags, cigs, cancer sticks, chaw
- *Modes of administration:* Inhalation, chewing, prescription gum, or patch

Site of Action

Nicotine acts as an agonist at the nicotinic receptor, a subtype of acetylcholine receptor. It acts as a stimulant to the CNS by releasing DA in the nucleus accumbens, the reward center of the brain (Di Matteo, Pierucci, Di Giovanni, Benigno, & Esposito, 2007).

Effects

Nicotine produces feelings of alertness; increases blood pressure, heart rate, and respiration; increases irritability; and decreases appetite. Nicotine is as least as addictive as heroin, cocaine, or alcohol.

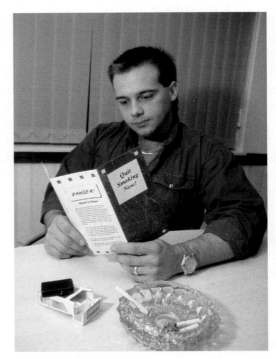

PHOTO 15.2 ■ Smoking is one of the greatest preventable hazards to health.
SOURCE: Dennis MacDonald/PhotoEdit. Used with permission.

Complications

Nicotine is still the leading cause of preventable, premature death in the world. The long-term health problems are related to the tars and other compounds released when burned. The most common complications are lung disease, cancer of the lung, and cardiovascular disease. People who chew tobacco are at higher risk for cancer of the mouth. Use of nicotine is more common among people with other mental disorders. Chronic smoking reduces longevity by an average of 13.2 years for men and 14.5 years for women (Cofta-Gunn, Wright, & Wetter, 2004).

Community education has resulted in a significant decrease in the use of nicotine by pregnant women. Unfortunately, most return to smoking within the first 6 months after the birth. Since secondhand smoke is a health risk for infants, further research is needed to determine the most effective way to help mothers prevent postpartum smoking relapse (Gaffney, 2006).

Withdrawal

Symptoms of withdrawal include craving, anxiety, restlessness, decreased concentration, overeating, irritability, frustration, constipation, and headaches. Nicotine gum and nicotine patches relieve withdrawal symptoms.

Overdose

Symptoms of nicotine overdose include heart palpitation, anxiety, and sleep disturbance.

Etiologies

Extensive research on the causes of substance dependence has yielded theories that combine biological and sociocultural components. It is obvious that there are multiple pathways for substance use disorders. The high risk factors are a genetic predisposition, an exposure to substances, and social reinforcement. Those individuals with the strongest predisposition may develop substance use disorders in any cultural setting where substances are available. Although the theories are presented separately, remember that they interact in ways that are not yet clearly understood.

Genetics

Substance-related disorders are heterogeneous. Many studies have focused on families in an attempt to determine whether a predisposition to alcoholism or substance abuse is inherited. Twins and adoptees have been studied to determine the role of genetics, and it has been found that alcoholism clearly runs in families, with inheritability estimates of 40% to 60%. This means that approximately half the risk for alcohol abuse disorders in the population can be explained by genetic factors.

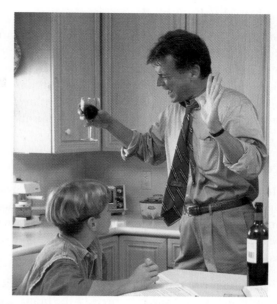

PHOTO 15.3 ■ Alcoholism runs in families because of a combination of genetic and environmental factors.
SOURCE: Tom & Dee Ann McCarthy/Corbis/Stock Market. Used with permission.

Early-onset alcoholism is a marker for a stronger genetic predisposition. Though we know there is an inheritable component, we do not know exactly what is inherited. It may be poor self-regulation, sensation seeking, or negative affect with a need to self-medicate (Kremer et al., 2005).

The genetic susceptibility is complicated and involves multiple genes. Each gene alone may not have power to cause

Chris: ❝ My uncle on my mother's side abused cocaine for many years. Alcohol abuse is prevalent all over my family—my father's sister, my mother's father, my father's mother, many of my father's uncles. So it's all over my family. ❞

alcoholism, but a group of genes acting together has a stronger influence. If the individual inherits a set of predisposing genes and encounters the necessary environmental influences, there will be a high probability that substance abuse disorder will result (Compton et al., 2005).

Tanya: "I talk to my husband a lot. He is a recovering alcoholic and we help each other out during times of stress because we each have the urge to drink under stress. I can't talk to my siblings or parents because they are all alcoholics who don't want to think they need help. My twin sister is very negative. She feels I am overexaggerating and I don't have a problem."

Genetic defects lead to deficiencies and imbalances in neurotransmitters, neuropeptides, neurotransporters, and receptors. These chemical changes may give rise to a wide range of behavioral disturbances and a variety of compulsive disorders.

Twin and adoption studies have demonstrated that up to 70% of the risk for becoming addicted to cocaine is due to genetic factors. Identifying the specific genes involved in cocaine dependence has not yet been accomplished (Dahl et al., 2005).

Neurobiology

Addiction to alcohol, drugs, and food share a mechanism involving the reward system in the brain. DA is not just the neurotransmitter that transmits pleasure signals; it may, in fact, be the master molecule of craving and addiction. Genetic defects may alter normal DA neurotransmission by:

- Interfering with the normal release of DA at critical receptor sites in the reward centers of the brain
- Changing the structure of DA receptors, resulting in decreased DA binding
- Decreasing the number of DA receptors, leading to decreased DA binding

Addictive substances such as alcohol, amphetamines, and marijuana temporarily offset or overcome these defects by releasing increased amounts of DA. Cocaine and MDMA (Ecstasy) block the reuptake of dopamine, resulting in increased levels in the synapse. Nicotine acts on the nicotinic acetylcholine receptors that facilitate release of DA. The opiates produce reinforcement independently of the DA system by acting directly on opioid receptors. Increased DA transmission in the basal ganglia, particularly the nucleus accumbens, is directly responsible for the exhilarating rush that reinforces the desire to get more of the substance. Thus, these substances move normal brain processes into an exaggerated state. Glucose probably has the same effect, thus causing a compulsive craving for food in some eating disorders. While DA is the primary neurotransmitter, it is believed that other neurotransmitters are involved, including GABA, glutamate, serotonin, norepinephrine, and endorphins (Berrettini & Lerman, 2005; Nader & Czoty, 2005; O'Malley, 2005).

Some individuals may begin with low levels of neurotransmitters. The first use of a substance corrects for this deficiency, which explains why people often enjoy their first experience with the alcohol or drug. The problem is that the psychoactive substance then creates an even greater deficiency of neurotransmitters, which contributes to craving for more of the substance.

Craving for a drug is a cardinal feature of addictive disorders and is significant because of its potential to trigger drug use and relapse. Craving is associated with the learned response that links the drug and its environment to an intensely pleasurable experience. The parts of the brain involved in this memory are the amygdala and the hippocampus. Stress and internal and external cues both prompt craving in people who abuse substances. Internal cues might be the feeling of anxiety, anger, depression, or frustration. External or environmental cues include drug-using friends, places where drugs are used, or seeing drug paraphernalia. Mental imagery of drug use creates significant activity in the nucleus accumbens and the amygdala (Kilts, Gross, Ely, & Drexler, 2004).

Compulsive use of drugs in addicted individuals occurs even when the drug is no longer perceived as pleasurable and even when there are adverse physical reactions to the drug. This process most likely involves the anterior cingulated gyrus. Drug *withdrawal* disrupts behavioral circuits in the frontal lobes, resulting in irritability, depression, and anhedonia. Symptoms of physical withdrawal persist for a short time after stopping long-term drug use. However, people report intense drug craving long after physical symptoms have subsided. That vulnerability to relapse can persist after years of abstinence implies that addiction causes long-lasting changes in brain function (Nestler & Self, 2004).

Drinking behavior is strongly influenced by the metabolism of alcohol. *Alcohol dehydrogenases* and *aldehyde dehydrogenase* are the enzymes that oxidize alcohol to acetaldehyde and acetate. High blood concentration of acetaldehyde causes extremely unpleasant flushing response—facial flushing and cardiac palpitations. Genes can either cause acetaldehyde to accumulate more rapidly or can delay the clearance of acetaldehyde, both of which protect against alcohol abuse through negative reinforcement. Fifty percent of Asian Americans lack the active form of the enzyme aldehyde dehydrogenase, as do many Sephardic Jews (Guindalini et al., 2005).

Drugs and alcohol affect brain functioning by inhibiting or facilitating certain kinds of processing. This results in a change of perception and a change in the length of time to process information. Crittenden and Claussen (2002) state that the exact effect of a particular substance depends on site of action, dosage, and frequency of use. Possible effects are:

- The person acts impulsively before processing in frontal lobes.
- The person does not respond to critically important stimuli because of slowed frontal lobe activity.
- The person has an overactive perception, resulting in excessive thoughts of threat and danger.
- The person has a decreased level of perception, resulting in an inability to see danger and initiate self-protective behaviors.

There is still much to learn about addiction. Researchers are looking at different roles that DA receptor subtypes play in creating and maintaining addiction. Other researchers have vaccines for substance abuse in clinical trials. It is important to remember that all genetic and neurobiological theories leave room for the substantial impact of environmental, social, and individual factors.

Intrapersonal Factors

For many years, intrapersonal theories were the only causative explanations for substance dependence, and they contributed to the moral perspective that exists in the general population today. These theories describe substance dependence as being determined by personality traits and developmental failures. More recent research has made these theories much less popular.

One hypothesis is that a person's basic nature is to search for altered states of consciousness. The result of this unconscious search is chemical dependence. Another hypothesis is related to a person's desire to seek out and discover new experiences. Impulsive personality traits are another consideration. Rebellion has also been proposed as an explanation for initiating the use of substances. Unlawful or undesirable behavior is one of the most effective means of expressing contempt or defiance of authority.

Personality traits are strongly influenced by genetic factors. Traits such as extraversion, impulsivity, risk taking, sensation seeking, and rebelliousness predict substance use (Kremer et al., 2005).

Behavioral Theory

Behavioral theory looks at the antecedents of substance use behavior, prior experiences with use, and the beliefs and expectations surrounding the behavior. This perspective considers which reinforcement principles operate in substance dependence. Consequences for continuing to use or deciding not to use, such as increasing pleasure or decreasing discomfort, are studied. Behavioral theorists also look at the activities associated with substance dependence, social pressures, rewards, and punishments.

Learning Theory

Learning theory states that chemically dependent people have learned maladaptive ways of coping. It is thought that substance dependence is a learned, maladaptive means of decreasing anxiety. Abusive behavior is viewed on a continuum from no use to moderate use, through excessive to dependent use. All these behaviors are learned responses. Learning theorists look at childhood exposure to role models, customs surrounding the use of chemicals, and the symbolic meaning of a drug. Risk factors include the degree of effort required to search out and obtain substances; the frequency and intensity of negative events while obtaining and using the substance; the availability of nondrug, pleasurable resources; and family context in terms of modeling, conflict, and degree of parental supervision.

Sociocultural Theory

Sociocultural theory considers how cultural values and attitudes influence substance use behavior. Cultures in which religious or moral values prohibit or extremely limit the use of alcohol or drugs have lower rates of chemical dependence.

Sociocultural theory is based on the idea that values, perceptions, norms, and beliefs are passed on from one generation to another. Alcohol is part of everyday life in some families; in other families, there is infrequent use or abstinence. The United States is a *drug-oriented society*. Advertisements offer medicinal cures not only for minor aches and pains but also for major health problems. Adolescents and young adults see their parents use various substances such as alcohol, caffeine, nicotine, antianxiety agents, and sedatives. With sanction from media advertising and parental examples, these young people see nothing wrong with trying various drugs.

Peer group pressure can cause drug use. Being in a peer group is important for adolescents and young adults. If some members are experimenting with drugs, other members are likely to follow suit.

One of the primary causes of substance abuse and dependence among African Americans and Hispanic Americans is sociocultural. Substance abuse is symptomatic of larger social problems. *Racism* creates a disparity in the socioeconomic systems of minority groups, who must manage the oppression that accompanies this inequality. Racism results in unemployment/underemployment and it is very difficult to live in poverty in a culture with a materialistic ethic. Racism also results in dense clustering in substandard housing, environmental pollution, inadequate health care, and lack of power. When all this is combined with the relatively excessive availability of alcohol and other drugs, it is not surprising that there is a high rate of substance dependence among young people from minority populations.

One example of sociocultural theory is seen in substance-related disorders among Native Americans who have lost their historical traditions. The federal government made them relocate to reservations, forcing subservience on them. The *stress of acculturation* has been very high. Economically, most residents of the reservations are chronically depressed. Native Americans suffer from extreme poverty, poor health, inadequate health care, housing problems, and transportation problems. Short-term relief through drinking or using drugs may appear to outweigh the long-term damage that results from substance dependence.

Gender-Bias Factors

Most substance abuse research studies prior to the turn of the century focused almost exclusively on male abuses, neglecting the prevalence and impact of substance use disorders in and on women. Presently, one third of American women regularly drink alcohol and about 2% meet the criteria for dependence.

One third of people who use crack cocaine in the United States are women (Boyd, 2003; Kilts et al., 2004).

It is perceived that men who get drunk with their friends are macho; women who drink to excess are slobs or unfit mothers. That makes women more likely to hide their problems and less likely to seek help. Men are more likely to leave chemically dependent women than women are to leave chemically dependent men. Women take less time than men to progress to alcohol-induced cognitive impairment and liver disease than do men (Baigent, 2003).

Women frequently have childhood and adult histories of physical, sexual, or emotional abuse and often state that addiction occurred as a response to severe stressors. Victimization and symptoms of posttraumatic stress disorder result in numerous negative symptoms and alcohol and drugs may be perceived as a way to cope with these problems. Feelings of alienation from significant others contributes to feeling lonely, unloved, unwanted, and depressed. Thus, when women's relationships fail or are dysfunctional, the use of substances often increases.

Psychopharmacological Interventions

Alcohol withdrawal is a serious medical problem, and the primary treatment goal is the prevention of delirium. Benzodiazepines are the medications of choice as they decrease withdrawal symptoms by preventing CNS hyperexcitability and prevent seizures. Dosage is determined by withdrawal symptoms. One of the following medications will be used: chlordiazepoxide (Librium), 25 to 50 mg, orally or IV, every 4 to 6 hours; diazepam (Valium), 5 to 10 mg, orally or IV, every 4 to 6 hours; clorazepate (Tranzene), 15 mg, orally, every 4 to 6 hours; or lorazepam (Ativan), 2 mg, as needed. These medications are titrated downward over a period of 5 days. High doses of thiamine are given during alcohol withdrawal to decrease the rebound effect of the nervous system as it adapts to the absence of alcohol. For clients with delirium, delusions, or hallucinations, antipsychotic medications may be used.

Craving for alcohol does not go away with abstinence. Several medications help with the craving sensations. Topiramate (Topamax), an anticonvulsant, reduces the reward effect of alcohol by decreasing the release of dopamine. Ondansetron (Zofran), an antinausea drug, helps modulate alcohol craving, especially for those who began drinking at a young age. It may be used alone or in combination with the sustained-release form of naltrexone (ReVia). The opiate antagonists naltrexone, acamprosate (Campral), and nalmefene (in clinical studies) have been shown to significantly decrease craving for alcohol and narcotics and lower the relapse rate. These medications interfere with the intoxicating effects in the brain by blocking the opiate receptors. People who take these opiate antagonists and drink or use narcotics report that they feel less "high," less

uncoordinated, and less intoxicated than usual. Side effects can include difficulty sleeping, nervousness, and gastrointestinal distress. Since these drugs can interfere with the use of narcotic analgesics in emergencies, the person must carry a medical alert card at all times. Some Alcholics Anonymous (AA) groups disagree with the use of naltrexone or acamprosate since the person is not "drug free," while other AA groups support the use of this medication (Kenna, Mcgeary, & Swift, 2004).

Health care providers in Europe and Australia routinely prescribe naltrexone (ReVia) to help clients manage alcohol craving; only 5% of clients in the United States are given naltrexone. It is believed that, in the United States, efforts to treat addiction with medications are hampered by prejudice and a public view that addiction is a disorder of self-control, not a disease (Dackis & O'Brien, 2003)

Some people suffering from alcoholism take disulfiram (Antabuse) as part of their rehabilitation treatment program. Disulfiram inhibits aldehyde dehydrogenase and leads to an accumulation of acetaldehyde if alcohol is ingested. The reaction occurs within 5 to 10 minutes and may last from 30 minutes to several hours. Symptoms include flushing, nausea and copious vomiting, thirst, diaphoresis, dyspnea, hyperventilation, throbbing headache, palpitations, hypotension, weakness, and confusion. In severe reactions, coma, seizures, cardiovascular collapse, respiratory depression, and death can occur. Disulfiram should be used only under careful medical and nursing supervision, and clients must understand the consequences of the therapy. Disulfiram is contraindicated for people with cardiovascular disease, depression, schizophrenia, or those who are pregnant. See Box 15.3 for client teaching regarding Disulfiram.

BOX 15.3	**Medication Teaching**

Disulfiram (Antabuse)

- Avoid all exposure to alcohol and substances containing alcohol, including food, liquids, and substances applied to the skin.
- Read all product labels to ensure that they do not contain alcohol.
- Common products that contain alcohol include mouthwash, cough syrups, shaving lotion, and cologne.
- If you are exposed to alcohol while taking disulfiram, you will experience a reaction within 5 to 10 minutes, and it may last from 30 minutes to several hours.
- Symptoms of a disulfiram reaction include flushing, nausea and severe vomiting, thirst, sweating, shortness of breath, hyperventilation, throbbing headache, heart palpitations, low blood pressure, weakness, and confusion. In a severe reaction, you may experience seizures, coma, and cardiac or respiratory arrest.
- Disulfiram takes 14 days to be removed from your body following discontinuation of the medication. Do not drink or become exposed to alcohol during this time.

Opiate overdose causes sedation and hypoventilation which can cause injury to any organ in the body. Naltrexone (ReVia) and naloxone (Narcan) reverse severe respiratory depression. The client must be monitored for recurrence of the respiratory depression for at least 2 hours after the last doses of these medications.

In Europe and in some places in the United States, distribution programs have been established to prevent deaths from opioid overdoses. Participants receive two doses of naloxone (Narcan), as well as comprehensive training to reduce overdose risk, administer naloxone, perform CPR, and call 911. Naloxone very rapidly reverses respiratory depression. It does not provide a high, so it is not likely to be abused or sold on the black market (Worthington, Markham, Galea, & Rosenthal, 2006).

Opiate withdrawal symptoms may be alleviated with clonidine (Catapres) and should be used under supervision in an inpatient detoxification center. Clonidine acts on the receptors in the brain to moderate the withdrawal effects. Since clonidine lowers blood pressure, vital signs should be carefully monitored.

Ultrarapid detoxification of opiates is a new treatment approach designed to almost eliminate the distressful symptoms of withdrawal. Rather than the 5 to 15 days with traditional detoxification procedures, ultrarapid detoxification can be accomplished within 4 to 6 hours. This approach, done in a hospital or surgical setting, uses heavy sedation or general anesthesia to ensure comfort during this procedure. The individual is then given naltrexone (ReVia), which blocks the opiate receptors and assists the receptors to begin to reestablish normal sensitivity. When the anesthesia is discontinued, the individual awakens being physically detoxified. The greatest advantage of this approach is humanistic; that is, it lessens the very distressing withdrawal symptoms of opiate addiction. The only risk is that of a reaction to the general anesthesia. This approach does not relieve the psychological withdrawal symptoms, and clients must agree to intensive follow-up programs to maintain their drug-free state (van den Brink, Goppel, & van Ree, 2003).

Methadone maintenance programs are used to treat *opioid craving*. The daily dose is titrated upward over a period of 2 weeks, with a daily maintenance dose of 60 to 80 mg. Unlike heroin, methadone can be taken orally, and its effects last 24, instead of 4, hours. Levomethadyl (Orlaam) is a longer-acting preparation that can be administered three times a week. Since it cannot be sent home with clients, they must ingest it at the clinic. Extreme care must be taken to protect children from accidentally ingesting methadone, as it may result in death to the child. The purpose of methadone is to reduce the craving to ward off withdrawal symptoms. The typical course of this narcotic substitution therapy program is 2 to 4 years, but some researchers believe lifelong maintenance may be necessary.

Opiate antagonists, such as naltrexone (ReVia) or the monthly IM version Vivitrol, are effective for withdrawal and craving. Another choice is buprenorphine (Subutex), started at a low dose and then titrated upward. Following this, clients are switched to buprenorphine and naloxone (Suboxone) on a maintenance schedule.

There are no FDA-approved medications for the treatment of *cocaine dependence*. Disulfiram (Antabuse) has been reported to reduce cocaine use in people who use cocaine and alcohol both. Cocaine interferes with glutamate neurotransmission in the reward centers of the brain. Modafinil (Provigil), a medication for narcolepsy that enhances glutamate, has been found to reduce the euphoria, withdrawal, and craving aspects of cocaine dependence (Dackis & O'Brien, 2003).

Propranolol (Inderal), a beta-blocker, has been found to significantly reduce relapse in people experiencing severe withdrawal symptoms. Topiramate (Topamax) and vigabatrin (Sabril), anticonvulsants, also reduce craving by increasing the levels of GABA in the reward system of the brain. There is some anecdotal evidence that gabapentin (Neurontin) may reduce craving in those who have a long history of cocaine addiction. Selegiline (Eldepryl, Carbex), a monoamine oxidase inhibitor, appears to help cocaine and methamphetamine craving (O'Brien, 2005b).

Overdose of benzodiazepines results in mild to moderate sedation. It is most fatal when these medications are combined with other sedating substances such as alcohol or sleeping pills. Intravenous flumazenil (Romazicon), a benzodiazepine antagonist, is given IV to counteract the sedation. Individuals with physical dependence on benzodiazepines may experience withdrawal symptoms and seizures when receiving flumazenil (Betten, Vohra, Cook, Matteucci, & Clark, 2006).

Sustained-release bupropion (Zyban), an antidepressant, is helpful for some individuals who wish to *quit smoking*. The dosage is 150 mg one time a day for 3 days, and twice a day thereafter. The client is instructed to pick a day to quit smoking approximately 3 weeks after beginning the medication. The smoker can then use nicotine replacement in the form of a patch, gum, or nasal spray to ease withdrawal symptoms.

Varenicline (Chantix) blocks nicotine receptors in the brain, which lessens withdrawal symptoms and limits the stimulation from nicotine. Naltrexone (ReVia) combined with a nicotine patch appears to reduce the weight gain that often accompanies smoking abstinence.

Researchers have found a new nicotine vaccine, NicVAX, that is safe and well tolerated. This vaccine works by triggering production of antibodies that bind to nicotine, creating a complex that is too large to pass through the blood–brain barrier (Hatsukami et al., 2005). See Box 15.4 for an overview of medications used to prevent relapse.

BOX 15.4	Medications Used to Prevent Relapse

Alcohol

- Topiramate (Topamax)
- Ondansetron (Zofran)
- Naltrexone (ReVia)
- Acamprosate (Campral)
- Disulfiram (Antabuse)

Opiates

- Methadone
- Levomethadyl (Orlaam)
- Naltrexone (ReVia, Vivitrol)
- Naloxone (Narcan)
- Buprenorphine (Subutex)
- Buprenorphine and naloxone (Suboxone)

Cocaine

- Disulfiram (Antabuse)
- Modafinil (Provigil)
- Propranolol (Inderal)
- Topiramate (Topamax)
- Vigabarin (Sabril)
- Gabapentin (Neurontin)
- Selegiline (Eldepryl, Carbex)

Nicotine

- Nicotine replacement
- Bupropion (Wellbutrin/Zyban)
- Varenicline (Chantix)
- NicVAX (nicotine vaccine)

BOX 15.5	Principles of Substance Addiction Treatment

- No single treatment is appropriate for all individuals.
- Treatment must be readily available.
- Effective treatment attends to multiple needs of the individual, not just her or his drug use. This may include medical services, family therapy, vocational rehabilitation, and social and legal services.
- Remaining in treatment for an adequate period of time is critical for treatment effectiveness.
- Individual or group counseling and other behavioral therapies are critical components of effective treatment.
- Medications are an important element of treatment, especially when combined with counseling and behavioral therapies.
- For people with dual diagnoses, both disorders should be treated in an integrated way.
- Medical detoxification is only the first stage of treatment and by itself does little to change long-term use.
- Treatment does not need to be voluntary to be effective.
- Recovery from addiction can be a long-term process and frequently requires multiple episodes of treatment.

SOURCE: National Institute on Drug Abuse. www.drugabuse.gov/DrugPages.

Multidisciplinary Interventions

No single treatment is appropriate for all individuals, and overcoming addiction is never an easy process. Effective treatment attends to the multiple needs of individuals, not just their drug use. Treatment approaches must address medical, psychological, social, vocational, and legal problems. Unfortunately, many of those who enter treatment relapse. But with medications and intensive, long-term support, many people can recover (Ehrmin, 2001). See Box 15.5 for principles of addiction treatment.

Treatment options include brief therapy, intensive outpatient or inpatient treatment, and residential treatment. Trained professionals at a community drug treatment center usually provide brief therapy. Clients learn specific behavioral methods for stopping or reducing substance use, such as goal setting, self-monitoring, and identifying high-risk situations. Outpatient-intensive programs allow clients to remain in their work and home settings while participating in treatment for 4 or 5 hours every day. It is appropriate for those who require intensive care but have a reasonable chance for abstinence outside a restricted setting. Inpatient treatment occurs in the emergency room and acute care inpatient units. Hospitalization is appropriate for those at risk for severe withdrawal syndromes, those who are with persistent mental illness, those

who are a danger to themselves or others, and those who have not responded to less intensive treatment efforts. Inpatient treatment usually lasts 3 to 7 days and offers a safe and structured environment for those who lack social and vocational skills and drug-free social supports to be abstinent in a less restricted setting. Inpatient programs are downsizing and closing as third-party reimbursement is rapidly decreasing.

Most older adults resist referral to chemical dependency programs and are more comfortable in senior-oriented programs. In addition, a significant number are unable or unwilling to leave their homes. Programs, therefore, must be specifically designed for older adults, including community outreach, home visitation, and social services. Substance abuse problems should be presented to them in the context of problems of adjusting to aging. They may need special approaches such as slow-paced therapy and emotionally supportive therapy rather than the confrontational style used with younger adult males. Social bonding with peers often improves outcomes.

Drug rehabilitation is the recovery of optimal health through medical, psychological, social, and peer group support for chemically dependent people and their significant others. **Abstinence** is merely stopping the intake of the drug; it does not imply that any other behaviors have changed. People who abstain often continue all their other unhealthy behaviors. In contrast, **sobriety** implies that not only have these individuals stopped using the chemical, but they have also achieved a centered or balanced state. Emotional growth is achieved through the development of positive values, attitudes, beliefs, and behaviors. Sobriety is the overall goal of alcohol and drug rehabilitation.

The **recovery model** is a vital part of rehabilitation that views chemical dependence as a chronic, progressive, and often fatal disease. The responsibility for recovery is on the client, and any attempt to shift responsibility to others, such as to family or friends, is confronted directly. Recovery is considered a lifelong, day-to-day process and is accomplished with the support of peers with the same addiction. Recovery programs typically are *12-step programs*, first introduced by AA, in which honesty is valued very highly. These programs are deeply spiritual, and recovery is thought to depend, in part, on faith in a higher power. See chapter 9 ∞ for more detailed information on 12-step programs. Clients are referred to AA, Cocaine Anonymous, or Narcotics Anonymous. Partners are encouraged to join Al-Anon, children are encouraged to join Alateen or Alatots, and adult children are encouraged to join Adult Children of Alcoholics (ACOA). (The 12 steps of AA are found in chapter 9 ∞, Box 9.2.) For those actively involved in 12-step programs, the rate of continuous abstinence is 44% for year 1, 83% for the second through the fifth years, and 90% for those involved for more than 5 years (Miller & Adams, 2005).

Treatment programs have traditionally been designed for men, and many people believe that women require different, gender-specific approaches. Believing that causes of substance abuse are poor self-esteem, relationship problems, and history of abuse and depression, treatment for women focuses on competence, strengths, and confidence. Confrontational models are less effective for women than are treatment approaches framed in terms of relationships. *Women for Sobriety (WFS)* is the first self-help support group founded specifically for women who are alcohol dependent. It is an emotional and spiritual growth program in which members use positive affirmation and share experiences to aid in the recovery process. The group process helps decrease the isolation and loneliness many substance-abusing women experience. Box 15.6 shows the 13 affirmations of WFS.

SMART Recovery offers free face-to-face groups and online mutual help groups. It is a nonreligious self-help group that may be appropriate for those who do not believe in a higher power, or those who do not want to mix their religious beliefs with substance recovery. The four points of the program are enhancing and maintaining motivation to abstain; coping with urges; problem solving; and lifestyle balance. While the SMART approach differs from the 12-step programs, it does not exclude them.

Family therapy helps family members identify situations in which they act as enablers. They then suggest alternative actions or statements that could be used in those situations. These new behaviors are practiced in a variety of settings. The family then moves on to making a contract with the client to use new, nonenabling strategies in the future.

Preventive education is another multidisciplinary intervention. Adolescents and preteens who have not used alcohol or other drugs need anticipatory guidance to help them cope with the inevitable choices they will have to make. Many community alcohol and drug projects and school-based prevention programs are helpful for parents and children and offer support groups and literature. The goal is to protect children from the many adverse consequences of smoking, drinking, and illicit drug use.

The need for *community education* continues. The medical community recognizes addictive disorders as brain diseases, but the concept of moral failure is still evident in the thinking of U.S. citizens. Our country has a higher investment in criminal justice than in treatment, including the denial of health insurance payment for addictive disorders. Some states offer treatment options in place of jail for nonviolent offenders. The cost of keeping a person in prison for a year is approximately $30,000, whereas treatment for a year costs $6,000 to $12,000. Nurses must continue to fight for innovative treatment programs for those

---

BOX 15.6	**Levels of the New Life Program and 13 Affirmations: Women for Sobriety**

Level I: Accepting Alcoholism as a Physical Disease

I have a drinking (life-threatening) problem that once had me.

Level II: Discarding Negative Thoughts, Putting Guilt Behind, and Practicing New Ways of Viewing and Solving Problems

Negative thoughts destroy only myself.
Problems bother me only to the degree I permit them to.
The past is gone forever.

Level III: Creating and Practicing a New Self-Image

I am what I think.
I am a competent woman and have much to give life.

Level IV: Using New Attitudes to Enforce New Behavior Patterns

Happiness is a habit I will develop.
Life can be ordinary or it can be great.
Enthusiasm is my daily exercise.

Level V: Improving Relationships as a Result of Our New Feelings About Self

Love can change the course of my world.
All love given returns.

Level VI: Recognizing Life's Priorities: Emotional and Spiritual Growth, Self-Responsibility

The fundamental object of life is emotional and spiritual growth.
I am responsible for myself and my actions.

SOURCE: Reprinted with permission from Women for Sobriety Inc., PO Box 618, Quakertown, PA 18951.

with substance use disorders. Effective drug treatment reduces crime, reduces the spread of infectious disease, and restores the ability of addicted people to be functional, contributing members of society rather than a drain on public resources (Barclay, 2004).

Alternative Therapies

Herbs and Nutrients

A nutritional supplement called SAMe (pronounced "sammy") may be effective in substance use disorders. SAMe (S-adenosylmethionine), a compound made by every cell in the body, helps produce DA, 5-HT, and NE. SAMe may be used for depression that accompanies withdrawal from psychoactive substances. It may also reverse some of the effects of alcoholic hepatitis and cirrhosis. The dose is 400 to 1,200 mg/day and is best taken 30 minutes before meals. SAMe should be used with caution in people who have a history of cardiac arrhythmias. SAMe levels in infants are naturally three to four times higher than in adults. Given this knowledge, the amount of SAMe passing to infants through breast milk may be inconsequential (Fontaine, 2005).

Herbs may also be useful in easing withdrawal symptoms. Chamomile is helpful during withdrawal from a number of substances. Evening primrose oil is used for alcohol withdrawal. Ginseng eases cocaine withdrawal, while valerian decreases the effects of benzodiazepine withdrawal. Milk thistle is thought to speed the production of new liver cells and bind to the outside of liver cells, slowing the entry of liver-damaging toxins. This appears to be effective in people with hepatitis and cirrhosis. Kudzu is in clinical trials for decreasing the craving for alcohol. Heantos, a mixture of 13 herbs, is in clinical testing for the treatment of heroin and cocaine addiction (Fontaine, 2005).

Omega-3 fatty acid is made up of DHA (docosahexaenoic acid) and EPA (eicosapentaenoic acid). DHA makes up one half of all fat in brain cell membranes, especially in the cortex and the photoreceptors of the retina. Excessive alcohol depletes the brain of omega-3 fatty acids, especially DHA, which contributes to cortical damage and visual impairment. The recommended dose is 2 to 4 g/day of fish oil. Taking the capsules at night and with orange juice reduces the fishy aftertaste.

Individuals who are malnourished from the effect of drugs and inadequate nutritional intake need to supplement all the known vitamins and minerals. These nutrients include free-form amino acid complex (1,500 mg/day) and L-cysteine or N-acetylcysteine (1,000 mg/day) for withdrawal and improvement in brain and liver function; glutathione 3,000 mg/day for decreasing the craving for alcohol; and B-complex vitamins for absorption of nutrients and formation of red blood cells. In addition to depleting the body of B-complex vitamins, alcohol also depletes magnesium, and vitamins C, D, E, and K. Caffeine depletes the body of biotin, inositol, potassium, thiamine, and zinc. Heavy caffeine users should replace these substances. Tobacco use depletes vitamins A, C, and E.

Health care professionals now advocate precursor amino acid loading in the diet to facilitate the restoration of neurotransmitters. Tryptophan is the precursor for serotonin, and tyrosine is the precursor for epinephrine. Two vitamins, ascorbic acid and folic acid, are necessary for the metabolism of tyrosine. Tropamine includes precursors for most of the neurotransmitters as well as substances that inhibit the destruction of neuropeptides. Tropamine may also decrease drug and alcohol craving.

Acupuncture

Acupuncture is an effective treatment for substance use disorders. It eases the symptoms of withdrawal and decreases the intensity of cravings. Acupuncture shows promise not only for cocaine addiction, but also for addiction to narcotics, amphetamine, steroids, antianxiety agents, nicotine, alcohol, and even food. In alcoholism, acupuncture relieves the symptoms of withdrawal and decreases the number of relapses. Acupuncture is a safe and relatively low-cost form of treatment (Lu, Lu, Lu, Lu, Lu, 2004).

Qigong

Qigong (pronounced "chee gong") is a Chinese discipline consisting of breathing and mental exercises combined with soft, slow, continuous circular movements. The softness of movements develops energy without nervousness. The slowness of movements requires attentive control that quiets the mind and develops one's powers of awareness and concentration. Li, Chen, and Mo (2002) studied the effectiveness of qigong therapy on detoxification of heroin addicts compared with medical and nonmedical treatment. Those in the qigong groups had fewer withdrawal symptoms over a shorter period of time than the other groups.

Guided Imagery

Imagery is a two-way communication between the conscious and unconscious mind and involves the whole body and all of its senses. In guided imagery, the images may be created by the therapist based on the needs of the client or by clients as a way to access inner resources. Wynd (2005) studied guided imagery as a treatment for quitting smoking. Both the control group and the imagery group received educational and counseling sessions. Two years after the intervention, 26% of individuals in the imagery group were abstinent from nicotine compared with 12% of the control group. Guided imagery, therefore, may be a useful tool for some individuals who wish to quit smoking.

Nursing Process

A CLIENT WITH A SUBSTANCE-RELATED DISORDER

ASSESSMENT

It is important that nurses in most clinical settings routinely screen clients for substance use, abuse, and dependence. Determining patterns of use allows for identification and treatment for people at risk.

People who abuse substances rarely seek treatment because they think they are drinking too much alcohol or using too many drugs. Typically, what brings them into the health care system are problems with their jobs, relationships, money, or the legal system. All who enter treatment are ambivalent about giving up the chemicals they have become dependent on. If clients are coerced into treatment, expect them to feel angry, controlled, humiliated, fearful, defensive, and mistrustful.

The nursing assessment should be conducted in a nonjudgmental and matter-of-fact way. Give positive recognition that it was a personal choice to come into treatment. State that the goal is not to force them into doing anything but rather to help achieve an assessment and understanding of the nature of their use of substances. Following the assessment, the nurse will be able to provide them with realistic feedback about their substance use behavior. Begin with less intrusive questions, such as "How many cigarettes do you smoke a day?" before asking questions about other substances. Follow with questions related to the use of prescription drugs. Then proceed to ask questions about the past and present use of alcohol and illegal drugs. Box 15.7 is an overview of a substance abuse assessment.

The Focused Nursing Assessment feature provides questions for assessing clients who are substance dependent. The assessment has a twofold purpose: to identify problems and to increase clients' awareness of the toll that substance use may be taking on their lives.

Clients being detoxified from alcohol abuse should be assessed on an ongoing basis using the *Clinical Institute Withdrawal Assessment (CIWA-Ar)* tool, which is described in Table 15.4 ■.

BOX 15.7	Substance Abuse History

- Assess for each substance
- Age begun
- Method of use (oral, smoking, inhaling, injecting)
- Amount and frequency of use
- Most recent use
- Withdrawal symptoms in the past
- Setting and circumstances of use (people, places, things, moods, and emotional states associated with use; how and where drugs are procured)
- Benefits of use
- Proportion of income or savings spent on drugs
- Financial consequences of drug use (overdue bills, credit card debts, does person sell drugs to offset cost)
- Relationship, vocational, social problems associated with use

Focused Nursing Assessment | Clients With Substance-related Disorders

Behavior Assessment	Affective Assessment	Cognitive Assessment	Social Assessment
When did you begin to have problems with substances?	In what way does your drug use decrease your: Anxiety? Boredom? Depression?	What kinds of things do you have difficulty remembering?	Who do you consider to be the most significant people in your life?
Have you ever missed work/school because of drug use?	What kinds of comments have others made to you about rapid mood swings?	Have you ever had blackouts?	Can you confide in these people?
What kinds of employment/school problems have you experienced?	What drug-abusing behavior has led you to feel: Guilty? Embarrassed? Ashamed? Humiliated?	Have you invented information or stories to make up for forgetting?	Which of these individuals abuse substances with you?
Have you missed family/social events because of drug use?		What reasons do you give others for your use of drugs?	Who knows about your substance abuse?
How hostile and argumentative do you become when using substances?		Have you experienced hallucinations?	Describe family arguments relating to your substance abuse.
Have you ever attempted to harm yourself or others while under the influence of drugs?		Do you believe you have a chemical dependence that is out of your control?	Who protects you from the consequences of your abuse?
			How has your sexual behavior changed with your substance use?
			Have you had periods in your life when you were drug-free? How long did these last?
			Have you ever received treatment for using drugs?

TABLE 15.4	Clinical Institute Assessment (CIWA-Ar)

Patient: _____ Date: /_____/_____/_____ Time: _____
                                                  Y   M   D   (24-hour clock, midnight = 00:00)

Pulse or heart rate, taken for 1 minute: _____ Blood pressure: _____

NAUSEA AND VOMITING—Ask, "Do you feel sick to your stomach? Have you vomited?" Observation.

0 no nausea and no vomiting

1 mild nausea with no vomiting

2

3

4 intermittent nausea with dry heaves

5

6

7 constant nausea, frequent dry heaves and vomiting

TREMOR—Arms extended and fingers spread apart. Observation.

0 no tremor

1 not visible, but can be felt fingertip to fingertip

2

3

4 moderate, with patient's arms extended

5

6

7 severe, even with arms not extended

PAROXYSMAL SWEATS—Observation.

0 no sweat visible

1 barely perceptible sweating, palms moist

2

3

4 beads of sweat obvious on forehead

5

6

7 drenching sweats

ANXIETY—Ask, "Do you feel nervous?" Observation.

0 no anxiety, at ease

1 mildly anxious

2

3

4 moderately anxious or guarded so anxiety is inferred

5

6

7 equivalent to acute panic states as seen in severe delirium or acute schizophrenic reactions

TACTILE DISTURBANCES—Ask, "Have you any itching, pins and needles sensations, any burning, or any numbness, or do you feel bugs crawling on or under your skin?" Observation.

0 none

1 mild itching, pins and needles, burning, or numbness

2 mild itching, pins and needles, burning, or numbness

3 moderate itching, pins and needles, burning, or numbness

4 moderately severe hallucinations

5 severe hallucinations

6 extremely severe hallucinations

7 continuous hallucinations

AUDITORY DISTURBANCES—Ask, "Are you more aware of sounds around you? Are they harsh? Do they frighten you? Are you hearing anything that is disturbing to you? Are you hearing things that you know are not there?" Observation.

0 not present

1 very mild harshness or ability to frighten

2 mild harshness or ability to frighten

3 moderate harshness or ability to frighten

4 moderately severe hallucinations

5 severe hallucinations

6 extremely severe hallucinations

7 continuous hallucinations

VISUAL DISTURBANCES—Ask, "Does the light appear to be too bright? Is its color different? Does it hurt your eyes? Are you seeing anything that is disturbing to you? Are you seeing things that you know are not there?" Observation.

0 not present

1 very mild sensitivity

2 mild sensitivity

3 moderate sensitivity

4 moderately severe hallucinations

5 severe hallucinations

6 extremely severe hallucinations

7 continuous hallucinations

HEADACHE, FULLNESS IN HEAD—Ask, "Does you head feel different? Does it feel like there is a band around your head?" Do not rate for dizziness or lightheadness. Otherwise, rate severity.

0 not present

1 very mild

2 mild

3 moderate

4 moderately severe

5 severe

6 very severe

7 extremely severe

TABLE 15.4	Clinical Institute Assessment (CIWA-Ar) continued

AGITATION—Observation.

0 normal activity

1 somewhat more than normal activity

2

3

4 moderately fidgety and restless

5

6

7 paces back and forth during most of the interview or constantly thrashes about

Total CIWA-Ar Score:

Rater's Initials:

Maximum Possible Score: 67

ORIENTATION AND CLOUDING OF SENSORIUM—Ask, "What day is this? Where are you? Who am I?" Observation.

0 oriented and can do serial additions

1 cannot do serial additions or is uncertain about date

2 disoriented for date by no more than 2 calendar days

3 disoriented for date by more than 2 calendar days

4 disoriented for place and/or person

The tool measures the severity of alcohol withdrawal based on 10 common signs and symptoms: nausea and vomiting; tremor; paroxysmal sweats; anxiety; agitation; tactile, auditory, and visual disturbances; headache; and orientation. The maximum score is 67, and clients who score higher than 20 should be admitted to a hospital.

Assessment: Behavior

Lack of control in using chemicals is the central behavior in addiction. Because alcohol and drugs decrease inhibitions, many substance abusers become hostile, argumentative, loud, boisterous, and even violent when they are under the influence of the chemical. Compulsive and long-term substance abusers are at higher risk for violence than are recreational or intermittent users. Other users become withdrawn, tearful, and socially isolated when they are under the influence.

Chris:

" With my drinking came a lot of problems. I got into a lot of fights in college and that just isn't me. I had my whole face shattered in a fight one time, so all this has been reconstructed, and that actually happened during a blackout. I got into a fight with somebody and he got the upper hand on me and actually beat me pretty bad, and I had to have plastic surgery on this whole side of my face. "

Ask clients whether they are having any difficulty at their jobs since frequent absences may be a problem. If workers abuse substances at noon, their productivity decreases in the afternoon. They often have interpersonal problems at work related to their chemically dependent behavior. They may

not get promoted or may lose a job, and frequent job changes are common.

People who abuse alcohol are very protective of their supply. They may hide bottles in different places throughout their home to ensure a steady supply. Family members may look for the supply in order to throw it out in the hopes that the person will give up drinking. Some resort to nonbeverage sources of alcohol in desperation. One woman had a blood alcohol level of .322 after drinking a 14-ounce bottle of hairspray mixed with water because of its denatured alcohol content. That was the equivalent of 14 ounce-and-a-quarter shots of 80-proof liquor (Carnahan, Kutscher, Obritsch & Rasmussen, 2005).

Users who obtain their drugs through prescriptions may be able to live normally without arousing suspicion, but those who use illegal drugs may have to alter their lifestyle. The latter group often becomes involved in a drug subculture in which self-protection, prostitution, theft, and burglary prevail. As a result of this kind of lifestyle, they often find themselves in legal difficulties.

See the Focused Nursing Assessment for sample questions to ask regarding clients' behavior.

Assessment: Affect

Some people use stimulants to overcome feelings of boredom and depression and believe that the substances will produce euphoria. Others use these substances to manage their anxiety and stress. The overall intention is to decrease negative feelings and increase positive feelings.

People who abuse substances are often *emotionally labile*. They may be grandiose or irritable at one moment and morose and guilty the next. When they try to control their use of drugs and fail, they experience feelings of guilt and shame. When the problem becomes public knowledge, they are likely to feel embarrassed and humiliated.

Ellen is a 29-year-old woman who was recently released from an outpatient detoxification facility. Ellen's older daughter came home from school and found her mother drinking. When the daughter tried to take the bottle from Ellen, Ellen slapped her across the face. Realizing what she had done, Ellen tried to grab her daughter to comfort her, but the girl ran away screaming, "I hate you!"

See the Focused Nursing Assessment for sample questions to ask regarding clients' affect.

Assessment: Cognition

Some people have *low self-esteem* prior to their chemical dependence. They may have turned to drugs as a way to feel better about themselves. Others develop low self-esteem as a result of problems with substance abuse. Grandiose thoughts may be an attempt for both groups to compensate for low self-esteem.

Denial is the major defense mechanism that helps maintain a chemical dependence. Denial, which is self-deception and an unconscious attempt to maintain self-esteem in the face of out-of-control behavior, enables a person to underestimate the amount of drugs used and to avoid recognizing the impact of abusing behavior on others. Denial results from cultural standards of what is or is not appropriate behavior. Supporting the denial is the use of projection, minimization, and rationalization. *Projection*, seeing others as being responsible for one's substance abuse, is heard in: "My three teenagers are driving me crazy. It's their fault I drink." *Minimization*, not acknowledging the significance of one's behavior, is heard in: "Don't believe everything my wife tells you. I wasn't so high that I couldn't drive." *Rationalization*, giving reasons for the behavior, is heard in: "I only use Valium because I'm so unhappy in my marriage." These defense mechanisms are considered consequences, not causes, of chemical dependence. They serve to protect self-esteem by giving an explanation that helps the person conform to cultural standards (Wing, 1996).

Alcoholic denial has many aspects, including denial of facts, denial of implications, denial of change, and denial of feelings. *Denial of facts* is the outermost layer of protection and the most frequently used form of denial. It functions to avoid negative consequences. It is heard in: "I have not been drinking," and "I only had one or two beers." *Denial of implications* is used when some threatening fact gets established and that fact is made public, as in a DUI (driving under the influence). It functions to avoid the image of failure and is heard in: "Okay, I had a few, but I wasn't drunk," "I only smoke pot," and "Your sister drinks more than I do." *Denial of change* helps people resist making any real change. It functions to protect them from assuming responsibility for their own behavior. It is heard in: "So, I'm an alcoholic, so what," "I'll try to stop," and "I wanted to stay sober, but I couldn't." *Denial of feelings* is aimed at shutting off feelings and protects people from being overwhelmed by strong emotions. It

is heard in: "It doesn't bother me" and "I'm not angry!" Denial can be a major obstacle to treatment, for no treatment will be effective until the individual acknowledges that the substance abuse is out of control.

Chris:

66 My life was just getting awful. I said I can't take it anymore and I said I needed help. I admitted I had a problem. That was the toughest thing I ever did was admit that I had a problem. 99

Blackouts are a form of amnesia for events that occurred during the drinking period. The person may carry out conversations and activities with no loss of consciousness, but have total amnesia for those activities the next day.

Chris:

66 When I was around the age of 14 I remember waking up the next morning not knowing what I did. My friends would call me—do you remember what you did last night? No, I have no idea. 99

See the Focused Nursing Assessment for sample questions to ask regarding clients' cognition.

Assessment: Interpersonal Relationships

Social values contribute to the problem of substance abuse in the United States. The mass media promote the desire for immediate gratification and self-indulgence. Complex family problems are solved in 30 minutes on television. All forms of media push medications for a wide variety of problems, contributing to the expectation of a pain-free existence. Values such as these indirectly support the use and abuse of chemical substances.

Effects on the Family

Substance abuse is a family problem, and the most devastating effect occurs when the abuser is a parent. Power struggles between abusing and nonabusing partners destroy couples and contribute to a *dysfunctional family system*. Family relationships begin to deteriorate, and family members become trapped in a cycle of shame, anger, confusion, and guilt. In some families, substance abuse is a contributing factor to emotional neglect and physical or sexual abuse. Often, family members and old friends will be abandoned for new relationships within the drug subculture. In other cases, chemically dependent people simply become more isolated as alcohol or drugs become the main focus of their lives. Some are successful in keeping their substance abuse hidden from their colleagues and most of their significant relationships.

Financial problems may arise from underemployment or unemployment as the compulsion to use chemicals takes precedence over work. However, many substance abusers continue to be employed. For those using illegal substances, the cost can be incredibly expensive. Illegal substance abusers may be criminally involved with the legal system. Some use prostitution or drug dealing as a way to pay for their drugs. Some become involved in minor crimes such as pocket picking or shoplifting to obtain money for the drugs. Yet others turn to robberies and burglaries to support the high cost of their habit.

Julian states: "I would spend all our rent money on cocaine but who cares. I'm the only one who works. She shouldn't get so upset. If she worked, then she would have a point."

Ineffective communication patterns contribute to anxiety and anger. In an attempt to create the illusion of normality, substance abuse is never discussed within or outside of the family system. This refusal to acknowledge there is a problem contributes to family denial. To avoid embarrassment, family members make excuses to outsiders for the user's behavior. A nonabusing partner may remain in a relationship because of emotional dependency, money, family cohesion, religious compliance, or outward respectability. Other nonabusing partners may threaten to or actually leave the abuser. At this point, the abuser promises never to drink or use again, the family is reunited, the promise is usually broken, and the family becomes locked into a dysfunctional pattern.

Codependency

Codependency is a relationship in which a non–substance-abusing partner remains with a substance-abusing partner. The relationship is dysfunctional—the nonabusing partner is overresponsible and the abusing partner is underresponsible. Codependents operate out of fear, resentment, helplessness, and hopelessness. They are obsessively driven to control the user's behavior and to solve the problems created by the user. When this is not effective, codependents become exhausted and depressed but are unable to stop the "helping" behaviors. They often suffer from low self-esteem and fear of abandonment. Codependents are *caretakers*, and this caretaking activity may be a compensation for feelings of inadequacy. Women may be more vulnerable to codependent behavior because they have been socialized to be responsible for the family and often feel they are expected to be loyal to their partner at all costs. As professionals, nurses must be careful not to blame women for the user's behavior (Martsolf, Sedlak, & Doheny, 2000; Stafford, 2001).

Codependents often engage in **enabling behavior**, which is any action by a person that consciously or unconsciously fa-

cilitates substance dependence. Enabling behaviors, such as making excuses for the partner with the employer and lying to others about the abuse, protect the substance abuser from the natural consequences of the problem. Enabling is a response to addiction, not a cause of addiction. The purpose of enabling is the family's instinctual desire to stay together. It is a process of compensating for the dysfunction in one family member and avoiding the issues that threaten the breakup of the family.

Children of Alcoholics

It is estimated that one of every eight Americans is a child of an alcoholic parent. Children who grow up in homes where one parent or both parents are alcoholics often suffer the effects their entire lives. Dysfunctional family roles develop around the impact of alcoholism. Despite mysterious events, nonsense language, and threats of impending doom, everyone in the family acts as if the situation were perfectly normal. It is extremely frightening to have a parent who switches from being a joking, pleasant person to a raging tyrant in the blink of an eye. It is terrifying to live with a drunken father who not only screams that he is going to kill the child, but also attempts to do just that. At the same time, the parent convinces the child that if it were not for what the child did, the parent would not be acting that way.

Parents preoccupied with addiction may jeopardize their children's health and safety. They may use the household budget for drugs. They may disappear for hours or days. Their ability to be emotionally and physically available to their children may be compromised. Their parental judgment is often impaired and, in some cases, children are exposed to criminal activity.

Very early in life, children of alcoholics learn to *keep the secret* and not talk about the alcohol problem, even within the family. They are taught not to talk about their own feelings, needs, and wants; they learn not to feel at all. Eventually, they repress all feelings and become numb to both pain and joy. The children become objects whose reason for existence is to please the alcoholic parent and serve his or her needs. Children of alcoholics are expected always to be in control of their behavior and their feelings. They are expected to be perfect and never make mistakes. However, within the family system, no child can ever be perfect "enough." Consistency is necessary for building trust, and alcoholic parents are very unpredictable. Children learn not to expect reliability in relationships. They learn very early that if you do not trust another person, you will not be disappointed.

Children of alcoholics tend to develop one of four patterns of behavior. The *hero*, often the oldest child, becomes the competent caretaker and works on making the family function. The *scapegoat* acts out at home, in school, and in the community. This child takes the focus off the alcoholic parent by getting into trouble and becoming the focus of conflict in the family. The behavior may also be a way to draw attention to the family in an unconscious attempt to seek help. The *lost child* tries to avoid conflict and pain by withdrawing physically and emotionally. The *mascot*, often the youngest child, tries to ease family tension with comic relief used to mask his or her own sadness.

In dysfunctional families, designated roles keep the family balanced. Each role is a way to handle the distress and shame of having an alcoholic parent. Every family member has a sense of some control, even though the roles do not change the family system's dysfunction.

Leticia, a 14-year-old high school student, had been an excellent student and suddenly her grades dropped dramatically. She tearfully confessed to her school counselor that personal problems were affecting her grades. Leticia explained that her father had a drinking problem but had been going to AA for several years. Three months ago, Leticia's father lost his job and was unable to get another. A month ago, he started a pattern of binge drinking. Leticia was reluctant to talk because she knew her mother would be furious if she knew Leticia had revealed the family secret. Leticia's mother was working overtime to keep the family going. When Leticia's mother was home, she fought constantly with her husband about his drinking. Her father tried to get Leticia to buy alcohol for him after her mother poured his supply down the drain. When Leticia tried to explain that she was too young to purchase alcohol, her father screamed at her, "Get out of my sight! You're useless!" When her father was sober, he tried to be Leticia's best friend. Leticia stopped bringing friends home because she didn't know what to expect. She was too nervous to do homework, always worrying about what her father might do. Leticia told the counselor, "I don't want him to be my friend. I don't even want him for a father anymore!"

Adult children of alcoholics grew up denying the stresses of their dysfunctional families. Denial becomes a frequent defense mechanism that only makes things worse as they proceed through life. The sense of total obligation to the alcoholic parent makes it extremely difficult for adult children to criticize the addicted parent.

Adult children of alcoholics have grown up without mature adult role models and without experiencing healthy family dynamics. They expect all relationships to be based on power, violence, deceit, and misinformation. They often have difficulty expressing emotion and receiving expressions of feelings. Some grow up to repeat the family pattern by either becoming addicted themselves or marrying an addicted person.

Adult children of alcoholics often feel a need to change others or to control the environment for the good of others. They typically deny powerlessness and try to solve all problems alone. They blame themselves for not being able to achieve what no one can achieve. Obsessions are common forms of defense, such as constant worrying, preoccupations with work or other activities that bring about good feelings, and compulsive achievement. The obsessive pattern covers the feelings of helplessness and blocks the feelings of anxiety, inadequacy, and fear of abandonment.

Social Morality

Most Americans have a moralistic attitude about substance dependence. Dependence is viewed as a sin or as the result of a weak will. Addicts are seen as totally responsible for their situation and are expected to use willpower to control themselves and become respectable members of society once again. Social class may also influence one's perspective of substance abuse. For example, nurses who have moralistic views may have difficulty accepting the disorder in a clergyperson yet have no reservations acknowledging alcoholism among gang members or the homeless population. It is very unfortunate when nursing students and nurses believe these cultural stereotypes. Moral judgment and stigma make therapeutic relationships impossible (Martinez & Murphy-Parker, 2003).

This moralistic perspective especially *stigmatizes women.* Men's drinking tends to be more public and more socially acceptable than women's, which often drives women's alcohol problems underground. Women are expected to be "ladylike" at all times, and when they drink too much or get high, they are quickly labeled "loose women," "sleaze bags," or "drunks." Most treatment programs are developed for and serve men. Often unacknowledged is the fact that women have different clinical courses and treatment needs than men. Mothers may avoid treatment for fear of triggering investigations by child welfare services and losing custody of their children. Another difficulty is that there may be no safe place for their children while they are in treatment.

Even more stigmatized by American society are *lesbian alcoholics.* They suffer as women in a male-dominated culture and also carry the double stigma of being lesbian and being alcoholic. Lesbian women have a higher rate of alcohol consumption than heterosexual women do. They also attempt suicide seven times more often and have higher rates of completed suicide than heterosexual, nonalcoholic women. In a homophobic culture, coming to terms with one's homosexuality and accepting a gay identity are very painful. It is thought that depression, alcohol use, and suicide among lesbians may be related to the effects of stigmatization (Drabble, Midanik, & Trocki, 2005).

Women who have been abused physically and sexually are at greater risk for becoming alcoholics than women who were not abused. It is believed that using alcohol may be an attempt to self-medicate while coping with the physical and emotional consequences of abuse. (Interpersonal violence is covered fully in chapter 22 ∞, and sexual abuse is covered in chapter 23 ∞).

High-technology Lifestyle

The digital revolution has transformed some young adult lives into a combination of excessive wealth, driving ambition, long work hours, and a pressure to perform. Illicit drug activity is booming among high-tech workers, and drugs are the latest "secret" of the industry—speed to work on, coke to play on, and smoking heroin to come down on. It is too early for formal research studies that quantify the problem, but there are obvious signs of its growth within the computer industry. See the Focused Nursing Assessment for sample questions to ask regarding interpersonal relationships.

Assessment: Cultural Influences

Tobacco continues to be the most frequently abused substance, causing the most health damage worldwide. The World Health Organization (2005) estimates that there are around 1.1 billion smokers in the world, about one third the global population aged 15 and older. Unless current trends are reversed, the use of tobacco will kill 10 million people every year by the 2020s.

The social consequences of chemical addictions are increasing in more and more countries, as well as in the United States. The problem has increased and become more complex with the arrival of hard drugs in third world countries. Many countries cannot cope with basic health needs, much less substance use disorders.

There are many different ethnic groups in the United States, each having unique values regarding the definition of substance abuse and how it should be regarded and treated. Sociocultural factors often determine the choice of the substance and the extent to which it is abused. The use of naturally produced drugs is deeply rooted in many cultures. In some contexts, such as in communion in Christian churches or in ceremonies of the Native American church, substances are considered sacred. The use of mind-altering drugs for treatment of medical conditions is legally permitted but controlled. In other circumstances, the use of these same drugs is considered criminal. In some cultures, alcohol is consumed as part of normal mealtime activities and used to celebrate social events and does not contribute to the development of substance-use problems.

Euro-Americans have the highest overall rates of alcohol consumption. Euro-American men are much more likely to be heavy drinkers, whereas only 8% of Euro-American women are classified as heavy drinkers. Heavy drinking among males is highest in the 18 to 29 age group. One third of women abstain (Naegle & D'Avanzo, 2001).

African American individuals abstain more and drink less than Euro-Americans. Only 4% of African American women are classified as heavy drinkers, and more than 50% abstain. African Americans are less likely than other ethnic groups to be dependent on marijuana. However, the leading cause of death among African American men between the ages of 15 and 34 is homicide, and alcohol or drugs are implicated in at least 70% of these incidents. African Americans are more likely to be arrested than to be treated for substance-related disorders (Boyd, Phillips, & Dorsey, 2003; Gil, Wagner, & Tubman, 2004).

Hispanic Americans are the largest minority population in the United States. Mexican Americans are the largest subgroup, followed by Puerto Rican and Cuban Americans. There are significant differences in the patterns of alcohol and drug use among the various subgroups. Puerto Rican Americans have the highest use of marijuana and cocaine, while among Mexican Americans, alcohol is the most abused substance. Hispanic American men typically increase their drinking from their 20s to their 30s, and then decrease it after age 40. The ability to consume large amounts of alcohol without appearing intoxicated is associated with *machismo*. Hispanic American women are similar to African American women in that nearly half abstain from any use of alcohol (Beals et al., 2005).

Alcohol use among Arab Americans is rare. One protective factor may be the influence of Islam, which condemns the use of alcohol. Little is known about substance abuse among this ethnic group. There is also not much data on Asian-Indian Americans. It appears that they are more prone to use alcohol or drugs after migration to a foreign country (World Health Organization, 2005).

The Europeans introduced alcohol to the Native American population. Because Native Americans are not homogeneous, there is considerable tribal variation in drinking patterns. In general, the magnitude of alcohol problems is greater among Native Americans than among other groups in the United States. The alcohol-related death rate for Native Americans is seven times that of the general population. The percentage of Native Americans who abstain is about the same as in the general population. Among those who do drink, however, there are significantly fewer light or moderate drinkers (23%) and over twice as many heavy drinkers. As with other cultural groups, the men drink more than the women do. Alcohol is associated with social situations, and there is little solitary drinking. Men tend to drink in groups and pass the bottle. It is considered rude or insulting to refuse the offer of a drink. Alcohol is the drug of choice for Native American youth, although marijuana and inhalants are also used more than in the general native population. The age of initiation has been steadily decreasing and is now around 11 or 12 years old. Hawk Littlejohn, the medicine man of the Cherokee Nation, Eastern Band, attributes this problem to the fact that Native peoples have lost the opportunity to make choices. They can no longer choose how they live or how they practice their religion. He believes that once people return to a sense of identification, they will begin to rid themselves of alcoholism (Novins & Baron, 2004; Spector, 2004).

Assessment: Age-specific Characteristics
Children and Adolescents

In American society, the use of alcohol and cannabis during the teen and young adult years is a common practice. For many, it is a stage of experimentation, with use decreasing with age. For others, use continues and expands until the stage of addiction is reached.

Adolescent substance use is related to many factors. If parents are users, there may be a genetic influence as well as a modeling influence. Research shows that all types of parental substance use are associated with children's substance use. Alcohol and drug use is often accepted in the teen peer group. Developmentally, adolescents may abuse substances as a means of rebelling against parents, in a search for identity, and in an effort to separate from the family. Other risk factors include sensation-seeking tendencies, risk-taking tendencies, and the availability of drugs. Some teens experiencing family dysfunction, problems in school, problems with peers, or emotional or physical trauma may feel overwhelmed and attempt to escape their pain through the use of substances. Some adolescents suffering from mental disorders try to self-medicate with alcohol or drugs (Silberg, Rutter, D'Onofrio, & Eaves, 2003).

The National Survey of American Attitudes on Substance Abuse XI: Teens and Parents (2006) found that parents are often unaware of the extent of their teens' drug and alcohol use. The survey found that:

- Eighty percent of parents believe that neither alcohol nor marijuana is usually available at teen gatherings, but 50% of their kids say they are available in at least some of the parties.
- Ninety-eight percent of parents say they are present during parties in their homes, while 33% of teens report that parents are rarely around.
- Teens report that their number one concern is drugs, followed by social pressures, academic pressures, and crime and violence. In contrast, parents believe that the number one concern of teens is social pressures, followed distantly by drugs and their future.

The nurse should teach parents of preadolescent and teenage children to look for evidence of substance use. Physical signs include frequent "colds" or "allergies" or other respiratory problems, unexplained frequent injuries, altered sleep pattern, and loss of appetite. Suspicious emotional signs include social isolation, sexual acting out, aggression, mood swings, and depression. Behavioral cues include changing friends to ones who have multiple problems, decline in school performance, problems with teachers, poor judgment, and loss of interest in hobbies or sports.

Peak initiation for alcohol and cigarette use is between the 6th and 9th grades. Initiation of marijuana peaks between the 9th and 11th grades, while other illegal drug initiation peaks between the 10th and 12th grades (National Institute on Drug Abuse, 2005).

Substance-related disorders progress more rapidly in adolescents than in adults. Adults may take from 2 to 7 years from the first use to full dependency. Teens may make this progression in 6 to 18 months. Alcohol and drug exposure during adolescence may be especially harmful to the still-developing brain. Research shows that the earlier the age at which young people take their first drink of alcohol, the greater the risk of developing serious problems. More than 40% of all people who drink alcohol between the ages of 11 and 14 become alcohol dependent. That is four times the rate (10%) for those who have their first drink at ages 20 and older (Chambers, Taylor, & Potenza, 2003).

The use of denial is often stronger since teens do not have years of negative consequences to highlight their substance use disorder. They also often experience developmental delays: Growth and development slows down, they fall behind in academics, their social skills stagnate, they experience poor impulse control, and they are intolerant of delayed gratification. They typically shift to a peer group composed solely of other drug-using adolescents. In a two-parent home, the roles may be polarized, with one parent being the enabler and the other parent the enforcer. This creates much family conflict and distress.

Twenty-three percent of teens have tried an illicit drug by the 8th grade. That number rises to 41% by 10th grade and 51% by 12th grade. One in five teens has abused a prescription painkiller to get high and one in eleven has abused over-the-counter (OTC) products such as cough medicine. Ease of access is the main reason teens are abusing prescription drugs. They do not have to go to a street dealer because the drugs are right at home in the medicine cabinet. Drug use increases from adolescence to young adulthood and then gradually declines (Compton et al., 2005).

For teens younger than 18, inhalants are the fourth most abused drug, after alcohol, tobacco, and marijuana. About 17% of adolescents in the United States say that they have sniffed inhalants at least once in their lives. Inhalant abuse is more common among early teens, with usage dropping off as they grow older. In addition, there is an extraordinary amount of online information on how to obtain, synthesize, extract, and ingest a wide range of hallucinogens. This Web-based information is proving to be of significant danger to vulnerable individuals.

Older Adults

Illicit drug use, such as cocaine or opiates, is more unusual in older adults than in young adults. Alcohol abuse, however, is a problem for 10% to 15% of older adults. Often, it is undiagnosed because in old age the symptoms can be subtle or atypical, or mimic symptoms of other geriatric illnesses. Clients may present with erratic changes in mood or behavior; malnutrition; bladder and bowel incontinence; gait disorders; and recurring falls, burns, or head trauma.

Older adults have less social, legal, occupational, and interpersonal consequences of their alcohol abuse because they are often not working, and many live alone. Two thirds of this group have had long-standing problems with alcohol and have multiple medical complications. One third develops the drinking problem late in life, often in response to bereavement, retirement, loneliness, relationship stress, and physical illnesses. Denial of substance abuse is common at all ages but may be more intense in older adults because of memory problems and the shame-based belief of this current generation that substance abuse is immoral. As the baby boomers enter old age, this shame-based belief may indeed change (Hall & Follette, 2002).

Older drinkers are more susceptible to physical complications from their alcohol intake. In addition, alcohol may potentiate prescribed or OTC medications, leading to a higher rate of confusion and accidents. Health care professionals often do not screen for alcohol use or abuse among older individuals. When assessment is conducted, women are less likely than men to be asked about their alcohol consumption (Stevenson & Masters, 2005).

Abuse of prescription drugs among the elderly is two to three times higher than the general population. Benzodiazepine dependence is most common and benzodiazepines may have been prescribed for long periods of time. Of individuals who have a history of long-term use (more than 1 year), 70% are older than 50 and often have physical health problems. Among older people who are institutionalized, the abuse is even more widespread. Benzodiazepine abuse in the elderly results in excessive daytime sedation; ataxia, which increases the risk of falls and accidents; and cognitive impairments such as attention and memory problems (Hall & Follette, 2002).

Assessment: Physical—Alcohol

Clients who are admitted with acute alcohol intoxication are easily identified by their behavior and cognitive symptoms. Not so easily identified are those who have long-term alcohol abuse and are admitted for gastrointestinal, cardiac, or respiratory problems. All clients, therefore, admitted to the acute care setting should be assessed for alcohol use and abuse in order to prevent severe alcohol withdrawal syndrome.

Physical assessment is a critical task, especially for clients who have a history of abusing alcohol. A complete physical assessment is necessary because alcohol affects so many body systems. Look first at the client's general appearance, take vital signs, and then examine the person in head-to-toe order.

Depending on the stage of alcoholism, the type of trauma the person may have been exposed to, poor hygiene, and malnutrition, you must examine for changes in the integrity of the *skin and scalp*. Ecchymosis, lacerations, color change, evidence of healed injuries, bumps, scars, and diaphoresis may be present. Bruises, lacerations, and numerous scars may be evidence of frequent trauma from bumps, falls, or fights. Decreased prothrombin production in advanced liver disease causes easy bruising. Dermatitis, seborrhea, and skin sensitivity to light result from vitamin B deficiencies. Spider an-

giomas are found on the face and sometimes on the chest of people with advanced liver disease. Diaphoresis may be a sign of impending withdrawal. Dependent edema may indicate liver problems. Statis dermatitis indicates the edema has been present for some time.

Observe the client's *head* for shape and symmetry of facial structures. Orbital ridges and bony areas around the eyes should be palpated for evidence of fractures. Advanced disease frequently causes facial edema or a "puffy face" with flushed cheeks and nose.

The *eyes* need to be inspected thoroughly. Icterus may be present in the sclera from hepatitis or cirrhosis. Extraocular movements are assessed to look for nystagmus and palsies of the lateral and conjugate gaze. When these signs are positive, Wernicke encephalopathy is suspected. Pupil shape, equality, and reactivity to light can be used to evaluate normal nerve function.

The *ear* canals need to be examined. Increased redness is an indication of infection. Since trauma is often seen in alcoholics, the ear canal is inspected for exudate, blood, and lesions.

The *mouth* is observed for signs of trauma and infection. Lip peeling and corner fissures are early signs related to vitamin B deficiencies. People who are homeless may have difficulty maintaining oral hygiene. Teeth need to be inspected for caries, cracks, and tenderness. Also check for missing teeth. Observe the gums for color, inflammation, consistency, bleeding, or retraction.

The *neck* is observed for color, skin texture, masses, symmetry, range of motion, and visible pulsations. Chronic alcoholism may lead to cardiomyopathy, with congestive heart failure causing increased venous pressure, which results in distended jugular veins.

Inspect the *chest* since debilitated substance abusers are at risk for pneumonia and tuberculosis. Note the rate and character of respirations. Auscultation can reveal breath sounds with lung consolidation. Gynecomastia is common with cirrhosis or chronic liver disease since the liver can no longer inactivate estrogen.

Observation of the *abdomen* may reveal bulging flanks indicative of abdominal fluid retention and tense glistening skin resulting from ascites. The abdomen is percussed to identify enlarged organs, fluid retention, gaseous distention, and masses. An enlarged liver, percussed as greater than 12 centimeters at the midclavicular line, can indicate alcoholic hepatitis or cirrhosis. Anorexia, nausea, vomiting, fever, and liver tenderness are all early signs of hepatitis. Later signs of hepatitis are pale stools, dark urine, and jaundice. Jaundice may be more readily identified on the abdomen because it is usually exposed less to the sun.

Portal hypertension may be indicated if there are dilated veins at the umbilicus, gastrointestinal bleeding, and hemorrhoids. Check for black or tarry stools or frank rectal bleeding. Esophageal varices, secondary to portal hypertension, are usually discovered when the person vomits bright red blood, passes red blood through the rectum, or has dark, tarry stools from the upper gastrointestinal tract. Esophageal varices make a person especially susceptible to life-threatening hemorrhage. Other signs of portal hypertension are dilated or varicose veins at the umbilicus and hemorrhoids.

The major areas observed when assessing *neurologic status* are consciousness, cognitive function, and motor function. Consciousness is assessed as the nurse converses with clients. Deviations may be observed in relation to arousability, responses to commands, and response to painful stimuli. Note the orientation to time, place, and person. Individuals suffering from Korsakoff syndrome may have intact intellectual functioning but an inability to retrieve long-term memory events or retain new information. Alcoholic dementia is characterized by impaired abstract thinking and judgment, personality changes, and impaired memory. Wernicke encephalopathy is characterized by ataxia, abnormal eye movements, and confusion.

Assessment: Physical—Drugs

Chronic use of sedatives/hypnotics/antianxiety agents results in a slower pulse and a slightly decreased respiratory rate and blood pressure. Urine tests remain positive for up to a week.

Chronic use of opioids causes a dry nose and mouth and a slowed gastrointestinal system. Those who inject the drug into the venous system may have puncture marks and thickened veins. Those who inject into the subcutaneous tissue may develop cellulitis and abscesses. Those who sniff opioids often irritate the lining of the nose which may progress into perforation of the nasal septum. The incidence of tuberculosis and HIV infection is high among intravenous users.

Urine tests for casual users of cannabis may test positive for 7 to 10 days after the last use. Those who have heavy use may test positive as long as 4 weeks after the last use. The irritation of the smoke can lead to a chronic cough and emphysema.

Cocaine remains in the urine for 1 to 3 days after a single dose, while those who use repeated doses may test positive for 7 to 12 days. Users are at higher risk for tuberculosis, HIV infection, and sexually transmitted infections. Those who snort cocaine often develop irritation of the lining of the nose, which may progress into perforation of the nasal septum. Since cocaine suppresses the appetite, the nurse may see weight loss and malnutrition. Cardiac problems and seizures are not uncommon.

Urine tests for amphetamines remain positive for 1 to 3 days after the last use. Clients may present with weight loss and malnutrition.

You may notice the odor of solvents on the breath or clothing of people who use inhalants. The eyes may be bloodshot and there may be a rash around the nose and mouth. Respiratory changes can range from a cough, to shortness of breath, to acute respiratory distress.

High levels of caffeine can cause agitation, sweating, rapid pulse, flushed face, and increased gastrointestinal activity.

Nicotine use can increase the risk of cancer, cardiovascular disease, and pulmonary disease. Signs of use include a tobacco odor, cough, and excessive skin wrinkling.

Central Nervous System Effects

An addicted brain is different physically and chemically from a normal brain. Substances of abuse alter the brain's reward system by artificially boosting DA effects. Cocaine blocks the DA transporter, leaving excess DA in the synapse, which keeps the pleasure circuit firing. Heroin and nicotine stimulate the release of DA. Amphetamines block DA transporters and stimulate the release of DA. Alcohol alters DA, 5-HT, glutamate, and GABA neurotransmission. Low levels of 5-HT are related to increased aggression. Long-term use of mind-altering drugs decreases the number of DA receptors. With fewer receptors, the drugs do not have the effect they originally did and higher doses are needed to get the same effect.

Withdrawal is also a result of the altered DA system. Withdrawal and abstinence deprive the brain of the only source of DA that produces a sense of pleasure. Without the drug, life seems not worth living. Abstinence allows DA receptors and the DA system to return to normal.

Professionals are concerned not just with the direct effects of alcohol and drugs on the brain, but also with residual effects that cause *craving* and a return to compulsive substance abuse. It is believed that each time a drug is used, specific brain structures are activated, leaving a memory trace that remains long after the drug has disappeared from the body. There is growing evidence that the cerebellum is involved in this learned memory association. Each incidence of drug use is paired with environmental cues of persons, places, and things, which then have the ability to trigger the same brain circuits even in the absence of the drug. Addicts begin to crave their drugs when they see, hear, or smell a reminder of past use. Brain imaging techniques have been able to measure changes in the amygdala, the anterior cingulate, and the prefrontal cortex in response to environmental triggers.

Cardiovascular Changes

Stimulants such as amphetamines and cocaine are associated with a number of cardiovascular complications as the result of serious vasoconstriction. These include intracranial hemorrhage, tachycardia, arrthymias, elevated blood pressure, and sudden cardiac death. Since nicotine causes similar changes, the harmful effects are increased if nicotine is used concurrently with stimulants.

Sexual Effects

A rapid increase in *sexually transmitted infections (STIs)* has been associated with substance abuse, especially crack cocaine.

Users of illegal substances may trade sex for the drug. Cocaine abusers often get involved in multiple-partner sex and are unable to consider safer sex practices when high. Since alcohol decreases inhibitions and judgment, there has been a rise in STIs among adolescents and young adults. Contaminated needles are a leading cause of the spread of hepatitis, HIV infection, and AIDS. As this problem grows, the premature death rate from drug abuse may approach that of alcohol abuse.

Substance-related disorders have a number of *sexual consequences*. Long-term *alcohol* abuse leads to erection problems for 40% of men, as well as ejaculation difficulties in 10% to 25% of men. Among women entering treatment for alcoholism, 70% to 80% have difficulty achieving orgasm, 30% to 40% have problems with sexual arousal, and 30% have lost their desire for sex. Alcohol slows the metabolism of estrogen leading to higher blood levels of estrogen, especially among postmenopausal women. This increased estrogen without opposing progesterone could increase the risk for uterine and breast cancer. People who use *marijuana* report enhanced sexual enjoyment with intensification of touch and perception. They have increased attentiveness to their partner, although sexual behavior remains the same. The initial use of *amphetamines* increases sex drive and sensations; long-term use leads to problems with arousal, function, and the sense of pleasure. Use of *hallucinogens* can create both extremely positive and extremely negative sexual effects. The heightened sensory-perceptual stimuli may enhance or intensify sex or create a terrifying experience. Sexual performance may be impossible because of intoxication. People using *opioids* find their desire for sex has been replaced with their desire for the drug. They also experience decreased sexual arousal and difficulties with orgasm/ejaculation (Johnson, Phelps, & Cottler, 2004).

Cocaine is associated with hypersexuality. Seventy percent of males and 30% of females report a strong link between cocaine use and a variety of sexual acting-out behaviors. Cocaine is a CNS stimulant that relaxes inhibitions, increases sexual fantasies, and increases sexual desire. High doses of cocaine can produce compulsive masturbation, multipartner marathons, group sex, and even sexual abuse of children. It is not uncommon for cocaine abusers to go on marathon binges of cocaine and sex (McElrath, 2005).

Intrauterine Substance Exposure

Many of the aforementioned chemicals cross the placental barrier and have harmful effects on unborn children. Prenatal substance use screening by primary care professionals has become an established public health priority, and women are advised to abstain completely during pregnancy.

Tobacco, the most abused substance by pregnant women, increases the flow of carbon monoxide to the fetus and decreases placental blood flow. Smoking is a risk factor for miscarriage, ectopic pregnancy, preeclampsia, abruptio placenta, placenta previa, and premature rupture of membranes. Effects on the infant include low birth weight, prematurity, higher risk for sudden infant death syndrome (SIDS), and an increase in respiratory illness, ear infections, and attention deficit hyperactivity disorder (ADHD) (Thapar et al., 2003).

Alcohol is the second most abused substance by pregnant women and causes **fetal alcohol spectrum disorder (FASD).** FASD is an umbrella term for abnormalities ranging from the subtle cognitive–behavioral impairments of alcohol-related birth defects (ARBDs) to the symptoms of fetal alcohol syndrome (FAS). It is believed that alcohol causes faulty CNS cell migration during fetal development. FASD is the third leading cause of birth defects in the United States, including heart defects, malformed facial features, and low IQ or cognitive impairment. Other effects are low birth weight, slow growth rate, hyperactivity, maladaptive behavior, and severe reading and math disabilities. Some children with FASD show improvement over time, but academic problems and behavioral disorders seem to persist for most of these children (Caley, Shipkey, Winkelman, Dunlap, & Rivera, 2006; Rasmussen, 2005).

Recent studies suggest that poverty and the use of cigarettes and alcohol while pregnant may be more responsible for fetal damage than cocaine. Cocaine is especially dangerous to the fetus if it is used during the first trimester of pregnancy when the brain is developing. Cocaine is such a potent vasoconstrictor that reduced blood supply to the fetus causes neurological abnormalities that may result in learning and behavioral problems. After birth, infants who had been exposed to cocaine before birth tend to experience abnormal sleep patterns, tremors, poor feeding, irritability, and sometimes seizures. Many of the effects disappear as the infant develops (Boyd et al., 2003).

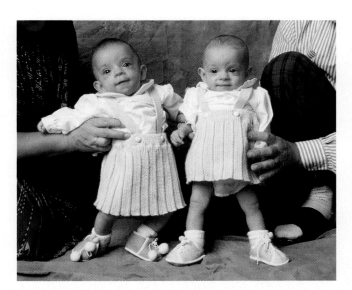

PHOTO 15.4 ■ Fetal alcohol syndrome. Fetal alcohol syndrome is the result of women consuming alcohol during pregnancy, and it can have many severe effects on the child; among them are physical malformations such as those shown here.

SOURCE: George Steinmetz/San Francisco AIDS Foundation. Used with permission.

Children who have been exposed to opioids prior to birth are very sensitive to noise and are irritable and tremulous. They may have uncoordinated sucking and swallowing reflexes, which cause feeding problems. Inhalants are associated with oral clefts, microcephaly, slowed growth, and developmental delay (Baigent, 2003).

DIAGNOSIS

After completing the assessment and appraising the knowledge base, you are ready to analyze and synthesize the information. Answer the following questions:

1. How does the client view substance abuse?
2. How does the client view alcoholics or addicts?
3. What is the client's concept of disease?
4. What does the client claim to want out of treatment?
5. Is the client being forced to seek treatment by family, employer, or the legal system?

The following are those diagnoses most commonly identified for clients with substance use disorders (North American Nursing Diagnosis Association, 2007). Nursing diagnoses relating to acute overdose and long-term physical complications of substance dependence are beyond the scope of this text. Refer to a medical–surgical text to review these diagnoses and the appropriate nursing responses.

- Risk for Self-directed Violence related to symptoms of drug/alcohol abuse or withdrawal
- Risk for Injury related to musculoskeletal, visual, auditory, or sensory disturbances from drug/alcohol intoxication
- Fear related to emotional responses to changes in sensory perception
- Ineffective Individual Coping related to using chemicals as a way to cope with life
- Ineffective Denial related to believing that there is no problem with the use of substances
- Powerlessness related to an inability to control the use of drugs
- Self-esteem Disturbance, Altered Role Performance related to lifestyle disrupted by substance abuse
- Social Isolation related to a lifestyle of substance abuse
- Spiritual Distress related to alienation from others; loss of faith in a higher being
- Dysfunctional Family Processes: Alcoholism related to codependent and enabling behavior; neglect or abuse of family members
- Sexual Dysfunction related to drug intoxication or long-term physical effects of alcohol abuse
- Deficient Knowledge related to parents' use of nicotine, alcohol, or other drugs; need for early prevention education

OUTCOME IDENTIFICATION AND GOALS

Based on the assessment data, the nurse selects outcomes appropriate to the nursing diagnoses. Broad outcomes are:

- Reduce or eliminate alcohol or drug use.
- Improve quality of life through abstinence.
- Improve quality of family life.

Client goals are specific behavioral measures which you, clients, and significant others identify as realistic and attainable. The following are examples of some of the outcomes appropriate to people who have substance-related disorders:

- Remains safe during the withdrawal process
- Acknowledges the reality of the disorder
- Acknowledges the negative consequences of substance-abusing behavior
- Identifies triggers to relapse
- Utilizes spiritual support resources
- Demonstrates improved problem-solving skills
- Improves levels of physical health and fitness
- Participates in self-help groups
- Family members participate in relapse prevention education
- Parents abstain from substance use/abuse

PLANNING

Once the nursing diagnoses, outcomes criteria, and goals have been identified, you develop the plan of care to assist clients toward a higher level of functioning and an enriched quality of life. Priorities of care for clients with substance use disorders are as follows:

- Maintain safety of client and others.
- Maintain abstinence.
- Assume responsibility for own behavior.

IMPLEMENTATION

Substance dependence is not hard to see, but it is hard to treat. Individuals may have had little control over development of the disorder but are solely responsible for their sobriety. Clients must become invested in and committed to long-term recovery. Intensive support from others is an important part of the treatment plan.

There are two phases of treatment: 1) crisis intervention as you assist clients through the detoxification phase; and

NURSING CARE PLAN for Clients With Substance-related Disorders

Preventing Violence
Nursing Diagnosis: Client at Risk for Other-Directed Violence

Outcomes: Client remains safe and does not harm others.

Some clients are at high risk for violence related to the psychotic effects of chemicals (hallucinations and delusions), impulsive behavior when intoxicated, and the process of withdrawal from chemicals (agitation, paranoia). Clients must be closely observed to prevent injury or suicide. Chapter 8 ∞ covers management of aggression in more detail.

Intervention	Rationale	Goal
Try to determine whether there is a history of violence.	History of violence is one of the best predictors of present or future violence	Verbalizes past history of violence
Alert all staff members and security if there is a risk for acting out and violent behavior.	Increased awareness to escalating aggression allows for early intervention.	Clients, family members, and staff remain safe
Decrease environmental stimuli.	This may help client regain self-control.	Regains self-control
Remove potentially dangerous items.	Some items could be used as weapons by an aggressive client.	Remains safe
Ask client and family members about situations that provoke violence.	Knowledge may help avoid triggers to aggression.	Identifies triggers
Encourage client to verbalize, rather than act out, violent feelings.	This reduces potential harm.	Reduces violent behavior
Assess for signs of self-inflicted harm.	Drug- or alcohol-altered thoughts may lead to self-harm.	Client remains safe

Managing Hallucinations
Nursing Diagnosis: Client at Risk for Disturbed Sensory Perception

Outcomes: Client verbalizes decreased hallucinations, and maintains contact with reality.

It is important that you stay with clients during this intense and often frightening experience. Isolating clients who are hallucinating often increases the intensity of the hallucinations. Chapter 8 ∞ covers management of hallucinations in more detail.

Intervention	Rationale	Goal
Maintain friendly eye contact and use client's preferred name.	This assists with contact with reality.	Responds appropriately to staff
Identify yourself and provide information about the surroundings in a calm, matter-of-fact voice.	This orients the client to person, time, place, and situation.	Verbalizes orientation
Identify any triggers for hallucinations that may be present in the environment.	Eliminating triggers may decrease hallucinations.	Responds appropriately to environmental stimuli
Clarify any misperceptions and reinforce perceptions that are reality based.	Sharing your perception of reality may lower anxiety levels.	Acknowledges other's perceptions

Responding to Anxiety and Fear
Nursing Diagnosis: Client at Risk for Fear

Outcomes: Client responds appropriately to environment, and verbalizes less anxiety and fear.

Anxiety may be heightened by the physical symptoms of alcohol or drug withdrawal. Changes in sensory perception caused by alcohol or drug intoxication may result in great fear for the client. Chapter 11 ∞ covers management of anxiety in more detail.

continued

NURSING CARE PLAN for Clients With Substance-related Disorders

Responding to Anxiety and Fear   *continued*
Nursing Diagnosis: Client at Risk for Fear

Intervention	Rationale	Goal
Assess level of anxiety from mild through panic.	This helps determine interventions necessary to reduce anxiety.	Verbalizes less anxiety
Assist client in identifying the source of the fear.	This helps determine the reality of the fear.	Verbalizes less fear
Explain sights, sounds, and smells in the environment.	This decreases misperceptions.	Verbalizes less fear
Explain all procedures and interventions before they occur.	This promotes orientation.	Verbalizes improved orientation

Overcoming Denial
Nursing Diagnosis: Client at Risk for Ineffective Coping

Outcomes: Client identifies personal adverse consequences of substance abuse, and accepts responsibility for own recovery.

An important nursing intervention is helping clients overcome denial and recognize the significance of the substance dependence. Keep in mind that it is very painful for clients to stop denying that alcohol and drugs are causing problems for themselves and others.

Intervention	Rationale	Goal
It is important that you see clients as primary sources for finding their own answers and solutions.	This helps them accept responsibility for own recovery.	Verbalizes responsibility
Help identify: ■ Situations in which abuse occurs ■ Type and amount of substances ■ Frequency of abuse	This provides a reality base.	Acknowledges the reality of substance abuse
Help identify the negative consequences of behavior and connect problems in life directly to chemical dependence.	Recognition of effects of abuse on self, family, work, and social situations will confront denial.	Acknowledges negative consequences
Introduce one-day-at-a-time philosophy.	This minimizes feelings of being overwhelmed.	Verbalizes an internal locus of control
Help identify strengths and abilities.	This decreases feelings of helplessness and hopelessness.	Verbalizes feelings of competence

Preventing Relapse
Nursing Diagnosis: Client at Risk for Ineffective Coping

Outcomes: Client identifies high-risk situations, identifies internal and external cues to use, develops strategies for preventing relapse, and maintains a substance-free lifestyle.

While attempting to help clients prevent recurrences of substance use, acknowledge the possibility that slips will occur, and develop strategies to limit the duration and intensity of any relapse episodes. It is believed that it takes 9–15 months to adjust to a lifestyle free of chemical use. Most treatment failures and relapses occur in the first 15 months after abstinence begins. There is also a lifelong vulnerability to relapse. Close to half the recovering people fail to maintain abstinence after a year—about the same proportion of people with diabetes and hypertension who fail to comply with their diet, exercise, and medications. With the limitations on the duration of intensive treatment programs, clients are often discharged well before the plan of care has been fully evaluated.

Recovery is abstinence from all drugs, not just the drug of choice. Once people have crossed the line from chemical use to chemical dependence, they can never return to controlled use without rekindling the addiction. A reasonably motivated client involved in an effective treatment program can have a better prognosis than previously thought. A variety of factors, such as social support, level of functioning before the addiction, and willingness to accept the need for lifestyle changes, influence the treatment outcome.

NURSING CARE PLAN for Clients With Substance-related Disorders

Preventing Relapse *continued*

Nursing Diagnosis: Client at Risk for Ineffective Coping

Intervention	Rationale	Goal
Ask client to identify high-risk situations, such as: ■ People (friends who use) ■ Places (bars) ■ Specific activities ("coke parties")	This is the first step in relapse prevention.	Identifies specific situations
Help client identify internal cues that trigger the urge to use: ■ Bodily sensations ■ Seeing drug paraphernalia	Cues activate substance wanting, seeking, and consumption.	Identifies specific cues
Help client identify any techniques in the past that led to success in avoiding substance use.	This builds on past successes.	Verbalizes positive coping behaviors
Develop strategies for avoiding or actively coping with triggers when faced with such situations, such as: ■ Self-statements regarding commitment to sobriety ■ Assertive skills ■ Relaxation techniques ■ Calling a friend or sponsor ■ Engaging in alternative activities	This helps clients anticipate and plan for problem situations.	Implements strategies
Plan a daily schedule, especially for days off work.	Having unstructured time is not helpful to people in early recovery. Having to change daily activities is a problem if there are no substitutes.	Creates a healthy balance of activities that prevents relapse
Teach client to identify early warning signals of impending relapse.	This helps client to seek support and help as early as possible.	Seeks interventions as early as possible

2) long-term abstinence. In this second phase, you coach clients in preventing relapse and improving general functioning. This is a lifelong commitment to sobriety.

Managing Alcohol Intoxication

Emergency management of acute alcohol intoxication is necessary to save lives. (Review Table 15.1 for signs of intoxication.) Clients must be given a priority status in the emergency department and quickly assessed for life-threatening situations requiring immediate response.

■ Blood alcohol levels (BALs) are generally obtained to determine the level of intoxication,

■ Be alert for complications of mixed addiction.

■ Monitor, record, and report alterations in vital signs since depression of the brain stem can lead to death.

■ Observe changes in skin color and nail beds and monitor arterial blood gases. Cyanosis is associated with depression in the hemoglobin-oxygen saturation.

■ Monitor fluid intake and output.

■ If there is evidence of ascites, place client in a semi-Fowler's position to relieve pressure on the diaphragm.

■ Provide a quiet environment to avoid excessive stimulation that could increase agitation.

■ Maintain room lighting to decrease the possibility of misinterpretation of stimuli and shadows.

■ Provide verbal reassurance and reality orientation as necessary.

■ If there is no one to stay in constant attendance, it may be necessary to restrain the client for protection from injury. Restraints, however, often increase confusion and agitation.

The desired outcome is that client's vital signs will stabilize within normal limits and agitation decreases.

Alcohol Withdrawal Syndrome

Refer back to the symptoms of alcohol withdrawal. Treatment of withdrawal is supportive, depending on the symptoms. Review the pharmacological interventions to ease withdrawal and alcohol withdrawal delirium.

- Monitor vital signs; if client experiences alcohol withdrawal delirium death may result from cardiovascular collapse or hyperthermia
- Provide comfort measures for tremors, sweating, and insomnia
- Orient to person, time, place, and situation
- Use strategies to protect from injury such as bed in low position, call light in reach, one-on-one observation if necessary
- Assess for suicide potential since withdrawal can worsen depression
- Monitor for seizures
- Make the environment meaningful:
  - Provide a clock and calendar
  - Introduce self each time you enter the room
  - Explain all procedures
  - Clarify misperceptions

Complete recovery from withdrawal may take as long as 2 or 3 weeks. An important component to successful treatment is consistent contact and development of a relationship with another person such as a nurse or nurse therapist.

The desired outcome is that the client remains free from injury; that orientation improves; and that agitation decreases.

Drug Intoxication and Withdrawal

Review Table 15.1 for signs of overdose and withdrawal. Refer to psychopharmacological interventions for the medical management of intoxication and withdrawal.

It is important that you monitor, record, and report alterations in vital signs. Overdose of drugs can lead to CNS depression, cerebral hemorrhage, and respiratory or cardiac arrest. MDMA, when combined with high levels of physical activity, can result in greatly increased body temperature. If the client is experiencing hyperthermia, a cooling blanket may be helpful. You will also need to maintain hydration. If the client has overdosed on an oral drug, activated charcoal or gastric lavage may be necessary. Refer back to the pharmacological interventions for drug intoxication.

The desired outcome is that vital signs stabilize and the client recovers physically.

Social Isolation

Many people have developed a lifestyle revolving around substance abuse. Their social interactions have been largely re-

stricted to drinking or using "buddies." Facilitate developing an appropriate social support system for clients and discuss the importance of regular social contacts. Help clients identify alcohol- and drug-free social activities. Group therapy is a treatment of choice in most programs. Clients learn to accept themselves as recovering individuals and help themselves while helping others. The group provides a sense of belonging and a source of friendships. Realizing that they are not alone, people feel less ashamed and despairing. Group members can also monitor one another for signs of relapse.

Refer clients and their families to self-help groups. Mutual support makes people feel useful and valuable. At the beginning of rehabilitation, you may need to monitor client attendance at group meetings. Within each category there are special interest groups, including AA meetings for nurses, AA meetings for gays and lesbians, and women's groups such as Women Reaching Women or Women for Sobriety.

Other groups affiliated with AA serve as support groups for families of those who abuse substances. Al-Anon is designed to help family members share common experiences and to gain an understanding of substance-related disorders. Alateen is another group designed to help the family and the person come to terms with the problem of substance abuse. ACOA helps people deal with past family issues and the impact of these issues on present life. If the family is to remain intact, expectations, role behaviors, and communication patterns must be assessed and modified, often with the support of appropriate 12-step groups.

The desired outcome is that the client participates in self-help groups and substance-free social activities.

Insufficient Physical Activity

Encourage clients to improve their physical health and fitness. Many will benefit from a regular exercise program, which will, in itself, reduce anxiety and depression. For some, exercise becomes a leisure activity to replace the activity of substance abuse. Exercise is also helpful in avoiding relapse. Physiologically, the brain is stimulated by endogenous endorphins instead of alcohol or other drugs. Those who get involved in running often describe the natural "high" of running as a replacement for the old "high" of drugs. Exercising with other people aids in socialization as new "drug-free" friendships are developed. Exercise also provides a focus and outlet for emotions and a sense of mastery over one's physical body.

The desired outcome is that the client participates in a meaningful exercise program.

Enhancing Motivation

Motivation is an internal or intrinsic state of readiness to change. Clients with high motivation at the beginning of treatment have improved outcomes and lower dropout rates than those who are coerced into treatment. Motivational problems are increasing in addiction treatment settings because more clients are identified by early interventions, are ambivalent, and are ordered by the court to attend. Those who do not accept that they have a substance abuse problem have little motivation to change.

Anyone could be labeled "in denial," "resistant to change," and "unmotivated" if asked to make a major change that one is not ready to make. You can consider your own life when others have "suggested" that you need to make a change. Some one may have told you to lose weight, stop smoking, eat a healthier diet, start an exercise program, manage your blood sugar, or lower your blood pressure. You can ask yourself, "How did I respond to this suggestion?" The **Stages of Change model** (Bierma, 2005; Sher & Erpler, 2004) helps you understand the process of change for yourself and your clients.

The first stage of change is one of precontemplation. People in this stage:

- Do not recognize that there is a problem,
- Do not recognize a need for change, and
- Have no plans for changing behavior in the immediate or near future.

The second stage of change is one of contemplatation. People in this stage:

- Think about change but have not initiated any new behaviors.

In the preparation stage, individuals:

- Identify a personal motivation for change,
- Make a commitment to change, and
- Design a plan of action.

The fourth stage, action, involves:

- Implementation of the plan, and
- Actually changing problem behavior.

Maintenance is the last stage, in which people:

- Sustain the behavioral change until it is integrated into their lifestyle.

You can ask yourself the following questions when assisting clients through the change process: What problem behaviors do clients exhibit? Where are these individuals in the change process? Are they making any attempts to modify their behavior? What are their beliefs and attitudes about changing the behavior? What are the reasons for changing? How important is it for them to make the change? The answers to these questions guide nursing interventions. Supporting client autonomy and choices results in better and longer lasting outcomes in substance abuse treatment.

The desired outcome is that the client verbalizes motivation to changes, progresses through the stages of change, and actively participates in treatment.

Spiritual Distress

Spirituality is that part of ourselves that deals with relationships and values and addresses questions of purpose and meaning in life. Chapter 1 ∞ presents spirituality in greater depth. In working with clients who abuse substances, you should identify the aspects of spirituality that enhance recovery. Often a person's life is in such disarray that she or he has lost track of her or his values and sense of purpose and meaning in life. Many clients feel a need for a power outside themselves that can provide a healing structure and restore hope. That strength may come from a higher power, an AA group, a sponsor, or a therapist. Supporting spirituality during treatment is actually helping addicted individuals replace a destructive approach to life with a life-enhancing one.

Many treatment approaches for chemical dependency have a strong spiritual basis and stress that people need to feel connected to a greater power. Review the 12 Steps of Alcoholics Anonymous in Box 9.2 ∞ in terms of the spiritual focus. Facilitate client use of meditation, prayer, communal worship, forgiveness, and other religious traditions and rituals. Refer clients to spiritual advisors of their choice. Some clergy are trained and skilled in substance abuse counseling and serve as a resource for people trying to find meaning in life.

Demonstrate hope by responding to clients' worth and dignity and viewing their substance use disorder as only one facet of the person. Encourage clients to realistically view themselves in the present after sorting through past experiences and to "let go" and move on. Promote anticipated positive experiences and the hope that life will be better without alcohol or drugs. Attitudes to be encouraged are hoping, having faith, trusting, anticipating the positive, looking forward to the future, and believing.

The desired outcome is that the client discusses purpose and meaning in life, identifies values guiding life direction, participates in personal spiritual activities, and verbalizes a sense of hope.

Codependency or Enabling Behavior

People who have substance use disorders must be treated in the context of their family and social systems. Encourage recognition that chemical dependency is a family disease and abstinence is affected by the family process.

When substance abuse becomes severe, conflict among family members often increases. Family relationships begin to deteriorate and the nonabusing family members feel trapped in a cycle of shame, anger, confusion, and guilt. Help nonabusing family members talk about feelings of pain and anger since they have most likely been prevented from expressing their feelings directly. Help them learn how to respect and take care of themselves, decrease their need for perfectionism, and "own" their full range of feelings.

By keeping the chemical dependency a secret, the family tries to compensate for the behavior of the substance abuser. Family members find themselves making excuses for the user's behavior to friends and even employers. Since family members are often unaware of their own codependent behavior, identify specific behaviors that enable their loved one to continue to abuse substances. Help family members acknowledge and change overresponsible behaviors, such as covering up for and protecting the client. This is a process of empowering family members to allow them to let go of responsibility for the abuser's choices.

The desired outcome is that the family members identify enabling behavior and seek support to limit enabling behavior.

Family Distress

The best available evidence at this time supports the inclusion of family within the treatment process. This inclusion can improve outcomes for both the substance abuser and other family members.

Behavioral Couples Therapy (BCT) is designed to intervene in the relationship interactions in which one member of the couple is addicted. Throughout the time of therapy, both individuals must agree to commit to the relationship, to staying together, and not threaten separation or divorce. BCT typically consists of 15 to 20 sessions over 5 to 6 months. BCT depends on the nonaddicted partner to build positive support for sobriety.

During this time, the couple agrees to only have certain discussions in the presence of the therapist. This includes talking about past drinking or drug use or discussion of fears about future use. When the couple is alone, they should focus on positive feelings and their commitment to the relationship. The nurse–therapist models specific behaviors and assigns them as "homework." Examples are:

- Catch Your Partner Doing Something Nice—Each person must notice and acknowledge one positive behavior on the part of the partner each day.
- Caring Day—Each person plans a special, caring activity to surprise the partner.
- Shared Rewarding Activities—Partners take turns to plan enjoyable activities, at or away from home, that involve both people. Children may be included in these activities (Downs & Miller, 2002).

Complementary/Alternative Therapies

How to Help Clients Meditate

Research has shown that people using meditation experience a significant decrease in tobacco, alcohol, and illicit drug use. All sitting meditative practices begin with finding a comfortable but erect position. The posture itself is a meditation. Slumping reflects low energy and passivity, while a ramrod-straight posture reflects tension and effort. It is easiest to meditate if the spine is straight and the body posture is symmetrical. Some people sit on the floor cross-legged using a firm cushion under their buttocks to support the spine. Others sit in a chair with a straight back with both feet on the ground. Many people use focus words or phrases such as *love, peace, let it be, relax, Our Father who art in heaven, Shalom,* or *Om.*

1. Pick a focus word or short phrase that is firmly rooted in your belief system.
2. Sit quietly in a comfortable position.
3. Close your eyes.
4. Relax your muscles.
5. Breathe slowly and naturally and, as you do, repeat your focus word, phrase, or prayer silently to yourself as you exhale.
6. Assume a passive attitude. Do not worry about how well you are doing. When other thoughts come to mind, simply say to yourself, "Oh, well," and gently return to the repetition.
7. Continue for 10 to 20 minutes.
8. Do not stand immediately. Continue sitting quietly for a minute or so, allowing other thoughts to return. Then, open your eyes and sit for another minute before rising.
9. Practice this technique once or twice daily.

SOURCE: Benson, H. (1997). *Timeless healing.* New York: Fireside Books.

The major goals are to help couples change dysfunctional ways of interacting, prevent relapse, and cope with relationship issues encountered in long-term recovery.

The desired outcome is that family members modify substance-related interactional patterns and utilize positive support for change.

Lack of Knowledge Among Family Members

Family members are considered collaborators in the treatment process. The nurse helps them collaborate with each other in an alliance against alcohol and drugs. Family members also need relapse prevention education to help identify triggers to relapse and coping strategies for dealing with trigger events. Provide suggestions in how they might develop and maintain "safe" social networks and "safe" recreational activities. Ask them to develop a list of a variety of leisure activities. Encourage them to try new activities even if they are not sure they will like these activities. The process of mutual problem solving often increases emotional intimacy among family members.

If the person who has abused substances has engaged in risky sexual behaviors, partners will need HIV/AIDS testing and education. They should also be tested for hepatitis B and C. If sexual problems exist or there are issues regarding betrayal, refer the couple for relationship or sexual therapy.

When working with parents or families, we must ask parents about their use of alcohol, nicotine, and other substances. We must help the adults of the family understand the influence of their behavior in terms of their children's attitudes and future behavior.

The desired outcome is that family members will verbalize their role in relapse prevention; if indicated, get tested for STIs; and verbalize an understanding of effect of modeling behavior on children's behavior.

Max says: "I attended AA for awhile and then I stopped because I felt I could handle it without the help. I was wrong. I was sober for 8 months. Then, one day it was warm outside and I had the taste for a cold beer. I figured that one beer wouldn't hurt. Well, that was the end of my sobriety and the beginning of my relapse."

Clinical Interactions   A Substance-abusing Client

Jim, age 34, has two daughters who live with his ex-wife. His parents are still living, and he has a twin sister and two older brothers. He has been living with his parents and has maintained a close relationship with all family members until recently, when his cocaine abuse problems worsened. He has recently entered a drug rehabilitation program. In the interaction, you will see evidence of:

- Grandiose thinking
- Use of cocaine to decrease anxiety about the family's response
- Denial
- Deterioration of family relationships
- Lack of control in the use of cocaine

NURSE: *"Would you tell me what led up to your coming into the program?"*

JIM: "Well, I was on my way to work and I had to stop and get more coke before I went in. I was on my bike going about 110 mph. I always push it like that—going real fast. I don't worry about it because I know I'll always get away with it. They all know who I am."

NURSE: *"Who is 'they'?"*

JIM: "The police. All I have to do is show them a picture of my dad and they know right away who it is—he was a fireman and battalion chief for years. I was always getting pulled over when I was a kid, and they would just take the booze and tell me to go home because they knew who I was because of my dad. So, anyway, I'm driving along and my bike runs out of gas, so I'm trying to push it to get some gas and I get too tired and just push it to the side of the road, lay down on it, and go to sleep. It must have been about 2 hours later when one of these roadside helper vans came by and woke me up. They filled my tank and by then it was too late to go to work and I knew I couldn't go home because I think my family had decided they were going to get me to go for some help. So I went into the city, met these guys I deal with all the time, and traded them my bike for an 8-ball [an eighth of an ounce of cocaine] and a little money so I could get something to eat."

NURSE: *"Are you saying that your family was aware of your drug use and that's why you came in for treatment?"*

JIM: "I don't really have a problem. I could quit any time, but they know there was something wrong. I had gotten to the point I would light up and smoke it in front of my sister."

NURSE: *"How did she react to that?"*

JIM: "She asked me not to do it in front of her. She didn't like the way it made me act. My mom even told me she didn't like the way I had been acting. She told me the other day that she had gotten to the point she didn't even know who I was anymore. She wanted her Jimmy back." [Hands the nurse a sheet of paper.] "I wrote this the other day. I don't know, maybe you'd like to read it and maybe not."

NURSE: *"Do you want me to read it?"*

JIM: "Well, yeah."

[This was a poem about cocaine where cocaine is an entity calling out to the client, promising euphoria, and taking away all his troubles.]

NURSE: *"You write about this taking away all your troubles and cares. Is that how you feel about using cocaine?"*

JIM: "When you're high, you don't care about anything."

NURSE: *"How do you feel when you don't have the high?"*

JIM: "Like going and getting more. Not now, though. I'm through. I've given it up and I'm not going to do it anymore."

NURSE: *"You sound pretty determined."*

JIM: "I am. I've got to get back to how I was before. My oldest daughter called me and told me she didn't like me the way I had become. She said I wasn't like her dad anymore. But she realizes now it was the drugs. She wants me to get better so I'll be more fun than I have been lately. I used to be a pretty friendly guy, smiled a lot, liked to have a good time. Before I came here, I usually just stayed at home and got high or was out trying to get more."

Using Research Evidence   Self-Care: Alcohol Addiction

Zakrzewski, R. F., & Hector, M. A. (2004). The lived experiences of alcohol addiction: Men of alcoholics anonymous. *Issues in Mental Health Nursing, 25,* 6177.

What is the study about?

Alcohol is the most widely used and abused drug in the United States. Statistics reveal that approximately 8% of the population meet the criteria for a diagnosis of alcohol dependence. Therefore, the purpose of this study was to identify themes in the experience of alcohol addiction as lived by male members of Alcoholics Anonymous (AA).

How was the study done?

This was a qualitative existential-phenomenological study of data from seven Caucasian male members of AA who were willing to share their experiences of alcohol use and abuse. These currently sober members participated in nondirective audiotaped interviews. Sobriety ranged from approximately 1 to 25 years, and these men ranged in age from 32 to 65. Participants were obtained through a modified version of the snowball method. The interview employed bracketing. Bracketing is a qualitative research technique of acknowledging the researchers' beliefs in an effort to separate the beliefs discussed by the study participants. The principal investigator (PI) reported himself to the participants as a recovering alcohol addict. This was done in an effort to eliminate or control any of the PI's biases from influencing further data analysis of the research participants' transcripts. The question to participants was: "Have you had the experience of alcohol addiction? If so, could you tell me about your experience?" Interviews lasted from 40 to 90 minutes. All interviews were transcribed verbatim and analyzed by the PI, secondary investigator, and research groups of fellow doctoral students using the methods of phenomenology.

What were the results of the study?

The following themes emerged from the bracketing interview, the lived experiences related by the PI: Time, Relation With Self, and Relations With Others. Time appeared to refer to three distinct stages: life before alcohol addiction, during alcohol addiction, and after alcohol addiction treatment. The theme of Relation With Self revolved around inner feelings and thoughts such as inadequacy, depression, and suicidal thoughts. The last theme, Relations With Others, evolved from the role that alcohol played in the PI's extended family, failed relationships while using alcohol, and how the PI had to learn again how to relate to others while maintaining sobriety.

As the participants described their lives, general themes emerged: Emotions, Control, Awareness, and a temporal ground centered in a Turning Point. (Temporal ground, referred to by all the participants, served as the time context of their experiences: before, during, and after their addiction to alcohol.) *Emotions* referred to their feelings before and throughout their addiction. Such feelings included inadequacy, insecurity, and low self-esteem or self-worth prior to using alcohol. Some participants spoke of pride and how drinking made them feel like they were men. Initially, the excessive use of alcohol made them feel better about themselves through a false sense of self worth. In the beginning, they described the drinking as fun, but eventually the fun became a nuisance. Some of the feelings prior to addiction continued into sobriety and abstinence. After they became

sober, some experienced more depression and insecurity; but they now see themselves in a more positive light. Some reported using other activities or hobbies as a substitute for drinking excessively. *Control*, the second theme, emerged as choice, control, and loss of control over drinking. Some equated the use of alcohol with survival. Loss of control emerged from discussions about arrests, fights, and physical abuse with others. Some described the use of alcohol as a paradox in their lives: Many drank to help cope with distress, yet they relinquished control over the drinking and encountered more distress. Out of control also meant drinking until they blacked out or lost memory. However, participants had no problem remembering how long they were sober—down to months, weeks, days, and hours. *Awareness* of others emerged from their relationships with their families, friends, and the PI. Some credited their loss of relationships as the catalyst to abstain from alcohol and lead a life of sobriety. Many participants reported divorces and failed relationships. Some recounted a family history of alcoholism and how their use of alcohol affected their own families.

Lastly, the Turning Point was identified as that significant time in their lives when they transitioned from using alcohol to being a recovering alcoholic. Achieving sobriety was described as the "turning point," "worst time of their lives," and/or their "rock bottom." Some participants thought of dying as a viable alternative to living free of alcohol. The participants also mentioned treatment programs. Some saw treatment as a way to assist them in feeling better about themselves, and some saw it as a pressure by others in their lives. All the participants, as members of AA, indicated the significance of spirituality, cohesion, and fellowship with other recovering addicts as important to their continuing recovery. All discussed how they had depended on another AA member during their recovery. Living without the use of alcohol was significant in improving the quality of life for most of the participants. In addition, the participants observed how participating in this interview was helpful in their recovery. Many only agreed to participate in the research provided the PI shared his experience of being a recovering alcoholic.

What additional questions might I have?

Would the results of the study be significantly different with women who are addicted to alcohol? Would the results differ with different racial or ethnic groups? What would be the results of a study exploring the phenomenon of alcohol addiction with persons choosing not to use AA as a treatment program?

How can I use this study?

This study can be significant for all nurses working with persons who live with alcohol addiction; it allows others to know what it is like to live with alcohol addiction. Nurses working with persons living with alcohol addiction need to encourage them to tell their own stories. In addition, the nurse may help them identify persons they would feel comfortable talking to about their life with alcohol use and abuse. Risk of relapse might be decreased if the person were helped to develop positive coping skills in lieu of excessive drinking. This study may also be useful to families trying to understand their loved ones' addiction to alcohol and related self-destructive behaviors.

SOURCE: Contributed by Dolores Huffman, PhD, RN, Associate Professor of Nursing, Purdue University Calumet, Hammond, Indiana.

EVALUATION

The future of drug and alcohol treatment is uncertain; the problems are great and the needs are many. There is increasing reluctance to expend resources on people who may show little gratitude and who seem to have brought their troubles on themselves. Programs often suffer from inadequate staff and unreliable funding. Waiting lists are long and the average

duration of treatment—days to several months—is generally thought to be insufficient. The few yearlong treatment programs available have a high success rate, but the current cultural value leans toward incarceration rather than treatment.

To complete the nursing process, you evaluate client responses to nursing interventions based on the selected outcomes. To build a Care Plan for a client with a substance-related disorder, go to the Companion Web site for this book.

ROAD: Assessment   Critical Thinking Questions

Go to the CD-ROM to assess Chris by answering the following critical thinking questions based on what you have **R**ead about Chris and **O**bserved on the videos.

1. Chris reveals data that confirm the need for a *thorough* substance abuse assessment. Review segment A of your student ROAD CD-ROM for chapter 15. What specific type of assessment is needed and why (provide rationale)?

2. Review segment B from your student CD-ROM for chapter 15.
   a. Identify the defense mechanism(s) you hear in Chris's statements. Support your answer.
   b. What key points does Chris verbalize that differentiate his drinking pattern from one of substance dependence versus one of substance abuse? Support your answer(s).

3. In your text's introduction to Chris, you learn that his substance abusing behaviors began during junior high school, increased in frequency, and were cumulative over time. You also learn from your text that substance dependency was a problem for many of his relatives. Listen to segment C of your student CD-ROM for chapter 15. What is your assessment of the issues that may have existed within Chris's family? Provide rationale for your answer.

4. Chris's reports that his substances of choice were alcohol, marijuana, and cocaine during his "drugging career." In your text you see quotes that give you insight into his pattern and frequency of use. As you listen to segment C of your student CD-ROM:
   a. What knowledge would you draw upon during an assessment to understand the *motivation* for Chris's behavior when he was under the influence of cocaine? Support your answer.
   b. What additional area of assessment is indicated for both Chris and his wife? Support your answer.

5. In the following statements on segment D of your student CD-ROM you learn of some physical changes Chris experienced during his substance abuse. Based upon Chris's substance abuse history and the information from your CD, identify the areas of physical assessment that would have been indicated as he entered addiction treatment and the rationale behind the chosen areas of physical assessment.

ROAD: Develop a Care Plan

Go to the CD-ROM to develop a care plan based on your assessment of Chris. Identify nursing diagnoses, outcomes, goals, and interventions.

SOURCE: Contributed by Susan Siwinski-Hebel, RN, MSN.

Focus Your Study

OBJECTIVES	KEY CONCEPTS
1. Outline information about the site of action, effects, complications, withdrawal, and overdose for commonly abused substances.	Review Table 15.1 for this information.

continued

---

2. Compare and contrast the different theories regarding the etiology of substance-related disorders.

- Genetics:
  - Half the risk for alcohol abuse can be explained by genetic factors.
- Neurobiology:
  - Dopamine (DA) may be the master molecule of craving and addiction.
  - Some substances increase the amount of DA and some block the reuptake of DA.
  - Increased levels of DA in the nucleus accumbens is directly responsible for the exhilarating rush that reinforces the desire to get more of the substance.
  - Craving is associated with the learned response that links the drug to the memory of an intensely pleasurable experience.
  - Drug withdrawal disrupts behavioral circuits in the frontal lobes resulting in irritability, depression, and anhedonia.
  - Drug and alcohol change perceptions and the length of time to process information.
- Intrapersonal factors:
  - Hypotheses include a search for altered states of consciousness, desire for new experiences, impulsive personality traits, and defiance of authority.
- Behavioral theory:
  - Theorists look at the activities associated with substance dependence, social pressures, rewards, and punishments.
- Learning theory:
  - Chemically dependent people have learned maladaptive ways of coping.
- Sociocultural factors:
  - The theory is based on the idea that values, perceptions, norms, and beliefs about substance use/abuse are passed on from one generation to another.
  - Peer pressure can cause substance abuse in adolescents and young adults.
- Gender-bias factors:
  - Women are more likely to hide their substance abuse problems and are less likely to seek help.

---

3. Discuss the psychopharmacological treatment of the symptoms of substance-related disorders.

- Alcohol withdrawal:
  - Benzodiazepines
  - Thiamine
  - Antipsychotics
- Alcohol craving:
  - Topiramate (Topamax)
  - Ondansetron (Zofran)
  - Naltrexone (ReVia)
  - Acamprosate (Campral)
  - Disulfiram (Antabuse)
- Opiate withdrawal:
  - Clonidine (Catapres)
  - Naltrexone (ReVia)
  - Buprenorphine (Subutex)
- Opiate craving:
  - Methadone
  - Levomethadyl (Orlaam)
  - Buprenorphine and naloxone (Suboxone)
- Cocaine:
  - Disulfiram (Antabuse)
  - Modafinil (Provigil)
  - Topiramate (Topamax)
  - Vigabatrin (Sabirl)
  - Gabapentin (Neurontin)
  - Selegiline (Eldepryl, Carbex)
- Benzodiazepine overdose:
  - Flumazenil (Romazicon)
- Nicotine dependence:
  - Bupropion (Zyban)
  - Nicotine replacement
  - NicVAX

---

4. Outline the different treatment options for a client with a substance-related disorder.

- Outpatient or inpatient therapy
- Recovery model
- 12-step programs
- Women for Sobriety
- SMART Recovery
- Family therapy
- Alternative therapies:
  - Herbs and nutrients
  - Acupuncture
  - Qigong
  - Guided imagery
- Preventive education
- Community education

---

5. Outline the assessment process for a client with a substance-related disorder.

- All who enter treatment are ambivalent about giving up the chemicals they have become dependent on.
- Assessment should be conducted in a nonjudgmental and matter-of-fact way.
- Give positive recognition that it was a personal choice to come into treatment.
- Begin with less intrusive questions before asking questions about their use of substances.
- Assessment has a twofold purpose:
  - To identify problems
  - To increase clients' awareness of the toll that substance use may be taking on their lives

6. Describe the impact of a substance-related disorder on the functioning of family members.

- Substance abuse leads to dysfunctional family systems, social isolation, financial problems, legal difficulties, ineffective communication, and codependency.
- Children learn to keep the secret about the substance abuse and eventually learn to repress all feelings in an effort to remain in control.
- Children tend to develop one of four patterns of behavior:
  - Hero—the competent caretaker
  - Scapegoat—becomes the focus of conflict in the family
  - Lost child—withdraws physically and emotionally
  - Mascot—uses comic relief to mask sadness

7. Use the nursing process to develop a comprehensive plan of care for a client with a substance-related disorder.

- Dealing with violence:
  - Observe closely to prevent injury or suicide.
  - Decrease environmental stimuli.
  - Remove potentially dangerous items.
- Promoting coping skills:
  - Substances have been used in the past as a coping strategy.
  - Help clients identify and discuss feelings; help them find meaning in and understand the personal significance in their disorder.
  - Teach problem-solving skills and provide vocational guidance.
- Overcoming denial:
  - Identify situations in which substance abuse occurs, the type and amount of substances used, and the frequency of the abuse.
  - Identify the negative consequences of substance abuse.
  - Identify strengths and abilities to decrease feelings of helplessness and hopelessness.
- Enhancing motivation:
  - Use the Stages of Change model to help clients understand motivation:
    - Precontemplation—no recognition of a need for change
    - Contemplation—thinking about changes but no new behaviors
    - Preparation—identify a personal motivation for change, make a commitment, and design a plan of action
    - Maintenance—sustain behavioral change until it is integrated into lifestyle
- Preventing relapse:
  - Impulse control training
  - Identify high-risk situations
  - Identify cues that trigger the urge to use
  - Develop strategies for coping with potential relapse
  - Develop a daily schedule of nonusing activities
  - Identify the early warning signals of impending relapse
- Decreasing isolation:
  - Refer to self-help groups.
  - Use group therapy.
  - Refer family to support groups.
- Supporting spirituality:
  - Discuss clients' sense of purpose and meaning in life.
  - Identify a power outside themselves to heal and restore hope. This may be a higher power, an AA group, a sponsor, or a therapist.
  - Facilitate clients' use of meditation, prayer, communal worship, forgiveness, and other religious traditions and rituals.
- Enhancing physical activity:
  - Help clients design exercise programs.
- Dealing with codependency or enabling behavior:
  - Help nonabusing family members discuss their pain and anger.
  - Help family members identify and change overresponsible behaviors that enable the substance abuse.
- Providing couples therapy:
  - Focus on positive feelings and commitment to the relationship.
  - Change interactional patterns.
  - Discussion of hurt and anger occurs only in the presence of the therapist.
- Educating the family system:
  - Help family identify safe social networks and safe recreational activities.
  - Help the family collaborate with each other in an alliance against alcohol and drugs.
  - Teach the adults that their behavior serves as a powerful model to their children.

continued

continued

7. Use the nursing process to develop a comprehensive plan of care for a client with a substance-related disorder.—*continued*

→

- Managing alcohol intoxication:
  - Priority status in emergency department
  - Vital signs, input and output
  - Quiet environment
  - Close observation
- Managing withdrawal syndrome:
  - Vital signs
  - Orient frequently
  - Protect from injury
- Managing drug intoxication and withdrawal:
  - Vital signs
  - Maintain body temperature and hydration

Explore MediaLink

For review questions, case studies, and other resources for this chapter see the Pearson Health MediaLink CD-ROM that accompanies this book and the Companion Website.

CD-ROM
- Audio Glossary
- NCLEX-RN® Review Questions
- ROAD to Critical Thinking: *Chris*
- Animations/Videos
  - How a Substance of Abuse Occupies a Receptor Site for a Neurotransmitter
  - Morphine (Astramorph PF, Duramorph, and other Opioids)
  - Cocaine Animation
  - Overdose Animation

Companion Website www.prenhall.com/fontaine
- Audio Glossary
- NCLEX-RN® Review Questions
- Case Study
  - Prescription Addiction
- Care Plan
  - Risk for Relapse
- Critical Thinking
  - Community Addiction
- MediaLink Application
  - Science of Addiction
- MediaLinks
  - Books for Clients & Families
  - Community Resources

NCLEX-RN® Review Questions

15-1. An intoxicated client, with injuries sustained from a motor vehicle accident, is admitted to the hospital at 10:00 p.m. What time of the following day will the nurse expect signs and symptoms of withdrawal?
1. 5:00 a.m
2. 10:00 a.m.
3. 5:00 p.m.
4. 10:00 p.m.

15-2. A nurse is teaching an adolescent group about substance abuse. Which of the following statements indicates that further teaching is necessary?
1. "If my parents are alcoholics, I could become one, too."
2. "Drinking beer gives my brother a feeling of power."
3. "Women become addicted more easily than men."
4. "Sometimes people drink so they feel accepted in groups."

15-3. Health care providers in Europe and Australia routinely prescribe the narcotic antagonist naltrexone (Trexan, ReVia) to help clients manage alcohol craving. Only 5% of clients in the United States are given naltrexone. The efforts to treat addiction with medications in the United States are hampered by:
1. Lack of research.
2. The need for universal health care.
3. Public view of addiction.
4. Required government support.

15-4. A client with a long history of cocaine abuse and frequent relapse episodes is hospitalized. Which of the following goals is a priority for this client?
1. Acknowledge association between substance use and personal problems.
2. Attend weekly Alcoholic Anonymous (AA) meetings.
3. Learn about the effects of cocaine on the body systems.
4. Practice adaptive coping strategies.

15-5. A client drank a liter of wine every day for the past year. The client has been arrested three times for driving while impaired. Which of the following terms should the nurse use to describe this client's behavior?
  1. Tolerance
  2. Intoxication
  3. Abuse
  4. Withdrawal

15-6. A client is admitted to the emergency department with needle marks on both arms. The spouse states that the client only uses heroin when feeling a great deal of stress at work. The spouse tells the nurse that the client only uses drugs on the weekend and can handle them. Which of the following assessments will the nurse make about the client and spouse relationship?

  1. Highly differentiated
  2. Triangulation
  3. Codependent behavior
  4. Dependent behavior

15-7. The nurse should initially focus on which of the following interventions when caring for a pregnant client with a substance abuse disorder?
  1. Accept client unconditionally.
  2. Confront the client's behaviors.
  3. List family responsibilities.
  4. Teach the effects of substance use.

See Appendix D for answers.

References

American Psychiatric Association. (2000). *Diagnostic and statistical manual of mental disorders* (4th ed., Text Revision). Washington, DC: Author.

Baigent, M. F. (2003). Physical complications of substance abuse. *Current Opinion in Psychiatry, 16*(3), 291–296.

Barclay, L. (2004). Top U.S. physician, lawyers tackle national drug policy. *Medscape Medical News 2004,* pp. 1–3. Retrieved April 28, 2004, from http://www.medscape.com/viewarticle/474247

Beals, J., Novins, D. K., Whitesell, N. R., Spicer, P., Mitchell, C. M., & Manson, S. M. (2005). Prevalence of mental disorders and utilization of mental health services in two American Indian reservation populations. *American Journal of Psychiatry, 162*(9), 1723–1732.

Berrettini, W. H., & Lerman, C. E. (2005). Pharmacotherapy and pharmacogenetics of nicotine dependence. *American Journal of Psychiatry, 162*(8), 1441–1451.

Betten, D. P., Vohra, R. B., Cook, M. D., Matteucci, M. J., & Clark, R. F. (2006). Antidote use in the critically ill poisoned patients. *Journal of Intensive Care Medicine, 21*(5), 255–277.

Bierma, J. R. (2005). The role of remotivation therapy in substance abuse prevention, treatment, and relapse prevention. In J. A. Dyer & M. L. Stotts (Eds.), *Handbook of remotivation therapy* (pp. 147–156). New York: Haworth Clinical Practice Press.

Boyd, M. R (2003). Vulnerability to alcohol and other drug disorders in rural women. *Archives of Psychiatric Nursing, 17*(1), 33–41.

Boyd, M. R., Phillips, K., & Dorsey, C. J. (2003). Alcohol and other drug disorders, comorbidity, and violence. *Archives of Psychiatric Nursing, 17*(6), 249–258.

Brady, K. T., & Sinha, R. (2005). Co-occuring mental and substance use disorders. *American Journal of Psychiatry, 162*(8), 1483–1493.

Caley, L. M., Shipkey, N., Winkelman, T., Dunlap, C., & Rivera, S. (2006). Evidence-based review of nursing interventions to prevent secondary disabilities in fetal alcohol spectrum disorder. *Pediatric Nursing, 32*(2), 155–162.

Carnahan, R. M., Kutscher, E. C., Obritsch, M. D., & Rasmussen, L. D. (2005). Acute ethanol intoxication after consumption of hairspray. *Pharmacotherapy, 25*(11), 1646–1650.

Carter, G. T., & Mirken, B. (2006). Medical marijuana: Politics trumps science at the FDA. *Medscape General Medicine, 8*(2), 1–4. Retrieved May 24, 2006, from www.medscape.com/viewarticle/531038_print

Chai, Y. G., Oh, D. Y., Chung, E. K., Kim, G. S., Kim, L., Lee, Y. S., et al. (2005). Alcohol and aldehyde dehydrogenase polymorphisms in men with type I and type II alcoholism. *American Journal of Psychiatry, 162*(5), 1003–1005.

Chambers, R. A., Taylor, J. R., & Potenza, M. N. (2003). Developmental neurocircuitry of motivation in adolescence: A critical period of addiction vulnerability. *American Journal of Psychiatry, 160*(6), 1041–1052.

Cofta-Gunn, L., Wright, K. L., & Wetter, D. W. (2004). Evidence-based treatments for tobacco dependence. *Evidence-Based Preventive Medicine, 1*(1), 7–19.

Compton, W. M., Thomas, Y. F., Conway, K. P., & Colliver, J. D. (2005). Developments in the epidemiology of drug use and drug use disorders. *American Journal of Psychiatry, 162*(8), 1494–1502.

Crittenden, P. M., & Claussen, A. H. (2002). Developmental psychopathology perspectives on substance abuse and relationship violence. In C. Wekerle & A. Wall (Eds.), *The violence and addiction equation* (pp. 44–63). New York: Brunner-Routledge.

Dackis, C., & O'Brien, C. (2003). Glutamatergic agents for cocaine dependence. *Annals of the New York Academy of Sciences, 1003,* 328–345.

Dackis, C., & O'Brien, C. (2005). Neurobiology of addiction: Treatment and public policy ramifications. *Nature Neuroscience, 8*(11), 1431–1436.

Dahl, J. P., Kampman, K. M., Oslin, D. W., Weller, A. E., Lohoff, F. W., Ferraro, T. N., et al. (2005). Association of a polymorphism in the Homer1gene with cocaine dependence in an African American population. *Psychiatric Genetics, 15*(4), 277–283.

Di Matteo, V., Pierucci, M., Di Giovanni, G., Benigno, A., & Esposito, E. (2007). The neurobiological bases for the pharmacotherapy of nicotine addiction. *Current Pharmaceutical Design, 13*(12), 1269–1284.

Downs, W. R., & Miller, B. A. (2002). Treating dual problems of partner abuse and substance abuse. In C. Wekerle, & A. Wall (Eds.), *The violence and addiction equation* (pp. 254–274). New York: Brunner-Routledge.

Drabble, L., Midanik, L. T., & Trocki, K. (2005). Reports of alcohol consumption and alcohol-related problems among homosexual, bisexual, and heterosexual respondents. *Journal of Studies on Alcohol, 66*(1), 111–120.

Ehrmin, J. T. (2001). Unresolved feelings of guilt and shame in the maternal role with substance-dependent African American women. *Journal of Nursing Scholarship, 33*(1), 47–52.

Eliopoulos, C. (2001). *Gerontological nursing* (5th ed.). Philadelphia: Lippincott.

Fletcher, C. E. (2004). Experience with peer assistance for impaired nurses in Michigan. *Journal of Nursing Scholarship, 36*(1), 92–93.

Fontaine, K. L. (2005). *Complementary & alternative therapies for nursing practice* (2nd ed.). Upper Saddle River, NJ: Prentice Hall.

Gaffney, K. F. (2006). Postpartum smoking relapse and becoming a mother. *Journal of Nursing Scholarship, 38*(1), 26–30.

Gil, A. G., Wagner, E. F., & Tubman, J. G. (2004). Associations between early-adolescent substance use and subsequent young-adult substance use disorders and psychiatric disorders among a multiethnic male sample in South Florida. *American Journal of Public Health, 94*(9), 1603–1609.

Gottschalk, C., Beauvais, J., Hart, R., & Kosten, T. (2001). Cognitive function and cerebral perfusion during cocaine abstinence. *American Journal of Psychiatry, 158*(4), 540–545.

Guindalini, C., Scivoletto, S., Ferreira, R. G. M., Breen, G., Zilberman, M., Peluso, M. A., et al. (2005). Association of genetic variants in alcohol dehydrogenase 4 with alcohol dependence in Brazilian patients. *American Journal of Psychiatry, 162*(5), 1005–1007.

Hall, M. L. R., & Follette, V. M. (2002). Substance abuse and interpersonal violence in older adults. In C. Wekerle & A. Wall (Eds.), *The violence and addiction equation* (pp. 220–235). New York: Brunner-Routledge.

Hatsukami, D. K., Rennard, S., Jorenby, D., Fiore, M., Koopmeiners, J., de Vos, A., et al. (2005). Safety and immunogenicity of a nicotine conjugate vaccine in current smokers. *Clinical Pharmacology and Therapeutics, 78*(5), 456–467.

Havassy, B. E., Alvidrez, J., & Owen, K. K. (2004). Comparisons of patients with comorbid psychiatric and substance use disorders. *American Journal of Psychiatry, 161*(1), 139–145.

Heise, B. (2003). The historical context of addiction in the nursing profession: 1850–1982. *Journal of Addictions Nursing, 14*, 117–124.

Hyman, S. E. (2005). Addiction: A disease of learning and memory. *American Journal of Psychiatry, 162*(8), 1414–1422.

Johnson, S. D., Phelps, D. L., & Cottler, L. B. (2004). The association of sexual dysfunction and substance use among a community epidemiological sample. *Archives of Sexual Behavior, 33*(1), 55–63.

Kenna, G. A., Mcgeary, J. E., & Swift, R. M. (2004). Pharmacotherapy, pharmacogenomics, and the future of alcohol dependence treatment. *American Journal of Health-System Pharmacy, 61*(22), 2380–2388.

Kessler, R. C. (2004). The epidemiology of dual diagnosis. *Biological Psychiatry, 56*(10), 730–737.

Kilts, C. D., Gross, R. E., Ely, R. D., & Drexler, K. P. G. (2004). The neural correlates of cue-induced craving in cocaine-dependent women. *American Journal of Psychiatry, 161*(2), 233–241.

Kremer, I., Bachner-Melman, R., Reshef, A., Broude, L., Nemanov, L., Gritsenko, I., et al. (2005). Association of the serotonin transporter gene with smoking behavior. *American Journal of Psychiatry, 162*(5), 924–930.

Li, M., Chen, K., & Mo, Z. (2002). Use of qigong therapy in the detoxification of heroin addicts. *Alternative Therapies in Health and Medicine, 8*(1), 50–54, 56–59.

Liska, K. (2004). *Drugs and the human body* (7th ed.). Upper Saddle River, NJ: Prentice Hall.

Lu, P. K., Lu, G. P., Lu, D. P., Lu, D. P., & Lu, W. I. (2004). Managing acute withdrawal syndrome on patients with heroin and morphine addiction by acupuncture therapy. *Acupuncture & Electrotherapeutics Research, 29*(3–4), 187–195.

Martinez, R. J., & Murphy-Parker, D. (2003). Examining the relationship of addiction education and beliefs of nursing students toward persons with alcohol problems. *Archives of Psychiatric Nursing, 17*(4), 156–164.

Martsolf, D. S., Sedlak, C. A., & Doheny, M. O. (2000). Codependency and related health variables. *Archives of Psychiatric Nursing, 14*(3), 150–158.

Mayfield, D. G., McCleod, G., & Hall, P. (1974). The CAGE Questionnaire. *American Journal of Psychiatry, 131*(10), 1121–1123.

McElrath, K. (2005). MMA and sexual behavior. *Substance Use & Misuse, 40*(9–10), 1461–1477.

Miller, N. S., & Adams, J. (2005). Alcohol and drug disorders. In J. M. Silver, T. W. McAllister, & S. C. Yudofsky (Eds.), *Textbook of traumatic brain injury* (pp. 509–529). Washington, DC: American Psychiatric Press.

Murphy-Parker, D., & Martinez, R. J. (2005). Nursing students' personal experiences involving alcohol problems. *Archives of Psychiatric Nursing, 19*(3), 150–158.

Nader, M. A., & Czoty, P. W. (2005). PET imaging of dopamine D2 receptors in monkey models of cocaine abuse. *American Journal of Psychiatry, 162*(8), 1473–1482.

Naegle, M. A., & D'Avanzo, C. E. (2001). *Addictions and substance abuse: Strategies for advanced practice nursing.* Upper Saddle River, NJ: Prentice Hall.

National Institute on Drug Abuse. (2005). Drugs of abuse information. Retrieved September 10, 2006, from www.drugabuse.gov/DrugPages

National Survey of American Attitudes on Substance Abuse XI: Teens and Parents. (2006). New York: The National Center on Addiction and Substance Abuse at Columbia University.

Nestler, E. J., & Self, D. W. (2004). Neuropsychiatric aspects of ethanol and other chemical dependencies. In S. C. Yudofsky & R. E. Hales (Eds,), *Essentials of neuropsychiatry and clinical neurosciences* (pp. 399–419). Washington, DC: American Psychiatric Publishing.

NIDA InfoFacts: High School and Youth Trends. (2005). *National institute on drug abuse.* Retrieved September 10, 2006, from www.drugabuse.gov/infofacts/HSYouthtrends.html

North American Nursing Diagnosis Association. (2007). *Nursing diagnoses: Definition and classification, 2007-2008.* Philadelphia: Author.

Novins, D. K., & Baron, A. E. (2004). American Indian substance use. *Journal of the American Academy of Child and Adolescent Psychiatry, 43*(3), 316–324.

O'Brien, C. P. (2005a). Benzodiazepine use, abuse, and dependence. *Journal of Clinical Psychiatry, 66*(Suppl. 2), 28–33.

O'Brien, C. P. (2005b). Anticraving medications for relapse prevention. *American Journal of Psychiatry, 162*(8), 1423–1431.

O'Malley, P. (2005). Ecstasy for intimacy: Potentially fatal choices for adolescents and young adults. *Clinical Nurse Specialist, 19*(2), 63–64.

Rasmussen, C. (2005). Executive functioning and working memory in fetal alcohol spectrum disorder. *Alcoholism, Clinical and Experimental Substance Research, 29*(8), 1359–1367.

Reoux, J. P., & Ries, R. (2001). Searching for new detoxification strategies. Retrieved September 10, 2006, from www.eurekalert.org/pub_releases/2001-09/ace-sfn091001.php

Sher, K. J., & Erpler, A. J. (2004). Alcoholic denial. In B. D. Beirman & J. Nair (Eds.), *Self-awareness deficits in psychiatric patients* (pp. 184–212). New York: W.W. Norton & Company.

Silberg, J., Rutter, M., D'Onofrio, B., & Eaves, L. (2003). Genetic and environmental risk factors in adolescent substance use. *The Journal of Child Psychology and Psychiatry, 44*(5), 664–676.

Snow, D., & Hughes, T. (2003). Prevalence of alcohol and other drug use and abuse among nurses. *Journal of Addictions Nursing, 14*, 165–167.

Spector, R. E. (2004). *Cultural diversity in health & illness* (6th ed.). Upper Saddle River, NJ: Prentice Hall.

Stafford, L. L. (2001). Is codependency a meaningful concept? *Issues in Mental Health Nursing, 22*, 273–286.

Stern, Y., & Sacheim, H. A. (2004). Neuropsychiatric aspects of memory and amnesia. In S. C. Yudofsky & R. E. Hales (Eds.), *Essentials of neuropsychiatry and clinical neurosciences* (pp. 201–238). Washington, DC: American Psychiatric Publishing.

Stevenson, J. S., & Masters, J. A. (2005). Predictors of alcohol misuse and abuse in older women. *Journal of Nursing Scholarship, 37*(4), 329–335.

Thapar, A., Fowler, R., Rice, F., Scourfield, J., van den Bree, M., Thomas, H., et al. (2003). Maternal smoking during pregnancy and attention deficit hyperactivity disorder symptoms in offspring. *American Journal of Psychiatry, 160*(11), 1985–1989.

van den Brink, W., Goppel, M., & van Ree, J. M. (2003). Management of opioid dependence. *Current Opinion in Psychiatry, 16*(3), 297–304.

Volkow, N. D., Chang, L., Wang, G., Fowler, J. S., Franceschi, D., Sedler, M. J., et al. (2001). Higher cortical and lower subcortical metabolism in detoxified methamphetamine abusers. *American Journal of Psychiatry, 158*(3), 383–388.

West, M. M. (2002). Early risk indicators of substance abuse among nurses. *Journal of Nursing Scholarship, 34*(2), 187–193.

Wing, D. M. (1996). A concept analysis of alcoholic denial and cultural accounts. *Advanced Nursing Science, 19*(2), 54–63.

World Health Organization. (2005). Substance abuse. World Health Organization. Retrieved September 10, 2006, from www.who.int/ substanceabuse.

Worthington, N., Markham, P. T., Galea, S., & Rosenthal, D. (2006). Opiate users' knowledge about overdose prevention and naloxone in New York City. *Harm Reduction Journal, 5*(3), 19.

Wright, V. L. (2003). A phenomenological exploration of spirituality among African American women recovering from substance abuse. *Archives of Psychiatric Nursing, 17*(4), 173–185.

Wynd, C. A. (2005). Guided health imagery for smoking cessation and long-term abstinence. *Journal of Nursing Scholarship, 37*(3), 245–250.

Zakrzewski, R. F., & Hector, M. A. (2004). The lived experiences of alcohol addiction: Men of alcoholics anonymous. *Issues in Mental Health Nursing, 25,* 6177.

Ziedonis, D. M., & Williams, J. M. (2003). Management of smoking in people with psychiatric disorders. *Current Opinion in Psychiatry, 16*(3), 305–315.

Chapter 16

Personality Disorders

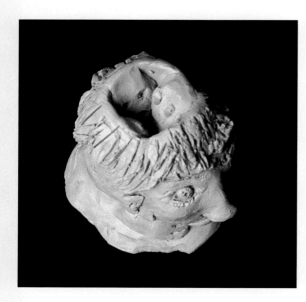

> ❝ *If I let you help me you'll want something in return. There's always a price. I give a little and you squeeze harder wanting more and more of me. You hold me so tight there's no way to get away. You're always there, never letting go. I don't want to talk or feel or look at what's making me sick. I just want to learn how to not feel and not think so I can get back to my old life.* ❞
>
> —Kay, Age 40

OBJECTIVES

After reading this chapter, you will be able to:

1. Compare and contrast the different symptoms of the personality disorders.
2. Outline the different theories regarding the etiology of the personality disorders.
3. Outline the assessment process for a client with a personality disorder.
4. Discuss the key points in effectively communicating with a person with a personality disorder.
5. Use the nursing process to develop a safe, comprehensive plan of care for a client with a personality disorder.
6. Develop illness management teaching plans for a client with a personality disorder and her/his family.

MediaLink www.prenhall.com/fontaine

Go to the Pearson Health MediaLink CD-ROM and the Companion Website at www.prenhall.com/fontaine for interactive resources for this chapter.

The ROAD to Critical Thinking   A Client Experiencing Borderline Personality Disorder

Travel this ROAD to understand Kylie and her condition.

Read about Kylie below and throughout this chapter.

Observe Kylie on the CD-ROM accompanying this book.

Assess Kylie by answering the questions at the end of this chapter.

Develop a Care Plan on the CD-ROM to address Kylie's condition.

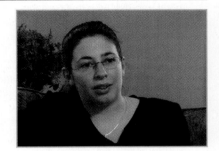

Kylie

Kylie was diagnosed with borderline personality disorder after a suicide attempt. She has had difficulty with relationships most of her life. She states that she was very good at masking her problems but when everything crumbled, her family was totally surprised. She recognizes that she lashes out at others impulsively and unreasonably.

Often borderline personality disorder is not diagnosed until a crisis occurs as the result of impulsive or self-destructive behavior.

Socially, individuals with this disorder have intense, unstable, and manipulative relationships.

You will meet Kylie on the video clip on your disc and throughout this chapter. At the end of the chapter you will find critical thinking questions relating to assessment and development of a plan of care for Kylie.

To understand the nature of personality disorders, it is helpful to review the concept of personality. Personalities develop as people adapt to their physical, emotional, social, and spiritual environments. *Personality* refers to stable patterns of thoughts, feelings, behaviors, and motivation. Personality determines how people cope with feelings and impulses, how they see themselves and others, how they respond to their surroundings, and how they find meaning in relationships and cultural values. Personality can also be thought of as a style of adaptive functioning. These patterns are noticeable in a variety of situations.

The psychobiological model of personality considers temperament and character. *Temperament*, heavily influenced by genetic variables, refers to the features of personality that are present in infancy. A person's temperament is highly stable over time. *Character*, heavily influenced by environmental variables, refers to enduring traits and behavior patterns. Those aspects of personality are the product of learning and interaction with the environment. Although these distinctions seem clear, the reality is that the separation of genetic and environmental influences is not possible (Gabbard, 2004).

A personality becomes *disordered* when the patterns are exaggerated, inflexible, and maladaptive. Personality disorders represent the extremes of normal variation of personality. The dysfunction may be a failure to establish personal identity, an inability to initiate or maintain intimate relationships, or a lack of social skills that interfere with cooperative relationships. Some people with personality disorders have intense emotional pain, whereas others seem invulnerable to painful feelings. Some are able to maintain relationships and careers, whereas others become functionally impaired.

Clients with personality disorders are among the most difficult to treat. Most will never enter a psychiatric hospital, seek or receive outpatient treatment, or undergo a diagnostic evaluation. Some will enter the mental health system through family pressure or because of a court order. With those who do come into the system, mental health professionals find their expertise tested. In most cases, the personality problems are **ego-syntonic**. Clients perceive their difficulties in dealing with other people to be external to them. Incapable of considering that their problems have anything to do with them personally, they will describe being victimized by specific others or by "the system." Some may develop an awareness of their self-defeating behavior but remain at a loss as to how they got that way or how to begin to change.

Personality disorders are diagnosed or coded on Axis II of the *Diagnostic and Statistical Manual of Mental Disorders* (4th ed., Text Revision) (DSM-IV-TR) (American Psychiatric Association, 2000). (See the DSM-IV-TR Classifications feature.) The personality disorders have a high degree of overlap, and many individuals exhibit traits of several disorders. Thus, individuals who receive any personality disorder diagnosis typically receive several. This lack of precision continues to be a criticism of the DSM-IV-TR. Some clinicians prefer to conceptualize personality disorders on a continuum from mild through moderate, to severe.

Typically, personality disorders become apparent before or during adolescence and persist throughout life. In some cases, the symptoms become less obvious by middle or old age. Studies show that personality disorders have an impact on an individual's quality of life (Chen et al. 2006).

| **DSM-IV-TR** | **Diagnostic Criteria for a Personality Disorder** |

A. An enduring pattern of inner experience and behavior that deviates markedly from the expectations of the individual's culture. This pattern is manifested in two (or more) of the following areas:
  1. Cognition (i.e., ways of perceiving and interpreting self, other people, and events)
  2. Affectivity (i.e., the range, intensity, lability, and appropriateness of emotional response)
  3. Interpersonal functioning
  4. Impulse control

B. The enduring pattern is inflexible and pervasive across a broad range of personal and social situations.

C. The enduring pattern leads to clinically significant distress or impairment in social, occupational, or other important areas of functioning.

D. The pattern is stable and of long duration and its onset can be traced back at least to adolescence or early adulthood.

E. The enduring pattern is not better accounted for as a manifestation or

consequence of another mental disorder.

F. The enduring pattern is not due to the direct physiological effects of a substance (e.g., a drug of abuse, a medication) or a general medical condition (e.g., head trauma).

SOURCE: Reprinted with permission from the *Diagnostic and statistical manual of mental disorders,* 4th ed., Text Revision (p. 689). Copyright 2000 American Psychiatric Association.

It is extremely difficult to estimate the incidence of personality disorders. Many people with personality disorders never come to the attention of the mental health system. Personality disorders are frequently diagnosed among the psychiatric client population.

KNOWLEDGE BASE

There are 10 personality disorders, grouped into three clusters. The disorders within each cluster have similar characteristics. The clusters are traditional but likely to be challenged as new information in behavioral genetics and developmental psychology alter the current understanding of the nature, origins, and treatment of personality disorders. The DSM-IV-TR clusters and corresponding disorders are as follows:

Cluster A

1. Paranoid (PPD)
2. Schizoid (SZPD)
3. Schizotypal (STPD)

Cluster B

4. Antisocial (APD)
5. Borderline (BPD)
6. Histrionic (HPD)
7. Narcissistic (NPD)

Cluster C

8. Avoidant (AVPD)
9. Dependent (DPD)
10. Obsessive–compulsive (OCPD)

People with diagnoses from **Cluster A personality disorders**, sometimes referred to as schizophrenia spectrum personality disorders, usually seem eccentric, and they exhibit

many withdrawal behaviors. People with diagnoses from **Cluster B personality disorders** seem dramatic, emotional, or erratic. They tend to be very manipulative in their behavior. People with diagnoses from **Cluster C personality disorders** seem anxious or fearful. Their behavior pattern is one of compliance. People with diagnoses from the anxious Cluster C improve more than those from the erratic Cluster B, who in turn improve more than those with the eccentric and withdrawn Cluster A disorders.

An additional category, *personality disorder not otherwise specified,* refers to those who do not meet criteria for any specific personality disorder. This category also includes disorders being researched, in this case passive–aggressive personality disorder and depressive personality disorder.

Cluster A Personality Disorders
Paranoid Personality Disorder

Behaviorally, people with **paranoid personality disorder (PPD)** are very *secretive* about their life. Confiding in other people is perceived as dangerous and is not likely to occur, even within family relationships. Paranoid people are hyperalert to danger, search for evidence of attack, and become argumentative as a way of creating a safe distance between themselves and others. They rarely seek help for their personality problems, and they seldom require hospitalization.

Affectively, paranoid people typically *avoid sharing their feelings* except for a very quick expression of anger. They may never forgive perceived slights and may bear grudges for long periods of time. There is a prevalent fear of losing power or control to others. These individuals experience a continuous state of tension and rarely are able to relax.

Cognitively, paranoid people are very *guarded* about themselves and secretive about their decisions. They expect to be used or harassed by others. When confronted with new situations, they look for hidden, demeaning, or threatening meanings to benign remarks or events, and they respond by criticizing others. For example, if there is an error in a bank statement, the paranoid person may say the bank did it to ruin his or her credit rating.

Socially, paranoid people have great difficulty with intimate relationships. They interact in a cold and *aloof manner,* thus avoiding the perceived dangers of intimacy. Because they expect to be harmed by others, they question the loyalty or trustworthiness of family and friends. *Pathological jealousy* of the spouse or sex partner frequently occurs.

Devin's boss has been critical of Devin's inability to get his work done in a timely fashion. Although Devin is constantly trying to hear what others are talking about and is easily distracted, he is unable to relate this behavior to his job difficulties. Instead he states, "People at work keep bothering me and talking to each other just to slow me down. They are trying to turn my boss against me. Every little thing I do or say is used against me."

Schizoid Personality Disorder

Behaviorally, people with **schizoid personality disorder (SZPD)** are *loners* who prefer solitary activities because social situations and interactions increase their level of anxiety. They may be occupationally impaired if the job requires interpersonal skills. However, if work may be performed under conditions of social isolation, such as being a night guard in a closed facility, they may be capable of satisfactory occupational achievement.

Affectively, people with SZPD are stable but have a limited range of feelings. Their *affect* is *blunted* or flat. Because they do not express their feelings verbally or nonverbally, they give the impression that they have no strong positive or negative emotions. However, if they are forced into a close interaction, they may become very anxious.

Cognitively, they could be described as having *poverty of thoughts.* The thoughts they do express are often vague. Some of their beliefs include, "It doesn't matter what other people think of me" and "Close relationships are undesirable."

Socially, they interact with others in a cold and aloof manner, have *no close friends,* and prefer not to be in any relationships. They are indifferent to the attitudes and feelings of others, and, thus, are not influenced by praise or criticism.

Charlie, age 34, lives alone in a residential hotel. He is employed as a night guard in a warehouse. He interacts minimally with the other night guards and always eats his meals by himself. He has no friends and no social contacts outside of work. He describes people as "replaceable." He visits his parents, who live a mile away, once a year.

Schizotypal Personality Disorder

Behaviorally, people with **schizotypal personality disorder (STPD)** have a considerable disability. With peculiarities of

thinking, appearance, and behavior that are not severe enough to meet the criteria for schizophrenic disorder, this disorder seems related to schizophrenia. It is assumed that in some people STPD will progress to schizophrenia. Some studies have shown a greater prevalence of this personality disorder among biological relatives of people with schizophrenia. Under periods of extreme stress and anxiety, people with STPD may experience transient psychotic symptoms that are not of sufficient duration to make an additional diagnosis (Keshavan et. al., 2005).

People with this disorder exhibit *odd speech.* It is coherent but often tangential and vague or, at times, overelaborate. Individuals prefer solitary activities and often experience occupational difficulties.

Affectively, they are typically constricted, and their affect may be *inappropriate* to the situation. Social situations create anxiety for those with STPD.

Cognitively, these individuals experience the most severe distortions of any of the personality disorders. The disturbances include *paranoid ideation* (suspicious of other people), ideas of reference, odd beliefs, and magical thinking. They may experience illusions such as seeing people in the movement of shadows. They usually have *difficulty making decisions.*

Socially, they fear intimacy and desire no relationships with family or friends. Thus, they are isolative and are usually *avoided by others.*

Carol, a 24-year-old unemployed single woman, lives in a rooming house. She keeps to herself, and most of the other boarders in the rooming house find her eccentric. Carol is preoccupied with the idea that her dead father was a movie star who left her a fortune with which her guardian absconded. Carol has a habit of saying odd things like, "So go the days of our lives." Most of the rooming house boarders avoid Carol because of her strange behaviors.

Cluster B Disorders

The three unstable disorders in this category—borderline, histrionic, and narcissistic—can barely be distinguished from one another. More so than with other disorders, the diagnosis may be influenced by personal bias, gender stereotypes, and cultural prejudices on the part of the professional.

Antisocial Personality Disorder

A diagnosis of **antisocial personality disorder (ASPD)** necessitates that the characteristics appear before the age of 15, and the client is usually given the diagnosis of conduct disorder. The diagnosis of ASPD is not applied until after the age of 18. In boys, the behavior typically emerges during childhood, whereas for girls it is more likely to occur around puberty. There are at least twice as many men as women diagnosed with ASPD. They are at risk for substance abuse, criminal behavior, and becoming victims of violence (Livesley, 2003).

DSM-IV-TR   Diagnostic Criteria for Personality Disorders: Clusters A, B, C

CLUSTER A (ODD–ECCENTRIC)
Paranoid Personality Disorder

A. A pervasive distrust and suspiciousness of others such that their motives are interpreted as malevolent, beginning by early adulthood and present in a variety of contexts, as indicated by four (or more) of the following:

1. Suspects, without sufficient basis, that others are exploiting, harming, or deceiving him or her
2. Is preoccupied with unjustified doubts about the loyalty or trustworthiness of friends or associates
3. Is reluctant to confide in others because of unwarranted fear that the information will be used maliciously against him or her
4. Reads hidden demeaning or threatening meanings into benign remarks or events
5. Persistently bears grudges, i.e., is unforgiving of insults, injuries, or slights
6. Perceives attacks on his or her character or reputation that are not apparent to others and is quick to react angrily or to counter-attack
7. Has recurrent suspicions, without justification, regarding fidelity of spouse or sexual partner

SCHIZOID PERSONALITY DISORDER

A pervasive pattern of detachment from social relationships and a restricted range of expression of emotions in interpersonal settings, beginning by early adulthood and present in a variety of contexts, as indicated by four (or more) of the following:

1. Neither desires nor enjoys close relationships, including being part of a family
2. Almost always chooses solitary activities
3. Has little, if any, interest in having sexual experiences with another person
4. Takes pleasure in few, if any, activities
5. Lacks close friends or confidants other than first-degree relatives
6. Appears indifferent to the praise or criticism of others
7. Shows emotional coldness, detachment, or flattened affectivity
8. Considers relationships to be more intimate than they actually are

SCHIZOTYPAL PERSONALITY DISORDER

A pervasive pattern of social and interpersonal deficits marked by acute discomfort with, and reduced capacity for, close relationships as well as by cognitive or perceptual distortions and eccentricities of behavior, beginning by early adulthood and present in a variety of contexts, as indicated by five (or more) of the following:

1. Ideas of reference (excluding delusions of reference)
2. Odd beliefs or magical thinking that influences behavior and is inconsistent with subcultural norms (e.g., superstitiousness, belief in clairvoyance, telepathy, or "sixth sense"; in children and adolescents, bizarre fantasies or preoccupations)
3. Unusual perceptual experiences, including bodily illusions
4. Odd thinking and speech (e.g., vague, circumstantial, metaphorical, overelaborate, or stereotyped)
5. Suspiciousness or paranoid ideation
6. Inappropriate or constricted affect
7. Behavior or appearance that is odd, eccentric, or peculiar
8. Lack of close friends or confidants other than first-degree relatives
9. Excessive social anxiety that does not diminish with familiarity and tends to be associated with paranoid fears rather than negative judgments about self

CLUSTER B (DRAMATIC–EMOTIONAL)
Borderline Personality Disorder

A pervasive pattern of instability of interpersonal relationships, self-image, and affects, and marked impulsivity beginning by early adulthood and present in a variety of contexts, as indicated by five (or more) of the following:

1. Frantic efforts to avoid real or imagined abandonment. Note: Do not include suicidal or self-mutilating behavior covered in Criterion 5.
2. A pattern of unstable and intense interpersonal relationships characterized by alternating between extremes of idealization and devaluation
3. Identity disturbance: markedly and persistently unstable self-image or sense of self
4. Impulsivity in at least two areas that are potentially self-damaging (e.g., spending, sex, substance abuse, reckless driving, binge eating)
5. Recurrent suicidal behavior, gestures, or threats, or self-mutilating behavior
6. Affective instability due to a marked reactivity of mood (e.g., intense episodic dysphoria, irritability, or anxiety usually lasting a few hours and only rarely more than a few days)
7. Chronic feelings of emptiness
8. Inappropriate, intense anger or difficulty controlling anger (e.g., frequent displays of temper, constant anger, recurrent physical fights)
9. Transient, stress-related paranoid ideation or severe dissociative symptoms

Histrionic Personality Disorder

A pervasive pattern of excessive emotionality and attention seeking, beginning by early adulthood and present in a variety of contexts, as indicated by five (or more) of the following:

1. Is uncomfortable in situations in which he or she is not the center of attention
2. Interaction with others is often characterized by inappropriate sexually seductive or provocative behavior
3. Displays rapidly shifting and shallow expression of emotions
4. Consistently uses physical appearance to draw attention to self
5. Has a style of speech that is excessively impressionistic and lacking in detail
6. Shows self-dramatization, theatricality, and exaggerated expression of emotion
7. Is suggestible, i.e., easily influenced by others or circumstances

Narcissistic Personality Disorder

A pervasive pattern of grandiosity (in fantasy or behavior), need for admiration, and lack of empathy, beginning by early adulthood and present in a variety of contexts, as indicated by five (or more) of the following:

1. Has a grandiose sense of self-importance (e.g., exaggerates achieve-

DSM-IV-TR Diagnostic Criteria for Personality Disorders: Clusters A, B, C *continued*

ments and talents, expects to be recognized as superior without commensurate achievements)

2. Is preoccupied with fantasies of unlimited success, power, brilliance, beauty, or ideal love

3. Believes that he or she is "special" and unique and can only be understood by, or should associate with, other special or high-status people (or institutions)

4. Requires excessive admiration

5. Has a sense of entitlement, i.e., unreasonable expectations of especially favorable treatment or automatic compliance with his or her expectations

6. Is interpersonally exploitative, i.e., takes advantage of others to achieve his or her own ends

7. Lacks empathy: is unwilling to recognize or identify with the feelings and needs of others

8. Is often envious of others or believes that others are envious of him or her

9. Shows arrogant, haughty behaviors or attitudes

Antisocial Personality Disorder

There is a pervasive pattern of disregard for and violation of the rights of others occurring since age 15 years, as indicated by three (or more) of the following:

1. Failure to conform to social norms with respect to lawful behaviors as indicated by repeatedly performing acts that are grounds for arrest

2. Deceitfulness, as indicated by repeated lying, use of aliases, or conning others for personal profit or pleasure

3. Impulsivity or failure to plan ahead

4. Irritability and aggressiveness, as indicated by repeated physical fights or assaults

5. Reckless disregard for safety of self or others

6. Consistent irresponsibility, as indicated by repeated failure to sustain consistent work behavior or honor financial obligations

7. Lack of remorse, as indicated by being indifferent to or rationalizing having hurt, mistreated, or stolen from another

CLUSTER C (FEARFUL–ANXIOUS)

Avoidant Personality Disorder

A pervasive pattern of social inhibition, feelings of inadequacy, and hypersensitivity to negative evaluation, beginning by early adulthood and present in a variety of contexts, as indicated by four (or more) of the following:

1. Avoids occupational activities that involve significant interpersonal contact, because of fears of criticism, disapproval, or rejection

2. Is unwilling to get involved with people unless certain of being liked

3. Shows restraint within intimate relationships because of the fear of being shamed or ridiculed

4. Is preoccupied with being criticized or rejected in social situations. Note: Do not include suicidal or self-mutilating behavior covered in Criterion 5.

5. Is inhibited in new interpersonal situations because of feelings of inadequacy

6. Views self as socially inept, personally unappealing, or inferior to others

7. Is unusually reluctant to take personal risks or to engage in any new activities because they may prove embarrassing

Dependent Personality Disorder

A pervasive and excessive need to be taken care of that leads to submissive and clinging behavior and fears of separation, beginning by early adulthood and present in a variety of contexts, as indicated by five (or more) of the following:

1. Has difficulty making everyday decisions without an excessive amount of advice and reassurance from others

2. Needs others to assume responsibility for most major areas of his or her life

3. Has difficulty expressing disagreement with others because of fear of loss of support or approval. Note: Do not include realistic fears of retribution.

4. Has difficulty initiating projects or doing things on his or her own (because of a lack of self-confidence in judgment or abilities rather than a lack of motivation or energy)

5. Goes to excessive lengths to obtain nurturance and support from others, to

the point of volunteering to do things that are unpleasant

6. Feels uncomfortable or helpless when alone because of exaggerated fears of being unable to care for himself or herself

7. Urgently seeks another relationship as a source of care and support when a close relationship ends

8. Is unrealistically preoccupied with fears of being left to take care of himself or herself

Obsessive–compulsive Personality Disorder

A pervasive pattern of preoccupation with orderliness, perfectionism, and mental and interpersonal control, at the expense of flexibility, openness, and efficiency, beginning by early adulthood and present in a variety of contexts, as indicated by four (or more) of the following:

1. Is preoccupied with details, rules, lists, order, organization, or schedules to the extent that the major point of the activity is lost

2. Shows perfectionism that interferes with task completion (e.g., is unable to complete a project because his or her own overly strict standards are not met)

3. Is excessively devoted to work and productivity to the exclusion of leisure activities and friendships (not accounted for by obvious economic necessity)

4. Is overconscientious, scrupulous, and inflexible about matters of morality, ethics, or values (not accounted for by cultural or religious identification)

5. Is unable to discard worn-out or worthless objects even when they have no sentimental value

6. Is reluctant to delegate tasks or to work with others unless they submit to exactly his or her way of doing things

7. Adopts a miserly spending style toward both self and others; money is viewed as something to be hoarded for future catastrophes

8. Shows rigidity and stubbornness

Behaviorally, actions may range from fairly mild to moderate to very severe. Predominant childhood manifestations are lying, stealing, truancy, vandalism, fighting, and running away from home. In adulthood, the pattern changes to failure to honor financial obligations, inability to function as a responsible parent, tendency to lie pathologically, and inability to sustain consistently appropriate work behavior. Persons with ASPD may engage in nonviolent sexual offenses, such as voyeurism or exhibitionism. A few commit violent crimes, such as sadistic acts and murder. People with ASPD conform to rules only when they are useful to them. Their behavior is often *impulsive* and they have difficulty delaying gratification.

When Norma Toliopoulos lived in Chicago she sold insurance for several different companies. She could easily charm clients into buying her products but she was an unreliable worker. She "talked a good game" but people soon discovered that she could not be trusted, since she lied constantly. She left Chicago in 1999 when the FBI began to investigate her for fraud. The next time her roommate saw her she was on television with a different name (Norma Khouri) speaking about the book she had just written. Her book was supposedly a true story of how she was best friends with a Muslim woman she had grown up with in Jordan and who was murdered by a relative for dating a Christian man. This book made her a celebrity as she was interviewed on National Public Radio, the "Today" show, and in the *New York Times*. In reality, Norma lived in Chicago since she was 3 years old, not in Jordan, and fabricated the entire book. Once again, she had conned everyone—publishers, media, and her friends.

Affectively, people with ASPD express themselves quickly and easily but with very little personal involvement. They can profess undying love one minute and terminate the relationship the next. In addition, they are very *irritable* and *aggressive*. They have no concern for others and experience no guilt when they violate societal rules.

Cognitively, people with ASPD are *egocentric* and *grandiose*. They make no long-range plans and they are extremely confident that everything will always work out in their favor because they believe they are more clever than everyone else. The disorder is ego-syntonic; they assume no responsibility for their actions, and they have no desire to change in any way.

Socially, these individuals are unable to sustain lasting, close, warm, and responsible relationships. Their sexual behavior is impersonal and impulsive. They *exploit others* in a cold and calculating way, while disregarding others' feelings and rights. With their quick anger, poor tolerance of frustration, and lack of guilt, they are often emotionally, physically, and sexually abusive to others (Beck, Freeman, & Davis, 2004).

Borderline Personality Disorder

Individuals with **borderline personality disorder (BPD)** exhibit a heterogeneous mixture of symptoms. In many ways, BPD would be more appropriately called *cyclical personality*

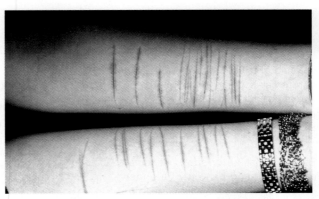

PHOTO 16.1 ■ Some people with borderline personality disorders engage in recurrent suicidal gestures or self-mutilating behaviors.
SOURCE: Dr. P. Marazzi/Science Photo Library Photo Researchers, Inc. Used with permission.

because of the erratic moods or an impulse control disorder because of unpredictable behavior.

Behaviorally, people with BPD are impulsive, unpredictable, and manipulative. They engage in such *self-destructive behaviors* as reckless driving, substance abuse, binge eating, risky sexual practices, financial mismanagement, and violence. Self-mutilation, suicide threats, and attempted suicide are maladaptive responses to intense pain or attempts to relieve the sense of emptiness and gain reassurance that they are alive and can feel pain. Physically self-damaging actions, such as cutting or burning, may be precipitated by threats of separation from others, by rejection, or by demands of parenting or intimacy. Self-mutilation is a *severity* marker for the disorder, and those who self-mutilate are at higher risk for suicide (Beck et al., 2004; Shedler & Westen, 2004). See chapter 8 ∞ for a full discussion of self-mutilation.

Kylie:

❝ My boyfriend was about to go off to flight school in the Air Force and was leaving me behind, and things were really up in the air. We'd been real on-again/off-again about whether we were going to get engaged or not. Right before he left, I opened up an e-mail in his account because I was going to look for his grandmother's e-mail address, and I found an e-mail from another girl that was not really that big of a deal. I just said this is going to lead to you cheating on me, and then you cheating on me is going to lead to us not getting engaged, then we won't get married, then I won't have a husband, then I won't have a family, then I won't have a job. And in 5 seconds I'd come to the conclusion that I didn't want to live anymore. So I just went in the bathroom and swallowed pills—like, drank them out of the bottle. ❞

Persons with BPD may *manipulate others* to act against them in a negative or aggressive way. They alternate between periods of competence and incompetence. Although they do not deliberately avoid responsibility, they cannot explain how such avoidance occurs. They may be arrogant and challenging one minute and eager to please and submissive the next.

Kylie:

❝ I never blame myself when things go wrong. Even if I know I'm wrong, I think I use to my advantage the fact that I can usually talk people under the table. I guess that's manipulation. I'm not proud of it, but I think sometimes in conversation, I can make people doubt their own name. ❞

Affectively, people with BPD are intense and unstable. They often have difficulty managing anxiety. Some are *anxious* most of the time, some have recurrent bouts of anxiety, and others experience intermittent panic attacks. People with BPD have difficulty tolerating and moderating strong feelings, which rapidly escalate to intense states of emotion. Irritation jumps to rage, sadness to despair, and disappointment to hopelessness. Their emotions are *labile* without apparent reason or stimulus. Anger is often the predominant feeling. Some individuals are incapable of caring for or loving others because of their feelings of inferiority. They might say they do not deserve to exist. In contrast, most have an inability to experience empathy in interactions with others or guilt for personal wrongdoing.

Cognitively, people with BPD are characterized by *identity disturbance*. Their self-descriptions tend to be vague and confusing. These individuals often suffer from changing identity and body image and changing sexual orientation, all of which may be indications of transient dissociative states. Some take on the identity of the people with whom they are interacting. Self-evaluation of abilities and talents alternates between grandiosity and deprecation. At times, they feel entitled to special treatment and, at other times, unworthy of anyone's attention. Believing that the world is dangerous and hostile, they feel powerless and vulnerable. Another cognitive characteristic is *dichotomous thinking*—things are either all good or all bad. For example, people with BPD are unable to see positive and negative qualities in the same person or in themselves at the same time. The result is a shifting view of the self, with rapidly shifting roles such as victim and victimizer, dominant and submissive. Psychotic episodes are common for some clients with BPD. These episodes may be brief or lengthy and are likely to result in repeated hospitalizations (Beck et al., 2004).

Socially, people with BPD have a history of intense, unstable, and *manipulative relationships*. Inside is a deprived, fragile child who may have grown up in a dysfunctional family. As adults, they desperately seek the love and nurturing they never received as a child. At the same time, they fear they will be abused and abandoned by others. This fear leads to rapid shifts

from extremes of dependency to extremes of autonomy. Desperate clinging alternates with accusations and fights, in a frantic effort to avoid abandonment. There is a great overlap between BPD and all the other personality disorders. Because symptoms vary in any given client at any given time, the disorder is difficult to diagnose and difficult to treat. Clients with BPD use a large amount of mental health resources, often present themselves in acute crisis, and frequently drop out of treatment programs. Two thirds of people diagnosed with BPD are female. Some professionals believe that the BPD diagnosis has become the negative catchall of psychiatric diagnoses. There is also a prejudice associated with this label and clients are seen as manipulative and noncompliant rather than as sick.

Other explanations for the high rate of occurrence among females include the stresses of being female in a sexist culture, gender differences for "normal" behavior, and differences in the socialization of boys and girls. Many people with BPD have been sexually abused as children. For these individuals, a better diagnosis might be atypical posttraumatic stress disorder or severe survivor syndrome, neither of which is a standard diagnosis in the DSM-IV-TR (Beck et al., 2004).

Histrionic Personality Disorder

Behaviorally, people with **histrionic personality disorder (HPD)** are most prominently characterized by *seeking stimulation* and excitement in life. Their behavior and appearance focus attention on themselves in an attempt to evoke and maintain the interest of others. They are seen as colorful, extroverted, and seductive individuals who seem always to be the center of attention. When they do not get their own way, however, they believe they are being treated unfairly and may even have a temper tantrum. They may resort to assaultive behavior or suicidal gestures to punish others.

Affectively, people with HPD are overly *dramatic*. Even minor stimuli cause emotional excitability and an exaggerated expression of feelings. They often seem to be on a roller coaster of joy and despair.

Kylie:

❝ If my fiancé and I were to call off the wedding date, which is not going to happen—but if that were to happen, anything could trigger—being in a store, hearing a song, because I would feel the hurt of a breakup a million times stronger than the average person. ❞

Cognitively, they are *self-centered*. They become overly concerned with how others perceive them because of a high need for approval. Thoughts include: "I need other people to admire me in order to be happy," "People are there to admire me and do my bidding," and "I cannot tolerate boredom." Histrionic people are guided more by their feelings

MediaLink

MediaLink Application, Borderline Personality Disorder

than by their thinking, which tends to be vague and impressionistic. The basic belief is: "I don't have to bother to think things through—I can go by my gut feeling."

Socially, they constantly seek assurance, approval, or praise from family and friends. There is often exaggeration in their interpersonal relationships, with an emphasis on acting out the *role of victim or princess*. People with HPD commonly have flights of romantic fantasy, though the actual quality of their sexual relationships is variable. They may be overly trusting and respond very positively to strong authority figures, who they think will magically solve their problems.

Leticia, a 25-year-old hairdresser, is popular with her clients. Leticia is very attractive, with long black hair and elegantly sculptured nails. She always wears the latest fashions and lots of jewelry. Leticia enjoys entertaining her customers with tales of exploits with the many men in her life. Recently, she told of meeting a handsome cowboy in a bar and deciding to go to Las Vegas with him for the weekend. She claimed he treated her like a queen, hiring a chauffeured limo, dining by candlelight, and dancing until dawn. However, Leticia doesn't plan to see the young man again because she lives by the motto, "So many men, so little time!"

Narcissistic Personality Disorder

Behaviorally, those with **narcissistic personality disorder (NPD)** strive for power and success. Failure is intolerable because of their *perfectionist standards*. They do what they can to maintain and expand their superior position. Thus, they may seek wealth, power, and importance as a way to support their image of superiority. Persons with NPD tend to be highly competitive with others they view as also superior.

Affectively, people with NPD are often labile. If criticized, they may fly into a *rage*. At other times, they may experience anxiety and panic and short periods of depression. They try to avoid feelings of blame and guilt because of intense fear of humiliation. When their needs are not met, they may react with rage or shame but mask these feelings with an aura of cool indifference.

Kylie:

❝ When I get angry, I go from zero to 60 in like zero seconds. I feel that a lot actually when I'm driving. It would not surprise me if I engaged in road rage. There have been times when I've come very close to just ramming into the back of someone's car. ❞

Cognitively, those with narcissistic personality disorder are *arrogant* and *egotistical*. They are even more grandiose than people with HPD. Persons with NPD exaggerate their accomplishments and talents. They expect to be noticed and treated as special whether or not they have achieved anything. Their feelings of specialness may alternate with feelings of

special unworthiness. They are preoccupied with fantasies of unlimited success, power, brilliance, beauty, and ideal love. Underneath this confident manner is very low self-esteem.

Socially, people with NPD have *disturbed relationships*. They have unreasonable expectations of favorable treatment and exploit others to achieve personal goals. Friendships are made on the basis of how they can profit from the other person. Romantic partners are used as objects to bolster self-esteem. They are unable to develop a relationship based on mutuality.

Santo, a 43-year-old attorney, lives in an expensive house and drives a foreign sports car. He thrives on letting others know how successful his law practice is and about all the luxuries it affords him. He pays meticulous attention to his appearance. He has had multiple affairs during his marriage and justifies these by saying that his wife is not living up to his expectations. He does not believe others have a right to criticize him and becomes irate if his wife makes requests of him.

Cluster C Disorders
Avoidant Personality Disorder

Behaviorally, *social discomfort* is the primary characteristic of people with **avoidant personality disorder (AVPD)**. Any social or occupational activities that involve significant interpersonal contact are avoided. The belief underlying this behavior is: "If people get close to me, they will discover the real me and reject me."

Affectively, these individuals are fearful and shy. They are easily hurt by criticism and devastated by the slightest hint of disapproval. They are distressed by their lack of ability to relate to others and often experience depression, anxiety, and anger for failing to develop social relationships.

Cognitively, people with AVPD are overly sensitive to the opinions of others. They have an *exaggerated need for acceptance*. The thought is: "If others criticize me, they must be right."

Socially, they are reluctant to enter into relationships without a guarantee of uncritical acceptance. Because unconditional approval is not guaranteed, they have few close friends. In social situations, people with AVPD are afraid of saying something inappropriate or foolish or of being unable to answer a question. They are *terrified of being embarrassed* by blushing, crying, or showing signs of anxiety to other people.

Other students consider Eric, a 22-year-old college senior, shy. Eric stays in his room studying and generally avoids parties. He has no real friends at college and spends his time watching television when he has no homework. Eric has a hard time in some of his classes, especially those that require him to speak in front of the group. He frets for hours over being embarrassed by something he might say that will make him look foolish. In class, Eric never sits next to the same person twice because this helps him avoid having to socialize. He has been admiring a girl named Jennie in his philosophy class, but he has never attempted to speak to her. Eric has been trying to find a way to ask Jennie out. However, everything he plans to say seems foolish. He is afraid Jennie will say no.

MediaLink Case Study, A Narcissistic Client

Dependent Personality Disorder

Behaviorally, dependence and *submissiveness* are the major features of **dependent personality disorder (DPD)**. People with DPD have difficulty doing things by themselves and getting things done on their own. They go to great lengths not to be alone and always agree with others to avoid rejection. With a strong need to be liked, dependent people volunteer to do unpleasant or demeaning things to increase their chances of acceptance. They avoid occupations in which they must perform independent functions.

Affectively, they *fear rejection* and abandonment. They feel totally helpless when alone. They are easily hurt by criticism and disapproval and are devastated when close relationships end. These fears contribute to a continuous sense of anxiety, and depression may develop.

Cognitively, people with DPD have a severe *lack of self-confidence* and belittle their abilities and assets. Unable to make everyday decisions without an excessive amount of advice and reassurance from others, they often allow others to make choices for them. They exercise dichotomous thinking, such as: "One is either totally dependent and helpless or totally independent and isolated."

Socially, those with DPD desire *constant companionship* because they feel helpless when they are alone. Passively resisting making decisions, they often force their spouses or partners into making important choices for them, such as where to live, where to work, with whom to socialize, and in what activities to participate.

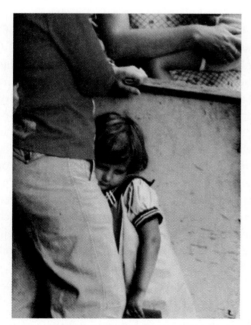

PHOTO 16.2 ■ Parental overprotectiveness may encourage dependence and interfere with the child's opportunities to learn skills that are necessary for more independent behavior.

SOURCE: Lester Sloan/Woodfin Camp & Associates. Used with permission.

Min, a 32-year-old homemaker, married at 18 and moved directly from relying on her parents to relying on her husband. She was unable to go to any stores alone and unable to drive. She relied on her husband to pick out her clothing because she felt she had no taste. She stayed in the marriage for 10 years, even though her husband was verbally abusive and had multiple affairs. When she separated from her husband, she felt devastated, even though it was a terrible relationship. Within a few months, Min remarried and felt very relieved to be taken care of again.

Obsessive–Compulsive Personality Disorder

Behaviorally, people with **obsessive–compulsive personality disorder (OCPD)** exhibit *perfectionism* and *inflexibility*. The need to check and recheck objects and situations demands much of their time and energy. They are industrious workers, but because of their need for routine, they are usually not creative. They may fail to complete projects because of the unattainable standards they set for themselves. No accomplishment ever seems good enough.

People with OCPD are polite and formal in social situations, where they can maintain emotional distance from others. They are protective of their status and material possessions, so they have difficulty freely sharing with other people.

Affectively, they are *unable to express emotions*. To alleviate the anxiety of helplessness and powerlessness, they need to feel in control. Total control means that emotions, both tender and hostile, must be held in check or denied. Life and interpersonal relationships are intellectualized. Emotional distance and blocking of feelings are attempts to avoid losing control over themselves and their environment.

Because defenses are rarely adequate to manage anxiety, people with OCPD develop a number of *fears*. They fear disapproval and condemnation from others and, therefore, avoid taking risks. They dread making mistakes. When mistakes occur, they experience a high level of guilt and self-recrimination, thus becoming their own tormentors. They also fear losing control. Rules and regulations are an attempt to remain in control at all times. Still fearful that things could go wrong, people with OCPD invent rituals to ensure constancy and increase their feelings of security. As they try to control fear with a narrow focus on details and routines, the need for order and routine escalates.

People with OCPD have three types of *cognitive* distortions: *perfectionism*, a need for certainty and a belief in an absolutely correct solution for every problem, *procrastination*, and *indecision*. Procrastination and indecision are common because a person with OCPD would rather avoid commitment than experience failure. Before making a decision, people with OCPD accumulate many facts and try to figure out all the potential outcomes of any particular decision. When a decision is finally made, they are plagued by *doubts* and fears that an alternative decision would have been better. Because they constantly strive to be perfect in all things, doing nothing is often considered better than doing something imperfectly. The underlying belief is: "I must avoid mistakes to be worthwhile."

Questioned about how they view themselves, people with OCPD say they are conscientious, loyal, dependable, and responsible—descriptions that conflict with an underlying low self-esteem and belief of inadequacy. *Socially*, their need for control extends to interpersonal relationships. Regarding themselves as *omnipotent* (all-powerful) and *omniscient* (all-knowing), they expect their opinions and plans to be acceptable to everyone else; compromise is hardly considered. Frequent demands on their families to cooperate with their rigid rules and detailed routines undermine feelings of intimacy within the family system. Because they view dependency as being out of control and under domination of the partner, they may abuse or oppress their partners so that an illusion of power and control can be maintained.

When interacting, people with OCPD have an overintellectual, meticulous, detailed manner of speaking designed to increase feelings of security. They unconsciously use language to confuse the listener. By bringing in side issues and focusing on nonessentials, they distort the content of the subject, which is a source of great frustration to the listener.

Jim, a 42-year-old midlevel executive for a food-processing plant, is always in trouble with the plant manager because he fails to get reports in on time. Jim blames his secretary for the problem, saying, "I can't get anything done right unless I do it myself." However, Jim's secretary promptly types exactly what he gives her. Jim then adds new details and reorganizes the report and she has to type a new version. Jim keeps all the drafts of the report and documents the time it takes for the secretary to type them. He stores these in a file that only he is allowed to use. Jim lost his "to do" list one morning and had his secretary help him try to find it for over half an hour. Jim yelled at the secretary when she suggested that he try to remember what was on the list.

Obsessive–compulsive personality disorder must be distinguished from obsessive–compulsive disorder (OCD), which was covered in chapter 11 ∞. In the past, it was thought that OCD was a more severe form of OCPD. Research indicates distinct differences between the disorders, with only 20% of people with OCD exhibiting characteristics of the personality disorder. People with OCD do not experience rigid patterns of many behaviors, the restricted affect, or the excessive passion for productivity that people with OCPD do. OCD is ego-dystonic, whereas OCPD is ego-syntonic (Eisen et al., 2006).

Personality Disorders Not Otherwise Specified

The label *personality disorder not otherwise specified* is used when a person does not meet the full criteria for any one personality disorder, yet there is significant impairment in social or occupational functioning or in subjective distress.

Depressive Personality Disorder

People with **depressive personality disorder** are persistently gloomy and unhappy and are unable to experience the feelings of pleasure, joy, or humor. They worry and obsess on negative subjects. Their view of the future is *pessimistic* and they are unable to believe that their lives will improve. They have low self-esteem, evidenced by their focus on their inadequacies and failures. This disorder occurs equally among women and men (American Psychiatric Association, 2000).

Passive–Aggressive Personality Disorder

Individuals with **passive–aggressive personality disorder** oppose and resist the expectations and demands of others. This persistent behavior occurs in work and social situations. Forms of passive–aggressive behavior include procrastination, forgetfulness, intentional inefficiency, chronic lateness, and no carryover of learning. Overtly, the behavior is passive and submissive, but beneath this façade is a great deal of hostility and resentment.

Passive–aggressive people are often seen as nice people, and it is only when their "victims" are completely frustrated, that their hidden defiance becomes apparent. They say they did not do it "on purpose" and present themselves as innocent and well intentioned. The victim feels guilty and avoids confrontation for fear of being called a nag.

Chronic forgetters are unable to say they do not want to do something. Instead, they passively agree to everything and then proceed to forget to do it. Eventually, others learn not to count on them to do anything important and thus they avoid tasks and responsibilities. *Procrastinators* are passively aggressive with their annoying delays and refusal to be held to a fixed date or time. They also trigger feelings of guilt in others by saying such things as, "Relax, you'll live longer!" Their hostility is passively expressed by keeping others waiting. People who are *chronically late* for appointments, dates, or social events are indirectly expressing their hostility for the person or persons kept waiting. They are also usually creative apologizers who have amazing excuses for their lateness. Those who have *no carryover of learning* express their aggression by never anticipating the needs of significant others or never learning from previous experience. Instead, they force the victim to make repeated requests each and every time. They may further manipulate victims by saying such things as, "Relax. If you want me to do something, just tell me!"

Table 16.1 ■ summarizes the characteristics related to types of disorders.

Comorbid Disorders

There is a high correlation between *substance abuse* and antisocial personality disorder. At times, it is difficult to separate these disorders, as substance abuse is itself an antisocial behavior that causes problems similar to those of the per-

TABLE 16.1	Characteristics of Personality Disorders			
Cluster	**Behavioral**	**Affective**	**Cognitive**	**Sociocultural**
A	Eccentric, craves solitude, argumentative, odd speech	Quick anger, social anxiety, blunted affect	Unable to trust, indecisive, poverty of thoughts	Impaired or nonexistent relationships, occupational difficulties
B	Dramatic, craves excitement, wants immediate gratification, self-mutilates	Intense, labile affect; no sense of guilt; anxious; depressed	Considers self special and unique, egocentric, identity disturbances, no long-range plans	Manipulates and exploits others; stormy relationships
C	Tense, rigid routines, submissive, inflexible	Anxious; fearful, depressed	Moralistic, low self-confidence	Dependent on others, avoids overt conflict, seeks constant unconditional love

sonality disorder. Thus, substance abusers are divided into two groups: *primary antisocial addicts,* whose antisocial behavior is independent of the need to obtain drugs, and *secondary antisocial addicts,* whose antisocial behavior is directly related to drug use.

Psychotic episodes or disorders often co-occur with schizotypal, borderline, and dependent personality disorders. Mood disorders co-occur more often with avoidant and borderline personality disorders; and anxiety, eating, and somatoform disorders co-occur with avoidant, dependent, and borderline personality disorders. The presence of personality disorders impedes the recovery from Axis I disorders (Zanarini, Frankenburg, Hennen, Reich, & Silk, 2004).

Recurrent *suicidal behavior* is characteristic of borderline personality disorder. Suicides are often associated with anger and often the result of impulsive behavior in the context of interpersonal relationship problems. Other factors contributing to suicide in persons with personality disorders include depression and substance abuse. A history of prior attempts is the strongest predictors of future attempts and suicide completion (Yen et al., 2004).

Some studies indicate a comorbidity of borderline personality disorder and posttraumatic stress disorder (PTSD) in combat veterans. There are two possible explanations for this co-occurence. First, individuals with BPD have limited ability to cope with traumatic events, which makes them more vulnerable to PTSD. Secondly, the trauma of war causes long-lasting changes in personality leading to a diagnosis of BPD (Axelrod, Morgan, & Southwick. 2005).

Etiologies

As with other psychiatric disorders, a number of theories have been offered to identify the causes of personality disorders. With continuing refinement of diagnostic criteria for each cluster of disorders, it will become possible to conduct useful research on specific populations that have been accurately diagnosed. In the past, wide differences in the application of

specific diagnostic labels precluded the gathering of reliable data. Since there was so little agreement about whether a person should be included in the category at the outset, it is easy to understand why the search for any common factors—in genetics, early experiences, family patterns, or any other variable—failed to yield results from which general conclusions could be drawn.

Remaining obstacles are the refusal to seek treatment on the part of the client and the relatively infrequent need for psychiatric hospitalization. Thus, research has usually focused on those individuals who seek therapy or those who are referred through the criminal system (most often with antisocial personality disorder).

There is no single cause of the personality disorders. Most likely, they arise from an interaction between biological factors and the environment. Just as one's biology or constitution can alter experiences in life, so, too, can many experiences alter one's basic biology. The brain constantly changes to absorb new experiences.

Genetics

Studies suggest a common genetic factor in schizotypal personality disorder and schizophrenia. Individuals in both groups have an equal probability of having a sibling with schizophrenia. This shared genetic vulnerability has led many people to consider schizotypal personality disorder as one of the schizophrenia spectrum disorders (Keshavan et al., 2005).

Extreme shyness beginning in infancy may be associated with Cluster C disorders. Overanxious children are more likely to be overprotected and vulnerable to developing dependent traits. It is critical, however, that labels not be attached to behavior that is developmentally appropriate (American Psychiatric Association, 2000).

A strong predictor of the development of antisocial behavior is antisocial personality disorder in one or both parents. This seems to be due to both genetic and environmental factors. There also appears to be a genetic link between antisocial and borderline personality disorders. It is believed that people with both disorders are born with an innate biological tendency to react intensely to low levels of stress (Paris, 2001).

Neurobiology

Some of the personality disorders are primarily disorders of impulse control. There may be problems with limbic system regulation. Brain imaging studies report reduced glucose utilization in the limbic system and the prefrontal cortex of people who exhibit impulsive aggression when compared to normal controls. People diagnosed with BPD and ASPD appear to have lower serotonin (5-HT) activity than control groups. The lower the 5-HT levels, the more likely the client is to self-mutilate, experience intense rage, and behave aggressively toward others. A concurrent high level of norepinephrine (NE) creates hypersensitivity to the environment and is related to aggressive behavior. Abnormalities in levels of dopamine (DA) may explain the psychotic episodes experienced by some clients with BPD and schizotypal personality disorder (MacFarlane, 2004; Ni et al., 2006).

Many people with personality disorders have a history of traumatic childhood events such as physical or sexual abuse. Trauma increases activity in the hypothalamic–pituitary–adrenocortical axis, which, with long-term stimulation, increases anxiety and self-destructive behavior. Childhood trauma may also reduce the volume of the hippocampus (Brambilla et al., 2004; Lee, Geracioti, Kasckow, & Coccaro, 2005).

Recent research has found that there may be a relationship between criminal behavior and physiological underarousal to stimulation. Heart rate, skin conductance, and electroencephalogram (EEG) readings are lower in people with ASPD than in those without the disorder. This underarousal can be interpreted in two ways: Either the person seeks inappropriate stimulation to counteract the underaroused state or it is a marker of low fear levels, which interferes with the anticipation of danger (Ratey, 2001).

Intrapersonal Factors

The idea that most children are *resilient* to adversity is critical for understanding the impact of negative events in childhood. Some aspects of resilience are biological. Children with positive personality traits and higher levels of intelligence are more adept at finding ways to cope with adversity. In contrast, children with negative personality traits and lower levels of intelligence experience more stress as they attempt to cope with adversity. Psychosocial aspects of resiliency are positive relationships, which buffer negative experiences. Thus, growing up in a dysfunctional family can be offset by attachments to competent extended family members.

People with Cluster A personality disorders have been studied minimally because they seldom request or are forced into treatment. Intrapersonal theory suggests that the pri-

mary defense mechanism is one of projection; that is, they project their own hostility on others and respond to them in a fearful and distrustful manner. It is also thought that they defensively withdraw from others for fear they will be hurt.

Intrapersonal theory explains ASPD as a developmental delay or failure. It is believed that people with ASPD have an underdeveloped superego, in that authority and cultural mores have not been internalized. Conformity to cultural expectations is situational and superficial, and there is an inability to experience guilt when rules are violated.

Individuals with BPD often think, feel, and behave more like toddlers than adults. When young children experience inadequate parenting, their basic needs and desires remain unsatisfied. Unmet needs lead to hostility toward those on whom their lives depend. At the same time, these children are terrified by the destructiveness of their anger. They begin to believe that they have been, or will be, abandoned, and the parents are unable to provide good experiences to balance the intense feelings of neglect. All of this contributes to adults who feel so utterly empty inside that they can never get enough attention and nurturing. At the same time, they are terrified of intimacy because of their fears of abandonment. This constant tension between need and fear leads to acting out feelings of rage and self-destructive behavior to manage the guilt.

Sociocultural Factors

Negative childhood experiences do not necessarily lead to mental disorders in adulthood. Risk factors may, however, increase the likelihood of negative outcomes. In community populations, psychosocial stressors contribute to pathology in only a minority of those who are exposed. In clinical populations, people with a variety of mental disorders report more psychosocial stressors during childhood than do those without mental disorders. In other words, most people are resilient to adversity but those who develop mental disorders have an underlying vulnerability to stress.

A variety of social conditions lead to low self-esteem, negative self-concept, and even self-hatred. When one is on the receiving end of social oppression, it is more difficult to develop self-esteem and a healthy identity.

Social expectations encourage some kinds of behavior and suppress others. Traditional societies are more tolerant of dependence, and people are expected to conform to family and group norms. Some believe that industrialization has contributed to a changing value system and that Cluster B personality disorders may be a response to society's increasing complexity. We have come to recognize current values such as these: Personal needs are more important than group needs, expediency is more important than morality, and appearance is more important than inner worth. Believing that survival depends solely on themselves, those with Cluster B personality disorders develop a value system of "Every person for herself or himself" and "Take care of number one first."

Family Theory

Many individuals diagnosed with personality disorders report dysfunctional families of origin. This may reflect some reality but may also reflect how distressed adults account for their present difficulties by blaming their parents. Multiple negative experiences in childhood are more likely to cause problems than one or two negative experiences. Abnormal parenting (abuse, neglect, overcontrol) may also be a risk factor for personality disorder.

The diathesis–stress model states that biology and social environment of the family interact in such a way as to produce personality disorders. For example, children who are born with a temperament of impulsivity and mood instability may be badly treated by family members. Other children who are born with an anxious temperament and who have problems with peer relationships may be overprotected or rejected by parental caregivers. Children with difficult temperaments come into conflict with peers and parents, increasing the likelihood of either social rejection or physical abuse.

People with ASPD are thought to come from families with inconsistent parenting that resulted in emotional deprivation in the children. Because of their own personality or substance abuse problems, parents may be unable to supervise and discipline their children, or they may even model antisocial behavior for the children. Others seem to come from healthy families and had good childhood experiences.

Family theorists view BPD as a dysfunction of the entire family system across several generations, with similar dynamics of blurred generational boundaries of the incestuous family (see chapter 23 ∞). BPD usually occurs in an enmeshed family system. With a high family value on children's loyalty to parents, adult children cling to their parents even after marriage. As a result, the marital couple is unable to bond with each other. When children are born, they are encouraged to cling, and normal separation behavior is discouraged. Often, the children end up in a caretaking role with parents and must assume a high level of family responsibility. During late adolescence, they are unable to separate from their parents because of an incorporated family theme that separation and loss are intolerable. It is within the third or fourth generation of enmeshed families that borderline traits develop into the personality disorder. Male children with BPD tend not to marry and remain connected with their families of origin. Female children with BPD often marry but tend to pick passive and distant partners who are enmeshed with their own families (Livesley, 2003; Magnavita & MacFarlane, 2004).

It is believed that a chaotic, depriving, abusive, or brutalizing environment is a major factor in the development of BPD. Research shows that 50% to 70% of clients diagnosed with BPD have a history of abuse. Tentative findings at this point indicate that the abuse began at an early age, that the child was neglected as well as abused, that sexual abuse was often combined with physical abuse, and that there was usually more than one perpetrator. It must be noted that abuse within the family is not a single incident but rather part of a dysfunctional family behavior pattern that is either chaotic or coercively controlling. Dysfunctional families distort all interactions and relationships (Livesley, 2003).

Gender-Bias Theory

Girls and boys are socialized very differently in America. Boys are encouraged to be independent, self-sufficient, active, and thinking rather than feeling individuals. Girls are taught to be dependent, submissive, passive, and feeling individuals who are more concerned with the needs of others than with their own needs. Such rigid role expectations can lead to identity difficulties. The same behaviors that may be considered acceptable in men (impulsiveness, expressing anger, argumentativeness, making demands) are labeled pathological in women. It is more likely that men are diagnosed as having antisocial personality disorder and women are diagnosed as having BPD when exhibiting similar behaviors. These differences in diagnoses reflect the real and unfortunate consequences of gender-role stereotyping in American culture (Sperry, 2004).

Psychopharmacological Interventions

Studies are being conducted on the effectiveness of medications in treating personality disorders. Medications are used to target specific symptoms or to treat comorbid Axis I disorders. Psychotic symptoms appear to respond to low doses of the antipsychotic agents. These medications are best used for relief of acute symptoms and are typically discontinued when the psychotic features disappear. A number of medications are being tried to decrease the impulsive, aggressive, and self-destructive behavior patterns of BPD. Selective serotonin reuptake inhibitors (SSRIs), clonidine (Catapres), and guanfacine (Tenex) diminish rage and rapid mood swings as well as decrease aggression and impulsive and self-destructive behavior. SSRIs are also used to treat obsessive ruminations in people with personality disorders. SSRIs include fluoxetine (Prozac), paroxetine (Paxil), and sertraline (Zoloft). Medications should be viewed as a means of controlling symptoms that are disabling. The overall treatment plan includes individual, group, family, and behavioral therapy. As more is learned about these disorders, improved techniques can be designed to better meet individual client needs (Keshavan, Shad, Soloff, & Schooler, 2004; Soler et al., 2005).

Alternative Therapies

There are no specific alternative therapies for individuals with personality disorders. Those who experience anxiety may find chamomile tea to be helpful. Yoga and meditation may also decrease levels of anxiety. People who have a concomitant mild or moderate depression may find St. John's wort or SAMe helpful. Vitamin B_{12} is necessary for the production of dopamine and serotonin, which may be lowered in depressive states. Omega-3 fatty acids are helpful in decreasing depression, which may be comorbid with the personality disorders.

Nursing Process

A CLIENT WITH A PERSONALITY DISORDER

ASSESSMENT

As with other psychiatric disorders, data collection serves as the starting point for the nursing process for clients with personality disorders. The main obstacle to assessment is the probability that the client will not perceive that a problem exists. If possible, interview family members for their perceptions of the problem. Exercise professional judgment in seeking information from others about their relationships with the client. Although the objective is to obtain a description of the client's functioning within various family and social contexts, the nurse must be certain that the client's rights are protected. By remaining alert to the potential for a breach of confidentiality, you can ensure that neither the legal nor the ethical limits of the professional domain are exceeded. The Focused Nursing Assessment feature lists assessment questions for clients with personality disorders. Table 16.2 ■ provides examples of how thoughts, behavior, and feelings relate to one another in the various personality disorders.

Assessment: Cluster A

Behaviorally, people diagnosed with Cluster A personality disorders are loners who prefer solitary activities. Their behavior is eccentric, at times argumentative, and they may exhibit odd speech. *Affectively*, they experience social anxiety and a blunted affect with bursts of quick anger. They have difficulty experiencing strong pleasurable emotions. In the *cognitive* area they have poverty of thoughts, lack insight, and have difficulty making sense of other people's behavior. In terms of *relationships* they have impaired or nonexistent relationships and occupational difficulties.

Assessment: Cluster B

People diagnosed with Cluster B personality disorders *behave* in dramatic ways to create excitement in their lives. They seek immediate gratification of their needs in an impulsive way. They are unable to soothe themselves when distressed. Their af-

fect is very intense and labile. They vacillate between anxiety, depression, and guilt. *Cognitively*, they are egocentric and consider themselves special and unique. They may experience identity disturbances. They lack empathy for others and have a tendency to externalize blame. With a power-oriented approach to *relationships* their interpersonal lives are stormy and chaotic. They tend to manipulate and exploit other people.

Assessment: Cluster C

Behaviorally, people diagnosed with Cluster C personality disorders are frightened, reserved, and submissive individuals. They will do almost anything to avoid being left alone. Rigid routines provide a sense of safety and they have great difficulty being flexible. *Affectively*, they are anxious, fearful, shamed, and depressed. *Cognitively*, they have low self-confidence, beliefs of inferiority, and are moralistically judgmental of others. In their *relationships* they are needy and dependent, constantly seek unconditional love, and avoid overt conflict with others. Some avoid other people because they feel like outcasts with little sense of belonging.

Assessment: Cultural Influences

When assessing for the presence of personality disorders, practitioners must consider the cultural context and life circumstances influencing ways of thinking, feeling, and behaving. For example, immigrants or refugees might be perceived as being suspicious or paranoid when, in reality, they are simply unfamiliar with American culture. They may also be perceived as cold, hostile, or indifferent as they struggle to blend in to the dominant society.

Some ethnic and cultural norms emphasize politeness and passivity, which might be misinterpreted as traits of dependent personality disorder. The concept of dependency is regarded differently in various parts of the world. In some cultures, adult children remain in the parental home until they are married. In other cultures, women are expected to be compliant and socially avoidant. In Japan, there is a disorder called taijin kyofusho, which is avoiding interpersonal relationships out of a fear of offending others. Histrionic behavior is more common in some cultures than in others. For

TABLE 16.2	Characteristics Related to Types of Disorders

Behavioral Characteristics

Impulsive	ASPD—difficulty delaying gratification; criminal behavior
	BPD—behavior unpredictable; self-destructive
Rigid	OCPD—perfectionism interferes with task completion
	AVPD—doesn't want to be embarrassed by trying new activities

Affective characteristics

Intense, unstable, inappropriate affect	BPD—affect instability; difficulty moderating strong feelings
	HPD—rapidly shifting and shallow expression of emotions; overly dramatic
	ASPD—irritable, aggressive
	PPD—quick expression of anger; bears grudges; pathological jealousy
Restricted, flat affect	SZPD—cold and detached
	STPD—inappropriate or constricted
	OCPD—unable to express emotions; fearful
	AVPD—fearful; shy

Cognitive characteristics

Hostile, paranoid world view	STPD, BPD—transient paranoid ideation
	PPD—hyperalert to danger; secretive
Negative sense of self	NPD—envious of others or believes others are envious of them
	AVD—views self as socially inept or inferior
	DPD—can't do things on own; lack of self-confidence in judgment or abilities
Lack of sense of self	BPD—unstable self-image or sense of self
Exaggerated sense of self	HPD—needs to be the center of attention
	NPD—grandiose sense of self-importance
	ASPD—egocentric and grandiose
Peculiar thought processes	Odd beliefs, magical thinking
	Poverty of thoughts (schizoid)

Social characteristics

Overly close relationships	BPD—unstable and intense; alternate between idealization and devaluation
	HPD—considers relationships to be more intimate than they actually are
	DPD—goes to excessive lengths to obtain nurturance and support from others
Distant/avoidant relationships	OCPD—excessively devoted to work to exclusion of friendships; unable to compromise
	PPD—argumentative; fear information and relationships will be used against them
	SZPD—doesn't want relationships
	STPD—only maintains contact with family
	AVPD—fears criticism, disapproval, or rejection from others
Lack of concern for other's needs	ASPD—indifferent to others' feelings; no remorse for hurting others
	NPD—unreasonable expectations of others; exploits others

SOURCES: Geiger, T. C., & Crick, N. R. (2001). A developmental psychopathology perspective on vulnerability to personality disorders. In R. E. Ingram & J. M. Price (Eds.), *Vulnerability to psychopathology* (pp. 57–102). New York: Guilford Press; Livesley, W. J. (2001). Conceptual and taxonomic issues. In W. J. Livesley (Ed.), *Handbook of personality disorders* (pp. 3–38). New York: Guilford Press; and Paris, J. (1999). *Nature and nurture in psychiatry.* Washington, DC: American Psychiatric Press.

PPD, paranoid; SZPD, schizoid; STPD, schizotypal; ASPD, antisocial; BPD, borderline; HPD, histrionic; NPD, narcissistic; AVPD, avoidant; DPD, dependent; OCPD, obsessive–compulsive

Focused Nursing Assessment   Clients With Personality Disorders

Behavior Assessment	Affective Assessment	Cognitive Assessment	Social Assessment
What is your usual pattern of daily activities?	Describe your usual mood.	Would you describe yourself as independent or dependent?	How do you usually relate to others?
What is your work history?	What happens when you feel frustrated?	What do you like about yourself?	When do you prefer to be alone? To be with others?
Describe your functioning at work/school.	Angry? Fearful?	What would you like to change about yourself?	Describe the differences between your business and social relationships.
Has anyone ever told you your behavior was a problem? If so, what did they tell you?	Happy? Peaceful?	What are your expectations for the future?	How many close relationships with others do you have? Describe the relationships.
Describe any problematic behavior you displayed as a teenager.	What causes you to be upset with others?		Are other people out to discredit or hurt you?
Describe both successful and unsuccessful attempts you have had in trying to modify your behavior patterns.	How do you react to criticism?		Are you able to say "no" to other people?
How do you resolve conflicts with others?	Do others ever describe you as detached, cool, or aloof? If so, what do they say?		
When did you have your last drink? When did you last use drugs?	How do you feel when you are with groups of people?		
	How often are you rejected or do you feel others reject you?		
	Would you consider yourself to be affectionate and empathetic toward others?		

example, Hispanic people tend to be more emotionally expressive than the British. Since personality is somewhat a reflection of one's culture, nurses must be careful not to inadvertently label normal behavior as pathological (McLean & McLean, 2004).

Personality disorders can be diagnosed in clinical populations all over the world. Social expectations of any given culture encourage some kinds of behavior and suppress others. Thus, if culture has some influence in shaping personality, these disorders should have different prevalence rates. For example, antisocial personality disorder is rapidly increasing in North America and has very low rates in certain East Asian societies such as Taiwan. It is thought that North American families increase risk factors by failing to discipline their children effectively. In contrast, the Taiwanese have a strong belief in discipline and suppress most of the impulsive behaviors in children and adolescents (Paris, 2001).

Assessment: Age-Specific Characteristics

Personality disorders may become apparent in childhood and adolescence. Those prone to Cluster A disorders may have poor peer relationships; social anxiety and withdrawal; underachievement in school; and peculiar thoughts, language, and fantasies. They may become victims of teasing because they appear "odd" or "eccentric." The first signs of avoidant personality disorder begin by early childhood. The remaining disorders are apparent by late adolescence or early adulthood (American Psychiatric Association, 2000).

Childhood behavioral disorders such as conduct disorder and attention deficit/hyperactivity disorder contribute to the development of adult antisocial personality disorder. The validity of borderline personality disorder in children and adolescents is a controversial topic. Some researchers believe that BPD in young people can be reliably diagnosed while others believe this is not possible (Westen, Shedler, Durrett, Glass, & Martens, 2003). See chapter 17 ∞ for more information on child and adolescent disorders.

Since personality, and therefore personality disorders, is relatively stable over time, the disorder persists into late life. There may be some modification of symptoms since impulsiveness decreases with age (Stevenson, Meares, & Comerford, 2003).

DIAGNOSIS

There are many potential nursing diagnoses for clients with personality disorders. In synthesizing the assessment data, consider how well clients are functioning in daily life, how stable their affect is, how they get along with others, and what their skills and talents are (North American Nursing Diagnosis Association, 2007).

- Risk for Violence, Self-directed, related to poor impulse control
- Self-mutilation related to poor impulse control
- Ineffective Coping related to intense, labile affect
- Anxiety related to fear of rejection, fear of separation, fear of embarrassment
- Deficient Knowledge related to diagnosis, outcomes, commitment to treatment
- Social Isolation related to inability to trust, odd behavior, fear of relationships
- Impaired Social Interaction related to manipulation, egocentricity, quick anger
- Ineffective Role Performance related to inappropriate affect, manipulation, inflexibility, highly dependent
- Disturbed Personal Identity related to vague self-descriptions, grandiosity, deprecation
- Interrupted Family Processes related to extreme dependency, fear of abandonment, exploitation of family members

OUTCOME IDENTIFICATION AND GOALS

Based on the assessment data, the nurse selects outcomes appropriate to the nursing diagnoses. Three broad outcomes are:

- Manage symptoms.
- Decrease the incidence of crises.
- Improve quality of life and adaptive functioning.

Client goals are specific behavioral prescriptions that the nurse, the client, and significant others identify as realistic and attainable. Be aware that many of these clients have a tendency to set broad, vague goals, such as 'feel better,' and may need assistance in being specific. The following are examples of some of the outcomes appropriate to people with personality disorders:

- Incidents of self-mutilation decrease
- Decrease in suicidal behavior
- Utilizes the problem-solving process
- Verbalizes an internal locus of control
- Interacts socially with others
- Verbalizes decreased anxiety
- Decreases perfectionistic behavior

PLANNING

Once the nursing diagnoses, outcome criteria, and goals have been identified, the nurse develops the plan of care to assist clients toward a higher level of functioning and an enriched quality of life. Priorities of care for clients with personality disorders are:

- Safety
- Managing crises
- Setting limits
- Improving socialization

IMPLEMENTATION

Individuals with personality disorders do not respond to therapy very easily and treatment tends to be prolonged—years rather than months. Building a relationship is critically important to any success. When clients are in acute distress they are more motivated to attempt changes. In the chronic phase, it is often very difficult for them to envision anything changing. Your role, as a nurse, is to provide support, respect, empathy, and validation. Over the course of time, ideally you become a role model for the client (Perseius, Ekdahl, Asberg, & Samuelsson, 2005).

Approach clients with *Cluster A* personality disorders in a gentle, interested, and nonintrusive manner that is respectful of the client's need for distance, privacy, and respites from interpersonal interactions. Demands for trust or self-disclosure may heighten anxiety and even precipitate a transient psychotic state. The staff needs to understand that clients' social withdrawal and lack of feeling or responses are self-protective rather than unappreciative. You demonstrate your trustworthiness through your actions. You should only make offers you are willing and able to follow through on. Try to be clear and consistent.

Clients with *Cluster B* personality disorders require much more patience and structure from nurses. The approach must be one of consistency and limit setting. It is critically important that staff members keep open and clear lines of communication with one another. Nurses working with these clients must know how to deal with problems of anger and dishonesty. Since some clients alternate between criticism and flattery, avoid personalizing clients' behavior.

Clients with *Cluster C* diagnoses will find it helpful when the nurse points out their avoidance behavior and secondary gains. Assertiveness training helps these clients manage their dependency and anger. Anxiety may lessen when they learn to modify their perfectionistic standards.

Three fundamental beliefs guide your approach in working with persons experiencing personality disorders. The first is *self-determination*. Clients are partners in treatment and have the right to choose their own course in life. Second, the focus is on *role functioning* while recognizing that not all symptoms will disappear. Third is *maintaining hope*. These clients are particularly susceptible to loss of hope for change and giving up on treatment.

Maintaining Boundaries

The boundaries between people are those edges that maintain a clear distinction between individuals. In terms of the nurse–client relationship, clear boundaries are designed to create an atmosphere of safety and predictability within which the nursing process can be implemented. Individuals experiencing identity confusion may be unclear about the norms of social and professional interaction. Teach them about physical, social, emotional, and sexual boundaries. Help them understand when they inadvertently or purposefully cross those boundaries.

Some individuals cannot separate their own experiences from those of others. Their self-image changes according to the reactions of others. Talk about how they adopt other's thoughts and feelings as their own. Teach them that when someone makes a personal comment to them, they have a choice of what they do with this comment. Ask them to imagine the comment as a brick. They can choose to accept the brick and build it into their wall of self-image. Alternatively, they can set the brick down, they can give it back, or they can throw it away. Point out the choices they have, for example, if someone says, "You are an ugly person." They can take that opinion and build it into their self-image and believe that they indeed are ugly. They can simply ignore the comment or tell themselves that the person must have a hidden agenda to say such a mean thing. Alternatively, they can give the "brick" back by saying, "I'm sorry you see me that way. I don't believe I am ugly." Help them establish and maintain their own boundaries. Begin with simply asking them to list their likes and preferences. Move on to goals they would like to achieve and decisions they need to make. Role-play situations in which their boundaries may be violated and how they may respond to this situation.

The desired outcome is that clients will respect others' boundaries and establish their own boundaries.

Teaching

Individuals with personality disorders are often puzzled by their problems and their inability to manage their lives. Telling clients the diagnosis is essential to establishing a relationship and validating their sense that their suffering is real. Many are relieved to learn that they have an identifiable disorder and that there is hope for change. It is helpful to teach them the nature and origin of personality and personality difficulties. Explore the way in which past events influence the way they think about themselves and others. Connect their patterns of thinking to their mood and emotions. Provide information on the treatment process including goal setting, commitment to change, and evaluation. Explain that changes occur slowly and the process will take time.

The desired outcome is that clients will verbalize an understanding of their disorder.

Modifying Cognitive Distortions

Clients with personality disorders have a number of cognitive distortions such as dichotomous thinking, overgeneralization, magnification, and suspiciousness. Help clients understand how these cognitive distortions relate to behavioral and social problems. Do not try to talk them out of their beliefs but rather suggest that each thought is just one of a number of possibilities. For clients who believe that others are especially looking at them, assign them to go to a shopping mall and sit and watch people. Ask them to analyze when individuals look at others and under what conditions. This exercise may help them recognize that they are not the focus of other people's attention (McLean & McLean, 2004).

As you identify specific cognitive distortions, ask clients to write these in a journal along with evidence against the thought. The client's thought may be that "People want to tease me and bully me." Evidence against that thought might be, "This happened when I was young but has not happened recently" or "These people do not tease or bully other individuals, so why would they want to do that to me?" The journal writing will help clients develop a range of alternative interpretations for core beliefs.

The desired outcome is that clients will identify cognitive distortions and develop a more adaptive thinking style.

Improving Family Communication

Personality disorders often have a negative impact on the family and friends surrounding the individual. It is important to include families in the treatment process. See chapter 2 ∞ for more information on family intervention. Families need information about the nature of the disorder, its course, and the available treatments. See Box 16.1 for topics to include in family education.

Teach friends and family members how to set limits with individuals who are manipulative. Family members tend to get drawn into dysfunctional interactions. Support them in setting limits and establishing consequences for manipulative behavior. Explain that they need to be consistent in what they will and will not tolerate. Teach friends and family how to set limits with individuals who are passive–aggressive. To avoid the "misunderstandings," you should have the person repeat back

NURSING CARE PLAN for a Client With a Personality Disorder

Enhancing Impulse Control
Nursing Diagnosis: Client at Risk for Ineffective Coping

Outcomes: The client will remain safe, tolerate distress without acting out, and develop adaptive ways to manage impulsive behavior.

The first priority of care is client safety. Dangerous behaviors such as self-mutilation or suicide or behaviors that threaten or endanger others, especially dependent children, are the first order of intervention. Take all suicidal thinking seriously. It is an indication clients are not feeling safe. The immediate goal of crisis management is to ensure safety of all involved and help clients manage emotions and impulses. Specific nursing interventions for clients who are suicidal are covered in chapter 21 ∞, and for those who self-mutilate in chapter 8 ∞.

Intense emotional pain and poor impulse control contribute to self-destructive behavior. The most helpful initial response is to talk in a calm, monotone voice, repeating a phrase such as: "You are with me. I will help you remain safe." Often, clients regress to an earlier age and thus your interventions should match the presenting age. For example, if they are acting like 3- or 4-year-olds in a rage, use a kind, soothing approach with simple, firm directions to contain the behavior.

Once clients are able to control behavior, there are a number of nursing interventions directed toward the goal of remaining safe and increasing impulse control. Clients need a great deal of support, reminding, and guidance from nurses before they are able to develop any consistency in new behaviors. They need to be encouraged to identify and use sources of support during this time. Remember that competency is often achieved by the gradual substitution of progressively more adaptive behaviors. For example, clients may be encouraged to seek help from a crisis center before engaging in self-harming behaviors. The next step is to develop alternative behaviors until the next scheduled therapy appointment. And finally, clients learn how to manage and tolerate distress without engaging in harmful behavior. With a gradual approach, change is not so overwhelming.

Intervention	Rationale	Goal
Establish a verbal or written hour-by-hour or day-by-day no-harm contract.	This sets limits on acting out behavior and helps clients assume responsibility for behavior.	Agrees to no-harm contract
Help clients identify and label feelings.	The client learns to recognize that self-destructive behaviors are responses to feelings and that these responses can be changed over time.	Self-monitors feelings
Help clients identify triggers and patterns in self-destructive behavior.	This helps improve insight into the problem.	Articulates improved insight
Encourage the use of a journal to: ■ Track changes in feelings ■ Identify specific stimuli causing the change	Journaling provides a more accurate recall and detail about relationship between mood, triggers, self-harm behavior, and effective coping strategies.	Utilizes journal to adapt behavior
Help them think through the consequences of impulsive behavior—to themselves and others.	Identifying consequences helps clients assume responsibility for behavior.	Identifies specific consequences
Brainstorm ideas on what other behaviors might be substituted for the harmful ones.	Brainstorming increases the number of options available.	Verbalizes more options
Ask clients to decide which response will be implemented the next time they feel like hurting themselves.	Clients need to learn how to tolerate dysphoric emotions, rather than acting impulsively.	Chooses option

Managing Crises
Nursing Diagnosis: Client at Risk for Ineffective Coping

Outcomes: Client regulates affect, organizes behavior, and thinks clearly.

Clients with borderline personality disorder often experience crises and when crises occur, they want attention right away and want problems fixed immediately. You may need to refer them to community-based emergency services when the crisis occurs outside of regular therapy hours. Symptoms of crises states include:

■ Affective dysregulation—rapid changes in affect; intense anger and rage
■ Behavioral dysregulation—impulsive behavior, regression, dissociation, self-harm
■ Cognitive dysregulation—decreased logical thinking, impaired information processing, decreased problem solving, transient psychotic features

continued

NURSING CARE PLAN for a Client With a Personality Disorder

Managing Crises *continued*
Nursing Diagnosis: Client at Risk for Ineffective Coping

Crises are best managed by helping clients contain their out-of-control feelings, behavior, and thinking. Use straightforward, concrete statements that demonstrate an understanding of the situation and how they are experiencing it. Encourage clients in crisis to temporarily avoid the situation or relationship that contributed to the crisis. Since safety takes a priority, the level of danger must be quickly assessed. Medication is often used to stabilize the client. Partial hospitalization or inpatient treatment might be necessary to ensure the safety of the client. If other people are at risk of being harmed by the client, notify authorities.

Intervention	Rationale	Goal
Quickly assess the level of danger in the crisis situation.	Safety takes a priority.	Remains safe
Partial hospitalization or inpatient treatment may be necessary.	This ensures the safety of the client.	Remains safe
If other people are at risk of being harmed by the client, notify authorities.	Safety takes a priority.	Remains safe
Use straightforward, concrete statements.	This demonstrates an understanding of the situation and how they are experiencing it.	Provides feedback on nurse's comprehension
Encourage client to temporarily avoid the situation or relationship that contributed to the crisis.	This defuses the anxiety and anger associated with the crisis.	Manages feelings appropriately

Stabilizing Affect
Nursing Diagnosis: Client at Risk for Impaired Adjustment

Outcomes: Client will moderate emotional lability and limit acting out behavior.

Some clients overreact to environmental stimuli and interpersonal interactions, which may lead to disruptive behavior. They need to learn to decrease their reactivity and contain their behavior. When they are criticized or frustrated, have them problem solve other ways to respond besides anger. Encourage them to write their feelings in a journal. Help them understand that their acting out behaviors are an attempt to escape from the strong emotions. Model appropriate verbal expression of intense feelings. Discuss and role-play assertive behavior in the context of intense emotions. At a time of low anxiety, encourage them to practice relaxation techniques so that they will be able to implement those strategies during times of high anxiety.

Intervention	Rationale	Goal
When criticized or frustrated, help them problem solve other ways to respond besides anger.	Anger is the usual response, which leads to increased conflict with others.	Responds in more effective ways
Encourage to write feelings in a journal.	Journal writing helps track progress on what response is most effective.	Uses journal for greater insight
Explain that acting out behaviors are an attempt to escape from strong emotions.	This establishes the link between feelings and behavior.	Verbalizes improved insight
Model appropriate verbal expression of intense feelings.	A "real life" example is more effective than a discussion.	Uses appropriate verbal expression of feelings
Role-play assertive behavior in the context of intense emotions.	Active learning is an effective teaching strategy.	Participates in role-play
At times of low anxiety, encourage them to practice relaxation techniques.	Practice increases their ability to implement these strategies during times of high anxiety.	Engages in relaxation techniques

NURSING CARE PLAN for a Client With a Personality Disorder

Reducing Fears of Rejection and Abandonment
Nursing Diagnosis: Client at Risk for Fear

Outcome: Client verbalizes decreasing fears of rejection and abandonment.

Individuals with schizoid and avoidant personality disorders are so fearful of embarrassment and possible rejection that they avoid social contact. Therefore, they have had little opportunity to learn that rejection is not inevitable. Discuss the validity of their fears. Use gradual exposure to social situations and have them note how other people respond to them. Ask them to deliberately set up small "rejections" so they can practice being rejected without being devastated. An example is that they must ask 10 different people to go out for a cup of coffee on a single day. The odds are slim that 10 people won't be available without prior notice. Therefore, some of these ten will reject the offer. Direct clients to keep notes about what happened and how they felt. When they manage that situation in a calm manner, you can design other practice situations. Fear prevents some clients from asking for help when it is needed. Have clients identify expectations that will occur should help be sought. They need to recognize that fear of rejection precludes seeking help. Use appropriate self-disclosure regarding situations in which you have sought help, to enable clients to recognize that asking for assistance need not result in rejection. Role-play with clients how to ask for help in a particular situation to increase the use of unfamiliar skills. After seeking help, have clients evaluate the situation in terms of their own feelings and the response of others. This helps them assess the reality of their anticipated fears.

People with dependent personality disorder are terrified of being abandoned and fearful that they will not survive if significant others leave them.

Intervention	Rationale	Goal
Explore core belief that if they become more competent they will be abandoned.	Insight depends on the identification of core beliefs and fears.	Acknowledges connection between belief and fears
Direct them to set up situations where they behave more competently.	Beginning with very small steps will encourage progress to the larger outcome.	In limited situations, able to act more competently
Ask client to identify an upcoming decision.	Problem solve using a real-life situation.	Identifies decision
Encourage client to use problem-solving process to make the decision.	They may not ask others for advice or reassurance. They must make the decision without input from others.	Makes an independent decision
Ask client to observe the reactions of others to this newly independent behavior.	The expectation is that they will be abandoned. The reality will most likely be quite different.	Identifies support and encouragement from others

Managing Anxiety
Nursing Diagnosis: Client at Risk for Anxiety

Outcomes: Client verbalizes less anxiety when moderating perfectionist behavior.

Some clients become perfectionists to guard against the anxiety of feeling inferior.

To help clients gain insight into the need for perfectionist behavior, comment on the link between this behavior and feelings of anxiety and helplessness.

For those who predict terrible catastrophes when mistakes are made, give the following assignment. Ask them to make three columns in their journals. In the first column, they list each predicted catastrophe. In the second column, they identify if the catastrophe did or did not occur. If the catastrophe occurred, the third column is devoted to their description of how they coped with the catastrophe. This intervention helps clients notice that much of what they fear will occur, in fact, does not occur. In addition, when catastrophes do occur, they may learn that they have more effective coping skills that they anticipated.

Intervention	Rationale	Goal
Explore fear of being judged inferior by others.	This helps client evaluate if this is a realistic appraisal of others' responses.	Discusses fear
Discuss abilities and limitations.	This helps client promote realistic self-appraisal.	Limits unrealistic expectations of self

continued

NURSING CARE PLAN for a Client With a Personality Disorder

Managing Anxiety   *continued*
Nursing Diagnosis: Client at Risk for Anxiety

Intervention	Rationale	Goal
Assign three purposeful, nonharmful mistakes a day such as setting the table incorrectly, giving wrong directions, and wearing two different socks. Encourage journaling to record feelings when mistakes occur.	This increases clients' sense of control over errors and helps them recognize that many mistakes are not serious.	Makes purposeful mistakes; identifies feelings in response
Provide feedback for positive changes.	This reinforces behavior.	Improves ability to accurately self-appraise
Help clients acknowledge that an anxiety-free life is impossible.	This helps them give up striving for perfection.	Verbalizes more realistic understanding of role of anxiety in life

Setting Limits
Nursing Diagnosis: Client at Risk for Impaired Social Interaction

Outcome: Client adheres to established expectations and routines of the outpatient or inpatient setting.

Many clients with personality disorders tend to test nurses and behave in a manipulative manner. To help you identify when this is occurring, consider how the following behaviors might be manipulative. The client appears helpless; lies; uses rationalization or minimization of responsibility for own behavior; engages in seductive behavior; abuses the use of emergency phone number of therapist; refuses to participate in agreed-upon therapy; compliments or flatters staff; asks for special privileges; makes demands of or threatens staff; gets other clients to confront staff; works on other clients' problems and not on own issues; uses role reversal with staff.

You must maintain a careful balance between being an authority figure while not being harsh or judgmental. If you try to be their "friend," you will be open to manipulation.

If you take a strong authority stance, you will create frequent power struggles. The best approach is straightforward and businesslike.

Pay attention to your own emotional responses to these clients. It is very easy to internalize the client's sense of chaos, anger, and frustration. In a residential home or inpatient unit, power struggles often develop, and the milieu becomes chaotic for everyone. Remaining therapeutic may require supervision or consultation from an unbiased colleague. One staff member may see a client as vulnerable and needy, while another might perceive the same client to be aggressive, provocative, and in need of clear limits. The client is an expert at playing one person off another in a manipulative attempt. Without outside supervision, debates among staff members can become highly personalized and polarize the staff into several factions.

Intervention	Rationale	Goal
Explain the expectations, structure, and routines of the clinical setting.	This decreases the opportunities for manipulation.	Verbalizes an understanding of unit milieu
Clearly state the consequences when expectations are not met.	Clients must be held accountable for own behavior.	Acknowledges potential consequences
Request clarification to determine the client's understanding.	This decreases use of manipulation through misunderstanding.	Verbalizes understanding
Working with the client, develop goals of treatment and behavioral contracts.	This reduces inappropriate behaviors.	With guidance, formulates goals and contracts
The focus is always on the client's behavior.	They tend to blame others for their problems.	Acknowledges self-responsibility

NURSING CARE PLAN for a Client With a Personality Disorder

Improving Self-Management
Nursing Diagnosis: Client at Risk for Ineffective Coping

Outcome: Clients will verbalize an internal locus of control, and implement more adaptive ways to manage affect and impulsive behavior.

The style of interaction in the nurse–client relationship must be one of respect and collaboration. It is helpful to use words such as "we" and "together" to promote a collaborative working relationship. At the same time you must recognize that clients are responsible for their own lives. Listen to clients' concerns and communicate your empathetic understanding of their situations. If verbal interactions are too intense, remain physically present without expecting verbal responses. Let clients know that you are there to help them but do not reinforce dependent behaviors. Recognize and support strengths and areas of competence without minimizing their pain and distress. Change is difficult and painful, and clients need to be supported and motivated to stay in treatment.

Intervention	Rationale	Goal
Encourage journal keeping regarding thoughts, feelings, and behaviors throughout the day.	People with personality disorders externalize responsibility for their behavior and feel like helpless victims.	Keeps daily journal
Review journal together. Point out examples of the causes and consequences of behavior.	This helps them understand how repetitive actions contribute to their day-to-day difficulties.	Identifies consequences in real-life situations
Discuss reasons that old patterns are not necessarily validated by current relationships.	There is a tendency to repeat old familiar patterns with all people they meet.	Identifies reasons to learn more effective coping patterns
Help clients explore the impact of their behavior on other people.	Often, clients are so caught up in their own lives that they disregard the reactions of other individuals.	Describes the responses of others
Ask clients to choose one distressful behavior they would consider changing.	Starting with a behavior that is distressful will increase motivation to change.	Identifies one behavior
Explore advantages and disadvantages of adapting their behavior.	Clients must explore both positions so change is not sabotaged.	Lists advantages and disadvantages
Encourage clients to use journaling to monitor the process. Review journal with clients on a regular basis.	Journal keeping will track progress on a daily basis.	Keeps daily journal

Improving Social Skills
Nursing Diagnosis: Client at Risk for Social Isolation

Outcome: Client interacts appropriately with others.

Interventions designed to decrease socially isolative behaviors and reward socially outgoing behaviors are often accomplished through social skills training, assertiveness training, and group therapy. The process of group therapy helps clients focus on interpersonal issues as well as individual issues. Clients not only get feedback from more than one person, they also have the opportunity to be therapeutic with other group members. Since clients with personality disorders have inadequate social skills, group therapy is one way to develop and foster better relationships with others, decrease real isolation, and increase the sense of feeling understood.

Intervention	Rationale	Goal
Respect clients' need to be distant or isolative, while encouraging and supporting interaction with others.	Forcing complex interactions beyond level of social skills defeats the purpose of interactions.	Interacts at a comfortable level
Help clients identify interpersonal problems resulting from social skill deficits.	This provides a motivation for changing old patterns of behavior.	Identifies problems in current life
Assist in identifying alternative ways to relate without seduction or intimidation.	Clients need to learn ways to socialize with others in an effective manner.	Discusses other ways to interact

continued

NURSING CARE PLAN for a Client With a Personality Disorder

Improving Social Skills   *continued*
Nursing Diagnosis: Client at Risk for Social Isolation

Intervention	Rationale	Goal
Role-play and provide feedback.	This helps them learn about the appropriateness of their responses.	Participates in role-playing
Encourage them to evaluate their behavior in social situations.	This allows for ongoing feedback from real-life situations.	Verbalizes increased insight into social behavior

Fostering Independent Functioning
Nursing Diagnosis: Client at Risk for Impaired Home Maintenance

Outcomes: Client acts on own behalf.

The goal of nursing interventions with clients who are helpless and dependent is to increase their coping skills and encourage independent functioning. Clients can choose environments that are less stressful and have a better fit with their personality traits. For example, people who are highly introverted will manage better in a very predictable environment and often do better when they can work alone. Clients who are highly extroverted respond best in an environment that presents challenges and a high level of interaction with others. The first step is to communicate to clients that you recognize their feelings of helplessness and fears of becoming more independent. This expression of empathy will help them be more collaborative in the problem-solving process. Explore dichotomous thinking, such as "One is either totally dependent and helpless or one is totally independent and isolated." Often clients view nurses as all-powerful rescuers who will make everything better. Carefully avoid rescuing behavior because it would reinforce the client's feeling of helplessness and the external locus of control. The next step is to help clients identify what would be different, what they would gain, and what they would lose if they were less helpless. Focus on one issue at a time. Begin with a fairly insignificant situation, and help them identify what they would like out of this situation. They can then problem solve ways to achieve their goals. With each subsequent use of the problem-solving process, their skills will increase, and they will become more confident in their ability to handle problems as they arise.

Intervention	Rationale	Goal
Communicate that you recognize feelings of helplessness and fears of becoming more independent.	This expression of empathy helps them be more collaborative in the problem-solving process.	Willing to collaborate
Explore dichotomous thinking such as, "One is either totally dependent and helpless or one is totally independent and isolated."	This cognitive distortion interferes with problem solving.	Identifies personal cognitive distortions
Avoid behavior that rescues clients from their problems.	Often clients view nurses as people who will make everything better. Rescuing behavior reinforces feelings of helplessness and external locus of control.	Verbalizes an internal locus of control
Focus on one fairly insignificant situation in which they feel helpless.	This prevents feeling overwhelmed by too many problems at once.	Verbalizes a sense of control over problems
Help them identify: ■ What would be different ■ What they would gain ■ What they would lose if they were less helpless	This prevents unconscious sabotage of change in behavior.	Identifies potential consequences when feelings of helplessness lessen
Help them problem solve ways to achieve their goals.	With each use of problem-solving process, skills increase.	Verbalizes more confidence in ability to handle problems as they arise

NURSING CARE PLAN for a Client With a Personality Disorder

Facilitating Decision Making
Nursing Diagnosis: Client at Risk for Decisional Conflict

Outcomes: Client utilizes the problem-solving process and makes own decisions.

Some clients have difficulty making decisions, so they do not make them. Some make impulsive decisions, while others procrastinate in deciding. Some want to make a perfect decision, while others refrain from making decisions to avoid the anxiety of failure. Some make decisions on the basis of immediate gratification of needs. All of these clients need to be encouraged to make their own decisions, thereby reinforcing a sense of competence and an internal locus of control. The problem-solving process is covered in more detail in chapter 7 ∞.

Intervention	Rationale	Goal
For those unable to make decisions: ■ Point out destructive effects of indecision. ■ Explain there are no absolute guarantees of the future for any of us. ■ Explore how many decisions in life can be remade.	This increases recognition that an imperfect decision may be less harmful than no decision. They often believe decisions are always final.	Verbalizes an understanding that most decisions are not "perfect"; verbalizes less anxiety when making decisions
For those making impulsive decisions: ■ Discuss the short- and long-term consequences of those decisions. ■ Teach problem solving. ■ Give feedback for decisions they make.	This helps them see that there are a variety of choices that can be made, tested, and evaluated. This reinforces positive changes in behavior.	Makes fewer impulsive decisions; utilizes problem-solving process

the instructions given before the person sets out to perform the task. Family members and friends should never take it for granted that the person has understood. To deal with a person who procrastinates, they should set a precise, never vague, deadline and establish a penalty for delays. The same is true for latecomers—a clearly set consequence is established for late behavior. Family and friends must consistently enforce all consequences in order to lessen the passive–aggressive behavior. Teach families how to solve problems and negotiate

BOX 16.1   Family Education

■ Personality disorders are long-standing and inflexible patterns of relating to the world and other people.
■ Affected people usually have little insight into their behavior.
■ Their loved one is handicapped but not disabled.
■ There are frequent comorbid conditions such as depression, anxiety disorders, psychotic episodes, and substance abuse.
■ Life stresses make clients more vulnerable to relapse.
■ Go slowly. Recovery takes time.
■ Maintain family routines as much as possible.
■ Do not ignore threats of self-harm.

Complementary/Alternative Therapies

How to Help Clients Relax

Throughout the day you may find hundreds of opportunities to integrate some deep breathing, relaxation, self-massage, and gentle movement techniques into usual activities. Try these techniques:

■ You are sitting at a stoplight. Take a deep breath.
■ You are just about to fall asleep or have just awakened. Breathe deeply and allow your whole body to become completely relaxed.
■ You are in the shower washing your hair. As you apply shampoo, massage your scalp vigorously; rub your ears, relax, and take several deep breaths.
■ As you apply lotion or oil to your body following your bath, do so with the intent of relaxing each muscle group as you gently massage your entire body.
■ You are watching television. During each commercial break, massage your hands, feet, and ears. Breathe deeply and relax.
■ You are vacuuming the house. Relax your shoulders, breathe deeply, and coordinate your movements with your breathing.

SOURCE: Adapted from Jahnke, R. (1997). *The healer within.* San Francisco: Harper San Francisco.

conflict. When family conflict arises, ask all members to identify specific behavior that triggers the conflict and to tell one another how they felt as a result of the conflict. Discourage the use of "you" language since that assigns blame and leads to further arguing. An example of a "you" statement is "You drive me crazy by wanting me by your side all the time." Teach the use of "I" language, in which all individuals assume responsibility for themselves. An example of an "I" statement is "I feel overloaded with your requests that I be with you so much of the time." Encourage each person involved in the conflict to explain what specific behavior change they would like to see and would be willing to make. Throughout this process provide clear direction and coaching to reduce emotional overreaction. Teach *empathic listening* and *responding* since most people with personality disorders have difficulty with this. The person who is listening concentrates on the other person's statements and tries to understand what the speaker is saying. The listener then restates what the other person has said, ensuring that the communication was clear and understood. The roles are then reversed and the process begins again. Your role is to explain and demonstrate the process and coach the family members as they learn empathic listening and responding.

The desired outcome is that clients and family members will respect each other's boundaries, increase empathetic listening, and negotiate conflicts.

EVALUATION

To complete the nursing process, you evaluate clients' responses to nursing interventions based on the selected outcomes. Personality traits are almost always too ingrained for radical change through therapy. Because the problems associated with personality disorders have been with most clients for their entire lives, clients respond to intervention strategies very slowly. You must define small steps toward the achievement of therapeutic goals. You can assist them most by helping them see how their behavior affects their lives so that they can learn to modify patterns enough to develop a more adaptive lifestyle. Some clients are in enough pain that they wish to grow and change. Others do not see that they have any problems and choose not to be involved in the therapeutic process.

Clinical Interactions | A Client With Borderline Personality Disorder

Enid, age 34, is an inpatient with a diagnosis of borderline personality disorder. She has been in and out of relationships with many different men and does not stay in a job for more than a year. She has a history of self-mutilation and numerous suicide attempts. During the past year, she has been writing love letters to her psychiatrist. She has just demanded one-to-one contact with her nurse. In the interaction, you will see evidence of:

- Attempted manipulation of the nurse
- Self-mutilation as a way to decrease anxiety
- Labile affect

ENID: "First, my doctor doesn't see me until after he sees all his other clients. Then you're too busy doing group. I just don't have anyone to talk to."

NURSE: *"Enid, I do one group per day, and I'm available most of the other hours of my shift. You need to deal directly with me, but if necessary, there are other staff members available."*

ENID: "But you are the only nurse who understands me. You are the only one I feel I can really open up to. I can't talk about my issues with anyone but you!"

NURSE: *"Enid, what is making you so upset?"*

ENID: "Do you promise not to tell anyone else if I tell you? You must promise me this! My doctor made me talk about the letters I've written him. They were beautiful. He sat there and read them to me like he was reading the newspaper totally devoid of the emotion they were written with. So I did this." [Enid pulls up her sleeves to reveal multiple new longitudinal superficial lacerations.] "Now you have to promise me not to tell anyone else!"

NURSE: *"I can't promise that. I will need to inform the other members of your treatment team. Any time there is a significant event or change in a client's status, that information needs to be shared. But why don't we talk about it first?"*

ENID: "You are just like all the others. You are going to betray me! How dare you!"

NURSE: *"If I failed to share this information, it would be unfair to you."*

Using Research Evidence   Suffering As a Component of Borderline Personality Disorder

Perseius, K. I., Ekdahl, S., Asber, M., & Samulesson, M. (2005). To tame a volcano: Patients with borderline personality disorder and their perceptions of suffering. *Archives of Psychiatric Nursing*, 19(4), 160–168.

What is the study about?

Borderline personality disorder (BPD) is a serious mental health problem, and persons with BPD might receive a better quality of care if clinicians understood how these persons experience their life situations and encounters with psychiatric care. Therefore, the purpose of this study was to analyze suffering as perceived by persons living with BPD.

How was the study done?

This qualitative study of suffering used a hermeneutic method applied to guided narrative interviews (and to autobiographical writings) with 10 Swedish clients (informants) diagnosed with BPD. The study was approved by a Research Ethics Committee. Its theoretical framework came from Eriksson's theory of health and suffering. All informants had been in psychosocial treatment for 12 months or longer for BPD. BPD was diagnosed using the *Diagnostic and Statistical Manual of Mental Disorders*, 4th edition, Axis II. Informants were 10 women between the ages of 22 and 49. Informants reported their own rates of suicide attempts and deliberate self-harm (DSH). In addition, informants revealed that they suffered (either currently or in the past) a variety of disorders, including depression (n = 9), anxiety disorders (n = 9), eating disorders (n = 3), and social phobia (n = 2). Many informants reported a history of substance-abuse disorder. Five informants reported 10 or more suicide attempts, one reported 5–10 attempts, and four reported fewer than 5. The median number of years in psychiatric care was 11.5, with a range of 4–14 years; over half had been associated with psychiatric services since childhood. Two informants reported more than 500 episodes of DSH; half the informants reported 100–500 DSH episodes, and three reported fewer than 100.

Data were obtained from individual narrative interviews and autobiographical writing. The interviews were guided, focusing on two areas: (1) personal experiences of symptoms, suffering, and life situation; and (2) perception of contacts and treatments in their psychiatric care. Questions were open-ended and followed a funnel approach, starting with broad questions such as "Can you describe what your life situation was like before entering the program?" and progressing to "Could you give an example. . .?" A semistructured questionnaire was used to collect sociodemographic and symptom data. All audiotaped interviews took place in the hospital and lasted 50–90 minutes. The first author of this study, who did not previously know the informants, obtained all interview data. Five informants volunteered autobiographical material that reflected their life situations and suffering. This material was obtained in the form of poems, diary excerpts, and diaries.

To analyze the data, the researchers used a hermeneutic approach inspired by Ricoeur and adapted to methods of interpretation in caring science. Validity of the analysis was enhanced by having the first and second authors independently interpret the texts, and then jointly reflect on the texts and discuss their interpretations. Finally, all the authors of the study discussed and reflected on the interpretations.

What were the results of the study?

This rigorous data analysis yielded three theme areas: (1) life on the edge, (2) the struggle for health and dignity—a balance act on a slack wire over a volcano, and (3) the good and the bad "act" of psychiatric care in the drama of suffering. Life on the edge was portrayed by participants discussing a life of constant falling and climbing—falling into "black holes with slippery walls with something creepy and disgusting crawling around the legs." Within this first theme, three subthemes were identified: the world of emotional pain and self-hate, the mask of normality, and the Janus (or dual) face. Pain and self-hate emerged from statements such as ". . .If you listen really carefully, you can hear me crying inside" or "I have not cut myself yet, but I'm counting my pills, which I collected for possible use in the future—98 sleeping pills, so I'm sure I will sleep well, and if I'm lucky never wake up again." The mask of normality appeared through statements such as "I'm a clown, a mask with sad eyes and close to tears all the time, but no one notices, or do you notice and keep quiet?" The Janus face represents BPD's rapid mood swings, typified by this entry: "After supper I phoned P and J. Then I and E were out walking. Still feel fat. I know that I'm not. I cut my wrist again."

The second theme was the struggle for health and dignity, a balance act on a slack wire over a volcano. Buffeted by shifts in feeling and mood, these informants seek balance while emotional pain and self-hate always bubble beneath. Informants spoke of feeling despairing and hopeless, at the mercy of impulses. Three contradictory subthemes emerged. The first subtheme was a fear of life and longing for death versus fear of death and longing for life, depicted through this informant's statement: "What happened? Why did I take these pills, when I really want to live? This feels like a failure that I'm alive. At the same time I felt scared; I could have died." The second subtheme was hopelessness and helplessness versus the will to struggle for change; these paradoxical feelings reflect both the darkness and pain inside and a strong will to struggle toward coping, competence, and control. The third subtheme was solitude and fear of relations versus longing for love and fellowship, a conflict between wanting love and feeling the self-hate that, they feel, disqualifies them for it.

The third theme area, the good and bad "act" of psychiatric care in the drama of suffering, included five subthemes: (1) feeling misunderstood and disrespected; (2) discontinuity and betrayal; (3) understanding, respect, and validation—the foundation of being helpful; (4) being helped toward acceptance, which initiates change; and (5) getting help in being responsible. The first subtheme was described as a feeling that no one seemed to care or listen, and that personnel were hostile; for example, "No one cared about what I said" and "She didn't talk to me, she talked right over my head." The second subtheme, discontinuity and betrayal, emerged when some informants described how therapists and attendants ended contact with them and turned them over to someone else, and how that felt like betrayal. The third subtheme was understanding, respect, and validation—the foundation of being helpful, and the beginning of relief. This subtheme was reflected in the statement, "Number one is to get respected, being treated like an equal. . . ." The fourth subtheme, being helped toward acceptance, which initiates change, is typified by this statement: "I'm trying to accept that life is like it is, and some days are good, and some are like hell;

continued

Using Research Evidence

Suffering As a Component of Borderline Personality Disorder *continued*

but I couldn't accept that before; just accepting it is easier to live with." The fifth subtheme, getting help in being responsible, was reflected when participants saw themselves as having responsibility for their own lives, which included their treatment, and for their struggle to have a healthy life.

What additional questions might I have?

How are the themes identified in this study relevant to persons living with other psychiatric disorders? How can nurses working with persons living with BPD use the results?

How can I use this study?

Nurses who genuinely help persons living with BPD will refrain from being judgmental. Nurses need to recognize the unique needs of the person, and the emotional struggle within these clients to live a healthy life. The research reinforces that all persons, regardless of their mental health concerns, desire to be understood, validated, and respected.

SOURCE: Contributed by Dolores Huffman, PhD, RN, Associate Professor of Nursing, Purdue University Calumet, Hammond, Indiana.

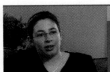

ROAD: Assessment

Critical Thinking Questions

Go to the CD-ROM to assess Kylie by answering the following critical thinking questions based on what you have **R**ead about Kylie and **O**bserved on the videos.

1. Your clinical rotation places you in a university-based student health clinic. Kylie comes to the clinic for treatment of an upper respiratory infection (URI). While conducting her health history, she openly states she was once admitted to a hospital for attempted suicide. She elaborates and shares that at the time she was fearful her boyfriend was going to abandon their relationship. You briefly review her chart as you are writing the clinic note. Under client information, there is a diagnosis of borderline personality disorder (BPD). Review your student ROAD CD-ROM segment A for chapter 16. Two weeks pass and Kylie returns to the clinic for follow-up to evaluate the efficacy of treatment for the URI. While you are auscultating lung sounds, you notice several circular, regular, pinkish-white healing scars on the inner aspect of her left arm that appear to be about a 1/2 cm in diameter. Upon asking Kylie about the marks, she states she burned herself while draining a pot of spaghetti.
   a. What concerns are elicited after observing the marks on Kylie's arm and compel you toward further assessment? Pro-

   vide rationale for your answer. (*Hint*—Refer to chapter 8 from the textbook for support in composing your answer.)
   b. How will you transition your nursing assessment to ask questions about your concerns? Support your answer.
   c. What are some points you would assess or specific questions you would ask Kylie?

2. What are you able to assess about the quality and stability of Kylie's relationship from the following statements? Review Kylie's statements on segment B of your student ROAD CD-ROM for chapter 16.

3. Review segment C of your student ROAD CD-ROM for chapter 16. What emotion is producing the physical sensations Kylie is voicing? What are the dangers to Kylie with this type of response? Provide rationale for your answers.

4. Based upon your earlier assessment of Kylie's relationships in question 2, what type of referral might you discuss with Kylie after hearing her response in segment D of your student ROAD CD-ROM? Support your answer.

ROAD: DEVELOP A CARE PLAN

 Go to the CD-ROM to Develop a care plan based on your assessment of Kylie. Identify nursing diagnoses, outcomes, goals, and interventions.

SOURCE: Contributed by Susan Siwinski-Hebel, RN, MSN.

Focus Your Study

OBJECTIVES	KEY CONCEPTS

1. Compare and contrast the different symptoms of the personality disorders.

- Cluster A:
  - Eccentric, craves solitude
  - Quick to anger, social anxiety
  - Indecisive, unable to trust
  - Impaired or nonexistent relationships, occupational problems
- Cluster B
  - Dramatic, craves excitement, wants immediate gratification, self-mutilates
  - Intense, labile affect
  - Egocentric, identity disturbances
  - Manipulates others, stormy relationships
- Cluster C
  - Rigid routines, inflexible
  - Anxious, fearful, depressed
  - Moralistic, low self-confidence
  - Dependent on others, seeks constant unconditional love

2. Outline the different theories regarding the etiology of the personality disorders.

- Personality disorders have no single cause. They likely arise from an interaction between biological factors and the environment.
- Neurobiological factors include limbic system and prefrontal cortex dysregulation, low levels of serotonin (5-HT), high levels of norepinephrine (NE), and abnormal levels of dopamine (DA). Traumatic childhood events may alter brain structure and function.
- Intrapersonal factors include projection of hostility, perfectionist standards, underdeveloped superego, and fear of abandonment.
- Social oppression and changing value systems may contribute to the development of personality disorders.
- Family factors include an inability to manage conflict, lack of individuation from the parents, and a chaotic and abusive environment.
- Gender-bias theorists consider rigid gender role stereotyping to be a factor in personality disorders.

3. Outline the assessment process for a client with a personality disorder.

- The main obstacle to assessment is the probability that the client will not perceive that a problem exists.
- Exercise professional judgment in seeking information from others about their relationships with the client. Although the objective is to obtain a description of the client's functioning within various family and social contexts, you must be certain that the client's rights are protected.

4. Discuss the key points in effectively communicating with a person with a personality disorder.

- Crises are best managed by helping clients contain their out-of-control feelings, behavior, and thinking:
  - Use straightforward, concrete statements that demonstrate an understanding of the situation and how they are experiencing it.
- Intense emotional pain and poor impulse control contribute to self-destructive behavior:
  - The most helpful initial response is to talk in a calm, monotone voice, repeating a phrase such as: "You are with me. I will help you remain safe."
  - Often, clients regress to an earlier age and thus your interventions should match the presenting age. For example, if they are acting like 3- or 4-year-olds in a rage, use a kind, soothing approach with simple, firm directions to contain the behavior.
  - Model appropriate verbal expression of intense feelings.
  - Clients who are manipulative respond best to a high level of structure and *clear ground rules*. Explain the reasons for the rules as well as the consequences when expectations are not met.

continued

continued

| 5. Use the nursing process to develop a safe, comprehensive plan of care for a client with a personality disorder. | ■ Cluster A disorders:
• Respect clients' need for distance and privacy through short-term interactions.
• Help them socialize with others.
• Teach them how to ask others for help.
■ Cluster B disorders:
• Your approach is one of consistency and limit setting.
• Help clients learn how to control impulsive behavior.
• Utilize principles of crisis intervention.
• Help them moderate labile emotions.
• Use journal keeping to help clients identify consequences of own behavior.
• Help them establish and maintain own boundaries and respect the boundaries of others.
• Help family and friends respond to manipulative behaviors.
■ Cluster C disorders:
• Point out avoidance and secondary gains when they occur.
• Engage clients in exercises that improve self-esteem.
• Recognize and support strengths and areas of competence.
• Teach the problem-solving process.
• Teach clients and families how to negotiate conflict. |
| 6. Develop illness management teaching plans for a client with a personality disorder and his/her family. | ■ Manage symptoms:
• Help them identify and label feelings (self-monitoring) in order to learn to recognize that self-destructive behaviors are responses to feelings and that these responses can be changed over time. This is the beginning of the problem-solving process.
• Let clients know that you are there to help them but do not reinforce dependent behaviors.
• Encourage them to keep a journal regarding their thoughts, feelings, and behaviors throughout the day. In reviewing the journal together, point out examples of the causes and consequences of behavior.
• Teach friends and family members how to set limits with individuals who are manipulative.
■ Decrease the incidence of crises:
• Refer to community based emergency services.
■ Improve quality of life and adaptive functioning:
• Function as a role model for clients.
• Clients need a great deal of support, reminding, and guidance from nurses before they are able to develop any consistency in new behaviors.
• They need to be encouraged to identify and use sources of support during this time.
• Clients can also choose environments that are less stressful and have a better fit with their personality traits. For example, people who are highly introverted will manage better in a very predictable environment and often do better when they can work alone. Clients who are highly extroverted respond best in an environment that presents challenges and a high level of interaction with others. |

Explore MediaLink

For review questions, case studies, and other resources for this chapter, see the Pearson Health MediaLink CD-ROM that accompanies this book and the Companion Website.

 CD-ROM
- Audio Glossary
- NCLEX-RN® Review Questions
- ROAD to Critical Thinking: *Kylie*
- Animations/Videos
  - Antisocial Personality Disorder–Parts 1 and 2

 Companion Website www.prenhall.com/fontaine
- Audio Glossary
- NCLEX-RN® Review Questions
- Case Study
  - A Narcissistic Client
- Care Plan
  - Self-mutilation
- Critical Thinking
  - Antisocial Behavior
- MediaLink Application
  - Borderline Personality Disorder
- MediaLinks
  - Books for Clients & Families
  - Community Resources

NCLEX-RN® Review Questions

16-1. A client who has paranoid personality disorder is participating in a treatment group. Which behavior should the nurse be most aware of as the client participates in the group?
1. Hypervigilance
2. Aloofness
3. Exploitative
4. Passive resistance

16-2. A psychiatric nurse is providing education about clients with personality disorders to medical–surgical nurses. One nurse asks, "What is the cause of personality disorders?" The nurse knows there is a need for further teaching if she hears which of the following statements?
1. "It is a brain disorder in which there is not enough serotonin."
2. "Personality disorders have a genetic component."
3. "Negative childhood experiences lead to personality disorders."
4. "This seems like too much or not enough of the normal personality traits."

16-3. A 19-year-old client is diagnosed with borderline personality disorder (BPD). The client has an eating disorder behavior consisting of eating and then purging. Which of the following is the best question to assess the client's nutritional status?
1. "Do you have a reason for purging?"
2. "What are your feelings about an acceptable weight?"

3. "Has food always been a problem?"
4. "What do you eat in a day?"

16-4. A client with a borderline personality disorder tells the nurse: "Everything bad happens to me. It is entirely my fault." What is the best response by the nurse to assist the client to reframe this negative thought?
1. "Do you believe that you are always at fault?"
2. "Let us examine what you mean by bad things."
3. "Everyone has bad things in life."
4. "Why are you so hard on yourself?"

16-5. In what phase of the nurse–client relationship should the nurse introduce the issue of termination to the client?
1. The termination phase
2. The orientation phase
3. The working phase
4. When the client is ready

16-6. The nurse is teaching assertiveness techniques to a group of clients diagnosed with a dependent personality disorder. Which of the following statements indicates that the teaching was not successful?
1. "I decided to use one of the assertiveness techniques."
2. "I am going to the library to get the book you suggested."
3. "I learned so much that I didn't know before."
4. "I appreciated the suggestion you made to me."

See Appendix D for answers.

References

American Psychiatric Association. (2000). *Diagnostic and statistical manual of mental disorders* (4th ed., Text Revision). Washington, DC: Author.

Axelrod, S. R., Morgan, C. A., & Southwick, S. M. (2005). Symptoms of posttraumatic stress disorder and borderline personality disorder in veterans of Operation Desert Storm. *American Journal of Psychiatry, 162*(2), 270–275.

Beck, A.T., Freeman, A., & Davis, D. D. (2004). *Cognitive therapy of personality disorders* (2nd ed.). New York: Guilford Press.

Brambilla, P., Soloff, P. H., Sala, M., Nicoletti, M. A., Keshavan, M. S., & Soares, J. C. (2004). Anatomical MRI study of borderline personality disorder patients. *Psychiatry Research, 131*(2), 125–133.

Chen, H., Cohen, P., Crawford, T. N., Kasen, S., Johnson, J. G., & Berenson, K. (2006). Relative impct of young adult personality disorders on subsequent quality of life. *Journal of Personality Disorders, 20*(5), 510–523.

Eisen J. L., Coles, M. E., Shea, M. T., Pagano, M. E., Stout, R. L., Yen, S., Crillo, C. M., & Rasmussen, S. A., (2006). Clarifying the convergence between obsessive compulsive personality disorder criteria and obsessive compulsive disorder. *Journal of Personality Disorders, 20*(3), 294–305.

Gabbard, G. L. (2004). Reflective function, mentalization, and borderline personality disorder. In B. D. Beitman & J. Nair (Eds.), *Self-awareness deficits in psychiatric patients* (pp. 213–228). New York: W.W. Norton & Company.

Keshavan, M. S., Duggal, H. S., Veeragandham, G., McLaughlin, N. M., Montrose, D. M., Haas, G. L., et al. (2005). Personality dimensions in first-episode psychoses. *American Journal of Psychiatry, 162*(1), 102–109.

Keshavan, M. S., Shad, M., Soloff, P., & Schooler, N. (2004). Efficacy and tolerability of olanzapine in the treatment of schizotypal personality disorder. *Schizophrenia Research, 71*(1), 97–101.

Lee, R., Geracioti, T. D., Kasckow, J. W., & Coccaro, E. F. (2005). Childhood trauma and personality disorder. *American Journal of Psychiatry, 162*(5), 995–997.

Livesley, W. J. (2003). *Practical management of personality disorder.* New York: Guilford Press.

MacFarlane, M. M. (2004). Systemic treatment of borderline personality disorder. In M. M. MacFarlane (Ed.), *Family treatment of personality disorders* (pp. 205–240). New York: Haworth Clinical Practice Press.

Magnavita, J. J., & MacFarlane, M. M. (2004). Family treatment of personality disorder: Historical overview and current perspectives. In M. M. MacFarlane (Ed.), *Family treatment of personality disorders* (pp. 3–39). New York: Haworth Clinical Practice Press.

McLean, P. D., & McLean, C. P. (2004). Family therapy of avoidant personality disorder. In M. M. MacFarlane (Ed.), *Family treatment of personality disorders* (pp. 273–303). New York: Haworth Clinical Practice Press.

Ni, X., Chan, K., Bulgin, N., Sicard, T., Bismil, R., McMain, S., & Kennedy, J. L. (2006). Association between serotonin transporter gene and borderline personality disorder. *Journal of Psychiatric Research, 40*(5), 448–453.

North American Nursing Diagnosis Association. (2007). *Nursing diagnoses: Definitions and classification, 2007 to 2008.* Philadelphia: Author.

Paris, J. (2001). Psychosocial adversity. In W. J. Livesley (Ed.), *Handbook of personality disorders* (pp. 231–241). New York: Guilford Press.

Perseius, K. I., Ekdahl, S., Asberg, M., & Samuelsson, M. (2005). To tame a volcano: Patients with borderline personality disorder and their perceptions of suffering. *Archives of Psychiatric Nursing, 19*(4), 160–168.

Ratey, J. J. (2001). *A user's guide to the brain.* New York: Pantheon Books.

Shedler, J., & Westen, D. (2004). Dimensions of personality pathology. *American Journal of Psychiatry, 161*(10), 1743–1754.

Soler, J., Pascual, J. C., Campins, J., Barrachina, J., Puigdemont, D., Alvarez, E., et al. (2005). Double-blind, placebo-controlled study of dialectical behavior therapy plus olanzapine for borderline personality disorder. *American Journal of Psychiatry, 162*(6), 1221–1224.

Sperry, L. (2004). Family therapy with a histrionic-obsessive couple. In M. M. MacFarlane (Ed.), *Family treatment of personality disorders* (pp. 149–172). New York: Haworth Clinical Practice Press.

Stevenson, J., Meares, R., & Comerford, A. (2003). Diminished impulsivity in older patients with borderline personality disorder. *American Journal of Psychiatry, 160*(1), 165–166.

Westen, D., Shedler, J., Durrett, C., Glass, S., & Martens, A. (2003). Personality diagnoses in adolescence. *American Journal of Psychiatry, 160*(5), 952–966.

Yen, S., Shea, M.T., Sanislow, C. A., Grilo, C. M., Skodol, A. E., Gunderson, J. G., et al. (2004). Borderline Personality Disorder criteria associated with prospectively observed suicidal behavior. *American Journal of Psychiatry, 161*(7), 1296–1298.

Zanarini, M. C., Frankenburg, F. R., Hennen, J., Reich, D. B., & Silk, K. R. (2004). Axis I comorbidity in patients with Borderline Personality Disorder. *American Journal of Psychiatry, 161*(11), 2108–2114.

Chapter 17

Disorders of Children and Adolescents

> *"Away From My Family"*
>
> —*George, Age 8*

Removed from home due to disruptive and assaultive behaviors toward family

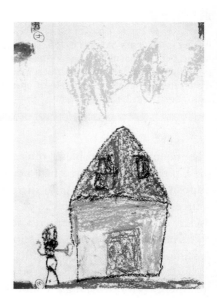

OBJECTIVES

After reading this chapter, you will be able to:

1. Compare and contrast the different theories regarding the etiology of disorders of children and adolescents.

2. Discuss the psychopharmacological treatment of the symptoms of childhood and adolescent disorders.

3. Outline the different treatment options for the disorders of children and adolescents.

4. Outline the assessment process for a client with a childhood or adolescent disorder.

5. Use the nursing process to develop a comprehensive plan of care for a client with a childhood or adolescent disorder.

6. Discuss the key points in effectively communicating with a person with a childhood or adolescent disorder.

7. Develop illness management teaching plans for a client with a childhood or adolescent disorder.

MediaLink www.prenhall.com/fontaine

Go to the Pearson Health MediaLink CD-ROM and the Companion Website at www.prenhall.com/fontaine for interactive resources for this chapter.

The ROAD to Critical Thinking

A Client Experiencing Oppositional Defiant Disorder and Attention Deficit Hyperactivity Disorder

Travel this ROAD to understand Ashley and her condition.

Read about Ashley below and throughout this chapter.

Observe Ashley on the CD-ROM accompanying this book.

Assess Ashley by answering the questions at the end of this chapter.

Develop a care plan on the CD-ROM to address Ashley's condition.

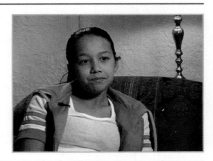

Ashley

Ashley is 13 years old and in the eighth grade. She has been diagnosed with oppositional defiant disorder and attention deficit hyperactivity disorder. She has been placed in the BD (behaviorally disordered) classroom because of arguing with teachers, fighting with peers, and skipping classes. She has since been suspended from school. You will meet Ashley on the video clip on your disc and throughout this chapter. At the end of the chapter, you will find critical thinking questions relating to assessment and development of a plan of care for Ashley.

The mental health problems of children and adolescents in the United States have reached a crisis state. Problems with oppositional, aggressive, and disruptive behaviors are the source of much distress to the child and to the family and society. One in 10 children and adolescents in the United States has a mental illness severe enough to cause impairment at school and in relationships with peers, friends, and family. Sadly, fewer than one in five of these children receive needed treatment. Nationally, high school students with mental illness have the highest rate of school dropout of any disability group. If left untreated, these disorders can lead to additional problems, including juvenile delinquency, substance abuse, and, for some, criminal activity.

Child and adolescent disorders presented in this chapter include attention deficit/hyperactivity disorder, oppositional defiant disorder, conduct disorder, Tourette disorder, bipolar disorder, Asperger disorder, pervasive developmental disorder not otherwise specified, and autistic disorder (see the DSM-IV-TR Classifications feature). Children who develop these disorders experience severe disruption in their social and emotional lives. Inattention, hyperactivity, and impulsivity characterize **attention deficit/hyperactivity disorder (ADHD)**. **Oppositional defiant disorder (ODD)** is a recurrent pattern of disobedient and hostile behavior toward authority figures. More severe in symptoms is **conduct disorder (CD)**, which is characterized by a persistent pattern of aggressive and destructive behavior with disregard for the rights of others and the norms of society. The term *disruptive behavior disorder* covers both ODD and CD. **Tourette disorder (TD)**

looks like ADHD with chronic motor and vocal tics. **Bipolar disorder** is characterized by the occurrence of one or more manic episodes and one or more depressive episodes. Autism spectrum disorders include Asperger disorder, pervasive developmental disorder, and autistic disorder. **Asperger disorder** involves severe impairment in social interactions and repetitive patterns of behavior and activities. Children with **pervasive developmental disorder (PDD) not otherwise specified (NOS)** have severely impaired social interaction and very limited verbal communication. Many consider this a milder form of autism. Social isolation, communication impairment, and strange repetitive behaviors characterize **autistic disorder**. Other child and adolescent disorders such as anxiety disorders, eating disorders, depression, and schizophrenia are discussed in chapters 11 through 14 ∞.

Mental disorders in this chapter overlap in terms of signs and symptoms and genetic similarities. Although the *Diagnostic and Statistical Manual of Mental Disorders* (4th ed., Text Revision) (DSM-IV-TR) encourages health care professionals to limit their diagnoses to one, most clinicians recognize that children and adolescents often have two or three of these problems concurrently. This chapter looks beyond the limitations of categories to the commonalities of the disorders presented here.

Child and adolescent disorders are polygenetic, caused by the coming together from both parents of a number of genes affecting dopamine (DA), serotonin (5-HT), and norepinephrine (NE) transmission. As the genetic load increases, the symptoms increase from the milder symptoms of ADHD

DSM-IV-TR   Attention Deficit/Hyperactivity Disorder

A. Either 1 or 2

1. Six or more of the following symptoms of inattention have persisted for at least 6 months to a degree that is maladaptive and inconsistent with developmental level:
   a. Often fails to give close attention to details or makes careless mistakes in school-work, work, or other activities
   b. Often has difficulty sustaining attention in tasks or play activities
   c. Is often easily distracted by extraneous stimuli
   d. Is often forgetful in daily activities
   e. Often does not seem to listen when spoken to directly
   f. Often avoids, dislikes, or is reluctant to engage in tasks that require sustained mental effort
   g. Often does not follow through on instructions and fails to finish school work, chores, or duties in the workplace
   h. Often has difficulty organizing tasks and activities
   i. Often loses things necessary for tasks or activities

2. Six or more of the following symptoms of hyperactivity-impulsivity have persisted for at least 6 months to a degree that is maladaptive and inconsistent with developmental level:
   a. Often fidgets with hands or feet or squirms in seat
   b. Often leaves seat in classroom or in other situations in which remaining seated is expected
   c. Often runs about or climbs excessively in situations in which it is inappropriate
   d. Often has difficulty playing or engaging in leisure activities quietly
   e. Is often "on the go" or often acts as if "driven by a motor"
   f. Often talks excessively
   g. Often blurts out answers before questions have been completed
   h. Often has trouble awaiting turn
   i. Often interrupts or intrudes on others

B. Some hyperactive-impulsive or inattentive symptoms that caused impairment were present before age 7 years.

C. Some impairment from the symptoms is present in two or more settings (e.g., at school and at home)

D. There must be clear evidence of clinically significant impairment in social, academic, or occupational functioning

DSM-IV-TR   Diagnosis Criteria: Conduct Disorder

A. A repetitive and persistent pattern of behavior in which the basic rights of others or major age-appropriate societal norms or rules are violated, as manifested by the presence of three (or more) of the following criteria in the past 12 months, with at least one criterion present in the past 6 months:

1. Aggression to people and animals
   a. Often bullies, threatens, or intimidates others
   b. Often initiates physical fights
   c. Has used a weapon that can cause serious physical harm to others (e.g., a bat, brick, broken bottle, knife, gun)
   d. Has been physically cruel to people
   e. Has been physically cruel to animals
   f. Has stolen while confronting a victim (e.g., mugging, purse snatching, extortion, armed robbery)
   g. Has forced someone into sexual acitivity

2. Destruction of property
   a. Has deliberately engaged in fire setting with the intention of causing serious damage
   b. Has deliberately destroyed others' property (other than by fire setting)

3. Deceitfulness or theft
   a. Has broken into someone else's house, building, or car
   b. Often lies to obtain goods or favors or to avoid obligations (i.e., "cons" others)
   c. Has stolen items of nontrivial value without confronting a victim (e.g., shoplifting, but without breaking and entering; forgery)

4. Serious violations of rules
   a. Often stays out at night despite parental prohibitions, beginning before age 13 years
   b. Has run away from home overnight at least twice while living in parental or parental surrogate home
   c. Is often truant from school, beginning before age 13 years

B. The disturbance in behavior causes clinically significant impairment in social, academic, or occupational functioning

C. If the individual is age 18 years or older, criteria are not met for Antisocial Personality Disorder.

SOURCE: Reprinted with permission from the *Diagnostic and statistical manual of mental disorders*, 4th ed., Text Revision. Copyright 2000 American Psychiatric Association.

DSM-IV-TR Diagnosis Criteria: Oppositional Defiant Disorder

A. The diagnosis of oppositional defiant disorder is made when negativistic, hostile, and defiant behavior is present for at least 6 months during which four (or more) of the following are present:
1. Often loses temper
2. Often argues with adults

3. Often actively defies or refuses to comply with adults' requests or rules
4. Often deliberately annoys people
5. Often blames others for his or her mistakes or misbehavior
6. Is often touchy or easily annoyed by others
7. Is often angry and resentful

8. Is often spiteful or vindictive
B. The disturbance in behavior causes clinically significant impairment in social, academic, or occupational functioning
C. The behaviors do not occur exclusively during the course of a Psychotic or Mood Disorder.

DSM-IV-TR Diagnosis Criteria: Tourette Disorder

The diagnosis of Tourette disorder is made when the following symptoms are present:

A. Both multiple motor and one or more vocal tics have been present at some time during the illness, although not necessarily concurrently.

B. The tics occur many times a day (usually in bouts) nearly every day or intermittently throughout a period of more than 1 year, and during this period there was never a tic-free period of more than 3 consecutive months.

C. The onset is before age 18 years.
D. The disturbance is not due to the direct physiological effects of a substance or a general medical condition.

DSM-IV-TR Diagnosis Criteria: Asperger Disorder

A. The diagnosis of Asperger disorder is made when the following symptoms are present:
1. Qualitative impairment in social interactions, as manifested by at least two of the following:
   a. Marked impairment in the use of multiple nonverbal behaviors such as eye-to-eye gaze, facial expression, body postures, and gestures to regulate social interaction
   b. Failure to develop peer relationships appropriate to developmental level
   c. A lack of spontaneous seeking to share enjoyment, interests, or achievements with other people
   d. Lack of social or emotional reciprocity

2. Restrictive and repetitive and stereotyped patterns of behavior, interests, and activities as manifested by at least one of the following:
   a. Encompassing preoccupation with one or more stereotyped and restricted patterns of interest that is abnormal either in intensity or focus
   b. Apparently inflexible adherence to specific, nonfunctional routines or rituals
   c. Stereotyped and repetitive motor mannerisms (e.g., hand or finger flapping or twisting, or complex whole-body movements)
   d. Persistent preoccupation with parts of objects.

3. The disturbance causes clinically significant impairment in social, occupational, or other important areas of functioning.
4. There is no clinically significant general delay in language (e.g., single words used by age 2 years, communicative phrases used by age 3 years).
5. There is no clinically significant delay in cognitive development or in the development of age-appropriate self-help skills, adaptive behavior (other than in social interaction), and curiosity about the environment in childhood.
6. Criteria are not met for another specific Pervasive Developmental Disorder or Schizophrenia.

through the most severe symptoms of autism. Figure 17.1 ■ illustrates this concept: comorbidity in the disorders increases as genetic loading increases. For example, although ADHD is a distinct clinical condition, it commonly occurs concomitantly with one or more of the other disorders, creating a distinctive set of problems. In addition, the same child may experience different disorders over time. For example, at age

4, Sam is diagnosed with ADHD. At age 6, he develops tics, and the diagnosis of Tourette disorder is made. By 8 years of age, he is defiant of authorities (ODD), and by 10, he has become extremely destructive and disruptive (CD).

In the general population, 85% to 90% of young people do not experience mental disorders. Of the remaining 10% to 15%, 7% to 11% have ADHD, 4% have oppositional defiant

DSM-IV-TR	**Diagnosis Criteria: Autistic Disorder**

A. The diagnosis of autistic disorder is made when the following symptoms are present:

1. Qualitative impairment in social interactions as manifested by at least two of the following:
   a. Marked impairment in the use of multiple nonverbal behaviors such as eye-to-eye gaze, facial expression, body postures, and gestures to regulate social interaction
   b. Failure to develop peer relationships appropriate to developmental level
   c. A lack of spontaneous seeking to share enjoyment, interests, or achievements with other people
   d. Lack of social or emotional reciprocity
2. Qualitative impairment in communication as manifested by at least one of the following:

a. Delay in, or total lack of, the development of spoken language (not accompanied by an attempt to compensate through alternative modes of communication such as gesture or mime)
b. In individuals with adequate speech, marked impairment in the ability to initiate or sustain a conversation with others
c. Stereotyped and repetitive use of language or idiosyncratic language
d. Lack of varied, spontaneous make-believe play or social imitative play appropriate to developmental level

3. Restricted repetitive and stereotyped patterns of behavior, interests, and activities, as manifested by at least one of the following:
   a. Encompassing preoccupation with one or more stereotyped

and restricted patterns of interest that is abnormal either in intensity or focus
b. Apparently inflexible adherence to specific, nonfunctional routines or rituals
c. Stereotyped and repetitive motor mannerisms (e.g., hand or finger flapping or twisting, or complex whole-body movements)
d. Persistent preoccupation with parts of objects

4. Delays or abnormal functioning in at least one of the following areas, with onset prior to age 3 years: (1) social interaction, (12) language as used in social communication, or (3) symbolic or imaginative play.
   a. The disturbance is not better accounted for by Rett Disorder or Childhood Disintegrative Disorder

---

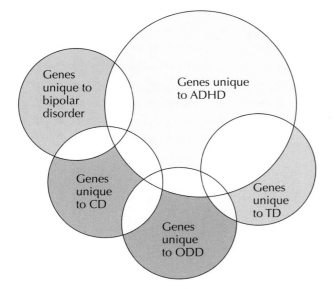

☐ Genes common to two or more disorders

Figure 17.1 ■ Diagram illustrating the concept of child and adolescent disorders as polygenetic disorders sharing some, but not all, genes in common with comorbid disorders.

SOURCE: Original concept by David E. Cummings, MD, 1998.

disorder, 5% to 6% have conduct disorder, 1% has Tourette disorder, 1% has bipolar disorder, 0.5% has Asperger disorder, 0.5% has pervasive developmental disorder, and 0.1% has autistic disorder. Nearly half the children with ADHD also have many of the other disorders. In addition, ADHD-like symptoms are sometimes manifestations of childhood-onset bipolar disorder. These disorders are so intertwined that it is often difficult to sort them out. Until more is known about these disorders, no diagnosis should be discounted because another disorder is present. Child and adolescent disorders are clear examples that health care providers must treat the symptoms the individual is experiencing, not the diagnosis (Canty-Mitchell, Austin, Jaffee, Qi & Swigonski, 2004; Chakrabarti & Fombonne, 2005; Nierenberg et al., 2005).

KNOWLEDGE BASE

Attention Deficit/Hyperactivity Disorder

Attention deficit/hyperactivity disorder (ADHD) is characterized by inattention, hyperactivity, and impulsivity. In spite of much publicity, the incidence of ADHD in the United States has not increased in 20 years. The 7% to 11% prevalence rate in the general population makes ADHD more common than cancer and many other disorders. More boys receive the diagnosis of ADHD than girls. It is believed that this happens because, in general, boys are more disruptive than girls. Girls with ADHD are less likely to misbehave, talk back to the teacher, or knock their desk over. The earlier the onset, the more likely ADHD will continue into adulthood.

There are three types of ADHD, each with different symptoms: (1) predominantly inattentive, (2) predominantly hyperactive/impulsive, and (3) combined. The combined type is the most common. A diagnosis of ADHD is made when a person displays at least six symptoms from either list, with some of the symptoms having started before age 7. See Table 17.1■ for a list of symptoms. For a valid diagnosis, symptoms of ADHD should be present in two or more settings (e.g., home and school/work), and the person's behavior must adversely affect social, academic, or occupational functioning (American Psychiatric Association, 2000).

ADHD can be thought of as an addiction to the present. Individuals with ADHD are unable to complete tasks that will provide a later reward. Immediate pleasure and gratification are their driving forces. An interesting perspective on ADHD suggests that persons with ADHD are hunters among farmers. This analogy serves to explain the *roaming* characteristics. The hunter thinks visually, is excited by the hunt, but becomes easily bored with mundane tasks. The hunter constantly monitors the environment and readily changes strategies at a moment's notice. Hunters are often very creative and people with higher levels of activity may have functioned better in hunter–gatherer societies. Although children with spectrum disorder are disruptive in school, which may disturb the teachers and classmates, there is no biological advantage to sitting quietly in a classroom. Although parents may be frustrated, it is helpful for them to remember the many hunters who have made positive changes in the world.

At one time, ADHD was considered strictly a childhood condition, outgrown in adolescence and of little consequence for adults. Research indicates, however, that the disorder persists into adulthood in 30% to 70% of affected individuals, often with serious consequences. ADHD is a known risk factor among adults for antisocial behavior, substance abuse, being involved in serious accidents, academic underachievement, and low occupational success. In adults, inattention is more persistent than hyperactivity or impulsivity. Physical hyperactivity often changes to verbal hyperactivity in adults (Nierenberg et al., 2005).

Deepak is a 9-year-old boy who has ADHD, as do his two siblings. He is hyperactive in school—climbing on desks and chairs. When he gets angry, he becomes aggressive toward his teacher and throws objects around the room. He states that he has nothing to look forward to and feels he does everything wrong.

TABLE 17.1	**Symptoms of ADHD**

Those with predominantly inattentive type often

- Fail to pay close attention to details or make careless mistakes in schoolwork, work, or other activities
- Have difficulty sustaining attention to tasks or leisure activities
- Do not seem to listen when spoken to directly
- Do not follow through on instructions and fail to finish schoolwork, chores, or duties in the workplace
- Have difficulty organizing tasks and activities
- Avoid, dislike, or are reluctant to engage in tasks that require sustained mental effort
- Lose things necessary for tasks or activities
- Are easily distracted by extraneous stimuli
- Are forgetful in daily activities

Those with predominantly hyperactive–impulsive often

- Fidget with their hands or feet or squirm in their seat
- Leave their seat in situations in which remaining seated is expected
- Move excessively or feel restless during situations in which such behavior is inappropriate
- Have difficulty engaging in leisure activities quietly
- Are "on the go" or act as if "driven by a motor"
- Have accidental injuries
- Talk excessively
- Blurt out answers before questions have been completed
- Have difficulty awaiting their turn
- Interrupt or intrude on others
- Experience peer rejection

Those with the combined type

- Have a combination of the inattentive and hyperactive–impulsive symptoms

SOURCE: American Psychiatric Association. (2000). *Diagnostic and statistical manual of mental disorders* (4th ed., Text Revision). Washington, DC: Author.

Oppositional Defiant Disorder

Oppositional defiant disorder is a recurrent pattern of disobedient and hostile behavior toward authority figures. Children with ODD are frequently disruptive, argumentative, hostile, irritable, and commonly annoy people. They often deliberately defy adult rules but tend to blame others for their own mistakes and difficulties. Such disruptive behavior occurs at a more frequent rate, at greater intensity, and for longer periods than the usual behavioral problems of peers. Disturbances in behavior lead to social problems with peers and adults and impaired academic functioning. For most of these individuals, the problem behaviors end in adolescence.

Ashley:

❝Interviewer: 'Who would you argue with in school?'
  Ashley: 'Teachers.'
  Interviewer: 'Would you only argue with them if they were wrong about something'?
  Ashley: 'No, just to argue. I love arguing and I feel good when I do it.'❞

Conduct Disorder

Conduct disorder (CD) is one of the more common diagnoses given to adolescents and is characterized by a persistent pattern of aggressive and destructive behavior with disregard for the rights of others and the norms of society. One third of teens with CD develop antisocial personality disorder, especially those with early onset and severe and wide-ranging symptoms. Though not all children with CD progress to antisocial personality disorder, virtually all have difficulties functioning as adults. See chapter 16 ∞ for a complete discussion of personality disorders (Kim-Cohen et al., 2005).

There are two subtypes of conduct disorder: (1) childhood-onset type, which is heritable; and (2) adolescent-onset type, which is influenced more by environmental factors. Both subtypes can be further described as mild, moderate, or severe. Individuals with childhood-onset type are usually male, are frequently physically aggressive to others, are more violent, and have disturbed peer relationships. Those with the adolescent-onset type are less likely to be physically aggressive and will have better peer relationships (American Psychiatric Association, 2000).

Children and adolescents with moderate and severe CD engage in significant and persistent antisocial behavior that violates the rights of others at home, in school, and in the community. Antisocial behavior may be solitary or it may occur in a peer group, such as a gang. Physical aggression is common, and cruelty to other people and animals may occur.

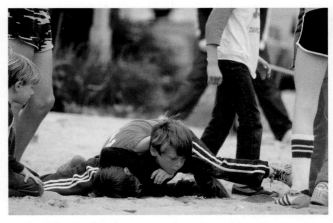

PHOTO 17.1 ■ Many fights among children are caused by their attributing hostile intent to others and then retaliating.
SOURCE: Catherine Ursillo/Photo Researchers, Inc. Used with permission.

Youths with CD may destroy other people's property, set fires, steal, and rob.

Fifteen-year-old Ruben has been admitted to a residential setting for aggressive behavior. His mother was raped when she was 15 years old, and Ruben is the result of the rape. His mother has been married and divorced twice. He has three younger siblings ages 11, 9, and 5 years. For the past several months, Ruben has been cutting school and getting into gang fights. He has been expelled for truancy and fighting. His mother was disciplining him by making Ruben go to work with her. He recently told his mother that if she continued to make him go to work, he would kill her. His younger siblings are afraid of him and his friends. He becomes very angry with anyone who does not agree with his views. He states that he is in the residential placement only because his mother is "crazy and a bitch." When asked about future expectations, he states, "to hang with friends and not go back to school."

Anger resulting from self-hatred, depression, and helplessness is directed outward. These youths lack guilt or remorse over their deviant behavior. Maladjustment to school, truancy, and dropping out of school are common. The unacceptable behavior and lack of social controls bring about social alienation, unless the youths are part of a similar group of teens. Relationships with peers and adults are manipulative and used for personal advantage.

Tourette Disorder

Clinically, Tourette disorder appears to be ADHD with chronic motor and vocal tics. Tourette disorder usually starts between 6 and 7 years of age. It can, however, begin as early as 1 year of age and as late as the teens. This is a disorder of the brain characterized by sudden, rapid, recurrent **motor tics** (involuntary movements) and **vocal tics** (involuntary vocalizations). These tics are further subdivided into simple and complex. Table 17.2 ■ summarizes the behaviors. Motor tics include eye blinking, facial grimacing, head jerking, neck

TABLE 17.2	Types of Tics	
	Vocal Tics	**Motor Tics**
Simple	Throat clearing	Eye blinking
	Sniffing	Shoulder shrugs
	Grunting	Facial grimacing
	Coughing	Head jerking
Complex	Animal sounds	Smelling objects
	Repeating words	Hopping
	Coprolalia	Touching people
	Stuttering	Pulling on clothes

movements, shoulder shrugging, and hand movements. Common vocal tics include throat clearing, grunting, coughing, sniffing, yelling, or screaming. A much smaller group of children exhibits **coprolalia**—the involuntary use of obscene words. More than half have obsessive–compulsive symptoms and 7% to 10% are diagnosed with obsessive–compulsive disorder (Teicher, Andersen, Navalta, Polcari, & Kim, 2004).

> When Jaycee was 6 years old, he developed a motor tic of rapid and recurrent eye blinking. At age 9, he developed a vocal tic of sniffing and was diagnosed with moderate ADHD. By age 12, Jaycee had frequent periods of eye blinking, side-to-side head turning, foot stamping, and repeatedly inserting his fingers into his mouth. He was able to voluntarily suppress these tics only for short periods. His tics increased in severity during periods of stress, anxiety, and fatigue.

An estimated 100,000 people in the United States have Tourette disorder, and as many as 1 in 200 have partial symptoms of the disorder. Tourette disorder is more frequent among males. It is thought that the dysfunction occurs in the caudate nucleus, part of the basal ganglia, an area of the brain that helps control movement.

Bipolar Disorder

Almost 50% of children first diagnosed with depression develop the bipolar form of a mood disorder. Bipolar disorder in adulthood is characterized both by manic episodes and by depressed episodes with intervals of normal mood. In contrast to the typical adult characteristics, children with bipolar disorder have moods that are more irritable, with explosive outbursts, and their cycles of mania and depression are far more rapid. The rapidity of the mood swings, occurring multiple times a day, is referred to as ultra-ultra rapid cycles. Most also experience recurrent rage-filled, and often violent, temper tantrums, which may last as long as an hour (Scheffer, Kowatch, Carmody, & Rush, 2005). Chapter 13 ∞ provides information

about bipolar disorders in adulthood. Psychotic symptoms, such as delusions and hallucinations, can occur in both the manic and the depressive phases of bipolar disorder. The content of these may reflect the current mood state.

> When Rachel experiences a manic state, she often talks about playing golf with Tiger Woods, winning, and being invited to play on the Olympic golf team. When she is clinically depressed, Rachel believes that her parents want to kill her to prevent her from becoming famous.

Bipolar disorder in children is an underidentified problem. It is estimated that one third of all the children in the United States who are diagnosed with ADHD also meet the criteria for bipolar disorder. Hyperactivity and distractibility are symptoms for both mania and ADHD. The distinguishing feature is elation and grandiosity, characteristic of the manic state.

Asperger Disorder

Asperger disorder involves severe impairment in social interactions and repetitive patterns of behavior and activities. People with Asperger disorder exhibit a variety of characteristics and the disorder can be mild or severe. By definition, those with Asperger disorder have a normal IQ and many exhibit exceptional skill or talent in a specific area. They often become obsessively preoccupied with a particular subject, which may lead to a career at which they may be successful as adults. Some experience bizarre obsessions. They are often viewed as eccentric or odd and easily become victims of teasing and bullying.

On the surface, language development seems normal, and children with Asperger disorder have extraordinarily rich vocabularies. They often, however, sound like little professors and have difficulty using language in a social context. Their attempts at conversation result in one-sided, long-winded lecturing (Perry, 2004).

> By 4 years of age, Westin was very interested in, and knowledgeable about, astronomy. He would pursue this interest at any opportunity. In conversations with peers, he inevitably brought the conversation or play around to stars and planets. He was quickly seen as a rather odd child. By age 10, he had significant social problems. He did not always respond to other people's facial expressions or gestures. He actively avoided eye contact and seemed to look through people. When interacting with others, he engaged in long monologues describing the history of the universe, in spite of repeated attempts by others to change the subject.

People with Asperger disorder are not solitary or withdrawn, but they put people off by their abrupt and awkward approaches. They may have difficulty making eye contact and may actually turn away at the same moment as greeting another person. They have a great deal of difficulty reading nonverbal cues and body language and very often have difficulty determining proper body space. As a result, social and occupational functioning are significantly impaired.

Autistic Disorder

Autistic disorder, or autism, is the most severe form of the autistic spectrum disorders, though severity varies from person to person. Autism is most likely many disorders with many distinct causes. Currently, 1 in every 175 school children are affected. There are twice as many boys than girls with autism. There has been some concern that the incidence of autism is increasing. What has changed over the past 20 years is the definition and characteristics of the disorder. These changes have resulted in more people fitting into the category and improved case finding strategies. There has also been some concern that childhood vaccines cause autism. Research shows that no association exists between autism and the measles, mumps, and rubella vaccine (Centers for Disease Control and Prevention, 2006; Wilson, Mills, Ross, McGowan, & Jadad, 2003).

Autism is characterized by a triad of impairments: social isolation, communication impairment, and strange repetitive behaviors. In infancy, the symptoms of autism may be subtle and almost unnoticeable, but it is unusually clear by age 2 or 3 that something is seriously wrong. The most striking feature of autistic disorder is profound social isolation. Children with autism dislike being touched or looking peo-

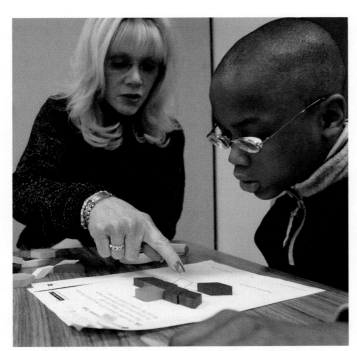

PHOTO 17.2 ■ Children with autistic disorder, like the child in this picture, are normal in physical appearance. The communication problems, autistic aloneness, and need to preserve sameness are readily apparent among children with autism, however.
SOURCE: Patrick White/Merrill Education. Used with permission.

ple in the eye, and they seem to take no pleasure in sharing experiences with others. They have little sense of human relations, or even their parents being their parents, and have difficulty experiencing affection and cannot anticipate the thoughts and actions of others.

Disturbances in motor behavior such as whirling, lunging, darting, rocking, and toe walking present a bizarre picture. Some behavior may be self-mutilative, such as head banging or hand biting. People with autism may throw tantrums for no apparent reason. They often *perseverate*, that is, show an obsessive interest in a single toy, activity, or person. They insist on sameness and resist changes in routine.

Language development is usually slow. What first seems a creative choice of words turns out to be the beginning of abnormal language patterning. Communication with others is seriously impaired. Children with autism may be mute, may make unintelligible sounds, or may say words repeatedly. They may be unable to name objects and cannot use or understand abstract language.

Two thirds of children with autism have IQ scores of 70 or less and the rest have normal or above average IQs. Ten percent of children with autism have unusual talents and are known as *savants*. Savants possess unusual talents that appear at an early age—an exceptional rote memory, a capacity for lightning-quick calculation, precocious musical talent or drawing ability, or the ability to name the day of the week corresponding to any calendar date. Although they possess rare talents, they may or may not be mentally ill in other respects. The movie *Rain Man*, in which Dustin Hoffman portrays a savant with unusual counting abilities, is a dramatic example of autism (Nair, 2004).

Special education costs for a child with autism are more than $8,000 per year while care in a residential setting costs $80,000 to $100,000 a year. Follow-up studies of children with autism have found that only 5% to 10% become independent as adults, 25% progress but require supervision, and the remainder continue to be severely impaired and in need of a high level of care (Centers for Disease Control and Prevention, 2006; Howlin, Goode, Hutton, & Rutter, 2004).

Comorbid Disorders

Depression is the most common comorbid condition of child and adolescent disorders. Early diagnosis of depression is crucial because depression impairs overall functioning. Depression is thought to arise from not feeling good enough, not feeling loved, and not feeling connected to others (DeJong & Frazier, 2003).

Children with autistic disorder and Asperger disorder are at higher risk for seizures. Various research studies put the risk at 7% to 42%. Most electroencephalographic changes are in the temporal and central brain areas (Reinhold, Molloy, & Manning-Courtney, 2005).

Studies show a high risk for *substance use disorders* for people with ODD, CD, and bipolar disorders. The potential for substance use disorders is high during adolescence, a time when individuals may begin to experiment with alcohol and drugs. Adolescents who continue to exhibit antisocial or delinquent behavior after age 15 are much more likely to develop substance problems. Researchers are currently asking the following questions: Is the association due to an attempt to self-medicate? Is the tendency to use substances something in the genes that is common to these disorders and substance use disorders? Does substance abuse trigger the genes for child and adolescent disorders? Are substance use disorders another variation of these disorders (Wilens et al., 2004)? See chapter 15 ∞ for further information on substance use disorders.

Ashley:

❝ I smoke cigarettes. I drink once in a while. The last time I drank was last week. I had brandy and Smirnoff. I drink in my room so my dad doesn't find out. I don't smoke marijuana or do other drugs. ❞

Comorbidity is associated with mental disorders and delinquent behavior in the adolescent population. Similar antecedents include family dysfunction, parental mental health problems, low academic achievement, relationships with other troubled peers, and chaotic neighborhoods. It is estimated that as many as 80% of youth incarcerated in juvenile correctional facilities have emotional illnesses. The juvenile justice system is beginning to respond to this problem and make efforts to provide mental health care. It is not easy to provide services for adolescents whose behaviors involve both the mental health system and the juvenile justice system (Shelton, 2004).

Etiologies

The cause of child and adolescent disorders is unknown, but it is likely that it involves genetic factors, anatomical abnormalities, neurotransmission problems, and environmental factors.

Genetics

Child and adolescent disorders are polygenic disorders. The candidates for further study include DA receptor genes D1, D2, and D4; DA transporter gene; monoamine oxidase gene; 5-HT genes; NE genes; gamma-aminobutyric acid (GABA) genes; and androgen receptor genes. Because these disorders are the result of many genes acting together, each of these genes individually exerts only a small effect on the disorders.

There is a genetic basis for ADHD in about 80% to 94% of the cases. In the other cases, ADHD is caused by trauma to the brain. Biological relatives of children with ADHD are at higher risk for the disorder. In 50% to 80% of monozygotic twins, both twins have ADHD. Among dizygotic twins, both twins have the disorder 30% of the time. Adoption studies suggest that the transmission is biological (Hudziak, Derks, Althoff, Rettew, & Boomsma, 2005; Voeller, 2004).

Monozygotic twins have a concordance rate of 50% to 60% for Tourette disorder, compared with only 8% for dizygotic twins. In one study of monozygotic twins who were discordant (only one twin affected) for Tourette disorder, the twin with the disorder consistently had a lower birth weight than the unaffected twin. In the monozygotic twins who both had Tourette disorder, the twin with the lower birth weight had a more severe tic disorder than the other (Teicher et al., 2004).

Monozygotic twin studies of people with bipolar disorder found a concordance rate of 60% and 90% for a milder form of the disorder. For those twins raised apart from each other, the concordance rate was 67%. Studies of Asperger disorder show that the incidence of the disorder in first-degree relatives is significantly greater. Twin and family studies show that the rate of heritability for autism is more than 90%. Families with one child who has autistic disorder are 50 to 100 times more likely than the general population to have additional children with the disorder. Men older than 40 are nearly 6 times as likely to father a child with autism as those under 30. It is thought this is associated with mutations or alterations in genetic imprinting (DeJong & Frazier, 2003; Ramoz et al., 2004; Reichenberg et al., 2006).

Ashley:

❝ I have one younger brother who has Down syndrome and ADHD and two older brothers. I don't see my two older brothers very often. My oldest brother is 16 and he's been in lockup for a week. My other brother is 14 and he's been in lockup for the past 6 months. ❞

Making genetic associations to human behavior and temperament is the most complex area of study in molecular genetics. The attempt to solve this puzzle will require massive testing of the entire human genome.

Neurobiology

Abnormalities in child and adolescent disorders have been observed in different brain regions. Structural brain imaging studies have shown size abnormalities of the frontal lobes, basal ganglia, corpus callosum, and parietal lobes. Small frontal lobes have been found to correlate with inability to change or transition from one activity to another. Researchers have also discovered that, in adults with autism, the brain is larger, and they are trying to find out where the extra tissue is concentrated (Voeller, 2004).

The results of functional imaging studies have shown low brain activity in the prefrontal cortex, the caudate nucleus, and parietal brain regions. In hyperactive adolescents, there is a delayed development of the frontal lobes. This may explain why much of the physical hyperactivity lessens or disappears in adulthood. The response inhibition system of the brain is located in the right prefrontal lobe and its underactivitation seems to be related to a lack of control. This means that children and adolescents with these disorders have greater problems than most in inhibiting or delaying a behavioral response. Prefrontal lobe dysfunction has been suggested as a potential biological deficit in antisocial behavior. The prefrontal area of the brain is responsible for motivation, mood regulation, and executive function. Abnormalities in this area contribute to impulsivity, short attention span, mood instability, difficulty planning or delaying gratification, and poor motivation, which are problems common to these disorders (Herpertz et al., 2005; Kaur et al., 2005).

Hyperactivity, impulsivity, and inattention suggest neurotransmission dysfunction. NE contributes to a person's ability to sustain attention and mental effort. DA is responsible for physical movement, reward-motivated behaviors, and body temperature regulation. It is thought that people with ADHD actually have an increase in the numbers of DA transporters, which reduces DA levels by taking the neurotransmitter back up into the transmitting cell. Abnormal variations may contribute to highs and lows in mood and physical and verbal hyperactivity. In some cases, it is thought that there are DA abnormalities in the frontal lobe and NE abnormalities in the parietal lobe—two sites for the process of attention. Others believe that the basic difficulty is related to the balance between DA and NE. Disturbances in 5-HT may contribute to problems in social relatedness and communication, ritualistic characteristics, and aggressive and impulsive behavior (Hunt, 2006).

Acetylcholine (ACh) and its nicotinic receptors influence learning and memory and are involved in emotional regulation. Recent studies suggest that **nicotinic dysregulation** may play a role in child and adolescent disorders. People with many of these disorders have a greater risk for and an earlier age of onset of cigarette smoking than other individuals. In addition, maternal smoking during pregnancy increases the risk for ADHD in children. In one study, adults with ADHD treated with commercially available transdermal nicotine experienced a significant improvement in their symptoms and neuropsychological functioning. Nicotine specifically improves attention and executive function problems and decreases aggression.

Recent studies of autism suggest that some individuals may have an autoimmune basis for the disorder. Immune abnormalities include problems in the numbers of T cells, abnormal B- and T-cell function, and poor antibody production. Autoimmune findings have also been demonstrated in Tourette disorder (Sweeten, Posey, & McDougle, 2003).

Nutritional Factors

Malnutrition is associated with antisocial behavior by impairing neurocognitive functioning. Sons of women who experienced inadequate nutrition during pregnancy had 2.5 times the normal rate of CD and antisocial personality disorder. Artificial food coloring and benzoate preservatives in food have an adverse effect on the behavior of young children. When these substances are removed from the diet, hyperactive behavior is significantly reduced. Other nutritional factors being explored are hypoglycemia, cholesterol, iron-deficiency anemia, and low zinc levels (Bateman et al., 2005; Liu, Raine, Venables, & Mednick, 2004).

Interpersonal Factors

The genetic and neurobiological factors do not exist in isolation, but rather interact with psychosocial factors in people's social, cultural, and physical environments. For example, abnormal brain structure and functions lead to cognitive deficits, which then lead to behavioral manifestations. The extent—and, to some degree, the nature—of the behaviors are influenced by social and psychological factors. These factors include people's experiences, which may or may not enable them to compensate for cognitive deficits or provide them with a low or high degree of motivation, which in turn affects their ability to cope. Even where biological factors are clearly implicated, the social and cultural environments determine whether the observed behaviors are desirable or undesirable. If the judgment is one of deviancy, the judgment itself has an effect on the self-image and behavior of the individual. Because biological and psychosocial factors are so intertwined, it is impossible to determine the extent of the affect of each.

Psychopharmacological Interventions

These child and adolescent disorders are neurobiological, disabling conditions for which a number of medications may be used to normalize the neurobiology. Medication must not be seen as a magic cure and must always be used in conjunction with multidisciplinary interventions. However, the change induced by medication frequently is striking. The purpose of the treatment plan is to help people become productive members of the community. Attempting this without trying to correct the problem with medications is like trying to teach reading to people with very poor vision and no glasses. People with poor vision would not be told that if they just tried harder they could read the blackboard. Yet, that is often what is said to children with these disorders, "Just try harder to sit still and pay attention."

Medication should be seen as providing a window of opportunity to allow other strategies to be more effective. There is clearly little point in attempting complex teaching strategies, behavioral management, or psychotherapy if children are excessively impulsive and unable to pay attention.

TABLE 17.3	Therapeutic Effects of CNS Stimulant Medications
Increase	**Decrease**
▪ Attention ▪ Accuracy ▪ Concentration ▪ Learning ▪ Memory ▪ Coordination ▪ On-task behavior	▪ Aggression ▪ Daydreaming ▪ Defiance ▪ Distractability ▪ Destructiveness ▪ Hyperactivity ▪ Mood swings

Stimulants are the most widely used drugs for treating ADHD. The therapeutic effects are listed in Table 17.3 ▪. The most commonly used stimulants are methylphenidate (Ritalin, Concerta, Metadate, Daytrana); dextroamphetamine (Dexedrine); amphetamine and dextroamphetamine (Adderall); and pemoline (Cylert). These drugs increase activity in parts of the brain that are underactive, improving attention and reducing impulsiveness, hyperactivity, or aggressive behavior. A newer, nonstimulant medication is atomoxetine (Strattera). Modafinil (Provigil) is used for the hypoactive form of ADHD and for narcolepsy.

Methylphenidate (Ritalin) increases the synaptic concentration of DA by blocking more than 50% of the DA transporters. The time to reach peak action in the brain is 60 minutes. It is rapidly metabolized and out of the body in 4 hours. Therefore, dosage may be as frequent as five times a day. The typical dose is 0.3 to 0.8 mg/kg given two to three times a day. Dextroamphetamine (Dexedrine) and amphetamine and dextroamphetamine (Adderall) increase the release of DA, thereby increasing the concentration in the synapse. Dexedrine and Adderall may be too stimulating for the hyperactive person but appropriate for the hypoactive form of ADHD. Modafinil (Provigil) blocks DA reuptake in the basal ganglia and reticular activating system (RAS).

Dosage and timing adjustments are critical to effective management. This can often make the difference between successful and unsuccessful management. See Table 17.4 ▪ for

TABLE 17.4	Medications for ADHD
Generic Name	**Trade Name**
Atomoxetine	Strattera
Dexmethylphenidate	Focalin, Focalin XR
Dextroamphetamine and Amphetamine	Adderall, Adderall XR
Methylphenidate	Concerta, Daytrana, Ritalin, Ritalin LA, Ritalin SR
Modafinil	Provigil

these drugs. Dosages should be titrated slowly to achieve the lowest satisfactory dose. The goal is to achieve a tolerable suppression of the symptoms. These disorders have ever-changing symptoms, so medications must be adjusted, increased, or decreased in a rational fashion.

Duration of side effects of the stimulant medications is short and lasts only for the duration of each dose, about 4 hours. Adverse reactions are usually dose related. Growth should be monitored during treatment with stimulants. Caution is indicated where there is an increase in blood pressure or heart rate or there are other cardiac abnormalities. Contraindications include marked anxiety, tension or agitation, glaucoma, and concurrent treatment with monoamine oxidase inhibitors (MAOIs). There is some evidence that atomoxetine (Strattera) may increase the risk for suicidal thinking in children and adolescents. The most common side effects are listed in Box 17.1, and client and family teaching information is provided in Box 17.2.

BOX 17.1	Side Effects of Stimulant Mediations

- Appetite suppression—most frequent side effect; often decrease over first few weeks.
- Abdominal pain/headaches—occasionally occur in first few days; rarely persist.
- Transient change in personality—some children become irritable, weepy, and agitated; more common with Dexedrine/dextroamphetamine.
- Sleep problems—too high a dosage too late in day may make it difficult for child to fall asleep.
- Rebound effect—some children become worse as drug wears off; more frequent doses may be necessary.
- Itchy skin, rashes, mood change, or nausea can occasionally occur.
- Tolerance and dependence can occur with Adderall dextroamphetamine/amphetamine and dextroamphetamine.

SOURCE: Cooper, P. (1999). ADHD and effective learning: Principles and practical approaches. In P. Cooper & Bilton (Eds.), *ADHD: Research, practice, and opinion* (p. 138–157). London: Whurr.

BOX 17.2	Medication Teaching

Stimulant Medications

- No caffeine; increases feeling jittery
- No cough medicine with ephedrine; increases feeling jittery
- Do not take on an empty stomach
- No drug "holidays"; this is a life problem, not an academic problem

Dexedrine/Adderall

- Do not eat or drink citrus foods within 1 hour of taking; interferes with absorption

Ritalin

- Antihistamines nullify effect

Because children and adolescents with these disorders have a variety of symptoms, other medications may be used. The symptoms that are most bothersome in terms of social and academic functioning are treated first. *Antidepressants* are used for depressed or manic mood states; *mood stabilizers* are used for mood swings, tantrums, and rage; *antipsychotic* agents are used for rage episodes, ODD, CD, Asperger disorder, and Tourette disorder. Antipsychotic medication improves the repetitive patterns of behavior and irritability in autism but has no effect on social withdrawal. The *antihypertensive* medication clonidine (Catapres) reduces the occurrence of motor tics in many of the people with Tourette disorder and may be a treatment option for ADHD. Other drugs under study for Tourette disorder include two antihypertensives—mecamylamine (Inversine) and guanfacine (Tenex)—and botulinum toxin (Botox). Initial studies have shown that the use of a *nicotine* patch may have a beneficial effect in relieving some symptoms of Tourette disorder. Studies are just beginning on modafinil (Provigil) for ADHD. Naltrexone (ReVia) has helped some people with autism decrease self-injury and improve cognitive processing (Teicher et al., 2004).

Multidisciplinary Interventions

Effective management of child and adolescent disorders is collaborative, involving education, nursing, medical, and psychological strategies, where appropriate. Day-to-day interaction is very much in the hands of the educator. These disorders often go undiagnosed until the child is enrolled in a school setting. As children begin school, issues of emotional and behavioral health and learning disorders become much more important.

School nurses are responsible for meeting the health needs of emotionally and mentally disabled students. The single most frequently used medication in schools is methylphenidate (Ritalin). As part of the zero-tolerance policy on drugs, students are not allowed to carry prescribed medication. The school nurse, typically, is responsible for administering medication during school hours.

Occupational therapists have recently introduced weighted vests as a noninvasive way to help children with ADHD and the autistic spectrum disorders. The vests add a few pounds of pressure to the joints and muscles, slowing down the child in an attempt to improve attention and the ability to stay seated and focused. The amount of weight and the wearing schedule is determined by the therapist.

Because of the impaired abilities in communication and social relatedness in children with Asperger disorder and autistic disorder, outcomes that are more positive are shown in children who receive early intervention services. The *LEAP* (Learning Experiences—Alternative Program for Preschoolers and Parents) intervention model focuses on children's social development. The theoretic basis of LEAP is social learning theory. Proponents believe that learning can take place through observation of others' behavior and the consequences of that behavior. Proponents recognize that children with developmental disorders need support and assistance to learn vicariously. Typically, developing peers serve as models in integrated preschool classrooms. The goal is to provide autistic children the opportunity to observe and imitate peer behavior in natural settings.

Floor time is a developmental approach to intervention with children who have severe difficulties in relating and communicating. This model is a child-directed play period in which the parents function as the first and primary play partners. Parents are challenged to follow their children's lead while creating situations that address emotional needs. For example, if a child's problem-solving abilities are limited, the parent may set up several problems during the course of a session (e.g., a toy is stuck in a hole or a part of a puzzle is missing). Through this playful process, it is hoped that children will be able to master developmental milestones.

TEACCH (Treatment and Education of Autistic and related Communication Handicapped Children) provides a lifelong continuum of services for individuals and families. Services include assessment, diagnosis, treatment, use of community resources, and supported employment and living situations. The goal of TEACCH is for the adult with the disorder to fit into the community as well as possible (Hudson & Dixon, 2003).

Alternative Therapies

Hyperactive children and children who avoid touch often benefit from positive physical contact with their parents. Touch is a primal need, as necessary for growth and development as food, clothing, and shelter. Touch can be thought of as a nutrient transmitted through the skin in many different ways: holding, cuddling, caressing, and massage. *Massage* is combined with *aromatherapy* when essential oils are used in the massage oil. Molecules of essential oils are so tiny they are quickly absorbed through the skin and enter the intercellular fluid and the circulatory system, bringing healing nutrients to the cells. Benefits are gained not only from the penetration of the oil through the skin, but also from inhalation of the vapor and from direct massage of the skin and muscles. Soothing oils are chamomile, lavender, clary sage, and marjoram. They have significant calming effects and are useful for children who are angry and aggressive. A whole body massage, a back massage, or a simple massage of the hands and feet may decrease anxiety and tension and increase the sense of well-being. The two most suitable essential oils for babies and small children are chamomile and lavender (Fontaine, 2005). See the Complementary/Alternative Therapies box and the procedure for hand massage.

Reflexology stimulates the natural healing processes of the body. Some people find this very useful for hyperactive children. After a few sessions, children will often treat their own hands when upset. However, too much work on the tip of the thumb or the great toe will overstimulate, rather than calm, the child.

Electroencephalographic *biofeedback* records information about brain wave activity from sensors placed on the scalp. The electrodes feed the information to a computer that registers the results on a visual monitor that produces a kind of video game of brain waves. When the person produces waves associated with concentration, the game speeds up. The game slows down when brainwaves associated with daydreaming are produced. This type of computer system is used for mind quieting and attention control in people with these disorders; it also makes learning control of attention and concentration more interactive and fun, especially for children (Fontaine, 2005).

Complementary/Alternative Therapies

How to Help Clients Decrease Anger and Frustration

Massage provides a valuable tactile approach, which, when combined with verbal approaches, communicates nurses' care and compassion. Children and adolescents with poor impulse control, short attention, and low tolerance for frustration may accept and benefit from hand massage (see Figure 17.2 ■).

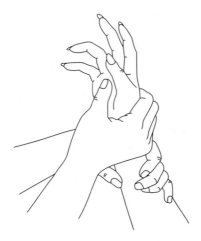

A

While holding the client's hand, place massage oil or lotion on the hand. Gently bend the hand backward and forward to limber the wrist. Grasp each finger and do range of motion exercises.

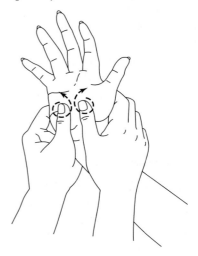

B

With the client's elbow resting on the table, hold the hand upright and massage the palm of the hand with the cushions of your thumbs, using circular movements in opposite directions.

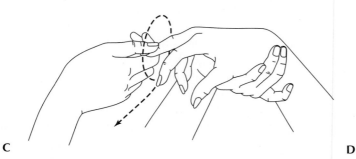

C

Massage each finger from the base to the tip, along all surfaces of the finger.

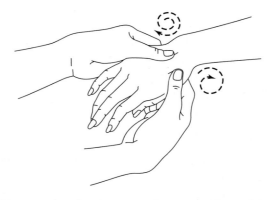

D

Use your thumbs to massage the wrist and top of the hand, using circular movements. Repeat three times. Repeat the entire procedure on the other hand.

Figure 17.2 ■ Procedure for hand massage.

SOURCE: Fontaine, K. L. (2005). *Complementary and alternative therapies for nursing practice* (2nd ed.). Upper Saddle River, NJ: Prentice Hall. Used with permission.

Repetitive transcranial magnetic stimulation (rTMS) uses a magnetic field that passes through the skull, which causes cells in the cerebral cortex to fire. rTMS shows promise as a drug-free option for ADHD and Tourette disorder (Acosta & Leon-Sarmiento, 2003).

Melatonin has been used to treat insomnia in people with autism. The melatonin not only improves sleep, but also decreases irritability and improves alertness and sociability. *SAMe* has been somewhat successful with mood changes secondary to these disorders. The amino acid *tyrosine* may help increase levels of dopamine (Williams, 2006).

Omega-3 fatty acids are critical for neural development and are important cognitive enhancers. In individuals with ADHD, a genetic dysfunction may interfere with ability to metabolize needed fats. Research shows abnormally low levels of omega-3 fatty acids in people with aggression and impulsivity. Omega-3 fatty acids can be found in salmon, tuna, trout, sardines, and anchovies. Flax is the best plant source of these acids. For people who dislike fish, fish oil capsules may be helpful (Brown & Gerbarg, 2000).

Nursing Process

CLIENTS WITH DISORDERS OF CHILDREN AND ADOLESCENTS

ASSESSMENT

No two children or adults present with these disorders in the same way. Different individuals experience different family and cultural environments and different complications and have different personalities and characteristics. This section on nursing assessment considers the behavior, affect, cognition, and interpersonal relationships common to these child and adolescent disorders.

Assessment: Behavior

Common to these disorders is **hyperactive behavior**. As early as the first few weeks of life, a child may show signs of hyperactivity. Infants sleep little, are active in the crib, and cry frequently. Sometimes, an infant manages to escape the confines of the crib to begin a journey of rapid, impulsive activity. Toddlers cannot sit still, and they leave a trail of destruction. The degree of activity may be comparable to that of peers, but the child with hyperactive behavior is unable to stop being active even when appropriate, as in not being able to sit down to eat. Older children frequently leave their classroom seats or constantly fidget in their chairs. They are in constant motion, with fingers or feet tapping, legs swinging, or wiggling in the chair. Adults may experience hyperactivity as a difficulty in relaxing or sitting still. They may often feel restlessness and have a powerful urge to move around. Not all adults are hyperactive and this symptom is least likely to persist in adulthood. A small group of individuals experience **hypoactive behavior**, in which they move much less than other children and may even seem lethargic. These children may be misdiagnosed with chronic fatigue syndrome.

People with child and adolescent disorders are often characterized by *impulsivity*. They do not stop to think before they speak or act. Most of us process our thoughts before we verbalize them. We may meet someone and think, "She's ugly," or "He's fat," but do not say those words aloud. Someone with a spectrum disorder will say their words even as they are thinking them and are sorry before they finish. They do not learn from these experiences because they cannot pause long enough to reflect before they act. Impulsive children have difficulty waiting their turn and often interrupt or intrude on others. In adults, impulsivity may lead to serious problems, such as impulse buying, foolish business investments, or hasty marriages.

Ashley:

> **❝** I love to pick on people. Well, not the slow kids because my brother's slow. Just the kids I don't like. I pick on the geeks. They are the ones that always do their homework and they always listen in class. If I see a geeky kid wearing a nice jersey, I beat him for it. I get him up against the corner, take it off, and tell him if he tells anybody I'll beat him up some more. **❞**

Obsessions (recurrent persistent ideas, thoughts, images, impulses) and **compulsions** (repetitive behavior performed in a stereotyped fashion) may be clinical manifestations of these disorders. People may engage in compulsive checking, touching, counting, or lining up. Rituals may develop related to "evening things up" such as running around a circle three times in one direction and then three times in the opposite direction to "unwind." Routines must be followed exactly; objects must be returned to their rightful place or the child will become agitated. Some children may spend hours in *repetitive behavior* such as stacking blocks or examining and fondling objects. In the more severe disorders, the child may exhibit repetitive physical movements such as clapping, hand flapping, finger snapping, rocking, dipping, and swaying.

Individuals tend to be *inflexible*. They have difficulty with transitions or changes and prefer sameness. They may even panic at the slightest change of a daily routine. Any request to change or to transition from one activity to another is perceived as a stressor and a threat. For example, if the parent asks the child to turn off the television and come to dinner, the response may be one of anger and the child quickly becomes oppositional and defiant. This oppositional behavior is defensive and arises out of an attempt to maintain control when experiencing stress. Adults with these disorders often become frustrated with changes in social plans. If the plan is to go to a specific movie that is then sold out, the response may be one of extreme frustration and anger.

Assessment: Affect

Affective symptoms include *labile mood*, that is, variations in mood characterized by rapid, wide swings of emotion and levels of arousal. Because these children have multiple difficulties in school and problems with family and friendships, they feel inadequate and frustrated. Some may internalize their feelings, becoming withdrawn and depressed. Others may act out these feelings, becoming aggressive, getting into fights, or impulsively striking out. They may seem like Jekyll and Hyde, moving in a split second from pleasant and compliant to angry, argumentative, and controlling.

Individuals with a spectrum disorder are extraordinarily irritable and most experience periods of explosive *rage* over which they have no control. They have tantrums for hours at a time, often for no obvious reason. They may be aware or unaware of the effects of their temper on other family members.

Assessment: Cognition

Inattention is a hallmark of child and adolescent disorders. Inattention or distractibility is defined as the inability to regulate attention or concentration during the performance of a task. Children with a spectrum disorder may be easily distracted by sights (movements of people around them, clouds moving in the sky), sounds (conversations, traffic noises), or internal thoughts that intrude on the task. Although most people have occasional problems with inattention, for these individuals, the problem is so pervasive that it interferes with their day-to-day lives and they often miss important information.

Maria issues an invitation to Jose by saying, "Come to dinner on Friday. It's a potluck and the party starts at 7." Jose shows up at 5 p.m. on Friday without a dish to share since all he heard Maria say is "dinner on Friday."

An extremely short attention span and distractibility are sometimes accompanied by *learning disabilities*. The ability to think abstractly, conceptualize, and generalize are disturbed, as is the ability to assimilate, retain, and recall. Even without learning disabilities, no learning can occur if the child is unable to pay attention. Compared with children without child and adolescent disorders, children with disorders have additional academic problems, underachieve at school, and are placed in special education more frequently.

A common frontal lobe problem is evidenced by difficulties with **executive function**, in which affected individuals are unable to set goals or plan. They are unable to anticipate what may happen and are unable to change plans when necessitated by the situation.

Before long, children begin to recognize that they cannot conform to the expectations of parents and teachers. Some children accept that these expectations are "correct," (internalize expectations) and their inability to achieve them results in loss of self-esteem, helplessness, and depression. This is more typical of girls. Others, more frequently boys, decide that parents and teachers are "wrong" (externalize expectations), develop a defiant attitude, and may act out their frustrations in a hostile manner.

Ashley:

❝ I've been on all the medications. None of them work. I have like six counselors and none of them are any good. They're all worthless. They're not going to help. Nothing will help. They should just let me be. I can control it sometimes. Like, if I really want to, I could. If I really don't, I don't. ❞

Assessment: Interpersonal Relationships

Child and adolescent disorders cause *impaired social interactions*. The primary cause of this difficulty is impulse control problems. For example, when children cannot wait their turn, interrupt and intrude on others, say whatever comes to mind, or explode in rage, their social inappropriateness leads to rejection by peers and social exclusion. The combination of intensity and inflexibility that these children bring to social interactions can only produce conflict with parents, siblings, friends, and teachers. The rejection may lead to low self-esteem, which in turn leads to further behavior of acting out. The lack of social experiences limits the possibilities for healthy interactions that might provide a sense of self-esteem.

Social interactions are severely impaired in those individuals with Asperger disorder or autism. There is an inability to share activities or interest with other people and a lack of social or emotional reciprocity that is the basis of interpersonal relationships. Nonverbal behaviors—such as eye contact—and body postures and gestures that regulate interactions are very difficult for these individuals. For those who are autistic, it is unlikely that they will be capable of adult intimate relationships (American Psychiatric Association, 2000).

As the symptoms become more severe and obvious to people outside the family, others start *blaming the parents* for having no control over the child. Because parents never know when a violent rage will occur, they describe themselves as walking on eggshells. When a rage attack occurs in public, strangers often feel free to give advice on parenting skills. Parents end up feeling criticized, humiliated, incompetent, and extremely angry. Over time, the family may withdraw socially to avoid exposing themselves and their children to public attention and possible ridicule.

Child and adolescent disorders predict multiple problems in adulthood. These problems include occupational problems, lowered educational level, higher rate of divorce/separation, and less contact with supportive others.

At age 38, Brian has been diagnosed with ADHD and is being treated with methylphenidate (Ritalin). He recalls being given some medication for about a year sometime in his early years of elementary school. He describes himself as a very lonely child who was constantly being teased by other children. He could not concentrate at school or home and his father repeatedly told him how inadequate he was. He says the teachers just passed him along so they would not have to teach him for a second year. Before being diagnosed and treated for ADHD, his fellow workers would make fun of him when he could not follow directions from the supervisor. They used to tell him he had a hamster for a brain and would try to provoke him into a physical fight.

Assessment: Cultural Influences

The prevalence of child and adolescent disorders is similar in other countries where the population has been studied. In those cultures with a fast tempo, such as the United States and Japan, the increase in environmental stimulation may contribute to an increase in inattention and overactivity. Immigrant youth from countries with a long history of war and violence may have learned to be aggressive for survival. Therefore, their problematic behavior is a result of reaction to their immediate social context.

Approximately 10% of children in the United States have serious emotional and behavioral disturbances. Many of these children, especially minority youth, receive no treatment or receive inappropriate or inadequate treatment. As with adults, children and adolescents should receive services in the least restrictive setting that is appropriate for their needs. In a study comparing placement for African American versus Euro-American youth, several differences were found. First, a disproportionate number of African American youth were in the mental health system. Second, the Euro-American youth had more substance abuse and emotional problems than the African American youth. Third, African American youth were more likely to be placed in correctional facilities and foster care, whereas Euro-American youth were more likely to be admitted to the hospital. Race and ethnicity may be determinants of the type of placement provided to American youth. More

information is needed about inequity in health care so that uniform levels of care are achieved (Shelton, 2004; Sheppard & Benjamin-Coleman, 2001).

Assessment: Physical

For those with bipolar disorder, manic or depressed episodes increase in response to seasonal variation and during periods of hormonal change that occur during the menstrual cycle in females. There is also difficulty in the thermoregulatory system, as evidenced by persistently low body temperature and asynchronization of circadian rhythms of appetite, energy production, and activity.

Children with bipolar disorders have difficulties with the integration of sensory information. They may overreact to normal social cues; for example, they might misinterpret a casual touch as a threatening gesture. In response, they can become hypervigilant and develop paranoid tendencies. The limbic system, or "emotional brain"—particularly the amygdala—dictates the response to the perceived threats in 100ths of a second, even before the stimulus reaches the cognitive centers of the brain. Dysfunction in the amygdala, in individuals with these disorders, contributes to inappropriate fear, rage, and anxiety.

The brain of people with autism registers sensory experiences too intensely sometimes and barely at all at other times. When overaroused by sensations (internal or external), the person reacts as if the stimulus is irritating or even threatening. Children with autism may shut down or try to get away from the stimuli by screaming, covering their ears, or running away. Often, overly sensitive to sounds, tastes, smells, and sights, they may prefer soft clothing and certain foods, and may be bothered by sounds or sights no one else hears or sees. At other times, they may be oblivious to what is occurring in the environment.

Sleep problems are common for individuals with these disorders. Those who have difficulty falling asleep describe the problem as not being able to "slow down and stop thinking." Others are restless sleepers who wake at the slightest noise and who are then unable to return to sleep. About one third of children with ADHD have nocturnal enuresis, or bedwetting, which is usually outgrown by the age of 10.

The Focused Nursing Assessment feature gives examples of assessment questions you may ask children or adolescents. The type of nursing assessment you conduct will depend on the child's or adolescent's growth and developmental level. Observations of behavior and interactions with others may be the most important tool you will use. Play and art therapy techniques are often used in the assessment process. Family members must also be assessed for accurate data. Teachers often provide valuable data for a total assessment picture. Nurses always learn from their clients. Listen very carefully to what it is like to have one or several of these disorders.

Focused Nursing Assessment	**Clients With Child and Adolescent Disorders**			
Behavior Assessment	**Affective Assessment**	**Cognitive Assessment**	**Social Assessment**	**Physiological Assessment**
Do your friends comment that your behavior is in any way unusual? Do you see your behavior as being different from that of others your age? Are there exact routines that you follow on a daily basis? Can you give me an example of ways you have gotten into trouble with your parents? Teachers? Other adults? Have you been in trouble with the police?	Do your moods or feelings seem to change frequently? Are there certain seasons of the year when you feel better or worse?	How well do you think you are able to concentrate? How difficult is it to get your attention? Do others say they have trouble understanding you? Who is responsible for the mistakes you make?	Has there been increasing conflict with your parents or siblings? Who do you get into physical fights with? Are you having any problems with school? Attendance? Academic performance? Interactions with your friends?	Do others comment that you seem clumsy? Do you dislike other people touching you? Do you seem to be more sensitive to sights and smells than others? (Observe use of eye contact, bizarre movements, use of personal space)

DIAGNOSIS

In synthesizing the assessment data, consider the following: How well are clients and families functioning in daily life? What are their skills and talents? How stable is their affect? How well are they able to communicate? How well do they interact with others? How well do they function at school? The following is a list of the common diagnoses applicable to children and adolescents and their families (North American Nursing Diagnosis Association, 2007).

- Risk for Violence, Directed at Others related to impulsive behavior, anger, antisocial behavior, lack of guilt or remorse over deviant behavior
- Risk for Injury related to overactivity, impulsive behavior
- Impaired Social Interaction related to motor and vocal tics, bizarre motor behaviors, difficulty using language in a social context, difficulty reading body language, impulsive behavior, inability to share pleasurable experiences with others
- Ineffective Individual Coping related to an inability to read nonverbal communication, inadequate listening skills
- Altered Thought Processes related to poor concentration, inability to focus attention, difficulties with executive functions
- Impaired Memory related to inattention, difficulties with executive function
- Self-esteem Disturbance related to low achievement in school, beliefs that others do not understand them, frequent criticism from others, inability to conform to the

expectations of parents and teachers, rejection from peers and adults
- Altered Family Processes related to intensified parent–child conflict, parents feeling criticized, humiliated, and incompetent

OUTCOME IDENTIFICATION AND GOALS

Based on the assessment data, you select outcomes appropriate to the nursing diagnoses. Broad outcomes are:

- Limit inappropriate behavior.
- Stabilize mood.
- Improve interpersonal relationships.

Client goals are specific behavioral prescriptions that you, the client, and significant others have identified as realistic and attainable. The following are examples of goals that may be pertinent to children and adolescents:

- Acknowledge the effect of your own behavior on social interactions.
- Improve social interaction skills, such as cooperation, assertiveness, trustworthiness, and responsibility.
- Acknowledge personal strengths.
- Identify factors that precipitate violent behaviors.
- Practice behaviors that generate self-confidence.
- Identify alternative ways to cope with problems.
- Stay on task.

NURSING CARE PLAN for Clients With Disorders of Children and Adolescents

Managing Anger
Nursing Diagnosis: Client at Risk for Ineffective Coping

Outcomes: Clients will identify triggers to angry outbursts and implement anger management strategies.

Children and adolescents with these disorders do not start the day planning on screaming obscenities at or threatening parents, teachers, or nurses. Instead, they get caught up in situations that seem beyond their control. When clients' anger begins to escalate, ask yourself: What is the source of frustration? What is the client capable of right now? What issues are essential to address right now? What situations should be avoided now? What situations can be adapted now? See chapter 8 ∞ for further information on managing clients who are aggressive.

Intervention	Rationale	Goal
Identify specific situations that may routinely lead to explosive episodes.	They get caught up in situations that seem beyond their control.	Lists common triggers
When trigger situations occur, de-escalate the behavior with diversional activities, physical exercise, or emotional/physical space.	This prevents out-of-control episodes.	Responds to de-escalation interventions
When calm, discuss nature and function of anger.	Appropriate use of anger leads to desirable, productive change.	Verbalizes function of appropriate anger
Discuss inappropriate use of anger that is too intense.	This level of anger leads to problems with other people.	Identifies expressions of inappropriate anger
Discuss physical sensation and usual thought patterns when anger begins, escalates, and lessens.	Recognizing cues is an important step in anger management.	Identifies personal anger cues
Teach self-calming procedures as listed in Box 17.3.	This controls escalating intensity of anger (Larson, 2005).	Uses a variety of self-calming techniques
Discuss actual and hypothetical situations in which clients see other people as hostile.	People who get angry quickly often see others as hostile, miss pertinent social cues in the here-and-now, and respond based on memories of similar situations.	Identifies past experiences
Role-play various responses to the above situations.	Replacing familiar responses with new responses takes a good deal of practice time.	Role-plays situations; practices new responses in real-life situations

Managing Hyperactivity
Nursing Diagnosis: Client at Risk for Fatigue

Outcomes: Client avoids environmental triggers to hyperactivity and establishes a balanced routine of activity.

Clients who are hyperactive or in a manic episode may become exhausted when excessive levels of activity are combined with decreased awareness of fatigue. When intervening, you must first get the person's attention by calling his or her name or lightly touching the arm.

Intervention	Rationale	Goal
If the environment (a person or situation) is overstimulating, redirect or remove the client to a quieter area.	This facilitates self-control.	Responds to redirection
Teach clients to avoid stimulating places such as school sporting events, dances, or shopping malls.	Clients who are in hypomanic or manic state will escalate in these situations.	Verbalizes need to avoid overstimulation
Limit intake of caffeinated food and fluids.	This facilitates self-control.	Chooses noncaffeinated food and fluids

continued

NURSING CARE PLAN for a Client With Disorders of Children and Adolescents

Managing Hyperactivity *continued*
Nursing Diagnosis: Client at Risk for Fatigue

Intervention	Rationale	Goal
Teach clients to establish a routine that includes a balance of structured time (school, homework, physical exercise) and quiet times.	Balance in lifestyle activities facilitates self-control.	Creates and posts list in visible place
Discuss need to take medications on prescribed schedule.	Failure to do so may contribute to hyperactive behavior.	Takes medications as ordered
When giving instructions or explanations, call by name or lightly touch the arm.	You must first get the person's attention.	Pays attention
Use simple, concrete language; ask to repeat what they heard; give one instruction at a time; give positive feedback.	Attention span is very short so instructions must be given in short steps.	Accomplishes task appropriately.

Setting Limits
Nursing Diagnosis: Client at Risk for Ineffective Coping

Outcomes: Client makes positive choices about behavior.

All children, and particularly those with mental disorders, benefit from clear, predictable routine and structure.

Intervention	Rationale	Goal
State rules and expectations clearly according to developmental level.	Clear, predictable routine and structure help clients maintain self-control.	Verbalizes an understanding of expectations
Establish logical and meaningful consequences for noncompliant behavior.	Consequences are different from punishment. Punishment is retaliatory rather than corrective. Consequences relate logically to the misbehavior.	Parents are able to institute this process
Provide frequent, immediate, and consistent feedback on behaviors.	This provides input to behavior to increase clients' level of insight.	Acknowledges feedback
Give client a choice between behaving in a correct manner or continuing with the misbehavior.	This fosters a sense of internal locus of control.	Opts to change misbehavior to appropriate behavior
Use time-outs with younger children— 3 to 10 minutes depending on developmental level.	A "boring" room provides safety for clients without stimulation or attention.	Calms down
Explain reason for time-out and what it is intended to do.	The reason is the actual misbehavior and intent is for child to cool off.	Verbalizes an understanding of the time-out; behavior becomes more appropriate

Improving Social Skills
Nursing Diagnosis: Client at Risk for Social Isolation

Outcomes: Clients will interact appropriately with others.

It is important to help children and adolescents with these disorders become socially integrated and not a disruptive influence in the family, school, or with peers. These individuals have found that any attention is better than no attention at all. Children sometimes learn that it is easier to get noticed by behaving in negative or foolish ways, than by being "good." The best thing you can do in these circumstances is to minimize the amount of attention given for negative behavior and to maximize the amount of attention given for positive behavior. Obviously, it is not always possible to ignore negative behavior. When necessary, deal with the behavior immediately, decisively, and as quietly as possible.

People who are impulsive may not stop to consider consequences before acting. They tend to become intrusive and interruptive and are totally unaware that their behavior is irritating to others.

NURSING CARE PLAN for a Client With Disorders of Children and Adolescents

Improving Social Skills *continued*
Nursing Diagnosis: Client at Risk for Social Isolation

Individuals with these disorders are often so aggressive and belligerent that they offend and alienate others. It is important to teach them the differences among passive, aggressive, and assertive behavior. Passive behavior is behavior in which people fail to express their needs and feelings and allow their rights to be violated by others. Aggressive behavior is inconsiderate of other's rights and feelings and destructive to interpersonal relationships. Aggressive behavior results in arguments and power struggles. Assertive behavior is asking for what one wants (respect for self) or acting to get it in a way that respects other people. Assertiveness is often associated with positive self-esteem. It is also an attitude that says, "Here I am, a person with unique gifts to give the world. Who are you? What do you bring?"

Assertiveness training is a program that teaches individuals ways to change negative self-concepts, reduce anxiety, identify strengths, and increase self-awareness. Assertiveness training typically includes discussion of ideas concerning assertiveness, practice of communication skills, making requests, refusing requests, giving and receiving positive comments, and handling criticism. Assertiveness training programs teach people how to manage anger.

Along with assertiveness training exercises, clients must learn how to resolve interpersonal conflict. As a nurse, you discuss and model the processes of compromising, negotiating, and dealing with frustration. Teaching the problem-solving process will help clients generate alternative solutions to problems and teaches children how to resolve their own problems. See chapter 7 ∞ for more detail on problem solving.

Intervention	Rationale	Goal
Teach social skills through discussion, modeling, and practice.	Social competence determines success as an adult.	Interacts appropriately with others
Discuss trustworthiness—do what you say you will do.	Trust is a necessary component of social relationships.	Acts in a trustworthy way with others
Discuss responsibility—acknowledge own contributions to situations in which they are involved. See chapter 9 ∞ for detail on social skills training.	Responsibility is a component of effective interpersonal relationships.	Acts in a responsible manner

Promoting Effective Communication Skills
Nursing Diagnosis: Client at Risk for Impaired Communication

Outcomes: Clients will communicate an understanding of nonverbal communication, actively listen to others, and give others an opportunity to speak.

Children and adolescents with mental disorders are often unable to read nonverbal communication. Because two thirds of communication is considered to be nonverbal, it is critical that they learn to observe, understand, and respond to nonverbal cues. They must also learn how to be a "self-observer," paying attention to what messages they are communicating nonverbally. (Review nonverbal communication in chapter 7 ∞.) If their listening skills are inappropriate, they must be *taught the body language of active listening*. Use the mnemonic device, **OFFER**, as a way to help them remember:

O = open posture
F = face person
F = lean forward
E = make eye contact
R = relax

Nonverbal children, such as those with autism, may be able to learn alternative ways to communicate. Young children may be able to use customized picture books to let others know their thoughts and needs. Pictures might include food choices, clothes to wear, activity choices, and activity schedules. The written and spoken word should accompany the picture. Some people with autism are able to "talk" with the assistance of a computer. A variety of products are available that, often, are covered by insurance or school districts.

Intervention	Rationale	Goal
Teach clients to repeat what they have heard the teacher or other person say.	Often they miss important information the first time around. Repeating what was heard will prevent problems.	Uses repetition to clarify understanding
Encourage them not to blurt out whatever comes to mind. Teach them to stop and process thoughts silently before speaking.	Unfiltered thoughts can indeed cause harm, even when harm in unintended.	Monitors own verbal expressions

continued

NURSING CARE PLAN for a Client With Disorders of Children and Adolescents

Promoting Effective Communication Skills   *continued*
Nursing Diagnosis: Client at Risk for Impaired Communication

Intervention	Rationale	Goal
Teach them to ask friends and family to let them know when they are talking too much.	They often have little perception of how they monopolize conversations.	Utilizes feedback from others to limit long monologues
Suggest a vibrating watch and set it for 3 minutes at the beginning of interactions.	This is a silent reminder to stop talking and give the other person a chance to talk.	Participates in give-and-take conversation

Enhancing Memory
Nursing Diagnosis: Client at Risk for Impaired Memory

Outcomes: Client utilizes techniques to improve memory.

A number of coping techniques can be taught to people who are experiencing short-term memory problems.

Intervention	Rationale	Goal
Use self-adhesive notes on mirrors, staircases, notebooks, dashboards, or any other place.	This provides visual reminders in places that catch one's attention.	Makes and responds to visual reminders
Use a tape recorder, electronic message system, or home answering machine to note assignments, due dates, appointments, etc.	Memory is "tweaked" when they listen to their messages.	Utilizes a memory enhancing system
Encourage a daily to-do list, which is done the night before or first thing in the morning. Break list down into periods such as before school, during school, after school, and the evening.	Written list will help client stay on task.	Accomplishes desired daily activities
Encourage leisure time and relaxation time in the daily list.	Learning is such a hyperfocused activity that they need frequent breaks to release build up of excess energy.	Takes time to relax; participates in leisure activities

Fostering Self-Esteem
Nursing Diagnosis: Client at Risk for Chronic Low Self-Esteem

Outcomes: Clients will verbalize positive qualities and celebrate achievements.

Self-esteem enhancement means that you support people's persistence, competence, and their overall ability to deal effectively with life's problems. These children need assistance to maintain a healthy self-esteem in the face of their difficulties. You further this assistance by giving them a sense of acceptance, belonging, and security.

In one study, preadolescents diagnosed with ADHD participated in a school-based, nurse-facilitated support group twice a week for 4 weeks. The experimental group focused on social skills training and self-esteem improvement. At the end of the study, the students in the experimental group scored significantly higher on perceptions of self-worth, physical appearance, acceptance by others, and athletic capabilities than the students in the control group (Frame, Kelly, & Bayley, 2003). Nurses in a variety of settings could establish and lead similar support groups to help children cope with self-esteem problems.

Intervention	Rationale	Goal
Encourage hobbies and interests at which they can be successful.	Success in leisure activities fosters positive self-esteem.	Participates successfully in leisure activities
Teach positive self-talk, e.g., "I can do this. I am a worthwhile person."	Identifying their strengths such as smart, funny, respectful, good at math, etc. fosters positive self-esteem.	Engages in positive self-talk

NURSING CARE PLAN for a Client With Disorders of Children and Adolescents

Fostering Self-Esteem   *continued*
Nursing Diagnosis: Client at Risk for Chronic Low Self-Esteem

Intervention	Rationale	Goal
Encourage self-reliance through responsibilities at home and at school.	Responsibilities help them feel needed and give a sense of purpose and achievement.	Assumes appropriate responsibilities for developmental age
Teach them that mistakes are okay.	Mistakes are a minor setback and an opportunity for learning.	Acknowledges mistakes and takes corrective actions
Celebrate their achievements.	As they develop better self-control, their self-esteem rises.	Acknowledges behavioral progress
Encourage daily self-evaluation. Ask the following questions: What have I tried that was new today? What have I done today better than before? Who are the people I have helped today? Who has helped me today? What gave me the most pleasure today?	Review of positive interactions and successes changes the focus from negative events to positive events that improve self-esteem.	Participates in accurate self-evaluation

Developing an Exercise Routine
Nursing Diagnosis: Client at Risk for Activity Intolerance

Outcomes: Clients will implement a daily exercise routine.

All children and adolescents behave and pay attention better under circumstances in which their needs for physical activity are met.

Intervention	Rationale	Goal
Encourage them to plan a daily schedule for physical activities.	Having a plan in place helps focus attention.	Develops a daily plan
Encourage them to keep an exercise diary or log.	A written review helps maintain the exercise program.	Keeps a daily log
Encourage them to find a friend who will exercise with them.	This is another way to stay on task with the exercise program.	Exercises with a friend
Encourage stretching exercises at times throughout the day.	Breaking up the routine of sitting at a desk fosters better attention and learning.	Does stretches periodically throughout the day
Encourage participation in competitive games.	This not only provides exercise but they also learn how to function as team members and how to play by the rules. This is a good venue for developing friendships.	Participates in games. Verbalizes an enjoyment of being a team member.

IMPLEMENTATION

Children and adolescents should not be "blamed" for their symptoms, nor do they "cause" their symptoms. They do, however, share responsibility for managing their symptoms along with their parents and the treatment team. As a nurse, your focus is on providing these clients with the tools necessary to take an increasing responsibility for symptom management.

Children experiencing such a range of difficulties need help in many aspects of their lives. The goal is to help clients function more effectively in their social and emotional lives and achieve balance in their behavior. That means you provide nurturing, compassionate care balanced with a strong emphasis on self-discipline, personal accountability, and social responsibility. Be verbally and physically assertive and provide consistent, confident messages without being demeaning to the client.

BOX 17.3 | **Teaching: Self-statements for Dealing With Anger**

Preparing for Instigation

- This is going to upset me, but I know how to deal with it.
- I can work out a plan to handle this.
- I can manage the situation. I know how to regulate my anger.
- There won't be any need for an argument.
- Easy does it. Remember to keep your sense of perspective.

Impact and Confrontation

- Stay calm. Just continue to relax.
- As long as I keep my cool I'm in control.
- I don't need to prove myself.
- I'm not going to let him get to me.
- There is no need to doubt myself. What he says doesn't matter.

Coping With Arousal

- My muscles are starting to feel tight. Time to relax and slow things down.
- I have a right to be annoyed, but let's keep the lid on.
- Time to take a deep breath.

- He would probably like me to get really angry. Well, I'm going to disappoint him.
- Let's try a cooperative approach. Maybe we are both right.

Reflecting on the Provocation: Conflict Unresolved

- Forget about the aggravation. Thinking about it only makes me upset.
- There are difficult situations, and they take time to straighten out.
- I'll get better at this with practice.
- Don't take it personally.
- Take a deep breath and think positive thoughts.

Reflecting on the Provocation: Conflict Resolved

- I handled that one pretty well. It worked!
- That wasn't as hard as I thought.
- It could have been a lot worse.
- I guess I've been getting upset for too long when it wasn't even necessary.
- I'm doing better at this all the time.

Helping children and families cope with autistic disorder is intense, with many specific interventions. Entire books are devoted to the subject. Hence, interventions designed for people with autism are beyond the scope of this text.

Family Stress

The desired outcome is that clients and families will use effective coping techniques, implement stress management techniques, conduct regular family council meetings, develop clear family rules, use positive and negative consequences, structure the home environment, and remain connected to extended family and friends.

These disorders profoundly change the life of the person with the disorder and the lives of those who care for her or him. Symptoms are often disruptive, and social impairments can stress the family system. The stress also contributes to increased rates of mood and anxiety disorders among family members. Parents of children with autism report more family problems, more marital problems, more depression, and more social isolation than parents of typically developing children or parents of children who are severely and persistently mentally ill. The greater the severity of the child's symptoms, the greater the degree of parental stress (Birnbaum et al., 2005).

Parents who use a style of escape–avoidance to manage their children's problems are at higher risk for depression, isolation, and relationship problems. Examples of this style of coping include hoping for miracles, fantasy solutions, distancing themselves or avoiding others, and food or drugs. Discourage the use of escape–avoidance patterns. Encourage parents to spend time with supportive peers. Help them face reality through the problem-solving process. It may be appropriate to refer parents to couples or family therapy.

Family members are an important resource to clients and professionals. Caregivers have the most immediate and consistent impact on their children's lives, and it is best to view them as part of the solution. The nurse must understand and empathize with the distress that relatives experience when trying to cope with the disruption created by their children and adolescents.

Suggest to parents that they not blame themselves or the other parent by helping them understand that "we do not get to choose the genes we get or the genes we give." It is very important that parents move on from "who or what is to blame" to "what can we do about this now."

Parents are often exhausted from sleepless nights and endless meetings with teachers and therapists. Teach stress management techniques to all family members. Examples of these techniques are:

- Good sleep habits
- Healthful eating
- Regular exercise
- Balance between work and play
- Avoidance of overload on time and energy
- Deep breathing, muscle relaxation, guided imagery

It is also important that parents make time for other children in the family who do not have a disorder. It is important that these children do not feel neglected or lost in the shuffle. Giving the other children positive attention may prevent them from acting out to get attention.

Suggest that the family schedule weekly family council meetings. In an atmosphere of give-and-take, every family

Clinical Interactions A Client With Bipolar Disorder and Oppositional Defiant Disorder

Seventeen-year-old Ben was brought to the hospital after his mom called the police and told them Ben was attacking her. Ben states that he often lives with his dad, which he much prefers. He verbalizes a lot of anger toward his mother. He says she did not treat him well growing up. She was always yelling at him and punishing him instead of giving him the love he needed and wanted. In the interaction, you see evidence of:

- Concrete thinking
- Dichotomous thinking
- Hyperactive behavior
- Hostility
- Flight of ideas
- Grandiose thinking

NURSE: *"Earlier in group, it was suggested that everyone write two goals they want to achieve when they go home. Would you like to work on that for a while?"* [offers pencil and paper]

BEN: "Yeah sure, that would be great." [tapping fingers, running fingers through hair] "Well, I already know what my short-term goals are. You see, when I go home I want to be close to my father. Like tell him stuff and talk with him." [His writing is scratchy and unclear] "I definitely want to be close to my dad. And I want to clean up the house. That helps me calm down. Oh yeah, I want to recycle." [laughs]

NURSE: *"Are you close to your dad now?"*

BEN: "Oh yeah. I live with him. I'm 17 years old. I'm not close to my mother though. I hate her right now, like I hate her actual being. I mean I love her unconditionally, but I hate her right now." [Starts a very fast rap song about all of the negative things his mom did to him as a child. Ends with him singing angrily how he wished she could have taught him and shown him love instead of anger.]

NURSE: *"You seem angry about how your mom treated you when you were growing up."*

BEN: "Yeah, well that's the way it was. Heck, she cares more about the kids she baby sits than me. And I do have another short-term goal. I want to get into the music business. You know, get into the studio." [tapping fingers, running fingers through hair, looking around]

NURSE: *"What are some ways you could get information about getting into the studio?"*

BEN: "Oh, I could look in the phone book." [writes that down] "Hmm, my friend Andy has connections. I could call him up and hook up with him." [writes that down]

NURSE: *"Those seem like good ways of starting."*

BEN: "Man, you help me so much." [smiling]

NURSE: *"Make sure you keep that paper so you can refer back to it. That way, if you forget what your plan is, you will have everything written down."*

BEN: [is distracted by other clients and starts laughing]

NURSE: *"In group, you mentioned you also wanted to go into the Navy eventually."*

BEN: "Yeah, maybe. I want to be a seaman. Or maybe go into the reserves. That's long term though, because you have to stay a while. And I don't want to stay in for 2 years."

NURSE: *"You would have to make that commitment if that is what you decide."*

BEN: "Yeah, I guess." [acts nonchalant]

NURSE: *"You said earlier that you also wanted to go to college."*

BEN: "You know what else I am going to do after that? A preacher." [nodding] "I was told at a young age that I would be a preacher. You know that flea market near here? Well, there was a psychic there once when I was a little shorty who said that is what I would do and I believe her. I do." [starts a rap about putting fear of the holy ghost into people] "Cuz I only have one life to live and I've got to keep going. Keep it going smooth. I used to drive an '84 Riviera. Then I sold it for $800. Then I bought an '86 Camaro yellow and black just like your name badge. Those are the colors of the gang I used to be in that I told you about."

NURSE: *"You have looked at your goals now. How do you feel about that?"*

BEN: "I feel great. I can't wait to get out of here." [Starts another rap. This time it makes no sense and is not understandable.] "Okay. I gotta go now. Thanks for talking to me."

---

member has the opportunity to discuss relationships with other family members and to discuss any functions of the household. Topics usually include household chores, daily schedules, and leisure activities. Other topics regarding family functioning are discussed as the need arises.

Help parents work together to establish clear and firm rules. One important rule is that all family members are expected not to hurt one another through words or actions. Other family rules vary according to each family. It is most helpful if the parents write out the list of rules with the attendant consequences for noncompliance. The consequences should be a two-tier system. If the child ignores the first con-

sequence, there is a second consequence until the first one is completed. The list should be posted in a visible location. Parents must be careful not to make the consequence difficult for themselves. If the consequence is harder on the parent than on the child, children become empowered in their misbehavior.

Parents must also learn to give positive reinforcement for appropriate behavior. Give praise and positive feedback when it is legitimate. The goal is to develop more positive, warm, and nurturing patterns of interaction within the family. Parents can help children participate in pleasurable activities with other children. They also should schedule parent–child fun as a way to reinforce positive experiences and feelings.

Using Research Evidence   Depression and ADHD

LeBlanc, N., & Morrin, D. (2004). Depressive symptoms and associated factors in children with attention deficit hyperactivity disorder. *Journal of Child and Adolescent Psychiatric Nursing, 17* (2), 49–55.

What is the study about?

Attention deficit hyperactivity disorder (ADHD) is a common developmental problem in children, and it is often associated with depression. This study compared ADHD-diagnosed children with other children for depressive symptoms. Also, the researchers investigated whether depression in children with ADHD might be influenced by individual and family factors.

How was the study done?

This was a quantitative study based upon Roy's Adaptation Model and using a convenience sample of 34 children diagnosed with ADHD and 34 non-ADHD children. All children were selected from normal classes in eight elementary classrooms in the Quebec City area, and parental consents were obtained. Children with ADHD were identified through school health records, which indicated that the child was medically diagnosed with ADHD by their pediatrician or psychiatrist. All participants' ages ranged from 7–12 years, and none had a history of mental retardation, physical disabilities, or chronic illness. Most children with ADHD (90.9%) were taking prescribed stimulants during the course of the study. Sociodemographic data (individual and family factors) were obtained through a parental questionnaire. The 15-minute Children's Depressive Inventory (CDI) was administered during school hours to obtain self-rated, symptom-oriented information on dimensions of depression. These dimensions included negative mood, interpersonal problems, ineffectiveness, anhedonia (feeling of not having fun at school or home), and negative self-esteem. Data were analyzed through frequency measurement.

What were the results of the study?

In the non-ADHD group, significantly more parents had more than 12 years of formal education (55% in the non-ADHD group and 28% in the ADHD group). The non-ADHD group's families reported a higher income, but a slightly lower employment level: 52% currently employed compared to 60% in the ADHD group. Results of the CDI showed that, in both groups, the children's most severe depressive symptoms were in the dimension of anhedonia. For both groups, the mildest symptom area was interpersonal problems. The overall CDI scores showed that depressive symptoms were significantly more common for children with ADHD. Of children living with ADHD, 14.7% endorsed the suicide item and indicated possible clinical depression; none of the non-ADHD children did so. Depression severity did not correlate significantly with child's age, parent's level of education, working status, presence of illness, family type, or income. Comparing the two groups of children, the researchers found no differences in the ways that depression severity might have been affected by individual or family factors.

What additional questions might I have?

Would the results have differed significantly with a larger, randomly obtained sample? Could the children in the ADHD group taking stimulants have experienced any side effects from their prescribed medications that affected their emotions and/or responses? Would the results of this study be different with another cultural group?

How can I use this study?

Nurses working with children diagnosed with ADHD should consider that the child might also be living with symptoms of depression. Young children should be assessed for both ADHD and depression, and appropriate referrals should be made as needed.

SOURCE: Contributed by Dolores Huffman, PhD, RN, Associate Professor of Nursing, Purdue University Calumet, Hammond, Indiana.

Because they are often very disorganized, these children and adolescents benefit from a structured home environment. Parents and children can establish the same routine every day, from waking to bedtime. There should be a place for everything, from school supplies and backpacks, to clothing and toys. Because they are so easily distracted, they should have a clean, quiet study area with no distractions from media or other family members. They should structure frequent, short breaks in homework to release pent up energy and improve concentration.

Families of children and adolescents with mental disorders are often socially isolated. They may be too fearful or ashamed to bring their children to social gatherings. It is important that parental and child support networks be developed. See Community Resources at the end of this chapter.

Families may need social services to help them cope with the tremendous financial strain. Mental disorders are not covered by insurance to the same degree as physical disorders. There may be a need for specialized childcare, which can be very expensive. Some parents may have to decrease the amount of outside employment to help their children.

The Serenity Prayer, an important piece of 12-step self-help groups, can also be used by all family members:

"God, grant me the serenity to accept the things I cannot change *(do not deny the disorder, meet it head on)*, the courage to change the things I can *(social and communication skills, medications)*, and the wisdom to know the difference."

EVALUATION

To complete the nursing process, the nurse evaluates clients' responses to nursing interventions based on the selected out-comes. It is seldom an all-or-nothing phenomenon, but rather an ongoing process of movement toward the goal of better health and improved quality of life.

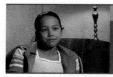

ROAD: Assessment

Critical Thinking Questions

Go to the CD-ROM to assess Ashley by answering the following critical thinking questions based on what you have **R**ead about Ashley and **O**bserved on the videos.

1. Ashley reacts to her life and problems at school in segment A of your student ROAD CD-ROM for chapter 17. Listen to her ver-balizations and observe her nonverbals to assess how she feels. Describe what you observed and your assessment of her emo-tional reaction. Provide rationales for your interpretation.

2. Ashley talks about her counseling relationships and her general outlook on life in segment B of your student ROAD CD-ROM for chapter 17. What is your assessment of Ashley's feelings about her life and herself? Support your answer(s).

3. Ashley continues talking in segment C of your student ROAD CD-ROM for chapter 17. Considering Ashley's comments from segments B and C, what additional assessment about Ashley's early life is important for you to evaluate? Provide rationales for your answer.

4. Ashley tells you about what she wishes she could do in her life in segment D of your student ROAD CD-ROM for chapter 17.

What insight do you gain about what Ashley values? Explain your answer.
The interviewer's reply to Ashley's statements about obtaining a college education and "being a" veterinarian or pediatri-cian is one of acknowledgement of the work and commit-ment required to achieve such goals. What type of therapeutic communication might you have used if you wanted to reinforce and promote Ashley's self-esteem and reinforce motivation to improve her behavior? Support your answer(s).

5. Ashley's doctor has prescribed atomoxetine (Strattera) for her di-agnosis of ADHD. Based on what you have learned about her emotional status and feelings, what specific adverse reaction will you assess for related to this medication? Explain.

ROAD: DEVELOP A CARE PLAN

 Go to the CD-ROM to Develop a care plan based on your assessment of Ashley. Identify nursing diagnoses, outcomes, goals, and interventions.

SOURCE: Contributed by Susan Siwinski-Hebel, RN, MSN.

Focus Your Study

OBJECTIVES	KEY CONCEPTS
1. Compare and contrast the different theories regarding the etiology of dis-orders of children and adolescents.	■ These disorders are the result of many genes acting together to alter neurotransmis-sion. ■ Small frontal lobes correlate with an inability to transition from one activity to an-other, lack of control over behavior, impulsivity, short attention span, and mood in-stability. ■ In some cases, artificial food coloring and benzoate preservatives in food contribute to hyperactive behavior in children.
2. Discuss the psychopharmacological treatment of the symptoms of child-hood and adolescent disorders.	■ The most commonly used stimulants are methylphenidate (Ritalin, Concerta, Meta-date, Daytrana); dextroamphetamine (Dexedrine); amphetamine and dextroamphet-amine (Adderall); and pemoline (Cylert). ■ A newer, nonstimulant medication is atomoxetine (Strattera). ■ Modafinil (Provigil) is used for the hypoactive form of ADHD and for narcolepsy.

continued

continued

3. Outline the different treatment options for the disorders of children and adolescents.

- School nurses are responsible for meeting the health needs of emotionally and mentally disabled students.
- Occupational therapists have designed weighted vests that seem to improve the attention of children with ADHD and autistic spectrum disorders.
- The LEAP program for preschoolers and parents focuses on children's social development.
- Floor time is a play process that helps children with autism master developmental milestones.
- TEACCH provides a lifelong continuum of services for individuals and families.

4. Outline the assessment process for a client with a childhood or adolescent disorder.

- Behaviors common to these disorders:
  - Hyperactive
  - Impulsive
  - Obsessions and compulsions
  - Inflexible
- Affect common to these disorders:
  - Labile mood
  - Explosive rage
- Cognition common to these disorders:
  - Inattention
  - Learning disabilities
- Difficulty with executive function
- Internalize or externalize expectations from others
- Interpersonal difficulties common to these disorders:
  - Impaired interactions with others related to interruptions, intrusions, rage, lack of social or emotional reciprocity, or withdrawal

5. Use the nursing process to develop a comprehensive plan of care for a client with a childhood or adolescent disorder.

- Managing anger:
  - Discuss the function of anger.
  - Identify triggers.
  - Recognize cues.
  - Teach self-calming techniques.
  - Role-play other responses.
- Dealing with hyperactivity:
  - Maintain a calm environment.
  - Establish daily routines.
- Setting limits:
  - Clearly state rules and expectations.
  - Provide frequent, immediate, and consistent feedback.
  - Establish logical consequences for misbehavior.
  - Time-outs are effective for younger children and usually last for 3 to 10 minutes.
- Contracting for behavior:
  - A contract consists of behavioral expectations, how these can be achieved, and the reward when the behavior is achieved.
  - Token economies are rewards for positive behavior utilizing concrete rewards such as a privilege or a favorite activity.
- Fostering social skills:
  - Maximize the amount of attention given for positive behavior.
  - Discuss likeability factors such as trustworthiness, responsibility, and a sense of humor.
  - Model these skills and have clients practice them.
- Providing assertiveness training:
  - Teach the difference between passive, aggressive, and assertive behavior.
  - Implement assertiveness training.
  - Teach conflict resolution.
  - Teach problem-solving process.
- Enhancing memory:
  - Teach the use of self-adhesive notes as reminders.
  - Make specific, daily to-do lists.
- Fostering self-esteem:
  - Celebrate their achievements.
  - Teach positive self-talk.
  - Encourage self-reliance.
  - Review daily achievements.
- Promoting exercise:
  - Plan daily physical activities.
  - Encourage keeping an exercise diary or log.
  - Find an exercise friend.
  - Design team games such as volleyball.

6. Discuss the key points in effectively communicating with a person with a childhood or adolescent disorder.

- Give instructions or explanations in simple, concrete language.
- Clearly state rules and expectations.
- Provide frequent, immediate, and consistent feedback.
- Promoting communication skills:
  - Teach clients the body language of active listening.
  - Ask clients to repeat what they have heard.
  - Teach clients to slow down and process silently before speaking.
  - Determine an environmental cue that they should give others an opportunity to speak.
  - For those who are nonverbal, use customized picture books to communicate. Pictures might include food choices, clothes to wear, activity choices, and activity schedules.

7. Develop illness management teaching plans for a client with a childhood or adolescent disorder.

- Encourage parents to spend time with supportive peers.
- Teach stress management techniques.
- Make time for other children in the family.
- Suggest family council meetings.
- Help parents set clear and firm rules.
- Teach parents how to provide positive reinforcement.
- Help parents establish a structured home environment.
- Encourage parental and child support networks.

Explore MediaLink

For review questions, case studies, and other resources for this chapter see the Pearson Health MediaLink CD-ROM that accompanies this book and the Companion Website.

DVD-ROM
- Audio Glossary
- NCLEX-RN® Review Questions
- ROAD to Critical Thinking: *Ashley*
- Animations/Videos
  - Autism: Case Study–Parts 1–4
  - Autism: What It Is–Parts 1 and 2

Companion Website www.prenhall.com/fontaine
- Audio Glossary
- NCLEX-RN® Review Questions
- Case Study
  - The Child With Autism
- Care Plan
  - Oppositional Defiant Disorder
- Critical Thinking
  - Psychopharmalogical Treatment for the Depressed Adolescent
- MediaLink Application
  - Parent Stress in Primary Caregivers of Psychiatrically Hospitalized Children
  - Books for Clients & Families
  - Community Resources

NCLEX-RN® Review Questions

17-1. An adolescent is admitted to the hospital with a diagnosis of conduct disorder. The parent asks why the adolescent gets into so much trouble. The nurse informs the parent that there are several thoughts about the cause of this disorder. Which of the following statements indicates that the parent needs more information about the causative factors of conduct disorder?
1. "Yes, my child fits in with the group so well."
2. "There is a cousin who also has this diagnosis."
3. "Drinking alcohol is a part of our family life."
4. "Since age 3, this child has been hard to manage."

17-2. A child diagnosed with attention deficit hyperactivity disorder (ADHD) is receiving methylphenidate (Ritalin, Concerta). The nurse recognizes which of the following behaviors as a therapeutic outcome of this medication?
1. Improved academic performance
2. Increased ability to concentrate
3. Less defiant behavior
4. Better manners

17-3. A school nurse is assessing a 5-year-old child. Which assessment finding should the nurse report to the child protection agency?
1. Marginalized family functioning
2. Marital disharmony in the family
3. Unexplained bruises on the child
4. Delay in developmental achievement

17-4. A nurse is providing counseling to a group of teenagers who have lost two friends in an automobile accident. One of the teenagers walks out of the group and states, "I don't want to talk about this, there is no fairness in life." The nurse recognizes this behavior as:
1. Denial.
2. Anger.
3. Bargaining.
4. Depression.

17-5. A 6-year-old boy with attention deficit hyperactivity disorder (ADHD) is acting aggressively toward the other children in a day care center. The best action for the nurse is to:
1. Tell the boy his behavior is bad.
2. Direct his mother to take him home.
3. Ignore the behavior.
4. Take him to another room to play out his feelings.

17-6. A teen, attending a substance abuse group, threatens other clients and swears at the nurse. Which response by the nurse is the most helpful to the client?
1. "What does the group think about this behavior?"
2. "Why are you angry at the group?"
3. "Sit down and join the group."
4. "I will tell the doctor about your anger."

17-7. A nurse is counseling a teenager with depression whose parent died 2 months ago. Before teaching the steps of the grief process to the client, the nurse should assess the client's current stage of grief. Which of the following statements indicates guilt?
1. "I feel upset with my friends who still have parents."
2. "I wish I had been nicer."
3. "I just feel like I can't do anything."
4. "I can't talk about the death."

See Appendix D for Answers.

References

Acosta, M. T., & Leon-Sarmiento, F. E. (2003). Repetitive transcranial magnetic stimulation (rTMS): New tool, new therapy, and new hope for ADHD. *Current Medical Research and Opinion, 19*(2), 125–130.

American Psychiatric Association. (2000). *Diagnostic and statistical manual of mental disorders* (4th ed., Text Revision). Washington, DC: Author.

Bateman, B., Warner, J. O., Hutchinson, E., Dean, T., Rowlandson, P., Gant, C., et al. (2005). The effects of a double blind, placebo controlled, artificial food colourings and benzoate preservative challenge on hyperactivity in a general population sample of preschool children. *Archives of Disease in Childhood, 89*(6), 506–511.

Birnbaum, H. G., Kessler, R. C., Lowe, S.W., Secnik, K., Greenberg, P. E., Leong, S. A., et al. (2005). Costs of attention deficit-hyperactivity disorder (ADHD) in the US. *Current Medical Research and Opinion, 21*(2), 195–205.

Brown, R. P., & Gerbarg, P. L. (2000). Integrative psychopharmacology. In P. R. Muskin (Ed.), *Complementary and alternative medicine and psychiatry* (pp. 1–66). Washington, DC: American Psychiatric Press.

Canty-Mitchell, J., Austin, J. K., Jaffee, K., Qi, R. A., & Swigonski, N. (2004). Behavioral and mental health problems in low-income children with special health care needs. *Archives of Psychiatric Nursing, 18*(3), 79–87.

Centers for Disease Control and Prevention. (2006). CDC examines autism among children. Retrieved November 14, 2006, from http://www.cdc.gov/ncbddd/fact/autims1.htm

Chakrabarti, S., & Fombonne, E. (2005). Pervasive developmental disorders in preschool children. *American Journal of Psychiatry, 162*(6), 1133–1141.

DeJong, S., & Frazier, J. A. (2003). Bipolar disorder in children with pervasive developmental disorders. In B. Geller & M. P. Delbello (Eds.), *Bipolar disorder in childhood and early adolescence* (pp. 51–75). New York: Guilford Press.

Fontaine, K. L. (2005). *Complementary and alternative therapies for nursing* (2nd ed.). Upper Saddle River, NJ: Prentice Hall.

Frame, K., Kelly, L., & Bayley, E. (2003). Increasing perceptions of self-worth in preadolescents diagnosed with ADHD. *Journal of Nursing Scholarship, 35*(3), 225–229.

Herpertz, S. C., Mueller, B., Qunaibi, M., Lichterfeld, C., Konrad, K., & Herpertz-Dahlmann, B. (2005). Response to emotional stimuli in boys with conduct disorder. *American Journal of Psychiatry, 162*(6), 1100–1107.

Howlin, P., Goode, S., Hutton, J., & Rutter, M. (2004). Adult outcome for children with autism. *Journal of Child Psychology and Psychiatry, 45*(2), 212–229.

Hudson, G. T., & Dixon, D. (2003). Autism: Challenges in diagnosis and treatment. *Clinician Reviews, 13*(7), 45–52.

Hudziak, J. J., Derks, E. M., Althoff, R. R., Rettew, D. C., & Boomsma, D. I. (2005). The genetic and environmental contributions to attention deficit hyperactivity disorder as measured by the Conners' rating scales—revised. *American Journal of Psychiatry, 162*(9), 1614–1620.

Hunt, D. (2006). Functional roles of norepinephrine and dopamine in ADHD. *Medscape Psychiatry & Mental Health, 11*(1). 1-6. Retrieved March 16, 2005, from http://www.medscape.com/viewarticle/523887_print

Kaur, S., Sassi, R. B., Axelson, D., Nicoletti, M., Brambilla, P., Monkul, E. S., et al. (2005).

Cingulate cortex anatomical abnormalities in children and adolescents with bipolar disorder. *American Journal of Psychiatry, 162*(9), 1637–1643.

Kim-Cohen, J., Arseneault, L., Caspi, A., Tomas, M. P., Taylor, A., & Moffitt, T. E. (2005). Validity of DSM-IV conduct disorder in 4 1/2–5-year-old children. *American Journal of Psychiatry, 162*(6), 1108–1117.

Larson, J. (2005). *Think first: Addressing aggressive behavior in secondary schools.* New York: Guilford Press.

LeBlanc, N., & Morrin, D. (2004). Depressive symptoms and associated factors in children with attention deficit hyperactivity disorder. *Journal of Child and Adolescent Psychiatric Nursing, 17*(2), 49–55.

Liu, J., Raine, A., Venables, P. H., & Mednick, S. A. (2004). Malnutrition at age 3 years and externalizing behavior problems at ages 8, 11, and 17 years. *American Journal of Psychiatry, 161*(11), 2005–2013.

Nair, J. (2004). Knowing me, knowing you. In B. D. Beitman & J. Nair (Eds.), *Self-awareness deficits in psychiatric patients* (pp. 159–183). New York: WW Norton & Company.

Nierenberg, A. A., Miyahara, S., Spencer, T., Wisniewski, S. R., Otto, M. W., Simon, N., et al. (2005). Clinical and diagnostic implications of lifetime attention-deficit/hyperactivity disorder comorbidity in adults with bipolar disorder. *Biological Psychiatry, 57*(11), 1467–1473.

North American Nursing Diagnosis Association. (2007). *Nursing diagnoses: Definitions and classification 2007-2008.* Philadelphia: Author.

Perry, R. (2004). Early diagnosis of Asperger's disorder. *Journal of the American Academy of Child and Adolescent Psychiatry, 43*(11), 1445–1448.

Ramoz, N., Reichert, J. G., Smith, C. J., Silverman, J., Bespalova, I. N., Davis, K. L., et al. (2004). Linkage and association of the mitochondrial aspartate/glutamate carrier SLC25A12 gene with autism. *American Journal of Psychiatry, 161*(4), 662–669.

Reichenberg, A., Gross, R., Weiser, M., Bresnahan, M., Silverman, J., Harlap, S., et al. (2006). Advancing paternal age and autism. *Archives of General Psychiatry, 63*(9), 1026–1032.

Reinhold, J. A., Molloy, C. A., & Manning-Courtney, P. (2005). Electroencephalogram abnormalities in children with autism spectrum disorders. *Journal of Neuroscience Nursing, 37*(3), 136–138.

Scheffer, R. E., Kowatch, R. A., Carmody, T., & Rush, A. J. (2005). Randomized, placebo-controlled trial of mixed amphetamine salts for symptom of comorbid ADHD in pediatric bipolar disorder after mood stabilization with divalproex sodium. *American Journal of Psychiatry, 162*(1), 58–64.

Shelton, D. (2004). Experiences of detained young offenders in need of mental health care. *Journal of Nursing Scholarship, 36*(2), 129–133.

Sheppard, V. B., & Benjamin-Coleman, R. (2001). Determinants of service placements for youth with serious emotional and behavioral disturbances. *Community Mental Health Journal, 37*(1), 53–64.

Sweeten, T. L., Posey, D. J., & McDougle, C. J. (2003). High blood monocyte counts and neopterin levels in children with autistic disorder. *American Journal of Psychiatry, 160*(9), 1691–1693.

Teicher, M. H., Andersen, S. L., Navalta, C. P., Polcari, A., & Kim, D. (2004). Neuropsychiatric disorders of childhood and adolescence. In S. C. Yudofsky & R. E. Hales (Eds.), *Essentials of neuropsychiatry and clinical neuroscience* (pp. 535–606). Washington, DC: American Psychiatric Publishing.

Voeller, K. K. S. (2004). Attention-deficit hyperactivity disorder (ADHD). *Journal of Child Neurology, 19*(10), 798–814.

Wilens, T. E., Biederman, J., Kwon, A., Ditterline, J., Forkner, P., Moore, H., et al. (2004). *Journal of the American Academy of Child and Adolescent Psychiatry, 43*(11), 1380–1386.

Williams, R. I. (2006). Evaluating the effects of aromatherapy massage of sleep in children with autism. *Evidence-Based Complementary and Alternative Medicine, 3*(3), 373–377.

Wilson, K., Mills, E., Ross, C., McGowan, J., & Jadad, A. (2003). Association of autistic spectrum disorder and the measles, mumps, and rubella vaccine: A systematic review of current epidemiological evidence. *Archives of Pediatric and Adolescent Medicine, 157*(7), 628–634.

Chapter 18

Gender Identity and Sexual Disorders

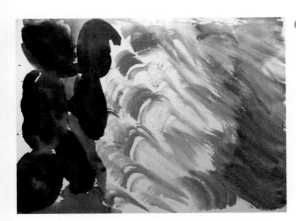

> *" The black clouds are my depression; the yellow, orange, and red, my hope. "*
>
> —Anna, Age 49

OBJECTIVES

After reading this chapter, you will be able to:

1. Compare and contrast the different theories regarding the etiology of gender identity and sexual disorders.

2. Outline the different treatment options for gender identity and sexual disorders.

3. Outline the assessment process for a client with a gender identity or sexual disorder.

4. Describe the use of the PLISSIT model for clients with a gender identity or sexual disorder.

5. Use the nursing process to develop a safe, comprehensive plan of care for a client with a gender identity or sexual disorder.

6. Develop teaching plans for a client with a gender identity or sexual disorder and his/her family.

MediaLink www.prenhall.com/fontaine

Go to the Pearson Health MediaLink CD-ROM and the Companion Website at www.prenhall.com/fontaine for interactive resources for this chapter.

All humans are sexual beings. Regardless of gender, age, race, socioeconomic status, religious beliefs, physical and mental health, or other demographic factors, we express our sexuality in a variety of ways throughout our lives.

Human sexuality is difficult to define. Sexuality is an individually expressed and highly personal phenomenon in which meaning evolves from objective and subjective experiences. Physiologic, psychosocial, and cultural factors influence a person's sexuality and lead to the range of attitudes and behaviors seen in humans. There are no normal, universal sexual behaviors. Satisfying or *normal* sexual expression can be described as whatever behaviors give pleasure and satisfaction to those adults involved, without threat of coercion or injury to others. The United States is a sexually multicultural society. We, as nurses, should work toward the goal of appreciating and affirming the rich sexual diversity among our clients.

KNOWLEDGE BASE

Sexual Health

Sexual health is an individual and constantly changing phenomenon falling within the range of human sexual thoughts, feelings, needs, and desires. A person's degree of sexual health is best determined by that individual, sometimes with the assistance of a qualified professional.

Sexual health includes *freedoms* and *responsibilities*. Sexually healthy people engage in activities that are freely chosen, including self-pleasuring and consensually shared pleasuring activities. Individuals also have freedom of sexual thought, feeling, and fantasies. Sexually healthy people are ethically motivated to exercise behavioral, emotional, economic, and social responsibility for themselves (Vision of Sexual Health, 2004). Box 18.1 lists characteristics of sexual health.

BOX 18.1	Characteristics of Sexual Health

- Knowledge about sexuality and sexual behavior
- Ability to express one's full sexual potential, excluding all forms of sexual coercion, exploitation, and abuse
- Ability to choose to be sexually active or not
- Ability to make autonomous decisions about one's sexual life within a context of personal and social ethics
- Experience of sexual pleasure as a source of physical, psychologic, cognitive, and spiritual well-being
- Capability to express sexuality through communication, touch, emotional expression, and love
- Right to make free and responsible reproductive choices
- Ability to access sexual health care for the prevention and treatment of all sexual concerns, problems, and disorders.

SOURCES: *Declaration of Sexual Rights*, by the World Association for Sexual Health, 1999, Adopted at the 14th World Congress of Sexology, Hong Kong and People's Republic of China. Retrieved January 28, 2006, from http://www.worlds exology.org. Sexual health—a new focus for WHO. (2004). *Progress in Reproductive Health Research, 67*, 1–8. Retrieved January 27, 2006, from http://www.who.int/en/

Sexual health care is a relatively new area of involvement for psychiatric–mental health nurses. Until recently, sexuality has not been viewed within the scope of treatment. Sexuality is increasingly recognized as an important component of a holistic approach to overall health status. Sexual health care is a legitimate and appropriate nursing concern. The close and often extended relationships that psychiatric–mental health nurses have with clients and families foster the rapport necessary to discuss this private area of client health status.

Gender and Transgender

Western culture is deeply committed to the idea that there are only two sexes or genders. Biologically speaking, however, there are many gradations running from female to male; this is known as **transgender**. In some cases, gender is clear, in some it is unclear, and in other cases there is a blending of both genders within the same individual. This diversity of gender represents normal variations in the human population.

Gender Identity

Gender identity is an individual personal or private sense of identity as female or male. Gender identity develops from an interaction of biology, identity imposed by others, and self-identity. A newborn is assigned a gender (identity imposed by others) according to the appearance of the external genitals (biology); by 3 years of age, the child says, "I am a girl" or "I am a boy" (self-identity). Gender identity can be viewed as a continuum. At one end of the continuum are those whose gender identity is congruent with their anatomic sex. In the middle are individuals who have both male and female gender identities. At the other end of the continuum are people whose gender identity conflicts with their anatomic sex. In addition, sexual identity is fixed for some people while for others it is more variable and changing.

Gender Roles

Gender roles are the roles a person is expected to perform as a result of being male or female in a particular culture. The expectation that people will exhibit certain behaviors because they are female or male is referred to as *gender role stereotyping*. Stereotypical images of people do not take into account individual differences. The danger of such stereotypes is that people take them seriously and act on them, ignoring the qualities and interests of individuals. In North American culture, gender roles are more strictly enforced for males than for females, and males are socially punished for female behavior.

Androgyny Flexibility in gender roles, is the belief that most characteristics and behaviors are human qualities that should not be limited to one specific gender or the other. Being androgynous does not mean being sexually neuter nor does it imply anything about sexual orientation. Rather, it describes

MediaLink   MediaLink Application, Standards of Care for Gender Identity Disorders

the degree of flexibility a person has regarding gender-stereotypic behaviors. Adults who can behave flexibly regarding their sexual roles may be able to adapt better than those who adopt rigid stereotyped gender roles.

Intersex About 1 in every 2,000 babies is born with an **intersex** condition in which there are contradictions among chromosomal gender, gonadal gender, internal organs, and external genital appearance. The gender of such an infant is ambiguous. What this means is that an intersexed person has some parts usually associated with males and some parts usually associated with females (Melby, 2002).

Transgender The medical profession considers transgender people to have a condition called *gender dysphoria* (strong and persistent feelings of discomfort with one's assigned sex) or **gender identity disorder**. For the transgender person, sexual anatomy is not consistent with gender identity. Those who are born physically male but are emotionally and psychologically female are called *male to female*, or MtF. Those who are born female but are emotionally and psychologically male are called *female to male*, or FtM. Many consider transgenderism a normal variation, and by no means a disorder.

Most transgender people report that they have felt gender dysphoria since earliest childhood. They often suffer for many years and try to hide the situation from family and friends for fear of being considered "crazy." Being transgendered puts women and men at extreme risk of being:

- Ridiculed and humiliated
- In constant jeopardy over getting and keeping a job
- Evicted without cause from restaurants and stores
- Denied housing
- Refused medical treatment, even to save a life (Lips, 2004)

As self-understanding and acceptance increase, many transgender persons live part time or full time as members of the other sex. Cross-dressing (dressing in the clothing of the desired gender) not only makes a person's outward appearance consistent with her or his inner identity and gender role, but also increases her or his personal comfort. A number of individuals decide to undergo sex reassignment surgery so their bodies match their gender identity. Most report a high level of satisfaction with the results of the surgery. Sexual orientation, pre- and postoperative, may be heterosexual, homosexual, or bisexual (Lawrence, 2005).

Cross-dressers **Cross-dressers** are typically males who cross-dress to express the feminine side of their personality. In most instances, cross-dressers are not interested in permanently altering their bodies through surgical means, especially because most of them are comfortable with their original birth genders. Most cross-dressers exhibit stereo-

typic masculine identity and behavior in their public and professional lives.

Cross-dressing is a conscious choice and may occur at home or in public settings. The frequency of the activity ranges from rarely to often. It is not unusual for cross-dressers to have a female name to go with the female personality and wardrobe. Cross-dressing occurs more frequently in cultures in which males are expected to be strong, independent, and unemotional protectors. If the social climate is one with rigid gender roles, some men may need to express their gentleness and dependence by creating a separate world and female persona within that social climate (Barnett & Rivers, 2004).

Often, these individuals do not tell their spouses about the cross-dressing before their marriage. Some are embarrassed and do not know how to bring up the subject. Others view the need to cross-dress as a problem and hope that it will disappear after the marriage takes place. Most wives eventually find out. For some women, the discovery raises doubts about their own sexuality and self-worth, and they may decide to end the relationship. Some women are not threatened by the cross-dressing but fear it will become public knowledge. Other women move on to full acceptance and understanding of their partner's cross-dressing.

Paraphilias

The DSM-IV-TR classifies **paraphilias** as a group of psychosexual disorders characterized by unconventional sexual behaviors as defined by the dominate culture. A person with paraphilia, usually a male, has learned to associate sexual arousal with some environmental stimulus, which triggers the unusual behavior.

Paraphilias have a strong obsessive–compulsive component. Affected individuals are often preoccupied with, and feel compelled to engage in, their particular sexual behaviors. One of the distinguishing characteristics of paraphilias is the person's inability to control or stop the behavior.

Noncoercive Paraphilias

Noncoercive paraphilias are unconventional sexual behaviors engaged in by oneself or with a consenting adult. Many people engage in mild forms of the noncoercive behaviors and consider them simply love play. According to the DSM-IV-TR, the behavior becomes pathological when it is severe, insistent, coercive, and harmful to self or others. There is a movement to remove the category of noncoercive paraphilias from the DSM-IV-TR by those who believe these behaviors are normal activities which have been labeled as pathological by conservative health care providers.

Fetishism Humans respond to a wealth of sexual stimuli. Some people are aroused by the strident beat of rock music, while others are aroused by romantic music. Some people prefer making love in a brightly lit room; others, by candlelight; still others, in the dark. Everyone associates sexual arousal with an individual set of stimuli.

An association or stimulus that is not typical for the culture is called a *fetish*. A fetish is the sexualization of a body part, such as feet or hair, or of an inanimate object, such as shoes, leather, or rubber. In **fetishism**, early associations of a particular object or body part with sexual arousal condition the person to respond sexually to that stimulus. Once the initial association is made, repeated viewing or use (fantasized or actual) of the part or object during sexual activity (usually masturbation) reinforces its arousing nature. For instance, a boy may get an erection after trying on his mother's panties. The erection is pleasurable. The next time the boy masturbates, he puts the panties on or fantasizes about them. With repeated experiences, seeing the panties or putting them on becomes a sexual stimulus.

LaDarius, a 24-year-old college graduate with a major in accounting, was unable to hold a job because of his foot fetish. LaDarius spent a considerable amount of time fantasizing about women's feet—bare feet, pretty feet, long and narrow feet—and how they looked, felt, tasted, and smelled. He fantasized at work, at the grocery store, and at the library (where he even went under tables to look at women's feet). LaDarius' fantasies made it impossible for him to work effectively or to maintain satisfactory interpersonal relationships with others. LaDarius refused to undergo therapy, preferring instead to pray that he would "get over it."

As with all people, fetishists' responses are highly individual. Fetishism is not considered a problem as long as it is not harmful and occurs in the context of consenting adult partners.

Transvestic Fetishism In contrast with cross-dressers, men who become sexually aroused by dressing in women's clothing are considered transvestic fetishists. Almost 3% of men report at least one episode of cross-dressing to obtain sexual excitement. They may wear female underclothes or may cross-dress completely. Like other fetishists, they have often undergone conditioning, and female clothing is an intense sexual stimulus. Many report great emotional stress if they try to resist the urge to cross-dress. Similar to other fetishes, cross-dressing is not considered a problem among consenting adult partners (Langstrom & Zucker, 2005).

Sexual Sadism and Sexual Masochism Sexual sadism and sexual masochism (S/M) is highly stigmatized in North American culture, and few people admit to being sexually aroused by receiving or inflicting emotional or physical pain. As much as 10% of the population may participate in some form of S/M activity, and all groups—heterosexual,

bisexual, homosexual—are represented. Physical behaviors include:

- Intense stimulation (scratching, biting, use of ice)
- Discipline (slapping, spanking, whipping)
- Bondage (holding down, tying down)
- Sensory deprivation (use of blindfolds, hoods, ear plugs)

Psychological behaviors include humiliation or degradation, such as verbally berating others or requiring them to perform menial acts. S/M behavior varies in intensity and in its significance in the lives of couples. Some couples engage in the behavior only during sex. Some integrate the roles throughout the relationship, but not at all times. Other couples attempt to live out the dominant/submissive roles continuously. Thus, S/M may be only a part of foreplay, or it may be a significant component of lifestyle. Most sadomasochists do not engage in S/M behavior unless the partner is willing. Typically, both participants agree to safety rules, and seldom is the behavior dangerous. Sadomasochists do not see the behavior as a problem and therefore do not wish to change.

A fairly new description, BDSM, has come out of the sexual and gender minority subculture. It is a combination of B/D (bondage and discipline), D/S (dominance and submission), and S/M. Thus BDSM refers to any or all of these behaviors. Participants find these activities highly erotic and emotionally charged. Often the activities are subtle and sensual and have little resemblance to pornographic material.

Autoerotic Asphyxia A noncoercive but often fatal sexual behavior is **autoerotic asphyxia**, sometimes referred to as hypoxyphilia. It is not categorized as a paraphilia in the DSM-IV-TR but, similar to paraphilias, it is a compulsive and unconventional sexual behavior. Also called head-rushing or scarfing, the autoerotic asphyxia behavior typically begins in adolescence and is primarily a male affliction. The person fashions a tourniquet-like device that constricts the neck (decreasing the blood and oxygen supply to the brain), masturbates, and, at the point of orgasm, releases the bonds to enhance the sensation or sexual high.

Tragically, this practice causes many deaths. The vagal nerve complex in the carotid artery is stimulated by pressure around the neck, slowing the heart rate and decreasing oxygen flow to the brain even further. The person becomes unconscious, slumps forward, and accidentally hangs himself. Many believe the cause of death is suicide, but family and friends cannot understand the reason for the suicide since these young men are not mentally ill or even troubled; the death is a tragic accident. Distinguishing features include evidence of sexual activity, the presence of various forms of sexually explicit materials, or a wide range of sexual paraphernalia such as bondage, hoods, and blindfolds.

MediaLink   Case Study, Sexual Sadism and Masochism

Coercive Paraphilias

People with coercive paraphilia become sexually aroused by including nonconsenting persons in their sexual acts. Coercive paraphilias are described in the legal code, and the sexual behavior is considered a criminal act.

Exhibitionism, Voyeurism, and Frotteurism Exhibitionists and voyeurs, who are almost exclusively men, have powerful urges to display their genitals to strangers (exhibitionism) or peep at unsuspecting women involved in intimate behaviors (voyeurism). Frotteurs rub up against others, often in a crowded train or elevator, to achieve sexual arousal. The frotteur does not attempt to engage in sex with the victim and has no desire to form a relationship. Many describe the urge to peep, expose, or rub themselves against others as something that just "happens" to them and therefore have difficulty assuming responsibility for their behavior (King, 2002).

Obscene Phone Calling A coercive sexual behavior, not categorized as a paraphilia in DSM-IV-TR, is obscene phone calling. Most women and many men have been victims of an obscene phone caller. The caller typically does not know the victim and becomes aroused when the victim reacts with disgust or shock or becomes upset. Some obscene callers breathe heavy, some make sexual noises, and some utter profanities. The caller may tell the victim that he is masturbating or may suggest they get together for sexual activity. Some pretend to have legitimate reasons for talking about sex (posing as researchers conducting a survey, for example) and continue until the victim is offended. The caller is sexually aroused by the combination of proximity (intimate conversation) and anonymity.

Pedophilia A pedophile is an adult who is sexually aroused by and engages in sexual activity with children. All sexual relationships between adults and children are criminal in North America. The courts consider these acts as nonconsensual because minors are presumed to have insufficient knowledge of the consequences of their acts to give meaningful consent. Pedophiliac activity can include exposure, voyeurism, explicit sex talk, touching, oral sex, intercourse, and anal sex. The child usually knows the pedophile, who may be a family member, neighbor, or friend. For a thorough discussion of the dynamics and consequences of the sexual abuse of children, see chapter 23 ∞.

Altered Sexual Function

The ability to engage in sexual behavior is of great importance to most people. Many individuals experience transient problems with their ability to respond to sexual stimulation or to maintain the response. A smaller percentage of people experiences lifelong problems. The problems may be generalized to all sexual interactions and settings or they may be situational, occurring in a specific setting or with specific types of sexual activity. It is often difficult to sort out the multiple factors contributing to an individual's or a couple's sexual problems.

Sexual Desire Disorders

For most people, sexual desire varies from day to day and over the years. Some people, however, report a deficiency in or absence of sexual fantasies and persistently low interest or a total lack of interest in sexual activity; these clients have *hypoactive sexual desire disorder*. Low desire may be related to relationship problems, other sexual problems, dissatisfaction or boredom with sexual activities, negative messages in childhood, fears, performance anxiety, negative expectations, inaccurate beliefs about sexuality, negative body image, exhaustion, or discordance for sexual orientation. The etiology is most often multifactorial, and treatment focuses on all related factors.

If both individuals in a relationship are similarly uninterested in sex, there really is no problem. More typically, there is a disparity of sexual needs, and the person with the greater desire becomes dissatisfied with the sexual relationship and often initiates seeking help. The key issue in the relationship is not frequency, but the dovetailing of partners' needs.

Sexual aversion disorder is a severe distaste for sexual activity or the thought of sexual activity, which then leads to a phobic avoidance of sex. It occurs in women and men. Intense emotional dread of an impending sexual interaction also can trigger the physiologic symptoms of anxiety: sweating, increased heart rate, and extreme muscle tension. The client then stops the sexual interaction or prevents it from beginning. The most common cause of sexual aversion disorder is childhood sexual abuse or adult rape. This severe trauma can lead to a phobic response to sexual activity (McCammon, Knox, & Schacht, 2004).

Linda and Mike, both 32 years old, dated all through high school and have been married for 12 years. Linda has a strong aversion to body secretions. She spends hours in the bathtub before she and Mike have sex. Although Mike wears a condom, Linda jumps up and out of bed before he has finished ejaculating, and runs to the bathtub.

Linda cannot identify any reasons for her feelings of disgust about body secretions and denies having a history of sexual abuse. She does, however, talk about feeling violated by Mike when he "talked me into sex" at age 18. Sometimes she refers to this first sexual experience as date rape.

Despite this problem, Linda and Mike refer to themselves as best friends. Linda has suggested that their marriage be conducted as a platonic relationship. Mike's not sure he wants to live that way the rest of his life. They are in counseling and want to learn how to enjoy one another sexually. They are learning how to be less genitally focused and to spend more time cuddling, stroking, and touching.

Sexual Arousal Disorders

Sexual arousal refers to the physiologic responses and subjective sense of excitement experienced during sexual activity. Lack of lubrication and failure to attain or maintain an erection are the major disorders of the arousal phase. In *female sexual arousal disorder*, the lack of vaginal lubrication causes discomfort or pain during sexual intercourse. The diagnosis of *male erectile disorder* is usually made when the man has erection problems during 25% or more of his sexual interactions. Some men cannot attain a full erection, and others lose their erection prior to orgasm. The pejorative term commonly applied to this condition, *impotence*, implies that the man is feeble, inadequate, and incompetent. The accurate term is *erectile dysfunction* (ED), which is objectively descriptive and not judgmental. By the age of 50, slightly more than half of all men report at least mild ED. Arousal disorder may also be diagnosed even when lubrication and erection are adequate if individuals report a persistent or recurring lack of subjective sexual excitement or pleasure (McCarthy & Fucito, 2005).

Paweena and Morufat, both 45 years old, sought counseling when Morufat found it impossible to achieve an erection. The first time he was unable to achieve an erection was 6 years ago. This was an emotionally traumatic experience for Morufat, who spent a considerable amount of time worrying that it would happen again. Eventually it did, and Morufat found that more and more often he was unable to attain an erection. About 6 months ago, he consulted a urologist. Nighttime penile tumescence study results showed normal functioning.

The couple was referred to a nurse–sex therapist, who discovered that Morufat had believed, from an early age, that sexual functioning stopped once the man reached age 49. In working with the couple, the nurse focused on providing sex education and experiential/sensory awareness training. Once it did not matter whether Morufat achieved an erection, his performance anxiety was decreased and he was able to attain a satisfactory erection.

Orgasmic Disorders

The pejorative term commonly applied in the past to women who did not experience orgasm, *frigid*, implies that the woman is incapable of responding sexually. The more accurate and objective term is *female orgasmic disorder*, which simply means that the sexual response stops before orgasm occurs. *Preorgasmic* women have never experienced an orgasm; *secondarily nonorgasmic* women have achieved orgasms in the past but do not currently experience them; and *situationally nonorgasmic* women achieve orgasms in some situations but not in others. Studies indicate that 10% to 15% of women are preorgasmic, and another 20% to 22% report irregular orgasms. Compounding the orgasmic difficulty is the associated anxiety. In the preoccupation with orgasm, the real goal of being sexual—mutual pleasuring and intimacy—is lost, and the interchange becomes one of anxiety, frustration, and anger (Heiman, 2007; McCammon et al., 2004).

Rapid ejaculation is one of the most common sexual problems among men. There are many definitions, with descriptions ranging from ejaculating before being touched, ejaculating before penetration, ejaculating with one internal thrust, to ejaculating within a minute or two of penetration. A more helpful description is the absence of voluntary control of ejaculation. The problem is best self-defined: A man is concerned about his ejaculatory control, or the couple agrees that ejaculation is too rapid for mutual satisfaction.

Some men have *male orgasmic disorder.* Men with this disorder can maintain an erection for long periods (an hour or more) but have extreme difficulty ejaculating, which is referred to as *retarded ejaculation.* In heterosexual intercourse, the difficulty may be limited to ejaculation in the vagina. Some men ejaculate after self-stimulation or manual or oral stimulation by the partner, whereas others have great difficulty ejaculating with any type of stimulation. This disorder is much less common than rapid ejaculation.

Sexual Pain Disorders

Women and men both can experience *dyspareunia*, pain during or immediately after intercourse. It is associated with many physiologic causes, especially those that inhibit lubrication. Thus, skin irritations, vaginal infections, estrogen deficiencies, and use of medications that dry vaginal secretions can cause women to experience discomfort with intercourse.

Pelvic disorders, such as infections, small lesions, endometriosis, scar tissue, or tumors, can result in painful intercourse. Engaging in painful intercourse can lead to *vaginismus*, an involuntary spasm of the outer one third of the vaginal muscles, because the body reflexively becomes guarded and tense. Similarly, in males, infection or inflammation of the glans penis or other genitourinary organs can cause pain with coitus. Also, some contraceptive foams, creams, or sponges can irritate either the vagina or the penis, causing pain.

Vaginismus makes penetration of the vagina painful and sometimes impossible. The woman often experiences desire, excitement, and orgasm with stimulation of the external sexual structures. Attempts at intercourse, however, elicit the involuntary spasm. She may have similar difficulty undergoing pelvic examination and inserting tampons or a diaphragm.

Vulvodynia is constant, unremitting burning that is localized to the vulva. Onset is acute. The girl or woman has problems in sitting, standing, and sleeping because of the intensity of pain. In contrast, *vestibulitis* causes severe pain only on touch or attempted vaginal entry. Half of all women with vestibulitis report lifelong dyspareunia. Women with either of these disorders report a negative impact on their sexual functioning and partner relationship, as well as their self-esteem and mental health (Metzger, 2005).

Problems With Satisfaction

Some people experience sexual desire, arousal, and orgasm and yet feel dissatisfied with their sexual relationships. These sexual problems are more commonly related to the emotional tone of the relationship than to the physiologic response. Because giving and receiving pleasure in a mutually intimate relationship are the primary goals of sex for most people, *dissatisfaction problems* may be more disturbing than other types of sexual dysfunctions.

At times, satisfaction problems may be situational. For example, one partner may choose an inconvenient time, or a partner may feel anxious and therefore cannot experience much pleasure or joy. Some people describe their problems as related to lack of extragenital satisfaction. These people describe how much they miss and continue to need all the touching and caressing of their earlier lovemaking experiences. Unfortunately, people who have been relating sexually for a long time often become genitally focused and neglect the rest of the body. One or both partners may feel touch starved, may long for more total body touching, and may become dissatisfied with sex.

Satisfaction problems are often related to relationship difficulties. The inability to communicate effectively in other relationship areas frequently results in sexual frustration. Partners who are angry at each other and make love without resolving the conflict may feel unhappy about the relationship despite having experienced arousal and orgasm. Couples who define their relationship in terms of rigid, unequal power and gender roles may have difficulty negotiating and compromising about sexual issues. Not infrequently, the person with the least amount of power feels helpless and dissatisfied with the sexual interchanges.

Lack of intimacy or a feeling of connectedness is understandably related to satisfaction problems. If one has sex with a stranger, the body may function well, but there is often a sense of something missing after the sexual experience. Making love to one person while feeling more attracted to, or in love with, another person can result in feelings of emptiness or disconnection. Even couples in a committed relationship may complain of lack of intimacy. Dissatisfaction issues include lack of romance, love, tenderness, and nurturance. Fulfillment of sexuality, then, depends on the ability to relate with a partner in an intimate and mutually pleasing manner that is compatible with values and chosen lifestyle.

Increased Sexual Interest

An increased interest in sex and sexual activity is symptomatic of the manic phase of bipolar disorder. Elevated mood is accompanied by a corresponding rise in sexual activity, variety of activity, and, often, number of partners. This behavior occurs despite contrary values and is out of the client's control. The end of the manic episode signals a return to the person's usual level of sexual interest and activity. Since memory is not impaired, the person may feel embarrassed and ashamed about uncontrolled sexual behavior during the manic episode.

Some adult survivors of childhood sexual abuse may go through periods of high sexual activity. This is often a desperate attempt to obtain the nurturance, love, care, and power they were denied in childhood. Having been sexualized at an inappropriately early age, some have learned to survive in a hostile environment by using their sexual availability to make contact with or control others.

Sexual Addiction

Frequency of sexual activity can be viewed on a continuum, with most people falling in the middle range. Some people have sex frequently in a way that enhances their lives; others have sex infrequently and report contentment and satisfaction. A sexual pattern that falls at either extreme of the continuum, however, can signal problems. At the low extreme are individuals who have great difficulty in choosing to be sexual; such people may have a **sexual dysfunction**. At the high extreme are people who have lost their ability to choose or control their sexual behavior; these people are sexual addicts.

Sexual addiction is a disorder in which the central focus of life is sex. People with this addiction spend 50% or more of all waking hours dealing with sex, from fantasy to acting-out behavior. Acting-out behaviors are often victimless (the partner is consenting) such as having affairs; overindulging in masturbation, fetishism, pornography, or commercial telephone sex; or visiting prostitutes. Victimizing behaviors (those with a nonconsenting partner) are less frequent. The incidence of sexual addiction is difficult to determine because of secrecy and shame, but it is estimated that 3% to 6% of the population may be affected. It is predominantly a male disorder with a gender ratio of 3:1 (Carnes & Wilson, 2002).

It is unethical to label people who do not conform to conventional moral codes as sexual addicts. Sexual addiction is not simply the frequent enjoyment of sexual behaviors. Many people engage in those behaviors without becoming sexual addicts. Rather, sexual addiction is a progressive disorder in which sex is used to numb pain. The payoff is the same as in any other addiction: an intensely pleasurable high, a short-lived release from pain, and an escape from the problems of daily life. The consequences are also the same in that the addict's life eventually becomes unmanageable. The components of sexual addiction are discussed in Box 18.2.

Sexual Problems Among Gay Men and Lesbians

Gay men and lesbians may have the same sexual dysfunctions that occur in the heterosexual population. Living in a homophobic culture with strict gender role expectations can cause additional pressures.

Men, whether gay or heterosexual (straight), may accept stereotyped male gender roles that can lead to ambivalence about intimacy and dependence. Because social norms re-

BOX 18.2	Components of Sexual Addiction

The components of sexual addiction have the hallmarks of obsessive–compulsive behavior.

1. *Preoccupation.* The person spends hours thinking or obsessing about sex. Preoccupation, in itself, gives a sexual high and is so time consuming that the person cannot fulfill work, school, or family responsibilities.
2. *Ritualization.* The individual engages in specific behaviors done just the "right" way and in the same sequence each time. Ritual behaviors include wearing certain clothing, taking certain steps to get ready, driving certain routes, or looking for partners only in a certain area. The ritual seems to control anxiety; once addicts begin a ritual, they cannot stop until the cycle is completed.
3. *Compulsivity.* The person cannot control sexual behavior, and this behavior becomes the most important aspect of life. Some demonstrate sexually compulsive behavior in a regular pattern; others resist for a time and then have a binge cycle.
4. *Shame and Despair.* At the end of the cycle, the person experiences guilt and shame at the loss of control. The pain of despair creates the need to begin the cycle all over again, because the addict seeks to relieve pain by getting high. Like other addicts, these individuals want to stop their behavior, promise to stop, try to stop, and are unable to stop without treatment.

quire that men be unemotional, competitive, and in control, two men in an intimate relationship may experience conflict if both try to be "macho men." The success of the relationship often depends on the partners' ability to negotiate and compromise on issues of power, control, dependence, tenderness, and nurturance. It is not uncommon for gay men to interpret sexual problems in relationships as a sign that the relationship is over, as opposed to seeing the dysfunction as a problem to be solved.

The most common sexual problem for lesbians, as for heterosexual women, is a lack of interest in sex. There are several differences between lesbian couples and heterosexual couples experiencing low sexual desire. Unlike heterosexual couples, lesbian couples do not typically withdraw from sex because of a lack of intimacy, a power imbalance, or rigid gender roles in the relationship. A lesbian couple is more likely to report that the nonsexual areas of their relationship are pleasing and agreeable and that there is minimal conflict about sex.

It is highly unlikely for lesbian couples to have difficulty with arousal, orgasm, or satisfaction. The explanation for this may be that lesbian couples spend more time making love and include more varied activities than do heterosexual couples (Nichols & Shernoff, 2007).

Etiologies

Human sexual behavior has been studied from various theoretical perspectives. The most significant are biological, intrapersonal, behavioral, interpersonal, and sociocultural theories.

A review of the various theoretical perspectives shows that human sexuality has been historically characterized by judgments and controversy that have inhibited sexual health care services. It is important for health care professionals to remember that all people to some extent deviate from some physical, social, behavioral, or emotional norm. Some are left-handed, some stutter, some are disabled, some are loners, and some are filled with fear. To achieve the highest level of professional practice, nurses must look beyond the characteristics and respond to the whole person.

Only in the past 40 years has human sexuality been scientifically studied from a multidisciplinary approach. With this knowledge came the beginnings of planned interventions for individuals suffering from a variety of sexual problems and disorders. Nursing has been an active participant in the evolution of treatment approaches and programs to provide sexual health care.

Biology

Those individuals who take a biological approach are concerned with the physiologic aspects of gender identity and sexual behavior. Some believe there is a neurological basis for gender differences and look to fetal exposure to sex hormones and adult levels of sex hormones as an explanation of gender dysphoria. They explore sexual dysfunctions to discover factors (e.g., organic disease, injury, medications, pain, or depression, or all) that interfere with the physiologic reflexes during the sexual response cycle.

It is clear from research over the past several years that the majority of sexual problems are physiologic in nature, initially. In middle age, for example, normal physiologic changes (such as decreased hormone production) may interfere with sexual pleasure and interest. Side effects of many medications or medical treatment may contribute to sexual problems. Arteriosclerosis, diabetes, and other medical problems can interfere with the ability to attain an erection. Not understanding the physical basis of the problem, people begin to experience anxiety, shame, or guilt and the stage is set for the emotional component for sexual problems.

There is no clear understanding of the etiology of transgender. Biological theory is based on animal studies because experimental research cannot be conducted with humans. When exposed prenatally to increased male hormones, experimental animals exhibit increased male behavior. Decreasing the levels of male hormones prenatally increases female behavior in animals. In humans, the male gonads develop and begin secreting androgen during weeks 8 to 12 of gestation. Differentiation of the hypothalamus to a male pattern, which occurs in months 4 to 5 of gestation, requires high androgen levels. Therefore, one explanation of transgender is that prenatal androgen levels were sufficient for the development of male anatomy but insufficient for differentiation in the brain. In transsexual persons who are anatomically female, the androgenic influences may have been high at the critical time of hypothalamic development, though not at the time of genital formation (Lips, 2004).

Intrapersonal Factors

Intrapersonal theorists view gender dysphoria, paraphilias, and sexual dysfunctions as problems occurring within the individual. Some view them as expressions of arrested psychosexual development, some seek an explanation in sexual guilt, some see the issue as one of self-punishment, and others see these as normal variations. People who grew up with rigid family and religious taboos about sex often experience guilt and anxiety about their adult sexual roles and behaviors. Inadequate sex education can lead to ignorance and anxiety about sexuality. Performance anxiety, negative self-concept, and negative body image are all seen as contributing to sexual problems. Problems to be solved during the treatment process include fears of:

- Intimacy
- Losing control
- Pain
- Pregnancy
- Sexually transmitted infections

Behavioral Theory

Behaviorists believe that gender dysphoria arises from social learning; that is, the child was rewarded in some way for adopting behaviors of the other sex. They believe paraphilias are learned responses; the person is conditioned to respond erotically to nonsexual objects or particular sexual acts. In the area of sexual dysfunctions, contributing factors include poor communication skills, lack of sexual experience with oneself or a partner, concern with sexual performance, and ineffective stimulation. The dysfunctions, too, are seen as learned responses.

Interpersonal Factors

Relationship difficulties may cause sexual problems. Negative patterns of communication or dislike or fear of one's partner inhibit sexual expression. Conflict over commonplace issues such as money, schedules, or relatives may lead to a loss of sexual interest. An inability to talk about preferences in initiating sex or determining sexual activities creates problems for some people. Fatigue and lack of time due to family and work obligations are other common causes. Likewise, sexual problems can contribute to relationship difficulties, especially when couples do not openly communicate about the situation. Misunderstanding leads to inappropriate guilt or anger and withdrawal from the relationship.

Sociocultural Factors

Ideas about sexuality and sexual behavior are based on cultural values and understanding. What is considered normal or abnormal depends on each group's specific viewpoint. The same behavior may be seen as positive in one culture and pathological in another. Each culture tends to incorporate ethnocentrism in its beliefs; that is, its members believe their particular sexual values and behaviors are superior and preferable to those of any other culture. Ethnocentrism encourages people to view the sexual behavior of other people as eccentric, exotic, and bizarre.

Consider the diversity of sexual values throughout the world. The Mangaia of Polynesia believe that young adolescents of both genders have high sexual drives. However, as they leave young adulthood, they expect their desire to rapidly decline. In contrast, the Dani of New Guinea believe that neither women nor men have high sexual drives and that the primary purpose of sex is for reproduction. Following the birth of a child, the husband and wife remain celibate for the next 5 years. Among the Sambrans of New Guinea, young boys around age 7 or 8 have sex with older boys. It is believed that the ingestion of semen is required for physical growth. This pattern of behavior changes to heterosexual interaction as the young men become adults.

Cultures in some parts of Africa and the Middle East practice ritual mutilation of the clitoris, which is referred to in the West as *female genital mutilation*. Because of serious medical complications and psychological trauma, the practice has been outlawed in many countries, though the laws are rarely enforced.

Among many cultures throughout the world, there is a third gender. Among the Zuni of New Mexico, this person is called a *berdache*, a male who assumes female dress, gender role, and status. Individuals with this third gender are often considered to have great spiritual power (King, 2002).

The sexual ethics of a culture reflect the culture's assumptions about the purpose of sex. In North American culture, sexual practices have been strongly influenced by the Judeo-Christian tradition, which historically considered procreation to be the primary purpose of sex. As a result, even modern North American culture is sexually intolerant and harshly critical of those whose gender identity or sexual behavior is not in the mainstream.

How people communicate about sexuality is culturally determined. In general, North American culture reflects Euro-American values, which include a negative view of public sexual communication, as evidenced by censorship and sex as taboo in general discussion. However, there are ethnic differences in communication patterns. African American people tend to be very expressive and communicate directly about sexual topics.

Latinos from the Caribbean and Central American cultures tend to use restraint in expressing their feelings, whereas those from Argentina and some other Latin American countries are emotionally expressive. Asian American individuals are often less verbally expressive, so nonverbal communication assumes even more importance. The gay and lesbian subculture has developed private words and expressions in reaction to the homophobia of the dominant culture (Hecht, Collier, & Ribeau, 2002; King, 2002; Ting-Toomey & Chung, 2002).

People with little tolerance for cross-gender behavior view transgender people and cross-dressers as deviants. The sexual acts of people with noncoercive paraphilia conflict with the traditional value of sex for procreation, and they, too, are made to feel like outcasts. Sociocultural theories regarding sexual dysfunctions focus on disturbed relationships between partners, negative early learning, and past or present traumatic events.

Multidisciplinary Interventions

Vulvodynia and vestibulitis are systemic problems that take some time and a lot of effort to overcome. A low glycemic diet—no sugar or white foods—is most helpful. It is also important to test for food allergies, as these seem to contribute to the inflammation. When the pain and inflammation are reduced, pelvic floor therapy by specially trained physical therapists is begun. Hands-on techniques include massage therapy and myofascia and pudendal nerve release. Vaginal dilators may be introduced for home use. An individual exercise program is designed to strengthen weak muscles and stretch tight muscles. Pelvic floor biofeedback measures the tension of the pelvic floor muscles and helps clients learn to relax and strengthen these muscles. Other techniques include pelvic floor electrical stimulation and perineal ultrasound.

Clients who have a true sexual addiction are usually referred to a 12-step–based recovery program. Like other 12-step programs, the initial standard is 90 meetings in 90 days. These groups are generally available in urban settings and have no associated financial cost. There is usually a sense of a "healing community" that includes others with similar hypersexual problems.

Oral medications have been the biggest breakthrough for ED. These medications work by relaxing smooth muscles in the penis, allowing arteries to expand and increase blood flow into the penis, causing an erection. These medications are sildenafil (Viagra), vardenafil (Levitra), and tadalafil (Cialis). Although research has been conducted using these medications for female sexual problems, the results have been inconclusive.

Androgen levels in women peak in early adulthood and decrease slowly with aging. Women in their 40s have approximately one half the level of androgen of women in their 20s. Testosterone has been linked to sexual desire and sexual frequency in menopausal women. It appears that testosterone therapy improves sexual function in women with low levels. Testosterone may be administered as a transdermal patch, a topical cream, or a sublingual pill.

The selective serotonin reuptake inhibitors (SSRIs) may be given for rapid ejaculation since a common side effect is the slow down in orgasmic response. The doses are usually lower than those given for depression.

Nursing Process

CLIENTS WITH GENDER IDENTITY AND SEXUAL DISORDERS

Historically, human sexuality has been shrouded in myth and controversy. This history has hindered both the delivery and the receipt of services that promote sexual health and well-being. Although scientific knowledge has expanded immensely during the past several decades, modern North Americans continue to view sex and sexuality with discomfort. Our confusion is complicated by our traditional religious and social values. Basic to nursing is the notion that the nurse's personal beliefs should not influence the quality of care given a client. If nurses hold negative, inappropriate, or stereotyped opinions and ideas, they must confront them before they can meet professional standards of care in helping clients attain optimal sexual health. It is easier for nurses to live up to this standard if they engage in value clarification before providing sexual health care. Giving nonjudgmental nursing care does not mean that the nurse has to agree with others' beliefs and values about sexuality. However, self-awareness can help psychiatric–mental health nurses respect their clients' sexual rights and needs. Box 18.3 provides a checklist for personal knowledge and attitudes about sex.

The nursing care of clients with gender identity and sexual disorders requires extensive background and experience. Although nurses at all levels of practice should aim to develop a trusting relationship and assess clients for sexual concerns, they should refer clients to a health care provider with special expertise in dealing with these complex issues. The actual diagnoses and interventions of these clients are best left to the providers with special expertise.

BOX 18.3	Nursing Self-awareness

Check Your Knowledge and Attitudes About Sex

Use this checklist periodically to assess changes in your knowledge and attitudes.

Knowledge

Circle True or False for each statement.

T F Women can and do have orgasms while sleeping.

T F It is dangerous to engage in intercourse during menstruation.

T F Sex drive usually diminishes after a vasectomy.

T F An older male may actually have some advantages over a younger male in sexual activity.

T F Masturbation is a relatively common practice of both women and men.

T F Females have two kinds of orgasm: clitoral and vaginal.

T F Children raised by same sex couples are very likely to become homosexual.

T F An adult male who has been castrated immediately loses his sex drive.

T F Intercourse should always be avoided during the last trimester of pregnancy.

T F Oral–genital stimulation is unhygienic.

Attitudes

Circle the letter corresponding to your level of agreement with each statement.

A: Strongly agree; B: Agree; C: Uncertain; D: Disagree; E: Strongly disagree

A B C D E   Sex education has caused a rise in premarital intercourse.

A B C D E   Extramarital relations are almost always harmful to a marriage.

A B C D E   Relieving tension by masturbation is a healthy practice.

A B C D E   Premarital intercourse is morally undesirable.

A B C D E   Parents should stop their children from masturbating.

A B C D E   Women should have sexual experience before marriage.

A B C D E   Homosexual and bisexual behavior should be against the law.

A B C D E   Seeing family members nude arouses undue curiosity in children.

A B C D E   Promiscuity is widespread on college campuses today.

A B C D E   Men should have sexual experience before marriage.

ASSESSMENT

Information about a client's sexual health status should always be integral to nursing assessment. The amount and kind of data collected depend on the context of the assessment; that is, the client's reason for seeking health care and how the client's sexuality interacts with other problems.

Including a sexual history as part of the general nursing history is important for some clients and not important for other clients. It is critical, however, at least to introduce the topic of sexuality to give permission for clients to bring up any concerns or problems. All nursing histories should at least include a question such as, "Have there been any changes in your sexual functioning that might be related to your illness or the medications you take?" Nurses might also facilitate communication by saying, "As a nurse, I'm concerned about all aspects of your health. People often have questions about sexual matters, both when they are well and when they are ill. When I take your history, sexual concerns are included to help plan a comprehensive treatment approach." For an

overview of past and current factors that may contribute to sexual problems, see Table 18.1 ▪. The Focused Nursing Assessment lists questions that can be part of a general nursing history. Some medications affect sexual desire or sexual behavior. See Table 18.2 ▪ for a description.

Assessment: Behavior

It is critical nurses not make assumptions about client behavior because assumptions interfere with accurate history taking. If you assume that all people do all things, you will be more open to clients than if you make assumptions about who is and who is not sexually active, how many partners they have, or if they do or do not masturbate. Imposing personal values on others is detrimental to the nurse–client relationship.

Assessment: Affect

Sexual problems can create affective responses such as guilt, anxiety, or fear, which interfere with the ability to experience

TABLE 18.1	Factors Contributing to Sexual Dysfunctions	
Type	**Past Factors**	**Current Factors**
Psychologic	■ Taught that sex is dirty ■ Childhood sexual abuse	■ Performance anxiety ■ Spectatoring ■ Fear of failure ■ Guilt, anxiety, or anger ■ Negative thoughts
Spiritual	■ Taught that sex is sinful ■ Childhood sexual abuse	■ Not feeling connected to partner ■ Lack of intimacy ■ Fear of intimacy
Sociologic	■ Punished as child for normal sex play ■ Lack of sex education	■ Failure to communicate ■ Relationship conflict
Physical	■ Trauma: abuse, rape	■ Illness/injuries ■ Organic disorders ■ Medications ■ Substance abuse ■ Failure to engage in effective sexual behavior

TABLE 18.2	Drugs and Related Sexual Side Effects						
Drug	**Sexual Side Effects**						
	Increased Sex Drive	**Decreased Sex Drive**	**Decreased Arousal**	**Retrograde Ejaculation**	**Inhibited Ejaculation**	**Painful Orgasm**	**Orgasm Problems**
Alcohol	Small amounts	Large amounts	Yes		Yes		
Amphetamines		May		Yes		Yes	
Antihypertensives		Yes	Yes		Yes		
Antipsychotics (atypical)	Yes	Yes		Yes		Yes	
Antipsychotics (conventional)	Yes	Yes	Yes	Yes			Yes
Anxiolytics (very few side effects)							
Beta-blockers	Yes	Yes					
Cocaine	Yes				Yes		Yes
Diuretics		Yes	Yes				
Hallucinogens (unpredictable side effects)		May	May				May
Heroin	Yes		Yes		Yes	Yes	
Lithium		Yes	Yes				
MAOIs			Yes	Yes			
Marijuana	Small amounts	Large amounts	Chronic use				
Mood stabilizers			Yes	Yes			
SSRIs		Yes				Yes	Yes
Steroids	Yes	Yes					
Tricyclic antidepressants		Yes	Yes		Yes	May	Yes

Focused Nursing Assessment · Clients With Gender Identity and Sexual Disorders

Affective Assessment	Behavioral Assessment	Cognitive Assessment	Sensation Assessment
To whom do you feel most intimate and connected?	Describe your level of satisfaction with the frequency of your sexual activity.	When you were growing up, how did you learn about sex?	Describe any physical discomfort you feel during sexual activity.
Describe the type of love and affection in this relationship.	Describe the positive aspects of your own sexual functioning.	How has your religion influenced your sexual values and behaviors?	To what degree do you experience pleasure during sexual activity?
In what way do you experience anxiety about sex?	Describe the negative aspects of your own sexual functioning.	What "shoulds/should nots," "musts/must nots" do you believe about your sexual behavior/relationships?	
In what way do you experience guilt about sex?	What concerns do you have about your future sexual functioning?	How rigidly were gender roles enforced in your family of origin?	
How depressed are you feeling?	What are your partner's concerns about current or future sexual functioning?	How are gender roles enacted in your present relationship/family?	
In what way does anger interfere with your sexual functioning?		Describe the negative thoughts you have about sex.	
Do you dislike or feel an aversion to any parts of your body?		Does the use of fantasy increase or decrease your sexual desire?	

pleasure and joy. Some people experience guilt when they simply enjoy sex, or when they participate in what they label "unusual" sexual activities, or guilt regarding the choice of the partner. Adults who have been sexually abused at any time of their lives may experience overwhelming anxiety when faced with the decision to engage in sex. Fears may include fear of pregnancy, of sexually transmitted infections, or of pain. Because vulnerability and intimacy are inherent in most sexual relationships, fear of these may lead to an avoidance of sex.

Fear of failure in sexual performance often becomes a vicious cycle; that is, fear of failure creates actual failure, which in turn produces more fear. "Spectatoring" is the detached appraisal of sexual performance or the body during a sexual act: "Am I going to lose my erection?" "Am I going to have an orgasm this time?" "My stomach is too flabby." "When did his thighs get that fat?"

Erectile problems may be threatening because the man often feels his whole sense of masculinity is at stake. Men tend to be dominated by a genital focus more than women are. Any difficulty in getting the penis to "perform" therefore results in feelings of humiliation and despair.

Assessment: Cognition

Cognitive factors relating to gender identity or sexual problems include the internalization of negative expectations and beliefs. Those with low self-esteem may not understand how another person could value and love them and find them sexually attractive. For those who have not yet accepted their sexual orientation or gender identity, this cognitive conflict may interfere with sexual relationships.

Assessment: Interpersonal Relationships

Sexual problems may also be symptomatic of relationship problems. Conflict and anger with one's partner are not conducive to positive sexual interaction. If there is a power imbalance in the relationship, the less powerful partner may lose interest in sex as a passive–aggressive way to achieve covert power. Some no longer feel physically attracted to one another or feel more attracted to someone else. Lack of intimacy and feeling like a sex object inhibit the feeling of communion and connection that is an important part of making love. Typically, couples have minimal insight into the association between their lack of sexual desire and their negative feelings and relationship problems.

Another factor in dysfunction is expecting one's partner to read one's mind about sexual needs and desires. Lack of sex education and failure to communicate may result in one or both partners not knowing how to please the other. Unless the partners experiment, sex may, in time, become boring. Disagreements in sexual frequency or sexual activities, or in both, may lead to further relationship conflict.

Assessment: Cultural Influences

Sexuality is regulated by the individual's culture. For example, culture influences the sexual nature of dress, rules about marriage, expectations of role behavior and social responsibilities, and specific sex practices. Societal attitudes vary widely. Gender role behavior varies from culture to culture. Attitudes about childhood sexual play with self or children of the same or other gender may be restrictive or permissive. Premarital and extramarital sex and homosexuality may be celebrated, tolerated, or unacceptable. Culture is so much a part of everyday life that it is taken for granted. We tend to assume that others share our own perspective, including those for whom we care. When we believe that our own culture is more important than, and preferable to, any other culture, we are expressing *ethnocentrism*. It is impossible to provide sensitive nursing care from an ethnocentric position.

Another cultural consideration is a very restrictive upbringing accompanied by inadequate sex education. Rigid gender role socialization may inhibit exploration of sexual activities, positions, toys, and other lovemaking behaviors. If a person's religious group believes that sex is only for procreating, there may be great difficulty in celebrating the pleasure and fun of a loving sexual relationship. In our current culture, the pressures of family and work often leave couples with too little time and not enough energy to enjoy sex.

Assessment: Physical

Health factors can interfere with a person's expression of sexuality. Physical changes brought on by illness, injury, or surgery may inhibit full sexual expression. Many prescription medications have side effects that affect sexual functioning. Most frequently, the effect is negative, but sometimes there is a positive effect. For example, antidepressants may slow ejaculation. This may be a problem for the man who finds himself suddenly feeling unable to ejaculate. If a man is experiencing rapid ejaculation, however, the antidepressant may "cure" this problem. The two antidepressants with the least negative sexual side effects are buproprion (Wellbutrin) and escitalopram (Lexapro). Some street drugs such as marijuana, amphetamine, and cocaine increase sexual drive and activity. Others, such as opioids and anabolic steroids, interfere with sexual functioning. Refer to Table 18.2 for information regarding the side effects of common medications.

Jared is seeing an advanced practice psychiatric nurse for clinical depression. After several weeks with no improvement, the nurse suggested he consider taking an antidepressant to lift his mood and facilitate the psychotherapy. Jared refused outright saying, "I took Prozac a couple of years ago and it caused me to lose my orgasms. I'm never taking that stuff again. I would rather be depressed than give up my sex life."

DIAGNOSIS

A number of nursing diagnoses are applicable to clients experiencing gender identity disorders and sexual problems (North American Nursing Diagnosis Association, 2007).

- Risk for Violence: Self-directed related to accidental injury or death when experimenting with autoerotic asphyxia
- Risk for Violence: Directed at Others related to engaging in coercive sexual paraphilias
- Personal Identity Disturbance related to transgender issues such as cross-dressing or transsexualism
- Pain related to extreme discomfort when vaginal intercourse is attempted
- Ineffective Sexuality Patterns related to the need to engage in noncoercive paraphilias when having a sexual encounter
- Ineffective Sexuality Patterns related to increased sexual interest during the manic phase of bipolar disorder
- Ineffective Sexuality Patterns related to lack of control over compulsive sexual behavior
- Sexual Dysfunction related to the presence of one or more sexual problems affecting a couple's intimate relationship
- Spiritual Distress related to lack of intimacy with partner; multiple fears; history of sexual abuse
- Deficient Knowledge related to a lack of comprehensive sex education when growing up; not knowing how to communicate about sexual needs and desires
- Altered Role Performance related to rigidity in gender role expectations and behavior

OUTCOME IDENTIFICATION AND GOALS

Based on the assessment data, you select outcomes appropriate to the nursing diagnoses. Broad outcomes are:

- Verbalize acceptance and self-respect regarding gender identity.
- Eliminate coercive behavior.
- Engage in consensual, healthy sexual interactions.

Once you have established outcomes, you and the client mutually identify goals for change. Client goals are specific behavioral measures by which you, clients, and significant others identify as realistic and attainable. The following are examples of some of the goals appropriate to people with gender identity issues and sexual problems:

- Remains safe
- Utilizes support systems
- Verbalizes less pain
- Verbalizes increased intimacy with partner
- Verbalizes increased sexual satisfaction

PLANNING

Once the you identify the nursing diagnoses, outcome criteria, and goals, the plan of care is developed to assist clients in reaching an enriched quality of life. The interventions you select are based on the data obtained from the client and the diagnoses, outcomes, and goals. Nurses require basic sex skills to help clients in the area of sexuality:

- Self-knowledge and comfort with their own sexuality
- Acceptance of sexuality as an important area for nursing intervention and a willingness to work with clients expressing their sexuality in a variety of ways
- Knowledge of sexual growth and development throughout the life cycle
- Knowledge of basic sexuality, including how certain health problems and treatments may affect sexuality and sexual function and which interventions facilitate sexual expression and functioning
- Therapeutic communication skills
- Ability to recognize the need of the client and family members to have the topic of sexuality introduced not only in written or audiovisual materials, but also in a verbal discussion

IMPLEMENTATION

The nurse can use the PLISSIT model developed by Annon (1974) to help clients with gender identity issues or sexual problems. The model involves four progressive levels represented by the acronym PLISSIT:

P	Permission giving
LI	Limited information
SS	Specific suggestions
IT	Intensive therapy

At each level, nurses provide additional guidance and information to clients and therefore require more specialized and specific knowledge and skill. All professional nurses should be able to function at the first three levels.

Permission Giving. Clients may feel that they need permission to be sexual beings, to discuss their gender identity, to ask questions, to show affection, and to express themselves sexually. Giving permission means that you, by attitude or word, let clients know that sexual thoughts, fantasies, and behaviors between informed, consenting adults are allowed. Giving permission begins when you acknowledge clients' spoken and unspoken sexual concerns and convey the attitude that these are important to health and healing.

For example, you might ask a client who is diagnosed with major depressive disorder the following question: "Many people who are depressed experience a loss of sexual interest. Has this been a problem for you?"

Limited Information. Clients need accurate but concise information. You might explain what is usual sexual behavior; how mental disorders and medications affect sexuality; or the affect of cultural expectations regarding gender role behavior. Continuing with the preceding example, you might say the following: "I notice that you have been taking antidepressant medication for 2 months. Although this medication improves mood and general functioning, there are often some sexual side effects, especially related to orgasms."

Specific Suggestions. At this level, you must have specialized knowledge and skill about specific interventions. Offer suggestions to help clients adapt sexual activity to promote optimal functioning. If you are working on a cardiac unit, need specialized knowledge about sexual readjustment during cardiac rehabilitation. If you are working with clients with spinal cord injuries, you need information about the sexual consequences of spinal injuries at various levels. If you are working with a client who has gender identity issues, you might say the following: "I'm not sure whether you are aware of support groups available in the area for people who are transgendered. I would like to give you a list of these groups, if you would like that information."

Intensive Therapy. At this level of intervention, nurses must have specialized preparation and knowledge of sexual and gender identity disorders. Nurses who function in the sex therapist role should meet the qualifications for practice as identified by the American Association of Sexuality Educators, Counselors, and Therapists (AASECT), which differentiates sex counseling from sex therapy. *Sex counseling* helps clients incorporate their sexual knowledge into satisfying lifestyles and socially responsible behavior. *Sex therapy* is a highly specialized, in-depth treatment to help clients resolve serious sexual problems. AASECT publishes a national directory of professionals, certified to provide sex education, counseling, or therapy. This directory is an excellent resource for nurses and clients.

Reducing Violence Against the Self

The most important nursing intervention regarding autoerotic asphyxia is community education. Warnings about autoerotic asphyxia should be routinely included in adolescent sex-education programs. Teenagers who practice it must be encouraged to seek immediate professional help. Parents should be taught to look for physical signs of trauma to the neck such as bruising, abrasions, pressure marks, or rope burns. Ropes, knotted sheets, knotted T-shirts, or the like hidden in the bedroom may be warning signs.

The desired outcome is that clients will verbalize the dangers of autoerotic asphyxia and remain safe.

Reducing Violence Against Others

Individuals who practice coercive paraphilias typically do not stop the behavior and usually end up in the criminal justice system. The court may or may not mandate therapy. Therapy for sex offenders is a specialized area that should not be undertaken lightly.

The desired outcome is that clients will identify sexual behaviors that are criminal offenses.

Although behavior-modification techniques, group therapy, and hypnosis are used, they are generally unsuccessful. In severe cases, male sex offenders are treated with the antiandrogen drug medroxyprogesterone acetate (Provera or Depo-Provera), which induces a reversible chemical castration. The drug reduces the male sex drive, erections, and ejaculation and decreases the obsessional focus on sex.

Promoting Comfort With Gender Identity

People who experience gender dysphoria have many possible options to manage the transgendered part of themselves. Physically they may undergo hormonal treatment, genital reassignment surgery, electrolysis, breast surgery, or other cosmetic surgery. They may decide to live in the other gender role part time or full time, prefer to have sex as a woman or as a man with a female, male, both, or neither. They may view themselves as female, male, both, a third gender, or a transgendered person. Interventions focus on promoting comfort with the chosen gender role.

The desired outcome is that clients will report increasing comfort and satisfaction with gender identity, and will negotiate cross-dressing behavior with partner.

Transgendered people are usually referred to therapists who specialize in this area or to gender identity disorder clinics. Because gender identity is stable, the goal of treatment with these individuals is to help them live and function in society in the preferred gender role. They need a great deal of support and assistance as they establish themselves in this new role. If their current job is not gender-role stereotyped, they may be able to remain in the same or a similar position. Others may need retraining programs to find acceptable employment. A multidisciplinary approach is most effective in helping them adjust to their situation. Family and friends need support and counseling to reintegrate this person into their lives as a person of the other sex.

If cross-dressing is a newly divulged secret to the partner, offer education and support. If the relationship is to continue, both partners must agree on where and how cross-dressing will take place. Some couples compromise; for instance, a husband may agree never to cross-dress in front of his wife, and she may agree to give him privacy. Some agree to limit cross-dressing to the home; others are comfortable going out in public with the partner cross-dressed. The long-term success of the relationship depends on the couple's ability to negotiate these issues.

Reducing Pain

Whenever pain is associated with intercourse, a thorough physical examination is necessary to find and treat the organic cause of the pain. During vaginal examinations, careful attention must be paid to tiny tears in the vaginal wall, which are often overlooked. Even very small tears can cause great pain during intercourse. Vaginismus is treated with education, dilators, and supportive psychotherapy. The initial treatment for vulvodynia and vestibulitis involves decreasing the inflammation. That is followed by pelvic floor therapy by specially trained physical therapists.

The desired outcome is that clients will verbalize less or no pain during sexual intercourse.

See Box 18.4 for guidelines for working with clients with sexual problems.

Education Regarding Noncoercive Sex Patterns

Once paraphilias are a programmed part of arousal, they are very difficult to deprogram. The response to certain sexual or erotic stimuli persists through life. A noncoercive, nonharmful paraphilia practiced with an adult, consenting partner requires no nursing intervention other than client and partner education and possible couple negotiation about the behavior.

The desired outcome is that clients and partners will establish parameters of behavior in mutual relationship.

Reinforcing Sexual Health

Clients in a manic episode often exhibit impulsive increase in their sexual activity. Explain to family members that such behavior is a symptom of the manic state, is not within the client's control, and is not an indication of a change in ethics and values. As much as possible, clients should be protected from sexual acting out until they are able to assume control over this behavior. Set firm limits on inappropriate verbal and physical sexual behaviors.

The desired outcome is that clients will decrease inappropriate sexual behavior.

Managing Compulsive Sexual Behavior

Sex addicts, just like other people with addictions, respond well to community-based programs. The cornerstone of recovery is a 12-step program modeled on the Alcoholics

BOX 18.4	Guidelines for Working With Clients With Sexual Difficulties

Male Orgasmic Disorder

Reestablish a climate of comfort and acceptance for sexual interaction. Encourage the client to masturbate and enjoy touch and body stimulation in general.

Premature Ejaculation

Instruct the client to stimulate the erect penis until the premonitory sensations of impending orgasm are felt. Then penile stimulation is abruptly stopped. This process is repeated to lower the threshold of excitability and make the client more tolerant of stimuli. Sometimes the client uses the squeeze technique: At the point of orgasm, the client squeezes the head of the penis with thumb and first two fingers for 3 to 4 seconds. This stops the urge to ejaculate.

Female Orgasmic Disorder

Instruct the client to avoid genital sex. Nongenital caressing exercises begin with the couple alternating as the initiator of a session of caressing, thus sharing responsibility for sexual interaction.

Next, genital stimulation is added to provide positive sexual experiences without intercourse. When intercourse is attempted, the woman is instructed to assume the superior position and insert the man's penis into her vagina. When setbacks occur, the couple is advised to rely on sexual techniques that do not involve intercourse. The woman is to place her hand lightly on her partner's to indicate her preference for contact. The emphasis is not on achieving orgasm but on learning erotic preferences.

The couple is instructed to use the side-by-side position, which enables both partners to move freely with emphasis on slow, exploratory thrusting. The goal is to develop an ability to enjoy pelvic play with the penis inside the vagina.

Vaginismus

Begin with a physical demonstration to the woman of her involuntary vaginal spasm by inserting an examining finger into her vagina. Then Hegar dilators in graduated sizes are inserted into the woman's vagina beginning with the smallest ones. After larger dilators are successfully inserted, she is instructed to retain the dilator for several hours each night. Most involuntary spasms can be relieved in 3 to 5 days with the daily use of dilators.

In addition to physical relief from spastic constriction, therapy is directed toward alleviating the fear that led to the onset of symptoms.

Vulvodynia and Vestibulitis

Clients with these conditions need a great deal of empathy and support because they have been living with acute pain for a significant period of time. Instruct them to use nonirritating substances to the vulva, such as Lipocream, Aquaphor, or even olive oil or Crisco. Testing for food allergies and environmental allergies is done because these may be contributing causes. Yoga and acupuncture may also be helpful.

Anonymous program. Partners and codependents are also referred to appropriate self-help groups. A variety of groups, such as Sexaholics Anonymous, Sex Addicts Anonymous, Sex and Love Addicts Anonymous, S-Anon, and Co-Dependents of Sexual Addicts, have been formed throughout the country.

The desired outcome is that clients will attend a 12-step program for sexual addicts.

Addressing Sexual Dysfunctions

Accurate identification of feelings is the first step in the problem-solving process, and clients may need help labeling the feelings they are experiencing. Following this step, help clients identify one anxiety-producing situation within their sexual interactions. At this stage, it is productive to focus diffuse anxiety on a manageable single situation or event. With the client, analyze the situation or event to discover negative anticipatory thoughts that may be the source of the anxiety. Together, review how the client has handled anxiety in the past and evaluate the range and effectiveness of this past coping behavior. It may be appropriate to help the client redefine the sensations of anxiety as sensations of sexual excitement, which is more likely to result in positive expectations. Together, explore alternative coping behaviors, and have the client evaluate their effectiveness after implementing them.

The desired outcome is that clients and partners will verbalize less anxiety, communicate effectively, utilize referral resources, and report a satisfying sex life.

Many adult survivors of childhood sexual abuse are periodically overwhelmed by anxiety, fear, and panic (see chapter 23 ∞).Refer adult survivors to support groups such as Incest Anonymous or VOICES, as well as individual therapy with a therapist who specializes in this field.

Good communication is an important part of a sexually fulfilling relationship. Apart from setting specific times to share feelings and beliefs, some couples need training in communicating more effectively. If they give ambiguous signals to indicate sexual interest, they must learn how to state their interest clearly. Some people expect their partners to "read their minds" about sexual needs and desires; these people need encouragement to assert their needs tactfully. Teach couples to avoid "you" language, which evokes a defensive response and results in arguments, and to use "I" language, which expresses personal thoughts, feelings, and needs. Some examples of accusatory "you" statements and answerable "I" statements are in Box 18.5.

If couples are able to reduce anxiety and improve communication but still have sexual problems, a referral is appropriate. Sexual disorders are explained in comfortable, lay terms on the Sexual Disorders Web site. Since most psychotherapists are not sex therapists, make a referral through

| BOX 18.5 | Asserting Sexual Needs Tactfully |

Couples involved in communications around emotionally difficult subjects such as sex convey messages more competently through "I" language than through the accusatory "you" language.

"You" Language

- "You only have sex on your mind. You're a pervert."
- "You keep grabbing at me like I'm always ready to go to bed with you."
- "You never pay attention to what turns me on. Are you dumb or hard of hearing?"

"I" Language

- "I'm concerned because we seem to have different expectations of how often we would like to make love."
- "I miss all the hugging and caressing we used to do even when we couldn't make love afterward."
- "I feel frustrated and hurt when it seems like I'm repeating myself. Maybe I'm not communicating my needs very clearly."

AASECT, mentioned earlier in this chapter. The common components of sex therapy are found in Box 18.6.

Reducing Spiritual Distress

Because the origin of spiritual distress is often a lack of intimacy or connection, the goal of nursing intervention is to help clients achieve and maintain a level of intimacy each partner finds comfortable. In the context of therapy, couples discuss their individual needs for closeness and identify barriers to intimacy. They are instructed to make three or four half-hour "dates" each week, during which they share warmth and intimacy. They spend some of the time discussing specific sexual issues; during other dates, the couple explores intimate, nonsexual

| BOX 18.6 | Common Components of Sex Therapy Programs |

- *Information and Education About Sexual Functions.* The therapist gives clients specific information about their particular needs. The therapist may assign books to read or discuss the information.
- *Experiential/Sensory Awareness.* The therapist helps clients recognize feelings of anxiety, anger, and pleasure by tuning into bodily cues. Clients focus on and describe feelings both in therapy sessions and at home. If they believe their genitals are ugly and unclean, the therapist assigns desensitization exercises at home for clients to explore and become familiar with their own bodies. Some clients need fantasy training if nonsexual thoughts interfere with sexual arousal.
- *Insight.* The therapist attempts to learn and understand what is causing and perpetuating the sexual problem. The goal is for clients to assume responsibility for their own behavior and recognize that change is possible.
- *Cognitive Restructuring.* Clients identify and reevaluate their fears about sexual interaction. The therapist encourages them to identify and eliminate negative self-statements and irrational expectations.
- *Behavioral Interventions.* Since the focus is on changing nonsexual behavior that contributes to sexual problems, the therapist may assign assertiveness training, communication training, stress-reduction exercises, and problem-solving techniques. Behavioral interventions include assigned pleasuring sessions to discover what is arousing and pleasing to the self and partner.

topics, such as hopes and expectations for the future. Couples should give these dates top priority, because a common way of avoiding intimacy is by not setting time aside for each other.

The desired outcome is that clients will set time aside for their intimate relationship and verbalize increased emotional intimacy.

| **Clinical Interactions** | **A Client With a Shoe Fetish** |

Dana and Keith have been married for 1 year. The nurse–sex therapist is meeting with them for the first time. When calling for the appointment, Dana told the nurse that Keith has a shoe fetish that she has grown to resent over the past few months. This interchange occurs after the first 30 minutes of the session. In this interaction, you see evidence of:

- The obsessive–compulsive component of the fetish
- Keith's dependence on shoes for sexual arousal

DANA: "Here's my problem with the shoes. He must have several hundred pairs of women's shoes and he can't get an erection unless there are women's shoes involved. Usually he wants me to wear them when we have sex."

NURSE: *"How do you feel about yourself, in relation to his shoe fetish?"*

DANA: "I feel like I'm just not enough of a woman for him. I mean, there must be something wrong with me that he doesn't get turned on by me. I feel inadequate."

KEITH: "You know it's not you. I've told you that a million times. I don't know why I need the shoes, but it's me, not you."

NURSE: *"Keith, tell me more about the shoes and your arousal."*

KEITH: "I have this collection of shoes and I just need Dana to wear them when we make love. What's so difficult about that? It's not like it hurts her. The shoes are all her size."

NURSE: *"What happens, Keith, if you try to have sex without shoes being involved?"*

KEITH: "Well, we tried once or twice but I just couldn't perform. I don't see why the shoes are such a big deal. I buy most of them at thrift shops, so it's not like I'm spending much money on them."

DANA: "Well, what about the times you want me to walk across your hands with very high spiked heels? That's weird."

NURSE: *"In addition to the shoes, it sounds like pain is part of what you need to become sexually aroused."*

Using Research Evidence   Self-care: Gay Men and Lesbians in Addiction Recovery

Matthew, C. R., Lorah, P., & Fenton, J. (2006). **Treatment experiences of gays and lesbians in recovery from addiction: A qualitative inquiry.** *Journal of Mental Health Counseling, 28,* 110–132.

What is the study about?

Gay men and lesbians are at higher risk for alcohol and drug addiction, and may experience substance use and addiction in unique ways. Therefore, this study sought to understand the experiences of gay men and lesbians in treatment for drug and alcohol addiction, and gain their perspective on whether it is vital, and if so, how vital, for a treatment program to address sexual orientation. Specifically, the research focused on what did and did not facilitate their recovery, and how mental health professionals might be failing to address their unique recovery needs.

How was the study done?

This was a qualitative phenomenological study that used purposive sampling to obtain narrative data from 10 participants. All participants responded to a recruitment announcement and reported a range of one to four treatment experiences for their addiction. Six women and four men were recruited, and the investigation was approved by a university's office of regulatory compliance. All participants identified involvement with Alcoholics Anonymous (AA) and had been in recovery from alcohol and/or drug addiction for at least 1 year. The researchers conducted semistructured 1-hour interviews by telephone. They asked a series of open-ended questions and encouraged participants to expand on relevant topics. The interviews were audiotaped, and tapes were transcribed by a professional transcriptionist. In addition, researchers and participants independently verified the accuracy of the transcripts. The researchers reviewed the narratives intensively to identify themes.

What were the results of the study?

Using a consensual qualitative method, the researchers identified 10 themes: 1) attention to gay and lesbian issues, 2) mixed versus gay-and-lesbian–specific programs/meetings, 3) importance of role models, 4) role of AA, 5) shame, 6) boundary issues, 7) interaction between sexual orientation and addiction, 8) suicide, 9) treatment as a safe space, and 10) issues related to family.
Attention to gay and lesbian issues included three subthemes: active homophobia from other clients and/or mental health workers, assumption of heterosexuality, and the need for counselors who would not wait for clients to broach the issue, but take the initiative to address substance abuse and sexual orientation directly. Participants wished for meetings and events that were *exclusively for gay men and lesbians*. Most participants saw value in *role models* who were both gay/lesbian and in recovery. For most, AA was a positive experience that was important to their recovery and continuing sobriety. Most participants addressed the theme of *shame* from both the perspective of sexual orientation and that of addiction. Shame was felt intensely, even after many years, and working through shame to self-acceptance was found to be vital for recovery. The theme of

boundary issues was pertinent to "coming out" with their sexual orientation as well as being open about their alcoholism and sobriety status. Boundary issues were seen as contributing to openness about sexual orientation, retarding openness, or making openness very difficult. Many participants discussed their fears of repercussions if they were honest about their sexuality, and pointed out how that fear left them conflicted during 12-step meetings, which emphasized honesty. All participants spoke to the theme of *interaction between sexual orientation and addiction* and saw these two issues as highly interdependent. Several participants referred to being gay or lesbian as a way to feed their addiction; comfortable socializing for them often took place in bars. They were clear that their sexual preferences did not cause their addiction but did influence how they experienced it and their recovery. The theme of *suicide* was raised by 6 of the 10 participants. All 6 had considered this option or knew of other gay men or lesbians who had. *Treatment as a safe space* centered on the belief that safety was vital for honesty, and honesty was important for recovery. Most participants greatly valued talking openly about who they were, both in treatment and in meetings, and pointed out that their recovery was aided by positive attitudes of mental health professionals. Some participants recommended that treatment facilities increase the sense of safety by employing openly gay and lesbian counselors. Interestingly, some participants revealed that they took their cues as to whether to disclose their sexual orientation by closely observing how the counselors treated minorities. The last theme, *family*, focused on issues that participants needed to address or did address in reference to their families. Here, concerns included families of origin, lesbian or gay partners, children and prior heterosexual marriages, and how well the facility staff understood the place of family in their lives. Some felt the facility staff could be more inclusive of the gay and lesbian family and others thought the staff were very helpful.

What additional questions might I have?

What is the effect of addiction on identity development? What themes would have emerged if the mental health workers shared a gay or lesbian lifestyle with the participants? What can be done to promote acceptance of gay men and lesbians in mental health settings?

How can I use this study?

Nurses need to be more aware of the uniqueness of gay men and lesbians living with addiction challenges. In this work, it is important to understand how sexual orientation in western culture may influence addictive behaviors. Nurses can serve as role models by accepting the differing lifestyles of all persons in treatment. In addition, it may be helpful for gay men or lesbians to be connected with gay or lesbian sponsors during their recovery. With both sexual orientation and addiction, the nurse needs to be aware of shame and possible suicidal ideation. Lastly, in working with this population, nurses may find it helpful to incorporate family oriented approaches or treatment plans.

SOURCE: Contributed by Dolores Huffman, PhD, RN, Associate Professor of Nursing, Purdue University Calumet, Hammond, Indiana.

Increasing Knowledge

Providing education for sexual health is an important component of nursing implementation. Many sexual problems exist because of sexual ignorance; many others can be prevented with effective sexual health teaching.

You can help clients understand their anatomies and how their bodies function. For example, understanding the anatomy of the clitoris may help a woman learn how her body is pleasing and causes arousal. The importance of open communication between partners should also be encouraged. Details about physiologic changes that occur throughout the life span should be provided as part of general health care. For example, you discuss the effects of puberty, pregnancy, menopause, and the male climacteric on sexual function at the appropriate times.

Although awareness is increasing regarding sexuality and sexual functioning, some people still hold certain myths and misconceptions about sexuality. Many of these are handed down in families and are part of beliefs in a particular culture. It is highly important that you learn about the beliefs clients hold and provide up-to-date information. Visit the Web site of the Sexuality Information and Education Council of the United States, which has a wealth of information on various aspects of sexuality.

The desired outcome is that clients will describe anatomy and physiology of sexual response and discuss beliefs related to sexuality.

EVALUATION

To complete the nursing process, you evaluate client responses in terms of outcomes you and the client established. It is seldom an all-or-nothing phenomenon, but rather an ongoing process of movement toward the goal of improved quality of life. If any outcomes have not been achieved, explore the reasons with questions such as the following:

- Were risk factors correctly identified?
- Did the client convey all significant fears and concerns about sexuality?
- Was the client more comfortable following discussions about sexual matters?
- Did the client understand the teaching?
- Was the teaching compatible with the client's culture and religious values?
- Was the client ready to deal with sexuality problems?

Focus Your Study

OBJECTIVES	KEY CONCEPTS
1. Compare and contrast the different theories regarding the etiology of gender identity and sexual disorders.	■ Biology: 　• Theorists are exploring fetal exposure to sex hormones as an explanation of gender dysphoria. 　• The majority of sexual problems experienced by individuals and couples are physiological. ■ Intrapersonal factors: 　• Factors include rigid family and religious taboos about sex; inadequate sex education; performance anxiety; negative self-concept; and negative body image. ■ Behavioral theory: 　• Gender dysphoria arises from social learning. 　• Paraphilias are learned responses. ■ Interpersonal factors: 　• Factors include relationship difficulties, negative patterns of communication, conflict, and fatigue. ■ Sociocultural factors: 　• Culture determines what sexual behavior is considered normal or abnormal.
2. Outline the different treatment options for gender identity and sexual disorders.	■ Pain disorders are treated with a low glycemic diet, pelvic floor therapy, vaginal dilators, and exercise. ■ Refer clients with sexual addiction to a 12-step program. ■ Erectile dysfunction is treated with sildenafil (Viagra), vardenafil (Levitra), and tadalafil (Cialis). ■ Testosterone may be prescribed for women with low levels. ■ SSRI antidepressants are used to treat rapid ejaculation. ■ Refer adult survivors of childhood sexual abuse to self-help groups. ■ Some transgender people undergo hormonal and surgical treatment to create bodies that match their gender identity.

continued

continued

| 3. Outline the assessment process for a client with a gender identity or sexual disorder. | ■ Nurses at all levels of practice should assess clients for sexual concerns.
■ The amount and kind of data collected depend on the context of assessment; that is, the client's reason for seeking health care and how the client's sexuality interacts with other problems. |

| 4. Describe the use of the PLISSIT model for clients with a gender identity or sexual disorder. | ■ P – Permission Giving. The nurse lets clients know that sexual thoughts, fantasies, and behaviors between informed, consenting adults is appropriate and healthy.
■ LI – Limited Information. The nurse provides accurate and concise information about sexuality, illness, and medication.
■ SS – Specific Suggestions. The nurse must have specialized knowledge and skill to intervene at this level. Offer suggestions to help clients adapt sexual activity to promote optimal functioning.
■ IT – Intensive Therapy. Nurses who function at this level should meet the qualifications for a sex therapist. This is in-depth treatment to help clients resolve serious sexual problems. |

| 5. Use the nursing process to develop a safe, comprehensive plan of care for a client with a gender identity or sexual disorder. | ■ People who engage in coercive paraphilias typically end up in the criminal justice system.
■ Transgendered people are usually referred to gender identity disorder clinics.
■ Help couples improve their communication skills.
■ Help clients achieve and maintain a level of intimacy each partner finds comfortable.
■ Refer to a sex therapist for complex sexual problems. |

| 6. Develop teaching plans for a client with a gender identity or sexual disorder and his/her family. | ■ Many sexual problems exist because of sexual ignorance and many others can be prevented with effective sexual health teaching:
  • Explain anatomy and physiology of sexual function.
  • Discuss myths and misconceptions clients may have.
■ The most important nursing intervention regarding autoerotic asphyxia is family and community education.
■ If cross-dressing is a newly divulged secret to the partner, offer education and support regarding gender identity and cross-dressing.
■ When appropriate, offer education to those couples engaging in noncoercive, nonharmful paraphilias.
■ Clients in a manic episode often exhibit impulsive increase in sexual activity. Teach the family that such behavior is a symptom of the manic state. |

Explore MediaLink

For review questions, case studies, and other resources for this chapter see the Pearson Health MediaLink CD-ROM that accompanies this book and the Companion Website.

CD-ROM
- Audio Glossary
- NCLEX-RN® Review Questions
- Animations/Videos
  - Gender Identity Disorder–Parts 1, 2, and 3

Companion Website www.prenhall.com/fontaine
- Audio Glossary
- NCLEX-RN® Review Questions
- Case Study
  - Sexual Sadism and Masochism
- Care Plan
  - Sexual Disorders and Communication
- Critical Thinking
  - Gender Identity Disorder
- MediaLink Application
  - Standards of Care for Gender Identity Disorders
- MediaLinks
  - Books for Clients & Families
  - Community Resources

NCLEX-RN® Review Questions

18-1. A client is upset after learning that a family member is arrested for exhibitionism. The nurse informs the client about the current theories related to the cause for this paraphilia. Which of the following statements indicates that the client requires more information?
  1. "The person who does this must have abnormal levels of hormones."
  2. "This behavior must result from not reaching normal developmental milestones."
  3. "Maybe the person who has this behavior was sexually abused."
  4. "This must be done by a person with a sexual dysfunction."

18-2. A client with a sexual arousal disorder asks the nurse if taking sildenafil (Viagra) is the only method to treat erectile dysfunction. What is the best response by the nurse?
  1. "It is the safest treatment for sexual arousal."
  2. "Taking Viagra is the only method that works."
  3. "Group therapy reduces the anxiety connected with erectile difficulties."
  4. "Reducing the pressure to perform only helps the woman."

18-3. A 70-year-old client who has had numerous affairs throughout his marriage tells the nurse, "The affairs helped me to have better sex with my spouse." What defense mechanism is this client using?
  1. Repression
  2. Denial
  3. Rationalization
  4. Suppression

18-4. The nurse uses the PLISSIT model to help clients with gender issues or sexual problems. Which of the following are the four progressive levels? (Select all that apply.)
  1. Permission giving
  2. Limited information
  3. Limited communication
  4. Specific suggestions
  5. Intensive therapy
  6. Cognitive therapy

18-5. A client tells the nurse that he has lost the desire to have sex with his wife. Further assessment reveals that the client is taking antihypertensive and antidepressant medication. Which of the following nursing diagnoses will the nurse select to identify the problem the client is experiencing?
  1. Sexual Dysfunction
  2. Ineffective Coping
  3. Ineffective Sexual Patterns
  4. Disturbed Body Image

18-6. A nurse is conducting a sexual awareness group of known pedophiles. What will the nurse emphasize as the primary focus of this group?
  1. Socialization
  2. Cognitive restructuring
  3. Insight
  4. Punishment

See Appendix D for answers.

References

Annon, J. (1974). *The behavioral treatment of sexual problems. Vol. 1, Brief therapy.* New York: Harper & Row.

Barnett, R., & Rivers, C. (2004). *Same difference.* New York: Basic Books.

Carnes, P. J., & Wilson, M. (2002). The sexual addiction assessment process. In P. J. Carnes & K. M. Adams (Eds.), *Clinical management of sex addiction* (pp. 3–19). New York: Brunner-Routledge.

Hecht, M., Collier, M. J., & Ribeau, S. (2002). *African American communication* (2nd ed.). Mahwah, NJ: Lawrence Erlbaum Associates.

Heiman, J. R. (2007). Orgasmic disorders in women. In S. R. Leiblum (Ed.), *Principles and practice of sex therapy* (4th ed., pp. 84–123). New York: Guilford Press.

King, B. M. (2002). *Human sexuality today* (4th ed.). Upper Saddle River, NJ: Prentice Hall.

Langstrom, N., & Zucker, K. J. (2005). Transvestic fetishism in the general population. *Journal of Sex & Marital Therapy, 31*(1), 87–95.

Lawrence, A. A. (2005). Sexuality before and after male-to-female sex reassignment surgery. *Archives of Sexual Behavior, 34*(2), 147–166.

Lips, H. M. (2004). *Sex and gender* (5th ed.). Mountain View, CA: Mayfield Publishing.

Matthew, C. R., Lorah, P., & Fenton, J. (2006). Treatment experiences of gays and lesbians in recovery from addiction: A qualitative inquiry. *Journal of Mental Health Counseling, 28*, 110–132.

McCammon, S. L., Knox, D., & Schacht, C. (2004). *Choices in sexuality* (2nd ed.). Cincinnati, OH: Atomic Dog Publishing.

McCarthy, B. W., & Fucito, L. M. (2005). Integrating medication, realistic expectations, and therapeutic interventions in the treatment of male sexual dysfunction. *Journal of Sex & Marital Therapy, 31*(4), 319–328.

Melby, T. (2002). Intersex interrupted. *Contemporary Sexuality, 36*(12), 1–6.

Metzger, D. A. (2005). When pleasure becomes a pain. Conference proceedings: *Women's Sexual Health.* The Berman Center and Northwestern University, Feinberg School of Medicine, Department of Obstetrics and Gynecology.

Nichols, M., & Shernoff, M. (2007). Therapy with sexual minorities. In S. R. Leiblum (Ed.), *Principles and practice of sex therapy* (4th ed., pp. 379–415). New York: Guilford Press.

North American Nursing Diagnosis Association. (2007). *Nursing diagnoses: Definitions and classification, 2007–2008.* Philadelphia: Author.

Ting-Toomey, S., & Chung, L. (2002). *Understanding intercultural communication.* Los Angeles, CA: Roxbury.

Vision of Sexual Health. (2004). *Contemporary Sexuality, 38*(7), 1–5.

Unit 4

Neurobehavioral Brain Disorders

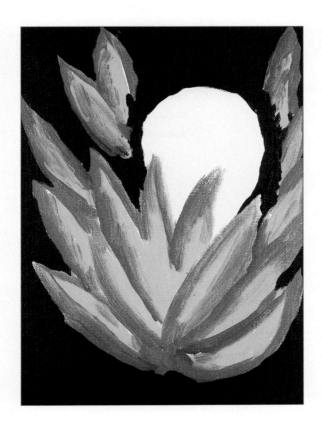

This is where I would like to be 5 years from now when I'm 20: In California.

—Rachel, Age 15

Chapter 19

Cognitive Impairment Disorders

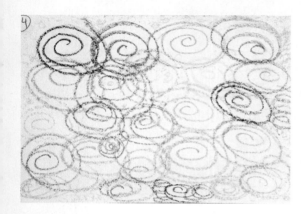

> *Lost in an unending maze*
> *Circling round and round*
> *Never stopping to ask questions*
> *Never slowing down*
>
> *The walls just seem to grow and grow*
> *With no end in sight*
> *Overlapping,*
> *Overflowing*
> *Drowning me in fright*
>
> *Alone am I*
> *On this crazy maze*
> *Alone*
> *Each night and day*
>
> *My biggest fear is*
> *To be alone,*
> *Alone*
> *With nowhere to go*

—Anna, Age 19

OBJECTIVES

After reading this chapter, you will be able to:

1. Distinguish between dementia and delirium.

2. Compare and contrast the etiologies of dementia and delirium.

3. Outline the different treatment options for dementia and delirium.

4. Outline the assessment process for dementia and delirium.

5. Develop teaching plans for a client with a cognitive impairment disorder and her/his family.

6. Use the nursing process to develop a safe, comprehensive plan of care for a client with a cognitive impairment disorder.

7. Discuss the key points in effectively communicating with a client with a cognitive impairment disorder.

MediaLink www.prenhall.com/fontaine

Go to the Pearson Health MediaLink CD-ROM and the Companion Website at www.prenhall.com/fontaine for interactive resources for this chapter.

The process of mental deterioration related to cognitive impairment disorders has a profound effect on individuals, their families, and society. This chapter presents dementia and delirium, the two most common forms, in which there are diffuse disturbances in cognitive performance. Causes, symptoms and outcomes differ in both.

Dementias are chronic, irreversible brain disorders characterized by impairment in memory, abstract thinking, and judgment, as well as changes in personality. Loss of autonomy, loss of dignity, and loss of the self result in despair of victims and families. *Alzheimer* disease is the most common cause of dementia. Vascular *dementia* is the second most common cause of dementia and results from ischemic events and hemorrhages in the brain. Hypertension is also a known risk factor for vascular dementia. *AIDS dementia complex* (ADC), which typically affects younger people, is another type of dementia and is caused by HIV infection of the brain. ADC occurs in approximately 15% to 25% of people with AIDS and its course is widely varied but progressively deteriorating. Symptoms include psychomotor slowing, decreased speed in processing information, impaired memory, and impaired executive functioning.

Lewy body dementia accounts for 15% to 25% of dementias. Visual hallucinations and delusions are far more common in individuals with Lewy body dementia than in those with Alzheimer disease (AD). *Frontal lobe dementias*, caused by a variety of brain diseases, are often misdiagnosed as mental disorders because personality, sociability, and executive function are prominently impaired (Ballard et al., 2004). Frontal lobe dementias are discussed in more detail in chapter 20 ∞, "Neuropsychiatric Problems."

Delirium is an acute, usually reversible brain disorder characterized by clouding of the consciousness (a decreased awareness of the environment), a reduced ability to focus and maintain attention, and altered perception. Delirium is the most common cognitive disorder (see the DSM-IV-TR Classifications feature). Statistics show that 10% to 42% of individuals hospitalized for a medical condition, 25% of inpatients with cancer, 51% of postoperative clients, and 30% to 40% of hospitalized AIDS clients develop delirium as a complication of their primary illness. The presence of delirium indicates that a medical illness is affecting the brain, and rapid medical intervention is needed to prevent irreversible deterioration or death. People with dementia are more susceptible to delirium (Trzepacz, Meagher, & Wise, 2004). For a comparison of dementia and delirium, see Table 19.1 ■. Take a look at the DSM-IV-TR criteria feature for dementia and delirium.

KNOWLEDGE BASE: DEMENTIA

Alzheimer disease accounts for 60% to 70% of late-onset dementia and affects about 4.8 million Americans. By the year 2050,

---

DSM-IV-TR | Diagnostic Criteria for Cognitive Disorders

Diagnostic Criteria for Delirium Due to . . .
[Indicate the General Medical Condition]

A. Disturbance of consciousness (i.e., reduced clarity of awareness of the environment) with reduced ability to focus, sustain, or shift attention.

B. A change in cognition (such as memory deficit, disorientation, language disturbance) or the development of a perceptual disturbance that is not better accounted for by a preexisting, established, or evolving dementia.

C. The disturbance develops over a short period of time (usually hours to days) and tends to fluctuate during the course of the day.

D. There is evidence from the history, physical examination, or laboratory findings that the disturbance is caused by the direct physiological consequences of a general medical condition.

Diagnostic Criteria for Dementia of the Alzheimer Type (DAT)

A. The development of multiple cognitive deficits manifested by both:

1. Memory impairment (impaired ability to learn new information or to recall previously learned information)
2. One (or more) of the following cognitive disturbances:
   a. Aphasia (language disturbance)
   b. Apraxia (impaired ability to carry out motor activities despite intact motor function)
   c. Agnosia (failure to recognize or identify objects despite intact sensory function)
   d. Disturbance in executive functioning (i.e., planning, organizing, sequencing, abstracting)

B. The cognitive deficits in Criteria A1 and A2 each cause significant impairment in social or occupational functioning and represent a significant decline from a previous level of functioning.

C. The course is characterized by gradual onset and continuing cognitive decline.

D. The cognitive deficits in Criteria A1 and A2 are not due to any of the following:

1. Other central nervous system conditions that cause progressive deficits in memory and cognition (e.g., cerebrovascular disease, Parkinson disease, Huntington disease, subdural hematoma, normal-pressure hydrocephalus, brain tumor)
2. Systemic conditions that are known to cause dementia (e.g., hypothyroidism, vitamin B_{12} or folic acid deficiency, niacin deficiency, hypercalcemia, neurosyphilis, HIV infection)
3. Substance-induced conditions

E. The deficits do not occur exclusively during the course of a delirium.

F. The disturbance is not better accounted for by another Axis I disorder (e.g., major depressive disorder, schizophrenia).

SOURCE: Reprinted with permission from the *Diagnostic and Statistical Manual of Mental Disorders,* 4th edition, Text Revision. Copyright 2000 American Psychiatric Association.

CD-ROM

Animations/Videos, PET/SPECT Dementia

TABLE 19.1	Dementia and Delirium Compared

Dementia	Delirium
Onset	
Onset of impairment generally slow and insidious	Onset usually sudden; acute development of impairment of orientation, memory, cognitive function, judgment, and affect
Essential feature	
Not based on disordered consciousness; however, delirium, stupor, and coma may occur	Clouded state of consciousness
Etiology	
Generally caused by irreversible alteration of brain function	Caused by temporary, reversible, diffuse disturbances of brain function
Course	
No diurnal fluctuations. The clinical course usually progresses over months or years, ending in death.	Short, diurnal fluctuations in symptoms. The clinical course is usually brief, although it may last for months. Untreated, prolonged delirium may cause permanent brain destruction and lead to dementia.
History	
Onset: Insidious	Onset: Sudden
Duration: Months to years	Duration: Hours to days
Course: Consistent deterioration with occasional lucid moments	Course: Fluctuating arousal
Motor signs	
None (until late)	Postural tremor, restless, hyperactive, or sluggish
Speech is usually normal in early stages, but word-finding difficulties progress	Slurred speech, reflecting disorganized thinking
Mental status	
Attention generally normal in early stages; inattention progresses	Attention fluctuates
Memory	
Memory impairment; recent memory affected before remote	Impaired by poor attention
Language	
Aphasia in later stages	Normal or mild misnaming of objects
Perception	
Hallucinations not prominent, although cognitive impairment may lead to paranoid delusions	Visual, auditory, and/or tactile hallucinations
Pronounced mood/affect	
Disinterested and/or disinhibited	Fear and suspiciousness may be prominent; anxiety, depression, anger, irritability, or euphoria may occur
Review of systems	
Extraneural organ systems usually uninvolved	History of systemic illness or toxic exposure
EEG	
Normal or mildly slow	Pronounced diffuse slowing of fast cycles related to state of arousal

between 11 and 16 million people will be stricken with AD. The current annual costs are approximately $200 billion in the United States, $3.9 billion in Canada, and €87 billion in Europe. It strikes 1 of 12 people older than the age of 65, 1 of 3 people older than age 80, and almost 1 of 2 people older than age 85. Onset usually occurs in late life but, in rare cases, the disorder appears at age 40 or 50. Slightly more women than men are affected, even when controlling for a longer life span (Wimo et al., 2004).

Approximately 15% to 20% of AD cases are inherited; this form is known as *familial Alzheimer disease* (FAD). Because FAD often begins at a much younger age than AD, it is also referred to as early-onset AD.

Mild cognitive impairment is often described as memory loss without dementia. In some cases, it may be a transitional state between normal aging and AD. In other cases, the cognitive impairment never worsens. If possible, it is important to distinguish between the two situations as knowledge of drugs that may delay the progression of AD advances (Modrego, Fayed, & Pina, 2005; Rose, 2005). See Table 19.2 ■ for comparison of normal aging and AD.

Because vascular dementia and AD have many of the same characteristics and because AD is more prevalent, AD is used as the model for dementia in this chapter. The average course of AD is 5 to 10 years, but the range may be 2 to 20 years. People who have early-onset AD often deteriorate more rapidly. The progression is roughly divided into three stages.

- *Mild:* typically lasts 2 to 4 years, during which people are alert and sociable but their forgetfulness begins to interfere with daily living.

- *Moderate:* often the longer stage of the disease. There is a deterioration of intellect, logic, behavior, and daily functioning. Diagnosis most often occurs during this stage. Day care or assisted home care may be necessary to ensure safety.

- *Severe AD:* may last 1 to 2 years or longer. People can no longer do basic self-care activities and usually require 24-hour care. They are extremely confused and lose most of their long-term memory and language skills.

Comorbid Disorders

Several reversible disorders simulate or mimic dementia. Referred to as **pseudodementias**, these include drug toxicity, metabolic disorders, infections, and nutritional deficiencies.

Chronic lung disease and heart disease can lead to cerebral hypoxia and symptoms of dementia. The most common cause of pseudodementia is depression, which is often overlooked by health care professionals. Up to 50% of people with AD experience a comorbid depression, which increases the level of disability and hastens death. It is imperative to recognize and differentiate such disorders from irreversible dementia. See Table 19.3 ■ for a comparison of depression and dementia. Only through recognition can appropriate treatment measures be initiated (Zubenko et al., 2003).

It is critical to identify and treat all other disease processes before a person is diagnosed with AD. Hamdy, Turnball, and Edwards (1994) developed a differential diagnosis tool based on the word *dementia:*

D   **Drugs and Alcohol.** Long-lived people often purchase many over-the-counter medications, have many medications prescribed, and sometimes borrow medication from friends.

E   **Eyes and Ears.** People who cannot hear or see well often appear confused.

M   **Metabolic and Endocrine Diseases.** Disruptions such as electrolyte imbalance, hypothyroidism, and uncontrolled diabetes may mimic dementia.

E   **Emotional Disorders.** Mood and schizophrenic disorders may be mistaken for AD.

N   **Nutritional Deficiencies.** These may mimic dementia.

T   **Tumors and Trauma.** Disorders of the central nervous system (CNS) may be confused with AD.

I   **Infection.** Infections of the urinary tract and pneumonia in long-lived people may lead to confusion. Clients may not have an elevated temperature.

A   **Arteriosclerosis.** A decreased blood flow to the brain, brain attacks, and multi-infarct dementia often mimic AD.

TABLE 19.2	Changes in Normal Aging and Changes in Alzheimer Disease Compared
Normal Aging	**Alzheimer Disease**
Recent memory more impaired than remote memory	Recent and remote memory profoundly affected
Difficulty in recalling names of people and places	Inability to recall names of people and places
Decreased concentration	Inability to concentrate
Writing things down is helpful in stimulating memory.	Inability to write; nothing stimulates memory
Changes do not interfere with daily functioning.	Changes cause an inability to function at work, in a social relationship, and at home.
Insight into forgetful behavior is preserved.	With progression, the person has no insight into changes that have occurred.

TABLE 19.3	Depression and Dementia Compared
Depression	**Dementia**
Relatively rapid onset	Insidious onset
Symptoms progress rapidly	Symptoms progress slowly
Able to recall recent events	Has difficulty recalling recent events
Has long-term memory	As disease progresses, loses long-term memory
"Don't know" answers are common	Uses confabulation rather than admitting "don't know"
Attention span normal	Impaired attention span
Affect is depressed	Affect is shallow and labile
Oriented to person, time, and place	Unable to recognize familiar people and places; becomes lost in familiar environments; disoriented as to time
Apathetic in relationship to ADLs	Struggles to perform ADLs and is frustrated as a result

Etiologies

Genetics

The cause of AD is unknown but is likely a combination of aging and genetic and environmental factors. Research continues in an effort to understand the biochemical events responsible for the destruction of brain cells and currently is focused on the role of chromosomes 1, 14, 19, and 21 and the *amyloid precursor protein* (APP) gene. *APP* is the precursor of beta-amyloid protein that accumulates into plaques in AD.

People with Down syndrome, which is caused by an extra copy of *chromosome 21* that includes the *APP* gene, are at high risk for lesions in the brain similar to those seen in AD. A reported 75% of persons with Down syndrome older than age 60 have dementia, with neurobiological changes post-mortem that are indistinguishable from those of AD (Krasuski, Alexander, Horwitz, Rapoport, & Schapiro, 2002).

It is not known how the genes and their various mutations cause AD. In FAD, the mutations of the *APP* gene that occur on *chromosomes 14* and *1* are the likely gene mutations. The defective gene on chromosome 14 is called *presenilin 1*, whereas the defective gene on chromosome 1 is referred to as *presenilin 2*. If a person inherits one of the presenilin-producing genes, they are likely to develop AD at an early age. These two defects account for approximately 50% of the cases of FAD (Schutte & Holston, 2006).

Chromosome 19 is the link to late-onset FAD and sporadic AD. Scientists are looking for the link between genes and the production of *apolipoprotein E* (Apo E). Apo E is associated with the transport of cholesterol and the formation of plaques in the brain. Apo E comes in three varieties: E2, E3, and E4. The E2 version of the gene protects people from getting AD, while E4 increases risk and causes AD to start at a younger age. Those with two copies of E4 are at a very high risk for AD. The risk from *E3*, the most common *Apo E* gene, falls in between, which gives individuals an intermediate risk for AD. Apo E plays a role in cholesterol transport, cerebral amyloid deposition, neuronal plasticity, and cholinergic activity.

Consensus is against *genetic testing* for AD. Tests are promising but lack the sensitivity and specificity for routine use. All the possible genetic mutations are also unknown, which limits the predictability of genetic testing. If testing is available in the future, it will be necessary to protect against genetic discrimination by employers and insurers.

Neurobiology

Pathophysiologic changes associated with AD are degenerative and result in gross atrophy of the cerebral cortex. As the disease destroys brain cells, two types of abnormalities occur: neurofibrillary tangles and amyloid plaques. *Neurofibrillary tangles* are thick, insoluble clots of protein inside the damaged brain cells or neurons. *Amyloid plaques*, found on the outside of dead and damaged neurons, consist of bits of dying cells mixed with beta-amyloid protein. The enzyme, beta-secretase, appears to play a key role in the building up of plaques. It is unclear which disease is more responsible for the disease process.

Galanin is a neuropeptide thought to play a role in the pathophysiology of AD. Galanin rescues neurons that are in distress by slowing the cells down and eventually immobilizing them so that repairs can be made. The destruction of cells in AD leads to twice the normal level of galanin as the condition worsens. Excess galanin inhibits memory, especially visual memory, which may explain why people with AD are easily lost in their own neighborhoods because they cannot remember landmarks. Drug antagonists to galanin do not cross the blood–brain barrier and must be directly injected into the brain. Researchers are trying to develop oral antagonists because of their potential to slow the progression of this disease (Counts et al., 2006).

The death of neurons in AD follows a specific pattern. The first nerves to die are in the *limbic system,* the center for emotion and memory. The limbic system interprets emotional responses from the cerebral cortex, and the hippocampus, a part of the limbic system, is involved in memory storage. Destruction of the hippocampus results in loss of recent memory. Remote memory loss occurs more slowly, possibly because the memories are stored in more than one location in the brain. AD often brings on depression related to limbic system damage, as well as damage to the locus ceruleus, which modulates mood and stress response.

The destruction of neurons spreads toward the surface of the brain, killing off nerve cells in the *cerebral cortex.* Various symptoms appear as the destruction spreads throughout the four lobes. See Table 19.4 ■ for symptoms related to CNS destruction. Computed tomography (CT scan) may show brain atrophy, widened cortical sulci, and enlarged cerebral ventricles. Positron emission tomography (PET) can detect AD-related abnormalities by the way certain sugars are processed in the brain, especially in the temporal and parietal lobes. Early AD is considered if glucose use is decreased in the areas where language processing and memory storage takes place.

AD causes a progressive loss of most neurotransmitters and a reduction of synaptic binding sites. Decreased serotonin (5-HT) in the brain is associated with increased aggressive behavior, anxiety, agitation, and psychosis. Decreased levels of dopamine (DA) lead to movement difficulties, blunted affect, and apathy. Lowered levels of acetylcholine

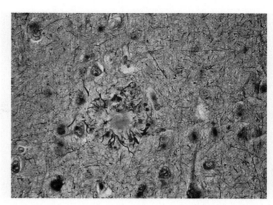

PHOTO 19.1 ■ This microscopic photograph illustrates senile plaques, which are found throughout the cortex and hippocampus of clients with Alzheimer disease.

SOURCE: Martin M. Rotker/Science Source/Photo Researchers, Inc. Used with permission.

(ACh) lead to memory difficulties, agitation, and psychotic symptoms. The balance between DA and ACh may also influence aggression in persons with AD. High levels of norepinephrine (NE) lead to anxiety, agitation, anorexia, and insomnia (Askin-Edgar, White, & Cummings, 2004).

Memory and learning are, to a certain extent, dependent on ACh. The enzyme choline-acetyl transferase (ChAT) synthesizes ACh from choline and acetyl coenzyme A. The enzyme cholinesterase (ChE) inactivates ACh. Individuals with AD have low levels of ChAT and ACh and high levels of ChE, compared with control groups. Researchers are seeking ways to raise and maintain ACh levels in those with AD (Dowling, 2004).

Glutamate (glu) is an excitatory neurotransmitter thought to be associated with learning and memory. Abnormally high amounts of glu may be responsible for the cell death that occurs in AD (Burbaeva et al., 2005).

TABLE 19.4	CNS Pathways of Destruction	
Area	**Function**	**Symptoms**
Limbic system	Memory, interpretation of emotion	Problems with recent and later remote memory; depression; apathy; unstable affect
Hippocampus	Memory storage	Decreased ability to learn; memory loss
Frontal lobe	Cognition, planning; motor aspects of speech; control of movement; control of outbursts; insight into own behavior	Problems with planning activities; inability to carry out skilled, purposeful movement; catastrophic reactions and emotional outbursts; delusions; inability to walk, talk, swallow
Parietal lobe	Sensory speech and ability to recognize written words; proprioception; ability to recognize objects and their function	Inability to recognize familiar places, people, and purpose of common household objects; expressive aphasia; agraphia; agnosia; hallucinations; seizures; falls
Temporal lobe	Memory, judgment, learning; ability to understand spoken words	Receptive aphasia; problems with memory and learning new concepts or activities
Occipital lobe	Ability to understand written words	Inability to read with comprehension; hallucinations

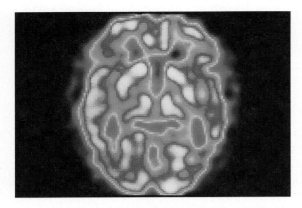

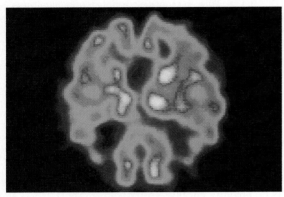

PHOTO 19.2 ■ PET scan of the brain (basal ganglia level) of a normal person and a client with Alzheimer disease. The scans show brain activity from low (blue) to high (yellow). Normal brain metabolic activity produces a roughly symmetrical pattern in the yellow areas of the left and right hemispheres (left). The patchy appearance of the client's scan indicates degeneration of brain tissue.

SOURCE: Tim Beddow/Science Photo Library/Photo Researchers, Inc. Used with permission.

Homocysteine is a metabolite of methionine, an essential amino acid. Elevated plasma homocysteine levels are associated with poor cognition, dementia, and AD. Further study may determine whether folate and vitamin B supplements, which reduce plasma homocysteine levels, can reduce the risk for AD (Seshadri et al., 2002).

Environmental Risk Factors

One environmental risk factor for AD is *traumatic head injury*. People who have experienced severe head injuries have a significant increase in the deposition of amyloid protein in the brain. The injury may decrease the functional reserves of the brain. It is also possible that damage to the blood–brain barrier allows entry of toxic products or somehow makes the brain more susceptible to the effects of aging (Lucas, Rothwell, & Gibson, 2006).

Protective Factors

Cigarette smoking may be a protective factor in both early- and late-onset AD. Smoking facilitates nicotinic receptor function and appears to delay signs and symptoms of AD.

The better educated people are, the less likely they are to experience dementia. It is believed that *mental stimulation* actually builds many more synapses between neurons, which allows individuals to better withstand the damages of disease. The same process is true for physical exercise. Drinking up to three glasses of wine daily is associated with a lower risk for AD. Intake of liquor or beer does not seem to provide protection (Larson et al., 2006; Ngandu et al., 2006).

Psychopharmacological Interventions

No known treatment can stop or reverse the mental deterioration of AD. The goals of medication are to improve ability or slow decline in cognition and activities of daily living (ADLs) with minimal side effects. Current medications either inhibit cholinesterase or regulate glu. Other drugs are used to manage symptoms such as anxiety, depression, or agitation.

Researchers are looking for ways to increase the amount of ACh in the brain. Because it is digested in the gastrointestinal tract, ACh cannot be taken orally. Three medications approved by the U.S. Food and Drug Administration (FDA) increase the availability of ACh in the synapses by inhibiting the enzyme cholinesterase responsible for the breakdown of ACh. These medications are donepezil (Aricept), rivastigmine (Exelon), and galantamine (Reminyl). Galantamine is a cholinesterase inhibitor that also includes nicotinic receptor–modulating activity.

Cholinesterase inhibitors do not cure AD but may slow the progression of the disorder. In some cases, this is almost as good as a cure: because AD usually strikes late in life, delaying its onset by a year would decrease the incidence and delay nursing home placement. Cholinesterase inhibitors are not effective for those with advanced AD. The side effects are usually transient, occurring at the onset of treatment, and include nausea, diarrhea, sweating, bradycardia, and insomnia. Taking the medication after breakfast may decrease side effects. Preliminary research suggests that angiotensin-converting enzyme (ACE) inhibitors may also slow the progression of AD (Ohrui et al., 2004).

Memantine (Namenda) has been approved for the treatment of moderate to severe AD. This new drug targets the excitatory amino acids such as glu. Excess glu is associated with neuronal nerve cell death found in the neurodegenerative disorders. The drug appears to correct the glu imbalance by acting as a receptor antagonist (Laustsen & Wimmett, 2005).

Because concomitant depression may increase functional disability, *antidepressant medications* are prescribed for people with depressive symptoms. Antipsychotic medications may decrease agitation, aggression, paranoid thinking, and poor impulse control. In 2005, the FDA issued a public health advisory regarding increased risk of death associated with the use of all second generation antipsychotics in elderly people with dementia. Clinicians must decide when the benefits of antipsychotics outweigh the potential harm. Selegiline (Eldepryl), a selective monoamine oxidase B inhibitor approved for motor dysfunction of Parkinson disease, may delay functional decline but does not improve cognitive performance. Citalopram (Celexa), a selective serotonin receptor inhibitor (SSRI) antidepressant, is helpful for behavioral disturbances and psychotic symptoms (DeDeyn et al., 2005).

Medication should not be overused to sedate and calm clients. For those clients experiencing sleep problems, the use of hypnotics is contraindicated because the medication does not improve sleep patterns and often increases confusion and sedation during awake periods. Medications used for agitation and aggression include trazodone (Desyrel), buspirone (BuSpar), carbamazepine (Tegretol), and valproate (Depakote).

Very early pilot studies suggest that intravenous immunoglobulin (IVIg) may slightly reverse the disease process in AD. IVIg is a combination of many antibiotics that is already in use for some autoimmune diseases. It is thought that antiamyloid antibodies in IVIg attach to beta amyloid and remove it from the brain.

Multidisciplinary Interventions

The most effective approach to AD occurs with the coordinated efforts of the multidisciplinary team. *Speech therapists* may be able to slow down the aphasic process and restore partial swallowing function. *Physical therapists* can maintain or increase range of motion, improve muscle tone, improve coordination, and increase endurance for exercise. *Occupational therapists* can provide additional sensory stimulation and self-care training programs. *Social workers* can provide individual or group therapy for families of people with AD; moreover, they can help with community resources or institutional placement. *Pastoral counselors* can help clients and families meet religious and spiritual needs.

A new hope for AD is *gene therapy*. Researchers remove genetic material from viruses and replace it with a gene that creates nerve growth factor, a chemical that keeps memory-related cells alive. Two holes are drilled in the upper skull and 40 billion carrier viruses are injected into the brain. The gene instructs cells to make nerve growth factor. Initial studies suggest that progression of AD can be significantly slowed. If research demonstrates a significant result, the procedure could become the treatment of choice (Tuszynski et al., 2005).

Alternative Therapies

Antioxidants

Antioxidants are a group of vitamins, minerals, enzymes, and herbs that help protect the body from naturally occurring free radicals. As the body goes through its normal processes, and oxygen is used to provide cellular fuel, some of the oxygen molecules lose one of their two electrons. When they do, the formerly stable oxygen molecules become dangerous free radicals that try to stabilize themselves by stealing another electron from stable molecules, thus damaging them and creating more free radicals. An excess of free radicals is, in part, responsible for the effects of aging and is implicated in degenerative conditions such as AD (Fontaine, 2005).

As people age, they produce fewer antioxidants and may benefit from dietary antioxidants such as vitamin C, vitamin E, carotenoids, the mineral selenium, and the hormone melatonin. Herbs with antioxidant properties include bilberry, ginkgo, grape seed extract, green tea, and flavonoids. Fruits and vegetables are the primary sources for antioxidants, though they are also available in the form of supplements. At the top of the list in providing antioxidants are fruits and vegetables with the deepest colors, such as prunes, raisins, blueberries, blackberries, raspberries, garlic, kale, cranberries, strawberries, spinach, broccoli, and beets (Berman & Brodaty, 2004).

Omega-3 Fish Oil

Omega-3 fish oil, an essential fat, especially the component DHA (ducosahexaenoic acid), is essential for optimal functioning of neuronal synapses in the brain. Good sources of omega-3 fish oil include salmon, mackerel, herring, sardines, and cod liver oil. Eating too many omega-6 vegetable fats, such as corn oil and other processed oils, makes the neuronal membranes rigid and can also destroy DHA. Low levels of DHA are a risk factor for low mental performance and AD.

Phosphatidyl Serine

Phosphatidyl serine (Ptd Ser) is a component of the nerve cell membrane that helps keep nerve cell membranes flexible. A dose of 300 mg/day for 1 month followed by 100 mg/day thereafter often improves memory. Ptd Ser from cow brains is rich in DHA and increases levels of DA and NE. As a supplement, it may be combined with ginkgo (Brown & Gerbarg, 2000).

Melatonin

Insomnia is a frequent problem among persons with AD. Melatonin, a hormone secreted by the pineal gland, plays a critical role in the regulation of the day–night cycle. As we age, we produce less melatonin, and for those with AD, the disturbance is even more pronounced. Studies have shown that melatonin is effective in inducing sleep and has no notable side effects. Slow-release melatonin often improves sleep pattern in people with AD.

Dehydroepiandrosterone

Dehydroepiandrosterone (DHEA) is a corticosteroid produced primarily in the adrenal glands. In addition to serving as a precursor to testosterone and estrogen, DHEA may be involved in regulating mood and one's sense of well-being. The method of action is unclear but it may stimulate gamma-aminobutyric acid (GABA) receptors or increase 5-HT levels. Since there is little known about long-term risks, it is probably best used under medical supervision. The usual dose is up to 90 mg/day.

SAMe

SAMe (S-adenosylmethionine), a compound made by every cell in the body, helps produce DA, 5-HT, and NE. In addition, SAMe (pronounced sam-ee) improves cell membrane flexibility. Low levels of SAMe have been found in persons with AD. SAMe should be used with caution in people who have a history of cardiac arrhythmia.

Lecithin

Lecithin is a major component of cell membranes. Nerve cells and the protective membranes surrounding the brain are largely composed of lecithin. High doses of lecithin may be helpful for people with AD. Most lecithin is derived from soybeans but, recently, egg lecithin has become popular.

Music Therapy

Neurohormone and neurotransmitter levels may change because of music therapy. One study of people with AD found that 30 to 40 minutes of music therapy in the morning, 5 days a week for 4 weeks, resulted in significant increases in serum melatonin concentration. Levels continued to rise even after the music therapy had been discontinued for 6 weeks. Some clinical effects were client ability to sing and learn new songs, an increased ability to follow rhythmic patterns, an ability to anticipate endings of phrases and songs, an improved ability to follow changes in tempo, and increased social interaction with peers and therapists (Kumar, Tims, & Gruess, 1999).

Touch Therapy

Management of agitation is one goal of alternative practices. Massage therapy relaxes and calms people with AD. One study evaluated the effect of therapeutic touch (TT) on 10 individuals with AD. A significant decrease in vocalization and pacing or walking was observed over time with the treatment of TT (Woods & Dimond, 2002).

Animal-Assisted Therapy

A nursing study investigated the use of fish aquariums in dementia-specific inpatient units. Increase in nutritional intake and significant weight gain was experienced in the residents exposed to the aquarium (Edwards & Beck, 2002).

KNOWLEDGE BASE: DELIRIUM

Delirium, an acute disorder of cognition and attention, has become increasingly recognized as a common and serious problem for hospitalized individuals. Delirium occurs in 10% to 40% of hospitalized elderly clients, in 30% to 40% of hospitalized people with AIDS, and in up to 60% of nursing home residents older than age 75. In the general hospital population, the rate is 10% to 30%. Nearly 80% of terminally ill people develop delirium near death (Trzepacz, Meagher, & Wise, 2004).

Delirium develops quickly and usually lasts about 1 week unless the underlying disorder is not corrected. Prompt medical attention is vital to prevent permanent brain damage or death. If the cause is not found and treated, death may occur in a matter of days or weeks. The course of the disorder fluctuates; that is, periods of coherence alternate with periods of confusion.

There are three subtypes of delirium:

- Hyperactive
- Hypoactive
- Mixed

Agitation, disorientation, hallucinations, delusions, and labile mood are evident in hyperactive delirium. Individuals with hypoactive delirium are confused, disoriented, and depressed. People with mixed delirium alternate between hyperactive and hypoactive states (Trzepacz & Kennedy, 2005).

Comorbid Disorders

Delirium occurs in people of all ages. However, the incidence increases with age because of the accompanying illnesses and medication use. Physiologic changes of aging, such as decreased blood flow to the liver and kidneys, predispose long-lived adults to delirium. People with AD are also predisposed to delirium because CNS function is already compromised. Other groups at high risk include people with terminal cancer and those with HIV/AIDS.

The term **pseudodelirium** is used to describe symptoms of delirium that occur without identifiable organic cause. The symptoms may occur because of sensory deprivation or because of the effects of psychosocial stress. Those most vulnerable to pseudodelirium have some pre-existing cerebral disease such as a mood disorder, anxiety, schizophrenia, and dementia.

Etiologies
Neurobiology

By affecting the CNS, many conditions may lead to delirium. Cerebral metabolism is dependent on sufficient amounts of oxygen, glucose, and metabolic cofactors. Brain hypoxia may result from pulmonary disease, anemia, or carbon monoxide poisoning. Decreased cerebral blood flow leads to ischemia of the CNS. *Ischemia* may result from cardiac arrhythmias or arrest, congestive heart failure, pulmonary embolus, decreased blood volume, systemic lupus erythematosus, or subacute bacterial endocarditis. Lack of glucose for cerebral metabolism occurs during a state of *hypoglycemia*. Certain metabolic cofactors are essential for cerebral enzyme actions. *Cofactor deficiencies* involve thiamine, niacin, pyridoxine, folate, and vitamin B_{12}.

Endocrine disorders of the thyroid, parathyroid, and adrenal glands are associated with delirium. Hepatic and renal failure may be contributing disorders. Fluid and electrolyte imbalance—particularly acidosis, alkalosis, potassium, sodium, magnesium, and calcium imbalances—are additional causes of delirium.

Toxicity from substances such as alcohol, sedatives, antihistamines, parasympatholytic agents, opioids, cerebral stimulants, digitalis, antidepressants, and heavy metals may also lead to a delirious state. (See chapter 15 ∞ for a thorough discussion of alcohol and drug abuse.) Other likely offenders include anticholinergic agents and analgesic agents, which induce CNS depression.

Any direct or primary CNS disturbance—trauma, infection, hemorrhage, neoplasm, or a seizure disorder—is likely to trigger delirium. In addition, drugs for the treatment of hypertension and Parkinson disease have been implicated in causing delirium.

Environmental Factors

The use of physical restraints may be a contributing factor to delirium. The use of restraints with older adults is often said to be for their personal safety and avoidance of harm. Yet restraint use has many negative affects, such as decreased mobility, skin breakdown, cardiac stress, agitation, confusion, and lowered self-esteem. Physical restraints can precede the onset of delirium, therefore precipitating this acute disorder.

Psychopharmacological Interventions

The medical treatment of delirium involves swift identification of the organic cause. Appropriate treatment requires removal of an offending substance, stabilization in the presence of trauma, administration of antibiotics for infection, or reestablishment of nutrition and metabolic balance. Medications used in managing substance withdrawal delirium are discussed in chapter 15 ∞.

Controlling the symptoms of delirium may be accomplished through administration of Haloperidol (Haldol) intravenously over a period of 1 to 3 minutes. When combined with lorazepam (Ativan), there is often a rapid reduction of delirium and severe agitation. Intramuscular (IM) administration of haloperidol (Haldol) has an unpredictable rate of absorption and is more likely to produce extrapyramidal side effects. The usual dose is 1 to 2 mg. Doses may be repeated every 20 to 30 minutes but should not total more than 5 mg every 15 minutes, with a maximum of 240 mg in a 24-hour period. The desired clinical effect is a person who is drowsy but arousable. Once the person is calm, 0.5 to 3 mg of haloperidol may be administered orally. If a client develops extrapyramidal symptoms, 25 to 50 mg of diphenhydramine (Benadryl) may be given intravenously (Trzepacz & Kennedy, 2005).

Nursing Process

A CLIENT WITH DEMENTIA

ASSESSMENT: DEMENTIA

Assessing clients with cognitive impairment disorders—specifically AD—can be a challenge to a nurse's ingenuity and patience. Some clients can respond appropriately when questions are asked simply and enough time is given. Others are so disoriented and confused that they are unable to answer questions; in these situations, the nurse must rely on family members to provide the necessary assessment data. Functional impairment, such as the ability to manage finances and household chores, is more accurately assessed with family members. See the Focused Nursing Assessment feature for clients with cognitive impairment disorders and their family members.

Assessment: Behavior

The most notable changes in behavior during mild AD are difficulties performing complex tasks, related to a *decline in short-term memory*. Persons may be unable to plan a meal, make a shopping list, or complete work assignments but they are capable of independent living. They recognize their confusion and are frightened by what is happening. Fearing the diagnosis, they attempt to cover up and rationalize their symptoms.

In moderate AD, behavior deteriorates markedly and client *safety* becomes an issue. The most common accidents are falls, followed by injuries resulting from difficulty using sharp objects. *Wandering behavior* poses a potential danger because persons with AD get lost easily and are unable to retrace their steps home.

During this stage, clients need assistance with the sequence of skills for ADLs. They also need help in dressing, toileting, and bathing. The inability to carry out skilled and purposeful movement or the inability to use objects properly is called **apraxia**. Also evident is **hyperorality**, the need to taste, chew, and examine any object small enough to be placed in the mouth. People in moderate AD must be protected from accidentally eating harmful substances such as soaps or poisons.

Although there may be a sharp increase in appetite and food intake, there is seldom corresponding weight gain. In contrast, some individuals have limited or no recognition of mealtimes or even food. Behavior in this stage is characterized

Focused Nursing Assessment | Clients With Cognitive Impairment Disorders

Behavior Assessment	Affective Assessment	Cognitive Assessment	Social Assessment
How much assistance is needed in: ■ Bathing? ■ Toileting? ■ Dressing? ■ Eating? Describe any difficulties in performing complex tasks at home and at work. Give me an example of something that has confused you recently. Have you ever become lost when you went out for a walk?	What kinds of things make you feel anxious? When do you feel sad? How often do you feel irritable? What are your major frustrations in life? How do you feel about growing older?	What month is it? What year is it? Who is the President of the United States? What is your telephone number (or address)? Where are you right now? Tell me your complete name. What did you do for activity this morning? What is the purpose of (show the objects to the client) a comb? Toothbrush? Pencil? Telephone book? Shoe? What is the meaning of the proverb "People in glass houses shouldn't throw stones"? What would you do if someone shouted "Fire!" right now?	How close do you feel to your family members? How do you handle disagreements?

by continuous, repetitive acts that have no meaning or direction. These repetitive behaviors—which may include lip licking, tapping of fingers, pacing, or echoing others' words—are referred to as **perseveration phenomena.**

Many long-lived adults, including those with AD, become disoriented at the end of the day; this is usually referred to as **sundown syndrome**. Orientation seems to decrease as daylight recedes. It becomes more difficult to distinguish shapes from shadows and to pinpoint the source of sounds in the environment. Sundown syndrome is more pronounced when clients are fatigued. Various behaviors relating to sundown syndrome include wandering, confusion, hyperactivity, restlessness, and aggression.

Disruptive, *agitated behavior* may occur during the moderate stage. Verbally agitated behaviors include outbursts or screaming. Physically agitated behavior includes pacing and resisting personal care. It may escalate into hitting, biting, or throwing things. Agitation and aggression often result from physical discomfort, sensory deprivation, or social isolation. Frequently, the person is unable to explain an unmet need such as pain, fecal or urinary urgency, constipation, anxiety, or depression (Kovach, Noonan, Schlidt, & Wells, 2005).

Almost 50% of clients with AD become withdrawn and *apathetic* as the disease advances. This is evidenced in passive behaviors such as decreased interaction with others, withdrawal from activities, less interest in a variety of experiences, and less willingness to try new activities.

Wandering is another problem at this time. Wandering may be a substitute for social interaction and thus is a way to alleviate loneliness and separation from others. Wandering may also be an expression of agitation, boredom, pain, or discomfort. Within a safe environment, wandering can be beneficial since it stimulates circulation and oxygenation and promotes exercise.

In the severe stage of AD, a syndrome like Klüver–Bucy syndrome develops, which includes the continuation of hyperorality and periodic binge eating. Behavior is also characterized by **hyperetamorphosis**, the need to compulsively touch and examine every object in the environment. There is a sharp deterioration in motor ability that progresses from an inability to walk to an inability to sit up and, finally, to an inability even to smile.

Assessment: Affect

In the mild stage of AD, anxiety and depression may occur as affected people become aware of and try to cope with noticeable deficits. They frequently experience feelings of helplessness, frustration, and shame in relation to their deficits.

Families of Clients With Cognitive Impairment Disorders

Behavior Assessment	Affective Assessment	Cognitive Assessment	Social Assessment
How much assistance is needed in activities of daily living?	Describe the degree of spontaneity to verbal and nonverbal stimuli.	Have there been changes in her or his ability to concentrate?	Is there a family history of organic brain disorder?
Tell me about her or his wandering away from home.	How anxious does she or he seem to you?	Describe any confusion about person, time, or place.	What are previous hobbies/interests? Family activities?
Is there difficulty in carrying out psychomotor activities?	How depressed does she or he seem to you?	Describe any suspicious thinking.	Who has been the primary caregiver?
Is she or he picking up and putting things in the mouth?	In what way is irritability increasing?	Describe any recent memory loss.	Describe the stresses in caregiving (emotional, physical, financial).
Does she or he touch everything in sight?	Does she or he have wide mood swings? Describe.	Describe any remote memory loss.	Describe the positive aspects of caregiving.
What kinds of repetitive movements does she or he make?		Does she or he make up answers when facts cannot be remembered?	What kinds of support systems are you able to use? Family? Friends? Religious? Self-help groups?
Describe her or his interactions with other people.		Is there difficulty in finding the right word for objects?	What kinds of discussions have taken place regarding placement?
Is she or he withdrawn? Agitated? Aggressive?		Has she or he lost the ability to read and write?	What other kinds of living arrangements are possible?
Are the behavior problems worse at night?		Is there an inability to identify familiar sounds?	Who is involved in making these decisions?
		Give me examples of irrational decision making.	How united is the family in providing care?
		Has she or he thought that strangers were family members? Please give examples.	

Diagnosis of these comorbid disorders is important because left untreated, they can worsen the symptoms of dementia.

In the beginning of AD, clients are less enthusiastic, less cheerful, and less affectionate. As the disease progresses into the moderate stage, there is an increased *lability* of emotions from flat affect to periods of marked irritability. Delusions of persecution may precipitate feelings of intense fear. *Catastrophic reactions*, resulting from underlying brain dysfunction, are common. In response to everyday situations, the person may overreact by exploding in rage or suddenly crying. In the severe stage, response to environmental stimuli continues to decrease until the person is wholly nonresponsive.

Assessment: Cognition

The primary cognitive deficit in mild AD is memory impairment with a *decrease in concentration*, an increase in distractibility, and the appearance of absent-mindedness. The ability to make accurate judgments also declines. People with early-onset AD may have difficulty managing their finances or may give away large amounts of money in response to radio and television solicitations. It is difficult to decide when to prevent them from driving. Because they are easily distracted, they may forget the meaning of road signs, may confuse the meaning of red and green lights, and may not look to see that no other cars are coming; they are also extremely accident prone. On the other hand, giving up driving privileges is a blow to a person's sense of autonomy and self-esteem.

Language skills begin to deteriorate in mild AD as individuals have problems thinking of what to say and language processing takes longer. They may have word-finding and object-naming difficulties. They have problems with complex conversations, rapid speech, and speech in noisy and distracting environments. At this stage, they may self-correct or apologize for communication problems.

In moderate AD, there is a progressive memory loss, which includes recent and remote memory. New information cannot be retained, and there is no recollection of what occurred 10 minutes or an hour ago. Loss of remote memory becomes obvious when there is no recognition of family members or recall of significant past events. This loss may be the most painful aspect of AD, erasing a whole lifetime of memories for that person.

Confabulation, the filling in of memory gaps with imaginary information, is an attempt to distract others from observing the deficit. Comprehension of language, interactions, and significance of objects is greatly diminished. During this stage, the person becomes completely disoriented in all three spheres of person, time, and place.

More than 50% of people with AD develop delusions, often involving themes of persecution. They may believe strangers are intending to harm them or are breaking into their home and stealing from them. Paranoia can also take the form of delusional jealousy and manifest with accusations of infidelity, which can be heartbreaking for the partner.

Holocaust survivors with AD can have flashbacks of old horrors. Their minds can no longer keep buried the tortured memories of concentration camps, gas chambers, and loved ones killed in front of them. Many things that trigger flashbacks, such as restraints, people yelling in pain, and being taken to the showers, are found in hospitals and nursing homes. Flashbacks are an especially tragic outcome for holocaust survivors.

Misidentification syndrome frequently occurs, in which familiar people are seen as unfamiliar and vice versa. They may even believe that people on television are actually present.

As the disease progresses, communication breakdowns become more frequent and more severe. Stressful and confusing situations compound the difficulty in understanding others or in expressing thoughts. An increase of **aphasia**—the loss of the ability to understand or use language—occurs and begins with the inability to find words and eventually limits the person to as few as six words. Concurrently, **agraphia**, the inability to read or write, develops. Finally, the inability to recognize familiar situations, people, or stimuli evolves; this is known as **agnosia**. *Auditory agnosia* is the inability to recognize familiar sounds such as a doorbell, the ring of a telephone, or a barking dog. *Tactile agnosia*, or **astereognosia**, occurs when the person is unable to identify familiar objects placed in the hand, such as a comb, a pencil, or a paintbrush. *Visual agnosia*, or **alexia**, occurs when the person can look at a frying pan, a telephone, or a toothbrush and have no idea what to do with these objects.

The following interchange illustrates the aphasic characteristics of AD. Pat is able to give a variety of descriptors but cannot think of the one necessary word.

Sue called her mother, Pat, to see how she was doing.

Sue: *"It sounds like you are eating, Mom. What are you eating?"*
Pat: *"I can't tell you."*
Sue: *"Is it hot or cold?"*
Pat: *"It's cold."*
Sue: *"Did you get it out of the refrigerator?"*
Pat: *"No, it's like bread."*
Sue: *"Is it a sandwich?"*
Pat: *"Sort of. I put butter on it."*
Sue: *"Is it crackers?"*
Pat: *"No. I used to buy a lot of it and put it in the freezer."*
Sue: *"Is it cookies?"*
Pat: *"No. Usually I have it for breakfast. I took the last slice."*
Sue: *"Is it coffee cake?"*
Pat: *"Yes, that's what it is."*

In the severe stage of AD, cognitive functioning declines severely. Clients may be oblivious to others in the home and may be unable to recognize themselves in the mirror. They may scream or yell spontaneously or be able to say only one word or be unable to say anything. In addition, there is no longer nonverbal response to internal and external stimuli; the person degenerates to a *vegetative state*.

Assessment: Perception

Hallucinations can occur in all of the senses, but visual hallucinations are the most common and occur in more than 20% of clients with AD. Persons with AD may have visions of animals, people from the past, or even of intruders. The hallucinations are distressing and are associated with more rapid cognitive decline. Hallucinations are associated with a 78% risk for death (Wilson et al., 2005).

Assessment: Interpersonal Relationships

There are at least two victims of AD: the person with the disease and the caregiver. Remember that, for every client, there is a family in distress. Spouses or partners may experience the loss of growing older together as planned, fear for one's own future, and the anguish of watching a life partner deteriorate. Children and siblings may wonder whether they will inherit the disease. AD has been called by some "death by a thousand subtractions" and by former First Lady Nancy Reagan as "the long goodbye."

While clients are still able to participate and make their wishes known, family members can seek their guidance regarding long-term plans. A living will or an advance directive may be formulated. A durable power of attorney for health care should be named as well as a durable power of attorney for financial matters.

Families are the primary providers of long-term care for people with dementia. Most often, the person is elderly. Elderly spouses, who are most likely to provide care, have limited strength and energy to meet the demands of the situation. Middle-age children, most typically daughters, must manage their own problems and the role reversal that occurs with a dependent parent. Caring for a person with dementia is among the most difficult family responsibilities and the one for which caregivers receive minimal support and training.

Concerns about intimacy and sexuality are important for most couples, regardless of sexual orientation. Most of us have been socially conditioned to think that old people are—or should be—nonsexual, especially old people with dementia. The reality is that sexuality ranges along a continuum of no interest to active, ongoing interest. Severity of the disease is not always the standard by which to judge the appropriateness of sexual behavior. Some healthy partners have no interest in continuing a sexual relationship with an ill partner. This may be in response to feeling more like a parent to the partner or feeling insignificant when not recognized by the ill person. Some healthy partners are interested in maintaining sexual intimacy but may be physically exhausted or feel guilty about being sexual with a partner who is unable to clearly consent. Other healthy partners express no interest in genital sex but remain interested in emotional intimacy (loving words) and physical intimacy (holding, kissing, stroking). Others are able to maintain all types of intimacy, including genital sex, and feel satisfied and joyful with the interaction. A satisfactory sex life is a comfort to these couples as their bodies remember and celebrate this pleasure.

Clients who attend day treatment programs or live in extended care facilities meet other people who also have AD. Some of these clients develop emotionally and physically intimate relationships with one another. Families may be happy that their loved ones have found a source of joy in an otherwise bleak world of confusion. As people with AD have no memory of their previous lives, this new romance is not a betrayal of the spouse or partner. Retired Supreme Court Justice Sandra Day O'Connor shared her views about her husband falling in love with another client at a facility for people with AD. Justice O'Connor stated that she was thrilled that her husband was relaxed and happy in the situation (Biskapic, 2007). Other families do not understand what is occurring and need education and support from the nursing staff to process the new situation.

The changes that occur in AD are frightening to family members, and witnessing the steady deterioration of their loved ones is extremely painful. Many families eventually become exhausted and have emotional, physical, and financial problems. Outside relationships may need to be forfeited. Custodial care in an appropriate facility may be necessary. Many couples, however, cannot afford day care early in the disease process or full-time nursing care late in the process. Finding the money to hire sitters or housekeepers can be stressful for the well partner (Beeson, 2003).

The nurse must also assess caregivers for caregiver burden. Consider multiple stressors when assessing caregivers. Questions to consider are:

- How is caregiving interfering with employment or other family roles?
- Can stress be decreased through anticipation and prioritization?
- Is respite care an option?
- What are the quality and extent of supportive relationships for the caregiver?
- Is there evidence of anxiety or depression?

Support for caregivers is essential at all times while caring for clients with AD.

Assessment: Cultural Influences

In the United States, Latin Americans and African Americans are at increased risk for AD. Latin Americans develop AD almost 7 years earlier than non-Latin Americans. The rate of cognitive decline is slower in African Americans than in Euro-Americans. In spite of this knowledge, research on the progression of AD in minority populations has been minimal. The rate for dementia in other countries is highest in Japan, followed by Italy, and then Hong Kong. In these countries, female family members are responsible for the care of their loved ones and there are few nursing home institutions (Barnes et al., 2006; Fung & Chien, 2002; Rose, 2005; Vellone, Sansoni, & Cohen, 2002).

Assessment: Physical

Deterioration of the CNS results in physical changes throughout the body. People with dementia may suffer from **hypertonia**, an increase in muscle tone that results in muscular twitching. While hyperactivity may occur, eventually there is a loss of energy and increasing fatigue with physical activity. The sleep cycle is impaired; there is a decrease in total sleep time and awakenings are more frequent. This disruption leads to sleep deprivation, which magnifies the already disturbed cognitive functions.

People with AD are susceptible to injuries from falls. About half the falls are secondary to problems such as orthostatic hypotension, postural instability, and impaired vision. Other falls are related to such factors as poor lighting or loose rugs. Some people will fall because of poor judgment, as in putting a chair on top of a table and climbing up to reach something. Because of changes in the CNS, people with AD have a decreased reaction time. Therefore, it is more difficult to regain balance when beginning to fall.

As the disease progresses, incontinence of urine and stool occurs. In the final stage, anorexia and difficulty swallowing leads to an emaciated physical condition. Very common to AD is immune suppression. Death usually occurs from pneumonia, urinary tract infection leading to sepsis, malnutrition, or dehydration (Kovach et al., 2005).

ASSESSMENT: DELIRIUM

Since nurses are the health care professionals who spend the most time with clients, they are usually the first to notice that the client's condition is worsening. Delirium must be identified in the early stages to prevent permanent damage and even death.

Assessment: Behavior

People with delirium generally display an alteration in psychomotor activity and poor impulse control. Some are apathetic and withdrawn, others are agitated and tremulous, and still others shift rapidly between apathy and agitation. Hyperactivity is typical of a drug withdrawal state, whereas hypoactivity is typical of a metabolic imbalance. Speech patterns

MediaLink Case Study, Caregiver Burden

may be limited and dull, or they may be fast, pressured, and loud. There may be a constant picking at clothes and bed linen as the result of an underlying restlessness. Bizarre and destructive behavior, which worsens at night, may occur as the person attempts to protect herself or himself or escape from frightening delusions or hallucinations. This behavior may take the form of calling for help, striking out at others, or even attempting to leap out of windows.

> Over the course of the past 2 days, Mary has exhibited abrupt behavioral changes. Sometimes, she seems apathetic and withdrawn, barely responding to questions or environmental stimuli. Most of the time, however, particularly at night, she becomes agitated and calls out loudly. She vacillates between being verbally aggressive and abusive and being very vulnerable and frightened, asking for help and whimpering like a small child. Much of the verbal content of her messages has to do with snakes that are in bed with her. She desperately keeps trying to remove these snakes from her bed linens.

Assessment: Affect

In the state of delirium, a person's affect may range from apathy to extreme irritability to euphoria. Emotions are labile; they can change abruptly and fluctuate in intensity. A person may be laughing and suddenly become extremely sad and tearful, reflective of the CNS injury. The predominant emotion in delirium is fear. Illusions, delusions, and hallucinations are vivid and extremely frightening.

> Mary is terrified by the visual hallucinations of snakes on her bed. She perceives her safety to be threatened and cries for help in removing the snakes. During a family interview, the nurse in charge learns that Mary has always been extremely frightened of snakes, which increases the impact of her hallucinations.

Assessment: Cognition

The primary cognitive characteristics of delirium are disorganized thinking and a diminished ability to maintain and shift attention. Disorganized thinking is evidenced by rambling, bizarre, or incoherent speech. Lack of judgment and reason severely impairs the decision-making process. Delirious people have difficulty focusing their attention and are easily distracted by environmental stimuli; therefore, interactions are difficult, if not impossible. Attention problems result in impairment in recent memory. Remote memory problems may result from changes in the neurotransmitters, making information retrieval difficult.

Another cognitive disruption is disorientation, which often results from attention deficits. Disorientation to time and place is common, whereas identity confusion is rare. Almost all people with delirium misperceive sensory stimuli in the environment. The result is usually visual or auditory illusions. For example, the person may believe that spots on the floor are insects. Visual hallucinations are also common and may involve people, animals, objects, or bright flashes of light or color. Delusional beliefs exist, supporting the illusions and hallucinations. These changes often extend into sleep, which may be accompanied by vivid and terrifying dreams (Trzepacz et al., 2004).

> Marie is an 18-year-old, extremely thin, anorexic client. Laboratory analysis reveals her blood glucose level to be 40 mg/dL. She is agitated and incoherent. Owing to her inability to think logically and to the fact that she is trying to communicate to others not actually present, she is unable to give a history. She is completely disoriented to time and place. In terms of orientation to people, she is able to state her own name but does not recognize the boyfriend who brought her to the hospital. In fact, she is convinced that Ron, a nurse, is her boyfriend.

Assessment: Interpersonal Relationships

Because of the sudden and often unexplained onset of delirium, families are usually anxious and frightened. They may not know how to respond to the agitation, pressured speech, destructive behavior, and labile moods. Equally confusing to families are the disorientation, illusions, hallucinations, and delusions. Because delirious individuals are unable to make decisions, family members must temporarily assume that responsibility.

Assessment: Physical

People with delirium experience a disturbance in the sleep cycle. Some have hypersomnia and sleep fitfully throughout the day and night. Others have insomnia and sleep very little, day or night. There are obvious signs of autonomic activity, including increased cardiac rate, elevated blood pressure, flushed face, dilated pupils, and sweating. Respiratory depth or rhythm may be altered because of brain stem depression or in an attempt to correct an acid–base imbalance that results from the underlying disorder.

Delirious individuals may experience irregular tremors throughout the body. Those in a resting position may have myoclonus, a sudden, large muscle spasm. Although they occur most frequently in the face and shoulders, these spasms, which are a result of irritation of the cerebral cortex, can happen anywhere in the body. If the hand is hyperextended, there will be an involuntary palmar flexion called asterixis. Generalized seizures may also occur.

> Kimora arrived at the emergency department confused and disoriented. Her family reports that she has not been eating and sleeping well and has lost 35 lb in the past 2 months. She is unable to concentrate or focus and her immediate recall is poor. She answers questions inappropriately and has very limited insight. She is experiencing visual hallucinations and picks at things in the air. Her potassium level is dangerously low at 2.9 mEq/L.

DIAGNOSIS

There are many potential nursing diagnoses for clients experiencing cognitive disorders. In synthesizing the assessment data, consider how well clients are functioning in daily life, what skills they still retain, how well they are able to communicate, and how the caregivers are coping (North American Nursing Diagnosis Association, 2007).

- Risk for Injury related to poor judgment, environmental hazards, wandering behavior
- Risk for Falls related to poor vision, postural instability
- Risk for Other-directed Violence related to labile emotions, aggressive behavior
- Fear related to catastrophic reactions, delusions of persecution, hallucinations
- Impaired Memory related to temporary or permanent CNS changes
- Impaired Verbal Communication related to aphasia, agraphia, agnosia
- Bathing/Hygiene/Dressing/Grooming/Feeding/Toileting Self-care Deficit related to an inability to sequence these skills
- Impaired Social Interaction related to distractibility, withdrawal, apathy
- Disturbed Sleep Pattern related to CNS changes
- Caregiver Role Strain related to fatigue, lack of support systems, increasing dependency of family member
- Anticipatory Grieving related to impending death during severe stage of AD

OUTCOME IDENTIFICATION AND GOALS

Once you have established diagnoses, select outcomes appropriate to the nursing diagnoses.

Broad outcomes are:

- Remains safe
- Utilizes remaining skills/abilities
- Returns to predelirium level of functioning

Client goals are specific behavioral measures by which you and significant others determine progress toward goals. The following are examples of some of the goals appropriate to people (and their caregivers) with cognitive impairment disorders:

- Improves orientation as delirium clears
- Participates in appropriate social activities

- Participates in a gentle exercise routine
- Establishes routines to decrease confusion
- Remains safe from harm
- Utilizes support groups and respite care

PLANNING

Once the nursing diagnoses, outcome criteria, and goals have been identified, you develop the plan of care to help clients and their families adapt to a progressive loss of function and abilities. Priorities of care are as follows:

- Maintaining safety
- Managing agitation
- Responding to catastrophic reactions
- Communicating
- Supporting the family

IMPLEMENTATION

Most clients with delirium will be in the acute care setting. In caring for these clients, all measures must be taken to ensure that permanent brain damage or death does not occur. Because delirium is acute and short-term, plans of care are directed toward short-term goals, with the long-term medical and nursing goal of correcting the underlying disorder. The neurological status of clients must be monitored on an ongoing basis. Clients benefit from nursing interventions designed to prevent or manage agitation, anxiety, and perceptual or cognitive disturbances. Whenever possible, interventions other than restraints, such as sitters, a foot or back massage, good lighting, and frequent observation, should be used to prevent delirious clients from harming themselves or others. Restraints often increase agitation and carry risks for injuries and are used only when other interventions fail.

More than 50% of people with AD live in the community. The goal of nursing intervention is to facilitate optimal quality of life for clients and caregivers and to manage problems as they arise. At the present time, there are no evidence-based nursing interventions that will prevent AD. Nursing care focuses on managing the symptoms the individuals experience. Home care can be a great challenge to families and health care professionals. The role of the nurse is to build therapeutic alliances with significant others and teach specific skills for caregiving. All of the following nursing interventions are skills to be taught to caregivers. In caring for clients with AD, patience and compassion are the guiding principles, with innovation and flexibility as the key elements. What works today may not work tomorrow. Because cognition underlies and directs behavior, client cognitive abilities guide the selection of

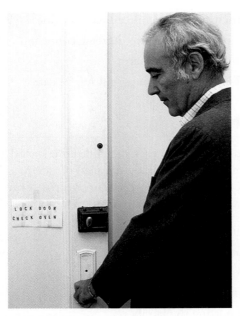

PHOTO 19.3 ■ People with dementia can remain active longer by using signs to prompt their behavior. This man is reminded to lock the door when he leaves his apartment.

SOURCE: Ira Wyman/Corbis/Sygma. Used with permission.

appropriate nursing interventions. Even though AD is progressive and eventually terminal, it is important to support and encourage clients to remain at the highest possible level of functioning (Schutte & Holston, 2006).

Agitation

Client difficulties in verbalization and cognitive deficits may lead to a lack of communication about basic needs. Using the need-driven approach, agitated behavior is considered an indicator of unmet need. When clients are hungry, thirsty, in pain, too hot, too cold, and so on, the only indication may be increased agitation, pacing, and shouting. It is most helpful if family and care providers can anticipate usual problems before they occur. Such anticipatory care should decrease agitation and improve comfort (Kovach, Noonan, Schlidt, & Wells, 2005).

Boredom, sensory deprivation, and loneliness may also increase agitation. Not being able to hear or see clearly decreases the ability to respond to environmental stimulation and cues. Ensure that glasses and hearing aids are in place during waking hours. Some clients experience visuospatial impairment and may walk into objects or people or may sit down when there is no furniture present on which to sit. Recognizing these difficulties is paramount to preventing injury (Miceli, 2005).

The desired outcome is that families anticipate client needs.

Difficulty Socializing With Others

Cognitive stimulation group therapy appears to improve both cognitive function and quality of life for people with early and moderate dementia. Groups usually meet once or twice a week. They may listen to lectures on politics, history, and the arts; hear live music; exercise; discuss current events; go out for coffee; or go shopping. Group members help each other find words, remember details, share memories, and laugh with one another. The social interactions are just as important as the cognitive stimulation. Clients with mild AD may find Internet discussion groups and chat rooms helpful.

Clients who live in nursing homes often experience limited interactions with others because they are unable to initiate conversations and activities. Lack of engagement with others may lead to boredom and agitated behaviors. It is important that staff plan frequent contact and organized activities (Kolanowski & Litaker, 2006).

The desired outcome is that the client maintains socialization.

Quality of Life

Life review or reminiscence therapy is a guided recollection in which clients are encouraged to remember the past and share their memories with family, peers, or staff. Reminiscence therapy focuses on strengths and does not encourage people to dwell on losses. It can raise self-esteem and increase social intimacy. Choose a comfortable setting and set aside adequate time when doing a life review. Use pictures and memorabilia as cues. Encourage verbal expression of feeling of past events. Comment on the feelings that accompany the memories in an empathic manner. Use direct questions to refocus back to life events if clients digress. By encouraging older adults to tell you about their lives, you can learn about hope, grief, achievement, and loss. It is a way you can communicate caring while helping them maintain their sense of identity.

Music therapy is used to reduce the effects of stress and improve the quality of life for clients with AD. Singing, drumming, or moving to music may decrease aggressive outbursts, reduce agitation, lessen anxiety, improve affect, and increase perceptual, motor, and verbal skills.

Pets, especially dogs, often seem to understand what their owners are feeling. For some clients, pets are a reason to get up in the morning. It is something to nurture, touch, and stroke. For stress relief, it apparently does not matter much whether the pet is a Labrador dog, a tomcat, or a canary. What is most important is the person's relationship with the pet. The contributions companion animals make to the emotional well-being of people with dementia include total acceptance; unconditional love and opportunities for affection; a reason to exercise; and functioning as a confidant.

When clients are no longer able to live at home, their families may look for residential care facilities. Three significant problems that manifest within traditional facilities are loneliness, helplessness, and boredom. They often have not served as home for people, but rather as institutions in which to store people. The basic concept of the *Eden Alternative*, a new approach to residential care, is quite simple: care facilities are viewed as habitats for human beings rather than institutions

NURSING CARE PLAN for Clients With Cognitive Impairment Disorders

Risk for Accidents/Trauma
Nursing Diagnosis: Client at Risk for Impaired Memory

Outcomes: The client remains safe.

The client should be prohibited from smoking or be provided with supervision to prevent burns or fires. Prescribed medications can become a hazard when clients take the wrong medication, too much medication, or the right medication at the wrong time. Since memory loss interferes with correct self-administration, it is often appropriate for caregivers to administer the medications. Rid the home of firearms and poisonous plants and put safety locks on cabinets containing harmful substances. Even early AD can impair driving to some extent, and the risk of accidents increases with increasing severity of the dementia. Family members or institutional staff members must be taught measures to reduce potential injury from wandering or becoming lost. Family members should assess the neighborhood for potentially dangerous areas such as busy streets, swimming pools, rivers, and bridges.

Many clients will require *safety measures* regarding impaired physical mobility, which might be evidenced by stiffness, awkwardness, and unsteadiness. Keep furniture in the same places and provide good lighting. Pad sharp corners, and discard throw rugs to minimize the likelihood of falls. If the client is unsteady, a supportive person should be nearby to help maintain balance. Handrails on staircases and in bathrooms provide additional support. If the client is unable to sit unassisted, a chair with a posey bar may be helpful.

Intervention	Rationale	Goal
Discuss the risks of driving with clients and caregivers.	Information directs appropriate decision making.	Refrains from driving when no longer safe
Explore transportation needs and possible alternatives.	Finding ways to get needs met may make it easier to give up driving.	Identifies alternative modes of transportation
Caregivers may need to lock the car keys in a cabinet, hide the garage door controller, and learn easily reversible ways to disable the car.	Client may not believe that driving is a dangerous activity.	Remains safe
Provide client with an ID bracelet and ID card.	Others will be able to contact family if client becomes lost.	Wears identification material
Have family register with the Safe Return program through the Alzheimer Association (800-621-0379).	Others will be able to contact family if client becomes lost.	Client is registered
Have family write out simple directions home, along with home phone number, and put in wallet or purse.	If client can still read and comprehend, this will increase ability to get home.	Follows direction to return home
Have family alert other people in the neighborhood to the situation.	This increases client's protection.	Neighbors verbalize an understanding of the situation
Yard should be fenced in with locked gates.	This increases client's protection.	Remains safe in yard
Doors to the house should be kept locked and an alarm system should be connected to the doors.	This prevents client from slipping out unnoticed.	Remains in the home unless accompanied by others
Day care centers and nursing homes can provide a dementia wander garden with designed paths and stimuli for all five senses.	This has been shown to improve attention and reduce stress (Detweiler & Warf, 2005). Wandering decreases with regular exercise.	Exercises in a dementia wander garden
Objects in the home that may be potentially dangerous must be locked up or removed including irons, power tools, paints, solvents, stove knobs, and cleaning agents. Water heater should be turned to a lower temperature and hot water faucets and knobs should be painted red.	Caregivers must minimize hazards in the home because people with AD suffer from poor judgment. Lower water temperature will prevent accidental burning.	Remains safe
Remove footstools, extension cords, throw rugs, table lamps, and other breakables. Keep night lights on at night.	These objects might trip the person or break if knocked over. This reduces hazards of falling during darkness.	Does not fall

continued

NURSING CARE PLAN for a Client With Cognitive Impairment Disorders

Catastrophic Reactions

Nursing Diagnosis: Client at Risk for Impaired Adjustment

Outcomes: Client remains calm and safe.

Catastrophic reactions may occur when clients feel overwhelmed and overstimulated. Rapid questions, excessive commands, and too much noise and activity can provoke the response. Criticism and conflict may also contribute. Clients may respond with anger, stubbornness, agitation, and combativeness. If they become physically abusive to their caregivers, steps should be taken to ensure the safety of clients, family, and staff.

Intervention	Rationale	Goal
Respond calmly and do not retaliate with anger.	Client's anger is often exaggerated and displaced.	Remains calm
Remove objects in the environment that may be used to harm self or others.	This reduces opportunities for physical harm.	Remains safe
Try to identify the triggers to the catastrophic reaction. Does client behave this way with everyone or only to specific people? Are they in pain and believe nothing is being done to help them?	Accurately identifying precipitating events increases the ability to prevent or minimize recurrence.	Triggers are identified
Remove client from upsetting situation or environment.	Impaired memory makes client forget what caused the immediate anger.	Calms down and verbalizes less anger
Avoid catastrophic reactions by: ■ Keeping requests relatively simple ■ Avoiding confrontation and deferring requests if client becomes angry ■ Being consistent and avoiding unnecessary change ■ Providing frequent reminders, explanations, and orientation cues ■ Ignoring inappropriate behavior that is not harmful ■ Avoiding crowds, strangers, confusion, and noise	Identifying and eliminating triggers may prevent these reactions.	Catastrophic reactions decrease or are eliminated

Confusion Related to Delirium

Nursing Diagnosis: Client at Risk for Acute Confusion

Outcomes: Client returns to predelirium level of orientation.

The primary cognitive characteristics of delirium are disorganized thinking and attention deficits resulting in confusion.

Since both sensory deprivation and sensory overstimulation can worsen symptoms, you will need to adjust the environment according to the client's response. This is often a process of trial and error. Intensive care units are noisy environments with beeps, alarms, pumps, and respirators. This ongoing noise level may overstimulate the confused person with delirium. On the other hand, a too-quiet environment may contribute to clients' intense focus on their altered perceptions and thoughts. In general, you should provide enough light at all times to minimize shadows that may contribute to illusions.

Following recovery, educate clients and their families about the apparent cause of the delirium. It is important that they and future health care providers are aware of risk factors that may lead to delirium in the future.

Intervention	Rationale	Goal
Provide frequent contact, reassurance, and repeat information.	This increases client's orientation.	Verbalizes improved orientation
Use brief, simple statements.	These are better understood than lengthy explanations.	Verbalizes understanding

NURSING CARE PLAN for a Client With Cognitive Impairment Disorders

Confusion Related to Delirium   *continued*
Nursing Diagnosis: Client at Risk for Acute Confusion

Intervention	Rationale	Goal
Provide information about what is happening and what can be expected to occur; include family in care.	This decreases fear of the unknown. This decreases family's sense of helplessness.	Verbalizes less fear
Provide client with glasses and hearing aids if appropriate.	Delirium is aggravated by visual and auditory impairment.	Level of delirium lessens
Provide a visible clock and calendar in the room.	This improves orientation.	Orientation improved
Instruct all who come in contact with client to remind them of where they are, the date and time, and what is happening.	Reorientation is consistently provided.	Orientation improved
Role-model how to interact with client.	This increases family's ability to participate in plan of care.	Interacts appropriately with client

Confusion Related to Dementia
Nursing Diagnosis: Client at Risk for Chronic Confusion

Outcomes: Client responds to reorientation interventions.

Caregivers of people with dementia can establish measures to decrease disorientation. Routinely and frequently orient clients to who, where, and what is happening, which allows them to become oriented without shame. It is helpful to repeat the date, the day of the week, the season, and the weather throughout the waking hours.

Intervention	Rationale	Outcome
Provide large-print calendars, clocks, and labels on objects in the environment.	These aids assist with orientation.	Verbalizes basic orientation to person, place, time, and situation
Minimize use of televisions and radios; be selective and avoid programs with intricate plots or frightening content.	Continuous noise from media may increase confusion. May be unable to distinguish reality from what is occurring on TV.	Reality orientation improved
Discuss topics meaningful to clients such as work, hobbies, children, or significant life events.	These topics promote identity.	Participates in discussion
Do not argue or persist in trying to convince clients of actual reality when they use confabulation.	Confabulation is used to reduce their shame or embarrassment about memory losses. Pointing out reality will only increase confusion and frustration.	Verbalizes less confusion

Difficulties With Self-Care
Nursing Diagnosis: Client at Risk for Ineffective Coping

Outcomes: Client experiences small successes and actively participates in ADLs.

Focusing on the strengths and abilities of people with dementia, as opposed to problems and disabilities, may counteract negative views held by some health care providers. This positive focus may also prevent excess disability. Caregivers should identify small, achievable goals on which they can build success as opportunities arise. Clients are often more capable than either they or their families realize, and there may be any number of simple tasks they could do by themselves. Performing *simple tasks* around the home keeps them busy and helps them feel good about themselves. Flexible consistency is the most effective approach when caring for people with dementia.

continued

NURSING CARE PLAN for a Client With Cognitive Impairment Disorders

Difficulties With Self-Care   *continued*
Nursing Diagnosis: Client at Risk for Ineffective Coping

Intervention	Rationale	Goal
Encourage activities and skills still present.	This maintains independence and gives sense of competency.	Does activities of daily living within range of competence
Try to follow familiar routines as much as possible, e.g., time of day for bath, preference for bath or shower.	This decreases confusion that occurs with changes in routine.	Follows routine of self-care
Encourage as much decision as possible in ADLs.	Increases sense of control and prevents disengagement that occurs when all responsibility is taken away.	Makes appropriate decisions
If necessary, give step-by-step directions with only one step at a time. Demonstrate the action and use verbal encouragement.	This decreases the confusion related to slowed thinking and distractibility.	Follows step-by-step directions
Lay out clean clothes in the order they are to be put on. Use Velcro tape instead of buttons and zippers.	This increases independence by decreasing the need for decisions and manipulation of complex closures on clothing.	Dresses self appropriately
Do ADLs "with" not "for" client as long as possible.	This maintains independence and sense of competency as long as possible.	Participates in ADLs

Inadequate Nutrition
Nursing Diagnosis: Client at Risk for Imbalanced Nutrition

Outcomes: Client maintains an adequate state of nutrition.

Clients with dementia may have difficulty eating because of apraxia which is the inability to perform purposeful movements or use objects appropriately.

Intervention	Rationale	Goal
Provide a balanced diet according to food categories.	This prevents nutritional deficiencies and prevents other related illness.	Eats balanced diet
Refer to community resources such as Eating Together or Meals-On-Wheels.	Complete, balanced meals are provided.	Uses resources
Maintain regular schedule of mealtimes.	This prevents confusion related to change.	Responds to routine mealtime
Make certain that dentures fit well.	Poor-fitting dentures interfere with chewing.	Able to chew food
Serve familiar foods.	New foods often increase confusion.	Eats willingly
Limit the amount of foods in front of client.	Client may have difficulty deciding which food to eat.	Eats willingly
Provide utensils with large built-up handles.	These are easier to use when coordination is poor.	Manipulates utensils to eat
Try using bowls rather than plates.	These are easier because food is not pushed off.	Feeds self from bowl
Do not rush eating process.	Impaired people eat slowly.	Feeds self given enough time
Ensure adequate fluid intake.	This prevents dehydration.	Remains hydrated
Weigh client weekly.	This provides an additional monitoring of status.	Weight remains constant

NURSING CARE PLAN for a Client With Cognitive Impairment Disorders

Difficulty Communicating

Nursing Diagnosis: Client at Risk for Impaired Communication

Outcomes: Client responds to appropriate communication.

Communication with clients is an extremely important nursing intervention. See Box 19.1 for ways to improve communication with clients. Attempts to communicate are more likely to be successful when environmental distractions and noise are kept to a minimum.

Intervention	Rationale	Goal
Begin each conversation by identifying yourself and addressing clients by name.	This gets their attention and orients them.	Attention improves
Speak slowly and distinctly, in a low tone of voice.	This conveys a sense of calm.	Remains calm
Use clear, simple sentences; ask one question at a time or present one idea at a time.	Client may be able to comprehend some words with less complex language.	Responds appropriately to simple sentences
Do not demean the person or use baby talk.	Clients can often comprehend the emotional tone of speech even when they can no longer understand the words.	Responds positively to a respectful approach
Ask closed-ended questions; give client time to respond.	These are easier to respond to than open-ended questions.	Answers yes/no questions
Provide necessary word when client is unable to recall word.	Client will often recognize the forgotten word when it is heard.	Acknowledges the correct word when hearing it
Use a direct address, as in "Mary, it is time to eat now."	Pronouns are often misunderstood.	Responds to direct address
Use nonverbal communication such as smiles, hugs, gestures, and handholding.	This conveys concern and caring, and reinforces verbal communication.	Responds positively to nonverbal communication
Treat client with respect and dignity at all times.	Clients are valued adult individuals worthy of respect.	Responds positively to respectful approach

Paranoid Accusations

Nursing Diagnosis: Client at Risk for Caregiver Role Strain

Outcomes: Client decreases use of accusations.

Many people with dementia develop delusions and may make paranoid accusations against family members.

Intervention	Rationale	Goal
Teach family that arguing or explaining does not help.	Discussion will not change client's mind about suspicions.	Family does not argue
Teach family that client's accusations are a cover up for forgetting where things have been placed.	Family needs to understand process to respond appropriately to client's memory loss.	Family verbalizes understanding
Help client locate lost object.	The location may solve immediate problem.	Decrease in family tension
Support client's feelings of anger and frustration.	Feelings behind accusatory statements must be acknowledged and supported.	Verbalizes feelings of support
Distract client with an alternative activity.	This decreases obsession with suspicious thoughts.	Participates in other activities

continued

NURSING CARE PLAN for a Client With Cognitive Impairment Disorders

Need for Exercise
Nursing Diagnosis: Client at Risk for Activity Intolerance

Outcome: Client remains as physically active as limitations allow.

Older people who *exercise* three or more times a week are less likely to develop AD. It also may delay the onset of symptoms. It is thought that exercise reduces amyloid plaques associated with AD. Exercise also decreases disruptive behaviors and wandering and increases appropriate interactions with others. Consistent, low-impact exercise will increase the oxygenation of the brain, slow the loss of motor function, and increase energy and feelings of well-being and accomplishment (Larson et al., 2006).

Intervention	Rationale	Goal
Provide regular exercise such as walking, group exercise, or dancing.	This decreases tension, maintains range of motion, and promotes sleep at night. Rhythmic motions may be a way to meet the need for the repetitive behavior that occurs in people with AD.	Exercises daily
Exercise with client.	This increases client's participation.	Exercises daily
Maintain exercise routine—same time, same exercises.	Regular schedule decreases confusion.	Exercises daily
If unsteady, have supportive person nearby.	This prevents falls and injuries.	Remains safe

Impaired Sleep Cycle
Nursing Diagnosis: Client at Risk for Disturbed Sleep Pattern

Outcomes: Client experiences at least 4 hours of uninterrupted sleep at night.

Because many clients with AD experience sleep problems, actions to *improve sleep* will benefit clients and families both. In a randomized, controlled sleep education study, participants were instructed to walk daily for 30 minutes, usually accompanied by a caregiver, and increase their daily light exposure by 1 hour using a light box. Clients reduced their number of nighttime awakenings, spent less total time awake, and experienced less daytime sleepiness than the control group (McCurry, Gibbons, Logsdon, Vitiello, & Teri, 2005).

Intervention	Rationale	Goal
Encourage client and family to keep a record of sleep patterns. Questions to be answered are: ■ How many daytime naps? ■ How many nighttime awakenings? ■ Medications? ■ Is pain interfering with sleep?	This establishes baseline data.	Establishes sleep record
Minimize napping during daytime.	Napping interferes with sleep cycle.	Naps less often
Schedule exercise 2 hours before bedtime.	Increased physical fatigue promotes sleep. Exercise too close to bedtime interferes with sleep.	Exercises each evening
Limit caffeine intake.	Caffeine increases CNS activity.	Consumes less caffeine
Ensure quiet environment.	Atmosphere must be conducive to sleep.	Environment is quiet
Provide comfort measures such as back or foot rubs.	Increased comfort is conducive to sleep.	Responds positively to comfort measures

- Reduce background noise.
- Speak only when you can be seen so your facial expression can provide visual cues to the meaning of your words.
- Address client by name.
- Speak slowly to compensate for decreased ability to process information.
- Ask only one question at a time and wait for the response.
- Give instructions one step at a time.
- When possible, demonstrate actions you want the person to take—miming and gestures can increase understanding.
- Pictures may increase understanding.
- Learn the limits of the person's attention span.
- Be quick with praise and encouragement.

for the frail and elderly. The approach uses animals, plants, and children to interact with residents, creating a "human habitat" that makes them feel more at home. Resident animals are part of the total environment. Children and teenagers come in and interact and build relationships with residents as opposed to the usual pattern of coming in, putting on a program, and leaving. The Eden Alternative empowers staff members to have more say in their daily routines and work patterns. It is really about liberating the spirit of the people who are living and working in adult day care services, assisted-living facilities, and residential care institutions (Thomas, 1998).

The desired outcomes are that the client verbalizes improved self-esteem and identity, participates in music therapy, and interacts with their companion animal, if appropriate.

Supporting the Family

The nurse must be an advocate for family caregivers. Families are often in need of teaching and counseling, support groups, and respite care. Help them locate local resources and develop support networks (see the Community Resources feature on your CD-ROM). Peer support through dementia caregiver groups lessens the alienation and the sense of inadequacy that caregivers often experience. Other benefits of support groups include caregiving tips, suggestions on negotiating with community agencies, and overcoming practical and emotional barriers to care. By decreasing caregiver burden, these groups may improve the quality of life for clients and their families. Other resources that might help include social service agencies, home health agencies, cleaning services, Meals on Wheels, transportation programs, geriatric law specialists, and financial planners.

In the early stage of the disease, clients and families should discuss end-of-life care issues. Advance directives regarding feeding tubes, respirators, hemodialysis, and cardiac resuscitation should be carefully discussed. The appointment of a durable power of attorney for health care decisions and for financial decisions should be made while the client is still able to participate in the decision-making process.

Family members experience three typical conflicts in caring for their loved ones with dementia. There are disagreements over the diagnosis and treatment plan, conflict over the quantity and quality of care, and different ideas about who should provide care and to what extent various family members share in the care. Family meetings are often necessary to help individuals express their views and for the family to gain consensus when possible.

Caregivers need breaks from a very stressful job. They may need assistance in developing coping strategies that deal directly with specific problems, as well as the multitude of emotions they are experiencing. Respite care provided by other family members or through adult day care programs may limit the sense of being overwhelmed by the combination of hard work and personal loss associated with caring for a person with AD. Discuss the need for periods of rest and recreation to prevent total emotional and physical fatigue of caregivers. Since clients are unable to provide positive feedback to caregivers, discuss how they might seek rewards and recognition apart from clients. Families must keep their expectations realistic. Their loved ones with AD will not get better, but with good caregiving, clients can maintain independence and dignity for a long time.

The desired outcome is that families will utilize support groups, use community resources, and access respite care.

Anticipatory Grieving

Since there are usually years of gradual losses for clients and family members who are touched by cognitive disorders, grieving is a long-term process. The severe stage of dementia indicates that death is not too far off in the future and anticipatory grieving occurs. Anticipatory grief is "real" grief, occurring at the same intensity as conventional grief. The phases are similar: recognition and acceptance of the impending death, the experience of emotional and physical pain, and the rebuilding of a life without the loved one.

Thoughts about the impending death are influenced by the family's prior experiences with death and loss. Other factors affecting the grieving process are the quality of the relationship before the diagnosis of dementia, the perceived ability to cope with the death, concurrent stressors, and the availability of social support systems. For those who have had primary caregiving duties, the death can cause ambivalence. On the one hand, there is a sense of relief that the often overwhelming responsibilities are ended. On the other hand, caregiving may have given direction and meaning to the caregiver's life and that is now ended. Those who work through these feelings are better able to adapt after the death.

Your role as a nurse is to provide emotional and spiritual support through the process of anticipatory grieving. Give family members permission to express their anxiety, anger, guilt,

MediaLink Critical Thinking, Caregiver Support Group

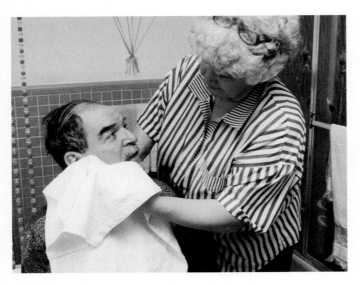

PHOTO 19.4 ■ Individuals who care for people with dementia assume an enormous burden. Respite programs attempt to provide assistance to these individuals.

SOURCE: Richard Falco/Black Star. Used with permission.

and sadness. Explore their beliefs about the purpose of life and death. Help them search for meaning in their past, present, and future losses. Sharing memories is a way of connecting with past meanings. Loving caretaking may involve the pres-

ent meaning in life. Finding a way to carry out their loved one's hopes and dreams may be the way to find future meaning in life. With anticipatory guidance, the family may be able to approach the death with a sense of dignity and peace.

The desired outcome is that families will discuss feelings regarding their loved one's impending death and verbalize past, present, and future meaning in life.

Complementary/Alternative Therapies

Interacting With a Pet

Individuals suffering from Alzheimer disease often have fewer episodes of anxiety, depression, and outbursts of verbal aggression when they are also able to interact with a companion pet or therapy animal. Caregivers can encourage interaction with the animal, such as a dog or a cat, when the individual seems to be more upset.

■ Note the physical and emotional signs of tension: Are the hands clenched? Body trembling? Restlessness? Unable to relax? Breathing more rapidly?

■ Encourage interaction with the animal for at least 20 minutes. You may have to join in to model appropriate interaction with the pet such as gentle play, stroking, petting, and talking to the animal.

■ Note any changes that would indicate less anxiety and less aggression.

Clinical Interactions   A Client With Dementia of the Alzheimer Type

Ray, 72 years old, has been experiencing symptoms of AD for the past several years. For the past year, he has been attending a day program for persons with AD. His daughter drops him off on her way to work and picks him up on her way home. If outside appointments must be scheduled during that time, the staff of the day program provides transportation. Ray's daughter has forgotten to inform the staff about Ray's appointment to have his hair cut. In the interaction, you will see evidence of:

■ Confusion with pronouns: Ray uses "we" to mean "I."
■ Difficulty comprehending even small changes in schedule
■ Loss of short-term memory
■ An inability to remember the word *barber*

NURSE: *"Ray, we are going to have lunch 30 minutes earlier today because it is the day for the music therapist to be here with us."*

RAY: "We go to lunch at 12."

NURSE: *"It is necessary to have lunch now."*

RAY: "We don't want to go now."

NURSE: *"Please come with me. It is time to go to lunch."*

RAY: "We won't go now."

NURSE: *"It's time to go to lunch."*

RAY: "We go at 12!"

NURSE: *"It's time for lunch."*

RAY: [throwing up his hands] "Okay, okay." [Ray eats and returns to the day room.]

RAY: "We have an appointment at 2 p.m."

NURSE: *"Can you tell me what that appointment is for?"*

RAY: "It's at 2 p.m."

NURSE: *"Do you know where you are supposed to go for the appointment?"*

RAY: "Main Street."

NURSE: *"Do you know where you are supposed to go on Main Street?"*

RAY: "Main Street. That's where we have to go."

NURSE: *"Can you give me any other hints as to where you are supposed to go?"*

RAY: "We need the wallet."

NURSE: *"You need your wallet. Is it a store?"*

RAY: "We need the wallet."

NURSE: *"Do you need to buy something?"*

RAY: "Hair."

NURSE: *"Hair. Did you make an appointment at the barbershop?"*

RAY: "Yes."

NURSE: *"I need to take you to your barbershop on Main Street at 2 p.m."*

RAY: "We have an appointment at 2 p.m."

NURSE: *"I will make certain that you get to your hair appointment by 2 p.m."*

EVALUATION

To complete the nursing process, you evaluate clients' responses to nursing interventions based on the selected outcomes. Although the long-term outcome for the person with dementia is certain, the road to that end can be made smoother with empathetic nursing care.

Using Research Evidence   Caring for the Delirious Client

Voyer, P., McCusker, J., Cole, M. G., & Khomenko, L. (2006). Influence of prior cognitive impairment on the severity of delirium symptoms among older patients. *Journal of Neuroscience Nursing, 38*, 90–101.

What is the study about?

Alarmingly, many nurses (75%) report that they cannot distinguish between dementia and/or delirium in older clients. Delirious elderly persons behave in unsafe ways that can contribute to increased falls and even deaths; and delirium calls for more supportive nursing care. Because this distinction is complex and challenging, the purpose of this study was to provide new data on the symptoms of delirium among older clients with prior cognitive impairment.

How was the study done?

This was a quantitative secondary-analysis study of data obtained in two concurrent research projects on delirium. This institutional review board–approved study used participants who were inpatients, diagnosed with delirium, and enrolled in a larger study at a university-affiliated primary care hospital. Consecutive clients 65 years or older, admitted to a hospital from its emergency department, had been screened within 48 hours of admission by a nurse researcher for the initial study's eligibility. Four hundred and forty-four participants had met the initial study's criteria, based on the Short Portable Mental Status Questionnaire and the confusion assessment method (CAM). From these participants, 71 individuals met the criteria for the secondary-analysis study due to a diagnosis of prior cognitive impairment as mild (n=24), moderate (n=23), or severe (n=24). That cognitive impairment was assessed using the Delirium Index (DI). In addition, these participants were admitted from long-term centers that provided information on their prior cognitive impairment as measured by the Informant Questionnaire on Cognitive Decline in the Elderly (IQCODE). This 71-client sample had a mean age of 85 years. The percentage of female participants was higher for all groups except the group with severe prior cognitive impairment. Cognition, current delirium, and functional autonomy were then measured as follows: In addition to the nurse researcher, a research assistant, blind to the results of the CAM, assessed cognition using the Mini-Mental State Examination and assessed severity of delirium using the Delirium Index (DI) and the Barthel Index (BI) to determine functional autonomy. To identify the client's global health status, a nurse researcher interviewed a family member, and from that interview assessed previous cognitive deficits by using the IQCODE, BI, and the Instrumental Activities of Daily Living. Medication and sociodemographic data were obtained from chart reviews. Statistical analysis included descriptive analyses (sociodemographic data), chi-square tests (among clients experiencing delirium, to determine whether the severity of the prior cognitive impairment was associated with the severity of the delirium symptoms), Fisher exact tests (marginal frequencies were less than 5), and a general linear model (comparison of mean scores on the DI).

What were the results of the study?

This study was guided by three hypotheses. Hypothesis 1: Among hospitalized older clients, symptoms of delirium are more severe in those with severe (as compared to mild) prior cognitive impairment. Mean DI scores supported hypothesis 1. Among these persons with delirium, severe prior cognitive impairment was coupled with more inattention, disorganized thinking, disorientation, and memory problems. Hypothesis 2: Among hospitalized older clients, risk of dying in hospital is greater for those with severe (as compared to mild) prior cognitive impairment. Data analysis revealed that severity of the symptoms of delirium did *not* appear to increase the risk of dying during the hospital stay. However, of the 71 clients in this study, at least 13% died during their hospital stay. Hypothesis 3: Among hospitalized older clients, severe symptoms of hypoactivity are more common with severe (as compared to mild) prior cognitive impairment. Data analysis did not support hypothesis 3: neither levels of consciousness nor of motor activities differed statistically among the three groups of clients. This finding underlines a weak relationship between symptoms of psychomotor agitation and symptoms of delirium. In addition, the data analysis identified several trends: As the severity of prior cognitive impairment increased, comorbidity level increased, cognitive deficit scores at admission decreased, functional autonomy decreased, and the number of prescribed drugs decreased.

What additional questions might I have?

Can the findings be generalized, since the study data were obtained from clients admitted to one hospital? Would a larger sample size have differing results? What specific nursing interventions could help to decrease the severity of delirium and enhance health outcomes? What impact could prescribed drugs have on the symptoms of delirium?

How can I use this study?

All nurses working with an older adult population need to be knowledgeable in distinguishing delirium from dementia. Nurses working in acute care settings need to assess risk factors for delirium among older adults and determine severity of presenting symptoms. In addition, nurses should not judge severe delirium only by activity level, but should pay special attention to thinking, orientation, and memory. Because the symptoms of delirium can fluctuate, it is critical to document the description of delirium episodes. In detecting these fluctuations, 24-hour chart reviews may be useful. Delirium can be better assessed by taking into account the severity of symptoms. Among this older population, nurses can increase safety and enhance quality of life by monitoring these clients closely.

SOURCE: Contributed by Dolores Huffman, PhD, RN, Associate Professor of Nursing, Purdue University Calumet, Hammond, Indiana.

Focus Your Study

OBJECTIVES	KEY CONCEPTS

1. Distinguish between dementia and delirium.

- Dementia:
  - Onset slow
  - Irreversible
  - Progression over months or years ending in death
  - Inattention progresses
  - Memory impairment beginning with recent memory
  - Aphasia
  - Paranoid delusions
- Delirium:
  - Sudden onset
  - Reversible; usually short term; if untreated may cause permanent brain damage
  - Hyperactive or hypoactive
  - Slurred speech
  - Attention fluctuates
  - Hallucinations

2. Compare and contrast the etiologies of dementia and delirium.

- Alzheimer disease results from neurofibrillary tangles and amyloid plaques in the brain.
- Vascular dementia results from ischemic events and hemorrhages in the brain.
- AIDS dementia complex is caused by HIV infection of the brain.
- Lewy body dementia and frontal lobe dementia are caused by a variety of brain diseases.
- Delirium is an acute, usually reversible brain disorder as a complication of a primary medical illness or as a response to surgery.

3. Outline the different treatment options for dementia and delirium.

- Dementia:
  - Medications that slow the decline in Alzheimer disease include cholinesterase inhibitors and memantine (Namenda).
  - Antidepressant medication may be given if the client is also suffering from depression.
  - Antipsychotic medications may decrease agitation, aggression, paranoid thinking, poor impulse control, and sleep difficulties.
- Delirium:
  - The medical treatment involves swift identification of the organic cause of delirium.
  - Haloperidol (Haldol) may be given IV to control the symptoms.

4. Outline the assessment process for dementia and delirium.

- Some clients can respond appropriately when assessment questions are asked.
- Ask simple questions and give enough time for the client to respond.
- If the client is too disoriented or confused, you must rely on family members to provide the necessary assessment data.

5. Develop teaching plans for a client with a cognitive impairment disorder and his/her family.

- Modify home environment to ensure safety from accidents, poor judgment, and wandering.
- Anticipate client's needs, thereby decreasing agitation.
- Help family locate local resources and develop support networks.
- In early stages of AD, help families and clients discuss end-of-life care issues.
- Locate respite care resources.
- Discuss anticipatory grieving.

6. Use the nursing process to develop a safe, comprehensive plan of care for a client with a cognitive impairment disorder.

- Catastrophic reactions occur when clients feel overwhelmed and overstimulated.
- Ensure safety of clients, family, and caregivers.
- Use orientation devices such as clocks and calendars; repeat time, date, season, location as necessary throughout the day.
- Support active participation in ADLs.
- Communicate slowly and clearly; introduce only one question/topic at a time.
- Maintain dignity.
- Foster socialization with others.
- Structure exercise routine.
- Institute activities that promote sleep.
- Improve quality of life with reminiscence therapy, music therapy, and pet therapy.

7. Discuss the key points in effectively communicating with a person with a cognitive impairment disorder.

- Decrease environmental distractions.
- Ensure that clients have glasses and hearing aids in place.
- Speak only when you can be seen by the client.
- Address by name.
- Ask simple questions and speak slowly.
- Provide enough time for clients to respond.
- Give instructions one step at a time.
- Routinely and frequently orient clients to who, where, and what is happening.
- Demonstrate actions you want the client to take.
- Pictures may increase understanding.
- Learn the limits of the client's attention span.
- Be quick with praise and encouragement.

Explore MediaLink

For review questions, case studies, and other resources for this chapter see the Pearson Health MediaLink CD-ROM that accompanies this book and the Companion Website.

CD-ROM
- Audio Glossary
- NCLEX-RN® Review Questions
- Animations/Videos
  - PET/SPECT Dementia
  - Parkinsonism
  - Extrapyramidal Signs: Tremor– Hands and Arms
  - Extrapyramidal Signs: Tremor– Grasping Tremor
  - Extrapyramidal Signs: Tremor– Lateral Tremor
  - Extrapyramidal Signs: Tremor– Akinesia and Pill Rolling

Companion Website www.prenhall.com/fontaine
- Audio Glossary
- NCLEX-RN® Review Questions
- Case Study
  - Caregiver Burden
- Care Plan
  - ICU Psychosis
- Critical Thinking
  - Caregiver Support Group
- MediaLink Application
  - Dementia: It's Not Always Alzheimer's
- MediaLink
  - Books for Clients & Families
  - Community Resources

NCLEX-RN® Review Questions

19-1. A client who developed delirium following surgery asks if having delirium is the beginning of Alzheimer disease. The nurse explains the differences between delirium and dementia. Which of the following statements by the client requires further teaching?
1. "So I developed delirium because I had surgery."
2. "If I have dementia I will slowly get worse."
3. "In dementia there are quick changes in the levels of consciousness, too."
4. "I might have developed permanent brain damage."

19-2. A client is diagnosed with vascular dementia. Which of the following explanations will assist the family to understand the cause of this type of dementia?
1. Blood vessels in the brain are bleeding.
2. Strands of protein are tangled together.
3. Acetylcholine production is decreased.
4. Fragments mix with molecules to make plaques in the brain.

19-3. Clients on the unit avoid the client with HIV dementia. Which of the following is an appropriate intervention for this group of clients?
1. Form an educational focus group on the unit.
2. Meet individually with the clients.
3. Form a social group on the unit.
4. Change the client's room.

19-4. An 80-year-old client who lives with her daughter tells the nurse, "No one lets me eat with them. I have to hide my food under the bed." The nurse plans a family meeting to discuss:
1. Family eating patterns.
2. Current living arrangement.
3. Cultural values of the family.
4. Adequate nutrition for the family.

19-5. The family is caring for their parent with Alzheimer disease. Which of the following topics should the nurse include in the family education? (Select all that apply.)
1. Management of the illness
2. Intellectually stimulating activities for the client
3. Nature of the cognitive impairment
4. Exercise regimens
5. Support services

19-6. A client with dementia has a disturbed sleep pattern. Which of the following interventions should the nurse utilize for the client?
1. Encourage TV watching during the day.
2. Give sleep medication.
3. Promote mild exercise.
4. Awaken the client when napping.

19-7. The nurse is working with families of clients with Alzheimer disease. One of the members says, "I feel so sad because my loved one is lost." The nurse can best facilitate group discussion on this issue by saying:
1. "Grieving for a lost relationship is a normal behavior."
2. "Are you experiencing anger about this?"
3. "How have others in the family dealt with these feelings?"
4. "You will not feel sad as soon as you can accept his illness."

See Appendix D for answers.

References

American Psychiatric Association. (2000). *Diagnostic and statistical manual of mental disorders* (4th ed., Text Revision). Washington, DC: Author.

Askin-Edgar, S., White, K. E., & Cummings, J. L. (2004). Neuropsychiatric aspects of Alzheimer's disease and other dementing illnesses. In S. C. Yudofsky & R. E. Hales (Eds.), *Essentials of neuropsychiatry and clinical neurosciences* (pp. 421–456). Washington, DC: American Psychiatric Publishing.

Ballard, C. G., Jacoby, R., Ser, T. D., Khan, M. N., Munoz, D. G., Holmes, C., et al. (2004). Neuropathological substrates of psychiatric symptoms in prospectively studied patients with autopsy-confirmed dementia with Lewy bodies. *American Journal of Psychiatry, 161*(5), 843–849.

Barnes, L. L., Wilson, R. S., Li, Y., Gilley, D. W., Bennett, D. A., & Evans, D. A. (2006). Change in cognitive function in Alzheimer's disease in African-American and white persons. *Neuroepidemiology, 26*(1), 16–22.

Beeson, R. A. (2003). Loneliness and depression in spousal caregivers of those with Alzheimer's disease versus non-caregiving spouses. *Archives of Psychiatric Nursing, 17*(3), 135–143.

Berman, K., & Brodaty, H. (2004). Tocopherol (vitamin E) in Alzheimer's disease and other neurodegenerative disorders. *CNS Drugs, 18*(12), 807–825.

Biskupic, J. A new page in O'Connors' love story. *USA Today,* (November 12, 2007).

Brown, R. P., & Gerberg, P. L. (2000). Integrative psychopharmacology. In P. R. Muskin (Ed.), *Complementary and alternative medicine and psychiatry* (pp. 1–66). Washington, DC: American Psychiatric Press.

Burbaeva, G. S., Boksha, I. S., Tereshkina, E. B., Savushkina, O. K., Starodubtseva, L. I., & Turishcheva, M. S. (2005). Glutamate metabolizing enzymes in prefrontal cortex of Alzheimer's disease patients. *Neurochemical Research, 30*(11), 1443–1451.

Counts, S. E., Chen, E. Y., Che, S., Ikonomovie, M. D., Wuu, J., Ginsberg, S. D., et al. (2006). Galanin fiber hypertrophy within the cholinergic nucleus basalis during the progression of Alzheimer's disease. *Dementia and Geriatric Cognitive Disorders, 21*(4), 205–214.

DeDeyn, P. P., Katz, I. R., Brodaty, H., Lyons, B., Greenspan, A., & Burns, A. (2005). Management of agitation, aggression and psychosis associated with dementia. *Clinical Neurology and Neurosurgery, 107*(6), 497–508.

Detweiler, M. B., & Warf, C. (2005). Dementia wander garden aids post cerebrovascular stroke restorative therapy. *Alternative Therapies in Health and Medicine, 11*(4), 54–58.

Dowling, J. E. (2004). *The great brain debate: Nature or nurture?* Washington, DC: Joseph Henry Press.

Edwards, N. E., & Beck, A. M. (2002). Animal-assisted therapy and nutrition in Alzheimer's disease.

Western Journal of Nursing Research, 24(6), 697–712.

Fontaine, K. L. (2005). *Complementary & alternative therapies for nursing practice* (2nd ed.). Upper Saddle River, NJ: Prentice Hall.

Fung, W. Y., & Chien, W. T. (2002). The effectiveness of a mutual support group for family caregivers of a relative with dementia. *Archives of Psychiatric Nursing, 16*(3), 134–144.

Hamdy, R. C., Turnball, J. M., & Edwards, J. (1994). *Alzheimer's disease: A handbook for caregivers* (2nd ed.). St. Louis, MO: Mosby.

Kolanowski, A., & Litaker, M. (2006). Social interaction, premorbid personality, and agitation in nursing home residents with dementia. *Archives of Psychiatric Nursing, 20*(1), 12–20.

Kovach, C. R., Noonan, P. E., Schlidt, A. M., & Wells, T. (2005). A model of consequences of need-driven, dementia-compromised behavior. *Journal of Nursing Scholarship, 37*(2), 134–140.

Krasuski, J. S., Alexander, G. E., Horwitz, B., Rapoport, S. I., & Schapiro, M. B. (2002). Relation of medial temporal lobe volumes to age and memory function in nondemented adults with Down syndrome. *American Journal of Psychiatry, 159*(1), 74–81.

Kumar, A. M., Tims, F., & Gruess, D. G. (1999). Music therapy increases serum melatonin levels in patients with Alzheimer's disease. *Alternative Therapies, 5*(6), 49–57.

Larson, E. B., Wang, L., Bowen, J. D., McCormick, W. C., Terri, L., Crane, P., et al. (2006). Exercise is associated with reduced risk for incident dementia among persons 65 years of age and older. *Annals of Internal Medicine, 144*(2), 73–81.

Laustsen, G., & Wimmett, L. (2005). 2004 drug approval highlights: FDA update. *The Nurse Practitioner, 30*(2), 14–29.

Lucas, S. M., Rothwell, N. J., & Gibson, R. M. (2006). The role of inflammation in CNS injury and disease. *British Journal of Pharmacology, 147*(Suppl 1):S232–S240.

McCurry, S. M., Gibbons, L. E., Logsdon, R. G., Vitiello, M. V., & Teri, L. (2005). Nighttime insomnia treatment and education for Alzheimer's disease. *Journal of the American Geriatrics Society, 53*(5), 793–802.

Miceli, D. G. (2005). Falls associated with dementia: How can you tell? *Geriatric Nursing, 26*(2), 106–111.

Modrego, P. J., Fayed, M., & Pina, M. A. (2005). Conversion from mild cognitive impairment to probable Alzheimer's disease predicted by brain magnetic resonance spectroscopy. *American Journal of Psychiatry, 162*(4), 667–675.

Ngandu, T., Helkala, E. L., Soininen, H., Winblad, B., Tuomilehto, J., Nissinen, A., et al. (2006). Alcohol drinking and cognitive functions. *Dementia and Geriatric Cognitive Disorders, 23*(3), 140–149.

North American Nursing Diagnosis Association. (2007). *Nursing Diagnoses: Definitions and Classification 2007–2008*. Philadelphia: Author.

Ohrui, T., Tomita, N., Sato-Nakagawa, T., Matsui, T., Maruyama, M., Niwa, K., et al. (2004). Effects of brain-penetrating ACE inhibitors on Alzheimer disease progression. *Neurology, 63*(7), 1324–1325.

Rose, K. M. (2005). Mild cognitive impairment in Hispanic Americans: An overview of the state of the science. *Archives of Psychiatric Nursing, 19*(5), 205–209.

Schutte, D. L., & Holston, E. C. (2006). Chronic dementing conditions, genomics, and new opportunities for nursing interventions. *Journal of Nursing Scholarship, 38*(4), 328–334.

Seshadri, S., Beiser, K. A., Selhub, J., Jacques, P. R., Rosenberg, I. H., D'Agostino, R. B., et al. (2002). Plasma homocysteine as a risk factor for dementia and Alzheimer's disease. *New England Journal of Medicine, 346*(7), 476–483.

Thomas, W. H. (1998). *Open hearts, open minds.* Acton, MA: VanderWyk & Burnham.

Trzepacz, P. T., & Kennedy, R. E. (2005). Delirium and posttraumatic amnesia. In J. M. Silver, T. W. McAllister, & S. C. Yudofsky (Eds.), *Textbook of traumatic brain injury* (pp. 175–200). Washington, DC: American Psychiatric Press.

Trzepacz, P. T., Meagher, D. J., & Wise, M. G. (2004). Neuropsychiatric aspects of delirium. In S. C. Yudofsky & R. E. Hales (Eds.), *Essentials of neuropsychiatry and clinical neurosciences* (pp. 141–187). Washington, DC: American Psychiatric Publishing.

Tuszynski, M. H., Thal, L., Pay, M., Salmon, D. P., U, H. S., Bakay, R., Patel, P., et al. (2005). A phase 1 clinical trial of nerve growth factor gene therapy for Alzheimer's disease. *Nature Medicine, 11*(5), 551–555.

Vellone, E., Sansoni, J., & Cohen, M. Z. (2002). The experience of Italians caring for family members with Alzheimer's disease. *Journal of Nursing Scholarship, 34*(4), 323–329.

Voyer, P., McCusker, J., Cole, M. G., & Khomenko, L. (2006). Influence of prior cognitive impairment on the severity of delirium symptoms among older patients. *Journal of Neuroscience Nursing, 38,* 90–101.

Wilson, R. S., Krueger, K. R., Kamenetsky, J. M., Tang, Y., Gilley, D. W., Bennett, D. A., et al. (2005). Hallucinations and mortality in Alzheimer disease. *Amercian Journal of Geriatric Psychiatry, 13*(11), 984–990.

Wimo, A., Winblad, B., Shah, S. N., Chin, W., Zhang, R., & McRae, T. (2004). Impact of donepezil treatment for Alzheimer's disease on caregiver time. *Current Medical Research Opinion, 20*(8), 1221–1225.

Woods, D. L., & Dimond, M. (2002). The effect of therapeutic touch on agitated behavior and cortisol in persons with Alzheimer's disease. *Biological Research for Nursing, 4*(2), 104–114.

Zubenko, G. S., Zubenko, W. N., McPherson, S., Spoor, E., Marin, D. B., Farlow, M. R., et al. (2003). A collaborative study of the emergence and clinical features of the major depressive syndrome of Alzheimer's disease. *American Journal of Psychiatry, 160*(5), 857–866.

Chapter 20

Neuropsychiatric Problems

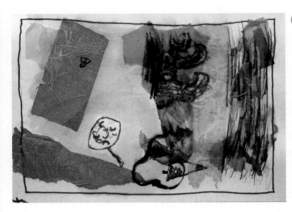

> *Clouds cover my face*
> *I can only feel my fear*
> *My eyes won't see, my lips won't breathe*
> *I'm lost in a lonely breeze*
>
> *I can only feel my fear*
> *It wraps its wretched claws too tight*
> *Knowing more than I*
> *And as fear laughs with delight*
> *Time passes slowly by*
>
> *Knowing more than I*
> *And not stopping to see if I care*
> *Time passes slowly by*
> *While I live in despair a little*

—Anthony, Age 17 (painting)
—Anna, Age 19 (poetry)

OBJECTIVES

After reading this chapter, you will be able to:

1. Discuss the psychiatric symptoms associated with disorders that cause central nervous system disruption.
2. Outline the different treatment options related to neuropsychiatric problems.
3. Outline the assessment process for neuropsychiatric problems.
4. Use the nursing process to develop a comprehensive plan of care for a client with a neuropsychiatric problem.
5. Develop teaching plans for a client with a neuropsychiatric problem and her/his family.

MediaLink www.prenhall.com/fontaine

Go to the Pearson Health MediaLink CD-ROM and the Companion Website at www.prenhall.com/fontaine for interactive resources for this chapter.

The focus of this chapter is on psychiatric problems associated with specific neurological disorders. The disorders presented in this chapter have variable causes, but all impose psychiatric disability to a greater or lesser extent. Helping you see the connection between central nervous system disruption and the psychiatric sequelae illustrates how the principles and skills of mental health nursing are basic to all nursing specialties. Anxiety, depression, delirium, dementia, psychosis, and aggression complicate the progression and treatment of these disorders. Psychiatric disorders must be considered on an ongoing basis since they can appear or resolve during the course of the illness (see Table 20.1■).

Other than a brief definition of each disorder, the concentration of this chapter is on the psychiatric components. Refer to a medical–surgical or neurology text for detailed information on other aspects of these disorders. Likewise, you will find more detail about these mental health problems in the anxiety, mood, schizophrenia, cognitive, and suicide disorders chapters. The disorders used to illustrate concepts of mental health nursing include degenerative disorders, dementias, epilepsy, multifocal disruptions, infections, and traumatic brain injury.

KNOWLEDGE BASE

Degenerative Disorders

Parkinson Disease

Parkinson disease (PD) is a degenerative disease of the basal ganglia that results in a progressive loss of dopamine (DA). It is the second most common neurodegenerative disorder after Alzheimer disease (AD). Muscle rigidity, difficulty initiating movement, resting tremor, weakness, gait disturbances, and a masklike face characterize the disorder. PD and the drugs used to treat it can also cause a range of psychiatric symptoms.

DA not only plays an important role in motor ability, but also is involved in the motivation to act. Apathy, or reduced motivation, results from low levels of DA. People lose interest in activities that were previously enjoyable. Apathy interferes with the ability to be productive and the interest to try new activities. As a result, persons with PD may become increasingly withdrawn.

Between 30% and 50% of people with PD have depression at some time during their illness. Symptoms include feelings of hopelessness, helplessness, decreased self-esteem, and disruptions in eating and sleeping. Risk factors for depression include female sex, early age at onset, greater right-sided symptoms, and gait instability. In some instances, depression appears before motor symptoms. Protective factors for depression include low level of disability, positive social support, effective coping strategies, and an internal locus of control (Aarsland & Ehrt, 2003).

About 40% of individuals with PD develop anxiety disorders; the most common are phobias, panic disorder, generalized anxiety disorder, and obsessive–compulsive disorder. Anxiety may occur with or without concurrent depression. As PD progresses, individuals may become anxious in situations that previously would not have caused anxiety. In some instances, anxiety is severe enough to cause serious disruption in a person's life (Askin-Edgar, White, & Cummings, 2004).

Cognitive disruptions are not apparent until late in the disorder. Between 25% and 40% of individuals develop dementia with profound memory loss, confusion, and disruption in day-to-day functioning.

TABLE 20.1	Psychiatric Symptoms of Neuropsychiatric Problems							
	Emotional Lability	Aggression	Anxiety	Depression	Cognitive Problems	Psychosis	Delirium	Dementia
Parkinson disease			X	X				X
Huntington disease	X	X	X	X	X	X		X
Pick disease		X			X			
Creutzfeldt–Jakob disease					X		X	X
Epilepsy	X			X	X	X		
Multiple sclerosis	X			X	X			
Brain attack	X			X	X			
HIV/AIDS	X		X	X	X		X	X
PANDAS	X		X					
Lyme disease				X	X			
Traumatic brain injury			X	X				X

The medications used to treat PD may cause behavior changes and psychiatric symptoms. This is related to the duration of time taking medications, higher doses over time, and the prescription of multiple medications. Many people experience vivid dreams and nightmares, so realistic as to be frightening. During the nightmare they may talk, scream, or make violent threatening movements referred to as REM behavioral disorder. Some develop hallucinations, which are usually visual and which may be threatening or nonthreatening. Others develop delusions, which are often paranoid. If the individual becomes extremely agitated and difficult to control, it is considered a medical emergency and admission to a safe environment is necessary until the medications are readjusted. These problems may be reduced or eliminated with a decreased dosage of antiparkinson medications (Matsui et al., 2006).

Huntington Disease

Huntington disease (HD) is a hereditary neurodegenerative disorder characterized by an excess of undesired movement and lack of muscle tone. As the disorder progresses, movements become uncontrolled, resulting in purposeless, rapid motions such as flexing and extending the fingers, raising and lowering the shoulders, or grimacing. The duration of this disorder is typically 15 years.

Psychiatric symptoms are among the most common features of HD and include affective and cognitive changes. About 30% of affected individuals develop severe irritability and episodic aggressive behavior. Some are unable to tolerate frustration, whereas others cannot delay gratification. Some obsess about a single request and become irritable when they are not accommodated. Irritability may alternate with apathy during which there is little desire to do anything. Families may label this behavior as laziness, not understanding that this is a symptom of the disease. Sadly, those with the disease may have little insight into this dramatic change in their personality (Sullivan, 2005).

Mood swings and bouts of depression are common for about 30% of those with HD. Bipolar disorder is a complication for 10% of people with HD. Anxiety over minor issues occurs early in the illness. Obsessive–compulsive symptoms occur in about 25% of clients. Other complications include generalized anxiety disorder and panic disorder (Tost, Wendt, Schmitt, Heinz, & Braus, 2004).

People with HD have a global decrease in cognitive functioning. The changes begin with slowed thinking, decreased concentration and problem solving, and deterioration in quality of work. Visual memory impairment occurs early, whereas verbal memory remains intact until late in the disease. For example, a person with HD may not be able to reproduce a design he or she saw, such as a square or a circle, but may remember words and stories. Orientation is usually intact until the late stages. Paranoid delusions are common, but hallucinations are much less common. Dementia appears in all people with HD, although the rate of progression and the extent of symptoms vary from individual to individual.

Frontal Lobe Dementias

Frontal lobe dementias, caused by a variety of brain diseases, are often misdiagnosed as mental disorders because personality, sociability, and executive function are prominently impaired. Frontal lobe dementias include Pick disease and Creutzfeldt–Jakob disease.

Pick Disease

Pick disease is a rare form of progressive dementia involving abnormal ballooning of neurons, accompanied by atrophy of the frontal and temporal lobes. The disorder usually begins in middle age with a life span of 2 to 10 years after diagnosis. There is no known cause, treatment, or cure.

Pick disease often begins with socially uninhibited behaviors and sudden changes in personality. Poor judgment, socially inappropriate interactions, and impulsive sexual behavior cause embarrassment to family and friends. Early in the disorder, behaviors may include illegal acts such as stealing, sex crimes, or aggression toward others. These behaviors may contribute to a misdiagnosis of a primary mental disorder (e.g., schizophrenic or mood disorders) rather than a dementia.

Other psychiatric symptoms include euphoria, jealous delusions, poor insight, a lack of concern for loved ones, and inattentiveness to surroundings. In interactions with others, individuals with Pick disease either lose attention to the conversation or simply repeat the words of the other person. As the disease progresses they may no longer recognize family and friends. Some experience hyperorality, the need to taste, chew, and examine any object small enough to be placed in the mouth. It is thought that a deficit of serotonin (5-HT) contributes to carbohydrate craving, overeating, and weight gain (Askin-Edgar et al., 2004).

Creutzfeldt–Jakob Disease

Creutzfeldt–Jakob disease (CJD) is a rare, fatal brain disorder that causes inevitable death within 2 to 12 months. CJD is the human equivalent of bovine spongiform encephalopathy or mad cow disease. There are two forms of CJD: (1) *classic*, which can arise spontaneously, be genetically transmitted, or be contracted via infection; and (2) *variant*, which is caused by eating diseased meat or cattle products or receiving infected blood products. An infectious agent unlike any known pathogen causes CJD. This newly discovered pathogen is called a prion, short for proteinaceous infectious particle. **Prions** are small particles that resist inactivation and are thought to transform normal protein molecules into infectious ones, eventually eating spongy holes in the brain, that destroy the person's ability to function (Ironside, Ritchie, & Head, 2005; Ludlam & Turner, 2006).

CJD has signs and symptoms similar to AD, except that the mental deterioration occurs very rapidly. Affected persons have a bizarre range of symptoms, such as hallucinations, seeing things upside down, ataxia, and hyperreflexia. Memory problems lead to confusion and disorientation. Speech becomes difficult for others to understand. Personality changes are obvious and there is a rapid decline into delirium and dementia. In the final stages, people lose all mental and physical function.

Epilepsy

Epilepsy is unprovoked, recurring seizures caused by sporadic electrical discharge of neurons in the cerebral cortex leading to a spectrum of problems. It is one of the most common neurological disorders in the United States. The association between epilepsy and schizophrenialike psychosis has long been noted. Psychotic symptoms are classified according to the phase of clinical seizures: *ictal* (the onset of an epileptic seizure) or *postictal* (after an epileptic seizure).

Ictal psychosis is usually brief, lasting hours to days. There may be a wide range of perceptual, behavioral, cognitive, and affective symptoms. Clients may experience hyperorality or stereotypic behaviors such as constant picking at clothing. They may become mute during the psychotic episode. Hallucinations and thought distortions are not uncommon. There is no change in the level of consciousness, and insight is usually maintained. Individuals with ictal psychosis often have amnesia for the episode (Tucker, 2004).

Postictal psychosis usually follows seizure clusters or a recent increase in seizure frequency and occurs in as many as 7% to 10% of clients. The psychotic episode occurs within a few hours to a few days following the last seizure. Cognitive symptoms include grandiose, somatic, or religious delusions and ideas of reference. There may be some clouding of consciousness. Perceptual symptoms involve auditory hallucinations. Affective symptoms may be either manic or depressive. Postictal psychosis disappears within a few days (Tucker, 2004).

Sam, age 19, has a history of temporal lobe seizures. He has experienced a recent increase in the frequency of his seizures. For the last several days he has been bothering the neighbors at all times of the day and night wanting to discuss religion and asking whether they have been saved. He explained his actions by telling everyone he was God. Even though the neighbors threatened to call the police, Sam wasn't worried because "who would call the police on God?"

Multifocal Disruptions
Multiple Sclerosis

Multiple sclerosis (MS) is a chronic inflammatory disorder of the central nervous system (CNS) caused by destruction of the myelin sheath. The resulting scar tissue slows or blocks transmission of nerve impulses. Symptoms of MS range from relatively benign, to somewhat disabling, to devastating.

Psychiatric symptoms, which may appear even before the typical neurological symptoms, include cognitive dysfunction and mood disorders. Cognitive impairment is present in 55% to 65% of persons with MS. Basic language skills and verbal intelligence is not affected. Decreased attention span and slowed information processing are common. Clients are able to encode and store memories but may not be able to spontaneously recall those memories. Given cues, people with MS are able to retrieve memories. Repeated presentations of new material result in improved learning. Executive functions may be interrupted, resulting in decreased judgment, loss of the ability to think abstractly, and loss of the ability to generalize (Hafler et al., 2005).

When people cannot control their laughing and crying, they are said to have labile affect. This occurs for about 22% to 29% of people with MS. Laughing or crying may be exaggerated or inappropriate to the situation or to the person's overall mood. As much as 10% of people with MS develop bipolar disorder, compared with less than 1% of the general population. In addition 60% of clients develop major depression sometime during their illness and disability. The suicide rate is almost eight times higher than that of the general population. Affective symptoms are not necessarily correlated with the degree of disability, suggesting that they are independent of physical and mental deficits (Asghar-Ali, Taber, Hurley, & Hayman, 2004).

Linnea was diagnosed with MS 3 years ago and with bipolar disorder 18 months ago. She has only very mild neurological symptoms with occasional tingling and numbness, mostly of the upper extremities. Her mother states that Linnea is more confused lately, is getting messages from the television (ideas of reference), and disappears for days at a time. Linnea says that she has periods of severe fear during which she stays in her car in parking lots, and is afraid to go home, to the police, or to the hospital. During one of these episodes, she stayed in a stranger's home and during another, she gave a stranger a ride home. Her family is very concerned because Linnea acts as if nothing is wrong and refuses to take responsibility for her behavior.

Brain Attack

Brain attack, also called a *stroke*, is a major cause of cerebrovascular dementia. Most occurrences of brain attack (77%) are thrombic or embolic, leading to ischemia of brain tissue. The remaining 23% is hemorrhagic. Psychiatric symptoms include cognitive impairment, apathy, disordered emotions, and mood disorders.

Cognitive impairment is the most frequent psychiatric symptom following brain attack. Individuals with left hemisphere destruction have difficulty with orientation, language, executive functions such as decreased judgment, and abstract thinking. Apathy is a frequent cognitive impairment that interferes with pleasure and activities of daily living (ADLs) and contributes to increased social withdrawal.

Affective problems include emotional lability, as demonstrated by pathological laughing and crying. These episodes may be excessive to the situation, may appear spontaneously, or may be in response to nonemotional events. Depression is the most common mood disorder, affecting 40% to 50% of people who have experienced a brain attack. Half of these people will experience major depression, and half will have a less severe form of depression (Lui, Lee, Ross, & Yeung, 2006). Interestingly, people who have primary depression may be at higher risk for brain attack. Depressed people have greater platelet activation and responsiveness than nondepressed individuals. Secretion of 5-HT by platelets produces aggregation or clumping of blood cells, which makes people with depression more susceptible to atherosclerosis, thrombosis, and vasoconstriction (Patterson & Kotrla, 2004).

George, who is 73 years old, has been admitted for major depression. He is upset that most of his children do not take care of him, except his youngest son, who "respects" him. He recently went to his granddaughter's birthday party and thought family members ignored him. He claims his wife is abusing him physically and mentally. On admission he states, "People think I'm nuts. I'm not nuts. I'm just angry that my gun and car were taken away. I've been robbed of my independence." Three days after admission, the staff noticed that George was having difficulty following verbal directions and was alternating between lethargy and agitation. He was noted to have difficulty swallowing food and liquids. His speech was slurred and he was drooling. Further assessment determined that George had experienced a brain attack.

Infections
HIV/AIDS

Direct involvement of the brain by human immunodeficiency virus (HIV) is known as **HIV/AIDS encephalopathy**. CNS involvement in HIV infection can result either from the direct effect of the virus on the brain or from secondary opportunistic infections and malignancies. HIV enters the brain by infecting monocytes that are able to cross the blood–brain barrier. This typically occurs early in the course of infection and initially it is usually asymptomatic. Later psychiatric manifestations include delirium, dementia, mood disorders, and anxiety disorders (Everall, Hansen, & Masliah, 2005).

Delirium is the most frequent psychiatric complication of acquired immune deficiency syndrome (AIDS) and affects as many as 40% to 65% of HIV-infected persons. Rapid recognition and treatment is necessary to prevent permanent brain damage.

Research indicates that 70% of individuals with AIDS will develop HIV-associated minor cognitive disorder. Abnormalities of minor cognitive disorder include impaired attention or concentration, mental slowing, impaired memory, personality change, irritability, or emotional lability. Since orientation and insight are preserved, clients become very concerned and depressed over their loss of functioning. As neurotoxicity continues, problems become more pronounced and as many as 20% to 30% of infected individuals will develop HIV-associated dementia, often referred to as AIDS dementia complex. At this point, individuals have difficulty processing information, impaired executive function, memory and learning problems, apathy, labile emotions, and inappropriate social behavior (Teicher, Andersen, Navalta, Polcari, & Kim, 2004).

Depression may be related to chronic stress such as social stigma, long-term physical discomfort and illness, and the prospect of eventual death. Between 10% and 20% of people with AIDS experience major depression, which is more likely to occur later in the infection (Gibbie et al., 2006; Moneyham et al., 2005).

Anxiety is a frequent problem among AIDS victims. It is estimated that as many as one third of clients will have an anxiety disorder sometime during their disability. The most common disorders are panic disorder, generalized anxiety disorder, and posttraumatic stress disorder.

Although AIDS affects all people regardless of age, sex, ethnicity, or sexual orientation, some populations may be at higher risk. One such group is persons who are severely and persistently mentally ill. The prevalence of HIV infection in the general population is 0.3% and 4% to 23% in severely and persistently mentally ill individuals. One risk factor is the high rate of alcohol and substance use in this population. Infection occurs directly through the sharing of contaminated needles. Substance use is also associated with unsafe sexual activities such as multiple partners, exchanging sex for money or drugs, and not using condoms. People with severe and persistent mental illness are also at higher risk because of poor judgment, ineffective problem-solving skills, sexual impulsivity, a tendency toward taking chances, low motivation to alter sexual behaviors, and transient social relationships (Carey et al., 2004).

Pediatric Autoimmune Neuropsychiatric Disorders

Pediatric autoimmune neuropsychiatric disorders (PANDAS) are a neurological complication associated with streptococcal infections in some children. The antibodies produced to fight the *streptococci* bacteria can trigger an autoimmune reaction. This reaction is most frequently directed against cells in the heart and joints (rheumatic fever), but in 20% to 30% of cases it reacts with the basal ganglia, causing antibody-mediated inflammation, leading to CNS dysfunction (Pavone, Parano, Rizzo, & Trifiletti, 2006).

There is some correlation between PANDAS and *obsessive–compulsive disorder* (OCD), *Tourette disorder*, and *attention deficit/hyperactivity disorder* (ADHD). (See chapter 17 ∞ for more information on these disorders.)

Some children develop these disorders simultaneously with or subsequent to the autoimmune reaction. A number of children, however, have ADHD, tic disorders, and OCD before the occurrence of streptococcal infection. It is thought that these mental disorders may reflect a vulnerability to PANDAS (Mell, Davis, & Owens, 2005).

The symptoms of PANDAS are a sudden and dramatic onset of OCD, ADHD, or Tourette disorder. Affected children are described as having changed overnight. They exhibit classic OCD symptoms such as excessive hand washing, nighttime rituals, checking behavior, and obsessions about death. They may develop tics and sudden uncontrollable movement, grunts, and facial grimaces. They demonstrate a peculiar "squirminess" in which they try very hard to sit still but constantly wiggle and fidget in their chairs. Other symptoms include separation anxiety, age-inappropriate behavior, and nighttime difficulties, including severe nightmares and new bedtime fears or rituals. More than 90% experience emotional lability with unprecipitated bouts of crying or hysterical laughter and increased irritability. In some children, PANDAS resolve; in others, the symptoms continue with less severity, and a few will have periods of acute symptom relapse (Mell et al., 2005).

Lyme Disease

A small percentage of people with Lyme disease develop CNS symptoms months to years after diagnosis and treatment. **Lyme disease** is a tick-borne infection that may affect the skin, joints, heart, eyes, and CNS. Lyme meningitis may occur within the first few months after infection. Symptoms include irritability, headache, lethargy, and cognitive dysfunctions (Halperin, 2005).

Late-stage Lyme disease CNS involvement leads to symptoms such as memory loss, naming problems, difficulty concentrating, fatigue, and depression. It is thought that these changes are the result of a diffuse inflammatory process in the basal ganglia and cerebral cortex. This process is an extremely rare complication and usually responds to antibiotic therapy (Halperin, 2005).

Traumatic Brain Injury

Traumatic brain injury (TBI) is defined as a head injury caused by accidents, or assaults. Causes of the injury vary with the developmental stage. Infants suffer TBIs when they experience shaken baby syndrome at the hands of an adult. Toddlers are at risk for TBIs from falls. Middle-school–aged children are at risk for sports-related injuries and older children experience TBIs from auto accidents (Keenan & Bratton, 2006).

In comparison with the general population, a higher percentage of people who have had traumatic brain injury develop psychiatric illnesses within a year. The period of greatest risk for TBIs is from the mid-teens through the mid-20s, be-

fore the onset of many major psychiatric disorders, contributing to the belief that the injury itself is associated with the onset of the psychiatric disorder. Behavioral, affective, and cognitive symptoms are more likely to prevent the return to work, school, and social activities than are the physical deficits related to the injury (Kao & Stuifbergen, 2004; Wongvatunyu & Porter, 2005).

Often a change in personality is reported after TBI. Behavior may be impulsive and disinhibited. Some have trouble with anger control. Depression is the most common complication and occurs in 39% of people with mild injury and in 77% of those with severe injury. Depressive symptoms usually begin within the first 6 months after injury. Anxiety symptoms occur in 24% to 28% of people with TBI. Anxiety disorders include posttraumatic stress disorder, panic disorder, and obsessive–compulsive disorder. There is also a high rate of sleep disorders, especially nightmares (Bay, Hagerty, Williams, Kirsch, & Gillespie, 2002; Koponen et al., 2002).

Cognitive changes include attention and concentration difficulties and short-term memory problems. Often, executive functions are disturbed, including judgment, insight, problem solving, planning, and information processing. Language problems are common.

Psychosis after TBI resembles schizophrenia. Reported rates range from 0.07% to 10%, with an increasing risk over time, compared with a rate of 0.8% of schizophrenia in the general population. The exact relationship between schizophrenia and TBI is unclear. It may be a result of a gene–environment interaction. The TBI (environment) may lower the threshold for development of schizophrenia in those with genetic vulnerability to the disorder. Another possibility is that early symptoms of schizophrenia, such as agitation or psychosis, might increase vulnerability to TBI. This vulnerability might be related to impaired attention or cerebellar dysfunction, or both (Corcoran, McAllister, & Malaspina, 2005).

People with TBI may be more susceptible to Alzheimer disease (AD). TBI may not cause AD but may reduce the time to onset of disease for those with a predisposition. People who have experienced severe head injuries have a significant increase in deposition of amyloid protein in their brains. The injury may decrease the functional reserves of the brain. It is also possible that damage to the blood–brain barrier allows entry of toxic products or somehow makes the brain more susceptible to the effects of aging (Corcoran et al., 2005).

Psychopharmacological Interventions

Medications are prescribed to manage the specific *psychiatric symptoms* people are experiencing. The preferred drug for depression in PD is paroxetine (Paxil), which eases depression without increasing motor fluctuations. Two antipsychotic medications, clozapine (Clozaril) and quetiapine (Seroquel), improve memory and concentration while decreasing psychiatric symptoms. Risperidone (Risperdal) and olanzapine (Zyprexa) are not prescribed because they worsen the symptoms of PD. People who take pramipexole (Mirapex) for PD are at significantly higher risk for hallucinations than those receiving ropinirole (Requip) (Aarsland & Ehrt, 2003).

When people with post–brain attack depression are given antidepressants, their depression eases, as does the cognitive and social impairment that complicates the recovery from brain attack. Nortriptyline (Aventyl or Pamelor) is a better choice than fluoxetine (Prozac) for individuals who have concurrent depression and medical illness. The side effects, such as nausea, anorexia, and weight loss, occur more frequently with fluoxetine in the elderly population.

A cholinesterase inhibitor, rivastigmine (Exelon), has been approved for use in the treatment of dementia. Early studies demonstrate effectiveness in treating moderate to severe memory loss in some individuals with TBI.

Multidisciplinary Interventions

Recently, deep brain stimulation has been tried for those people with PD who no longer respond to medication. Electrodes are implanted in deep subcortical nuclei and provide intermittent stimulation. Potential side effects include bleeding, seizures, infections, paresthesia, and hallucinations (Pahwa et al., 2006).

Alternative Therapies

Oxidative stress and generation of free radicals have an important role in the etiology of PD. Antioxidants may be helpful, along with traditional therapies. The two antioxidants under study are coenzyme Q(10) and melatonin (Mayo et al., 2005; Shults, 2005).

One study assessed the usefulness of group exercise programs for people with advanced HIV/AIDS. One group did aerobic exercise twice a week for 8 weeks; another group did t'ai chi for the same period, and the control group did not exercise. The individuals in the exercise groups demonstrated significant improvement in physical functioning and quality of life (Galantino et al., 2005).

Pilates exercises are controlled movements sometimes moving the body only by inches. These small motions seem to be helpful for persons with PD. Anecdotal evidence shows a reduction in symptoms, especially muscle rigidity and balance.

Nursing Process

CLIENTS WITH NEUROPSYCHIATRIC PROBLEMS

ASSESSMENT

In addition to a complete physical assessment, a careful history is needed from the client and family members. To maintain clients' sense of self-determination, the mental status assessment should begin with family members present and progress to an individual interview. If possible, the nurse must gain clients' permission to share information with the family. Emphasis is on openness and full disclosure, which is essential in the management of future deterioration, if that is the likely outcome.

Client assessment includes ADLs. Obtaining information from family members may more accurately assess functional impairment because the client may be unaware of

Focused Nursing Assessment | Clients With Neuropsychiatric Problems

Behavior Assessment	Affective Assessment	Cognitive Assessment	Social Assessment
Describe any difficulties in performing complex tasks at home, school, or work.	What kinds of things make you feel anxious?	What year is it? Month?	How close do you feel to your family members?
Give me an example of something that has confused you recently.	When do you feel sad?	What is your telephone number? Address?	How do you handle disagreements?
Do you find yourself repeatedly checking or counting things?	How often do you feel irritable?	What would you do if you found a stamped, addressed envelope on the sidewalk?	
How much help do you need in ADLs?	What are your major frustrations?	Which one of the following objects does not belong in this group: car, dog, wagon, truck?	
		Do you hear voices that others say they do not hear?	

impairments. Assessment of ADLs covers hygiene and grooming, household chores and responsibilities, quality of schoolwork or outside employment, and management of finances. Clients may appear in immaculate condition because of attentive caregivers, yet not be able to shop, cook, bathe, dress, or pay bills without total assistance.

Psychiatric symptoms or mental disorders may occur or remit during the course of the neurological illness and must be assessed on an ongoing basis. See the Focused Nursing Assessment feature for some general questions. Questions that are more specific can be found in the chapters on anxiety, mood, schizophrenic, and spectrum disorders.

Assessment: Behavior

Clients with these neuropsychiatric disorders may alternate between social withdrawal and socially uninhibited behavior. Because of cognitive limitations, their behavior is often impulsive. They often lose interest in activities previously enjoyed. Most of these clients develop some level of difficulty with ADLs. Some experience severe irritability and episodic aggressive behavior. Clients and families may become socially isolated when they fear reactions from other people when they are out in public (Kao & Stuifbergen, 2004).

Assessment: Affect

Apathy, or reduced motivation, leads to more severe deficits in ADLs. Some persons develop *alexithymia*, which is the inability to identify and articulate feelings. Others have a labile affect, experiencing sudden and easily provoked changes in mood. They may be happy one moment, and angry or anxious the next. A general sense of hopelessness is fairly common.

Assessment: Cognition

Attention is not a single process. The components of attention are alertness, ability to selectively attend to incoming information, and the capacity to focus. When clients have attention problems, you must determine which of these components are disrupted. On assessment, you are likely to find slowed information processing, interrupted executive function, poor insight, and loss of short- and long-term memory. As the disease or infection continues, dementia is likely to develop.

Assessment: Interpersonal Relationships

Family life is often radically altered when a family member has one of these conditions. Family members are the primary providers of care. Hopes and expectations for the future are suddenly changed. Communication problems leave clients and caregivers feeling frustrated and misunderstood.

Assessment: Cultural Influences

In most of these neuropsychiatric disorders, it is unknown why one person develops the disorder and another does not. Some have a genetic component, such as PD, HD, CJD, and brain attack. Others, such as seizure disorders, MS, HIV/AIDS, PANDAS, TBI, and Lyme disease have a much stronger environmental risk. Most likely, most of these neuropsychiatric disorders are caused by a combination of environmental and genetic factors.

PD is one of the most common neurodegenerative disorders in the United States and Canada. The racial distribution is unclear. Some studies indicate similar frequency of PD for Euro-Americans and African Americans. Other studies suggest that the frequency is higher among Euro-Americans. Among the Japanese and some Europeans, there is a higher rate of young-onset PD.

Little is known about the impact of race and culture on HD. It is less frequent in Japan, China, Finland, and Africa. The variant form of CJD is related to the presence of infected cattle, which is then consumed by humans living in that geographical area. All but one case have been in the United Kingdom. MS is more common in Euro-Americans

---

Families of Client With Neuropsychiatric Problems

Behavior Assessment	Affective Assessment	Cognitive Assessment	Social Assessment
Has there been a sudden change in behavior?	How anxious does she or he seem to you?	Have there been changes in her or his ability to concentrate?	Describe interactions with other people.
Is it difficult to get her or him involved in activities?	How depressed does she or he seem to you?	Describe any confusion about person, time, or place.	Does she or he embarrass you in social situations?
How much assistance is needed in ADLs?	In what way is irritability increasing?	Describe any recent or remote memory loss.	What are previous hobbies/interests? Family activities?
Is she or he withdrawn? Agitated? Aggressive?	Does she or he laugh and/or cry inappropriately?	Give me examples of irrational decision making.	What kinds of discussions have taken place regarding the future?
Does she or he have bizarre, uncontrolled physical motions?		Is there any evidence of delusions?	Who is involved in making these decisions?

of northern and central European ancestry. Groups that are resistant to MS include American Indians, Chinese, Japanese, and Lapps.

The adult ticks that cause Lyme disease depend on the presence of deer for survival. The number of deer in any given area determines the population of ticks. As many as 92% of cases are found in 10 states: Connecticut, Rhode Island, New Jersey, New York, Pennsylvania, Delaware, Massachusetts, Wisconsin, Minnesota, and Maryland.

Assessment: Age-Specific Characteristics

The average age of onset of PD is 60 years of age, with 80% of all affected persons developing the disorder between 40 and 70 years of age. About 5% of those with PD are diagnosed between the ages of 30 and 40, which is referred to as young-onset PD. It is highly unusual for someone younger than the age of 30 to be diagnosed with this disorder, but there are a few cases of juvenile onset before the age of 20 (Askin-Edgar et al., 2004).

The average age of onset of HD is 40 years. However, 10% develop the disorder before the age of 20 and 25% develop it after the age of 50. CJD affects most people in their 60s. The average age of onset for the variant type of CJD is younger, with an average age of 29 years. Variant CJD has a longer duration: the average is 16 months before death. Pediatric autoimmune neuropsychiatric disorder is, by definition, a childhood disorder. The average age of onset is between 10 and 11 years. MS has long been thought to be an adult disorder. It is only recently that clinicians have discovered juvenile MS (Pena et al., 2006).

Epilepsy has the highest occurrence in individuals younger than age 20. The next highest age group is older than 70 years. It is possible to determine the cause of epilepsy in only less than half of the cases. Common causes include congenital brain malformations, high fevers, head trauma, brain tumors, and brain attacks.

DIAGNOSIS

Based on the assessment data, the nurse develops any number of nursing diagnoses for the child or adult client. In synthesizing the assessment data, consider how well clients are functioning in daily life (North American Nursing Diagnosis Association, 2007).

- Acute Confusion related to clouding of consciousness, disorientation, and sensitivity to environmental stimulation
- Anxiety related to chronic or terminal prognosis, emotional lability, impaired cognitive abilities
- Family Coping: Potential for Growth related to caretaking responsibilities, support of all family members, development of effective coping strategies

- Altered Thought Processes related to decreasing judgment, memory loss

OUTCOME IDENTIFICATION AND GOALS

Once you have established diagnoses, select outcomes appropriate to the nursing diagnoses. In many of these situations, there is a steady or intermittent progression downward in terms of functional abilities. In these cases, the overall outcome is maximizing the remaining strengths and keeping clients as comfortable as possible.

Client goals are specific behavioral measures by which you and significant others determine progress toward outcomes. The following are examples of some of the goals appropriate to people with neuropsychiatric disorders:

- Improved orientation as delirium clears
- Establishes routines to decrease confusion
- Remains oriented to person, time, and place
- Completes ADLs appropriate to functional level
- Improved levels of anxiety and depression
- Interacts appropriately with others

PLANNING

Once the nursing diagnoses, outcome criteria, and goals have been identified, develop the plan of care to help clients function more effectively in their physical, social, and emotional lives.

IMPLEMENTATION

Most nursing interventions appropriate to these clients are discussed in the chapters on anxiety (chapter 11 ∞), mood (chapter 13 ∞), cognitive (chapter 19 ∞), and child and adolescent disorders (chapter 17 ∞). When working with people who are experiencing neuropsychiatric disorders, review and integrate that knowledge. Physical nursing care is discussed in medical–surgical and neurological nursing texts.

Caregiver Strain

Effective family nursing interventions depend on the nurse's understanding of the effects of neurological disorders on family caregivers. The goal is to identify and reduce any negative perceptions, improve coping skills, and increase social supports.

NURSING CARE PLAN for a Client With Neuropsychiatric Problems

Managing Delirium
Nursing Diagnosis: Client at Risk for Acute Confusion

Outcomes: Client remains safe and verbalizes improved orientation.

The neurological status of clients experiencing delirium must be monitored on an ongoing basis. Clients benefit from nursing interventions designed to prevent or manage agitation, anxiety, and perceptual or cognitive disturbances.

Intervention	Rationale	Goal
Whenever possible, interventions other than restraints, such as sitters, should be used to prevent delirious clients from harming themselves or others.	Restraints often increase agitation and carry risks for injuries and are used only when other interventions fail.	Remains safe
Provide frequent contact and reassurance. Use brief, simple statements.	This improves orientation. Lengthy explanations are confusing to the client with delirium.	Responds appropriately to contact
Give client and family information about what is happening and what can be expected to occur in the future.	Education will lessen fear of the unknown.	Verbalizes an accurate understanding of the situation
Do not ask clients questions they are unable to answer.	This decreases clients' frustration with current cognitive status.	Verbalizes less frustration
Provide a written schedule of ADLs and daily activities.	This improves orientation.	Refers to written schedule
Give clients their glasses and hearing aids if appropriate.	Delirium is aggravated by visual and auditory impairment.	Uses glasses and hearing aids
Provide a visible clock and calendar.	This improves orientation.	Refers to clock and calendar throughout the day
Adjust the sensory environment according to clients' response. This is often a process of trial and error.	Sensory deprivation and sensory overstimulation both can worsen symptoms.	Remains oriented

Coping With Anxiety
Nursing Diagnosis: Client at Risk for Anxiety

Outcomes: Client utilizes calming techniques and verbalizes less anxiety.

Calming techniques such as muscle relaxation and deep breathing are useful for managing the physiological dimensions of anxiety.

Intervention	Rationale	Goal
Teach clients to take a deep breath through the nose, inhaling to the count of 5, and then exhaling to the count of 5.	Deep breathing replaces the shallow breathing that highly anxious people adopt unconsciously and prevents hyperventilation.	Uses deep breathing to prevent feeling overwhelmed when anxious
Teach clients to focus on and relax specific muscle groups. Have them practice twice a day for 20 minutes. It will be several weeks before they experience significant benefit.	This helps them recognize when their bodies are tightening up in response to anxiety.	Uses progressive relaxation to manage anxiety
Problem solve other calming techniques such as: ■ Take a walk. ■ Read a book. ■ Rub a worry stone. ■ Talk with a friend. ■ Sing a song.	Changing their sensory experiences or getting involved in activities may decrease anxiety.	Chooses and utilizes calming techniques

continued

NURSING CARE PLAN for a Client With Neuropsychiatric Problems

Coping With Anxiety *continued*
Nursing Diagnosis: Client at Risk for Anxiety

Intervention	Rationale	Goal
Teach positive affirmations such as: ■ I am calm and happy. ■ My breathing is slow and even. ■ I am very relaxed.	This counteracts the negative cognitions that accompany anxiety.	Repeats positive affirmations several times a day

Enhancing Memory
Nursing Diagnosis: Client at Risk for Impaired Memory

Outcomes: Client utilizes memory aids and accomplishes ADLs with minimal direction from others.

Help clients and families establish daily routines so that particular times of day may trigger the memory of what needs to be accomplished at what times.

Intervention	Rationale	Goal
Make lists or post notes regarding the daily schedule of activities and chores.	This assists with short-term memory loss.	Utilizes lists or notes
Handheld electronic devices are appropriate for some clients. They may need a cueing strategy to remind them to check the electronic device.	Some clients may find these devices too complicated to use. Those who have "grown up" in the electronic age may find these devices familiar and helpful.	Utilizes electronic memory devices
Suggest an alarm watch set for specific times.	This may trigger memory for activities or chores.	Utilizes alarm watch
For clients who have impaired verbal memory, suggest nonverbal cues such as: ■ Find or draw pictures of the series of steps in a procedure such as morning self-care. ■ These pictures should be posted in the place the activity is done.	Nonverbal cues will assist them in recall.	Copes with problems related to memory loss

Responding to Apathy
Nursing Diagnosis: Client at Risk for Hopelessness

Outcomes: Client identifies benefits of improved motivation.

Low motivation and apathy often interfere with recovery because there is no drive to change what is not working well.

Intervention	Rationale	Goal
Ask clients to: ■ Identify personal goals. ■ Link specific behavior change to attainment of these goals.	An internal locus of control will contribute to increased motivation in an effort to improve the situation.	Verbalizes responsibility in making changes in life
Help clients identify and compare the costs and benefits of changing versus not changing behaviors.	This focuses attention on the goals. It is best to start with behaviors that must be increased in frequency rather than with decreasing problematic behaviors.	Clarifies benefits of changing behaviors

NURSING CARE PLAN for a Client With Neuropsychiatric Problems

Teaching Skills
Nursing Diagnosis: Client at Risk for Ineffective Role Performance

Outcomes: Client increases level of functioning.

Through assessment you determine where clients are having difficulty in daily skills. The next step is teaching clients the particular skills they need. Skills training can be used for self-care activities such as grooming, home maintenance skills, shopping, or money management. In addition, skills training can be used to improve conversation skills, assertive skills, medication management, symptom management, and coping with stress.

Intervention	Rationale	Goal
Model the behavior.	Seeing the behavior in action promotes learning in comparison to simply discussing the behavior.	Able to imitate the modeled behavior
Help clients practice the skill by predesigned role-play.	Active participation improves comprehension and retention of new skills.	Engages in role-play
After the role-play, acknowledge successful behaviors and offer corrective feedback on less successful behaviors.	Feedback is a necessary part of learning new skills.	Acknowledges feedback
Assign clients practice in the real world.	This reinforces new skills.	Practices new skills
Together, evaluate what occurred during the practice sessions.	Evaluation is an important step when learning new skills.	Reviews what occurred during practice sessions

Clinical Interactions   A Client With Traumatic Brain Injury

George, 18 years old, was admitted to the acute care psychiatric unit following a violent outburst against his mother in which he beat her with a radio and then threw it out the front window. George experienced TBI 4 years ago in an automobile accident. He does not work or go to school. George states that he tries to avoid contact with his parents by walking around the neighborhood because he cannot drive or by just staying in his room. In this interaction, you see evidence of:

- Poor impulse control
- Aggressive behavior
- External locus of control

GEORGE: "I just want to get out of here." (Sitting on the bed fidgeting with the blankets)

NURSE: *"What do you plan on doing once you get out of the hospital?"*

GEORGE: "I'm going to go find Nicky. She was a girl here and she is the only one who is nice to me. She's my only friend."

NURSE: *"It seems sad that you only have one friend."*

GEORGE: "No one likes me." (Looking down with a sad expression)

NURSE: *"I like you."*

GEORGE: "You do?" (looks up with a smile)

NURSE: *"Yes, and it sounds like from group this morning that other people like you too."*

GEORGE: "I guess. Why don't you come and lay with me on the bed." (patting the bed, smiling). "Do you think my face is full of acne? Do you want to feel my head? Part of my skull is gone since I was 14. I want out of here."

NURSE: *"Do you know the reason you are in the hospital, George?"*

GEORGE: "Yes." (pause). "I hit my mother. I know I shouldn't have hit her but she doesn't care about me and she doesn't listen to me."

NURSE: *"You think that by hitting her, she will care about you and listen to you?"*

GEORGE: "I don't know." (looking down)

NURSE: *"Do you usually want to hit someone when you are upset?"*

GEORGE: "No, I don't think so." (looking down, clenching blankets, rocking)

NURSE: *"What do you do when you're upset and you don't hit anyone?"*

GEORGE: "I walk a lot. I don't want to hit anyone—I just do."

It is important to listen to each family member's perspective of the disease process and prognosis. Point out discrepancies in expectations and provide education regarding realistic prognosis. Normalizing the family's experience involves addressing family fears and helping the family adjust to the life changes that occur. It may be appropriate to introduce the family to other families undergoing similar experiences. Peer groups help families in problem solving and decreasing caregiver distress and social isolation. Equalizing caregiving tasks involves reducing disproportionate caretaking burdens on individual family members. Discuss possible options to the family that will assist them to make decisions about care of their loved ones. If appropriate and desired, help family arrange for respite care.

The desired outcome is that families will verbalize an accurate perception of prognosis, care for their own needs, and use support systems.

EVALUATION

To complete the nursing process, evaluate client responses to nursing interventions based on the selected outcomes. With appropriate planning and consistent implementation, clients will remain safe, reasonably oriented, and emotionally stable.

Using Research Evidence | Psychological Sequela of Traumatic Brain Injury

Bay, E., Hagerty, B. M., Williams, R. A., Kirsch, N., & Gillespie, B. (2002). Chronic stress, sense of belonging, and depression among survivors of traumatic brain injury. *Journal of Nursing Scholarship, 34,* 221–226.

What is the study about?

Traumatic brain injury (TBI) affects 5.3 million Americans and is associated with neurobehavioral, mood, and cognitive changes. After moderate and severe TBI, many persons suffer depression. The purpose of this study was to investigate whether depression post-TBI could be explained in part through three variables associated with clinical depression: chronic stress, interpersonal relatedness, and cognitive burden.

How was the study done?

This was a quantitative cross-sectional and exploratory study using a nonprobability sample that sought data from 75 mildly to moderately injured persons living with TBI, and from their significant others. All participants were residing in the community, had been living with TBI for up to 2 years, and had a significant other willing to take part in the study.

Of these adults, 91.7% were White; 48% were female and 52% male. Almost 71% experienced TBI as a result of a motor vehicle accident; 64% had been unconscious for less than an hour. A history of alcohol or drug problems was reported in 13% of the participants, and a previous head injury in 16%. Of this sample, 41% were currently taking prescribed antidepressants, 20% reported a preinjury psychiatric disorder such as anxiety or depression, and 8% had experienced suicidal thoughts within the year before the TBI. The sample was equally divided between mild and moderate TBI.

Data were collected in the presence of the principal researcher in a single 90-minute period, although that span might vary based on participant's schedule, level of fatigue, etc. The person living with TBI and the significant other provided demographic data, and they each answered questions about the severity of the brain injury—duration of unconsciousness and length of posttraumatic amnesia (PTA)—data confirmed retrospectively from their charts. To measure the injury's severity, researchers used the following tools: PTA, Glasgow Coma Scale (GCS) score, and duration of unconsciousness. Tools used to measure symptoms of depression were the Center for Epidemiological Studies Depression Scale (CES-D) and the Neurobehavioral Functioning Inventory (NFI) depression subscale. Postinjury stress was measured by the Perceived Stress Scale. To assess interpersonal relatedness, researchers used two instruments: the Interpersonal Relationship Inventory (IRI) and the Sense of Belonging Instrument—Psychological. To measure cognitive burden, researchers used a battery of six measures assessing directed attention and short-term memory.

What were the results of the study?

As approved by an institutional review board, the study tested three hypotheses: (1) Postinjury chronic stress is positively related to post-TBI depressive symptoms. This hypothesis was supported; postinjury chronic stress was significantly and positively related to post-TBI depression. (2) Interpersonal relatedness (postinjury sense of belonging and social support) is inversely related to post-TBI depressive symptoms. This second hypothesis was partially supported: Postinjury depression was not significantly related to social support since time of injury; however, it was significantly related to sense of belonging. (3) The cognitive burden that TBI places on processing speed and accuracy is positively related to post-TBI depressive symptoms. This final hypothesis was not supported: Variations in depression or stress were not explained by scores on the tests of directed attention and short-term memory.

What additional questions might I have?

Would the same or similar results have resulted from a study with a larger sample size? Would different results emerge from a sample of persons living with TBI for longer than 2 years?

How can I use this study?

After TBI, nurses need to educate families and significant others about the importance of identifying and managing stressors during the postinjury recovery phase. In addition, the nurse should encourage and plan interventions that assist persons living with TBI to feel a sense of belonging within the family unit and the community.

SOURCE: Contributed by Dolores Huffman, PhD, RN, Associate Professor of Nursing, Purdue University Calumet, Hammond, Indiana.

Focus Your Study

OBJECTIVES	KEY CONCEPTS

OBJECTIVES

1. Discuss the psychiatric symptoms associated with disorders that cause central nervous system disruption.

KEY CONCEPTS

- Parkinson disease:
  - Apathy
  - Depression
  - Anxiety disorders
  - Dementia
  - Hallucinations
  - Delusions
- Huntington disease:
  - Irritability, episodic aggression
  - Apathy
  - Depression, bipolar
  - Memory impairment
  - Delusions
  - Dementia
- Pick disease:
  - Socially uninhibited behaviors
  - Changes in personality
  - Poor insight, lack of judgment
  - Hyperorality
- Creutzfeldt–Jakob disease:
  - Rapid mental deterioration
  - Memory problems leading to confusion and disorientation
  - Delirium
  - Dementia
- Epilepsy:
  - Ictal psychosis: lasts a few days, with stereotypic behaviors and hallucinations
  - Postictal psychosis: lasts a few days, with delusions, hallucinations, manic behavior, and depression
- Multiple sclerosis:
  - Decreased attention, slowed information processing
  - Disrupted executive functions
  - Major depression, bipolar
  - Higher suicide rate
- Brain attack:
  - Apathy
  - Emotional lability, depression
  - Confusion
  - Disrupted executive functions
- HIV/AIDS encephalopathy:
  - Delirium
  - Dementia
  - Disrupted executive functions
  - Apathy
  - Labile emotions
  - Inappropriate social behavior
  - Depressions
  - Anxiety
- Pediatric autoimmune neuropsychiatric disorders:
  - Obsessive–compulsive disorder
  - ADHD
  - Tourette disorder
  - Emotional lability
- Lyme disease:
  - Irritability
  - Lethargy
  - Cognitive dysfunction
  - Memory loss
  - Decreased concentration
  - Depression
- Traumatic brain injury:
  - Change in personality
  - Depression

1. Discuss the psychiatric symptoms associated with disorders that cause central nervous system disruption.—*continued*

→

- Anxiety
- Cognitive changes
- Psychosis
- Increased risk for Alzheimer disease

2. Outline the different treatment options related to neuropsychiatric problems.

→

- Parkinson disease:
  - Paroxetine (Paxil)
  - Clozapine (Clozaril)
  - Quetiapine (Seroquel)
  - Ropinirole (Requip)
  - Deep brain stimulation
- Post–brain attack:
  - Nortriptyline (Aventyl or Pamelor)
- Dementia:
  - Rivastigmine (Exelon)

3. Outline the assessment process for neuropsychiatric problems.

→

- Obtain a careful history from client and family members.
- Assess ADLs.
- Assess for impulsive behaviors, irritability, and aggression.
- Assess for alexithymia, labile mood, and hopelessness.
- Assess for attention problems, disrupted executive function, and memory loss.
- Assess for changes within the family system.

4. Use the nursing process to develop a comprehensive plan of care for a client with a neuropsychiatric problem.

→

- Provide frequent contact and orientation.
- Use brief, simple sentences.
- Give clients their glasses and hearing aids if appropriate.
- Make certain there is a visible clock and calendar in the room.
- Use calming techniques such as muscle relaxation and deep breathing.

5. Develop teaching plans for a client with a neuropsychiatric problem and her/his family.

→

- Listen to each family member's perspective of the disease process or injury and prognosis for the client.
- Point out discrepancies in expectations.
- Provide information about what is happening and what can be expected to occur in the future.
- Normalize the family's experience by addressing fears and helping the family adjust to the life changes that occur.
- Refer to self-help groups.
- Provide a written schedule of daily activities.
- Teach skills by modeling the behavior, practice, and feedback until there is mastery of the skill.
- If appropriate and desired, help families arrange for respite care.

Explore MediaLink

For review questions, case studies, and other resources for this chapter see the Pearson Health MediaLink CD-ROM that accompanies this book and the Companion Website.

CD-ROM
- Audio Glossary
- NCLEX-RN® Review Questions
- Animations/Videos
  - T-cell Destruction by HIV

Companion Website www.prenhall.com/fontaine
- Audio Glossary
- NCLEX-RN® Review Questions
- Case Study
  - Traumatic Brain Injury
- Care Plan
  - Intervention for the Client With a Neurological Disorder
- Critical Thinking
  - Psychiatric Problems Associated With Neurological Disorders
- MediaLink Application
  - Overview of Neuropsychiatric Lyme Disease
- MediaLinks
  - Books for Clients & Families
  - Community Resources

NCLEX-RN® Review Questions

20-1. Which of the following assessment results would the nurse expect to find in a client with Pick disease?
1. Poor insight and lack of judgment
2. Memory problems leading to confusion
3. Delusions and hallucinations
4. Decreased attention and slowed information processing

20-2. A client is in the late stages of Parkinson disease. He states that he wants to be left alone and does not want visitors. In planning for treatment strategies the nurse should focus on:
1. Encouraging the client to have visitors.
2. Suggesting to the doctor the need for antidepressant medication.
3. Telling the client he cannot deny friends and family from visiting him.
4. Respecting the client's decision.

20-3. What distinctive symptoms do clients with Huntington disease manifest? (Select all that apply.)
1. Cognitive changes
2. Severe irritability

3. Inability to tolerate frustration
4. Heightened insight into their behavior
5. Ability to remember words and stories

20-4. A delirious client is physically restrained. The restraining intervention and the safety of the client is the responsibility of the:
1. Nurse who is assigned to care for the client.
2. Nursing assistant under the supervision of the nurse.
3. Physician who ordered the restraints.
4. Health care professional who applied the restraints.

20-5. During a family education session, the nurse focuses on the care of the client diagnosed with dementia. The nurse should counsel the family on the need to:
1. Understand the potential for the client wandering from the home.
2. Encourage the client to be socially active.
3. Prepare the client for increased mobility.
4. Plan the grief process for loss of self.

See Appendix D for answers.

References

Aarsland, D., & Ehrt, U. (2003). Basal ganglia diseases and geriatric psychiatry. *Current Opinion in Psychiatry, 16*(2), 621–627.

Asghar-Ali, A. A., Taber, K. H., Hurley, R. A., & Hayman, L. A. (2004). Pure neuropsychiatric presentation of multiple sclerosis. *American Journal of Psychiatry, 161*(2), 226–231.

Askin-Edgar, S., White, K. E., & Cummings, J. L. (2004). Neuropsychiatric aspects of Alzheimer's disease and other dementing illnesses. In S. C. Yudofsky & R. E. Hales (Eds.), *Essentials of neuropsychiatry and clinical neurosciences* (pp. 421–456). Washington, DC: American Psychiatric Publishing.

Bay, E., Hagerty, B. M., Williams, R. A., Kirsch, N., & Gillespie, B. (2002). Chronic stress, sense of belonging, and depression among survivors of traumatic brain injury. *Journal of Nursing Scholarship, 34*(3), 221–226.

Carey, M. P., Carey, K. B., Maisto, S. A., Gordon, C. M., Schroder, K. E., & Vanable, P. A. (2004). Reducing HIV-risk behavior among adults receiving outpatient psychiatric treatment. *Journal of Consulting and Clinical Psychology, 72*(2), 252–268.

Corcoran, C., McAllister, T. W., & Malaspina, D. (2005). Psychotic disorders. In J. M Silver, T. W. McAllister, & S. C. Yudofsky (Eds.), *Textbook of traumatic brain injury* (pp. 213–229). Washington, DC: American Psychiatric Press.

Everall, I. P., Hansen, L. A., & Masliah, E. (2005). The shifting patterns of HIV encephalitis neuropathology. *Neurotoxicity Research, 8*(1–2), 51–61.

Galantino, M. L., Shepard, K., Krafft, L., Laperriere, A., Ducette, J., Sorbello, A., et al. (2005). The effect of group aerobic exercise and T'ai Chi on functional outcomes and quality of life for persons living with Acquired Immunodeficiency Syndrome. *Journal of Alternative and Complementary Medicine, 11*(6), 1085–1092.

Gibbie, T., Mijch, A., Ellen, S., Hoy, J., Hutchison, C., Wright, E., et al. (2006). Depression and neurocognitive performance in individuals with HIV/AIDS. *HIV Medicine, 7*(2), 112–121.

Hafler, D. A., Slavik, J. M., Anderson, D. E., O'Connor, K. C., DeJager, P., & Baccher-Allan, C. (2005). Multiple sclerosis. *Immunological Review, 20*(4), 208–231.

Halperin, J. J. (2005). Central nervous system Lyme disease. *Current Neurology and Neuroscience Reports, 5*(6), 446–452.

Ironside, J. W., Ritchie, D. L., & Head, M. W. (2005). Phenotypic variability in human prion diseases. *Neuropathology and Applied Neurobiology, 31*(6), 565–579.

Kao, H-F. S., & Stuifbergen, A. K. (2004). Love and load: The lived experience of the mother–child relationship among young adult traumatic brain-injured survivors. *Journal of Neuroscience Nursing, 36*(2), 73–81.

Keenan, H. T., & Bratton, S. L. (2006). Epidemiology and outcomes of pediatric traumatic brain injury. *Developmental Neuroscience, 28*(4-5), 256–263.

Koponen, S., Taiminen, R., Portin, R., Himanen, L., Isoniemi, H., Heinonen, H., et al. (2002). Axis I and II psychiatric disorders after traumatic brain injury. *American Journal of Psychiatry, 159*(8), 1315–1321.

Ludlam, C. A., & Turner, M. L. (2006). Managing the risk of transmission of variant Creutzfeldt–Jakob disease by blood products. *British Journal of Haematology, 132*(1), 13–24.

Lui, M. H. L., Lee, D. T F., Ross, F., & Yeung , S. (2006). Psychometric evaluation of the center for epidemiological studies depression scale in Chinese poststroke older adults. *Journal of Nursing Scholarship, 38*(4), 366–369.

Matsui, H., Udaka, F., Tamura, A., Oda, M., Kubori, T., Nishinaka, K., et al. (2006). Impaired visual acuity as a risk factor for visual hallucinations in Parkinson's disease. *Journal of Geriatric Psychiatry and Neurology, 19*(1), 36–40.

Mayo, J. C., Sainz, R. M., Tan, D. X., Antolin, I., Rodriguez, C., & Reiter, R. J. (2005). Melatonin and Parkinson's disease. *Endocrine, 27*(2), 169–178.

Mell, L. K., Davis, R. L., & Owens, D. (2005). Association between streptococcal infection and obsessive–compulsive disorder, Tourette's syndrome, and tic disorder. *Pediatrics, 116*(1), 56–60.

Moneyham, L., Murdaugh, C., Phillips, K., Jackson, K., Tavakoli, A., Boyd, M., et al. (2005). Patterns of risk of depressive symptoms among HIV-positive women in the southeastern United States. *Journal of the Association of Nurses in AIDS Care, 16*(4), 25–38.

North American Nursing Diagnosis Association. (2007). *Nursing diagnoses: Definition and classification, 2007–2008.* Philadelphia. Author.

Pahwa, R., Factor, S. A., Lyons, K. E., Ondo, W. G., Gronseth, G., Bronte-Stewart, H., et al. (2006). Practice parameter: Treatment of Parkinson disease with motor fluctuations and dyskinesia. *Neurology, 66*(7), 983–995.

Patterson, J. C., & Kotrla, K. J. (2004). Functional neuroimaging in psychiatry. Neuropsychiatric aspects of Alzheimer's disease and other dementing illnesses. In S. C. Yudofsky & R. E. Hales (Eds.), *Essentials of neuropsychiatry and clinical neurosciences* (pp. 109–138). Washington, DC: American Psychiatric Publishing.

Pavone, P., Parano, E., Rizzo, R., & Trifiletti, R. R. (2006). Autoimmune neuropsychiatric disorders associated with streptococcal infection. *Journal of Child Neurology, 21*(9), 727–736.

Pena, J. A., Montiel-Nava, C., Ravelo, M. E., Gonzalez, S., & Mora, L. C. E. (2006). Multiple sclerosis in children. *Investigacion Clinica, 47*(4), 413–425.

Shults, C. W. (2005). Therapeutic role of coenzyme Q(10) in Parkinson's disease. *Pharmacology & Therapeutics, 107*(1), 120–130.

Sullivan, F. R. (2005). Use of remotivation therapy with persons who have Huntington's disease. In J. A. Dyer & M. L. Stotts (Eds.), *Handbook of remotivation therapy* (pp. 89–101). New York: Haworth Clinical Practice Press.

Teicher, M. H., Andersen, S. L., Navalta, C. P., Polcari, A., & Kim, D. (2004). Neuropsychiatric disorders of childhood and adolescence. In S. C. Yudofsky & R. E. Hales (Eds.), *Essentials of neuropsychiatry and clinical neurosciences* (pp. 535–606). Washington, DC: American Psychiatric Publishing.

Tost, H., Wendt, C. S., Schmitt, A., Heinz, A., & Braus, D. F. (2004). Huntington's disease. *American Journal of Psychiatry, 161*(1), 28–34.

Tucker, G. J. (2004). Neuropsychiatric aspects of seizure disorders. In S. C. Yudofsky & R. E. Hales (Eds.), *Essentials of neuropsychiatry and clinical neurosciences* (pp. 293–313). Washington, DC: American Psychiatric Publishing.

Wongvatunyu, S., & Porter, E. J. (2005). Mothers' experience of helping young adults with traumatic brain injury. *Journal of Nursing Scholarship, 37*(1), 48–56.

Unit 5

Violence

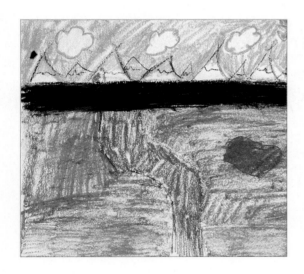

> *As I walk through obstacles, my problems lie behind.*
>
> *I am hoping to cross the mountains to see what future I can find.*
>
> *I must pass through the fog because my life is unclear.*
>
> *So I can pass through the dangers I always have feared.*

—Kenny, Age 12

Chapter 21

Suicide

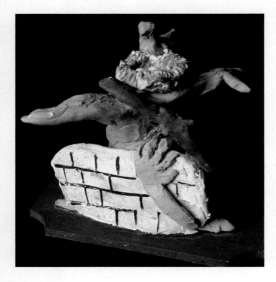

66 *A lifetime of fear and hiding behind a wall that no one could get through. The wall kept me alive. It blocked everything so I could survive. Now people want the wall to come down. Without the wall my only choice is the gun. The tree of life with 3 eggs in the nest: My children. How do I fit them into a life where my only choices are the wall or the gun?* 99

—Kay, Age 40

OBJECTIVES

After reading this chapter, you will be able to:

1. Identify risk factors and reasons for suicide.
2. Discuss the theories regarding the causes of suicide.
3. Outline the assessment process for a suicidal client.
4. Use the nursing process to develop a safe, comprehensive plan of care for a suicidal client and her/his family.
5. Discuss the key points in effectively communicating with a suicidal client.
6. Develop teaching plans for a suicidal client and her/his family.

MediaLink www.prenhall.com/fontaine

Go to the Pearson Health MediaLink CD-ROM and the Companion Website at www.prenhall.com/fontaine for interactive resources for this chapter.

The ROAD to Critical Thinking   A Client Contemplating Suicide

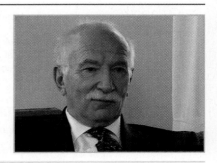

Travel this ROAD to understand Everett and his condition.

Read about Everett below and throughout this chapter.

Observe Everett on the CD-ROM accompanying this book.

Assess Everett by answering the questions at the end of this chapter.

Develop a Care Plan on the CD-ROM to address Everett's condition.

Everett

Everett is 71 years old and lives with his wife. He has three grown sons and six grandchildren. He states that he has been depressed since the age of 2 years. He remembers having suicidal thoughts when he was in the third grade. In spite of his continuing depression, he achieved a high level of education and had a career as a school principal. When the level of depression became more severe, he re-signed. He has been hospitalized several times for intensive treatment. You will meet Everett on the video clip on your disc and throughout this chapter. At the end of the chapter, you will find critical thinking questions relating to assessment and development of a plan of care for Everett.

Suicide is a worldwide, national, local, and familial problem. Although the definitions of suicidal behavior and suicide overlap, there are slight differences. **Suicidal behavior** can be defined in two ways:

1. The behavior and thoughts leading up to the act of suicide
2. The act of taking one's own life

The word **suicide** is defined in the following three ways:

1. The act of taking one's own life
2. A person who takes her or his own life
3. The result—survival or death—described as either attempted or completed

Worldwide, almost 2 million suicides occur every year. It is the third leading cause of death in young people in the United States and the leading cause of death in young adults in China, Sweden, Australia, and New Zealand, among other countries. Every 15 minutes, another American commits suicide, totaling 30,600 people a year. The reported numbers in the United States are low because many suicides are reported as accidental deaths. The actual rate may be three to five times higher. Even with underreporting, suicide is the eighth leading cause of death in the general population. The effect of these statistics becomes even greater when we recognize that for every suicide, 8 to 25 are unsuccessful attempts. There are more than four male suicides for every female suicide. However, at least twice as many females as males attempt suicide (Simon, 2004; Swann et al., 2005). Such data can also be viewed on the Centers for Disease Con-trol and Prevention (CDC) resource link provided on the Companion Web site for this book.

More than 90% of suicide victims have a psychiatric disorder at the time of death. Most psychiatric clients, however, do not commit suicide. People who are severely and persistently mentally ill often commit suicide because of years of pain, frustration, and low self-esteem, which contribute to demoralization and depression. Spiritually, they may perceive themselves as hopelessly damaged and lose all sense of purpose and meaning in life.

Nurses have higher rates of suicide than the general population and suicide is one of the top five causes of death among nurses. The most common method chosen by nurses is drug overdose, and nurses have easier access to drugs than most people in the general population. Knowing how drugs work and how much to take may increase the lethality of the suicidal behavior. The daily stress of caring for people suffering from violence and trauma, serious illness, and impending death may be a risk factor for suicide in nurses. Male physicians have a suicide rate of 1.5 to 3 times higher than other men and female physicians are 3 to 5 times more likely to kill themselves than are other women (Joiner, 2005; Pompili et al., 2006).

KNOWLEDGE BASE

There are various *philosophies* about suicide, from believing it is wrong to believing it has value. See Box 21.1 for details of these philosophies.

BOX 21.1 | Philosophies About Suicide

Suicide Is Wrong

- Suicide does violence to the dignity of human life.
- Suicide is an irrevocable act that denies future learning or growth.
- It is only for God to give and to take away human life.
- Suicide does violence to the natural order of things.
- Suicide adversely affects the survivors.

Suicide Is Sometimes Permissible

- Suicide is permissible when the person's life is unbearable.

Suicide Is Not a Moral or Ethical Issue

- Suicide is a fact of life that can be studied like other life events.
- Suicide is a morally neutral act in that every person has a free will and the right to act according to that will.

Suicide Is a Positive Response to Certain Conditions

- When life ceases to be enjoyable, people have the right to end their lives.
- There are certain times in life when death is less an evil than dishonor.
- Some suicides are demanded by society as a way of dispensing justice.

Suicide has Intrinsic Positive Value

- Suicide has a positive value when it is the way people can enter the meaningful afterlife they desire.
- Suicide has a positive value because it is a way in which people can be immediately reunited with valued ancestors and loved ones.

Reasons

People attempt and commit suicide for hundreds of reasons. The following are a few:

- Some are driven by delusions or command hallucinations.

- Because of depressed feelings related to a chronic or terminal illness, some see no hope for the future.

- For some, suicide is a relief from intolerable and inescapable physical or emotional pain.

- Some individuals have experienced so many losses that life is no longer valuable.

- Some have been beset with multiple crises, which have drained their internal and external resources.

- For some, suicide is the ultimate expression of anger toward significant others.

An attempt at suicide can be precipitated by many factors. It has various meanings to the potential victims and to the survivors. Despite this variety, potential suicide victims have a number of characteristics in common that can alert the nurse to the danger of suicide. *Previous suicide attempts* and a sense of *hopelessness* or *desperation* are the most powerful clinical predictors of suicide.

Assisted Suicide

Assisted suicide (euthanasia) by a physician has received increased attention over the past decade. Among the public, support for the "right to die" has grown steadily: 60% of the population supports euthanasia for people with terminal illness. At issue is whether a dying individual should have the right to request and receive euthanasia from physicians. Legal safeguards include multiple requests from the person over a 2-week period, witnessed and documented discussion of treatment options and hospice care, confirmation of the terminal condition by another physician, and psychiatric assessment that the person is not impaired by mental illness (Schwarz, 2003).

Those who are against the issue believe that the greater good for the society demands keeping the prohibitions in place. It is seen as a form of medical killing in violation of social, ethical, and medical traditions, which would turn physicians from healers into killers. There is concern that it will be applied in an involuntary way against elderly, poor, handicapped, or otherwise disadvantaged people. A further concern is that some individuals will be pressured to end their lives as an economic sacrifice for their families. The American Nurses Association opposes nurse participation in assisted suicide, believing that such actions are a breach of the Code for Nurses and the ethical traditions of the nursing profession. In contrast, the Oregon Nurses Association supports a person's right to self-determination and believes that nurses have a primary role in end-of-life decisions (Schwarz, 2003).

Little research has been done regarding nurses' responses to dying people who request assisted suicide, or euthanasia. In one study, 30% of terminally ill clients asked the oncology nurse for large amounts of drugs (for intentional self-overdose) and 25% asked for injections to end their lives (euthanasia). Nurses in this study indicated that they had a need to discuss these end-of-life situations, but in reality had few, if any, discussions with their peers and supervisors. It is important that further research be conducted on nurses' responses to such requests (Ersek, 2004; Fontana, 2002; Matzo & Schwarz, 2001).

In 2001, the Netherlands became the first country to legalize euthanasia, after 30 years of debate. Euthanasia has been tolerated for years, but most Dutch citizens wanted a legal framework to protect participating physicians. In 1994, Oregon passed the Death with Dignity Act, which made it legal for physicians to provide a prescription for lethal drugs for terminally ill clients who request them. In 1997, the United States Supreme Court recognized state decisions in the matter of physician-assisted suicide. This meant that battles must be fought in each state. These are not just legal debates, but also moral, medical, social, political, and religious debates. In 2002, Oregon was involved in new litigation with the federal government. The attorney general authorized federal drug-enforcement agents to identify and punish physicians who prescribe federally controlled drugs to help terminally ill clients die. A U.S. District Court overturned this directive, but the debate goes on (Ersek, 2004).

Those who support assisted suicide believe that a change in the law is necessary based on reasons of compassion and freedom of choice in the face of intolerable suffering. The desire to have medical help to end one's life is seen as an extension of the right to refuse to be sustained on life support systems or to request not to be resuscitated. Many people with life-threatening illnesses are already taking matters into their own hands and ending their lives, with or without help and regardless of laws. Most people have no one with whom they can discuss these issues and no place to turn for advice. Proponents believe that everyone has the right to open dialogue, counseling, and the involvement of family, partners, and friends regarding the wish to die when continued living is intolerable.

Comorbid Disorders

Although most people with mental disorders do not attempt suicide, more than 90% of people who do commit suicide have a diagnosable mental illness at the time of death. Among people with schizophrenia, 20% to 40% attempt suicide and 10% to 13% commit suicide; suicide is the leading cause of death in young people with schizophrenia.

For those with mood disorders, the suicide rate is 20%; for those with personality disorder, the rate is 5% to 10%; and 7% of people with alcohol dependence die by suicide. People with more than one of these disorders may be at very high risk for attempting or completing suicide (Fortune & Hawton, 2005; Simon, 2004).

Remember, people are at risk for suicide throughout the course of treatment for their mental disorder. In some cases, the risk increases as individuals improve. This transient greater risk may be because the person has the energy and the capacity to act on self-destructive plans made earlier in the course of their illness.

People with chronic medical diseases are more likely to commit suicide than those with acute illnesses or without illness. At greatest risk are people with progressive diseases such as cardiovascular disease, chronic obstructive pulmonary disease, seizure disorder, and moderate to severe pain. Moreover, people who take a large number of medications may, as a direct result of the chemical effects on the body, experience a depressive episode that leads to suicide. Substance abuse is a contributing factor for some suicidal people, particularly older men who live alone and have few or no support systems. The use of chemicals may be an attempt to self-medicate to control the symptoms of depression, or it may be a way to overcome inhibitions about the actual act of suicide (Moscicki & Caine, 2004). See Box 21.2 for a list of factors contributing to suicidal behavior.

BOX 21.2	Factors Contributing to High Suicidal Risk

- Euro-American
- Elderly people, especially men, followed by adolescents and college students
- People who are isolated without support systems
- Individuals who are recently unemployed
- Recent loss of a significant relationship
- Separated, divorced, or widowed people
- Social isolation, including rural location
- Presence of a substance use disorder
- Presence of a mental disorder
- Feelings of failure and hopelessness
- Presence of a gun in the home
- Previous suicide attempts
- Positive family history of completed suicide

Everett:

❝ Earlier in my life, my wife said I just wasn't functioning. I have to say that I was medicating myself. I had an MD friend who gave me sample medications. And if he said, take two or three a day, I thought if you took six or nine or twelve a day you would get better faster. And so I misused those. I also drank from morning 'til evening. Not drunk, but I think it was a protection from the depression. It was alcoholic drinking. ❞

Causes of Suicide

Suicide is a complex act, and a variety of factors contribute to the behavior. The degree of influence of each factor varies from individual to individual. When risk factors are combined, the likelihood of suicidal behavior is greater, either because internal restraints decrease or excess stress increases suicidal impulses.

Genetics

Adoption studies in the United States and Denmark indicate that there may be a genetic factor in suicidal behavior. Individuals who were adopted at birth and later committed suicide had significantly more biological relatives who had committed suicide than the control group. It is believed that this genetic factor may be an inability to control impulsive behavior, and that either environmental stress or a mental illness may drive the impulsive behavior toward suicide (Mann, Bortinger, Oquendo, Currier, Li, & Brent, 2005).

Neurobiology

Recent research indicates that the primary neurobiological factor in suicide is a disturbance related to serotonin (5-HT) dysfunction. 5-HT is the constraining and anti-impulsive neurotransmitter. Sufficient 5-HT may be related to people's tolerance for adversity, the ability to resist impulsive urges,

MediaLink · Case Study, The Suicidal Client

and the means to find solutions to problems. In people who attempt or commit suicide there is a significant *decrease* in 5-HT, irrespective of the primary psychiatric diagnosis. As levels of 5-HT decrease, people become more impulsive, more aggressive, and lose control more quickly. Interestingly, 5-HT levels increase during pregnancy, and pregnant women are at very low risk for suicide. The fetus produces much of the excess 5-HT, which may be self-protective, by inhibiting self-destructive behaviors by the mother (Joiner, 2005).

Suicide risk is also related to past traumatic brain injury. Aggressive, impulsive children and adults are more likely to sustain a head injury, and head injuries can cause impulsive and aggressive behavior. The final decision to commit suicide may be an impulsive act that is the result of powerful biological processes.

Interpersonal Factors

Suicide may result when people experience social isolation and become alienated from society, family, and friends. Another factor is rapid social change resulting in the loss of previous patterns of social integration. People who have difficulty adapting to the demand of new roles are more likely to view suicide as a solution to their problems.

Loss is closely related to suicide. Certainly, the impact of any loss depends on the significance the person attributes to that loss. Whenever the most important and significant aspects of a person's life are threatened or destroyed, suicide is likely to be considered. Women's motives tend to be interpersonal, that is, related to painful or lost relationships. Men's motives tend to be intrapersonal, that is, related to financial problems or the loss of a job.

Behavioral Theory

Behavioral theorists believe that suicide is often a learned problem-solving behavior. They consider the reinforcements prior to and following attempted suicide. The internal reinforcement is that the behavior itself serves to decrease anxiety. Following the suicidal behavior, the external reinforcement is that the person is removed from the stressful environment and freed from daily pressures. Significant others who were critical may now become supportive. These types of reinforcement are essential in the repetition of suicidal behavior.

Nursing Process

A CLIENT CONTEMPLATING SUICIDE

ASSESSMENT

The nurse may be apprehensive about assessing people who are at risk of attempting or committing suicide. The nurse's reasons may include fear of giving the person the idea of suicide, fear of being incorrect, fear of the person's reaction, and reluctance to discuss a taboo subject. It is important to recognize that *the nurse cannot give the idea of suicide to anyone.* By late childhood or early adolescence, every person knows that suicide is an option for solving problems. Most youngsters, without being actively suicidal, have thoughts of suicide in times of stress. An example is a child who is angry with his or her parents and thinks, "If I went out and got run over by a car, they'd be sorry they were so mean to me!" Many adults have considered which method they would choose if they were to commit suicide. Thus, even though the topic is taboo under most social conditions, most people have thought about and formed an opinion about suicide.

When assessing people for suicidal potential, use specific words such as "kill yourself" or "commit suicide." Using a more vague term, such as "want to hurt yourself," may cause some suicidal people to respond negatively. They may not want to cause themselves pain, but they do want to kill themselves. People need to know what you are talking about, and you cannot risk

misunderstandings. You might introduce the topic of suicide by saying something like, "Often, when people are feeling very upset or depressed, they have thoughts of killing themselves. Have you had any thoughts of wanting to kill yourself?"

It is also important to assess for protective factors (see Box 21.3) against suicidal acts. Protective factors include a social support system, problem-solving and coping history, a sense of responsibility to children, pregnancy, hopefulness, fear of suicide, fear of social disapproval, and moral objections to suicide. The more protective factors an individual has, the less likely it is that they will act on suicidal thoughts at vulnerable times.

You may find yourself struggling with ambivalence about suicide. The conflict centers on the issue of a person's right to choose his or her time to die and method of dying. Many people have thought about the conditions under which they would choose not to live, such as with a chronic or terminal illness. Having considered suicide, you may question whether

BOX 21.3	Protective Factors

- Intact, positive support systems
- Active religious affiliation or faith
- Presence of dependent young children
- Ongoing supportive relationship with a caregiver
- Absence of a mental disorder or substance abuse
- Living close to medical and mental health resources
- Problem-solving and coping skills

she or he has the right to prevent another person's suicide, or you may not experience this conflict at all because you believe that all suicide should be prevented.

Assessment: Behavior

Suicide is not a random act. It is a way out of a problem, dilemma, or unbearable situation. Suicide is an attempt to escape from unbearable suffering. People contemplating suicide often make subtle or even overt comments that indicate as much. They may mention all the pressure and stress they are experiencing and how helpless they feel. Some may discuss beliefs concerning life after death. Verbal cues are such statements as:

- "It won't matter much longer."
- "Will you miss me when I'm gone?"
- "I can't take this much longer."
- "The pain will be over soon."
- "I won't be here when you come back on Monday."
- "You won't have to worry about the money problems much longer."
- "The voices are telling me to hurt myself."

Certain behaviors may indicate suicidal intentions. Obtaining a weapon such as a gun, a strong rope, or a collection of pills is a strong indicator of impending suicide. Often, people contemplating suicide begin to withdraw from relationships and become more isolated. There may be a change in school or work performance. An increased tendency toward accidents might indicate initial suicidal behavior. Some may show a sudden interest in his or her life insurance policy, whereas others may make or change his or her will and give personal belongings away. Signs of substance abuse may also be present.

Everett:

❝ When I was in the third grade, I wrote a suicide note. My suicide was going to be going into the woods and not coming out. And I left my worldly possessions to my brother and other things to other people that I thought they should have. Well, my father found the note before I took off and said, 'What's the meaning of this?' and I said, 'That's what I want to do.' And he destroyed the note and said, 'This is foolishness. Stop this foolishness and get on with whatever you were doing.' ❞

Behavioral characteristics also include choosing a method for suicide. **Lethality** is measured by four factors:

1. The degree of effort it takes to plan the suicide
2. The specificity of the plan
3. The accessibility of the weapon or method
4. The ease by which one may or may not be rescued

Everett:

❝ After I got out of the hospital, I had a very serious attempt of suicide. I ingested cyanide. We were using it in the flower shop where I worked. I just took some. I felt that there was no hope for the future—why continue, it was time to end it. I was unconscious for a period of time and very, very surprised that I was still part of the world when I came out of the unconsciousness. And also feeling more despair because now I couldn't even make good on a suicide attempt. ❞

More people kill themselves with guns than by all other methods combined, and death by firearms is the fastest growing method of suicide. More than half the teenagers who commit suicide shoot themselves with a gun kept at home. An important social issue is the alarming increase in the number of guns purchased in the United States. Individual Americans now own 200,000,000 (two hundred million) guns, which is more than double the number held in 1969. Those who are most vulnerable to impulsive suicide are clearly the most affected by availability of guns. The dramatic increase in suicide in children and adolescents is almost solely due to easy availability of guns (Simon, 2004).

Studies show that people who live in a home in which there is a gun are five times more likely to experience a suicide than people who do not have a gun in the home. Most gun owners state that they keep a gun in their home for "protection" or "self-defense." Only 2% of gun-related deaths in the home are the result of a homeowner shooting an intruder. In contrast, 3% of gun-related deaths are accidental child shootings, 12% are the result of adult partners shooting one another, and 83% are the result of a suicide, often by a young person (Simon, 2004).

The next most commonly used methods for committing suicide are cutting/stabbing; hanging; and poisoning by liquids, solids, and gases such as carbon monoxide. The suicide methods most often chosen by younger children are hanging and jumping from a window or in front of a car.

Assessment: Affect

Remember, people who are suicidal are afraid. They fear that no one cares. They may not introduce the topic because they fear being judged or considered weak or "crazy." When nurses are confronted with their own fears about discussing suicide, they should remember that no nursing intervention will be effective unless the suicide threat is assessed. If the person is not suicidal, asking the questions will do no damage. But if the person is suicidal and the topic is not discussed, the person has been abandoned while in a dangerously vulnerable position. Remember, the answers you get depend on the questions you ask.

All the affective characteristics indicative of depression may be associated with people who are suicidal. These include feelings of desolation, guilt, failure, shame, and loss of emotional attachments. A pervading sense of hopelessness has the highest association with suicide. Life is seen as intolerable, with no hope for change or improvement. Some people, when faced with intolerable humiliation, such as scandals or criminal charges, commit what is called a "shame" suicide. In these situations, death is preferable to humiliation.

Trevor, age 13, was admitted to the acute care unit after telling his school counselor that he wished he were dead. Trevor states that he has been depressed since his father was hit by a car and killed a year ago. He says that his mother is working a lot and he hardly gets to see her. His best friend moved away 6 weeks ago and his dog recently died. He states that he has been thinking about suicide for a few weeks. He feels like a failure and has no hope that the future will be any better.

People have a high degree of ambivalence before making the final decision to commit suicide. An internal conflict exists between the wish to die and the wish to live. If the part that wants to live can be adequately supported during this struggle, the balance may shift in favor of life. Once the decision has been made to commit suicide, conflict and anxiety cease, and the person may appear calm and untroubled. Others may interpret this change in the affective state as an improvement. What appears to be a change for the better in fact may be an indication of the decision to die.

Assessment: Cognition

Suicidal behavior has a variety of cognitive components. Suicidal people tend to think dichotomously, that is, all-or-none reasoning such as good or bad, right or wrong. This rigid cognitive style makes it difficult for people who are suicidal to problem solve. Recurring thoughts of self-blame, negative self-evaluation, and dire expectations of the future contribute to a hopeless outlook. When people choose to die, they are so distorted by pain—physical, mental, or emotional—that the world is reduced to a solitary alternative. There seems to be only one answer: to die.

Another cognitive component involves fantasies. Unable to see the finality of death, suicidal people sometimes have fantasies about continuing on after death. They may talk about being able to see how people will react to their death or how their children will grow up. Others have expectations about meeting up with departed loved ones after death. Many people eagerly look forward to this reunion with family and friends.

A smaller percentage hopes or believes a suicide attempt will force a solution to interpersonal problems. For some, it is a cry for help. In either case, the suicidal behavior is a form of manipulation. They are so desperate that they can see no other method to resolve problems or get the necessary help.

People with sensory or thought disorders may be potentially suicidal. Command hallucinations are common and may often direct the person to commit suicide. At first, the person may be frightened by the voices, but later the person may be compliant and carry out the command. People with delusions of control or persecution may also be at risk for suicide. If these delusions cannot be managed with treatment, they may believe the only way to escape those who are controlling or persecuting them is to die. It is the ultimate method of getting relief from their extremely painful thoughts.

Ryan has heard voices for a long time. The voices tell him to die and he will go to heaven. He also sees angels telling him to go to heaven. He has made a couple of suicide attempts. He comes into the clinic saying, "I am thinking evil thoughts. If this pain in my ear gets worse, I will kill myself." The only thing standing in the way of suicide is his fear that he might go to hell.

For those rescued from their suicidal behavior, there is often a change of mind. Either they return to the ambivalent state of thought or they decide they do want to live. Throughout their lives, however, they remain at higher risk for suicide than the general population. It seems that once the decision to die was made in the past, that decision might be easier to make again.

Assessment: Interpersonal Relationships

People who attempt or commit suicide are often in periods of high stress in their lives. Stressors include under- or unemployment, family disruption, rejection by a significant other, abrupt changes in career responsibilities, and recent catastrophic events. They often have a limited social network, and when their attempts to get support fail, their level of distress increases. When people either have not developed their own coping skills or have exhausted their ability to cope, suicide may be a last, desperate attempt to cope with stress and resolve problems. Parents who have lost a child to a violent death may be so devastated that suicide seems like the only option. This group must be carefully assessed for suicide potential (Murphy, Tapper, Johnson, & Lohan, 2003).

Social pressures and a lack of resources often result in depression in adolescents who are gay, lesbian, bisexual, or transgendered (GLBT). They are vulnerable to all the stressors of adolescence and the many stressors related to a stigmatized sexual orientation. GLBT youth feel ostracized from the dominant culture because of an absence of role models and distorted media presentations. They may suffer intimidation, ranging from ridicule to threats and physical violence from beatings to rape. For reasons of acceptance and personal safety, GLBT youth hide from their families and the community in which they live. Given this type of social climate, it is no surprise that lesbian and gay youths are six times more likely to commit suicide than heterosexual youths (Huygen, 2006).

When teenage suicides are publicized by the news media or when there are television dramas about suicide, the rate of adolescent suicide increases several weeks after the event. Suicides that are inspired by suicides in this way are called **copycat suicides**. Copycat suicide seems to be an adolescent phenomenon and girls are more susceptible than boys. The potential copycat appears to be a troubled adolescent who empathizes with the pain of the suicidal person and is easily influenced by the media.

Some people who are suspicious by nature, or who are prone to violence as a method of coping with feelings, may combine homicide–suicide. The perpetrator, usually a male, commits one or more homicides and shortly thereafter commits a violent suicide. Homicide–suicide often occurs within a family. Most cases are adults who are spouses or partners; however, children may also be victims.

On May 27, 2006, Dr. Edward Van Dyk threw his two sons, ages 4 and 8, off a 15th floor hotel room balcony and then jumped to his death. The family was in Florida celebrating their 10th wedding anniversary. Mrs. Van Dyk told police that they had some marital problems but nothing that would indicate such a drastic action (George & Haas, 2006).

Whatever way the act of suicide is committed, it has a traumatic effect on the family and friends of the victim. In addition to grief, these people must cope with the stigma and cultural taboos associated with suicide. Family and friends are frequently unaware of the danger signs and respond to the suddenness of the death with shock and bewilderment. Some people respond with anger toward the victim and the event. Others feel betrayed and abandoned. Because society assumes that all survivors must feel guilty and responsible for the suicidal behavior, those who do not experience guilt may wonder why and may feel guilty about not feeling guilty. Some survivors experience a sense of relief when a suicide ends the physical or mental suffering of a loved one. Other survivors blame themselves with such thoughts as, "If only I had done (had not done), this would not have happened." Shame and guilt cast family members in the role of murderers, when in truth they, too, are victims. The death of a child, in particular, puts extreme strain on the parents. Because they were unable to protect their child, they may be overwhelmed with feelings of guilt and powerlessness (Simon, 2004).

Many survivors are plagued with real or imagined images of the death scene. Families must also cope with other people seeking details about the death, with others' inability to acknowledge the death, or others even blaming them for the death. Some people develop obsessions about their own suicide. Family survivors enter a higher risk category for suicide; about 20% of them will exhibit suicidal behavior themselves. Having a loved one die is traumatic at any time; having a loved one die as a result of suicide can be overwhelming.

Assessment: Cultural Influences

Suicide continues to be an urgent problem in all countries of the world, especially among the youth, where suicide may be the second or third leading cause of death. Acts of suicide relate to a range of social, political, and psychological factors. Philosophies about suicide are deeply rooted in cultural traditions. Because it is highly stigmatized and illegal in many places, suicide is thought to be grossly underreported.

Unlike the rate in almost every other country in the world, the rate of suicide in China is higher in women than in men. Rates are also higher in rural areas than in urban centers. Rapid changes in society and the economy are related to the increasing rate of suicide. Suicides in Japan are linked to job loss, corporate bankruptcy, and mounting debt. Group suicide pacts have become an increasing problem in Japan. In India, thousands of students are believed to commit suicide over exams each year. High school exams are crucial because exams determine who qualifies for the university (Beautrais, 2003; Phillips, Yang, Li, & Li, 2004).

Euro-Americans have the highest rates of suicide in the United States. The peak age for females is around age 50. For males, the suicide rate continues to increase throughout life; those older than 65 have the highest suicide rate of all groups. Rural men in all age groups have about twice the suicide rate of those men who live in urban areas. Some factors are greater access to firearms and physical and social isolation (Singh & Siahpush, 2002).

Native Americans are not a culturally homogeneous population. There are wide variations in the suicide rates of different Native tribes. For example, the Chippewa have the lowest rate, with 6 suicides of 100,000 people, and the Black Feet have the highest rate, at 130 of 100,000. The suicide rate for Alaskan natives is twice that of the general population of the United States. Suicide rates in the Canadian Indian population are more than three times the rate of the same age group of non-Indian Canadians. Tribes that have maintained traditions have the lowest rates. High rates of suicide are related to multiple factors, such as the breakdown of traditional values, enforced residence on reservations, geographic isolation, isolation of children from their families of origin, inadequate housing, high unemployment, extreme poverty, and a high incidence of alcoholism (Pumariega, Rogers, & Rothe, 2005).

Hispanic Americans are at highest risk for suicide during young adulthood. It is probably the stress of acculturation because the suicide rates are higher in the United States than in their countries of origin. Stressors include language barriers, discrimination, poverty, and educational disadvantages (Pumariega et al., 2005).

Asian Americans are one of the fastest growing ethnic groups in the United States. Having never been treated with the same courtesy given to immigrants from Europe, they have a long history of discrimination. Typically, the suicide rate increases with age among Asian Americans.

More African Americans attempt and complete suicide than previously thought. The misconception has been that suicide is rare because of cultural and religious beliefs that date to slavery times. A recently completed landmark study documents that rates are similar to those of Euro-Americans. Caribbean-American blacks have a higher rate of suicide than African Americans. This may be related to more recent immigration resulting in higher frustration with discrimination (Joe, Baser, Breeden, Neighbors, & Jackson, 2006).

In general, individuals with strong religious beliefs have a lower rate of suicide. Similarly, cultures with strong religious faith have low suicide rates. Islamic tradition regards suicide as morally wrong and in some Islamic countries, suicide is against the law (Dervic et al., 2004).

Judaism has a general prohibition against taking one's own life, based on two religious reasons. The first is that people belong to God and therefore have no right to destroy that which is not theirs. The second reason is that people are created in God's image, and suicide is the destruction of the divine image. In Christianity, the commandment against murder has been interpreted to apply to taking one's life. Suicide offends God, who offers life as a gift, and suicide offends the human community (American Psychiatric Association Practice Guidelines, 2003).

Assessment: Age-Specific Characteristics

In the United States and Canada, suicide rates vary dramatically by age groups. Although suicide occurs at all stages throughout life, people continue to be surprised when they learn about suicide in a child younger than 12. The fact is, children as young as age 3 to 5 have been known to commit suicide. Suicide is the fourth leading cause of death for children 10 to 14 years old (an increase of 100% since 1950) and the third leading cause of death for young people 15 to 24 years old (tripled since 1950). The risk for suicide among young people is greatest among Euro-American males. The suicide rate for African Americans 10 to 14 years old has increased the most (233%), while the rate for African American 15 to 19 years old increased 126%. In addition, 20% of students in grades 9 through 12 have seriously thought about attempting suicide, 16% have made a specific suicide plan, and 8% actually attempt suicide in any given recent year (Norton, 2005).

In addition to these general causes of suicide, there are causes that are more specific for various age groups. Some of the reasons children commit suicide are to escape from physical or sexual abuse, a chaotic family situation, feeling unloved or constantly criticized, anticipation of disciplinary action, humiliation in school, and the loss of significant others.

TABLE 21.1	Suicide and Homicide as Leading Causes of Death According to Age, Sex, and Ethnicity							
Group	1-4	5-9	10-14	15-24	25-34	35-44	45-54	55 and Over
All males	H-4th	H-4th	S-3rd H-4th	H-2nd S-3rd	S-2nd H-3rd	S-5th H-6th	S-5th	S-8th
All females	H-4th	H-4th	H-4th S-5th	H-2nd S-4th	H-4th S-6th	S-4th	S-8th	
African American Males	H-2nd	H-3rd	H-2nd S-4th	H-1st S-3rd	H-1st S-5th	H-5th S-7th	H-8th	
African American Females	H-2nd	H-3rd	H-2nd S-7th	H-2nd S-6th	H-4th S-9th	H-6th		
Euro-American Males	H-4th	H-4th	S-3rd H-4th	S-2nd H-3rd	S-2nd H-3rd	S-4th H-7th	S-4th	S-8th
Euro-American Females	H-4th	H-4th	S-4th H-6th	S-2nd H-4th	S-3rd H-5th	S-4th	S-6th	S-10th
Native People Both Sexes	H-4th	H-2nd S-9th	S-2nd S-3rd	S-2nd H-3rd	S-5th H-3rd	H-7th H-6th	S-10th	
Asian American Both Sexes	H-4th	H-4th	H-3rd S-5th	S-2nd H-3rd	S-3rd H-4th	S-4th H-6th	S-5th H-7th	S-9th

H = homicide
S = suicide
If no rank of death listed, it was not among the top 10 leading causes of death.

SOURCE: CDC, 2000.

Adolescents may commit suicide for the same reasons children do. Additional age-specific causes include the absence of meaningful relationships, difficulties in maintaining relationships, sexual problems, and acute problems with parents. Additional suicidal factors for college students include competition for success, anxiety over academic work, and academic failure signifying a loss of parental love or esteem.

People who are 65 and older have the highest suicide rate of all age groups. They comprise only 13% of the population, but they account for 25% of all suicides. In the United States, someone 65 years or older commits suicide every 95 minutes, most frequently with firearms. Suicide rates for men are relatively constant from ages 25 to 64, but increase significantly after age 65, and men account for 83% of suicides among persons 65 years of age and older (Bruce et al., 2004).

Suicide among older adults may be related to a change in status from autonomy to dependency, accompanied by decreased participation in social activities. Many changes experienced by older adults may contribute to a higher incidence of suicide. Those who experience illness that results in a lower level of functioning may become suicidal. Other factors include loneliness and social isolation, loss of partner and friends, loss of work deemed important by the culture, and outliving resources.

Table 21.1 ■ describes suicide and homicide as leading causes of death according to age, gender, and ethnicity.

Nurses and the families of clients should not expect that an accurate assessment will prevent all suicides. This expectation would contribute to unrealistic guilt when a person does commit suicide. Not all victims exhibit cues before their deaths; many people cannot be correctly identified before they kill themselves. This is not intended to minimize the importance of a suicide assessment; it is to establish realistic professional expectations. If a person is intent on suicide, it is difficult to intervene effectively. However, if a person is ambivalent, intervention may save that person's life. Therefore, it is always vital to perform a suicide assessment for those at risk.

See the Focused Nursing Assessment feature for specific questions to ask when assessing a person's potential for suicide. Box 21.4 describes the levels of suicide severity.

Focused Nursing Assessment   Clients With Suicidal Potential

Behavior Assessment	Affective Assessment	Cognitive Assessment	Social Assessment
Are you thinking about suicide?	How would you describe your overall mood?	What will your suicide accomplish for you?	What kinds of losses have you sustained during the past year? Relationships? Separations? Divorce? Deaths? Jobs? Roles? Self-esteem?
By what method would you commit suicide?	What kinds of things make you feel guilty?	What will your suicide accomplish for others?	
Do you have the means on hand?	In what areas of life do you feel like a failure?	What would have to change for you to decide to live?	
Have you done a practice session of the suicide?	What does the future look like to you?	What are your thoughts about death?	What kinds of stress have you been under during the past six months?
When do you plan to commit suicide?	To what degree do you feel hopeless or out of control of your life?	Is there a way for you to continue on in life after death?	Which people are able to provide support for you?
Have you tried to kill yourself before?	To what degree do you feel hopeful about the future?	Do you hope to meet dead loved ones after you die?	Have any of your friends or family members committed suicide? What is the anniversary date? What thoughts and feelings do you have about this suicide?
How have things been going at school/work for you?	What part of you wishes to die?	How well do you think you solve problems?	
Are you still interested in visiting with friends?	What part of you wishes to live?	Do you hear voices that others say they do not hear?	
Who depends on you to take care of them?	What will other people think of you if you commit suicide?	What do the voices say to you?	Who will benefit from your suicide? How?
How much have you been drinking lately?		Is suicide a way for you to escape control or persecution by others?	
How often do you use street drugs?			
Have you made or changed your will recently? Have you checked your life insurance policy?			
What kinds of personal belongings have you given away?			
Have you planned your funeral?			

BOX 21.4	Levels of Severity of Suicide

Nonexistent

■ No identifiable suicidal ideation

Mild

■ Suicidal ideation of limited frequency, intensity, and duration
■ No plan for suicide
■ Mild dysphoria
■ Good self-control
■ Few risk factors
■ Identifiable protective factors

Moderate

■ Frequent suicidal ideation with limited intensity and duration
■ Some specific plans
■ No intent to die
■ Good self-control
■ Limited dysphoria
■ Some risk factors
■ Identifiable protective factors

Severe

■ Frequent, intense, and enduring suicidal ideation
■ Specific plans
■ Some intent to die
■ Method is available/accessible
■ Impaired self-control
■ Severe dysphoria
■ Multiple risk factors
■ Few protective factors

Extreme

■ Frequent, intense, and enduring suicidal ideation
■ Specific plans
■ Clear intent to die
■ Method is available/accessible
■ Impaired self-control
■ Severe dysphoria
■ Multiple risk factors
■ No protective factors

SOURCE: Rudd, M. D., Joiner, T., & Rajab, M. H. (2004). *Treating suicidal behavior* (2nd ed.). New York: Guilford Press.

DIAGNOSIS

Based on the assessment data, you develop any number of nursing diagnoses. For a person who is suicidal, the most obvious nursing diagnosis is:

■ Risk for Violence, Self-directed related to active suicidal plan, method available, multiple risk factors, and no protective factors (North American Nursing Diagnosis Association, 2007)

If a person has committed suicide, the family may become your client—in the short-term, as in the emergency room, or for a longer period, in a community or home setting. Possible nursing diagnoses may be:

■ Ineffective Family Coping, Compromised, related to the suicide of a family member
■ Spiritual Distress related to questions regarding the death, anger at the deceased, or a struggle with the sense of life's injustices

OUTCOME IDENTIFICATON AND GOALS

Based on the assessment data, you select outcomes appropriate to the nursing diagnoses. The outcome in a suicidal crisis is simply to keep the person alive. The outcome for families of suicides is that the family will remain functional as a unit and as individuals.

Client goals are specific behavioral measures by which you, clients, and significant others determine progress to-

ward goals. The following are examples of some of the other goals appropriate to people who are suicidal:

■ Utilizes the problem-solving process
■ Discusses personal philosophy of death
■ Verbalizes a sense of hopefulness regarding the immediate future
■ Identifies realistic protective factors

PLANNING

In planning nursing care, use the following questions to guide the process:

■ Is the client suicidal? At what level of severity?
■ What is the degree of lethality of the plan?
■ Must the client be in a protected environment?
■ What is the extent of protective factors?

Priorities of care for clients who are suicidal are:

■ Remains safe from self-injury
■ Verbalizes a decrease in suicidal thoughts and related behaviors
■ Develops a no-suicide contract

IMPLEMENTATION

Suicidal ideation and behaviors are managed within the context of the nurse–client relationship. It is critical to establish rapport and demonstrate empathy with clients who are suicidal.

NURSING CARE PLAN for a Client Contemplating Suicide

Maintaining Safety

Nursing Diagnosis: Client at Risk for Self-Directed Violence

Outcomes: Client does not harm or kill self.

When clients are severely or extremely suicidal, the first priority of care is client safety. If clients are not in the hospital, someone must remain with them at all times until they can be moved to a safe environment. It is difficult to ensure client safety in the emergency room, on medical-surgical units, and in intensive care units. Equipment can be used to harm oneself. Windows may be able to be opened or broken. If they are not seriously ill, suicidal clients may simply walk off the unit and disappear. Most acute care facilities either ask family members to stay with the client at all times or provide a "sitter" to ensure client safety in these nonpsychiatric settings.

Clients should never be lectured about the negative consequences of suicide. The goal is to protect clients who are suicidal until they are able to protect themselves. Through active intervention, it is hoped that clients will be able to develop alternative solutions to the difficulties fostering their suicidal intentions.

Contracts are verbal or written agreements with clients not to act on suicidal impulses. They may be called no-harm contracts, **no-suicide contracts,** or contracts for safety. It is unknown at this time how effective they are in preventing suicide. Contracts are probably only as reliable as the state of the therapeutic alliance. A contract without a therapeutic alliance is meaningless. People who are determined to kill themselves may agree to a contract to avoid detection of their suicidal intent. Rejection of a no-harm contract is generally a more certain indicator of a person's suicide risk status than acceptance of the contract.

Never use a no-harm contract as a substitute for ongoing suicide assessment and maintaining environmental safety. Contracts are adjunct to other safety interventions. No-harm contracts are not appropriate for clients who are agitated, psychotic, or highly impulsive or for those under the influence of intoxicating substances.

Intervention	Rationale	Goal
Remain with the client at all times until she or he can be moved to a safe environment.	Protecting the client until able to protect self is a necessary form of client advocacy for the person who is suicidal.	Remains safe
Have the client taken immediately to the hospital for evaluation and possible admission. If family is unable to ensure safety, call for police escort.	Admission may be the only immediate intervention to prevent suicide.	Remains safe
Remove as many dangerous objects as possible (e.g., pocket knives, glass articles, belts, shoelaces, razors, curling irons, pills).	Objects that could be used to harm oneself must be removed to protect client.	Remains safe
When administering medications, make certain client swallows all of them.	It is necessary to prevent stockpiling of medications for a future suicide attempt.	Swallows all medication
Check on client's whereabouts and status every 10–15 minutes. Maintain an irregular schedule of observation. If client is acutely suicidal, provide constant observation.	Frequent observation can prevent a suicide plan from being implemented. If the schedule is regular, client can determine the best time to attempt suicide.	Remains safe
Gently explain to client that you will protect her or him until able to resist suicidal impulses.	Ambivalent client will experience relief of conflict and anxiety when staff assumes control.	Verbalizes less conflict and anxiety

Promoting Problem Solving

Nursing Diagnosis: Client at Risk for Decisional Conflict

Outcomes: Client identifies other solutions to problems other than suicide.

Suicidal people feel overpowered by life's problems. They may say, "Suicide is the only thing I can do." Your role is one of active participation in problem solving.

continued

NURSING CARE PLAN for a Client Contemplating Suicide

Promoting Problem Solving   *continued*
Nursing Diagnosis: Client at Risk for Decisional Conflict

Intervention	Rationale	Goal
Listen carefully and take all suicide talk seriously.	Serious attention conveys caring and helps to establish rapport.	Acknowledges concern and care
Do not try to talk client out of suicidal intentions.	Client may interpret this as evidence you do not understand or you do not believe reasons are valid.	Acknowledges concern and care
Use the problem-solving process regarding the reasons for suicide: ■ Have client write out list of reasons to live and reasons to die. ■ Have client describe the goal she/he hopes to achieve. ■ Remind client that suicide is only one of several possible alternatives. ■ Develop a list of alternatives to meet client's goal. ■ Discuss potential outcomes of suicide (e.g., "What is the likelihood that you will injure yourself seriously if your attempt is not successful?" and "Will death be the most successful method of meeting your goal?"). ■ Discuss potential outcomes of other alternatives.	A written list may help client conceptualize the conflict more clearly. A specific goal will help focus problem solving. Counterbalance the belief that suicide is the only alternative. Potential negative outcomes may not have been considered (e.g., permanent bodily damage or nonachievement of goal). This supports the part that wishes to live by focusing on other ways to meet goal, which will decrease feelings of helplessness.	Develops a list Identifies goals Lists alternatives Projects outcomes
Focus on things that may help client resist suicidal impulses: ■ Discuss death; what it means to client, feelings about death, and what client thinks it will be like. ■ Focus on the list of reasons to continue living. ■ Discuss meaningful network systems of family and friends. ■ Discuss impact of suicide on survivors (e.g., grief, anger, shame, guilt, and increased risk that they will commit suicide).	Suicidal people often have not thought past the act of self-injury, that is, the reality and finality of death. Strengthening the wish to live will weaken the wish to die and decrease internal conflict. Focusing on available support systems will decrease feelings of isolation and helplessness. Suicidal people often have not considered the impact of their suicide on family members. This external focus and concern may decrease the impulsive behavior.	Discusses death Develops a list Identifies support systems Discusses impact of suicide on others

Preventing Future Suicidal Behavior
Nursing Diagnosis: Client at Risk for Ineffective Coping

Outcomes: Client identifies potential problems and plans appropriate measures to manage anticipated problems.

Intervention	Rationale	Goal
Discuss with client and family that recurrences of suicidal thoughts and behavior may happen.	Education about suicide will decrease the denial process of future problems and promote earlier intervention.	Identifies potential problems
Encourage client and family to read books about suicide.	This broadens their understanding.	Discusses understanding of suicide

NURSING CARE PLAN for a Client Contemplating Suicide

Preventing Future Suicidal Behavior   *continued*
Nursing Diagnosis: Client at Risk for Ineffective Coping

Intervention	Rationale	Goal
Assist client in developing a crisis care card including: ■ Write out names and phone numbers of competent and willing family and friends. ■ Write out numbers of community resources such as hotlines, mental health emergency centers, and local emergency departments. ■ Write out reasonable, nonsuicidal responses to problems. ■ Make a list of activities that have helped in the past.	Knowledge of availability of resources and support systems may help client resist the impulse to commit suicide and provide the family with needed assistance.	Plans appropriate measures to manage anticipated problems

Supporting Families of Successful Suicides
Nursing Diagnosis: Client at Risk for Dysfunctional Grieving

Outcomes: Families will discuss the effect of suicide, express anger appropriately, and identify plans to manage anticipated problems.

When a client commits suicide, you must quickly intervene to support the family through the crisis. The taboo against suicide makes it difficult for survivors to discuss the situation.

Intervention	Rationale	Goal
Provide the opportunity for family to discuss the death.	Other family members and friends may avoid the issue because of discomfort. Most family members have a desperate need to talk in an environment of acceptance and understanding.	Discusses impact of suicide
Allow family to express anger at the victim for abandonment and anger at themselves for not being able to prevent the suicide.	This normalizes anger as an important part of the grieving process. There may have been no opportunity to prevent the death.	Processes anger
Help family anticipate future difficulties (e.g., holiday times, anniversary of the death, and suicidal ideation and behavior in other family members).	Anticipatory guidance will decrease the impact of expected difficulties.	Plans measures to manage anticipated problems
Refer family to a survivors of suicide support group.	Sharing with others who have had similar experiences provides support and resolution of feelings.	Attends a group
If family issues remain unresolved, refer for family therapy.	More intensive therapy may be necessary to intervene with complicated family issues.	Participates in family therapy

Within the context of the *therapeutic alliance*, explore and manage thoughts and feelings.

Sense of Desperation and Hopelessness

The nurse is a keeper of hope. It is a privilege to be intimately present with other human souls at some of their darkest moments. Hope is meaningfulness and dignity and a way of relating to oneself and others. Hope is also a way of being with clients. People who are suicidal feel very hopeless. They may need to borrow the nurse's hope until they can regain their own. The nurse sees clients not only as they are at the given moment but also as they can be. They need to hear about their

---

Using Research Evidence   Adolescents and Suicide

Park, H. S., Schepp, K. G., Jang, E. H., & Koo, H. Y. (2006). Predictors of suicidal ideation among high school students by gender in South Korea. *Journal of School Health, 76*(5), 181–188.

What is the study about?

Gender appears to be an important factor in suicidal thoughts and behavior in the adolescent population in South Korea. The purpose of this research study was to identify, in each gender, factors that would predispose to suicidal thoughts or protect against them. These factors have implications for suicide screening and prevention in this age group.

How was the study done?

Over a 2-month period, this quantitative, cross-sectional study was done with 1,334 volunteer high school student participants in six high schools located in three South Korean cities. The schools granted permission after they had approved the proposal and its measures for protection of human subjects. From each school, the researchers randomly selected either three or six classrooms of grade 10–12 students. To protect confidentiality, data were obtained through questionnaires without identifiers. *Historical variables* were assessed by asking questions regarding abuse, previous suicidal attempts, history of depression in self and/or family, and hostility. The experience of childhood physical abuse was measured by a single item asking students, "When you were growing up, how often did any adult do any hitting of you with something or physically attack you?" Sexual abuse was measured by asking, "When you were growing up, how often did any adult ever try to have sex with you or sexually attack you against your will?" Students were asked about any suicidal attempts during the past year. Students were also asked to report any depression treatment during the past year and/or any history of family depression. In addition, depression was measured using the Center for Epidemiologic Studies Depression Scale. Hostility was measured using a subscale of the Symptom Checklist 90—Revision. *Behavioral variables* were obtained by requesting data on sexual orientation, cigarette use, alcohol use, drug use, and whether the student experienced Wang-tta (being a victim of school bullying). *Psychosocial–environmental variables* were obtained by asking about economic status, parental divorce, and parental alcohol abuse. *Protective variables* included academic performance, communication with family and friends, and self-esteem. Self-esteem was measured through the Rosenberg Self-Esteem Questionnaire.

What were the results of the study?

During the two weeks before the study, thoughts of suicide had occurred to 48 males (7.3%) and 78 females (11.9%). Similarly, a higher proportion of females reported *ever* having suicidal thoughts. For the males, all of the historical variables were predictive of thoughts of suicide. Historical variables indicative of suicidal thoughts in females included childhood physical abuse two or more times, history of attempted suicide, history of treatment for depression, and history of family depression. For males, behavioral variables predicting suicidal thoughts were smoking, drinking, drug use, Wang-tta, sexual orientation, and sexual behavior. Behavioral predictors in females were Wang-tta and bisexual orientation; suicidal thoughts were not associated with any psychosocial–environmental variables. In males, the predictive psychosocial–environmental variables were parental divorce and parental alcohol abuse.

Overall, the strongest predictors of suicidal thoughts among adolescent males were history of suicidal attempt, depression, hostility, smoking, parental alcohol abuse, less communication with friends, and lower self-esteem. One historical variable was very strong: Among males, an adolescent with past suicide attempts was 17.6 times more likely to report thoughts of suicide. For females, the strong predictors of suicidal thoughts were depression, hostility, sexual orientation, and self-esteem. Males and females who had high depression scores had significantly more thoughts of suicide than adolescents with low scores.

What additional questions might I have?

How were these results affected by the fact that all participants were volunteers? How representative of all adolescents was the study? For measuring certain variables such as abuse, did using a single question limit reliability and validity? Why are psychosocial–environmental factors less likely to predispose a Korean female adolescent than her male counterpart to suicidal thoughts? What is the significance of smoking in males as related to suicidal thoughts? What cultural considerations should be acknowledged prior to generalizing this study to populations?

How can I use this study?

Nurses need to continue to be involved in education and programs that prevent childhood abuse. Nurses, especially school nurses, need to recognize that adolescent males with a history of attempting suicide should be closely observed and receive treatment for depression and/or behavioral challenges. Schools might well offer students screening for depression and programs in hostility management. In addition, school nurses might offer programs on the impact of bullying behavior on classmates. Female adolescents who have a bisexual orientation should be observed closely for suicidal thoughts. All adolescents should be encouraged to communicate their emotions; males especially may need to develop an emotional voice through effective communication techniques.

SOURCE: Contributed by Dolores Huffman, PhD, RN, Associate Professor of Nursing, Purdue University Calumet, Hammond, Indiana.

own competence and about their ability to grow and change, especially in times of discouragement and hopelessness.

The desired outcome is that the client verbalizes an increased sense of hope.

EVALUATION

To complete the nursing process, you evaluate client responses to nursing interventions based on the selected outcomes.

When clients are successful at suicide, nurses can ask themselves several questions to resolve any unnecessary self-blame and guilt:

- Did I take the client's suicidal intentions seriously?
- Did I provide as safe an environment as possible?

- Was the client willing to find alternative solutions?
- Do I have a right to prevent all suicides?
- Does the client have a right to determine her or his own death?
- Am I the only one who is blaming myself?
- What do I need to do to feel less guilty about this death?

It is necessary for staff members to discuss their feelings and responsibilities in regard to a client's suicide. They will find it helpful to explore concepts of life and death, as well as their moral obligations. If feelings of guilt and failure are not thought about and expressed, individual staff members may project anger and blame onto others or even onto the dead client.

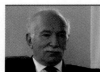

ROAD Assessment: **Critical Thinking Questions**

Go to the CD-ROM to assess Everett by answering the following critical thinking questions based on what you have **R**ead about Everett and **O**bserved on the videos.

1. You meet Everett while attending an open meeting of a local Depression and Bipolar Support Alliance Group. As the guest speaker for the meeting, you have been offered an opportunity to speak confidentially about his experiences. Everett reveals his feelings at the time he tried to commit suicide. Review his comments on segment A or your student ROAD CD-ROM for chapter 21. What is your assessment of his feelings and emotional state at that time in his life?

2. Everett tells you about his physician's response to a phone call he placed when he was having active suicidal ideations. You hear about this interchange in segment B of your chapter 21 student ROAD CD-ROM as he talks about alerting his doctor.
   a. What aspect of the physician–client relationship was successfully established and helped to promote a successful no-harm contract? Explain your answer.
   b. What is your understanding of the rationale behind the statements the doctor made to Everett? Support your answers.

3. Everett recalls his thinking prior to and after his suicide attempt and the impact upon his family in segment C of your student ROAD CD-ROM for chapter 21.
   a. What is your assessment of the cognitive component he expresses in this segment? Support your answer.
   b. What is your assessment of the prevailing affective component he expresses in this segment? Support your answer.

4. In responding to a client who, like Everett, voices intent to act upon suicidal thoughts, what nursing intervention(s) could you immediately implement? Explain your approach and provide rationales.

5. Discuss the prognosis you would assign to Everett's risk of suicide after considering his background and the knowledge you have gained from studying chapter 21, as well as the chapter 21 ROAD CD-ROM segments. Support your answer(s).

ROAD: DEVELOP A CARE PLAN

Go to the CD-ROM to Develop a care plan based on your assessment of Everett. Identify nursing disgnoses, outcomes, goals, and interventions.

SOURCE: Contributed by Susan Siwinski-Hebel, RN, MSN.

Focus Your Study

OBJECTIVES

KEY CONCEPTS

1. Identify risk factors and reasons for suicide.

- Persistent psychiatric disorder
- Previous suicide attempts
- Sense of hopelessness or desperation
- Chronic medical disease
- Elderly men
- Adolescents and college students
- Young persons who are gay, lesbian, bisexual, or transgendered

2. Discuss the theories regarding the causes of suicide.

- Genetics:
  - There may be a genetic factor regarding the inability to control impulsive behavior that may drive a person toward suicide.
- Neurobiology:
  - As levels of serotonin (5-HT) drop, people become more impulsive and aggressive.
  - Traumatic brain injuries can cause impulsive and aggressive behavior.
- Interpersonal factors:
  - Isolation and alienation from society, family, and friends
  - Significant loss
- Behavioral theory:
  - Suicide is a learned problem-solving behavior.

3. Outline the assessment process for a suicidal client.

- Use specific words such as "kill yourself" or "commit suicide."
- Listen for verbal cues such as "I can't take this much longer."
- Assess for delusions or command hallucinations.
- Ask about the plan and if the means are already available.
- Assess for presence of other disorders such as depression, schizophrenia, or substance abuse.
- Ask about goals they hope to achieve with suicide.
- Assess for the presence of protective factors such as a good social support system, problem-solving and coping history, sense of responsibility to children, hopefulness, and moral or religious objections to suicide.

4. Use the nursing process to develop a safe, comprehensive plan of care for a suicidal client and her/his family.

- Maintaining safety:
  - Remain with client until a safe environment can be provided.
  - Ensure environmental safety.
  - Closely observe those who are acutely suicidal.
  - Obtain a no-harm contract.
- Promoting problem solving:
  - Write out list of reasons to die and to live.
  - Establish goals the client hopes to achieve with death.
  - Remind client that suicide is only one option.
  - Write out list of alternatives to meet goals.
  - Discuss potential outcomes of suicide and alternative.
  - Identify resources that will help them choose life.

5. Discuss the key points in effectively communicating with a suicidal client.

- Use specific words to avoid any misunderstanding.
- Introduce the topic of suicide.
- Identify the fears the client is experiencing.
- Remember, the answers you get depend on the questions you ask.
- Support the part of the client who wishes to live.

6. Develop teaching plans for a suicidal client and her/his family. →

- Preventing future suicidal behavior:
  - Discuss possibility of recurrence.
  - Develop a crisis care with support people's phone numbers; community resources; reasonable, nonsuicidal responses to problems; list of helpful activities.
- Supporting families of successful suicides:
  - Provide opportunities to discuss the death.
  - Support expressions of anger.
  - Anticipate future difficult times or situations.
  - Refer to a survivors of suicide group.
  - Refer to family therapy.

Explore MediaLink

For review questions, case studies, and other resources for this chapter see the Pearson Health MediaLink CD-ROM that accompanies this book and the Companion Website.

CD-ROM
- Audio Glossary
- NCLEX-RN® Review Questions
- ROAD to Critical Thinking: *Everett*

Companion Website www.prenhall.com/fontaine
- Audio Glossary
- NCLEX-RN® Review Questions
- Case Study
  - The Suicidal Client
- Care Plan
  - Assessing Suicide Attempts
- Critical Thinking
  - Assessing the Client for Suicide Potential
- MediaLink Application
  - "If You Are Thinking About Suicide, Read This First"
- MediaLinks
  - Books for Clients & Families
  - Community Resources

NCLEX-RN® Review Questions

21-1. A client who attempted suicide 5 years ago with an overdose was brought to the emergency department (ED) by a friend. The client states, "I just don't feel like living anymore. No one would care if I lived or died." What question should the nurse ask next?
  1. "Do you have a plan for suicide at this time?"
  2. "What major losses have you experienced in the past 6 months?"
  3. "Have you experienced any major life crises in the past 6 months?"
  4. "Do you feel angry, overwhelmed or hopeless?"

21-2. The mental health nurse is giving a presentation in a rural community to increase the awareness of suicide risks. Which of the following population groups has a high risk for suicide and is an appropriate target audience? (Select all that apply.)
  1. Divorced or single middle-aged females
  2. Elderly men with a terminal disease
  3. Women with borderline personality disorder
  4. Nurses who work on a pediatric oncology unit
  5. Adolescent males on a football team

21-3. The guardian of a client diagnosed with paranoid schizophrenia is concerned that the client is at risk for suicide. The nurse should assess which of the following behaviors as a significant sign that the client is contemplating suicide?
  1. The client refuses to take the prescribed antipsychotic medication.
  2. The client accuses the guardian of poisoning the food.
  3. The client states, "Everything goes to the cat when I die."
  4. The client has been asking how to load a gun.

21-4. Which of the following client statements indicates a positive outcome to treatment for suicidal behavior?
  1. "I am thankful for my husband and children."
  2. "It helps me feel better to talk about possible ways to commit suicide."
  3. "I know my family realizes that I should never be left alone."
  4. "It's a lot harder to deal with my pain than it would be to face my death."

21-5. A client admitted to the hospital for a recent suicide attempt has been taking antidepressants as prescribed and attending group therapy. The client is sleeping 6 hours per night and reports a significant improvement in mood. The client states, "I have lots of things to do when I get home and I don't really need to be in the hospital anymore." Which of the following responses by the nurse would be most appropriate?
1. "Are you still having thoughts of suicide?"
2. "Are you willing to sign a 'no-harm' contract before you leave?"
3. "How would you rate your mood on a scale of 1 to 10?"
4. "How can we be sure you won't hurt yourself when you go home?"

21-6. The nurse is leading a group for depressed clients who have attempted suicide in the past. Which of the following topics is not appropriate to discuss in this group?
1. Community resources including phone numbers for mental health centers and hotlines
2. Alternative coping behaviors that have been successfully used in the past
3. Movies that dramatize suicidal behavior
4. National statistics and books about suicide

See Appendix D for answers.

References

American Psychiatric Association Practice Guidelines. (2003). *Practice guideline for the assessment and treatment of patients with suicidal behaviors.* Washington, DC: American Psychiatric Press.

Beautrais, A. L. (2003). Suicide and serious suicide attempts in youth. *American Journal of Psychiatry, 160*(6), 1093–1099.

Bruce, M. L., Ten Have, T. R., Reynolds, C. F. 3rd., Katz, I. I., Schulberg, H. C., Mulsant, B. H., et al. (2004). Reducing suicidal ideation and depressive symptoms in depressed older primary care patients. *JAMA, 291*(9), 1081–1091.

Dervic, K., Oquendo, M. A., Grunebaum, M. F., Ellis, S., Burke, A. K., & Mann, J. J. (2004). Religious affiliation and suicide attempt. *American Journal of Psychiatry, 161*(12), 2303–2308.

Ersek, M. (2004). The continuing challenge of assisted death. *Journal of Hospice and Palliative Nursing, 6*(1), 46–59.

Fontana, J. S. (2002). Rational suicide in the terminally ill. *Journal of Nursing Scholarship, 34*(2), 147–151.

Fortune, S. A., & Hawton, K. (2005). Deliberate self-harm in children and adolescents. *Current Opinion in Psychiatry, 18*(4), 401–406.

George, J., & Haas, B. (2006). Man throws 2 boys to deaths. *Chicago Tribune.* May 28, 2006.

Huygen, C. (2006). Understanding the needs of lesbian, gay, bisexual, and transgender people living with mental illness. *Medscape General Medicine, 8*(2), 1–5. Retrieved May 10, 2006, from http://www.medscape.com/viewarticle/529619

Joe, S., Baser, R. E., Breeden, G., Neighbors, H. W., & Jackson, J. S. (2006). Prevalence of and risk factors for lifetime suicide attempts among blacks in the United States. *JAMA, 296*(17), 2112–2123.

Joiner, R. (2005). *Why people die by suicide.* Cambridge, MA: Harvard University Press.

Mann, J. J., Bortinger, J., Oquendo, M. A., Currier, D., Li, S., & Brent, D. A. (2005). Family history of suicidal behavior and mood disorders in probands with mood disorders. *American Journal of Psychiatry, 162*(9), 1672–1679.

Matzo, M. L., & Schwarz, J. K. (2001). In their own words: Oncology nurses respond to patient requests for assisted suicide and euthanasia. *Applied Nursing Research, 14*(2), 64–71.

Moscicki, E. K., & Caine, E. D. (2004). Opportunities of life: Preventing suicide in the elderly. *Archives of Internal Medicine, 164*(11), 1171–1172, 1179–1184.

Murphy, S. A., Tapper, V. J., Johnson, L. C., & Lohan, J. (2003). Suicide ideation among parents bereaved by the violent deaths of their children. *Issues in Mental Health Nursing, 24,* 5–25.

North American Nursing Diagnosis Association. (2007). *Nursing Diagnosis: Definition and classification* (2007-2008). Philadelphia: Author.

Norton, K. (2005). Suicide prevention program promotes early recognition and treatment of mental illness. *NAMI Advocate, 3*(4), 9–10.

Park, H. S., Schepp, K. G., Jang, E. H., & Koo, H. Y. (2006). Predictors of suicidal ideation among high school students by gender in South Korea. *Journal of School Health, 76*(5), 181–188.

Phillips, M. R., Yang, G., Li, S., & Li, Y. (2004). Suicide and the unique prevalence pattern of schizophrenia in mainland China. *Lancet, 364*(9439), 1016–1017.

Pompili, M., Rinaldi, G., Lester, D., Girardi, P., Ruberto, A., & Tatarelli, R. (2006). Hopelessness and suicidal risk emerge in psychiatric nurses suffering from burnout and using specific defense mechanisms. *Archives of Psychiatric Nursing, 20*(3), 135–143.

Pumariega, A. J., Rogers, K., & Rothe, E. (2005). Culturally competent systems of care for children's mental health. *Community Mental Health Journal, 41*(5), 539–554.

Schwarz, J. K. (2003). Understanding and responding to patients' requests for assistance in dying. *Journal of Nursing Scholarship, 35*(4), 377–384.

Simon, R. I. (2004). *Assessing and managing suicide risk.* Washington, DC: American Psychiatric Press.

Singh, G. K., & Siahpush, M. (2002). Increasing rural-urban gradients in US suicide mortality, 1970–1997. *American Journal of Public Health, 92*(7), 1161–1167.

Swann, A. C., Dougherty, D. M., Pazzaglia, P. J., Pham, M., Steinberg, J. L., & Moeller, F. G. (2005). Increased impulsivity associated with severity of suicide attempt history in patients with bipolar disorder. *American Journal of Psychiatry, 162*(9), 1680–1687.

Chapter 22

Interpersonal Violence

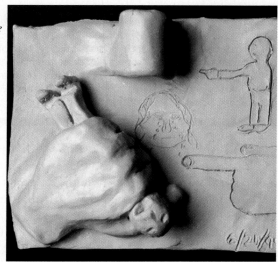

" *A tunnel is nothing but walls. You go into a long tunnel and all you see behind you and in front of you are more walls. You lose track of how long you've been there and you don't know how long it will take you to get out. If you do get out, what will be on the other side?* "

—*Kay, Age 40*

OBJECTIVES

After reading this chapter, you will be able to:

1. Describe the types of abuse that are likely to occur at each point in the life span.

2. Discuss the mental health implications for a victim of interpersonal violence.

3. Discuss the different theories regarding the etiology of interpersonal violence.

4. Outline the assessment process for a client experiencing interpersonal violence.

5. Use the nursing process to develop a safe, comprehensive plan of care for a client experiencing interpersonal violence.

6. Develop teaching plans for a client experiencing interpersonal violence and her/his family.

7. Discuss the key points in effectively communicating with a person experiencing interpersonal violence.

MediaLink www.prenhall.com/fontaine

Go to the Pearson Health MediaLink CD-ROM and the Companion Website at www.prenhall.com/fontaine for interactive resources for this chapter.

The ROAD to Critical Thinking

A Client Experiencing Interpersonal Violence

Travel this ROAD to understand Sara and her condition.

Read about Sara below and throughout this chapter.

Observe Sara on the CD-ROM accompanying this book.

Assess Sara by answering the questions at the end of this chapter.

Develop a Care Plan on the CD-ROM to address Sara's condition.

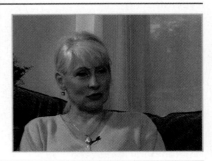

Sara

Sara was in a long-term relationship with a man for 9 years, the last 5 years of which she was a victim of abuse. As his cocaine and alcohol addiction worsened, he became increasingly out of control. He accumulated many weapons and would use them to intimidate and control Sara. Sara's fears kept her immobilized and she was unable to leave the relationship. When she finally was able to leave, she not only lost her home, she also lost her job because she was employed by him. Now, some years later, Sara still does not feel completely safe. Her name is not on her lease or on her utilities. She gets her mail in another town at the back of a convenience store. She believes she needs to continue in this way to protect herself. You will meet Sara on the video clip on your disc and throughout this chapter. At the end of the chapter, you will find critical thinking questions relating to assessment and development of a plan of care for Sara.

Healthy People 2010, published by the U.S. Department of Health and Human Services (2000), describes interpersonal violence as a significant problem in the United States. Interpersonal violence—violence between family members or friends—occurs at all levels in society. The myth is that violence occurs only among the poor and undereducated, but the reality is that violence occurs among the middle and upper classes and professional elite as well. See Box 22.1 for myths and facts about interpersonal violence. In the past, these problems among wealthy or prominent people were kept hidden from the public. With an increase in national concern, however, more publicity is being given to cases of interpersonal violence at all socioeconomic levels. These objectives can be viewed on the *Healthy People 2010* Web site, which can be accessed through a resource link on the Companion Web site for this book.

In this chapter, the word **family** refers to any one in these three categories: (1) those related by birth, adoption, or marriage; (2) those in an intimate relationship; and (3) those in a domestic (i.e., sharing the same household) relationship. Although the image or fantasy of the American family is one of happiness and harmony, this ideal is often in conflict with the underlying reality of violence. The home is the most frequent place for violence of all types. Women and children are more likely to be assaulted, raped, and killed by people who claim to love them. Perpetrators of violence do to intimates in their homes what they would not dare do any place else. The American culture does not condone violence in schools, at work, or on the streets, but it continues to "allow" it within the privacy of the family. It is time to cancel hitting licenses for all people.

BOX 22.1   Myths and Facts About Domestic Violence

Myth: Family violence is rare.
Fact: Every year, 10 million Americans are abused by a family member.

Myth: Family violence is confined to mentally disturbed or sick people.
Fact: Fewer than 10% of all cases involve an abuser who is mentally ill. The vast majority of abusers seem to be totally normal and are often charming, persuasive, and rational.

Myth: Violence is trivial—a joking matter.
Fact: A woman is beaten every 15 seconds in the United States, and 2,000 to 4,000 women are murdered by their husbands or boyfriends every year. Every year, 2.5 million children are abused, and 1,200 die from the abuse. There are 1 million cases of elder abuse annually.

Myth: Family violence is confined to the lower classes.
Fact: Social factors are not relevant. There are doctors, ministers, psychologists, and nurses who beat their family members. Violence occurs at least once in two thirds of all marriages.

Myth: All members of the family participate in the family dynamics; therefore, all must change in order for the violence to stop.
Fact: Only the perpetrator has the ability to stop the violence. A change in the victim's behavior will not cause the abuser to become nonviolent.

Myth: Family violence is usually a one-time event, an isolated incident.
Fact: Violence is a pattern, a reign of force and terror. It becomes more frequent and severe over time.

Myth: Abused women like being hit; otherwise, they would leave.
Fact: Abused women are forced to stay in the relationship for many reasons. The perpetrator dramatically escalates the violence when a woman tries to leave.

BOX 22.2	Types of Abuse

Emotional Abuse

Frequent belittling or demeaning; words or behaviors that undermine sense of self, competence, safety; psychological intimidation; accusations; demand obedience to every order; destruction of property, pets

Physical Abuse/Battering

Hitting, punching, grabbing, shoving, slapping, kicking, biting, hit with objects, use of weapons

Sexual Abuse

Inappropriate sexual behavior, including peeping, touching, rape, use of objects, forced sex with other people or animals

Social Abuse

Isolation from actual and potential support systems; controlling use of time and space; continual watching/spying

Economic Abuse

Little or no access to assets; minimal input into family expenditures

Neglect

Physical

Failure to provide adequate food, shelter, sleeping arrangements, clothing, and general physical care

Emotional

Failure to nurture, love, support; failure to validate self-worth

Medical

Failure to provide adequate medical care, especially when serious or life threatening

Educational

Failure to enroll child in school or alternative means of education; failure to get child to school; failure to assist child in completing educational tasks; generally applied to child under age 11

Abandonment

Leaving child alone without adequate supervision; abandoning child, throwing child out of home, not allowing a runaway to return home

---

Abuse, interchangeable with the term *violence* in this chapter, refers to a pattern of behavior that dominates, controls, lowers self-esteem, or takes away freedom of choice. It is systematic persecution of another individual, ranging from subtle words or actions to violent battering—acts of commission. Abuse also includes various types of neglect—acts of omission. See Box 22.2 for definitions of types of abuse.

The incidence of interpersonal violence can only be estimated. Studies often include only those people willing to respond to surveys. Typically underrepresented in such studies are those who do not speak English, the very poor, the homeless, and those who are hospitalized or incarcerated at the time of the survey. The actual rates of violence are probably much higher than reported. One in four violent crimes reported to the police involves interpersonal violence (Crane & Constantino, 2003).

In all 50 states, nurses are required by law to report suspected incidents of child abuse, and in every state, there is a penalty—civil, criminal, or both—for failure to report child abuse. In addition, not reporting child abuse is considered nursing malpractice. State laws vary for reporting the abuse of adults and the elderly. Forty-three states have mandatory reporting laws for elder abuse, with the other seven states saying elder abuse "may" be reported. In 1994, the Violence Against Women Act made it a federal crime to cross state lines to assault a spouse or domestic partner. This act was renewed and funded in 2000 and in 2006. Interpersonal violence is now considered a violent crime, against which the victim has the right to be protected and for which the perpetrator can be arrested and prosecuted.

KNOWLEDGE BASE

Sibling Abuse

The form of violence that is most unrecognized occurs between siblings. Many people assume it is natural and even appropriate for children to use physical force with one another. Parents say things like, "It's a good chance for him to learn how to defend himself," "She had a right to hit him; he was teasing her," and "Kids will be kids." With these attitudes, children learn that physical force is an appropriate method of resolving conflict among themselves. Children who are hit by their parents have more than double the rate of violence against siblings than children whose parents did not hit them. Hitting children increases the probability that they will be violent. Parents should not be complacent about sibling aggression; siblings cause 3% of all child homicides in the United States. Even though violence decreases with age, studies indicate that 63% to 68% of adolescent siblings use physical violence to resolve conflict (Marleau, 2005).

Closely related to sibling abuse is peer abuse, which occurs at the junior high school level. Unlike at any older age, at this level there is more female-to-male violence than male-to-female violence. Boys of this age still obey what their parents have told them: "Don't hit girls." Junior high school girls, however, feel empowered to hit boys when they tease, and the schools ignore this form of peer violence. Ultimately, young men abandon what they were told and strike back. We must tell young girls very clearly that, if a boy teases them, a kick in the groin is *not* appropriate and that there are other ways to defend themselves.

Child Abuse

Each year, approximately 2.8 million American children experience at least one act of physical violence, and 1.4 million are otherwise abused or neglected. Around 90% of these children have been abused in multiple ways. Children who live in homes in which a parent is being abused are 1,500 times more likely than the national average to be abused (Edwards, Holden, Felitti, & Anda, 2003).

Acts of violence against children range from a light slap, to severe beating, to homicide. Hitting or spanking children is condoned and even approved as being necessary and good for the child. Many parents, however, do not realize the underlying messages they are giving to the child by hitting (Straus, 1994):

- If you are small and weak, you deserve to be hit.
- People who love you hit you.
- It is appropriate to hit people you love.
- Violence is appropriate if the result is good.
- Violence is an appropriate method of resolving conflict.

Studies have not demonstrated that spanking is an effective method of discipline beyond the initial effect. Only nonphysical interventions, such as time-outs, are effective in the long run in helping children modify their unwanted behavior. When spanking is not effective, some parents increase physical punishment in an effort to maintain control and demand obedience. See Box 22.3 for myths that surround the use of spanking.

Parental violence often becomes habitual in that it occurs periodically or regularly. In extreme cases, it ends in the death of the infant or child. Child victims are helpless captives because they are dependent on the adults in the family. Abused children often try to please the abusive parent and may become overly compliant to all adults. They may avoid peers and withdraw from outside contacts. It is not unusual for child victims to act out with aggressive behavior later, during adolescence.

In the United States, **homicide** is one of the five leading causes of death before the age of 18. In fact, 61% of children who are killed by their parents/caretakers are younger than the age of 4, and 40% are younger than 1 year old. Most of these deaths are from head or abdominal injuries from battering in response to colic in the infant, toilet training difficulties in the toddler, and children with special needs. A small percentage of children are killed because they are unwanted, as the result of mercy killings, at the hands of a mentally ill parent, or in retaliation when one parent kills the child to inflict hurt on the other parent. Compared with other developed countries, the United States has the highest rate of child homicide at all ages (Friedman, Horwitz, & Resnick, 2005; Patton, 2003).

BOX 22.3	**Myths That Surround the Use of Spanking**

Myth: Spanking is harmless.
Fact: Spanking makes parenting more difficult because it reduces parents' ability to influence their children, especially when the children are teens and are too big to control by physical force. Also, authority figures should be trusted and respected, not feared.

Myth: I was spanked, and I'm okay.
FACT: You made it despite being hit; hitting increases the probability that you are more likely to use aggression to handle conflicts.

Myth: If you don't spank, your children will be spoiled or run wild.
Fact: Nonspanked children are better behaved than are children of parents who spank. Nonspanking parents tend to pay more attention to their children's behavior and tend to do more explaining and reasoning, which helps children develop internal controls.

Myth: Spanking is needed as a last resort.
Fact: If spanking is done at all, "last resort" may be the worst since parents are usually very angry and act impulsively. It teaches children that being extremely angry justifies hitting.

Myth: Parents spank rarely or only for serious problems.
Fact: Parents who spank tend to use this method for almost any misbehavior; many do not even give the child a warning—they spank before trying other things.

Myth: It is unrealistic to expect parents to never spank.
Fact: It is no more unrealistic to expect parents to not hit a child than to expect that husbands not hit their wives or that a supervisor never hit an employee.

SOURCE: Adapted from Straus, M. A. *Beating the devil out of them: Corporal punishment in American families.* Second Edition. New Brunswick, NJ: Transaction Publishers, 2001.

In May 2005, Nicole Harris was charged with first-degree murder in the death of her 4-year-old son who she said would not stop crying. She admitted to wrapping an elastic band around the boy's neck and choking him until he stopped struggling.

In November 2004, William Boesel was charged with the murder of his 1-month-old baby. He confessed that he squeezed the baby around the abdomen with his hands, shook him, slapped him with an open hand, and struck his legs with a fly swatter. The coroner's office reported injuries in the rectal area that indicated possible sodomy.

Shaken baby syndrome is one of the most serious yet frequently overlooked forms of child abuse. It involves vigorous shaking of babies while held by the extremities or shoulders, which causes whiplash-induced intracranial and intraocular bleeding. It is estimated that one third have significant and permanent brain damage and one third of the victims die. Not recognizing the dangers, many parents shake rather than hit the child, mistakenly believing it is less violent.

Clydell, a 19-year-old father, was found guilty of murdering his 2-month-old son. He sobbed uncontrollably at his sentencing, saying that he never meant to hurt his son—he just wanted him to stop crying. He didn't know that picking the baby up and shaking him would kill him.

Neglect is the most frequently reported type of child maltreatment. It differs from abuse in that it is an act of omission that results in harm. Neglect includes lack of adequate physical care, nutrition, and shelter. It also includes unsanitary conditions that often contribute to health and developmental problems. Lack of human contact and nurturance is considered emotional neglect.

In February 2005 Eric Bare and Deborah Cameron were arrested for unreasonable restraint of a child. They would put their 11-year-old daughter in a chain-link dog kennel for days at a time as discipline, letting her out only for school and chores. The kennel was assembled over a floor drain in case the girl had to urinate.

Although it is rare, each year more than 300 parents are killed by their children in the United States. This accounts for 1.5% to 2.5% of all homicides. Victims and perpetrators both tend to be Euro-American, with 30% of the perpetrators younger than age 18. The most frequent situation, 90% of cases, is one in which the teen has been severely abused or the mother is a victim of abuse. The adolescent's attempts to get help have failed and the family situation becomes increasingly intolerable before the murder. A critical factor is the easy availability of guns in the home. The other 10% of cases involve either a severely mentally ill child who experiences hallucinations and delusions or a dangerously antisocial child who has extreme conduct problems (Ewing, 1997).

In May 2005, a teen about to graduate from high school killed his grandparents, his mother, and his two friends and then wounded his younger sister before committing suicide. The death came hours after a family party to celebrate his graduation. School authorities said no one had seen any indication that he was a troubled teen.

Munchausen syndrome by proxy (MSBP) often goes unrecognized as a form of child abuse. A parent, often the mother, persistently lies about symptoms the child is experiencing or actually induces symptoms in the child with the intent of keeping in contact with health care providers and hospitals. For example, she may add blood to a child's emesis, urine, or feces; purposefully create wounds and infect them; or even inject feces, poisons, or other toxins directly into the bloodstream. In a sense, the child is doubly abused, by the parent's action and by frequent hospitalizations, extensive medical testing, and even a number of surgeries. Approximately 10% of cases are fatal. The mother often seems to be a very concerned and loving parent, and it may take months or years and multiple "illnesses" before the manipulation is discovered. The victims are often young because older children would be more likely to tell health care professionals the truth about their so-called symptoms. The motivation for this type of child abuse is unknown. It is thought that women with a history of childhood abuse, who feel unloved and insecure, may seek love and support from their children's health care providers. As the mother is consulted and included in the care, she receives the secondary gains of attention and support. Other thoughts are that some mothers may be expressing anger through MSBP or may be using the sick child to develop a closer relationship with her adult partner (Adshead & Bluglass, 2005).

On January 16, 2004, Tracie Fleck was arrested on 10 felony counts of child abuse. Police arrested her after she was video-taped tampering with her 21-month-old daughter's intravenous (IV) tube. Health care professionals became suspicious when the child continued to develop infections after treatment. The child was admitted to the hospital on January 4 and within the next several days suffered a series of four acute infections. Infectious-disease physicians traced her infection to fecal matter in the girl's IV tube.

Intimate Partner Violence— Heterosexual

Although no class, ethnic group, religion, or age group is immune from interpersonal violence, 76% of victims are women. If the abused are mothers of dependent children, their children are likely to be victims also. Female partner abuse in heterosexual relationships is the most widespread form of family violence in the United States. It is thought that one woman in four is physically abused by her partner, and that 3 to 4 million women are severely assaulted every year. Half the women who are abused suffer beatings several times a year. The other half may be beaten as often as once a week. The intensity and frequency of attacks tend to escalate over time. If verbal and emotional assaults were included, the numbers would be much higher. Violence is the single largest cause of injury to women in the United States, with 20% of emergency department visits resulting from physical abuse. Three to four battered women are killed every day in the United States (Daniels, 2005; Zlotnick, Johnson, & Kohn, 2006).

In July 2004, a man doused his girlfriend and three small children with gasoline inside a car. He then set them ablaze with a lighter as he drove. All five died after the car crashed in flames.

In December 2004, Martin Kracht confessed to strangling his mother, his wife, and his infant son. His wife had reported several instances of battery, resulting in a separation.

In March 2004, Moua Her was charged with domestic assault after being accused of choking and cutting his wife. Only 4 months later, in July, his wife was found on the garage floor with a butcher's knife in her neck. She had been stabbed 63 times.

It is estimated that there are between 100,000 and 150,000 heterosexual male partners who are abused by women who initiate the violence. They are generally not recognized as "real" victims, and when they do tell others, they are criticized for not standing up for themselves or for not fighting back.

MediaLink Critical Thinking, Spousal Abuse

Homicide is the ultimate expression of male control over females. Of women who are murdered, 50% are killed by a past or current husband or lover. At least two thirds of these women have been abused by their murderer before their death. Most have previously turned to the police and courts for help. The risk of death increases as the victims resist or try to take control over their lives by leaving the abuser. In the case of a joint homicide–suicide, the perpetrator is almost always male and the victim is almost always female.

Women sometimes kill their husbands or lovers, almost invariably in response to years of abuse. Those victims who kill typically have suffered more frequent abuse with serious injuries, have been threatened with death, and have fewer coping resources than battered women in general. They most often murder their partners in self-defense, fearing for their lives and the lives of their children. One third of the murders occur during the course of battering incidents. The remainder occurs while the abuser is asleep or otherwise preoccupied. Battered woman syndrome is a permissible legal defense in all 50 states (Loeber, LaCourse, & Homish, 2005).

Overwhelmingly, the first acts of partner violence occur in dating relationships. Physical abuse occurs among as many as 30% to 50% of college students and in 10% to 35% of high school students who are dating. Sadly, many victims and offenders interpret violence as a sign of love. Hitting is not the sole form of abuse. Text messaging a person every few minutes is a common form of control by teen perpetrators. Common reasons teens and young adults give for the violence is betrayal and jealousy. Boys and girls are just as likely to be perpetrators or victims of physical abuse. Girls are more likely to have their hair pulled, be punched, and be sexually violated. Boys are more likely to be pinched, slapped, scratched, and kicked (Amar & Gennaro, 2005; Close, 2005).

For early warning signs of teenage dating violence, see Box 22.4.

BOX 22.4	**Early Warning Signs of Teenage Dating Violence**

The teenage perpetrator:
- Believes that men should be in control and women should be submissive
- Is jealous and possessive of his girlfriend, won't let her have friends, and checks up on her
- Tries to control his girlfriend by giving orders and making all the decisions
- Threatens his girlfriend with violence
- Uses or owns weapons
- Has a history of losing his temper quickly and fighting
- Brags about mistreating others
- Blames his girlfriend when he is violent; says she provoked him and made him do it
- Has a history of abusive relationships

Intimate Partner Violence— Homosexual

Until very recently, there has been a public minimization or denial of physical abuse in lesbian and gay relationships. This denial has been supported by the myths that women are not violent people and that men can defend themselves. In reality, violence does occur in some gay and lesbian families, for the same reasons it occurs in heterosexual families: to demonstrate, achieve, and maintain **power** and **control** over one's partner. In addition to physical or emotional abuse, the violent partner may use homophobic control—the threat of telling ("outing") family, friends, neighbors, or employers about the victim's sexual orientation.

In the United States, interpersonal violence is the third largest health problem for gay men, following substance abuse and HIV/AIDS. It is estimated that 20% to 25% of coupled gay men and lesbians are victims. Men rarely talk about being victims for fear of being considered feminine if they admit that their partners are hurting them. Looking at violence in same-sex relationships demonstrates clearly that violence is not a gender issue but rather a power issue (Freedberg, 2006; Heintz & Melendez, 2006).

Homophobia and hatred of homosexuals in the United States contributes to difficulties of battered lesbians and gays. They are cut off from the usual support systems available to heterosexual victims such as specialized counseling services and shelters. Most state laws regarding domestic violence exclude gay men and lesbians with the use of terms such as "spouse" and "battered wife." Minority gay men and lesbians and those who live in rural areas are even more isolated than their counterparts. Because same-sex partnerships are not recognized as "legitimate," victims have no access to the legal system. Often, being victimized by one's lover is less frightening than being victimized by the legal system. Fear of being identified as gay or losing custody of children adds to the silence about the violence. Members of lesbian and gay communities are making an attempt to intervene with, and support, victims.

Elder Abuse

Two million elderly people are mistreated each year nationwide. Most cases go unreported due to shame, self-blame, or multiple fears (Pearsall, 2005). Elder abuse is any deliberate action or negligence that harms elderly people. Physical abuse is the nonaccidental use of physical force that results in bodily injury, pain, or impairment. Some older adults may have their basic physical needs neglected and suffer from dehydration, malnutrition, decubiti, urine burns, and oversedation. Families may deprive them of necessary articles, such as glasses, hearing aids, and walkers. Emotional neglect can mean leaving a person for long periods or failing to provide social contact. Some older people are psychologically abused by verbal assaults, threats, intimidation, humiliation, or harassment. Remarks such as "One of these days I am going to poison your food and you won't know when" are considered psychological abuse.

Families may violate an older person's rights by refusing appropriate medical treatment, forcing isolation or unreasonable confinement, denying privacy, providing an unsafe environment, or demanding involuntary servitude. Some elders are financially exploited by their relatives through theft or misuse of property or funds. Others are beaten and even sexually abused or raped by family members.

Perpetrators of elder abuse may be spouses, children, grandchildren, nieces, nephews, or some other caretakers. The abuse is most likely to be inflicted by a person with whom the victim lives. Those elders with mental or physical disabilities are at greatest risk. A number of factors contribute to abuse of older adults. Perpetrators may have personal problems such as lack of support in caring for the older family member, alcohol or drug addiction, or a family history of violence. Family factors include unresolved previous conflicts and power struggles. The perpetrator may be retaliating for previous abuse at the hands of the elder person. Elderly people are often resistant to intervention because they fear that losing a caregiver will mean they will be put in an institution.

> In December 2004, police found an 88-year-old woman living in a filthy, unheated house. The victim told police that her 53-year-old caregiver, William James, hit and kicked her all the time and that he had refused to feed her for 3 days.

Abuse of Pregnant Women

Pregnancy is a time of increased risk for abuse. There are more incidents of violence during pregnancy than of hypertension, gestational diabetes, or placenta previa, all of which are screened for regularly. Indeed, 16% to 25% of women report abuse during pregnancy. Pregnant teens have a higher rate of abuse than pregnant adults. It is not unusual for the violence to continue into the postpartum period. A history of abuse is one of the strongest predictors of abuse during pregnancy. Nonpregnant women are usually beaten in the face and chest. But pregnant women tend to be beaten in the abdomen, which can lead to miscarriage, placenta abruptio, fetal loss, premature labor, fetal fractures, pelvic fractures, rupture of the uterus, and hemorrhage. Battering during pregnancy is associated with severity of abuse. The man who beats his pregnant partner is an extremely violent and dangerous man. Battering during pregnancy is also a risk factor for eventual homicide of the female partner (Kearney, Haggerty, Munro, & Hawkins, 2003; Tan & Gregor, 2006).

The timing of the first prenatal visit is often related to abuse status. Abused women are twice as likely to delay prenatal care until the third trimester. Many abused women report that the abuser forced them to avoid prenatal care by denying them access to transportation.

Physical abuse during pregnancy may be related to ambivalent feelings about the pregnancy, competition for attention with the developing fetus, increased vulnerability of the woman, increased economic pressures, and decreased sexual availability. Unfortunately, abuse of pregnant women is often overlooked by health care professionals, even when the victim appears in the emergency department with bruises, cuts, broken bones, and abdominal injuries.

> In February 2004, Donnelle Thurman was charged with assaulting his pregnant girlfriend. He woke her up and started talking to her about the dog they had owned which she had given to a shelter. He pulled her out of bed, backed her in a corner, and hit her for 20 to 30 minutes while she pleaded with him that her stomach was hurting. His response was that he guessed she would lose the baby like he lost his dog.

Emotional Abuse

Although the focus of violence in this chapter is on physical abuse, it must be remembered that emotional abuse is often equally as damaging. Words can hit as hard as a fist, and the damage to self-esteem can last a lifetime. Emotional abuse involves one person shaming, embarrassing, ridiculing, or insulting another either in private or in public. It may include destruction of personal property or the killing of pets in an effort to frighten or control the victim. Such statements as, "You can't do anything right," "You're ugly and stupid—no one else would want you," and "I wish you had never been born" are devastating to self-esteem.

Stalking

The term "stalking" has become not only a part of the American vocabulary but also a new classification of crime. All 50 states have passed stalking laws. **Stalking** is the act of following, viewing, communicating with, or moving threateningly toward another person. Property damage and assault may accompany stalking. Most victims are exposed to a number of different stalking behaviors by the same perpetrator, such as:

- Unwelcome mail, phone calls, and visits
- Harassment at work or home
- Following on the street
- Threatening or using violence
- Making threats against family members
- Damaging property
- Ordering items and charging to victim's account
- Spreading rumors and lies

In the United States, 8% of women and 2% of men have been or will be stalked at some time in their lives. The average duration of the stalking is 2 years. Women are far more likely to be victims, and men are far more likely to be perpetrators (Amar, 2006).

Domestic stalking occurs when a former partner, a spouse, or a family member threatens or harasses a person. The stalker often makes it clear that the victim is his "property." The stalker is usually motivated by a desire to continue the relationship, which can evolve into an attitude of "If I can't have her/him, no one can." In some cases, the stalker is angry and retaliating against the victim whom he perceives as rejecting him. Frequently, there is a history of violence, and the stalking often ends in a violent attack on, or killing of, the victim (Muscari, 2005).

Victims often feel trapped in an environment filled with anxiety, stress, and fear that often result in their having to make drastic changes in how they live their lives. Most victims seek legal counsel, seek restraining orders, change their phone numbers and daily travel routes, avoid going out of their home, and increase their home security.

After 3 years of living together, Gwen left Brian because of his moodiness, violent temper, and infidelities. Shortly after Gwen moved out, Brian would leave threatening notes on her car windshield and would call her constantly at work and at her new apartment threatening to kill her if she would not marry him. Gwen would often find that her tires had been flattened and, on more than one occasion, Brian attempted to run her off the road. Gwen filed a restraining order but the stalking continued. Gwen was afraid to go out of the house because Brian would just seem to show up wherever she was. It took Brian beating up Gwen for authorities to notice. Brian screamed in court that he would kill Gwen for what she had done to him. The stalking had gone on for over a year.

Cyberstalking refers to the use of the Internet, e-mail, or other electronic communications to stalk another person. It is a serious problem that is likely to become more widespread. Similar to other forms of stalking, cyberstalkers wish to establish control over the victim. In many cases there was a prior relationship between perpetrator and victim, but there are also a number of situations of cyberstalking by strangers. With the anonymity and lack of direct confrontation with electronic media, some individuals feel empowered to stalk via electronic media. A common form of cyberstalking is repeated: sending of threatening or harassing messages. Some perpetrators post "supposed messages" from the victim on bulletin boards or in chat rooms, thus tricking other Internet users into further harassment of the victim. For example, a perpetrator "posted information on the Web claiming her 9-year-old daughter was available for sex. The Web posting included their home phone number with instructions to call 24 hours a day. They received numerous calls" (Reno, 1999, p. 8).

Comorbid Disorders

The effect of living in a climate of fear and uncertainty contributes to an increased risk for several mental disorders.

Problems associated with child abuse include depression, substance abuse, self-mutilation, eating disorders, and dissociative disorders. Conduct disorder is nine times as likely to occur in abused adolescents as in the nonabused population. Between 60% and 85% of abused children and adults are at risk for posttraumatic stress disorder (PTSD). The intensity of PTSD symptoms is commensurate with the severity of the battering episodes and injuries. Depression is common and women are at high risk for suicide. Alcohol and drugs may be used to self-medicate the physical and emotional pain. Family violence has the worst mental health outcomes of any form of interpersonal violence because there is no safe and supportive place for retreat. Even civilians caught up in a war still experience the family as a place of safety and security (Records & Rice, 2005; Scheiman & Zeoli, 2003).

Sara:

❝ I developed PTSD as a result of abuse. I have an extreme sense of hypervigilance. I startle very easily. All kinds of everyday noises will fry my nerves. A siren—I'll jump off the ground if I hear a siren. Even after I left him, at night I'd go into this state of red alert because my body was expecting this madman to come through the door and do something horrific as he did practically every single night. So I expected it even though intellectually, I knew I was safe. ❞

Research suggests that there is an association between violence and premature infants. This may be a result of direct physical abuse causing the onset of labor or death of the fetus. It is believed that premature delivery may also be related to the psychosocial stress of the abuse.

Etiologies

Interpersonal violence is easy to describe but difficult to explain. There is no single cause of this type of violence. It results from an interaction of biology, personality, relationship, and societal factors that have an impact on individuals and families.

Neurobiology

Researchers believe that genes and neurotransmitters may contribute to violent behavior. Although a genetic predisposition may make certain behaviors more likely, it does not make them inevitable. Serotonin (5-HT) plays an important role in mood and aggressive behavior. 5-HT calms us through inhibitory control over aggression. Abnormally low levels of 5-HT result in a lack of control, loss of temper, and explosive rage.

Childhood abuse and neglect lead to permanent alterations in the parts of the central nervous system known to be stress responsive. Corticotropin-releasing factor (CRF) is a major regulator of the endocrine, autonomic, immune, and behavioral stress responses. It is thought that stress early in life results in sensitization of the brain to even mild stressors in adulthood, thus contributing to mood and anxiety disorders long after the abuse or neglect has stopped (Griffin, Resick, & Yehuda, 2005).

Intrapersonal Theory

Intrapersonal theory suggests that the cause of violence lies in the personality of the abuser. It is thought that people who are violent choose not to control their expressions of anger and hostility. This lack of self-regulation leads them to over-respond to stress. Poor problem-solving skills and the belief that aggression is a legitimate response to conflict intensify the violence (Close, 2005).

As many as 80% of male abusers grow up in homes in which they were abused or observed their mothers being abused. Sometimes these children try unsuccessfully to intervene, and sometimes they just try to get out of the way. Typically, they are afraid to go for help because of the code of family secrecy regarding the abuse and because they recognize that they too will be abused if they tell. Some children "externalize" their responses and become aggressive to siblings and peers, destructive, and noncompliant with adults. Some children "internalize" their responses and become fearful and withdrawn. Both of these responses contribute to a delay in social development by being unpopular and rejected or by being too anxious to participate in activities.

This early emotional deprivation contributes to an adult who is very needy of nurturance and support. They come to adult relationships with unrealistic demands for time and attention. As the relationship develops, they discourage their partners' relationships with other people because of low self-esteem and fear of abandonment.

Social Learning Theory

Social learning theory proposes that violence is a learned behavior and people are conditioned to respond aggressively and violently. Young boys are encouraged to demonstrate strength and dominance rather than empathetic and caring attributes. Children learn about violence from observation, from being a victim, and from behaving violently. If the use of violence is rewarded by a gain in power or a reduction in anxiety, the behavior is reinforced. If there is immediate negative reinforcement within the family, a decrease in violent behavior will result. Learning to abuse is the first step in the battering process but it does not necessarily lead vulnerable individuals to abuse. The social environment affects how the potentially abusive person behaves. In other words, the person must have the opportunity to abuse without negative consequences. There is the perception that he can "get away with it." Although learning may have occurred and opportunity is present, the potentially abusive person makes a conscious choice to abuse. The batterer is solely responsible for the violence (Tremblay & Nagin, 2005).

In addition to family models, the media provide many models of violence to which children are exposed. Some movies and television shows demonstrate that "good" people use force to achieve "good" ends. Many of the stories make no attempt to justify the use of force for "good" ends; they simply present endless, senseless acts of cruelty by one human being upon another. With these types of family and media examples, children develop values that tolerate, and even accept as normal, everyday violence between people.

Gender-Bias Factors

The sexist structure of the family and society is important in interpersonal violence. The cultural value is that men have a right to keep women subordinate through power and privilege. Men abuse because they believe they have a right to do so and because they can get away with it. Violence is a power issue. Victims are sometimes labeled as codependent in the abusive relationship, but such labeling is just another way of blaming the victim for the abuse. Women are sexualized as objects, restricted in state and federal participation in decision making, dehumanized with labels, controlled over the rights to their own bodies, and demeaned in value (Downs & Miller, 2002).

The sexist economic system helps entrap women, who often are forced to choose between poverty and abuse. It is difficult for women to find advocates and solutions within the male-dominated legal, religious, mental health, and medical systems. Society sanctions male violence by neglecting female victims. What remains unacknowledged is that women are being murdered on a regular basis, not by strangers, but by husbands and lovers.

MediaLink

Care Plan, Care Plan for a Victim of Abuse

Nursing Process

CLIENTS EXPERIENCING INTERPERSONAL VIOLENCE

Nurses must be involved in the prevention, detection, and treatment of interpersonal violence. Developing the knowledge base and the ability to identify factors that contribute to family violence will help you to promptly detect and accurately diagnose the problem. Male perpetrator–female victim is used as the model for ease in reading.

Focused Nursing Assessment — Victims of Interpersonal Violence

Behavior Assessment	Affective Assessment	Cognitive Assessment
What types of things cause conflict within your family? How is this managed or resolved? Who in your family loses control when angry? Have you been emotionally abused by someone in your family? Have you been slapped? Hit? Punched? Thrown? Shoved? Kicked? Has anyone forced you to have sexual activities? Have you attempted to leave the relationship in the past? What occurred then?	Who do you view as responsible for the use of physical force within the family? How much guilt are you experiencing at this time? Are you afraid of your partner/parent/sibling or anyone else? Tell me about your fears: Financial problems? Child care problems? Loneliness? Further physical injury? Do you feel safe living in your home? How hopeless do you feel about your situation?	Do you believe or hope the violence will not recur? What are your beliefs about keeping the family together? Describe your personal strengths and abilities. What are the rules about using physical force within your family?

ASSESSMENT

Given the incidence of abuse, it is logical to assume that you will encounter victims in a variety of clinical settings. Although one third of all women's visits to emergency departments are caused by interpersonal violence, less than 10% of the violence is identified. Women are treated for the immediate injury or complaint and dismissed without assessing for the life-threatening condition—abuse—that caused the immediate injury.

During the assessment of every client, in all types of health settings, one or two introductory questions should be asked. In assessing a child, say, for example, "Moms and Dads try to help their children learn how to behave well. What happens to you when you do something wrong?" Or ask, "What is the worst punishment you ever received?" In assessing adolescents for dating violence you may ask, "Is hitting okay when your boyfriend/girlfriend flirts with other people or catches you flirting with someone else, or if you get hit first?"

In assessing adults, you may begin with this approach: "One of the sources of stress in our lives is family disagreement. Could you describe how disagreements affect you? What happens when you disagree?" If the responses to these questions are indicative of violence, a focused nursing assessment must be conducted. The Focused Nursing Assessment feature provides questions to guide nursing assessment. Obviously, the assessment questions must be adapted to the client's age, gender, and family situation.

For clients who do not speak English, it is important to use a non–family member who speaks their language to as-

sist in the assessment process. The use of a non–family member helps ensure client confidentiality and safety. Immigrants may need to be reassured that reporting of abuse will not change their immigrant status.

Assessment: Behavior

Violence is the deliberate and systematic pattern of abuse used to establish power and control over the victim through fear and intimidation. The behavior is always intentional. Perpetrators choose to be violent and give themselves permission to be violent. Perpetrators are not out of control, as is commonly assumed. They may be enraged or cool and calculating, but in either case they have made a choice. The victim cannot "make them do it." Generally, perpetrators of interpersonal violence are law abiding and are dangerous only to their loved ones.

To the victim, violence often happens without warning and without a buildup of tension. A pattern of violence usually develops. Frustration or stress may precipitate the first incident. If the victim immediately refuses to accept the violence and seeks outside help, there are often no further episodes. If the victim submits to the violence, then physical force, without the stimulus of frustration or stress, becomes a way of relating, and the pattern becomes resistant to change. A typical cycle occurs when conflict escalates into a violent episode, after which the perpetrator begs for the victim's forgiveness. The victim stays in the system because of promises to reform. With the next episode of conflict, the **cycle of violence** begins again and becomes part of the family dynamics. See Table 22.1 ■ for a description of the cycle of violence.

Social Assessment	Physiological Assessment
How did your parents relate to each other?	Is there a history of unexplained injuries?
What type of discipline was used when you were a child?	Is there evidence of trauma such as bruises, burns, bites, punctures, irregular areas of hair loss, or old scars?
Describe your relationships with people outside your basic family unit.	Are there any fractured bones or dislocated joints?
Who can you turn to for support in times of stress?	Does the client have problems with mobility?
Are you kept alone for long periods of time?	Is there any evidence of internal injuries such as abdominal distention, absent bowel sounds, persistent vomiting, injury to organs, or hypovolemic shock?
What types of contact have you had with the legal system: Phoned police? Restraining order? Obtained a lawyer? Court cases? Protective services?	Does the client complain of abnormal sensations, numbness, or pain?
If family members are present, what is the quality of their interactions?	Assess for signs of neglect-poor hygiene, cleanliness, proper clothing for the weather, over- or undermedication.
	Assess for sexual abuse such as sexually transmitted infections, dysmenorrhea, pelvic inflammatory disease, or genital or rectal tearing.
	Is growth and development normal for the client's age?

Sara:

" I could never tell when he would fly into a rage or become angered or just become unstable. He would sit in the corner and take weapons out of the storage cabinet and look at them and fondle them. He would point the gun in my direction while telling me how beautiful it was. Then he would look at me with a sort of demonic grin and say, 'Oh, does this make you nervous?' "

The abuser is the most powerful person in the life of the victim. The abuser's purpose is to enslave the victim, while simultaneously demanding respect, gratitude, and love. Control over the victim is established by repetitive emotional abuse that instills terror and helplessness. Threats of serious harm or threats against other family members keep the victim in a constant state of fear. To have complete domination, the abuser isolates the victim. She often is forced to give up work, friends, and family. He may stalk her, eavesdrop, and intercept letters and phone calls. Control and scrutiny of the victim's body and bodily functions further destroy her sense of autonomy. She is shamed and demoralized when told what to eat, when to sleep, what to wear, when to go to the bathroom, and so on. For a victim who has been deprived long enough, the hope of a meal, a bath, or a kind word can be a powerful reward. All this abusive behavior alternates with unpredictable outbursts of physical violence.

TABLE 22.1	The Cycle of Violence	
Perpetrator		**Victim**
Tension-building phase		
Moody, withdraws affection, isolates victim, name-calling, verbally abusive, destroys property		Attempts to calm partner, nurturing, stays away from support systems, passive, feels as if walking on eggshells
Battering phase		
Pushing, shoving, hitting, other acts of violence		Protects self any way possible; someone else calls police; victim leaves
Contrition phase		
Says sorry, begs forgiveness, promises never again		Agrees to stay or return; attempts to stop legal proceedings; hopeful

SOURCE: Adapted with permission from Dutton, D. G. (1998). *The abusive personality*. New York: Guilford Press.

Such domestic captivity of women, along with traumatic bonding to the batterer, often goes unrecognized.

There are clues that you must recognize that would indicate the possibility of interpersonal violence. One behavior to look for is the man speaking for the woman in response to questions about the injury. She may seek his approval before answering questions. He may criticize or correct her answers. Often, he may not want health care professionals to talk to the woman alone. You must ask questions related to abuse when the woman is by herself and away from significant others. Make certain that no one can walk into the room or overhear what is said.

Further assessment is needed if the victim says her partner has problems with alcohol or drug abuse or has a history of violent behavior. If she has concerns about the safety of her children or expresses a fear of returning home, more in-depth assessment must be completed.

Assessment: Affect

Violent people are often extremely jealous and possessive. They view other family members in terms of property and ownership and believe that they are entitled to control others. Abusers use violence to prove to themselves and others that they are superior and in control. The use of physical force temporarily obliterates their sense of inadequacy and compensates for a lack of internal resources.

Victims may be immobilized by a variety of affective responses to the abuse, such as anxiety, helplessness, and depression. Feelings of self-blame may be expressed in such statements as, "If I hadn't talked back to my mother, she wouldn't have hit me," and "If I were a better wife, he wouldn't beat me." Guilt can contribute to depression, which further immobilizes victims and keeps them from leaving or seeking help for the family system.

Fear contributes to women's inability to leave abusive relationships. Often threatened with death at the idea of leaving, they live in fear of physical reprisal. Fearing loneliness, some women may believe that being in a bad relationship is better than being alone. Also, leaving the relationship does not necessarily ensure the end of the abuse. The abuser is often most dangerous when threatened with or faced with separation. Some choose to kill when they believe that death is better than divorce. See Box 22.5 for reasons why people stay in or return to abusive relationships.

Sara:

" I was afraid to stay and also afraid to leave. I was well aware of the fact that most people who try to leave these types of situations are at the most risk when they try to leave. And that's the highest incidence of mortality, when people are leaving these situations and shortly thereafter. What finally enabled me to leave was that my pain became greater than my fear. "

Fear also contributes to the inability to leave a partner in an abusive gay or lesbian relationship. Because many couples

---

BOX 22.5	Why Do They Stay? Why Do They Go Back?

Fear

They fear physical reprisal if they resist, they fear being found and beaten again, or they fear their children will be hurt. Those who attempt to leave risk suffering worse violence and even death.

Learned Helplessness

They believe they have no choices and no control and they have come to believe that violence is an accepted way of life.

Traumatic Bonding

Traumatic bonding results from alternating good and bad treatment and is worsened by an absence of autonomy.

Emotional Dependency

They are convinced that they are weak and inferior and do not deserve better treatment. The thought of potential autonomy is frightening because of their insecurity.

Financial Dependency

They may not have a source of income. If the abuser is arrested, he may lose his job and the family will have no income. They have been taught that they have to be submissive in exchange for financial support.

Guilt/Shame

They have been convinced that they provoked the abuse and often feel guilt over the failure of the relationship. There may be family/religious/cultural values against divorce or separation. They may feel shame about remaining in the abusive relationship.

Severe Depression

Severe depression often accompanies abuse. Victims who are depressed do not have the energy to take action.

Isolation

They have few, if any, friends and little support from extended family. The abuser often allows no phone or mail contact, no use of a car, and may even confine the victim in the home.

Children

Victims may believe two parents are better than one. They may have been threatened with loss of custody or the abuser may threaten to harm or kidnap the children.

Hope

They hope that if they change in the way the abuser wants them to, the abuse will stop. They continue to hope that the abuser will keep promises and stop the assaults.

share close friends within the same community, victims may fear shaming their partners. They may also fear friends will either deny the problem or take the abuser's side. Homophobia contributes to the victim's reluctance to seek help. Calling the police may result in ridicule or hostile responses from the officers. Victims may not seek help from family members to avoid reinforcing negative stereotypes about homosexuality, which might exacerbate the family's homophobia.

Assessment: Cognition

Many abusive people have perfectionistic standards for family members. An unrealistically high standard results in rigidity and an obsession with discipline and control. Inflexibility hinders the abuser's ability to find alternative solutions to conflict. Some abusers have a self-righteous belief that they have a prerogative to use physical force to make others comply with their wishes. Many abusers lack an understanding of the effect of their behavior on the victims and may even blame their abusive behavior on the victims, evidence of the use of denial, projection, and an external locus of control. See Box 22.6 for examples of how people "explain" their violent behavior.

BOX 22.6	How Perpetrators Explain Violent Behavior

Denial

Denial of all or part of their violent behavior—"It never happened."

Forgetting

Blanking out their behavior—"I can't remember."

Minimization

Minimizing the extent, frequency, and effects—"It was just . . ." or "It was only . . . ."

Removal of Self

Separation of the sense of self from the abusive behavior—"I'm not a violent person."

Event Without Intention

Abuse has an independent dynamic of its own—"If she hadn't ducked down, she wouldn't have been hit in her face. She would have only been hit in her belly."

Excuses

Accepts the blame but not the responsibility—"I was abused as a kid, that's why I do it" or "I couldn't help it, I had too much to drink."

Justifications

Accepts the responsibility but not the blame—"You're a lousy mother—I'll teach you to keep these kids quiet."

Confessions

These can be with or without remorse. Confessions become normalized as part of a violent way of life—"I didn't mean to hit you so hard."

Abusers shape reality for and create significant cognitive distortions in their victims. Using fear and isolation, abusers construct a reality in which the victim is defective, incompetent, lazy, careless, ugly, undesirable, promiscuous, stupid, and bad. The abuser then justifies the abuse as punishment for these negative traits.

Many parents who abuse their children suffered emotional deprivation or abuse when they were children. As parents, they may lack information about the normal growth and development of children and therefore have unrealistic expectations. Anger may turn to violence when a child is unable to meet the parent's unreasonable demands.

Victims of abuse often begin with or develop low self-esteem. They begin to believe the violence itself is evidence of personal worthlessness. Some victims even absolve the abuser from responsibility by blaming violent behavior on a high level of stress or too much alcohol.

Assessment: Interpersonal Relationships

The abuser's family history is important in understanding interpersonal violence. Much of adult behavior is determined by childhood experiences within the family system. The experience of violence in the family of origin teaches that the use of physical force is appropriate. Children may cope with exposure to abuse by identifying with either the aggressor or the victim. Often, these children grow up to become another abuser or adult victim. In addition, the media provide ample opportunity for children to see violence and learn to identify with and tolerate violent behavior.

The violent family is often socially isolated. In some families, the isolation precedes the violence. In others, the isolation is in response to the violence. Family members, ashamed of what is occurring, withdraw from interactions with others to avoid the humiliation that might occur if the violence became known.

Abused women experience significant stress when they leave their abusers. Women who are forced to flee from their abusers to seek safety must give up their homes, their jobs, their system of childcare, and perhaps financial security. Women who experience these significant life changes and have few supportive networks are at risk for problems such as depression and posttraumatic stress disorder.

Sara:

66 I've had to rebuild my life from scratch. I left my job because it was directly tied into his business. I did the financial end of his business. We were together for 9 years and I was entitled to absolutely nothing when it came to my leaving him. I lost a lot of myself and I lost people from my life who stayed in contact with him. I went into a downward spiral of depression when I realized how much I had lost and just how much danger I had been in. 99

Assessment: Cultural Influences

Violence is a complex behavior, and, like all behaviors, it occurs in the context of culture. Severe and ongoing interpersonal violence has been documented in almost every country in the past 25 years. Most victims are females. In a study of 90 societies throughout the world, wife beating was present in 75 societies. There appear to be four cultural factors that are strong predictors of wife abuse. The strongest factor is (1) gender economic inequality, followed by (2) male authority and decision making in the home, (3) divorce restrictions for women, and (4) a pattern of using physical violence for conflict resolution. The more women are dependent on men, the more vulnerable they are to violent action with no options for escape (Desjarlais, Eisenberg, Good, & Kleinman, 1995).

The United States has a higher rate of intrafamily homicide than the overall rate of homicide in European countries such as England, Germany, and Denmark. Women of all racial and ethnic backgrounds are exposed to acts of violence by their male partners. The rate of violence for American women is 22%. In addition, 29% of African American women are abused and 37% of American Indian women are abused. Risk factors include low socioeconomic status, unemployment/underemployment, and financial hardship. Euro-American children are more likely to be abused by a biological parent, whereas other American children are more likely to be abused by someone other than a parent. African American mothers use more physical and verbal punishment than Euro-American mothers but they also have behaviors that are more nurturing, which may serve as a buffer to the punishment (Daniels, 2005; Fontes, 2005).

Immigration is very disruptive to families. The greater the difference between the culture of origin and the new environment, the longer lasting the culture shock. If the immigrant family had negative experiences with authorities in their native country, they may wish to avoid contact with the police or social service agencies. If they are undocumented immigrants, they may fear that their illegal status will be discovered if they report interpersonal violence.

Assessment: Physical

Unexplained bruises, abrasions, lacerations, burns, fractures, knife wounds, or old injuries in various stages of healing should alert you to the possibility of abuse. The size, shape, and appearance of all injuries must be carefully documented. Be aware that some victims use makeup, clothing, or hair to cover injuries. See the Focused Nursing Assessment feature for indicators of physical abuse.

DIAGNOSIS

There are a number of nursing diagnoses for victims and perpetrators of interpersonal violence (North American Nursing Diagnosis Association, 2007). Priority must be given to critical and serious physical injuries. The severity and potential fatality of the situation must be considered, as well as the needs of dependent children and legal issues surrounding the case. The care of physical injuries or physical neglect is beyond the scope of this text. Refer to a medical–surgical nursing text for this information.

- Interrupted Family Process related to an inability to manage conflict without violence
- Risk for Other-directed Violence related to a history of physical force with family or intimate friends
- Impaired Parenting related to abuse or neglect of children with ineffective parenting skills
- Powerlessness related to feelings of being dependent on the abuser
- Chronic Low Self-esteem related to feeling responsible and guilty for being a victim of interpersonal violence
- Social Isolation related to control by perpetrator and shame regarding family violence

OUTCOME IDENTIFICATION AND GOALS

Based on the assessment data, you select outcomes appropriate to the nursing diagnoses. Two broad outcomes are:

- Victims remain safe.
- Abusive behavior ends.

Client goals are specific behavioral prescriptions that you, the client, and significant others have identified as realistic and attainable. The following are examples of goals that may be pertinent to victims and perpetrators of violence:

- Remains safe and free from harm
- Develops an escape plan
- Manages conflict appropriately
- Verbalizes an internal locus of control
- Verbalizes an understanding of normal growth and development of children
- Implements appropriate and safe parenting techniques
- Utilizes community resources

PLANNING

Once the nursing diagnoses, outcome criteria, and goals have been identified, the nurse develops the plan of care to assist clients toward a safer and more predictable level of life functioning. Priorities of care are:

- Prevention of violence
- Safety
- Community advocacy

IMPLEMENTATION

Most victims of violence would like it to end, but they may not know how to seek the help they need. It is extremely important that you are nonjudgmental in your interactions with all family members. Initially, clients may be unwilling to trust you because of family shame and fears of being accused for remaining in the violent situation. It is vital that you do not impose your own values by offering quick and easy solutions to the very complicated problem of violence. Your approach should be a *survivor-centered approach.* This is not a group of specific techniques but rather a perspective or way of seeing and understanding the context in which women and children live, recognizing the cultural values that underlie domestic violence. Using this approach, speak up and say that violence is wrong and will not be tolerated.

Treatment of families experiencing violence requires a multidisciplinary approach, with a broad range of interventions. Nurses, social workers, physicians, family therapists, vocational trainers, police, protective services personnel, and lawyers must coordinate to intervene effectively in a violence situation.

Crisis State Related to Violence

The desired outcome is that the client returns to a precrisis (or higher) level of functioning.

Crisis intervention is an intensive, short-term counseling process based on assessment and diffusion of volatile violence situations. It is a time-limited approach to problem identification designed to promote the victim's return to a precrisis level of functioning within 4 to 6 weeks. Intervention is directed toward developing rapport with the victim, clarifying the presenting problems, and enhancing the victim's existing problem-solving ability. See chapter 9 ∞ for more detailed information on crisis intervention.

Crisis intervention focuses on the immediate problem and seeks an answer to the question, "Why have you come for help now?" A precipitating event of major consequence usually has occurred within a few days of seeking therapy. The primary point of crisis intervention is self-help on the part of the client, with assistance from the nurse. Successful crisis resolution leads to growth and an increased ability to cope in the future. Failure to resolve the issues contributes to decreased adaptation and perhaps problems in the future.

Violence Within the Community

The desired outcomes will be that communities will lower the incidence of interpersonal violence, protect victims of violence, and provide long-term resources for victims of violence.

Primary prevention includes educating the general population on the existence of interpersonal violence and its devastating effects. Nursing interventions include parent education, family life education, dating violence awareness and conflict resolution programs in schools, referral for appropriate child or elder care, establishing support groups, and educating fellow nurses about the problem of violence. It is important to challenge the belief that violence is a normal part of loving relationships. You can challenge gender stereotypes while exploring egalitarian relationships, social power, and personal power.

As a professional, you can monitor the media and keep the pressure on to decrease the amount of violence that is portrayed. It is tragic that some young people's popular music contains messages that support violence against females. Similar to the seat belt campaign, state and federal campaigns should be developed for zero tolerance against interpersonal violence.

Secondary prevention includes working with people who are victims or who have seen their loved ones beaten, and making referrals for multidisciplinary intervention. Teen victims and perpetrators of dating violence benefit from peer support and feedback in a group format. This allows them to learn from one another as well as provide support to other victims. Teach people the importance of confronting friends when they behave aggressively toward one another. Explain that it is important to send the message that violence is not socially acceptable.

Nurses must be community advocates in supporting hotlines, crisis centers, and shelters for victims of violence. Battered women's shelters need volunteer nurses to help support their programs. Violence information flyers should be available in health care facilities. Public women's bathrooms should have local violence hotline numbers posted in an easily visible site. On the political level, nurses must make their voices heard in regard to policies and laws affecting children, women, and older people. Questions to guide the evaluation of nursing practice include the following:

- What action have I taken to decrease violence in the media?
- Have I been an advocate for gun control?
- Have I confronted the use of physical punishment within families?
- Have I volunteered to teach parenting classes at grade schools and high schools?
- Have I written to legislators to protest funding cuts in programs designed to help children, women, and older people?

NURSING CARE PLAN for a Client Experiencing Interpersonal Violence

Maintaining Safety
Nursing Diagnosis: Client at Risk for Trauma

Outcomes: Client remains safe, and implements safety measures when dating.

In the initial contact with family members, ensure their physical safety as much as possible. It is critical to assess the level of danger for the victim; homicide may be a real possibility if previous threats have been made. If an adult is being abused, it is likely that children are being abused. Even if the children are not being physically abused, witnessing violence can be devastating. It is also important to assess the level of danger for the abuser. The severity and duration of the violence are the factors that contribute the most directly to victims killing their abusers in self-defense. If the level of danger is high, protective services or the police should be contacted for emergency custody placement or removal to a shelter.

You should help women develop a "safe plan" or "escape plan" to use when their safety is threatened. The goal is to escape before violence occurs. Young people should design their own safety dating plan. Refer young people to Break the Cycle—Empowering Youth to End Domestic Violence at http://www.breakthecycle.org or 888–988–8336. This group provides interpersonal violence education, information, and help to people ages 12 to 24. The earlier people learn that violence is not an option, the more self-protective they can be. The most common legal intervention is in civil law that is a restraining or protective order. The police evict the abuser from the family home and order him not to have contact with the victim. Hiring an attorney to get a protective order costs almost $2,000. Many people cannot afford such fees. There are restraining order clinics that help people obtain orders for themselves, but they are the exception, not the rule. Thus, legal protection is not equally accessible for all individuals.

There are two types of protective orders: a temporary protective order lasts only 2 weeks, whereas a permanent protective order lasts 12 months. Research shows that women with temporary protective orders experience more psychological abuse such as harassment, stalking, and threats than those without protective orders. Women with permanent protective orders are 80% less likely to be physically abused than those without protective orders (Holt, Kernic, Lumley, Wolf, & Rivara, 2002).

Intervention	Rationale	Goal
Safe plan: ■ Decide on a quick, safe exit from the home. ■ Determine a safe place to go and teach it to the children. ■ Put important documents in a secure location (birth certificates, orders of protection, money, medications, list of important phone numbers, few days clothing). ■ Have an extra set of car keys.	Exact and careful preplanning will aid escape during a time when anxiety and fear are at a high level.	Formulates escape plan
Safety dating plan: ■ Consider double-dating the first few times when going out with a new person. ■ Before leaving, know the exact plans for the date. ■ Inform parents or friend of these plans. ■ Establish an expected time home. ■ Explain that drugs or alcohol heighten danger. ■ Never leave a party with someone you have just met. ■ If uncomfortable, assert yourself and leave the situation. ■ Keep cell phone fully charged.	Careful preplanning and informing others of those plans may prevent dating violence. Substances decrease one's ability to react to threatening or dangerous situations.	Remains safe

Managing Anger
Nursing Diagnosis: Client at Risk for Other-Directed Violence

Outcomes: Client demonstrates effective anger management techniques, and verbalizes responsibility for own feelings and behavior.

NURSING CARE PLAN for a Client Experiencing Interpersonal Violence

Managing Anger   *continued*
Nursing Diagnosis: Client at Risk for Other-Directed Violence

Family interventions also include helping identify methods to manage anger appropriately. All family members must assume responsibility for their own behavior. Most abusers do not seek treatment unless it is court ordered or there are custody issues involved. It is frustrating to intervene with abusers who deny the reality of or the responsibility for their anger and violence.

Compared with other forms of murder, it is much easier to pick up a gun and kill someone in anger. The federal *Gun Control Act of 1968* prohibits anyone who has been convicted of a felony from owning or possessing a firearm or ammunition. The 1996 amendment to the act prohibits anyone who has been convicted of a misdemeanor involving interpersonal violence from owning or possessing a firearm or ammunition. There are no exceptions to this law including police or military personnel, although the National Rifle Association is challenging this law. Violation of this act results in 10 years in prison and a fine of $250,000.

The presence of a gun in the home means that a woman is 7.2 times as likely to be a victim of homicide by a spouse, an intimate partner, or a close relative. Encourage all clients to remove guns from the family home. If you would like to know how your individual state rates in terms of gun safety and interpersonal violence you may access this information at:

http://www.bradycampaign.org/facts/factsheets/report%20cards.

Intervention	Rationale	Goals
Suggest appropriate expression such as talking out anger as it occurs, physical exercise, striking safe, inanimate object (pillow, couch, punching bag).	When people can use alternative expression of anger, the use of violence will decrease.	Implements alternative strategies to manage anger
Help family establish limits and definite consequences if violence recurs.	Setting and enforcement of limits may lead to the extinction of violence.	Enforces limits on violence
Group therapy for perpetrators: ■ Responsibility for aggression is always placed on the aggressor. ■ Discuss issues such as patriarchal and power view of relationships. ■ Using genograms or family maps, look for a family history of violence. ■ Examine types of abuse. ■ Examine each member's specific abusive behaviors and the effect on their victims. ■ Role-play diversional activities. ■ Develop an emergency phone list.	Acknowledging responsibility is the first step in changing behavior. Those who see women and children as property are at higher risk to use violence for control. Reconnecting with own past feelings of being a victim may increase empathy for those who are currently victims. Perpetrators must acknowledge that violence is always a conscious choice. Diversional activities can be used when they feel they are losing control.	Verbalizes an understanding that anger can be controlled Decreases or eliminates the use of violence against others

Improving Communication
Nursing Diagnosis: Client at Risk for Decisional Conflict

Outcome: Client utilizes effective communication techniques.

Families experiencing violence often have poor communication skills. Nursing interventions can be designed to improve the family members' communication. Chapter 2 ∞ discusses family communication and family competency in more detail.

Intervention	Rationale	Goals
Teach communication skills: ■ Active listening with feedback ■ Clear and direct communication ■ Communication that does not attack personhood of family members	Improved communication skills will enable family to resolve issues before they escalate to the point of violence.	Communicates more directly and clearly; family members actively listen to one another
Discuss how disagreement in a family is inevitable.	Counteracts the myth that happiness will occur only where there is no conflict.	Identifies the normality of conflict
Explore with the family the democratic process in conflict resolution and decision making.	The more democratic the family structure in decision making and conflict resolution, the less likely that violence will occur.	Verbalizes understanding of democratic process
Using a minor, nonemotional family problem, have family solve the problem in a democratic manner.	Once the process is learned, family can transfer this knowledge and ability to solve other problems.	Uses democratic process

continued

NURSING CARE PLAN for a Client Experiencing Interpersonal Violence

Empowering Victims
Nursing Diagnosis: Client at Risk for Hopelessness

Outcome: Client verbalizes feelings of empowerment, and acts on own behalf.

One of the primary goals of therapy is empowering victims. The process of violence removes all power and control from a person, resulting in low self-esteem, anxiety, depression, and somatic problems. The following principles are basic to the empowerment of victims:

- A commitment to the belief that women and men are inherently equal
- An egalitarian approach to the nurse–client relationship in which the client is viewed as an equal partner rather than a helpless recipient of nursing interventions
- That a victim cannot keep the partner/parent from being violent by trying to "do better"
- Interventions that focus on the enhancement of the victim's power
- An emphasis on the victim's strengths and abilities
- That everyone deserves relationships that are nonviolent
- Respect for the victim's ability to understand her or his own experiences
- Family interventions that change destructive roles and expectations within the family system
- A willingness to state clear value positions about interpersonal violence

Intervention	Rationale	Goals
Help client identify past dependency relationships.	Identifying patterns will help client focus on how she maintains her own feelings of powerlessness.	Identifies past dependent relationship(s)
Help formulate a list of ways she is dependent on abuser (e.g., emotional and economic areas of dependency).	High levels of dependency make it difficult for victim to leave abuser without intense support.	Formulates list of dependencies
Help client identify intrapersonal and interpersonal strengths.	Recognition of strengths will decrease feelings of helplessness.	Identifies strengths
Help client identify aspect(s) of life under her control.	Feelings of control will decrease feelings of powerlessness.	Identifies situations of control
Provide assertiveness training. Caution client if she is still in an abusive situation, that assertive behavior may escalate the violence.	Continued submission to violence often escalates episodes of violent behavior.	Utilizes assertive techniques
Avoid trying to convince adult victims to leave their abuser. Be willing to support clients in their pain, rather than telling them what to do about their problems. Support and affirm positive choices and decisions they make.	For the most adaptive outcome, adult victims must be their own rescuers and take charge of their own safety and protection plan. If they need help with this process they must be taught to ask for that help directly.	Takes responsibility for self; verbalizes feeling more in control of situations
Refer to community resources for financial aid, legal aid, or job training.	This will decrease dependency on abuser.	Follows through on referrals

Improving Parenting Skills
Nursing Diagnosis: Client at Risk for Impaired Parenting

Outcomes: Client implements nonviolent discipline measures, and spends enjoyable family time together.

Parents who are physically abusive need help in developing and improving their parenting skills. Teach and encourage positive discipline, which includes:

- Tell children what is allowed as well as what is not allowed.
- Offer choices rather than threats.
- Requests should be realistic and age appropriate.
- Choose your battles—do not argue over every small transgression.
- Acknowledge and reward appropriate behavior.
- Spend enjoyable time together.

Parents need support in implementing, practicing, and evaluating these new skills. They need to help their children develop their own self-control as they manage each developmental stage.

NURSING CARE PLAN for a Client Experiencing Interpersonal Violence

Improving Parenting Skills *continued*
Nursing Diagnosis: Client at Risk for Impaired Parenting

Intervention	Rationale	Goals
Express concern for all family members, including parents.	When parents understand the nurse is also concerned about them, they will be more willing to become actively involved in treatment.	Acknowledges concern and care
Give recognition for positive parenting skills.	Recognition of positive aspects will increase parents' feelings of worth and engages them in the learning process.	Identifies areas of strengths in parenting
Share your understanding that the use of violence is a desperate attempt to cope with their children.	Confirming that they care about their children will increase the likelihood of their active participation in the treatment process.	Identifies need to cope more effectively
Discuss with parents how they were punished as children.	Violence is often transgenerational.	Discusses childhood experiences
Teach parents about normal growth and development of their children.	Unrealistic demands on children often result in violence in an attempt to have children comply beyond their developmental ability.	Verbalizes knowledge of growth and development
Help parents identify parenting tools other than physical force that are age appropriate for their children.	Lack of alternative skills contributes to increased use of violence.	Identifies alternative skills
Refer to community resources (e.g., crisis hotlines, Parents Anonymous, family therapy, group therapy).	Alternatives to violence can be discussed and role-played with other parents.	Parents make a nonviolent contract such as, "We don't believe in using violence to get our way and we will not do so in the future."
Encourage parents to have a few hours away from the children during the week.	This often lowers the level of stress and tension in the home.	Takes short breaks when necessary while providing for child safety
Recommend the family schedule family nights once every week or two. All electronic devices such as TVs, computers, video games, and cell phones should be shut down. Encourage families to play games, take walks, talk together, or have a story time.	These occasions allow members to reconnect through activities fostering new feelings and new behaviors in the family.	Schedules and implements family activities

Developing Support Networks
Nursing Diagnosis: Client at Risk for Caregiver Role Strain

Outcomes: Client cares for elderly family members in appropriate ways.

Support the elder person and caretakers in identifying and expanding social support networks that may decrease the level of stress within the household. These outside individuals may be able to help with activities of daily living (ADLs), transportation, financial advice, and assistance with personal problems.

continued

NURSING CARE PLAN for a Client Experiencing Interpersonal Violence

Developing Support Networks   *continued*
Nursing Diagnosis: Client at Risk for Caregiver Role Strain

Intervention	Rationale	Goals
Assist caregivers in exploring their feelings about the older person in their care.	Unexplored and unresolved negative feelings contribute to the potential for violence.	Discusses feelings
Help caregivers identify situations that are disturbing to them.	These situations may contribute to neglect or abuse.	Discusses disturbing situations
Determine the caretakers' ability to meet their loved one's needs and provide appropriate teaching.	Ensure safety of the elderly person.	Implements safe care for their loved one
Encourage family to formulate alternatives for coping with elderly person in the home: ■ Investigate day care centers. ■ Investigate extended care centers. ■ Enlist help from other family members. ■ Investigate short-term respite care so family can take a vacation.	Decreasing stress of total care for elderly person will decrease use of violence in the home.	Develops and implements plans to provide relief
Provide community resource information.	There are a number of agencies that offer senior service assistance.	Follows through on referrals

■ Have I spoken out on the need to increase the number of bilingual/bicultural counselors, lawyers, nurses, and physicians to attend to the cultural needs of families?

All nurses should evaluate their professional obligations and practice in counteracting those aspects of society that foster violence. Interpersonal violence is a mental health problem of national and international importance, and nurses should be leaders in helping prevent it in future generations.

Evaluation

Nurses in long-term settings or within the community have an opportunity to evaluate the effectiveness of the multidisciplinary treatment plan over an extended period of time. When violence no longer exists within the family system, the plan has succeeded. Sharing in the process of family growth and adaptation can be a tremendous source of professional satisfaction.

Using Research Evidence   Men Who Batter

Tilley, D. S., & Brackley, M. (2003). **Men who batter intimate partners: A grounded theory study of the development of male violence in intimate partner relationships.** *Issues in Mental Health Nursing, 26,* 281–297.

What is the study about?

In the United States, approximately 25% of females and 7.6% of males are identified as victims of intimate-partner violence, including spousal abuse. The number of victims might be reduced if we understood risk factors related to this aggressive behavior. Therefore, the purpose of this study was to develop a grounded theory of the development of intimate-partner violence by male partners, emerging from the point of view of the male batterer.

How was the study done?

This qualitative, grounded-theory study was based on a pilot study that had identified the context of violence in the lives of male batterers. The present study used semistructured face-to-face audiotaped interviews to discuss the men's experience of victimizing their intimate partner. Interviews were conducted at the site of the Batterers' Intervention and Prevention Program (BIPP). From a larger group of men completing that program, a purposive sample of 16 men volunteered to participate in this study that was approved by the institutional review board. The men were not in prison, and agreeing to participate in the study did not affect their position in the BIPP. Participants were requested to complete a demographic survey and take part in a 1-hour interview. These narrative data were synthesized via constant comparative analysis, to identify concepts and relational statements that might explain the intimate-partner violence.

What were the results of the study?

Data analysis yielded 22 large concepts, listed here from least to most prevalent: power and control, social isolation, desensitization to violence, relationships with mothers, violence as a private problem, parenting, ambivalent relationships, objectification of

Using Research Evidence   Men Who Batter   *continued*

females, immaturity, lack of awareness, mistrust, traditional views of women's roles, financial concerns, jealousy, justifying violence, minimizing violence, mutual violence, childhood exposure to violence, ineffective anger management, ineffective conflict resolution within the intimate relationship, use or abuse of alcohol or drugs, and social and familial influences. Interestingly, none of these men had used social isolation to maintain control.

Through the process of selective coding, researchers identified a major concept as families living in chaos. Many of the men came from chaotic families. These chaotic families had a history of fathers who abused alcohol and used physical violence with their spouses and children. The researchers posit that these participants and their intimate partners seem to have transferred the chaos from their upbringing to their current family and intimate relationships. The findings from this study are congruent with existing literature regarding intimate-partner violence. However, the grounded theory that emerged, called the Violent Families Paradigm, shifts away from a long-held view that considered the victim and batterer separately.

What additional questions might I have?

Is the Violent Families Paradigm relevant to other societal concerns? Are there specific developmental periods in a boy's life when he is more vulnerable to fallout of family violence? Why do siblings raised in the same family environment have differing experiences as adults with intimate-partner violence?

How can I use this study?

The results of this study have significant implications for nurses in health education. Previously, many educational programs for the prevention of domestic abuse have focused on educating women about its signs and symptoms. However, an additional focus should be avoiding family violence because it can contribute to future violence in intimate-partner relationships. In addition, intimate-partner violence may be reduced through programs that help boys and young men manage anger and avoid alcohol and drugs.

SOURCE: Contributed by Dolores Huffman, PhD, RN, Associate Professor of Nursing, Purdue University Calumet, Hammond, Indiana.

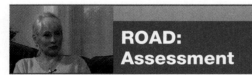

ROAD: Assessment   Critical Thinking Questions

Go to the CD-ROM to assess Sara by answering the following critical thinking questions based on what you have **R**ead about Sara and **O**bserved on the videos.

1. Sara is at a safe house for women who are victims of interpersonal violence. She talks about her abuse during her interview, which can be heard on segment A of your student ROAD CD-ROM for chapter 22 . What dynamics are present between Sara and her abuser as disclosed in this interaction? Support your answer.

2. While talking with Sara she tells you that she was afraid to leave her partner and at times thought that the abuse would go away if she was a *better* person or if he didn't drink so much. Sara also believed that she should have done a better job of being his girlfriend, meeting his needs, and handling the finances for his business. Sara tells you that she never spoke to anyone about what was going on in the relationship. He didn't like her spending time with the friends she had before they met and when they did socialize it was only with his friends. What is your assessment of Sara's cognitions while she lived in the abusive relationship? Explain your answer.

3. Sara voices the following in segment B of your student ROAD CD-ROM for chapter 22. What diagnosis might you find recorded on Axis I of Sara's DSM-IV-TR formulation? Support your answer with the corresponding signs and symptoms that you assess are present within her statements. (Hint: Refer to the appendices and chapter 11 in your text to help your respond to this question).

4. In screening for interpersonal violence (IPV) as part of your nursing practice: (*Hint:* Use the following Web site, http://endabuse.org/programs/healthcare/files/nursing.pdf, in addition to the knowledge you have gained from studying chapter 22, to assist you in answering the following questions)
   a. Discuss the nursing approach you would use to screen clients for IPV.
   b. Provide an example of how you would introduce screening for IPV to a client.
   c. Give an example of a verbal statement you could use that conveys trust, promotes an open-ended response, and targets the client's disclosure about IPV.

5. Many medical records that contain an assessment for IPV expose documentation shortcomings that ultimately render the evidence inadmissible in legal proceedings. Health care providers can improve their efforts to document evidence and strengthen an IPV victim's case. Identify two things that you can incorporate into your nursing practice and/or nursing documentation of IPV. (*Hint:* Use information found in the focused nursing assessment for IPV in chapter 22 and the Web site, http://www.ncjrs.org/txtfiles1/nij/188564.txt to assist you in formulating your answer.)

ROAD: DEVELOP A CARE PLAN

 Go to the CD-ROM to develop a care plan based on your assessment of Sara. Identify nursing diagnoses, outcomes, goals, and interventions.

SOURCE: Contributed by Susan Siwinski-Hebel, RN, MSN.

Focus Your Study

OBJECTIVES

KEY CONCEPTS

1. Describe the types of abuse that are likely to occur at each point in the life span.

- The form of violence most unrecognized occurs between siblings.
- Homicide is one of the five leading causes of death before the age of 18.
- Physical abuse occurs among as many as 30% to 50% of college students and 10% to 35% of high school students who are dating.
- Seventy-six percent of victims of heterosexual intimate partner violence are women. This is the most widespread form of family violence in the United States.
- Violence occurs in some gay and lesbian families for the same reasons as in heterosexual families—that is, to maintain power and control over the partner.
- Two million elderly people are mistreated each year in the United States.
- Pregnancy is a time of increased risk for abuse.

2. Discuss the mental health implications for a victim of interpersonal violence.

- Problems associated with child abuse include depression, substance abuse, self-mutilation, eating disorders, and dissociative disorders.
- Conduct disorder is nine times as likely to occur in abused teens as in the nonabused population.
- The majority of abused children and adults develop posttraumatic stress disorder.
- Abused adults are at risk for depression, anxiety disorders, substance abuse, and suicide.

3. Discuss the different theories regarding the etiology of interpersonal violence.

- Neurobiology:
  - Abnormally low levels of serotonin (5-HT) result in a lack of control, loss of temper, and explosive rage.
- Intrapersonal theory:
  - Perpetrators have a lack of self-regulation that leads them to overreact to stress.
  - The majority of perpetrators grew up in violent homes, leading them to externalize or internalize their responses to this violence.
- Social learning theory:
  - Violence is a learned behavior and people are conditioned to respond aggressively and violently.
  - The media provide many models of violence to which children and adults are exposed.
- Gender-bias factors:
  - Violence is a power and control issue.
  - Women are blamed for being victims of violence.
  - Women are often forced to choose between poverty and abuse.

4. Outline the assessment process for a client experiencing interpersonal violence.

- One third of all women's visits to the emergency department are caused by interpersonal violence.
- Behavior:
  - Perpetrators choose to be violent, are not out of control, and are often only dangerous to their loved ones.
  - Typical cycle is: conflict escalates into violence, perpetrator begs for victim's forgiveness, victim stays because of promises to reform, violence recurs.
  - In the clinical setting, the perpetrator may speak for the victim, correct her answers to questions, and refuse to leave her alone with the health care provider.
- Affect:
  - Perpetrators are often extremely jealous and possessive.
  - Victims are often immobilized by helplessness, depression, self-blame, and fear.
- Cognition:
  - Perpetrators have a self-righteous belief in use of physical force and blame the victim for the violence.
  - Parents who abuse their children often have unrealistic expectations about normal growth and development of children.
- Interpersonal relationships:
  - Violent families are often socially isolated.

5. Discuss the key points in effectively communicating with a person experiencing interpersonal violence.

- In all clinical settings, clients should be asked one or two introductory questions related to abuse.
- Ask children, "Moms and Dads try to help their children learn how to behave well. What happens to you when you do something wrong?"
- Ask adolescents, "Is hitting okay when your boyfriend/girlfriend flirts with other people or catches you flirting with someone else, or if you get hit first?"
- Ask adults, "One of the sources of stress in our lives is family disagreement. Could you describe how disagreements affect you? What happens when you disagree?"
- If the responses to these questions are indicative of violence, a focused nursing assessment must be conducted.

6. Develop teaching plans for a client experiencing interpersonal violence and her/his family.

- Primary prevention in the community includes educating people about interpersonal violence and challenging stereotypes underlying violence.
- Secondary prevention includes working with victims, supporting crisis centers and shelters, and interacting with law makers to protect victims of violence.
- Work with the family in ways to manage their anger appropriately.
- Teach parents positive discipline strategies for various developmental levels.
- Teach the family basic communication and conflict resolution skills.
- Teach adolescents and young adults about safe dating plans.

7. Use the nursing process to develop a safe, comprehensive plan of care for a client experiencing interpersonal violence.

- Help victims develop a safe or escape plan and obtain a protective order.
- Empower adult victims to advocate for themselves and maintain their own safety.
- Crisis intervention helps victims identify problems and enhance problem-solving abilities.
- Help caretakers of the elderly find social support and respite care.
- Refer clients to community resources.
- In all 50 states, nurses are required by law to report suspected incidents of child abuse.
- In every state, there is a penalty—civil, criminal, or both—for failure to report child abuse.
- Not reporting child abuse is considered nursing malpractice.
- The majority of states have laws regarding the reporting of elder abuse.

Explore MediaLink

For review questions, case studies, and other resources for this chapter see the Pearson Health MediaLink CD-ROM that accompanies this book and the Companion Website.

CD-ROM
- Audio Glossary
- NCLEX-RN® Review Questions
- ROAD to Critical Thinking: *Sara*

Companion Website www.prenhall.com/fontaine
- Audio Glossary
- NCLEX-RN® Review Questions
- Case Study
  - Interpersonal Abuse
- Care Plan
  - Abuse in a Cultural Context
  - Care Plan for a Victim of Abuse
- Critical Thinking
  - Spousal Abuse
- MediaLink Application
  - Why Do Women Stay in a Violent Relationship?
  - Sexual Trauma Survival
- MediaLinks
  - Books for Clients & Families
  - Community Resources

NCLEX-RN® Review Questions

22-1. Which of the following individuals is at highest risk for physical abuse?
1. A 20-year-old college student on a first date with her sister, her sister's fiancé, and his friend
2. A 16-year-old male who is the oldest of four children being raised by a single mother
3. A 30-year-old female who receives repeated unwelcome emails from a stranger
4. A 17-year-old pregnant woman who did not seek prenatal care until her seventh month

22-2. Which of the following behaviors does the school nurse recognize is an indicator that a school-age child has been physically abused?
1. The child acts obediently when a parent scolds him to be quiet.
2. The child sits quietly with a friend in the school yard instead of playing kickball.
3. The child bullies other children and threatens them to "keep quiet about it or else."
4. The child tells other children that they will get a "time-out" if they continue to misbehave.

22-3. A client who has been physically abused asks the nurse, "What makes people so violent toward others?" Which of the following is the best response to this question?
1. "It is difficult to give one specific reason for violent behavior."
2. "Hormones are the primary reason for violence in men."
3. "If women were more agreeable, there wouldn't be any violence."
4. "Violence is inherited from a person's family."

22-4. A 63-year-old man with Alzheimer disease is brought to the emergency department (ED) with pressure sores and severe dehydration. Upon further assessment, the nurse notices bruises on the client's neck, arms, and legs. Which of the following questions should the nurse ask the client's wife?
1. "What kind of support do you have at home to care for your husband?"
2. "Have you considered placing your husband in a nursing home?"
3. "How often do you turn your husband while he's in bed?"
4. "How long do you leave your husband at home alone?"

22-5. Which of the following nursing diagnoses is the most important for a homosexual client who has been repeatedly physically assaulted by his partner?
1. Powerlessness related to feelings of dependence on significant other
2. Risk for Injury related to history of abuse by significant other
3. Chronic Low Self-esteem related to guilt and shame for being a victim of abuse
4. Social Isolation related to control by the significant other and feelings of inadequacy

22-6. A student health nurse employed by a university is concerned about the increase of dating violence reported on campus. The nurse should be concerned if which preventive measure was included in a safety presentation for women in the dormitory?
1. Before going on a date, make sure your cell phone is fully charged.
2. Always inform a friend or family member who you are with and when you expect to return.
3. If you are uncomfortable in a situation, always ask a male student to drive you home.
4. Never drink from a glass that was left unattended or given to you by someone else.

22-7. A nurse came to work with a black eye and swollen lip. Her coworkers have noticed that her boyfriend calls her at least 10 times during her 12-hour shift. She has refused all invitations to go out with her coworkers, saying that her boyfriend will be there to pick her up and he doesn't like to wait for her. What is the most helpful response by the coworkers?
1. Convince the nurse to leave her boyfriend.
2. Encourage the nurse to get a restraining order against her boyfriend.
3. Enlist her parents' aid in getting her away from the boyfriend.
4. Encourage the nurse to talk to a professional.

See Appendix D for answers.

References

Adshead, G., & Bluglass, K. (2005). Attachment representations in mothers with abnormal illness behaviour by proxy. *British Journal of Psychiatry, 187*(10), 328–333.

Amar, A. F. (2006). College women's experience of stalking. *Archives of Psychiatric Nursing, 20*(3), 108–116.

Amar, A. F., & Gennaro, S. (2005). Dating violence in college women. *Nursing Research, 54*(4), 235–242.

Close, S. M. (2005). Dating violence prevention in middle school and high school youth. *Journal of Child and Adolescent Psychiatric Nursing, 18*(1), 2–9.

Crane, P. A., & Constantino, R. (2003). Is email interaction feasible for intervention with women and children exposed to domestic violence? A literature review. *Topics in Advanced Practice Nursing eJournal, 3*(3), 1–8.

Daniels, K. (2005). Violence and depression. *Journal of Psychosocial Nursing, 43*(1), 45–51.

Desjarlais, R., Eisenberg, L., Good, B., & Kleinman, A. (1995). *World mental health.* New York: Oxford University Press.

Downs, W. R., & Miller, B. A. (2002). Treating dual problems of partner abuse and substance abuse. In C. Wekerle & A. Wall (Eds.), *The violence and addiction equation* (pp. 254–274). New York: Brunner-Routledge.

Edwards, V. J., Holden, G. W., Felitti, V. J., & Anda, R. F. (2003). Relationship between multiple forms of childhood maltreatment and adult mental health in community respondents. *American Journal of Psychiatry, 160*(8), 1453–1460.

Ewing, C. P. (1997). *Fatal families.* Thousand Oaks, CA: Sage.

Fontes, L. A. (2005). *Child abuse and culture.* New York: Guilford Press.

Freedberg, P. (2006). Health care barriers and same-sex intimate partner violence. *Journal of Forensic Nursing, 2*(1), 15–24, 41.

Friedman, S. H., Horwitz, S. M., & Resnick, P. J. (2005). Child murder by mothers. *American Journal of Psychiatry, 162*(9), 1578–1587.

Griffin, M. G., Resick, P. A., & Yehuda, R. (2005). Enhanced cortisol suppression following dexamethasone administration in domestic violence survivors. *American Journal of Psychiatry, 162*(6), 1192–1199.

Heintz, A. J., & Melendez, R. M. (2006). Intimate partner violence and HIV/STD risk among lesbian, gay, bisexual, and transgender individuals. *Journal of Interpersonal Violence, 21*(2), 193–208.

Holt, V. L., Kernic, M. A., Lumley, T., Wolf, M. E., & Rivara, F. P. (2002). Civil protection orders and risk of subsequent police-reported violence. *JAMA, 288*(5), 589–594.

Kearney, M. H., Haggerty, L. A., Munro, B. H., & Hawkins, J. W. (2003). Birth outcomes and maternal morbidity in abused pregnant women with public versus private health insurance. *Journal of Nursing Scholarship, 35*(4), 345–349.

Loeber, R., LaCourse, E., & Homish, D. L. (2005). Homicide, violence and developmental trajectories. In R. E. Tremblay, W. W. Hartup, & J. Archer (Eds.), *Developmental origins of aggression* (pp. 202–219). New York: Guilford Press.

Marleau, J. D. (2005). Birth order and fratricide. *Medicine, Science, and the Law, 45*(1), 52–56.

Muscari, M. E. (2005). What should I do when a client is being stalked? *Medscape Ask The Experts Advance Practice Nurse.* Retrieved February 4, 2005, from http://www.medscape.com/viewarticle/502450

North American Nursing Diagnosis Association. (2007). *Nursing diagnoses: Definitions and classification (2007–2008).* Philadelphia, PA: Author.

Patton, S. B. (2003). Understanding the murder of children and intervening to reduce the risk. *Topics in Advanced Practice Nursing eJournal, 3*(3), 1–8.

Pearsall, C. (2005). Forensic biomarkers of elder abuse. *Journal of Forensic Nursing, 194,* 182–186.

Records, K., & Rice, M. J. (2005). A comparative study of postpartum depression in abused and nonabused women. *Archives of Psychiatric Nursing, 19*(6), 281–290.

Reno, J. (1999). Cyberstalking: A new challenge for law enforcement and industry. Retrieved January 5, 2001, from http://www.usdoj.gov/criminal/cybercrime/cyberstalking.htm

Scheiman, L., & Zeoli, A. M. (2003). Adolescents' experiences of dating and intimate partner violence. *Journal of Midwifery and Women's Health, 48*(3), 226–228.

Straus, M. A. (1994). *Beating the devil out of them: Corporal punishment in American families.* Lexington, MA: Lexington Books.

Tan, J. C., & Gregor, K. V. (2006). Violence against pregnant women in northwestern Ontario. *Annals of the New York Academy of Sciences, 11*(1087), 320–338.

Tilley, D. S., & Brackley, M. (2003). Men who batter intimate partners: A grounded theory study of the development of male violence in intimate partner relationships. *Issues in Mental Health Nursing, 26,* 281–297.

Tremblay, R. E., & Nagin, D. S. (2005). The developmental origins of physical aggression in humans. In R. E. Tremblay, W. W. Hartup, & J. Archer (Eds.), *Developmental origins of aggression* (pp. 83–106). New York: Guilford Press.

U.S. Department of Health & Human Services. (2000). *Healthy people 2010.* Retrieved June 2, 2004, from http://www.health.gov/healthypeople/lhi/lhiwhat.htm

Zlotnick, C., Johnson, D. M., & Kohn, R. (2006). Intimate partner violence and long-term psychosocial function in a national sample of American women. *Journal of Interpersonal Violence, 21*(2), 262–275.

Chapter 23

Sexual Violence

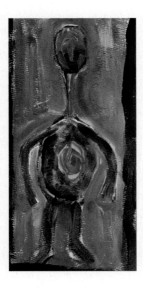

“ *Trauma*

split off
to endure

left with parts
to pull together

an internal family
to work with

separate feelings
with a united force

to win

to heal ”

—Heather, Age 30

OBJECTIVES

After reading this chapter, you will be able to:

1. Discuss the theories regarding the etiologies of rape and childhood sexual abuse.
2. Describe the short- and long-term implications for victims of sexual violence.
3. Outline the assessment process for a victim of sexual violence and her/his family.
4. Use the nursing process to develop a comprehensive plan of care for a victim of sexual violence and her/his family.
5. Develop teaching plans for a victim of sexual violence and her/his family.

MediaLink 🖲 www.prenhall.com/fontaine

Go to the Pearson Health MediaLink CD-ROM and the Companion Website at www.prenhall.com/fontaine for interactive resources for this chapter.

Sexual violence includes criminal behaviors such as sexual harassment, rape, and child sexual abuse. It is defined as the use of threat, intimidation, force, and exploitation of authority with the goal of imposing one's will on a nonconsenting person for the purpose of personal gratification that may or may not be predominantly sexual. Sexual violence is, first and foremost, an act of violence, hatred, and aggression. Like other acts of violence (assault and battery or murder), there is a violation of, and injury to, the victims. The injuries may be physical or psychological. Victims are overwhelmed and overpowered and violated as human beings. During the harassment, attack, or abuse, victims are not only out of control of their situation, but also are assaulted in the most vulnerable dimension of the self. Sexual violence is not an occasional, isolated incident experienced by people in extraordinary situations. Sexual violence is a widespread problem, taking place in a broad social context, which allows and even encourages it to occur. When we encourage gender role differences that accentuate masculine aggression and feminine passivity and when we confuse sexual activity with sexual violence, we create a climate of tolerance of sexual violence in our society.

SEXUAL HARASSMENT

Sexual harassment in the workplace and in schools has always existed as a hidden crime. Only recently has it been recognized for what it is—discrimination against, and violation of, individuals. People frequently do not report harassment because they do not expect to be believed and fear that they will be accused of contributing to the problem. Nurses are not immune to sexual harassment as they practice their profession. Studies have found that 60% to 80% of staff nurses report multiple incidents of sexual harassment, most frequently by clients, followed by coworkers and physicians (Hibino, Ogino, & Inagaki, 2006; Lanza, Zeiss, & Rierdan, 2006).

Sexual harassment is unwanted and unwelcome sexual behavior that interferes with everyday life. It is one end of the continuum of sexual violence against individuals; the other is rape. Sexual harassment behavior includes:

- Sexual teasing, jokes, remarks, or demeaning comments
- Making sexually stereotypical comments
- Showing offensive pictures
- Asking invasive questions regarding a person's personal life
- Persistent pressure for dates
- Letters, telephone calls, or e-mails of a sexual nature
- Sexual gestures

- Deliberate touching, cornering, or pinching
- Invasive watching
- Pressure for sexual favors
- Actual or attempted rape

Adolescent peer sexual harassment includes these behaviors and:

- Calling someone gay or a lesbian in a malicious manner
- Spreading sexual rumors
- Flashing someone or exposing one's naked buttocks ("mooning") to someone
- "Spiking"—pulling down someone's pants
- "Snuggies"—pulling underwear up at the waist so it goes in between the buttocks

The United States Equal Employment Opportunity Commission (EEOC) is the government agency that interprets and enforces employment laws. In 1980, the EEOC issued a position statement clearly stating that sexual harassment is considered a form of sexual discrimination and, therefore, an unlawful employment act. Although most cases of sexual harassment have traditionally involved a male harasser and a female victim, the EEOC also determined that the sexual harasser, as well as the victim, can be either a man or a woman. Research indicates, however, that most harassers are male and that the behavior is more about dominance than about sex.

There are two distinctive categories of sexual harassment: quid pro quo and hostile environment. *Quid pro quo* (translated as "this for that") means that an employer or other person of authority suggests that he or she will give the victim this job, promotion, or salary, in return for that sexual favor. This form of sexual harassment is the most well known. *Hostile environment* sexual harassment is unwelcome sexual conduct that has the purpose or effect of creating an intimidating, hostile, or offensive working environment. This type of sexual harassment can involve supervisors, coworkers, and even customers or vendors. The intent of the law is to give people the opportunity to work in an environment that is free from sex-based discrimination, taunts, jeers, and insults.

Sexual harassment can lead to severe stress in the victims. Many victims experience depression, isolation, feelings of powerlessness, helplessness, fear, restlessness, inability to concentrate, somatic complaints, sexual problems, and loss of self-esteem. At its most severe, harassment resembles the other sexual traumas of rape and child sexual abuse and may result in posttraumatic stress disorder. Filing a complaint of sexual harassment is never easy. Regardless of the outcome, the investigation can be extremely stressful for all people involved (Palmieri & Fitzgerald, 2005). See Box 23.1 for the harassment response steps.

BOX 23.1	Steps Toward Harassment Prevention and Response

- Give verbal notice to the offender. Respond directly and simply; for example, "I don't like it and I want you not to do it again."
- Give stronger warnings and notice that you will report the behavior; for example, "If this happens again, I'm going to discuss this with human resources."
- Issue a written warning.
- Keep a detailed record of the behavior you find objectionable, when it occurred, and what you did in response.
- Make an informal harassment inquiry—discuss the situation with your supervisor or human resources person. The goal is not punishment but problem solving, education, and consciousness raising.
- File a formal complaint within the organization. At this point, the harasser faces serious personal and professional damage. The situation cannot be kept completely confidential and the company or school is obliged to investigate.
- File a complaint with the EEOC in the United States: 800-669-4000.
- In Canada, file a complaint with the Canadian Human Rights Commission: 613-995-1151. It is highly advisable to have an attorney at this point.
- Go to court. This tends to be a long, painful battle. It may be settled before trial.

RAPE

Rape is a crime of violence. It is second only to homicide in its violation of a person. The issue is not one of sex but of force, domination, and humiliation. If you think rape is about sex, you have confused the weapon with the motivation. **Rape** refers to any forced sexual activity; the key factor is the absence of consent. Forcible rape by juveniles in both the United States and the United Kingdom has been on the increase, and teens now account for 18% to 20% of rapes (Murphy & Page, 1999).

KNOWLEDGE BASE: RAPE

Victims

There is no typical rape victim. Of reported rapes, however, 90% to 95% of the victims are female and 90% of the perpetrators are male. Given these percentages, this chapter utilizes the male rapist and female victim as the model. One can be a victim of rape at any age, from childhood through old age. Police records indicate that a woman is raped every 6 minutes in the United States. Experts believe that 80% of rapes are unreported. It is believed that one of every three or four American women will be raped or sexually assaulted at least once in her lifetime. In addition, 50% of victims are raped by a spouse, partner, relative, or friend (Rauch & Foa, 2004; Stermac, Dunlap, & Bainbridge, 2005).

Perpetrators

Of all rapes of women on college campuses, 50% are *date rapes*. Women very rarely report rapes when they know their attackers, especially if they are or were in a dating relationship with the attacker. The victim is often blamed by herself and others for being naive or provocative. A cultural value slow to die is: If a woman accepts a date and allows the man to pay all the expenses, she somehow "owes" him sexual access and has no right to refuse. For ways to minimize the risk of date rape, see Box 23.2.

Certain drugs are called "rape drugs" because they can be used to overpower and incapacitate victims to facilitate a sexual assault. Rohypnol is a benzodiazepine drug that is illegal in the United States. Gamma-hydroxybutyrate (GHB) has euphoric and sedative effects. Ketamine is a dissociative general anesthetic used by veterinarians. These drugs are often slipped into a victim's drink without the victim's knowledge or consent. When dissolved, they are colorless, odorless, and often tasteless. All three of these drugs can be fatal when mixed with alcohol.

Traditionally, husbands have not been charged if they raped their wives. It was not until 1974 in the United States and 1991 in Great Britain that the first cases of marital rape were prosecuted. In 1993, **marital rape** became a crime in all 50 states. Some states, however, still have exemptions from prosecuting husbands for rape. Marital rape is the most prevalent and underreported form of rape; 2 million instances are estimated to occur each year in the United States. Between one third and one half of battered women are raped by their partners. The attacks range from assaults that are relatively quick to those that involve sadistic, torturous episodes that last for hours. In some instances, wives are forced to have sex with other people while their husbands watch. Women who are raped by their husbands or partners are less likely to report the assault or to seek professional help (Rauch & Foa, 2004).

BOX 23.2	Minimizing the Risk of Date Rape

- Be cautious in relationships based on dominant-male, submissive-female stereotypes. Date rapists usually have macho attitudes and believe women to be inferior.
- Be cautious when a date tries to control your behavior—who you can meet, where you can go, what you can do. This indicates a need to dominate and control and increases your vulnerability by isolating you.
- Do not drink any drink at a party that you have set down.
- Do not stay in a situation in which you feel uncomfortable.
- Be very clear in your communication. If a simple no is not respected, leave or insist he leave. Speak forcefully.
- Avoid giving mixed messages. For example, do not say no and then continue petting.
- Do not go to a place that is so private that help is not available.

Some men who rape their wives see the rape as punishment for perceived wrongs. Others believe they have a right to sex on demand and that when sex is refused they have a right to take it. For other perpetrators, rape is a way to assert power and control. Some may even try to impregnate their wives to ensure that they will not leave the relationship. Others become angered over pregnancy and increase the level of violence in an attempt to abort the fetus.

The myth of male rape has been that it occurs only where heterosexual contact is not possible, such as in prisons or in isolated living conditions. As more *male rape* victims report the crime, however, this myth is being debunked. It is estimated that 5% to 10% of all sexual assault victims are men. Male victims as a group are more likely to have been beaten and are more reluctant to reveal the sexual component of their assaults. Homosexual victims fear police prejudice, and heterosexual victims feel shame and confusion regarding their own sexuality. Male rape is not a homosexual attack. Just as in female rape, the issue is one of *violence* and *domination* rather than of sex. Some perpetrators are gay males who coerce partners or dates into sexual activity by use of threats or intimidation, as in date rape. Other perpetrators are heterosexual males who rape other males as a way of punishing and degrading them. Often, the assaults involve more than one offender. This type of assault can occur among prison inmates or as part of gay bashing. Inmates who are sexually assaulted are often viewed by the public as deserving of their fate because of the crimes they have committed against society. Similarly, many people believe that gay men deserve to be raped as punishment for their "perverse" lifestyle (Lips, 2004; Walker, Archer, & Davies, 2005).

Comorbid Disorders

As a direct result of the rape, survivors may experience post-traumatic stress disorder (PTSD) or may turn to alcohol or drugs to numb the emotional pain. Survivors are more likely to experience major depressive disorder, anxiety disorders, eating disorders, and sexual problems. They are more likely to attempt suicide than are individuals who have not been raped (Faravelli, Giugni, Salvatori, & Ricca, 2004; Ullman, Filipas, Townsend & Starzynski, 2005).

Etiologies

Theorists in many disciplines have studied the crime of rape in an effort to understand the causes and develop preventive measures. Most agree that rape is a crime of violence generated by issues of power and anger rather than by sex drive.

Intrapersonal Factors

Most convicted sex offenders do not have major mental disorders. Many do meet the criteria for antisocial, schizoid, paranoid, and narcissistic personality disorders. Rapists are typically

young; 80% are younger than 30, and 75% are younger than 25. Most report having been sexually and physically abused as children or adolescents (Sexual Abuse Statistics, n.d.).

The causes of rape are many, but the dynamics of the act are that perpetrators abuse their own and others' sexuality as a method of discharging anger and frustration. From this perspective, there are five types of rape: anger rape, power rape, sadistic rape, gang rape, and date/acquaintance rape (McCabe & Wauchope, 2005).

Anger rape is distinguished by physical violence and cruelty to the victim. Believing that he is the victim of an unjust society, the rapist takes revenge on others by raping. He uses extreme force and viciousness to debase the victim. The ability to injure, traumatize, and shame the victim provides an outlet for his rage and temporary relief from his turmoil. Rapes occur episodically as the rage builds up and he strikes out at others to relieve his pain.

In **power rape**, the intent of the rapist is not to injure someone but to command and master another person sexually. The rapist has an insecure self-image, with feelings of incompetence and inadequacy. The rape becomes the vehicle for expressing power and strength. Seeing the victim as a conquest, the rapist temporarily feels omnipotent.

Sadistic rape involves brutality, bondage, and torture as stimulants for the rapist's sexual excitement. For the rapist, the assault is erotic. He plans very carefully, and the process of rape may be ritualized. The victims are often murdered after being raped.

Gang rape involves a number of perpetrators and may be part of a group ritual that confirms masculinity, power, and authority. Age of the perpetrators may range from 10 to 30 years, but the offenders are most typically adolescents. Victims are usually the same age as the group members.

Date rape, or **acquaintance rape**, is forced sexual activity by a perpetrator known to the victim. Typically, it involves less physical violence and more coercion and deception. Even during the high school years, it is estimated that 30% of female students are sexually or physically abused in their dating relationships.

Interpersonal Factors

Most rapists do not have normal interpersonal involvements. Preoccupied with their own fantasies, they want to control and dominate others rather than engage in mutually satisfying relationships. With this model in mind, a rapist sees no need for consent to sexual activity, particularly from a wife or partner. The husband may view the rape as merely a disagreement over sexual behavior. If the wife has said she does not want to engage in sex and the husband uses force, her control and autonomy have been violated. When sex occurs without consent, it is rape.

MediaLink   Care Plan, The Victim of Domestic Violence

Sociocultural Factors

The acceptance of interpersonal violence in a culture contributes to a higher incidence of rape. Societal approval of the use of intimidation, coercion, and force to achieve a goal promotes an excessive level of violence. Violent behavior is an expression of power and strength, and individual rights are disregarded.

Aggression is learned through three primary sources: family and peers, culture/subculture, and the mass media. The modeling effect occurs when potential offenders see rape scenes and other acts of violence against women in real life or in the media, in slasher and horror films, in violent pornography, video games, and degrading music lyrics. The media contribute to the process of desensitization; with repeated exposure, viewers become numb to the pain, fear, and humiliation of sexual aggression (Hues-

mann, Moise-Titus, Podolski, & Eron, 2003; Martino et al., 2006).

Gender-bias Factors

From the gender-bias perspective, rape is the result of long and deeply rooted socioeconomic traditions. Worldwide, men dominate most political and economic activities, and women are viewed as subservient and relatively powerless. At the furthest extreme, women are viewed as property. Sexual gratification is not the prime motive in rape; rather, sex is used to establish or maintain *control* of one person by another. When women are considered inferior to men, tacit approval is given for coercion and force. These stereotypes support the false beliefs that, at times, women deserve to be raped, that they may want or need to be raped, and that rape does not cause them much physical or emotional damage.

Nursing Process

A CLIENT WHO HAS EXPERIENCED SEXUAL VIOLENCE

ASSESSMENT

Rape victims must be assessed physically from head to toe for any serious or critical injuries that may have resulted from the assault. Critical injuries have the highest priority of care.

Before any further medical intervention occurs, clients must be informed of their right to have a rape crisis advocate with them during the assessment process. The victim must also be informed of their rights to:

- Having family or friends present during the questioning and examination
- Having their personal physician notified
- Privacy during the assessment and treatment process
- Confidentiality maintained by all members of the staff
- Gentle and sensitive treatment
- Detailed explanations of and give consent for all tests and procedures, including photographs
- Referrals for follow-up treatment and counseling

In the 1990s, *Sexual Assault Nurse Examiner (SANE)* programs were established throughout Canada and the United States to improve the community response to sexual assault victims. The retraumatization of victims in the medical setting in the past included long waits in busy public areas; not being allowed to eat, drink, or urinate to avoid destroying

evidence; and being examined by health care professionals untrained in procedures for collection of forensic evidence.

A SANE is a registered nurse who has advanced education and clinical preparation in forensic examination of sexual assault victims. SANEs provide respectful and prompt emergency medical–legal treatment. They offer victims compassionate care for physical and psychological trauma both. SANEs know what forensic evidence to collect and how to document injuries and other legal evidence. SANE programs provide improved medical and legal response to sexual assault victims (Stermac et al., 2005).

As a nurse, you must respect the victim's autonomy in order to prevent revictimization. Give the client as much control as possible through every step of the assessment and treatment process. With the victim's permission, perform a vaginal or rectal examination to determine necessary treatment and to provide evidence for legal action. With permission, take photographs of the injuries for legal documentation. The physical assessment process must be carefully documented in writing to assist with possible prosecution of the perpetrator. See the Focused Nursing Assessment feature for guidance in the assessment process of people who have been raped.

Rape is a violent act against an innocent person. It changes lives forever because once people become victims they never again feel completely safe. The victim's response to this act of violence is referred to as **rape-trauma syndrome**. Some rape survivors do not develop major symptoms in response to the trauma, whereas as many as 25% continue to have signs of impairment a year after the assault. A variety of factors contribute to the response, including age or developmental state, history of prior victimization, the relationship to the offender, precrisis coping abilities, and the ability to use support resources. Response factors related to the rape itself include severity of the rape, duration, frequency, number of offenders, and degree of violence. Environmental factors contributing to a rape victim's response are quality and continuity of social supports and community attitudes and values (American Psychiatric Association, 2000).

Assessment: Behavior

Many victims of rape do not report the crime. Sometimes this is due to guilt or embarrassment about what has occurred. Other victims are fearful of how their families or the police will react. Some perpetrators threaten victims by saying they will return to rape them again if the police are notified. Because many of the crimes are committed by acquaintances, friends, dates, or husbands, victims fear they will not be believed.

Some victims respond immediately with agitated and nonpurposeful behavior. They are brought to the emergency department emotionally distraught and unable to respond to questions about what has occurred. Their level of anxiety may be so high that they may not be able to follow simple directions. Some rape victims may shower or bathe before notifying the police or going to the hospital. This cleaning-up behavior is often an attempt to regain control of oneself and counteract the feelings of helplessness induced by the rape.

Most victims appear in good control of their feelings and behavior immediately after the rape. This appearance of outward calmness usually indicates a state of numbness, disbelief, and emotional shock. They may say such things as, "This whole thing doesn't seem real," "I must be dreaming. This couldn't have happened," and "I just can't believe this has happened to me." You must recognize that underneath the calmness is acute distress. If you assume that the calmness implies no distress, you will overlook the person's need for emotional support and intervention.

There may be long-term behavioral characteristics of the rape-trauma syndrome. Some survivors are prone to crying spells that they may or may not be able to explain. Some may have difficulty establishing or maintaining personal relationships, especially with people who remind them of the perpetrator. Many develop problems at work or school. Some report nightmares and have difficulty sleeping. Others develop secondary phobic reactions to people, objects, or situations that remind them of the rape. Sexual dysfunction is not unusual. A woman who is a survivor of partner rape suffers additional problems. Often, she must continue to interact with her rapist because she is dependent on him. She may be forced to pretend, to herself and to family members and friends, that the rape never occurred. Until it becomes more socially acceptable and legally feasible to report rape by an

intimate partner, many of these survivors will suffer in silence.

Assessment: Affect

Victims of rape have immediate and long-lasting emotional trauma. After a period of shock and disbelief, many experience episodes of fear. Fear can result from a stimulus directly associated with the attack, such as a penis, the act of oral sex, or a person who looks like the offender. There are also fears of rape consequences such as pregnancy; sexually transmitted infections, especially HIV; talking to the police; and testifying in court. In addition, there are fears related to potential future attacks, which underlie fears of getting close to men, of being alone, and of being in a strange place. Typically, the level of fear peaks around the third week, but it may take a long time for the level to decrease.

Depression frequently develops within a few weeks of the assault. This posttrauma depression usually lasts about 3 months, and it is not unusual for the survivor to experience suicidal ideation. For some, the depression will develop into a major depressive disorder necessitating medical intervention.

Rape victims feel physically and emotionally violated, and unclean and contaminated. The loss of control over their bodies and their autonomy leads to feelings of helplessness and vulnerability. They may feel alienated from friends and family, particularly if there is not a strong supportive network. Anger is a healthy response to the violation that has occurred, but the energy of anger must be appropriately discharged so the person does not become obsessed with fantasies of revenge.

Assessment: Cognition

During the rape, some victims use the defense mechanism of depersonalization or dissociation to cope with the attack. By perceiving the attack as "not really happening to me," a victim protects a sense of integrity. Other victims rely on denial to block out the traumatic experience. The use of these defense mechanisms may continue through initial treatment and should be supported until the person is able to face the reality of the attack.

Jaime, a graduate student at the local university, was brought to the hospital by the police who found her running down the street half-clothed. In the hospital, she was able to tell the staff that she had been raped by her date, Jovan, another graduate student. She exhibited outward calmness but kept repeating, "This cannot have happened to me. My friends introduced us and he seemed so nice." She was unable to decide who to call to take her back to the dorm or what to tell her friends about what had happened.

If victims are in a state of emotional shock, they will have great difficulty making decisions. Uncertain of how their significant others will react to the situation, they may hesitate

Focused Nursing Assessment | Clients Who Have Been Raped

Behavior Assessment	Affective Assessment	Cognitive Assessment
Nursing observations: Is the client able to respond verbally to questions? Is the client able to follow simple directions? Have you bathed, douched, changed clothes, or done any self-treatment before coming to the hospital?	Could you explain ways in which you are experiencing any of the following emotions? ■ Disbelief ■ Shame ■ Embarrassment ■ Humiliation ■ Helplessness ■ Vulnerability ■ Anxiety ■ Fear ■ Guilt ■ Anger ■ Depression	Nursing observations: Is there any evidence of the use of defense mechanisms? Describe the client's attention span. Can you tell me where you are? What is today's date? Can you describe what occurred? Have you been informed of your rights? Who have you informed about the rape? Family? Friends? Police? Do you need help in telling others about the rape? In what way, if any, do you feel responsible for the attack?

to tell family or friends. They need a great deal of support in using the problem-solving process to make decisions.

There may be a period during which victims blame themselves for the rape. This self-blame may be heard in such statements as, "If only I had taken a different way home," "I should have been able to escape because he didn't have a gun," and "If I were a better wife, he wouldn't have raped me." Remember that the victim is never to blame for this violent crime.

Some survivors develop obsessional thoughts about the rape, which may be severe enough to interfere with daily functioning. Some experience flashbacks, some have violent dreams, and others may be preoccupied with thoughts of future danger. Rape profoundly affects a person's beliefs about the environment. If the assault occurred in the home, the normal feeling of safety within the home will most likely be destroyed. Belief in an inability to protect themselves in the future may lead to social withdrawal or phobic avoidance. Young female survivors, especially, may generalize their fear to the point that it applies to all men or all strange men. Women who have been raped by their husbands often state that their ability to trust the husband or any other man has been destroyed. Box 23.3 describes the phases of response to rape.

Assessment: Interpersonal Relationships

Families of rape survivors experience many of the same thoughts and emotions as the victims themselves. They may talk about guilt, doubts, fear, anger, hatred of the perpetra-

BOX 23.3 | Phases of Response to Rape

Anticipatory Phase

■ Begins when the victim realizes the situation is potentially dangerous
■ The victim may think about how to get away, may reason or argue with the offender, and recall advice people have given about rape.
■ Use of dissociation, suppression, or rationalization to preserve the illusion of invulnerability
■ Possible physical action

Impact Phase

■ The period of actual assault and immediate aftermath
■ Intense fear of death or serious injury
■ Expressive styles:
■ Open expression of feelings—crying, sobbing, pacing
■ Controlled style—numbness, shock, disbelief

■ Compound reaction—reactivated symptoms of previous conditions, for example, psychotic behavior, depression, suicidal behavior, substance abuse
■ Somatic reactions—tension headache, fatigue, increased startle reaction, nausea, gagging

Reconstitution Phase

■ Outward appearance of adjustment with an attempt to restore equilibrium
■ Life activities are renewed, but superficially and mechanically
■ Periods of anxiety, fear, nightmares, depression, guilt, shame, vulnerability, helplessness, isolation, sexual dysfunctions

Resolution Phase

■ Anger at the assailant, at society, and at the judicial system
■ The need to talk to resolve feelings
■ The survivor seeks family and professional support

Social Assessment	Physiological Assessment
Who do you think are your most available support systems? Family? Friends? Clergy? Rape advocate?	Have physical injuries such as scratches, bruises, and cuts been recorded and photographed?
Are you in need of temporary shelter?	Have fingernail scrapings been taken and preserved?
May I provide you with information about available counseling?	Has blood typing been done?
	Have smears been taken of the mouth, throat, vagina, and rectum for detection of sexually transmitted infections?
	Have combings been made of the pubic hair and preserved?
	Has genital trauma been recorded and photographed?
	Has rectal trauma been recorded and photographed?
	Have semen specimens been preserved?
	If applicable, when was the client's last menstrual period?
	Has the clothing been inspected and preserved?

All questions in the Physiological Assessment section are nursing observations; they are not asked of the client.

tor, and feelings of helplessness. They must be educated about the nature and trauma of rape and the immediate and potential long-term reactions of the survivors. They require direction in how to best support the survivor so that they neither overprotect nor minimize the impact of the rape.

Many families believe the cultural *myths* that have surrounded the crime of rape for a long time. Some of these myths are:

- "Good girls" do not get raped.
- Women ask to be raped by the clothes they wear, such as going braless or wearing short skirts and tight tops.
- Women ask to be raped by going to their date's apartment on the first date.
- The average healthy woman can escape a potential rapist if she really wants to.
- A woman who is stuck-up and thinks she is too good deserves to be taught a lesson.
- If a woman engages in petting and lets things get out of hand, it is her own fault if she is raped.
- Women cry rape after they have consented to sex with a friend.
- Among males, only homosexuals are raped.
- Any man could resist rape if he really tried.
- Men are not as affected by rape as are women.

Sexual problems are one of the longest lasting effects of rape. Nearly all adult rape survivors feel the need to withdraw from sexual activity for a period. For some, a period of celibacy is necessary to reestablish control and autonomy. Others may choose abstinence because they feel unclean or contaminated. Both the survivor and the sex partner must understand that the need for closeness and nondemanding physical contact continues. Expressing caring and affection through nonsexual touching minimizes the partner's feelings of rejection and reduces the survivor's feelings of self-blame and uncleanliness.

Assessment: Cultural Influences

Rape occurs cross-culturally and is one of the most underreported crimes worldwide. Global statistics show that at least one in every five women experiences rape or attempted rape during her lifetime. Rape is a significant concern for women in all cultures. Many societies believe that women, not men, are responsible for rape. Female rape victims are sometimes more scorned than their male perpetrators on the premise that the men could not control themselves but the women should have been able to avoid the rape. People cling to stereotyped and prejudicial views of victims of sexual violence, which compounds the agony of the victims (Sivagnanam, Bairy, & D'Souza, 2005).

In societies where young women's worth is equated with virginity, the consequences of rape are especially disastrous. Their ruined reputation cannot be revised. In some countries, women are forced to marry their rapist to erase the stigma of "spoiled goods." Others turn to prostitution to survive, and some commit suicide. Women victims are blamed rather than perpetrators punished. In some instances, women may even be killed by male family members to cleanse the family (Fontes, 2005).

Throughout history, rape has been a part of war and civil strife. The right to rape women and children has been seen as the booty of war for the victors. Wars in Bangladesh, Bosnia, Kuwait, Somalia, South Africa, and El Salvador give evidence of many cases of systematic and repeated rape of civilian and refugee women. Torture of political prisoners is also gender based, with women being raped repeatedly by different men. Involuntary prostitution or female sexual slavery has a long history, and recent attention has been drawn to this problem in the Philippines, Thailand, Nepal, Burma, and India.

Rape is also used as a weapon of ethnic cleansing as enemies humiliate the women and attempt to exterminate a particular group. Unwanted impregnation results in botched abortion, psychological torture, unwanted children, stigmatized children, and abandoned children. Unfortunately, many of these women also suffer subsequent persecution from their own families and societies. They may be thought to have dishonored their family, questions are raised concerning their consent to sex, and they are no longer marriageable.

Assessment: Physical

Rape usually results in a number of physical injuries. The victim may be beaten, stabbed, or shot. Profuse bleeding and trauma to vital organs may be critical problems. Nongenital physical injuries occur in about 46% of rape cases. Most likely, the vagina or rectum will be sore or swollen. There may be tearing of the vaginal or rectal wall from forceful insertion of the penis or a foreign object. The throat may be traumatized from forced oral sex (Palmer, McNulty, D'Este, & Donovan, 2004).

Female victims of childbearing age may become pregnant because of the rape. The adult pregnancy rate associated with rape is estimated to be almost 5%. Victims of all ages and of both sexes may contract a sexually transmitted infection from the perpetrator, via any mucous membrane area such as the vagina, rectum, mouth, or throat. This transmission rate ranges from 4% to 30% (Rauch & Foa, 2004).

DIAGNOSIS

The assessment process provides the data from which you develop your nursing diagnoses. The health care team must quickly establish physical and mental status priorities. The team must then give attention to the long-range physical, emotional, social, and legal concerns of the survivor.

The nursing diagnosis for clients who have been raped is Rape-trauma Syndrome. If clients suffer from reactivated symptoms of a previous physical illness or mental disorder, or if they rely on alcohol or drugs to manage their trauma, they are given the more specific nursing diagnosis of Rape-trauma Syndrome: Compound Reaction. The nursing diagnosis of Rape-trauma Syndrome: Silent Reaction is applied when the client experiences high levels of anxiety, an inability to discuss the trauma, abrupt changes in relationships with men or changes in sexual behavior, and the onset of phobic reactions.

OUTCOME IDENTIFICATION AND GOALS

Based on the assessment data, you select outcomes appropriate to the nursing diagnosis. The primary long-term outcome is that survivors return to their precrisis level of functioning (minimal expectation) or achieve a higher level of functioning.

Once you have established outcomes, you and the client mutually identify goals for change. The following goals demonstrate that the crisis of rape has been resolved in an adaptive manner:

- Control over remembering—decreased flashbacks and nightmares
- Affect tolerance—feelings can be felt, named, and endured without overwhelming arousal or numbing
- Symptom mastery—anxiety, fear, depression, and sexual problems decrease and are more tolerable
- Reconnection—increased ability to trust and attach to others
- Meaning—has discovered some tolerable meaning to the trauma; feels empowered

PLANNING

Once nursing diagnoses, outcome criteria, and goals have been identified, the nurse develops the plan of care to assist clients in managing the traumatic crisis of rape. Priorities of care are:

- Treating acute physical injuries
- Supporting the individual through the crisis

IMPLEMENTATION

Difficulty Making Decisions

Help the clients identify immediate concerns and prioritize them. Focusing on immediate problems lessens the client's confusion and feelings of being overwhelmed. Next, help the client use the problem-solving process. Clients must be empowered to make their own decisions and act on their own behalf. Restoring personal choice is a primary antidote to rape trauma. Informed choices help clients regain control and autonomy, both of which were violated during the rape.

The desired outcome is that the client identifies immediate concerns and uses the problem-solving process to make own decisions.

Flashbacks

Calming techniques such as muscle relaxation and deep breathing are useful for managing flashbacks. Deep breathing replaces

NURSING CARE PLAN for a Client Experiening Sexual Violence

Supporting Coping Behaviors
Nursing Diagnosis: Client at Risk for Rape Trauma Syndrome

Outcomes: Client talks about the rape, and copes effectively with the crisis.

Rape is both a personal and family crisis. It is important to support clients and families until they are able to cope with the reality of the assault. Discuss beliefs about postcoital contraception and abortion if appropriate. Pregnancy may result from rape, and clients must have information about available options. The most common medical intervention is a course of hormonal treatment. Elevated doses of oral contraceptive or DES (diethylstilbestrol) may be administered if the woman chooses to prevent conception. Mifepristone (RU-486) is a chemical that greatly diminishes the chance that a fertilized ovum will be implanted or that a placenta will develop. Inform clients about the need for follow-up medical evaluation and treatment for sexually transmitted infections, including a test for HIV.

Intervention	Rationale	Goal
Give victim ample time to respond to simple questions.	Anxiety decreases the ability to perceive input, thereby slowing down the response time.	Responds to simple questions
If client is unable to express feelings, acknowledge the difficulty (e.g., "I understand that it is difficult for you to describe your feelings right now. That's okay. You may be able to talk about them later.")	Support coping styles until client is able to acknowledge the reality of the situation.	Copes in best fashion as able
Communicate your knowledge and understanding of the usual emotional responses to rape (e.g., "People usually experience a number of feelings such as anxiety, fear, embarrassment, guilt, or anger.")	Client needs reassurance that these feelings are a normal reaction to rape.	Identifies and expresses feelings about the rape
Encourage client to talk about the rape. Listen patiently and supportively.	Emotional arousal of the trauma contributes to an intense pressure to talk. Compulsive retelling is a natural way the victim is gradually desensitized to the trauma.	Talks about the rape
Identify specific coping behavior used during the rape (e.g., screaming, fighting, talking, blacking out). Reassure client that responses were all that was possible under the degree of fear that rape induces (e.g., "I know you handled the situation right because you are alive.")	Identifying behavior as an adaptive mechanism to survive increases self-esteem and decreases feelings of guilt.	Identifies adaptive behavior
Identify distortions related to self-blame or guilt. Repeatedly tell client it was not her fault.	Beliefs of personal responsibility and fault interfere with resolution of the syndrome.	Identifies self as a victim
Assist client to identify who to tell and how to tell about the rape.	Victims often fear how family and friends will respond to the situation.	Uses significant others for support

Enhancing Spirituality
Nursing Diagnosis: Client at Risk for Spiritual Distress

Outcomes: Client verbalizes meaning of the rape in her life, and uses spiritual support systems.

People who experience rape often have spiritual distress because their world is no longer safe.

continued

NURSING CARE PLAN for a Client Experiencing Sexual Violence

Enhancing Spirituality *continued*
Nursing Diagnosis: Client at Risk for Spiritual Distress

Intervention	Rationale	Goal
Explore ways to adapt personal environment. Encourage them to enlist assistance of family and friends in this endeavor.	This improves sense of security.	Verbalizes a sense of increased security and sense of connectedness to others
Help clients search for meaning in the trauma (e.g., "What does it mean to you that the rape happened? What purpose is there in your suffering? How might you find peace and strength again?")	This reestablishes a purpose in life.	Verbalizes meaning from the trauma of the rape
Help them identify spiritual support systems.	This increases feelings of connectedness to others.	Contacts identified individuals
If appropriate, refer to a religious counselor of their choice and support their use of meditation, prayer, or other religious traditions and rituals.	Religious support is a necessary part of healing for some victims.	Utilizes resources

the shallow breathing that occurs in highly anxious states and prevents hyperventilation. The goal is to provide clients with a skill response so that they can get through the flashback without feeling overwhelmed.

Guided imagery can be used to gain control over remembering the rape, the goal being to reduce the frequency of flashbacks. Instruct clients to assume a comfortable position and close their eyes. Make suggestions that induce relaxation such as describing peaceful images or slow, gentle breathing. Ask clients to imagine surrounding the flashback with a pink bubble. Then have clients let go of the bubble and watch the bubble float off into the universe and disappear. With practice clients will be able to initiate this process at the first sign of an unwanted flashback.

The desired outcome is that client uses self-calming techniques and has control over remembering.

Need for Community Resources

Provide a written list of referrals of community resources before clients are discharged from the emergency department. Sexual assault advocacy programs address a wide range of victim needs, including crisis counseling and emotional support to victims and their families. Crisis intervention counseling can help minimize the long-term emotional and spiritual impact of sexual assault. See the Community Resources feature on the Companion Website for a list of national resources that can provide local referrals.

Group therapy provides an opportunity for clients to meet with other survivors of rape in a safe, supportive, and egalitarian setting. In this therapeutic environment, client feelings are validated as normal reactions to the assault and clients receive confirmation of their survival behaviors. Support groups may help moderate depression by providing an opportunity to speak openly and network with other survivors and supportive people. Clients may be able to redirect the energy that is often spent on anger and pain into compassionate acts of supporting others. The long-term goal of support groups is to help survivors understand their distress and take charge of their own recovery. Recovery is accomplished by counteracting self-blame, sharing grief, and affirming self and life.

The desired outcome is that client utilizes community resources.

EVALUATION

The long-term goal of intervention is to help rape victims return to their precrisis level or achieve a higher level of functioning. The road to recovery is profoundly personal and uniquely individual. Finally, it is the victim/survivor who determines whether recovery is complete.

Recovery from sexual violence includes clients' ability to demonstrate effective coping strategies, modification of lifestyle and environment as necessary, a decrease in negative feelings, and a decrease in physical symptoms. Spiritual coping is evidenced by their discovery of some tolerable meaning to the trauma and to themselves as trauma survivors.

Childhood Sexual Abuse

Childhood sexual abuse is defined as inappropriate sexual behavior, instigated by a perpetrator, for purposes of the perpetrator's sexual pleasure or for economic gain through child prostitution or pornography. Behavior ranges from exhibitionism, peeping, explicit sexual talk, touching, caressing, masturbation, oral sex, vaginal sex, and anal sex, to forcing children to engage in sex with one another or with animals.

Childhood sexual abuse must be distinguished from natural and healthy sexual exploration during childhood. It is natural that children of similar age and developmental status explore one another's bodies by looking and touching, often referred to as "playing doctor." This is not considered problematic behavior.

Childhood sexual abuse does not discriminate. It occurs in all ethnic, religious, economic, and cultural subgroups. Affinity systems—immediate family, relatives, friends, neighbors, clergy members, scout leaders, coaches—account for 75% to 80% of the abuse. Heterosexual male perpetrators account for most of the reported cases. Children with mental retardation or physical disability are 4 to 10 times more vulnerable to sexual victimization than nondisabled children because disabled children may have difficulty asserting their rights or informing an adult protector. Although father–daughter incest is reported most, it is believed that **sibling incest** is the most widespread. Some siblings turn to each other for emotional nurturance and acceptance. In other instances, a sibling uses coercion or violence to perpetrate (National Center for Victims of Crime, 2004; Valente, 2005).

In March of 2006, Neil Lofquist was arrested and charged with sexually assaulting his 8-year-old daughter 2 days before her death and again the night he allegedly choked, stabbed, and dunked her head in a toilet.

Sexually abused children and adult survivors of childhood sexual abuse (hereafter referred to as adult survivors) are crying out for help. A few cry out loudly in protest, but most cry inwardly in silence. It is thought that as many as one in three girls and one in seven boys are abused sexually before the age of 18. Many of these are single incidents. Boys are more frequently molested outside the family system than are girls. The period of abuse tends to begin and end at a younger age in boys and is less likely to be disclosed (Valente, 2005).

Childhood sexual abuse is a major health problem in the United States. Most cases are probably unreported. Health care professionals, and families, have used denial to cope with ambiguous evidence of the cultural taboos of incest and sex with children. To respond appropriately to cues that signal sexual abuse, you must understand the characteristics and dynamics of the perpetrators, victims, and families involved. A note of caution must be added: With increased publicity, there is a real danger of a witch hunt developing. Any hint or accusation of sexual abuse may be interpreted as absolute proof of guilt. Individuals and families have been destroyed by rumors and false accusations. You must assess carefully and maintain a balance between the extremes of denial and automatic belief of guilt.

KNOWLEDGE BASE: CHILDHOOD SEXUAL ABUSE

Types of Offenders

Some offenders prefer girls; others prefer boys; and some abuse both, as long as the victim is a child. Some are interested in adolescents or preteens, some in toddlers, and some in infants. Some offenders do not abuse until they are adults, but more than half start in their teens.

Juvenile Offenders

Many, if not most, cases of juvenile offenses are unreported. Family members often want to protect and shield the young offender. At other times, the behavior is rationalized as adolescent male experimentation. Between 50% and 60% of juvenile offenders were sexually abused as children; they gradually develop offending behaviors as they reach adolescence. The other 40% to 50% show high rates of other delinquent behaviors, and most are diagnosed with conduct disorder. Generally, these individuals have problems in all areas of their lives (Johnson, 2000). (See chapter 17 ∞ for information on conduct disorder.)

Compared with nonabused teen sex offenders, those offenders who were child victims tend to be younger at onset of abusing behavior, to have more victims, and to have male victims. Juvenile offenders may seek victims within or outside the family system. The type of sexual offense often parallels their experiences of abuse. Sexuality and aggression are closely linked in the thoughts and actions of these young people. The most frequent offense is sexual touching, which may

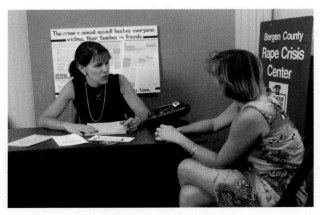

PHOTO 23.1 ■ Rape crisis centers offer women support in dealing with sexual assault.
SOURCE: R. Sidney/The Image Works. Used with permission.

escalate to rape and other sex crimes (Andrade, Vincent, & Saleh, 2006; Ryan, 2000).

Just as most juveniles who commit delinquent acts do not go on to adult criminal behavior, most juveniles who commit sexual offenses and receive treatment do not continue molesting behavior. For those in treatment, the sexual relapse rate is only 10% to 15%. This information is not meant to minimize the seriousness of their offenses, the impact on victims, and the nature of their psychological disturbances but to recognize the differences between adolescent and adult offenders (Brown, 2000).

Male Offenders

One research project that studied fathers who abused their daughters established five types of incestuous fathers. *Sexually preoccupied* abusers (26% of the fathers) have a conscious and often obsessive sexual interest in their daughters. Many of them regard their daughters as sex objects, in some cases as early as birth. *Adolescent regressors* (33% of the fathers) become sexually interested in their daughters when they begin puberty. These men sound and act like adolescents around their daughters. *Self-gratifiers* (20% of the fathers) are not sexually attracted to their daughters per se, and during the abuse, they fantasize about someone else. In effect, they are simply using their daughters' bodies. *Emotional dependents* (10% of the fathers) see themselves as failures and feel very lonely and depressed. They see their daughters as romantic figures in their lives. *Angry retaliators* (10% of the fathers) abuse out of anger, either at the daughter or at the mother. This type of offender is most likely to have a criminal history of assault and rape (Schetky, 1999).

Female Offenders

Female perpetrators have been largely overlooked but are responsible for about 10% of sexual abuse cases. The most common types of sexual abuse by women are fondling, oral sex, and group sex.

Female sex offenders fall into four major types. *Teacher–lovers* are older women who teach children about lovemaking. *Experimenter–exploiters* are often females who had no sex education growing up. Babysitting is often an opportunity to explore younger children. Many of the girls in this group do not even realize what they are doing or that it is inappropriate. *Predisposers* usually come from a family with a long history of physical and sexual abuse. These families have been dysfunctional over many generations. *Women coerced by males* are those who abuse children because men have forced them to abuse. Usually, they have been victims as children and are easily manipulated and intimidated (McCloskey & Raphael, 2005).

Recently, a number of female teachers have been accused of having sexual relationships with their male adolescent students. Cognitively, the accused teachers understand that it is not right

but they justify it by saying they are giving the gift of love. At this time, no one knows how common teacher–lovers are.

Pamela Turner, 27, a physical education teacher, was arrested for having sex with a 13-year-old student at his home and in the school over a 2-month period.

Laurie Augustine, 42, a high school library aide, was sentenced to 9 years in prison after pleading guilty to having sex with three 17-year-old students. The sexual liaisons took place in the school, in motels, and in cars.

Mary Kay Letourneau, 33, served 7 years in prison for having a sexual relationship with a 12-year-old student.

Internet Offenders

Some sexual perpetrators use the Internet to sexually abuse children or adolescents. About half of Internet offenders are strangers who locate and meet the victims online. Half are family and acquaintance offenders who use the Internet to store or circulate sexual pictures of victims or even advertise or sell victims. Most at risk for meeting offenders in Internet chat rooms are 14- through 15-year-old girls. Most offenders are honest about the fact that they are adults who are interested in having a sexual relationship with the teen. There is a concerted attempt by law inforcement to pose as minors on the Internet to catch potential sex offenders. Unfortunately these proactive investigations are only able to stop a few offenders because of personnel and time constraints (Mitchell, Finkelhor, & Wolak, 2005; Mitchell, Wolak, & Finkelhor, 2005; Wolak, Finkelhor, & Mitchell, 2004).

Comorbid Disorders

Having suffered sexual abuse in childhood is often a hidden feature of adult mental disorders. As much as 60% to 70% of psychiatric clients have a history of abuse. Repeated trauma in childhood distorts the personality. Since child victims cannot protect themselves, they must adapt to the trauma as well as they can. Behaviors that were originally adaptive become symptoms in adulthood. These people have a bewildering combination of symptoms, including anger, depression, anxiety, insomnia, suspicion, eating disorders, substance abuse, self-mutilation, and sexual dysfunction. Adult survivors often collect many different diagnoses before the underlying problem of PTSD is correctly identified (Kaplow, Dodge, Amaya-Jackson, & Saxe, 2005; Kreidler, 2005).

Etiologies

There is no single cause of childhood sexual abuse. Rather, the abuse results from a combination of personality, family, and cultural factors.

Intrapersonal Factors

There are many types of perpetrators of childhood sexual abuse. Some traits are contradictory, and there is no agreement on a composite personality. Certain characteristics apply to many people, not just abusers. The descriptions are guidelines for assessment, not proof that the person actually committed sexual abuse.

Perpetrators usually have low self-esteem and feel more secure in interactions with children than with adults. Some were emotionally deprived as children and therefore have a great need for constant, unconditional love, which is more easily obtained from children than from adults. Some perpetrators are described as lacking impulse control and the ability to experience feelings of guilt. Others are described as rigid and overcontrolled, whereas others are dominant and aggressive.

If perpetrators were themselves sexually abused as children, they may have learned to associate all feelings of love with sexual behavior. Most people who were sexually abused as children do *not* go on to sexually abuse others. However, some victimized children develop offending behavior in late childhood, adolescence, or adulthood. Most likely, a number of factors are involved in why some abuse and others do not. The world of abuse is composed only of victims (powerless) and perpetrators (powerful). Victims become perpetrators in an unconscious attempt to master the trauma of their own experiences and take over the power. The move from victim to offender may also result when anger and hostility are externalized and projected onto new victims.

Family Systems Theory

Family systems theory considers structure, cohesion, adaptability, and communication patterns of families in which children are being sexually abused. Refer to chapter 2 ∞ for more detailed information on families.

Family structure is usually hierarchical according to age, roles, and distribution of power. Typically, the adults, who are older, assume the parental roles and are the most influential. The structure of incestuous families, however, is often different as the result of dysfunctional boundary patterns. An adult may move "down" in the structure or a child may move "up" in terms of roles and influence (boundaries). If the father moves downward, he assumes a childlike role and

is cared for and nurtured like a child in the family. In this position, the father assumes little parental responsibility. He may then turn to the daughter, as a "peer," for sexual and emotional gratification. As another example, the daughter may move upward and replace the mother in the hierarchy. The mother does not usually move downward but rather moves out of the structure by distancing herself emotionally or physically from the family. As the daughter assumes the parental role and responsibilities, the father may turn to her for fulfilling his emotional and sexual needs.

Family cohesion refers to the degree of emotional bonding that occurs within a family. At one end of the cohesion continuum is the family system that is disengaged; that is, the family members are isolated and alienated from one another. At the other end of the continuum is the enmeshed family system, in which the members are immersed in and absorbed by one another. The healthiest family systems function between these two extremes. Sexual abuse in families usually occurs in an enmeshed family. The need to be overinvolved in each other's lives is accompanied by intense fears of abandonment.

Family adaptability is also described along a continuum. At one extreme is the rigid family system and at the other end, the chaotic family system. Families involved in sexual abuse tend to function at either end of the continuum. Rigid family systems have strict rules and stereotyped gender role expectations, with minimal emotional interaction. Children have no power and authority, even over their own bodies. They are not allowed to question or protest inappropriate sexual behavior. In contrast, chaotic family systems have either no rules or constantly changing rules. Within the chaotic system, there may be no assigned roles or no rules regarding appropriate sexual behavior, which may contribute to the incidence of sexual abuse.

Communication patterns within the family system may contribute to the occurrence of sexual abuse. Incest depends on keeping the secret within the family. In family systems that avoid conflict, accusations of sexual abuse are not tolerated. Peace must be kept at all costs.

Nursing Process

A CLIENT WHO HAS EXPERIENCED CHILDHOOD SEXUAL ABUSE

ASSESSMENT

Childhood sexual abuse is a process, not just an event. Not all children become symptomatic following sexual abuse— some may never have symptoms and some may not have

trouble until adulthood. A single traumatic experience does not usually lead to mental disorders. To the extent that other life experiences are positive, children are likely to have no or few long-term effects. To the extent that other life experiences are also negative, the effects of the sexual abuse are amplified.

There is no identified "sexual abuse syndrome," and reactions vary greatly from one person to another. The effects of sexual abuse are most severe when the incidents are frequent

Focused Nursing Assessment | Victims and Survivors of Childhood Sexual Abuse

Behavior Assessment	Affective Assessment	Cognitive Assessment
Child Victim		
Are there signs of regressive behavior in the child?	Do you get enough love from other family members?	How would you describe the family's problems?
Is the child exhibiting clinging behavior?	Tell me about the fears you may have if any family secrets are told: Not being believed? Being blamed for the problems? Your parents will not love you? Your parents will be taken away? You will be moved to a foster home? Physical punishment?	Who do you believe is responsible for these problems?
Does the child have friendships with other children?		What happens or might happen when you tell the family secrets?
Has there been any sexual acting out on the part of the child?		Are you able to separate your mind from your body while you are being hurt?
Has the child ever run away or threatened to run away?		
Has the child ever attempted suicide?		
Adult Survivor		
When growing up, who had which type of responsibilities in the home?	Describe the relationships in your family of origin.	Have you always remembered the abuse or was there a period of amnesia?
How were family secrets kept within the family?	In what ways do you continue to blame yourself for the childhood abuse?	What are the things you value most about yourself?
When you were young, who was (were) the closest family member(s) with whom you had any sexual activity?	Describe those people in your life who you are able to trust.	Do you have concerns about your sexual orientation?
Describe any self-mutilating behavior.	In what situations do you feel angry and out of control?	
Describe your present state of sexual functioning.		

and occur over a long period, the activities are wide ranging and extensive, there is more than one perpetrator, the relationship to the perpetrator is close, and sexual abuse is combined with physical and emotional abuse. There are behavioral, cognitive, and physical problems, as well as difficulties with emotional stability and interpersonal relationships during childhood, adolescence, and adulthood.

When assessing children, remember that some will exhibit most of the symptoms presented in this chapter, others will exhibit only some, and still others will exhibit none of the symptoms. The nurse must appreciate the power of secrecy and how difficult it is for adult survivors to disclose such information, especially for men, who, in our society, are expected to be anything other than victimized. Routine questions on nursing histories may provide an opportunity for survivors to share their pain and obtain treatment as adults. See the Focused Nursing Assessment feature for the types of questions to ask of both child victims and adult survivors.

Assessment: Behavior

Typically, adult perpetrators initiate sexual behavior in a manipulative or coercive manner. Often, the adult misrepresents the abuse as a game or "fun" activity. The behavior usually follows a progression of sexual activity, from exposure and fondling to oral, vaginal, or anal sex. Secrecy is imposed on the child by persuasion or threat. The abuser may say such things as, "If you tell, you'll be sent away," "If you tell, I won't love you anymore," "If you tell, I will kill you," and "If you tell, I'll do the same thing to your baby brother." Children know adults have absolute power over them, so they obey. When they have been threatened with abandonment or harm, they frequently choose to protect others. When asked, "Why didn't you tell sooner?" the answers are, "I didn't know who to tell," "I was scared," or "I did tell and no one believed me."

Between the ages of 3 and 12, Tamika's father sexually abused her. At the age of 7, Tamika told her mother. Besides not believing her, her mother washed her mouth out with a bar of soap for telling filthy lies.

Sometimes, adult perpetrators use grooming behaviors to prepare or persuade victims to comply with the abuse. **Grooming behaviors** are used to gain the trust of children or family members before the abuse begins. Behaviors include hanging out with and participating in activities with the children, babysitting for the parents, or buying gifts for the children or other family members.

Social Assessment	Physiological Assessment
Child Victim	Smears of mouth, throat, vagina, and rectum for sexually transmitted infections
Who are your friends? Do they come over to play at your home?	HIV testing
Who are the people in your life who hurt you?	Throat irritation
	Genital irritation or trauma
	Rectal irritation or trauma
	Chronic vaginal and/or urinary tract infections
Adult Survivor	
Describe the most important relationships in your life.	Weight and nutritional status
Has it been easier for you to maintain superficial relationships as opposed to intimate relationships?	Sleeping problems
In what ways do you need to be in control in relationships?	Evidence of substance abuse
In what ways have you been abused as an adult? Emotionally? Physically? Sexually?	Evidence of self-mutilation

All questions in the Physiological Assessment section are nursing observations; they are not asked of the client.

Some children who have been sexually abused form a clinging attachment to one or both parents. Some become extremely affectionate inside and outside the family system, while others have problems with impulse control and aggression toward others. Some children isolate themselves at school or in the neighborhood and limit most of their interactions to family members. They may act out sexually, by initiating oral or genital sex with other children or adults, for example. Some children, in an effort to master their trauma and regain a sense of personal control, victimize others as they were victimized. In addition, sexually abused children often engage in self-destructive behaviors such as head banging, self-mutilation, and suicide (Salter et al., 2003). See Box 23.4 for behavioral characteristics of children who have been abused.

Adolescent victims may run away from home to escape an intolerable situation. Because they have learned, at home, that sexual behavior is rewarded by affection, love, and attention, some turn to prostitution. Others are forced into prostitution as a way to support themselves while living on the streets. Adolescents may unconsciously seek to repeat the trauma as a way of mastering it. This repetition may take the form of revictimization or perpetrating against others.

Some adult survivors engage in self-mutilation, as in cutting, slashing, or burning themselves. It is important to understand the meaning of such behavior. For some, the pain of self-mutilation proves their existence and reassures them that they are alive and real. Self-mutilation may be a plea for

---

BOX 23.4 — **Sexual Behavior Clues of Abused Children**

Clues include sexual behavior that:
- Is with children of different ages or different developmental levels; the wider the age range, the greater the concern
- Is significantly different from other children of the same age
- Continues in spite of the child's having been given consistent and clear messages to stop
- Occurs in public or other places where the child has been told is not acceptable
- Is adult-type activities with other children; other children may complain about it
- Is initiated by the child toward an adult that is in the manner of adult–adult sexual contact
- Increases in frequency, intensity, or intrusiveness

SOURCES: Burton, J. E., & Rasmussen, L. A. (1998). *Treating children with sexually abusive behavior problems*. New York: Haworth Press; Damon, L. L., & Card, J. A. (1999). Incest in young children. In R. T. Ammerman & M. Hersen (Eds.), *Assessment of family violence: A clinical and legal sourcebook* (2nd ed.). New York: John Wiley & Sons; and Johnson, T. C. (1999). Development of sexual behavior problems in childhood. In J. A. Shaw (Ed.), *Sexual aggression* (pp. 41–74). Washington, DC: American Psychiatric Press.

nurturance, as they come to the emergency department seeking care. Others nurture them by cleaning up the wounds after self-mutilating. For those who dissociate, self-mutilation may be a way to stop the dissociation with physical pain. Other adult survivors self-mutilate as a form of self-punishment and as a way to decrease feelings of guilt. And finally, some self-mutilate as a way to reduce emotional pain through the feeling of physical pain. It is important to understand the function of the behavior in order to replace it with healthier behaviors that satisfy the same need. (See chapter 8 ∞ for further information on self-mutilation.)

There are a number of possible sexual effects for adult survivors. Sexual behaviors are a trigger for some abuse survivors who only develop symptoms once they become sexually active. Some have a very strong aversion to sex and are filled with terror in sexual situations. Some are sexually inhibited and experience discomfort with sexual thoughts, feelings, and behaviors. Some engage in compulsive sexual behavior, perhaps as an unconscious way to validate their shame and guilt or a way to feel powerful. Other sexual symptoms include anger or disgust associated with touch, feeling emotionally distant during sex, experiencing intrusive sexual thoughts or images, and experiencing orgasmic, erectile, or ejaculatory difficulties. Many adult survivors go through a period of celibacy as they try to manage fear, anger, and distrust.

Assessment: Affect

Behind a facade of dominance, perpetrators often feel weak, afraid, and inadequate. They inappropriately view the child as a safe and less threatening source of caring than an adult. They are unable to distinguish between nonsexual and sexual affection for children. Lack of empathy for the victim is typical of perpetrators. Many perpetrators experience intense pleasure based on their sense of power and domination.

Child victims experience many fears. They fear if they tell another adult, they will not be believed, and they fear that they will be blamed. If the abuse is occurring within the family, they may have fantasies of being rejected by family members. They may fear that the family will be separated, especially if this threat was made by the abuser.

Children often feel responsible for the adult's behavior and ashamed that they have not been able to stop the abuse. Secrecy and guilt keep these children isolated, causing them to feel alienated from their peers. The feeling of powerlessness is extremely prevalent because what the victim says and does makes no difference. The associated rage typically does not emerge until adolescence. When the suppressed *rage* comes to the surface, it may be directed against the self in self-defeating and self-destructive ways.

Many adult survivors continue to believe they were to blame for the abuse and should have been able to resist the adult. This self-blame often contributes to depression and

anxiety and to panic attacks. Distrusting and fearing men, many survivors have multiple fears relating to sexual interactions. For some, anger is the only emotion experienced and expressed, all other feelings being severely repressed. Many adult survivors continue to hate their perpetrators, as well as nonabusing significant adults for not protecting them.

Assessment: Cognition

Cognitive distortions are self-statements perpetrators use to deny, minimize, justify, and rationalize their behavior. In addition, they have an impaired capacity for empathy or bonding with children. They view their victims as objects and they focus primarily on their own pleasure and satisfaction.

Secrecy and silence are used by perpetrators to escape accountability. When secrecy fails and the child victims or adult survivors begin to talk to others about the abuse, perpetrators usually attack the credibility of the victims and try to make sure no one will listen. Perpetrators make such statements as, "It never happened. She's lying," "He's exaggerating some innocent touching," and "Even if it did happen, it's time to forget the past and move on." Other perpetrators acknowledge the abuse but minimize the impact with statements such as, "We didn't have intercourse, so it really wasn't sex" and "She didn't really mind; in fact, we have a very close relationship," and "It was just a game, I would never have forced myself on her." Others use the defense mechanism of projection and blame the child for the abuse, as evidenced by such statements as, "She's a very provocative child, and she seduced me" and "If he hadn't enjoyed it so much, I wouldn't have continued."

Some child victims use denial to cope with the trauma. Acknowledging the abuse would mean acknowledging that the world is dangerous and that those who are supposed to protect and nurture failed and caused harm. Other victims minimize the impact and say it was not important, saying things like, "It's not so bad; it only happens once a month" and "It's all right because it stopped when I was 11 years old."

Frequently, dissociation is the victim's major defense. The mind is "separated" from the body, so the victim is not emotionally present during the sexual attack. It prevents the feelings attached to the trauma from reaching conscious awareness in order to survive the trauma. Dissociation is evidenced by such statements as, "I put myself in the wall, where he couldn't reach all of me" and "When he would come into my room, I would close my eyes and go to my favorite place. Only my body stayed on the bed; the rest of me wasn't there." When sexual abuse is severe and sadistic, the victim may develop dissociative identity disorder (DID). (See chapter 11 ∞ for a discussion of DID.)

There is widespread belief that the mother always knows when her husband is sexually involved with one or more of the children. In reality, mothers are often unaware of the sexual abuse. Some deny any evidence of the abuse because they feel inadequate to cope with the family problems. Others use denial because they fear their husbands' retaliation against them if the accusation of incest is brought into the open. Denial may be a defense mechanism used by women who fear financial, social, and emotional problems if their husbands are removed from the family. When cues to sexual abuse are discovered, some women question their own thinking processes. Believing their husbands are incapable of this type of behavior, they, therefore, believe something must be wrong with themselves.

Cherenia has recently become somewhat suspicious that her husband Joe may be sexually abusing their daughter. In response to her fears, she says the following things to herself: "You must really have a dirty mind, Cherenia. How could you possibly think those things about Joe? He's a very good husband. He works hard and loves all of us. He goes to church every week, and everyone knows what a good family man he is. How could you even consider that he might be doing something so awful? You must be really sick, Cherenia."

It is not unusual for adult survivors to have total amnesia for the childhood sexual abuse. In such a case, amnesia is considered a defense mechanism in response to the trauma and is more likely to occur when the abuse began at a very young age. Recall of the abuse may be triggered by a significant life event, such as marriage or pregnancy, or during the process of psychotherapy.

Self-blame contributes to low self-esteem in adult survivors. They feel worthless and different from other people. Survivors often feel alienated from or even hate their bodies. They may believe they are only sex objects to be used and abused by others. They may suffer from flashbacks and nightmares. Many adult survivors have very little sense of self since their boundaries were so profoundly violated as children. This makes them more vulnerable to revictimization as adults.

Confusion about sexuality is very common among male survivors. Victimization of a male carries a hidden implication of being less than a man. Heterosexual survivors fear that the abuse has made, or will make, them homosexual. Intense homophobia and/or hypermasculine behavior may be an effort to disprove their fears. Gay survivors worry that their sexual preference may have caused the abuse. Remember that childhood sexual abuse is not related to adult sexual orientation.

Assessment: Interpersonal Relationships

Many adult survivors have difficulties with relationships. Superficial relationships are usually much easier than intimate relationships. As children, these adults learned that those who love you are the ones who hurt you, and that living in a family is not safe. There is a sense of betrayal by those they are dependent upon, a sense of powerlessness since they could do nothing to stop the abuse, and finally, a sense of stigmatiza-

tion when they incorporate the shame and guilt that has been communicated to them. As a result, in adulthood they may be incapable of trusting others and feel trapped by intimate relationships.

Sasha, age 19, describes her relationship with her father when she was 12 years old in this way: "I don't remember how it started, but my father conned me into soaping up his stomach, testicles, and erect penis when he was in the bathtub. This took place at his apartment when my brothers and I went there for the weekend. I didn't particularly enjoy it, but my father encouraged it. I got completely turned off by it when he offered to do it to me. One time, while I was sleeping on the bed, I woke up from a violent shaking of the bed. I was dressed in a shirt and shorts. I realized my father was rubbing his penis between my thighs and feeling on my vagina. I didn't let him know I was awake, and I turned slightly, hoping he would stop. I never wore that tee shirt or shorts again. I've never told anyone. Even my father doesn't know that I know. I think my experiences have had a deep effect on my relationships. Every time I get close to a man, I become afraid. I think what I'm most afraid of is being used. My childhood experiences seem to bother me the most when my friends talk about their childhood with their fathers and how they were 'Daddy's little girl.' Feelings of rage, anger, and total disgust burn deep inside me."

There is a significant connection between being sexually abused as a child and being revictimized as an adult. This in no way implies, however, that an adult survivor is responsible for being abused, as there is never a legitimate excuse for emotional or physical violence. Adults who were sexually abused as children become victims again in adulthood for many reasons. One thing a person learns from sexual abuse is how to be abused. In order to survive, children teach themselves to endure assaults. They learn they cannot protect themselves. They learn to keep the abuse a secret and to "forgive and forget" each violent incident. All of these survival techniques make them vulnerable to abuse in adulthood.

Assessment: Cultural Influences

Sexual abuse of children is an international public health problem; rates are similar in industrialized and nonindustrialized countries both. Any consideration of sexual abuse must take into account cultural views of appropriate and inappropriate sexual behavior. The aspects of culture relating to child sexual abuse include family structures, moral and religious principles, and child rearing practices. Other aspects include the relative value of interdependence, treatment of sexuality, gender roles, and interpersonal boundaries. The ways in which communities view violence and sexual assault, and the action that is taken when these occur, reflect cultural values. It is only when we understand cultural diversity that we are able to develop effective prevention programs (Fontes, 2005; Warne & McAndrew, 2005). Box 23.5 gives some culture-specific information on child sexual abuse.

BOX 23.5	Culture-specific Characteristics of Sexual Abuse

Euro-American Individuals

- The keeping of family secrets is a traditional value.
- Sex is a taboo subject.
- Many believe that satisfying one's own needs at the expense of others is a moral right.
- Sexual domination may be a manifestation of power.

African American Individuals

- Prevalence appears to be the same as for Euro-Americans.
- They are more likely to be physically abused and less likely to be sexually abused than Euro-American or Latino children.
- Many have had negative encounters with the criminal justice system and/or social service agencies, which impedes reporting of child sexual abuse.
- They may be reluctant to identify an African American perpetrator and turn him over to a system that administers harsher legal consequences to African Americans for criminal behavior.

Puerto Rican Individuals

- The reaction to sexual abuse is often geared toward maintaining the family's homeostasis; family loyalty is very important.
- If the daughter is a victim, the mother is perceived as being responsible.
- The popular beliefs are that sexually abused males become homosexuals and sexually abused females are considered promiscuous.

Mexican American Individuals

- There is a tendency for perpetrators to be more closely related to the victim.
- Both boys and girls are more likely than African American children to report rectal penetration.
- Boys are less likely to report abuse than girls.

Asian, Pacific Island, and Filipino American Individuals

- Sexuality is seldom discussed openly.
- Family structure is authoritarian and children are expected to be obedient to all authority figures.
- Physical abuse is more common than sexual abuse.
- When the child discloses, the family often directs its anger at the child and intervening adults; family will deny the abuse to save the family's reputation.
- Children may recant stories of sexual abuse, thus sacrificing their individual needs for family integrity.

American Jews

- They often have traditional gender roles.
- They believe that family togetherness provides a safe haven from inevitable persecution.
- Sexual abuse is seen as "the way of the gentiles," which burdens victims who anguish about revealing the family secret.

SOURCES: Abney, V. D., & Priest, R. (1995). African Americans and sexual child abuse. In L. A. Fontes (Ed.), *Sexual abuse in nine North American cultures* (pp. 11–30). Newbury Park, CA: Sage; Comas-Diaz, L. (1995). Puerto Ricans and sexual child abuse. In L. A. Fontes (Ed.), *Sexual abuse in nine North American cultures* (pp. 31–66). Newbury Park, CA: Sage; Featherman, J. M. (1995). Jews and sexual child abuse. In L. A. Fontes (Ed.), *Sexual abuse in nine North American cultures* (pp. 128–155). Newbury Park, CA: Sage; Huston, R. L., et al. (1995). Characteristics of childhood sexual abuse in a predominantly Mexican American population. *Child Abuse & Neglect, 19*(2), 165–176; Lefley, H. P. (1999). Transcultural aspects of sexual victimization. In J. A. Shaw (Ed.), *Sexual aggression* (pp. 129–166). Washington, DC: American Psychiatric Press; and Okamura, A., Heras, P., & Wong-Kerberg, L. (1995). Asian, Pacific Island, and Filipino Americans and sexual child abuse. In L. A. Fontes (Ed.), *Sexual abuse in nine North American cultures* (pp. 67–96). Newbury Park, CA: Sage.

Assessment: Physical

The obvious physical signs of sexual abuse in a child are the presence of a sexually transmitted infection, irritated or swollen genitals or rectal tissue, or both. Chronic vaginal or urinary tract infections with no known medical cause may be indicators that the child is being sexually abused. Among female victims, 12% to 24% become pregnant because of the abuse. The pregnant adolescent victim often has only vague stories regarding the father of her baby (Kawsar, Anfield, Walters, McCabe, & Forster, 2004; Rodgers, Lang, Twamley, & Stein, 2003).

Hure Hester, 35, was arrested for molesting a 13-year-old girl who became pregnant. The victim told police that he was her mother's boyfriend and she did not tell anyone because she was afraid of him. A DNA test indicated that Hester was the father of the newborn.

Some children will, consciously or unconsciously, attempt to abuse their bodies to either prevent or stop the sexual abuse. The child may gain a great deal of weight, hoping to become so unattractive that the abuser will leave the child alone. If an older child is being abused, a younger sister may become anorexic in an attempt not to mature and experience the same abuse. This lack of care for the body may continue into adult life in an unconscious attempt to maintain distance and avoid intimate relationships.

Corticotropin-releasing hormone (CRH) is associated with the "fight or flight" response to a threat. Animal studies demonstrate that traumatic experiences early in life change how the CRH gene is expressed in the brain. Increased CRH in the amygdala contributes to a chronic sense of fear that accompanies depression, anxiety, and PTSD in victims and survivors. Because there is an oversecretion of CRH, certain stressful life events may trigger symptoms in adult survivors. There is an accompanying increase in glucocorticoids that may also be neurotoxic to the hippocampus. Stress also increases the turnover of norepinephrine, which may affect areas of the brain involved in the regulation of emotion and memory (Bremmer et al., 2003).

Adult female survivors may have concerns about having a "normal" child and fears regarding pregnancy. For some, it is a difficult decision to bring a child into the world. Labor and delivery can be very difficult because, once again, their body is out of control and in pain. If health professionals are aware of the history of childhood sexual abuse, they can be more supportive during labor and delivery.

DIAGNOSIS

There are many potential nursing diagnoses for victims, survivors, and families suffering from childhood sexual abuse. In synthesizing the assessment data, consider how well clients are functioning in daily life. The following is a list of common diagnoses for victims, survivors, and families of child sexual abuse (North American Nursing Diagnosis Association, 2007):

- Child victim diagnoses:
  - Ineffective Individual Coping related to being a victim of sexual abuse
  - Powerlessness related to being helpless to stop the abuse
  - Posttrauma Syndrome related to being a victim of sexual abuse
  - Social Isolation related to keeping the family secret of sexual abuse
- Family diagnoses:
  - Interrupted Family Processes related to disruption of the family unit when parental abuse is discovered
- Adult survivor diagnoses:
  - Posttrauma Syndrome related to being an adult survivor
  - Spiritual Distress related to asking questions about fairness and justice in life or not being protected by a supreme being
  - Chronic Low Self-esteem related to self-blame for the abuse
  - Social Isolation related to difficulty in forming intimate relationships, mistrust of others
  - Sexual Dysfunction related to the trauma of the abuse

OUTCOME IDENTIFICATION AND GOALS

Based on the assessment data, you select outcomes appropriate to the nursing diagnoses. The long-term outcome is that children and adult survivors of child sexual abuse develop a higher level of functioning and an improved quality of life.

Once you have established outcomes, you, the client, and the family mutually identify goals for change. Goals are specific behavioral measures by which you, clients, and signifi-

cant others determine progress toward healing. The following are examples of some of the goals appropriate to people who have experienced childhood sexual abuse:

- Remains safe and free from harm
- Utilizes a variety of therapies to express feelings about the sexual abuse
- Verbalizes improved self-esteem
- Manages negative emotions in an appropriate manner
- Verbalizes a feeling of connectedness to significant others
- Verbalizes improvement in sexual functioning
- Utilizes community resources

PLANNING

Nurses are mandated by law to report any suspected child sexual abuse. Although as a culture we say that we protect our children, we do not in reality live out this value. We do not invest many of our energies—time, caring, and money—in the prevention of childhood sexual abuse. Our present approaches to treatment and to the social control of sexual abuse are not yet effective enough that we can be assured of the long-term safety of children. As nurses, we must all become active in the battle to stop child sexual abuse.

IMPLEMENTATION

The priority of care with child victims is to ensure the safety of the child. It is important that children feel personally safe and also that they are kept safe from further emotional damage in interactions with others. Civil authorities such as child protective services generally investigate complaints of abuse by a family member. Sexual abuse complaints are also referred to the police. If the investigation finds sufficient evidence, criminal prosecution of the alleged perpetrator may follow.

Protective services will implement one of four plans if they find that a child has been sexually abused by a family member:

1. The most frequent option is one in which the abuser is removed from the family. The nonabusing parent must be able to protect the child from any contact with the abuser.
2. When the nonabusing parent is unable to protect the child, both the child and the abuser are removed from the home. This option maximizes the safety of the child and decreases the child's feelings of responsibility.
3. In a few cases in which families have not used physical violence, where there is no substance abuse, and someone can ensure the child's safety, the family may be allowed to remain intact while participating in intensive therapy.
4. In a few instances, the child may be removed from the family when that appears to be the safest option.

NURSING CARE PLAN for a Child Victim

Collaborating With Families
Nursing Diagnosis: Client at Risk for Interrupted Family Process

Outcomes: Family will communicate clearly, establish appropriate boundaries, and demonstrate competency in family

Throughout the process of family intervention, you collaborate with family members in problem solving and attaining and maintaining positive relationships.

Intervention	Rationale	Goal
Help each family member write list of individual and family goals for treatment.	Writing a list increases each member's participation in therapy.	Formulates list
Help family identify individual and family strengths.	If able to identify strengths, they will feel more optimistic about change rather than feel defeated at the outset.	Identifies strengths and verbalizes hope for the future
Help family identify how the family perpetrator crossed generational boundaries by discussing roles and role reversals.	Crossing of boundaries is a contributing factor in sex abuse, because parent and child related to one another as peers.	Identifies appropriate roles according to the generation of each family member
Discuss ways that parents can maintain generational boundaries and appropriate power structure in the family.	Parents need to assume the responsibility for parenting all their children.	Parents function in parental roles and children function in age-appropriate roles
Help family members communicate directly with one another.	New and more effective communication styles are needed to improve family system functioning.	Communicates directly with family members
Discourage secrecy within the family.	Secrecy contributes to lack of trust and supports sex abuse.	Communicates openly with family members
Discuss ways rigid family systems can increase flexibility of roles and rules.	Rigid family systems are a contributing factor in sex abuse.	Rules and roles are more flexible
Discuss ways the chaotic family can organize appropriate roles and formulate consistent rules.	When parents have increased sense of competency and authority, they will parent more effectively.	Formulates consistent rules and roles
Teach family the problem-solving process.	Increasing alternative coping skills increases level of family functioning.	Uses the problem-solving process
Help family anticipate management of developmental transitions within family.	Anticipatory guidance may prevent future problems.	Verbalizes understanding of developmental phases of family
Refer to family therapy if appropriate.	More intense intervention is needed in some families.	Follows through on referral

Managing Flashbacks
Nursing Diagnosis: Client at Risk for Rape Trauma Syndrome

Outcomes: Client will utilize techniques to manage intrusive thoughts and flashbacks.

Adult survivors also need to learn skills for managing negative emotions, thoughts, and memories.

Intervention	Rationale	Goal
Teach muscle relaxation and deep breathing.	Deep breathing replaces the shallow breathing that occurs in highly anxious states and prevents hyperventilation.	Utilizes calming techniques to get through flashbacks without feeling overwhelmed
Teach sensory counting; name one thing clients can see in the room, one they can hear, and one they can sense in their bodies. Repeat and increase number.	This is a powerful self-help technique for managing memory flooding.	Utilizes sensory counting

NURSING CARE PLAN for a Child Victim

Managing Flashbacks
Nursing Diagnosis: Client at Risk for Rape Trauma Syndrome

Teach guided imagery: ■ Find a comfortable position and close eyes. ■ Make suggestions such as peaceful images or slow, gentle breathing. ■ Ask them to imagine surrounding the flashback with a pink bubble. ■ Have them let go of the bubble and watch it float off into the universe and disappear.	Used to gain control over flashbacks of the rape.	With practice, able to initiate this process at the first sign of an unwanted flashback

Promoting Self-Esteem
Nursing Diagnosis: Client at Risk for Chronic Low Self-Esteem

Outcomes: Client will verbalize feelings of empowerment, utilize positive affirmations, and practice assertive communication.

In working with adult survivors, remember that they have been robbed of a sense of power and feel detached from others. Recovery includes restoring power and control. Be sure to avoid becoming a "rescuer," as that might send the message that clients are not capable of acting for themselves. Also, be careful not to set yourself up as a powerful authority because that might recreate the type of relationship in which the abuse occurred. The most helpful approach is being ally, collaborator, and supporter as clients struggle through the healing process. Point out ways they have taken control of their lives, and help them identify situations in which they are able to make self-respecting choices. As Glaister and Able (2001, p. 193) describe the appropriate nurse therapist, "It was essential they find someone who could be present, who could understand, who could listen, and who could provide information on what to expect and on ways to grow. They needed supporters to step aside and allow them to be in control of their healing." Interventions are designed to increase self-esteem. Adult survivors have a continuous internal monologue of negative statements like, "You're weak, stupid, incompetent, unlovable, and unattractive."

Intervention	Rationale	Goal
Help clients become aware of the frequency and intensity of negative thoughts.	Negative statements become self-administered abuse and keep the adult survivor weak and powerless.	Verbalizes a conscious awareness of frequency of negative thoughts
Teach them to consciously replace negative thoughts with positive affirmations.	Often difficult at first, it becomes easier with practice.	Uses positive affirmations and verbalizes an improved self-esteem
When interacting with others, teach them to state their own opinions, interests, and needs directly and clearly.	Self-esteem is enhanced through the use of assertive skills.	Implements assertive skills
If others are demanding of them, teach clients to calmly and rationally set limits on this behavior.	Protection of self will increase feelings of self-control and power.	Verbalizes improved sense of control

Providing Spiritual Support
Nursing Diagnosis: Client at Risk for Spiritual Distress

Outcomes: Client will express a sense of hope and of meaning and purpose in life, and develop healthy relationships with others.

Betrayal by abusing adults is a spiritual issue. As nurses, we sometimes ignore a client's need for spiritual healing. Especially with adult survivors, you must support **spiritual recovery**. The sense of purpose in life is disrupted for victims and survivors. They also experience a loss in faith in a divine being as well as in other people. They are consumed with spiritual questions like, "Why did it happen to me?" "What's wrong with me?" and "Am I some evil person?" When people are sexually abused, they must struggle with questions of a God or some higher power that either overlooked their pain and did not respond or did not even see their pain at all. It is not unusual for survivors to be angry with the Divine and hold God responsible for the abuse. This anger may in turn trigger fear and guilt for hating someone so powerful.

continued

NURSING CARE PLAN for a Child Victim

Providing Spiritual Support

Nursing Diagnosis: Client at Risk for Spiritual Distress

Spirituality includes a *sense of connectedness to others*. Survivors must begin the long journey of developing trusting relationships. They need to experience human contact and the warmth of the nurse–client relationship. Approach each client individually and remember that the paths of human spirituality are as varied as the people taking them. Life events often shape belief systems in dramatic ways. The crisis and trauma of sexual abuse challenges victims and survivors to reflect on their values, beliefs, and their search for meaning. Approach each person with a sense of compassion and *encourage this spiritual reflection*. When requested, refer clients to religious/spiritual counselors who understand the emotional issues surrounding sexual abuse and who are sensitive to the need of survivors to work slowly through their spiritual struggles.

Intervention	Rationale	Goal
Encourage survivors to place responsibility for the abuse where it belongs—100% with the offender.	If they fail to do this, they will continue to be paralyzed by self-blame and guilt.	Identifies perpetrator's responsibility
Assist survivors to fully experience the rage and grief from their past sexual abuse.	Enables them to move on to self-forgiveness and more complete healing.	Expresses rage and grief in appropriate manner

Managing Anxiety

Nursing Diagnosis: Client at Risk for Anxiety

Outcomes: Client will verbalize decreasing anxiety.

Because adult survivors are often anxious, interventions to reduce anxiety are also necessary. Chapter 11 ∞ covers the management of anxiety in more detail.

Intervention	Rationale	Goal
Teach progressive relaxation and controlled breathing.	These techniques often prevent full-blown panic attacks.	Utilizes techniques to manage level of anxiety
When they are relaxed, instruct them to imagine a scene in which they feel safe and comfortable.	Returning to a safe place in their mind helps them remain in control.	Verbalizes control over episodes of anxiety
Teach clients to practice these techniques several times a day.	Practice facilitates the usefulness of these techniques.	Practices daily

Unfortunately, this decision may place additional guilt on the child.

Providing Adjunct Therapies

An important goal of nursing intervention is to facilitate the child's ability to talk and to think about the abuse with decreasing anxiety. The desired outcome is that the client will participate in available therapies, and express feelings.

It is up to the nurse to create a safe and predictable environment in which the child feels supported. Nurses should make it clear to the child that they understand that talking about the abuse is difficult. Plan interventions that encourage effective release in a supportive environment. Child victims must be able to experience a range of emotions. *Play therapy* helps these children play out traumatic themes, fears, and distorted beliefs. It is a nonthreatening way to process thoughts and feelings associated with the abuse, both sym-

bolically and directly. *Therapeutic stories* present the traumatic issues of abuse, link victims' feelings and behavior, and describe new coping methods. *Journal writing* can help children over age 10 cope with intrusive thoughts and feelings. They often choose to bring their journal into the one-to-one sessions with their therapist.

Art therapy provides an opportunity to *express feelings* for which there are no words. Art therapy helps adults in the healing process. Making group murals to express both individual progress and a sense of unity among clients can be very effective. Sitting and looking at soothing art works may be effective in reducing anxiety. *Music therapy*, combined with movement or dance, may be a way for clients to experience very early memories. *Anxiety may be lessened* by singing or humming a song, or playing a musical instrument. Journal writing is used more than any other expressive therapy and can be expanded to include poetry, songs, and plays.

The focus on *traumatic stress therapy* treats the trauma while acknowledging the process and result of victimization. *Developmental therapy* focuses on the "gaps" in the personality that occurred during the abuse process, such as trust issues, identity issues, and relationship issues. *Loss therapy* focuses on helping survivors identify and grieve over things lost during childhood sexual abuse, such as innocence, trust, nurturing, and memories.

Group therapy allows survivors to share their feelings and experiences with others who believe their stories. The group setting fosters mutual understanding and decreases the sense of isolation. Many adult survivors find self-help groups to be supportive in the process of healing. They are given a better idea of how their behavior affects others while helping others makes them feel more competent. They are reassured by seeing others recover. The Community Resources feature on the Companion Website lists national groups designed for survivors as well as perpetrators of child sexual abuse.

Promoting Sexual Health

Sexual healing is important for many adult survivors. It is an empowering process that enables the survivors to reclaim their sexuality as positive and pleasurable. This process may take several months to several years. It is usually not undertaken until the more general issues such as depression, anger, self-blame, and self-destructive behaviors are resolved. The program of recovery is best guided by a sex therapist with expertise in working with adult survivors. For survivors caught up in compulsive and addictive sexual behaviors, participation in 12-step recovery programs is often essential.

The desired outcome is that client will discuss age-appropriate sexual behavior, and verbalize improved sexual functioning.

EVALUATION

Nurses in the acute care setting may not have the opportunity for long-term evaluation. Short-term evaluation focuses mainly on identifying child victims and adult survivors and referrals to appropriate community resources. Nurses in long-term or community settings have the opportunity to evaluate the effectiveness of the multidisciplinary treatment plan over an extended period.

Clinical Interactions | A Child Victim of Sexual Abuse

Kylie is 10 years old and has been admitted for getting into physical fights at school, out of control behavior in the classroom, and talking about wishing she were dead. Her mother has substance abuse problems and the mother's boyfriend sexually abused Kylie. She lives with her father and stepmother. In the interaction, you see evidence of:

- Suicidal ideation
- Self-blame
- Mother's disbelief of abuse
- Limited peer relationships

KYLIE: "My stepmom brought me here. She couldn't take the way I was acting."

NURSE: "Could you tell me more about that?"

KYLIE: "I wanted to kill myself." [looking to see how the nurse is reacting] "I thought that all the bad things that had happened to me were my fault. Sometimes I think life is not worth living."

NURSE: "Could you help me understand what you mean by 'bad things'?"

KYLIE: "What I mean is . . ." [looking down] "I was sexually abused by my mom's boyfriend."

NURSE: "And you feel responsible for the abuse?"

KYLIE: "Yes."

NURSE: "Kylie, you are not responsible for what he did to you."

KYLIE: "That's not what my mom said." [shaking her head] "When I first told her what was going on she said I was lying. And then when she found out the whole truth, she blamed me for the abuse. I thought my mom would be on my side and leave him. That's what moms are for, to be there for kids and protect them." [angry voice]

NURSE: "Earlier you said that life is not worth living. Tell me more about those feelings."

KYLIE: "I wanted to kill myself a couple of times so far. The last time was the night I told my mom about the abuse. I felt very angry when she didn't believe me, so I took my jump rope and I put it around my neck and wanted to strangle myself. Unfortunately, my mom saw me and she took my jump rope away."

NURSE: "What would your suicide accomplish for you?"

KYLIE: "Well, I would be safe and free from all the people that I don't like at my school."

NURSE: "You are saying your problems would be resolved by killing yourself?"

KYLIE: "Right."

NURSE: "What would have to change for you to decide to live?"

KYLIE: "I want to forget all the bad things that happened to me. I also want to have more friends at school. I don't think the kids like me. They ignore me all the time. I feel kind of lonely at school."

Using Research Evidence   The Impact of Sexual Assault

McFarlane, J., Malecha, A., Gist, J., Watson, K., Batten, E., Hall, I., & Smith, S. (2005). Intimate partner sexual assault against women and associated victim substance use, suicidality, and risk factors for femicide. *Issues in Mental Health Nursing, 26,* 953–967.

What is the study about?

Very little is known concerning the occurrence and health effects of intimate partner sexual assault. Therefore, the purpose of this study was to provide additional knowledge about how sexual assault affects women's health. The study compared women physically *and* sexually assaulted by a partner to those nonsexually assaulted by a partner: It compared their risk factors for femicide and suicide. Also, the researchers aimed to establish the frequency of substance use following sexual assault.

How was the study done?

This second component of a two-part quantitative study included 148 women who experienced intimate partner sexual assault and/or physical abuse and were involved with the special family-violence unit of a district attorney's office. The study included women who identified themselves as African American (n=49), White (n=39), and Latino/Hispanic (n=60). The study received approval from an institutional review board. Sexual assault was defined as a positive response to any one of the five questions on the Severity of Violence Against Women Scale (SAVAWS). Questions asked whether an intimate partner had: 1) made you have sexual intercourse against your will, 2) physically forced you to have sex, 3) made you have oral sex against your will, 4) made you have anal sex against your will, or 5) used an object on you in a sexual way. Demographic data were obtained; then a researcher interviewed each participant about the participant's use of nicotine, alcohol, and/or illegal drugs following (and attributed to) the first and subsequent episodes of sexual assault. The Danger Assessment Scale [sic] was used to determine each woman's risk of becoming a femicide victim. Independent t-tests and chi-square analyses tested whether the women assaulted both physically and sexually differed in demographics from women who were nonsexually assaulted. Descriptive statistics and relative risk analyses were used to assess the reports of substance use following sexual assault(s). Two-way analysis of variance was done to test for differences in mean scores on risk for femicide. For each risk factor for femicide from the first study, relative risk analysis was used to distinguish those women physically and sexually assaulted from those nonsexually assaulted.

What were the results of the study?

Of the 148 women, 68% (n=100) reported sexual assault(s) during a relationship. There were no significant demographic differences between women who had been assaulted physically and sexually and those who were nonsexually assaulted. Among the women who were sexually assaulted, women who reported more than one sexual assault were more than three times as likely to acknowledge beginning or increasing substance use. Only these women reported using illicit drugs, usually crack or cocaine. The most frequently reported abused substance was alcohol. The sexually assaulted women had significantly increased risk factors for femicide. No significant differences were found between ethnic groups; nor was there an interaction between sexual assault and ethnicity. Suicidal ideation or attempts within 90 days of reporting the assault were 5.3 times more likely among women in the sexually assaulted group. Alcohol use was attributed to the sexual assault by 10% of the women reporting one sexual assault and 27% of women reporting more than one. Beginning or increasing drug use was attributed to the sexual assault by none of the participants who reported one sexual assault and 9% of those who experienced more than one. Nicotine use was attributed to sexual assault(s) in 10% of women who experienced one sexual assault and 22% of the women who reported more than one. Data analysis from the Danger Assessment Screen [sic] found that 22% of the sexually assaulted women had suicidal ideation or attempted to commit suicide, compared to 4.2% of the women not reporting sexual assault. Compared to physically abused women, women who also reported sexual assault had significantly more risk factors for femicide. In addition, women experiencing sexual assault(s) reported a high frequency of threats to harm children as well as murder threats to the woman.

What additional questions might I have?

Would the results have been significantly different with women who were not involved in seeking assistance from the justice system? How were the results affected by the use of self-report? Were the women who reported only physical assault also experiencing an increase in initiating or using illicit substances? What is the relationship of childhood assault to their current experiences of assault? What was the mental health history of the participants in this study in regard to traumatic events and suicidal ideation?

How can I use this study?

Nurses need to screen for both physical and sexual assault and be cognizant that women having these experiences are at increased risk for femicide and suicide. Nurses must develop skills in assessment and intervention of intimate partner violence in all areas of nursing practice. Among women who have experienced sexual assaults, nurses should assess for drug and alcohol use and suicidal ideation. Programs need to be devised to assist these women to explore substance abuse as possibly related to their experience of sexual assault. Nursing education needs to include information on the interconnectiveness of sexual assault, substance abuse, the risk for femicide, and threats to the family.

SOURCE: Contributed by Dolores Huffman, PhD, RN, Associate Professor of Nursing, Purdue University Calumet, Hammond, Indiana.

Focus Your Study

OBJECTIVES

KEY CONCEPTS

1. Discuss the theories regarding the etiologies of rape and childhood sexual abuse.

- Rape:
  - Eighty percent of rapists are under the age of 30 and many have been sexually and physically abused as children or adolescents.
  - Anger rape—use of extreme force and viciousness as a way of releasing rage on others
  - Power rape—intent is not to injure but to master another person sexually
  - Sadistic rape—violence is a stimulus for rapist's own sexual excitement
  - Gang rape—group ritual used to confirm masculinity and power
  - Acquaintance rape—forced sexual activity by a person known to victim
  - Acceptance of interpersonal violence and a view of women as subservient in a culture contributes to a higher incidence of rape
- Childhood sexual abuse:
  - Disrupted family structure, cohesion, and adaptability
  - Lack of empathy for victim
  - Sense of power and domination
  - Perpetrators deny, minimize, justify, and rationalize their behavior.

2. Describe the short- and long-term implications for victims of sexual violence.

- Behavior after rape:
  - Agitated and nonpurposeful behavior
  - Some appear outwardly calm when feeling numbness and emotional shock
  - Longer-term: crying spells; difficulty with relationships, school or work difficulties, nightmares, phobias
- Affect after rape:
  - Fear
  - Depression
  - Helpless, vulnerable
- Cognition after rape:
  - Depersonalization or dissociation
  - Difficulty with decision making
  - Self-blame
  - Obsessive thoughts
- Behavior after childhood sexual abuse:
  - Clinging attachment to adults
  - Sexual acting out behavior
  - Self-destructive behaviors
  - Teens may run away
- Affect after childhood sexual abuse:
  - Many fears
  - Self-blame
  - Powerlessness
  - Rage
- Cognition after childhood sexual abuse:
  - Denial to cope with trauma
  - Dissociation
  - Amnesia
  - Low self-esteem
  - Flashbacks

3. Outline the assessment process for a victim of sexual violence and her/his family. →	■ Rape:
	  • Provide immediate physical assessment for any serious or critical injuries.
	  • Following physical stabilization, inform clients of their right to have a rape crisis advocate with them for the assessment process.
	  • If a SANE nurse is available, have that nurse assigned to rape victims.
	  • Respect clients' autonomy to prevent revictimization.
	■ Child sexual abuse:
	  • Reactions vary greatly from one person to another.
	  • Respect the power of secrecy and how difficult it is for children and adult survivors to disclose information about the abuse.
	  • Assess for self-mutilation.
	  • Assess for self-blame.

4. Use the nursing process to develop a comprehensive plan of care for a victim of sexual violence and her/his family. →	■ Victims of rape:
	  • Support defense mechanisms and coping behaviors.
	  • Encourage victim to talk about the assault.
	  • Help victim use problem-solving process.
	  • If appropriate, discuss beliefs about postcoital contraception.
	  • Help victims search for meaning in the trauma and help them identify spiritual support systems.
	■ Childhood sexual abuse:
	  • Ensure child's safety.
	  • Report suspected child sexual abuse.
	  • Collaborate with family in problem solving and attaining and maintaining positive relationships.
	  • Support clients as they struggle to regain a sense of power and control.
	  • Replace negative self-statements with positive affirmations.
	  • Support clients in developing trusting relationships.
	  • Encourage spiritual reflection.
	  • Initiate adjunct therapies such as play therapy, therapeutic stories, journal writing, art therapy, music therapy, traumatic stress therapy, developmental therapy, and loss therapy.

5. Develop teaching plans for a victim of sexual violence and her/his family. →	■ Explain the usual reactions to victimization such as fear and depression. ■ Teach the family about the nature and trauma of rape or sexual abuse and the immediate and potential long-term reactions of the survivors. ■ Teach family how to best support the survivor so that they neither overprotect nor minimize the impact of the rape. ■ Explain the cultural myths regarding rape and teach the realities of rape. ■ Teach skills for managing flashbacks and calming techniques such as muscle relaxation, deep breathing, guided imagery, and sensory counting.

Explore MediaLink

For review questions, case studies, and other resources for this chapter see the Pearson Health MediaLink CD-ROM that accompanies this book and the Companion Website.

CD-ROM
- Audio Glossary
- NCLEX-RN® Review Questions
- Animations/Videos
  - Sexual Abuse Interview—Parts 1, 2, and 3

Companion Website www.prenhall.com/fontaine
- Audio Glossary
- NCLEX-RN® Review Questions
- Case Study
  - The Rape Victim in the Emergency Department
- Care Plan
  - The Victim of Domestic Violence
- Critical Thinking
  - Crisis Management for Rape Victims
- MediaLink Application
  - Domestic Violence: Before It Occurs; Primary Prevention of Intimate Partner Violence and Abuse
- MediaLinks
  - Books for Clients & Families
  - Community Resources

Review Questions

23-1. A high school teacher offers a 15-year-old student a ride home from an extracurricular activity. The teacher turns onto a deserted rural road and begins to manipulate the student's penis until he ejaculates. The student is embarrassed by his inability to stop his response and asks the teacher to take him home. He does not report the incident because of his feelings of shame and guilt. Which of the following types of rape is described in the above scenario?
  1. Sadistic rape
  2. Power rape
  3. Anger rape
  4. Acquaintance rape

23-2. Which of the following behaviors would lead a nurse to suspect that a child has been sexually abused?
  1. The child touches the nipples of another child the same age.
  2. The child questions a parent about how babies are put in a woman's stomach.
  3. The child continues to masturbate at school when told it is not appropriate to do so.
  4. The child clings to a parent when the nurse begins a physically examination of the child.

23-3. A 40-year-old male is accused of sexually abusing his 6-year-old niece while helping her out of the swimming pool. The man denies touching his niece in a sexual way. Which of the following factors is present if no sexual abuse occurred?
  1. The niece was persuaded by her uncle to let him touch her between the legs.
  2. The niece was confused because she had been told that no one should ever touch her between the legs without her permission.

  3. The uncle justified touching her between the legs by saying that he wanted to make sure she didn't slip and fall while getting out of the pool.
  4. The uncle showed no compassion or concern for his niece's allegations that he touched her inappropriately between the legs.

23-4. The nurse notified child protective services about the sexual abuse of a 10-year-old child by an unidentified family member. Which of the following options would best ensure the safety of this victim?
  1. The victim is removed from the home and placed in foster care.
  2. Both the victim and the abuser are removed from the family.
  3. The victim remains in the home and the family begins intensive treatment.
  4. The abuser is removed from the family.

23-5. A nurse is teaching victims of sexual violence and their families about available community resources. The nurse recognizes that more education is needed if a member of this class asks about joining which of the following organizations?
  1. Survivors of Incest Anonymous
  2. National Center for Victims of Crime
  3. Safer Society Foundation
  4. Men Can Stop Rape

See Appendix D for answers.

References

American Psychiatric Association. (2000). *Diagnostic and statistical manual of mental disorders* (4th ed., Text Revision). Washington, DC: Author.

Andrade, J. T., Vincent, G. M., & Saleh, F. M. (2006). Juvenile sex offenders: A complex population. *Journal of Forensic Sciences, 51*(1), 163–167.

Bremner, J. D., Vythiingam, M., Vermetten, E., Southwick, S. M., McGlashan, R., Nazeer, A., et al. (2003). MIR and PET study of deficits in hippocampal structure and function in women with childhood sexual abuse and posttraumatic stress disorder. *American Journal of Psychiatry, 160*(5), 924–932.

Brown, S. M. (2000). Healthy sexuality and the treatment of sexually abusive youth. *SIECUS Report, 29*(1), 40–46.

Faravelli, C., Giugni, A., Salvatori, S., & Ricca, V. (2004). Psychopathology after rape. *American Journal of Psychiatry, 161*(8), 1483–1485.

Fontes, L. A. (2005). *Child abuse and culture.* New York: Guilford Press.

Glaister, J. A., & Able, E. (2001). Experiences of women healing from childhood sexual abuse. *Archives of Psychiatric Nursing, 15*(4), 188–194.

Hibino, Y., Ogino, K., & Inagaki, M. (2006). Sexual harassment of female nurses by patients in Japan. *Journal of Nursing Scholarship, 38*(4), 400–405.

Huesmann, L. R., Moise-Titus, J., Podolski, C. L., & Eron, L. D. (2003). Longitudinal relations between children's exposure to TV violence and

their aggressive and violent behavior in young adulthood. *Developmental Psychology, 39*(2), 201–221.

Johnson, T. C. (2000). Sexualized children and children who molest. *SIECUS Report, 29*(1), 35–37.

Kaplow, J. B., Dodge, K. A., Amaya-Jackson, L., & Saxe, G. N. (2005). Pathways to PTSD, part II: Sexually abused children. *American Journal of Psychiatry, 162*(7), 1305–1310.

Kawsar, M., Anfield, A., Walters, E., McCabe, S., & Forster, G. E. (2004). Prevalence of sexually transmitted infections and mental health needs of female child and adolescent survivors of rape and sexual assault attending a specialist clinic. *Sexually Transmitted Infections, 80*(2), 138–141.

Kreidler, M. (2005). Group therapy for survivors of childhood sexual abuse who have chronic mental illness. *Archives of Psychiatric Nursing, 19*(4), 176–183.

Lanza, M. L., Zeiss, R., & Rierdan, J. (2006). Violence against psychiatric nurses. *Contemporary Nurse, 21*(1), 71–84.

Lips, H. M. (2004). *Sex and gender* (5th ed.). New York: McGraw-Hill.

Martino, S. C., Collins, R. L., Elliott, M. N., Strachman, A., Kanouse, D. E., & Berry, S. H. (2006). Exposure to degrading versus nondegrading music lyrics and sexual behavior among youth. *Pediatrics, 118*(2), 430–441.

McCabe, M. P., & Wauchope, M. (2005). Behavioral characteristics of men accused of rape. *Archives of Sexual Behavior, 34*(2), 241–253.

McCloskey, K. A., & Raphael, D. N. (2005). Adult perpetrator gender asymmetries in child sexual assault victim selection. *Journal of Child Sexual Abuse, 14*(4), 1–24.

McFarlane, J., Malecha, A., Gist, J., Watson, K., Batten, E., Hall, I., & Smith, S. (2005). Intimate partner sexual assault against women and associated victim substance use, suicidality, and risk factors for femicide. *Issues in Mental Health Nursing, 26,* 953–967.

Mitchell, K. J., Finkelhor, D., & Wolak, J. (2005). The Internet and family and acquaintance sexual abuse. *Child Maltreatment, 10*(1), 49–60.

Mitchell, K. J., Wolak, J., & Finkelhor, D. (2005). Police posing as juveniles online to catch sex offenders. *Sex Abuse, 17*(3), 241–267.

Murphy, W. D., & Page, I. J. (1999). Adolescent perpetrators of sexual abuse. In J. A. Shaw (Ed.), *Sexual aggression* (pp. 367–389). Washington, DC: American Psychiatric Press.

National Center for Victims of Crime. (2004). Retrieved March 1, 2006, from http://www.ncvc.org

North American Nursing Diagnosis Association. (2007). *Nursing diagnoses: Definitions and classification, 2007–2008.* Philadelphia: Author.

Palmer, C. M., McNulty, A. M., D'Este, C., & Donovan, B. (2004). Genital injuries in women reporting sexual assault. *Sexual Health, 1*(1), 55–59.

Palmieri, P. A., & Fitzgerald, L. F. (2005). Confirmatory factor analysis of posttraumatic stress symptoms in sexually harassed women. *Journal of Traumatic Stress, 18*(6), 657–666.

Rauch, S. A. M., & Foa, E. B. (2004). Sexual trauma. In B. T. Litz (Ed.), *Early interventions for trauma and traumatic loss* (pp. 216–240). New York: Guilford Press.

Rodgers, C. S., Lang, A. J., Twamley, E. W., & Stein, M. B. (2003). Sexual trauma and pregnancy. *Journal of Women's Health, 12*(10), 961–970.

Ryan, G. (2000). Perpetration prevention. *SIECUS Report, 29*(1), 28–34.

Salter, D., McMillan, D., Richards, M., Talbot, T., Hodges, J., Bentovim, A., et al. (2003). Development of sexually abusive behavior in sexually victimized males. *Lancet, 361*(9356), 471–476.

Schetky, K. H. (1999). Sexual victimization of children. In J. A. Shaw (Ed.), *Sexual aggression*

(pp. 107–128). Washington, DC: American Psychiatric Press.

Sexual Abuse Statistics. (n.d.). Retrieved October 29, 2005, from http://www.prevent-abuse-now.com/stats.htm

Sivagnanam, G., Bairy, K. L., & D'Souza, U. (2005). Attitude towards rape. *Medical Journal of Malaysia, 60*(3), 286–293.

Stermac, L., Dunlap, H., & Bainbridge, D. (2005). Sexual assault services delivered by SANES. *Journal of Forensic Nursing, 1*(3), 124–128.

Ullman, S. E., Filipas, H. H., Townsend, S. M., & Starzynski, L. L (2005). Trauma exposure, posttraumatic stress disorders and problem drinking in sexual assault survivors. *Journal of Studies on Alcohol, 66*(5), 610–619.

Valente, S. M. (2005). Sexual abuse of boys. *Journal of Child and Adolescent Psychiatric Nursing, 18*(1), 10–16.

Walker, J., Archer, J., & Davies, M. (2005). Effects of rape on men. *Archives of Sexual Behavior, 34*(1), 69–80.

Warne, T., & McAndrew, S. (2005). The shackles of abuse: Unprepared to work at the edges of reason. *Journal of Psychiatric and Mental Health Nursing, 12*(6), 679–686.

Wolak, J., Finkelhor, D., & Mitchell, K. (2004). Internet-initiated sex crimes against minors. *Journal of Adolescent Health, 35*(5), e11–e20.

Chapter 24

Community Violence

Contributed by Leslie Rittermeyer, PsyD, RN

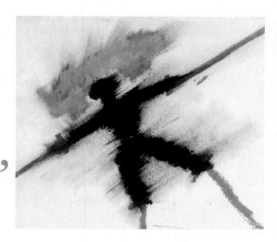

66 *Nights come*
Dreams advance
Terror strikes
Then loneliness

Emptiness consumes me
Hopelessness surrounds me
Despair drowns me

I'm lost in a hollow wheel
With no light showing me the way 99

—Kate, Age 19 (drawing)
—Anna, Age 19 (poetry)

OBJECTIVES

After reading this chapter, you will be able to:

1. Discuss the theories regarding the etiologies of violent behavior.

2. Outline the process for assessing the potential for violent behavior.

3. Use the nursing process to develop a comprehensive plan of care for addressing community violence.

4. Develop teaching plans to prevent community violence.

5. Discuss the key points in effectively communicating with a person who is at risk for violent behavior.

MediaLink www.prenhall.com/fontaine

Go to the Pearson Health MediaLink CD-ROM and the Companion Website at www.prenhall.com/fontaine for interactive resources for this chapter.

The prevalence of violence in American culture is significant. In the United States, 5 of every 10 people will be exposed to a major trauma sometime in their life (Litz, 2004). We live in a culture that promotes, supports, and sometimes encourages—even romanticizes—violence. According to the U.S. Department of Justice (2005) there is a violent crime committed every 23.1 seconds and a property crime committed every 3.1 seconds. Violence is a common theme in computer games, movies, television dramas, and the lyrics and visual images of music videos. Acts of violence remind us that communities cannot be complacent and must act together to make our schools, workplaces, and neighborhoods safer environments in which to work and play.

Whether it occurs in school or in the neighborhood, violence aimed at children and adolescents continues to be a concern. Many children die as a result of gun violence and many more are seriously wounded. Children who witness or become victims of physical assault are at higher risk for an acute stress response (Skybo, 2005).

This chapter focuses primarily on perpetrators of violence who are children and adolescents because they represent the majority. Youth also reflect the social, economic, moral, and ethical problems in society. The hope is that prevention strategies directed toward youths will decrease the level of epidemic violence throughout the United States. (For treatment aimed at victims and survivors of violence, see chapter 25 ∞ on terrorism.)

KNOWLEDGE BASE

Types of Violence

Affective Violence

Affective violence is the verbal expression of intense anger and emotions. It is bullying, ugly taunts, disrespect, alienation, scapegoating, and physical threats, which many people experience every day. The primary goal is to injure the target. Typically, the behavior is impulsive, in response to interpersonal stress, and is frequently expressed while under the influence of alcohol and drugs.

Predatory Violence

Predatory violence includes **hate crimes** which are also referred to as *bias crimes*. Hate crimes are motivated by bias and hatred of minority groups. People, who typically do nothing to provoke the attack, are harassed, tortured, and even killed just because they are different. Hate crimes occur in rural, suburban, and urban communities alike, targeting racial or ethnic minorities, religious minorities, and gay, lesbian, bisexual, or transgendered (GLBT) people. Following the terrorists attacks of September 11, 2001, there were scattered incidents of violence against people presumed to be from Muslim countries.

Many perpetrators of hate crimes are youthful thrill seekers who commit the crime for the thrill associated with the victimization. A part of this reflects the desire to live up to friends' expectations and to prove toughness and/or heterosexuality to friends. Some perpetrators are driven by racial or religious ideology or ethnic bigotry. They reflect negative cultural attitudes and justify their actions as righteous responses.

Perpetrators of hate crimes often plan the acts beforehand, frequently get pleasure from the violent act itself, and feel little, if any, remorse. Hate crimes may end in murder. Take two recent notable examples: the torture and crucifixion-style killing of Matthew Shepard, a homosexual college student in Wyoming, and the dragging death of James Byrd, Jr., an African American adult male, in Texas.

On February 2, 2006, Jacob Robida, age 19, walked into a popular gay tavern known for its quiet atmosphere. He asked the bartender if he was in a gay bar. When told that he was, he shoved several of the patrons to the ground, then pulled a hatchet from his sweatshirt and swung at their heads. Jacob then pulled out a handgun and began shooting at everyone. Three people were severely injured.

Many teens live in a violent world. Some are victims of violence that is common in their environment, such as drive-by shootings, but are also at an increased risk for violence unique to their minority status. Ideally, the school setting could offer a temporary haven where all students feel safe. The reality, however, is that hate crimes often occur during school hours. Gay youth report being verbally abused and physically harassed. Gay adults do not fare much better and report being the target of verbal harassment, threats, property vandalism, and physical assault as the result of their sexual orientation. Another form of predatory violence involves the phenomenon of **stalking**, which can be viewed on a continuum from nondelusional to delusional. In nondelusional stalking, there is a relationship between the victim and the perpetrator, which tends to be or has been one of close interpersonal involvement. (See chapter 22 ∞ for information on stalking and domestic violence.) At the delusional end of the continuum, the relationship exists only in the mind of perpetrators who may have a delusion that a famous person is in love with them (erotomanic delusion). Stalkers may also be motivated by religious delusions or hallucinations directing them to target a particular person. There is often a preoccupation with the victim that becomes consuming and ultimately could lead to the victim's death.

In between these two extremes of stalking is a mixture of relationships. The victim and perpetrator may have dated only one or two times; the victim may have only smiled or said hello in passing; or they may be in some way socially or vocationally acquainted. In some instances, the stalker may make obscene or harassing phone calls or send letters professing love or knowledge of the victim's movements. The behavior may eventually move to threats and menacing comments. At some point, stalkers may make their identity known by appearing at the victim's work or residence. One group of researchers who studied the legal punishments for stalking found that many stalking cases are dropped by the courts. This leniency is unfortunate because stalkers are prone to repeat their behavior, and often have orders of protection against them (Jordan, Logan, & Walker, 2003).

Cyberstalking refers to the use of the Internet, e-mail, or other electronic communications to stalk another person. It is a serious problem that is likely to become more widespread. Similar to other forms of stalking, cyberstalkers wish to establish control over the victim. In many cases, there was a prior relationship between perpetrator and victim, but there are also a number of situations of cyberstalking by strangers. Electronic harassment of adults is not a federal crime and is not a crime in most states. The U.S. Department of Justice does not yet publish aggregate statistics on any types of stalking crimes.

There are a small number of psychiatric clients who stalk, threaten, or harass health care staff. Those who engage in this type of predatory violence typically limit their behavior to oral or written threats or unwanted telephone calls.

Types of Homicide

Burgess and Dowdell (1999) have identified four types of *personal-cause homicide*: nonspecific homicide, revenge homicide, patricide/matricide homicide, and authority killing. Personal-cause homicides are not driven by material gain or sexual intention, unlike other types of homicide, which are motivated by a need for money, political concerns, organized crime or gangs, or violence for pleasure.

In **nonspecific homicide**, only the perpetrator, who seems to want as many victims as possible, knows the motive. The crime often becomes a massacre with little regard for the value of life. The crime, although planned, is often unorganized, with no arrangements for escaping the police.

On February 29, 2000, in Mount Morris Township, Michigan, a 6-year-old boy went to school, told first-grade student Kayla Rolland that he did not like her, and then shot her with a handgun he brought from home. Prior to the shooting, the boy was reportedly made to stay after school nearly every day for incidents of violent behavior.

On March 13, 2005, in Milwaukee, Wisconsin, long-time church member Terry Ratzman fired randomly into his congregation, killing seven church members before killing himself. No one who knew him could give an explanation for his actions. He was known as a gentle man.

On May 21, 2006, Anthony Bell opened fire at a church, fatally wounding four people before abducting his wife, whom he later killed at another location.

On Febuary 14, 2008, at Northern Illinois University, Steven Kazmierczak burst into a lecture hall brandishing several guns and shooting randomly at students and faculty. Within several minutes, five students and the gunman were dead and 16 people were wounded.

Perpetrators of **revenge homicide** retaliate for real or imagined offenses brought on by the victim. Depending on the event that triggered the act of revenge, there may be multiple victims. Perpetrators of revenge homicide are often the victims of bullying, teasing, humiliation, and physical assault. Killing those who torment them is an act of revenge. The murder is prearranged and organized, including plans for escaping the scene of the crime. A recent stressful event or the accumulation of long-term stress often motivates these individuals.

On March 24, 1998, in Jonesboro, Arkansas, 11-year-old Andrew Golden and 13-year-old Mitchell Johnson sat on a hill 100 yards from a school. As the children and teachers left the building in response to a false fire alarm, they fired 22 rounds of ammunition, killing five, and wounding 15, people.

On March 5, 2001, in Santee, California, 15-year-old Charles Andrew Williams opened fire from a bathroom at his high school, killing two, and wounding 13, people. Other students said he was picked on all the time because he was "scrawny." Peers called him "freak," "dork," and "nerd."

On March 22, 2005, in Red Lake, Minnesota, a 15-year-old boy shot both his grandparents and then drove to his high school and, while laughing and waving, killed seven classmates before killing himself. He was described by his relatives as a loner who was often teased.

Patricide/matricide homicide may be in response to many years of physical and sexual abuse or from a defiance of rules, a dare from a peer group, or other causes not related to parental behavior. Typically, children and adolescents who kill parents flee the scene only to be captured fairly quickly. Of all youths who commit murder each year in the United States, only 8% murder one or both parents. Juveniles who have killed a parent are typically Euro-American, middle-class boys who have had little contact with law enforcement. Some are loners anxious for acceptance by peers and adults. Others kill as the result of a family-related argument. Less often, parents are killed for money, possessions, or freedom.

In January 2005, 29-year-old Kenneth Allen and 18-year-old Kari Allen stabbed their mother to death and then lured their grandmother to their apartment where they smothered her with a plastic bag. Later that day, they went to their grandfather's home and beat him to death with a hammer. Taking their relatives' cash and credit cards, they headed to Las Vegas. When they were pulled over for speeding, they acknowledged the murders, which they said they did to get their grandparents' money.

Steven Michael Tomporowski, an 18-year-old high school dropout, was stopped by the police in Kentucky in February of 2004. Police discovered that Steven shot his father and uncle to death in a Wisconsin farmhouse and then lured his mother to the home and killed her as she walked in the door.

The morning of October 6, 2004, 36-year-old Steven Gobillot was killed by police in the home where his parents lived and where he grew up. He drove from Illinois to New Jersey where he killed both his parents. Steven had no criminal record and the neighbors described him as a most wonderful guy. They described his family—his wife and three young children—as one of those "ideal" families.

Those who commit an **authority killing** frequently do so in response to real or imagined offenses. The targets may be individuals or a building or structure that symbolizes authority. The killer may desire to commit suicide or die at the hands of police to attain martyrdom for the murders.

> On May 26, 2000, 13-year-old Nathaniel Brazill was sent home for throwing water balloons. He returned with a handgun, went into an English class, and shot and killed his teacher, Barry Grunow.

Settings of Community Violence

Violence occurs in all the usual places people turn to for security—home, workplace, school, and neighborhood. (Family violence is discussed in chapter 22 ∞).

Workplace Violence

Workplace violence has become a major social and economic problem, with thousands of people a year victims of crime on the job. The majority of workplace homicides are committed by strangers or intruders and are related to robbery. Those at highest risk are those working in law enforcement, working alone or in small numbers, working late at night, working in restaurants or gas stations, and driving a taxi. Workplace homicides not related to robbery are acts of domestic violence or stalking, or acts by disgruntled former or current employees (Ray & Ream, 2007).

> In 2003, Salvador Topin, a disgruntled former employee in Chicago, Illinois, returned to his workplace and shot six fellow workers.
>   In February, 2006, Jennifer San Marco killed her neighbor at a Santa Barbara condominium complex. She then went to the mail processing center, where she formerly worked, and shot five people to death before committing suicide.

Violence in hospitals has grown along with violence in society. In a survey of emergency nurses, 86% reported that they have been the victim of violence. Only about half of these incidents are reported. Risk factors for violence in the emergency department include long wait times, 24-hour accessibility of the emergency department, and lack of armed and visible security guards (Ray & Ream, 2007).

School Violence

Although the nation's schools are safer than ever and the crime rate has decreased, the legacy of the killings at schools across the country—including Oregon, Colorado, Virginia, Arkansas, Pennsylvania, Mississippi, Illinois, and Kentucky—looms large in the minds of Americans. **School violence** is the occurrence of violent crime at school as well as on the way to and from school. The Gun Free Schools Act of 1994 required schools to expel for at least one year any student who brings

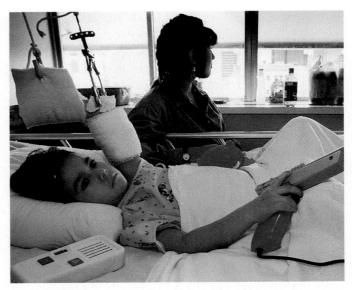

PHOTO 24.1 ■ Societal influences on children's behavior are pervasive. This 3-year-old boy received a gunshot wound during a drive-by shooting. Still, the boy plays with a toy pistol while recuperating in his hospital bed.
SOURCE: Rick Hunter/Corbis/Sygma. Used with permission.

a firearm to school as well as referring the student to the criminal justice or juvenile justice system.

One school-related problem behavior that has increased rather than decreased is bullying, which is intentional and chronic infliction of physical or psychological pain. One study of 3,530 third-, fourth-, and fifth-grade students found that 22% of these children were involved in bullying either as a victim, bully, or both (Glew, Fan, Katon, Rivara, & Kernic, 2005). Today's bully is more violent and can spread hate fast and wide on the Internet, 24 hours a day, 7 days a week. i-SAFE America (n.d.), a nonprofit Internet-safety advocacy group, reported that 42% of American children have been bullied while online and 35% have been threatened online.

Bullies often continue their antisocial behaviors throughout their lifetimes. They may be involved in dating or marital violence or workplace harassment.

Street Violence

Teens are much more likely than adults to be victims of **street violence**. No longer can they expect to be safe at school or in their neighborhoods. Violent **gangs** operate in the majority of all medium and large cities, and small towns are not exempt. Most, or all, gang members are involved in drug sales and in a variety of serious and violent crimes. Many acts of violence are the result of bad drug deals, infringement on drug territory, or an event perceived as disrespectful by a rival gang member—referred to in gang slang as *dissing*. In the past, fists may have established the gang leader. Now it is settled by flying lead. Innocent bystanders are often harmed or killed by violent gang members by being victims of drive-by shootings, cross-fire gang shootings, and murder as part of gang initiation.

Comorbid Disorders

It is common for youths with conduct problems to also display symptoms of attention deficit/hyperactivity disorder (ADHD) and conduct disorder.. These diagnoses are covered in detail in chapter 17 ∞. This co-occurrence is often associated with an early onset of aggression and impairment in personal, interpersonal, and family functioning. Exposure to community violence, through witnessing violence or being victimized, is significantly related to posttraumatic stress disorder (PTSD). See chapter 11 ∞ for more information on PTSD. It appears that as many as one third of children and teens exposed to community violence develop PTSD. Traumatic experiences, such as violence in the community, challenge people's basic belief that the world is safe, predictable, and controllable. When these basic assumptions are called into question, feelings of helplessness and hopelessness are likely to emerge.

Etiologies

Community violence is easy to describe but difficult to explain. There is no single cause of this type of violence. It results from an interaction of neurobiological, personality, and societal factors that have an impact on individuals and groups of people.

Some people believe that violence within the community is related to *a lack of something* such as discipline, religion, mothers at home, involved fathers, poverty, fair play, or rights of all sorts. Others believe that violence is related to an *excess of something*, such as welfare, permissiveness, attention, material goods, or rights of all sorts. Only where there are a number of risk factors does violent behavior occur.

Neurobiology

Neurobiological theorists propose that genes and neurotransmitters may contribute to causing violent behavior. Although a genetic predisposition may make certain behaviors more likely, it does not make them inevitable. Serotonin (5-HT) exerts inhibitory control over aggression and is inversely correlated with the level of aggression. Low levels of 5-HT are implicated in a lack of control, a loss of temper, and explosive rage. The relationships of dopamine (DA) and norepinephrine (NE) to aggression are less clear. Dopamine appears to be inversely correlated with aggression. Norepinephrine may be correlated with affective aggression through its sensitizing effects, which prepare a person to respond to threatening environmental stimuli (Pihl & Benkelfat, 2005).

The association between hormones and violence is more subtle and complex than formerly thought. Hormones are consequences as well as causes of behavior. In other words, hormones do not switch behaviors on or off. At times, hormones may change the probability that certain behaviors that can be labeled *aggression* will occur in particular situations by people with a history of psychosocial risk factors. Low cortisol has been associated with greater antisocial behavior. The male brain is organized by testosterone in such a way that males are more apt to react aggressively to annoyances and offenses. Much of the testosterone effects on aggression may involve 5-HT. It is also believed that mood may alter levels of testosterone. In sporting events, testosterone levels rise in the victors and fall in the losers. This may result from the individual's experience of dominance (Pihl & Benkelfat, 2005). Studies have shown that a higher number of minor physical anomalies of the mouth, ears, eyes, head, hands, and feet are found in groups of individuals with chronic violent antisocial behavior. Minor physical anomalies are considered indicators of disruption in fetal development. It is thought that the central nervous system may also be affected because it develops at the same time as the affected organs. Further research will be needed to determine whether a person is at higher risk for the development of violent delinquency as a result of atypical brain development.

Learning Theory

Learning theory proposes that violence is a learned behavior and people are conditioned to respond aggressively and violently. Children learn about violence from observation, from being victims, and from behaving violently themselves (Bandura, 1977). If the use of violence is rewarded by a gain in power, the behavior is reinforced. If there is immediate negative reinforcement from individuals and institutions within the community, a decrease in violent behavior will result.

Aggression, as a way of interacting with others and solving problems, is learned very early in life and usually is learned very well. The payoff in the experience of power and control often is high, so that, despite occasional or even more frequent punishment, it is difficult to unlearn—and so the behavior persists. This is probably why most interventions and rehabilitation programs that target adolescents and young adults have been unsuccessful.

Contextual Sensitivity Hypothesis

The **contextual sensitivity hypothesis** is based on the belief that human behavior is highly sensitive to social contexts. Certain social contexts are considered toxic because they contribute to violent perpetration and victimization. This toxicity can be understood from the perspective of socioeconomic factors, parent/family factors, and peer influences.

Socioeconomic Factors Community violence is associated with economic inequality. Extremes of poverty and racism contribute to the trauma of children and become breeding grounds for violence, as evidenced by a higher incidence of violence in poor communities. In the United States, 1 in 10 adults and 1 in 5 children live in poverty. Poverty is not an equal-opportunity condition: African American and Latino children, as well as children from mother-only families, are disproportionately poor. Families who are struggling to just put food on the table may have minimal time to supervise the children, who are then more likely to act out.

Poverty also affects the child's chance for school success. Poor academic performance, expulsion, and dropout rates are common indicators of unsuccessful youth functioning. The more children and adolescents are turned off by, and turned away from, the school system, the more they tend to associate with and seek approval from antisocial peers. Those who are subjected to racism experience humiliation, powerlessness, and rage and may act out in retaliatory violence. Racism and poverty create chaotic environments, making children vulnerable to violence as victims, witnesses, and perpetrators (Shelton, 2000).

Parent and Family Factors Research has shown that youths who engage in high levels of **antisocial behavior** are much more likely than other youths to have a biological parent who also engages in antisocial behavior. This association is thought to reflect the genetic transmission of predisposing temperament, the modeling of aggression, and the lack of control over expression of negative emotions. It is also believed that ineffective and inconsistent discipline and poor supervision contribute to antisocial behavior in children (Herrenkohl, Hill, Hawkins, Chung, & Nagin, 2006).

Childhood abuse and neglect places children at increased risk for violent criminal behavior. Child abuse and neglect often occur in chronically dysfunctional families, and it may be difficult to disentangle the effect of abuse and neglect from the effect of other stressors. Children living in abusive and neglectful families may also experience parental separations, poor physical and emotional health of their caretakers, and the need to cope with financial and social problems.

Peer Influences All children tend to make friends with peers who are similar to themselves. This becomes socially significant when antisocial children form groups and reinforce one another's antisocial behavior. By adolescence, violence can be the membership card for entry into some adolescent peer groups. Most studies that compare the relative effects of parental supervision and peer deviance find that peer deviance is a stronger predictor of delinquency than the family.

Nursing Process

A Client Experiencing Community Violence

Development of the knowledge base and the ability to identify factors that contribute to community violence will help you to promptly detect and accurately diagnose the problem.

It is also important to focus on potential perpetrators of community violence. The section on implementation suggests steps you can take to prevent violence and other troubling behaviors and to intervene and get help for troubled individuals. In the words of Carol Easley Allen, PhD, RN (2000, p. 2), we must all "advocate for a peaceful society, remove sources that teach violence to children, impose strict controls on firearms, provide resources to support family economic stability, and ensure access to care for victims of violence."

ASSESSMENT

Assessment: Behavior

Individuals are more likely to commit crimes when exposed to situations in which they model certain behaviors that they see others doing or being rewarded for. Corporal punishment, the hitting or spanking of children, gives the message that violence is acceptable. Children are spanked when parents are usually very angry and, thus, children learn that extreme anger justifies abuse. As was discussed in chapter 22 ∞, other underlying messages are if you are small and weak, you deserve to be hit; people who love you hit you; and violence is appropriate if the result is good. Being hit as a child increases the probability that aggression will be used to handle conflicts in the child's life. The inherent message is that authority figures should be feared, not trusted and respected. The message of violence is continued in some school systems. In those states where teachers are allowed to hit children, there is a significantly higher rate of student violence. Abuse that is persistent and continues from childhood to adolescence seems to have the most effect on individuals (Ireland, Smith, & Thornberry, 2002).

Several studies have shown that children who witness violence display more internalizing (withdrawn, anxious, depressed) behavior, whereas those who are victims display more externalizing (aggressive, disruptive) behavior. Those children who witness community violence watch from the sidelines, recognizing their own inability to change the situation. This sense of helplessness contributes to internalizing behavior. On the other hand, children who are victimized by community violence are more likely to learn aggressive, externalizing behavior as a means of self-protection or a way of relating to others.

At one end of the continuum of violent behavior are the numerous citizen militias and other assorted individuals who believe that violence targeted against representative members of groups is a legitimate protest. The most dramatic example of this type of community violence in the United States is the Oklahoma City bombing of the federal building in 1995.

Assessment: Affect

Violent people often have been denied normal emotional experiences as they were growing up. Hearing messages such as, "Big boys don't cry" and "The past is the past, just let it be" denies children the opportunity to experience emotional support from their caregivers. Some children, especially boys, are expected not to show any emotion, not to talk about feelings, and most of all not to cry. What usually stops most of us from striking out is empathy, imagining the hurt that the victim would feel. The process of denying one's feelings makes it impossible for some individuals to learn how to relate to others empathetically. The pressure to bottle up emotions leads some people to commit violence against the self—substance abuse and suicide—and violence against others—assault and homicide.

When people have little bonding with others and live an isolated life, they must rely on their internal psychological and social world. In the case of violent people, that internal world is filled with bitterness, resentment, and rage. There is no supportive network to correct or modify the misperceptions of people in their environment. This situation can precipitate violent acting out.

Assessment: Cognition

Thinking drives behavior, and violent individuals think of violent solutions to perceived offenses against them. They may live in an inner fantasy world with frequent thoughts of anger, revenge, and justifiable rage. They may rationalize their behavior or project their anger by saying, in essence, "You were disrespectful to me; that is why I had to blow your head off." Crime-prone persons are more likely to display cognitive deficits and distortions and have a tendency to process information incorrectly when making decisions. Crime is a convenient way to satisfy their individual needs, which take precedence over societal responsibilities (Ward & Stewart, 2003). Some perpetrators believe that if they commit violent acts they will become famous. The Columbine killers—in videos found after their deaths—basked in the attention they knew would come their way, even discussing which movie director should be entrusted to tell their story, Steven Spielberg or Quentin Tarantino (Burgess & Dowdell, 1999).

Assessment: Interpersonal Relationships

Violence in the United States is gender related. Males inflict violence on other males both overtly and covertly. Males are more likely to be involved in wars, physical battery, and economic and cultural subjugation of male minorities, gay men, and lower-class men. "Might makes right" in playgrounds, athletic fields, homes, and boardrooms. Boys are expected and permitted to push, pull, threaten, bully, and hurt each other. Many researchers who study violence believe that only hurt people hurt others. In other words, there is some systematic "hurting" of boys that underlies and contributes to the prevalence of violent acting out by males.

The myth that boys are "naturally" violent is dangerous. Although it is known that boys are most likely to be the perpetrators of violent crime, they are also the frightened victims of those acts. It is not only biology that makes boys violent, but also the environment in which they are raised. Boys are bombarded daily with professional wrestling, movie heroes who solve their problems with guns, and an ever-growing stream of hard-core violent video games. And then our culture calls this "healthy" adult masculinity. Boys say they are forced to lead a double life: strong and brave on the outside, yet full of worries and agitation on the inside (Pollack, 2000).

Concern is increasing that violence in girls is on the uprise. The arrest of girls has dramatically increased in the past few years. Although this seems to be an alarming statistic, its meaning is not clear. Societal attitudes toward crime are less tolerant and some crimes that previously were labeled as status or noncriminal have been relabeled as criminal offenses. The phenomenon of zero tolerance has also affected how society views violent crime. What used to be a schoolyard fight between two girls now is prosecuted as a violent offense. Although the reasons for this increase in violence among girls are unclear, it is certainly a trend worth watching.

Assessment: Cultural Influences

More people kill themselves with guns than by all other methods combined, and death by firearms is the fastest growing method of suicide. The use of guns in violent interactions increases the likelihood that one or more participants will be killed. Because firearms with greater firing power are increasingly available, lethality has also increased. More than half the teenagers who commit suicide shoot themselves with a gun kept at home. An important social issue is the alarming increase in the number of guns purchased in the United States. Two hundred million guns are now in the hands of individual Americans, which is more than double the number held in 1969. Those who are most vulnerable to impulsive suicide or murder are clearly most affected by availability of guns. The dramatic increase in the suicide rate in children and adolescents is almost solely due to the availability of guns (Simon, 2004).

The leading cause of death for persons in the United States varies according to age and ethnic group. At highest risk are African American males and at lowest risk are Euro-American females and males. These data support the earlier discussion regarding the impact of racism and poverty on violent behavior.

Cross-culturally, males are more physically aggressive than females. They assault more frequently and severely and commit more homicides. In the United States, Spain, and Russia, teen crime associated with gangs is a significant problem. Youth unemployment is a contributing factor to violence in Jamaica, St. Lucia, and South Africa. An increase in juvenile crime is associated with rapid political change and modernization in South Africa, Russia, Slovenia, and Jamaica (Hoffman & Summers, 2001).

Violence against the self is not common in Latin American countries, compared with other countries. Latin Americans do not kill themselves, but they do kill each other. The rate of homicide, however, is much higher than in North America or Europe. Among men in Guatemala, homicide is the most frequent cause of death. Homicide is the second leading cause of death in Ecuador, Mexico, Brazil, El Salvador, Venezuela, Paraguay, Panama, and other countries. The epidemic of violence is traced to guerrilla warfare, drug lords, poverty, inequalities, and social unrest. Violence is now the number one health priority in Latin America (Arboleda-Florez & Weisstub, 2000).

Given the incidence of community violence, it is logical to assume that you will encounter potential perpetrators in a variety of clinical settings. Violence can be inflicted by very different types of people in many different types of settings. There are clues, however, that you must recognize that would indicate the possibility of a violent outburst. See Box 24.1 for risk fac-

---

BOX 24.1	Risk Factors for Violent Behavior

- Truancy, suspension, and expulsion from school
- Little or no parental or adult supervision
- Is a loner and has few or no friends
- Mistreats animals
- Is a victim of neglect, abuse, or both
- Has been bullied
- History of aggressive and violent behavior
- Has made serious threats of violence
- Psychosis
- Romantic obsessions or erotomanic delusions
- Chemical dependency
- Depression and suicidality
- Pathological blaming, feelings of persecution
- Impaired neurological functioning
- Personality disorder
- Interest in firearms, bombs
- Affiliation with gangs

---

tors for violent behavior. Box 24.2 describes work-related behavior that is cause for concern regarding workplace violence.

The Focused Nursing Assessment feature is designed to assess children and adolescents so that problems can be identified early. Early warning signs are just that—indicators that a child may need help. Nurses must assess the situation and get help for the child before problems escalate. It is important, however, to avoid inappropriately labeling or stigmatizing because individuals appear to fit a specific profile. Early warning signs should not be used as a rationale to exclude, isolate, or punish a child. It is important to be aware of false cues—including race, socioeconomic status, cognitive or academic ability, or physical appearance. Children who are at risk for violence typically exhibit multiple warning signs, repeatedly, and with increasing intensity.

Focused Nursing Assessment　Potential Child/Teen Perpetrators

Behavior Assessment	Affective Assessment	Cognitive Assessment
How does this child/teen manage stress? Is there evidence of positive coping skills?	Is there an inappropriate expression of feelings?	Does this child experience uncontrolled anger?
Are there patterns of impulsive or intimidating behavior?	Does this child/teen believe that she or he is picked on and persecuted?	Is there a lack of responsibility for own behavior and a pathological blaming of others?
Is there a history of discipline problems?	Are there excessive feelings of isolation and rejection from peers?	Is there low interest in school and poor academic performance?
Is there a past history of violent and aggressive behavior? ·	Are there signs of depression?	Does the child show a strong interest in firearms and other weapons?
Is there an expression of violence in writings and drawings?	Is the child suicidal?	
Is there access to, possession of, and use of firearms?		
Does this child use alcohol and/or drugs?		
Have there been serious threats of violence?		
Is there evidence that the child is affiliated with a gang?		

BOX 24.2	Cues for Workplace Violence

- Attendance problems
- Increased demands for supervisor's time
- Decreased productivity
- Inconsistent work patterns
- Poor on-the-job relationships
- Blames others for life problems
- Unusual or changed behavior
- Preoccupation with weapons
- Substance abuse on the job
- Continual excuses

Imminent warning signs indicate that a person is very close to behaving in a way that is potentially dangerous to self or others. These signs require an immediate response. No single sign can predict that a dangerous act will occur. Usually, they are presented as a sequence of serious, hostile threats or behaviors directed at peers, family, staff, or other individuals. Imminent warning signs may include:

- Serious physical fighting with family or peers
- Severe destruction of property
- Severe rage for seemingly minor reasons
- Detailed threats of lethal violence
- Possession or use of firearms or other weapons
- Other self-injurious behaviors or threats of suicide

DIAGNOSIS

Based on assessment data, the nurse formulates nursing diagnoses for the potential perpetrators of community violence. Some examples of possible nursing diagnoses with this population are (North American Nursing Diagnosis Association, 2007):

- Risk for Loneliness related to excessive feelings of isolation and rejection from peers
- Self-esteem Disturbance related to beliefs of being bullied by others
- Fear related to being a victim of being teased, bullied, ridiculed, or humiliated
- Impaired Social Interaction related to an intolerance for diversity among peers and prejudicial attitudes
- Risk for Violence to Others related to threats of violence, past violent behavior, uncontrolled anger, and possession of firearms or other weapons

OUTCOME IDENTIFICATION AND GOALS

Based on the assessment data, you select outcomes appropriate to the client's current state and the identified nursing diagnoses. The broad outcome is: decrease in the incidence of community violence.

Client goals are specific behavioral prescriptions that you, the client, and the client's significant others identify as realistic and attainable. The following are examples of goals appropriate to potential perpetrators of community violence:

- Verbalizes an internal locus of control
- Relates appropriately to several peers
- Verbalizes an improved self-esteem
- Accepts responsibility for own behavior

Social Assessment	Physiological Assessment
Are there environmental risk factors such as poverty, parental stress, or a dangerous neighborhood?	Is the growth and development normal for the child's age?
Has the child been a victim of being teased, bullied, ridiculed, or humiliated?	Are there any minor physical anomalies of the mouth, ears, eyes, head, hands, or feet?
Has the child been a victim of violence?	Is there any impaired neurological functioning?
Is there an intolerance for diversity among peers and prejudicial attitudes?	Is the child experiencing a psychosis?

- Attends school or work
- Improves academic performance
- Interacts with others with less prejudicial behavior
- Exhibits no threats of violence and no violent behavior

PLANNING

Once the nursing diagnoses, outcome criteria, and goals have been identified, the nurse develops the plan of care to assist clients toward more adaptive ways of problem solving and better ways of relating to others. The plan should also encourage clients to identify potential support systems and ways to use them to their advantage. Priorities of care for clients who are perpetrators of violence are:

- Provision of a safe environment
- Development of a therapeutic alliance based on trust and rapport
- Treatment of underlying mental health problems
- Anger management
- Provision of adult supervision
- Identification of support systems
- Provision of needed social services
- Continuity in education

IMPLEMENTATION

Everyone has a personal responsibility for reducing the risk of violence. Nurses must take steps to maintain order, demonstrate mutual respect and caring for one another, and ensure that children who are troubled get the help they need.

NURSING CARE PLAN FOR A CLIENT EXPERIENCING COMMUNITY VIOLENCE

Providing a Safe Environment

Many of the children and adolescents at risk for perpetrating violent crimes are in nonsupervised and unsafe home and community situations. As reported earlier, many are victims of neglect and abuse. It is well documented that these issues predispose children to the development of low self-esteem, anger problems, posttrauma problems, and substance abuse problems, all of which chip away at their ability to adapt and cope. Following a basic-human-needs framework, it is extremely important, for treatment to be effective, to provide a safe environment for the client. This is true whether the child is institutionalized or being treated in the community.

The desired outcome is that the client remains free from harm, verbalizes feeling safe, verbalizes feeling cared for, and is under appropriate and caring adult supervision.

Nursing intervention should be aimed at first assessing the child's safety needs and intervening accordingly. The assessment should consider both immediate needs and future safety needs. It does not do much good to treat a child in a safe environment and return them to an unsafe environment. Multidisciplinary approaches are important. Being aware of the array of community resources is vital so that the appropriate referrals can be made. Children will be best served when there is coordination of care among all appropriate agencies. It is also important that these clients enter into a therapeutic alliance with someone they can trust. Many young perpetrators of violence are loners and alienated from others and desperately need someone who is their advocate. This does not mean accepting verbal or physical threats or failing to set limits. It calls for the nurse to respond in a caring, honest, consistent way.

Managing Anger

Because violence-prone children often experience explosive outbursts, they need to learn *coping skills* to help them avoid aggression in the future. Giving choices to the child who is acting out is often effective.

The desired outcome is that the client utilizes nonviolent expressions of anger, and self-calming techniques.

"There are two quieter places you may go to: your room or the deck. Which one would you like?" Each time a choice is given, the child must pause and consider the options. Each pause decreases the amount of energy behind the anger. Giving choices also helps children feel they have some control in the situation. It is best to intervene before the behavior escalates to out-of-control aggression. Assist in identifying the source of the anger, and establish the expectation that the child can control the behavior. Direct the child to seek assistance before lashing out with aggressive behavior. If appropriate, provide physical outlets for the expression of anger or tension. Help the child identify the benefits of expressing anger in an adaptive, nonviolent way, as well as identify the consequences of inappropriate expression of anger. Teach the child calming measures, such as deep breathing and self-controlled time-outs, when beginning to feel aggressive.

Setting Limits

When working with children and adolescents who have limited self-control, it is critical to *set appropriate limits*. Limit setting reinforces the predictability of the environment. Learning about and accepting external limits assists these individuals in developing internal controls. If the child or adolescent is institutionalized, the staff should adopt a *solution focus* rather than a *problem focus*, such as "What can we do to solve this problem?" rather than "What is the cause of this problem?"

When unwanted behavior occurs, staff should help children identify clearly what the desirable, positive alternative is, in behavioral terms. You may find it helpful to develop *behavioral contracts* with some children. The contract, which is mutually created, has clear behavioral expectations, states how these are to be achieved, and relates achievement to particular rewards. Consequences for inappropriate behavior must be immediate, logical, and appropriate to the child's age. *Time-out procedures* are used as a cooling-off period and provide the necessary time for reflection. Time-outs should be no longer than 1 minute per year of development. During this time, the child receives no attention and no environmental stimulation. A time-out is always accompanied by a clear statement of the reasons the time-out is necessary and a statement of the desirable alternative behavior. After it is over, review the incident with the child, who then returns to the normal milieu.

The desired outcome is that the client acknowledges when own behavior is out of control, utilizes behavioral contracts and/or time-outs, and demonstrates improved behavioral self-control.

Facilitating Self-Responsibility

The goal of the interventions is to help children overcome their defensiveness and tendency to blame others. Children who are at risk for becoming violent often are unable or unwilling to accept responsibility for their choices and behaviors. The nurse may hear, "She started it," or "I couldn't help it, he made me do it." Even young children can be taught the concept of good choices versus bad choices. The nurse needs to *establish reasonable and meaningful consequences* for good and bad decisions both. Excuses are not accepted for bad choices and the focus returns to the child's personal decisions regarding behavior. If self-esteem is low or the child does not have good coping skills, a defensive coping stance is often assumed. Nursing intervention should aim to provide positive and honest feedback, help the child develop insight about how others perceive them, and assist them in connecting their behavior to their feeling of inadequacy.

The desired outcome is that the client acknowledges ownership for feelings and behavior, does not ridicule others, learns to interact without taking a defensive stance, and accepts honest praise and criticism.

Improving Socialization

The inability to develop empathy for others decreases a child's social sensitivity and leads to peer disapproval and conflict. Because they are unable to put themselves in another's place, they demonstrate little or no empathy unless it is to manipulate someone. They often have no concept of how they have hurt another's feelings.

Because some of these children have learned violence from being treated disrespectfully, it is helpful if you role-play positive interactions. Treat the child with warmth, friendliness, humor, empathy, and unconditional positive regard. Minimize the amount of attention given for negative behavior and maximize the amount of attention given for desirable and positive behavior. A kindergarten through 12th-grade program called *Resolving Conflict Creatively Program (RCCP)* may be instituted in the clinical setting. The goal of RCCP is to help children learn to care about others, resolve conflicts nonviolently, solve problems cooperatively, value diversity, make responsible decisions, confront prejudice, and take positive, meaningful action. See the Community Resources feature on the Companion Website for address information.

Some violence-prone individuals alienate their peers by interrupting others, intruding in particular situations, invading personal space, and treating others' property as if it were their own. When youths experience conflict with peers or adults, they often refuse to back down, even on little points. It is important that the nurse *avoid power struggles*, which can be damaging to a child's self-esteem. It is better to act as a role model to teach children how to negotiate differences and how to admit to errors.

Nursing interventions are also directed at helping these children establish and maintain social relationships. Being a *role model* is an effective way to demonstrate social skills such as giving and receiving compliments, sharing, conflict resolution, and personal boundary issues. Because violence-prone children often use anger to control people, they may become abusive, aggressive, or threatening. *Feedback* and *consequences* must be immediate to avoid reinforcing this inappropriate behavior.

As the nurse, you should structure the child's environment to allow for success. It is very important to clearly state the rules and expectations. It is important to provide frequent, immediate, and consistent feedback regarding appropriate and inappropriate social behavior. You may select particular peers to interact with the child. It is best to begin with one-on-one interactions. You might suggest the child work with one child at the computer, another child while problem solving, and a different child in free play. As the child's social skills improve, two or more children can be included in each of the groups.

The desired outcome is that the client uses problem solving to resolve conflict, negotiates differences with others, and utilizes feedback to modify antisocial behaviors.

Involving the Community

Cooperative community action is needed to halt the violence in schools, in the workplace, and on the street. Because of their expertise in working with residents and leaders, community health nurses are often called on to collaborate in the development of community action programs. Nurses can help community leaders study violence-prevention programs that have already been established. Nurses can encourage neighborhoods to become active participants in community safety. Nurses may also conduct educational programs targeted at people who are at risk for becoming perpetrators of violence (Riner & Flynn, 1999).

The desired outcome is that communities will institute violence-prevention programs.

The Centers for Disease Control and Prevention (CDC) has published a 216-page guide called *Best Practices in Youth Violence Prevention*. This publication can serve as a sourcebook as you become involved in family, neighborhood, and school violence-prevention programs. For a free copy, call 888-252-7751. See Box 24.3 on tips for parents in preventing violence. See Box 24.4 for tips for peer education for preventing school violence.

BOX 24.3 **Family Education**

Tips for Parents

- Involve your child in setting rules for appropriate behavior at home.
- Spend time with your child.
- Talk with your child about the violence she or he sees—on television, in video games, and possibly in the neighborhood. Help your child understand the consequences of violence.
- Teach your child how to solve problems. Praise your child when she or he follows through.
- Help your child find ways to show anger that do not involve verbally or physically hurting others. When you get angry, use it as an opportunity to model these appropriate responses for your child—and talk about it.
- Note any disturbing behaviors in your child. Get help for your child.
- Listen to your child if she or he shares concerns about friends who may be exhibiting troubling behaviors. Share this information with a trusted professional such as the school nurse, principal, or teacher.

BOX 24.4 **Tips for Peer Education**

- Listen to your friends if they share troubling feelings or thoughts. Encourage them to get help from a trusted adult. Share your concerns with your parents.
- Participate in violence-prevention programs such as peer mediation and conflict resolution. Use your new skills in other settings, such as the home, neighborhood, and community.
- Break the deadly code of silence. Work with your teachers and administrators to create a safe process for reporting threats, intimidation, weapon possession, selling drugs, gang activity, graffiti, and vandalism. Use the process to report.
- Help to develop and participate in activities that promote student understanding of differences and that respect the rights of all.
- Be a role model—take personal responsibility by reacting to anger without physically or verbally harming others.

SOURCE: Adapted from Dwyer, K., Osher, D., & Warger, C. (1998). *Early warning, timely response: A guide to safe schools.* Washington, DC: U.S. Department of Education.

EVALUATION

To complete the nursing process, you evaluate client responses to nursing interventions based on the selected outcomes. It is very important to remember that the underlying social and clinical predicaments for these types of problems are serious and many layers of interventions may need to be used. Working with these types of clients can be frustrating and sometimes discouraging. If, through evaluation, you find that some interventions fail to achieve the outcomes, it will be necessary to design new ones and reevaluate.

Using Research Evidence | Stress and Inner-City Adolescents

Canty-Mitchell, J. (2001). Life change events, hope, and self-care agency in inner-city adolescents. *Journal of Child and Adolescent Psychiatric Nursing, 14*, 18-31.

What is the study about?

It is well known that minority adolescents living in an inner-city experience disproportionately high rates of social and health problems. However, research concerning inner-city adolescents coping with numerous stresses has revealed little about their self-care agency or about protective factors such as hope. Therefore, the purpose of this study was to investigate, in inner-city adolescents, the relationships among life change events, hope, and self-care agency.

How was the study done?

This was a quantitative study using Dorothea Orem's Nursing Theory of Self-care as an organizing framework. The specific questions were: 1) What are the relationships among life change events, hope, and self-care agency? 2) Are there relationships between basic conditioning factors and self-care agency? and 3) Is self-care agency predicted by basic conditioning factors, life change events, or hope? This study received approval from a university's human subjects committee and school board's principals. A volunteer convenience sample of 91 males and 111 females was recruited from a traditional inner-city public high school (80%) and an alternative high school (20%). The alternative school provides an education for students with behavior problems who have been expelled or suspended from the traditional high school. All students were enrolled in grades 9 through 12. Ethnic/racial makeup of the sample consisted of African American (85%), Haitian (5%), Jamaican or other Caribbean (5.5%), Hispanic (2.3%), and Native American (2%). Students receiving parental consent (response rate: 32.6%) were administered four instruments, all developed by nurse researchers. The instruments were designed to measure basic conditioning factors, life change events, hope, and self-care agency. The instruments were: Adolescent Life Change Event Questionnaire (ALCEQ), The Miller Hope Scale, Denyes Self-care Agency Instrument (DSCAI), and a form for demographic and general information. Questionnaires were completed within the school environment and took an average of 30 minutes per subject. Results were analyzed using descriptive statistics, correlations, and multiple regression.

What were the results of the study?

There were five research hypotheses for this study. The first hypothesis was, "There is a negative relationship between life change events and self-care agency." This hypothesis was not supported. The results showed no significant correlation between life change events and self-care agency. The second hypothesis was, "There is a negative relationship between life

change events and hope." The results indicated that there was no significant correlation between life change events and hope. The third hypothesis was, "There is a positive relationship between hope and self-care agency." The statistical analysis supported this hypothesis. There was a positive and significant correlation between hope and self-care agency. High hope scores were related to high self-care agency scores regardless of the number of life change events. In addition, self-care agency scores for traditional school students were significantly higher than those of students in the alternative school. No significant difference was found based on the gender or among adolescents experiencing health problems and those without health problems. The fourth hypothesis was, "There is a positive relationship between basic conditioning factors and self-care agency." This hypothesis was largely unsupported, except for relationships between perceived health status and self-care agency. The fifth hypothesis was, "Life change events, hope, and basic conditioning factors are significant predictors of self-care agency in inner-city adolescents." Multiple regression analysis revealed that, in this sample of students, the greatest predictors of self-care agency were hope, health status rating, and alternative school attendance. Sample participants were more likely to be able to engage in self-care behaviors if they had higher scores on the hope scale, higher ratings on perceived health status, and were not enrolled in the alternative school program. The phenomenon of hope was determined to be a significant factor in the power and ability of these young people to engage in self-care practices. Many of these adolescents may use hope to assist them in coping with numerous family, social, and environmental life changes that they encounter.

What additional questions might I have?

How different might the results have been if the sample consisted of those students not agreeing to participate in the study? What are the underlying factors causing students enrolled in an alternative school program to have less hope and self-care agency? Were there any specific life change events that supported these inner-city adolescents in their self-care and hope?

How can I use this study?

Nurses working with adolescents living in a multiple-stress environment need to be aware that hope may be an important coping factor. In addition, adolescents who appear to be hopeless may need additional help in making health-promoting decisions. These adolescents should be encouraged to involve themselves in programs that use hope-inspiring strategies. They may cope with life changes better if they see an adult who models positive regard.

SOURCE: Contributed by Dolores Huffman, PhD, RN, Associate Professor of Nursing, Purdue University Calumet, Hammond, Indiana.

Focus Your Study

OBJECTIVES	KEY CONCEPTS

OBJECTIVES

KEY CONCEPTS

1. Discuss the theories regarding the etiologies of violent behavior.

- Neurobiology:
  - Low levels of serotonin (5-HT) are implicated in a lack of control, loss of temper, and explosive rage.
  - Much of the testosterone effects on aggression may involve 5-HT.
- Learning theory:
  - Violence is a learned behavior and people are conditioned to respond aggressively and violently.
- Contextual sensitivity hypothesis:
  - Community violence is associated with economic inequality.
  - Family antisocial behavior is a combination of genetic transmission of predisposing temperament, the modeling of aggression, the lack of control over expression of negative emotions, ineffective and inconsistent discipline, and poor supervision.
- Four types of personal-cause homicides:
  - In nonspecific homicide, only the perpetrator, who seems to want as many victims as possible, knows the motive.
  - Perpetrators of revenge homicide retaliate for real or imagined offenses brought on by the victim.
  - Patricide/matricide homicide may be in response to childhood abuse, defiance of rules, arguments, or for money or possessions. Describe violence in the workplace, in school, and on the street.
  - The targets in authority killing may be people or buildings that symbolize authority in response to real or imagined offenses.

2. Outline the process for assessing the potential for violent behavior.

- The nurse will encounter potential perpetrators in a variety of clinical settings.
- Assess for risk factors for violent behaviors:
  - Past history of aggressive and violent behavior
  - Serious threats of violence
  - Psychosis
  - Romantic obsessions or erotomanic delusions
  - Chemical dependence
  - Depression and suicidality
  - Pathological blaming, feelings of persecution
  - Impaired neurological functioning
  - Personality disorder
  - Interest in firearms, bombs
  - Affiliation with gangs
- People who are at risk for violence typically exhibit multiple warning signs, repeatedly, and with increasing intensity.
- Imminent warning signs include:
  - Serious physical fighting with family or peers
  - Severe destruction of property
  - Severe rage for seemingly minor reasons
  - Detailed threats of lethal violence
  - Possession or use of firearms or other weapons
  - Other self-injurious behaviors or threats of suicide

3. Use the nursing process to develop a comprehensive plan of care for addressing community violence.

- Provide a safe environment:
  - Assess for immediate and future safety needs.
  - Refer to appropriate community resources.
- Manage anger:
  - Establish the expectation that the child can control the behavior.
  - Give limited choices when client is angry to help person feel there is some control over the situation.
  - Provide physical outlets for the expression of anger or tension.
  - Identify the benefits of expressing anger in nonviolent ways.
  - Identify the consequences of inappropriate expression of anger.
- Set limits:
  - Adopt a solution focus to problem solving.
  - Identify desirable behavior.
  - Behavioral contracts are helpful with some children.
  - Time-outs should be no longer than 1 minute per year of development.
- Facilitate self-responsibility:
  - Teach the concept of good choices versus bad choices.
  - Establish meaningful consequences for both good and bad decisions.
  - Provide positive and honest feedback.
- Improve socialization:
  - Treat child with warmth, friendliness, humor, empathy, and unconditional positive regard.
  - Minimize the amount of attention given for negative behavior.
  - Maximize the amount of attention given for positive behavior.
  - Avoid power struggles.
  - Gradually include other children in the socialization process.
  - Implement the Resolving Conflict Creatively Program.
- Involve the community.
  - Collaborate with community members in implementing violence-prevention programs.
  - Develop teaching plans to prevent community violence.
  - Community health nurses collaborate in the development of community action programs.
  - Identify community action programs that have been established and tested elsewhere.
  - Encourage neighborhoods to become active participants in community safety.
  - Conduct educational programs targeted at people who are at risk for becoming perpetrators of violence.

4. Develop teaching plans to prevent community violence.

- Community health nurses often collaborate in the development of community action programs.
- Nurses may conduct educational programs targeted at people who are at risk for becoming perpetrators of violence.

5. Discuss the key points in effectively communicating with a person who is at risk for violent behavior.

- Give limited choices to the child who is acting-out.
- Utilize Resolving Conflict Creatively Program where children learn to:
  - Care about others.
  - Resolve conflicts nonviolently.
  - Solve problems cooperatively.
  - Value diversity.
  - Make responsible decisions.
  - Confront prejudice.
  - Take positive, meaningful action.
- Avoid power struggles.
- Role-model social skills such as giving and receiving compliments, sharing, conflict resolution, and personal boundary issues.

Explore Medialink

For review questions, case studies, and other resources for this chapter see the Pearson Health MediaLink CD-ROM that accompanies this book and the Companion Website.

CD-ROM
- Audio Glossary
- NCLEX-RN® Review Questions

Companion Website www.prenhall.com/fontaine
- Audio Glossary
- NCLEX-RN® Review Questions
- Case Study
  - Prevention Programs in the School Setting
- Care Plan
  - Violence in the School Setting
- Critical Thinking
  - Crisis Intervention for School Violence
- MediaLink Application
  - Human Trafficking and Ritual Abuse-Torture
  - Screening Community Children for Family Violence
- MediaLinks
  - Books for Clients & Families
  - Community Resources

NCLEX-RN® Review Questions

24-1. The nurse is aware that changing levels of hormones and neurotransmitters may contribute to violent behavior. The nurse is most concerned about a potential for violence if a client has elevated levels of which of the following?
1. Serotonin
2. Testosterone
3. Dopamine
4. Cortisol

24-2. Which of the following population groups are most likely to be victims of murder, rape, robbery, or aggravated assault?
1. Children in elementary schools
2. Older adults living alone
3. Adolescent females in high school
4. Young adult male gang members

24-3. A high school freshman has been teased and taunted about his small size by senior class members. He has no close friends and usually sits alone when eating lunch in the cafeteria. When he fell down in physical education class, the other students laughed and called him "klutz." The school nurse should provide further teaching if the nursing student selected which of the following nursing diagnoses for this student?
1. Loneliness related to rejection from peers and feelings of isolation
2. Risk for Other-directed Violence related to history of violent behaviors
3. Self-esteem Disturbance related to being teased about small size
4. Fear related to being taunted and humiliated by peers

24-4. The nurse plans to teach employees in the community about methods of preventing workplace violence. The nurse will begin teaching the groups of employees who are at highest risk. Which of the following groups should the nurse teach first? (Select all that apply.)
1. Court judges
2. Nurse practitioners
3. Flight attendants
4. Gas station attendants
5. Taxi drivers

24-5. An adult client is pacing and yelling. Which of the following is the best response by the nurse?
1. "Why do you feel angry?"
2. "What are you doing?"
3. "Who are you angry with?"
4. "When did these feelings begin?"

See Appendix D for answers.

References

Allen, C. E.. (2000, April). Veterans, victims and violence. *The Nation's Health*, 2.

Arboleda-Florez, J., & Weisstub, D. N. (2000). Conflicts and crises in Latin America. In A. Okasha, J. Arboleda-Florez, & N. Sartorius (Eds.), *Ethics, culture, and psychiatry* (pp. 29–46). Washington, DC: American Psychiatric Press.

Bandura, A. (1977). *Social learning theory*. Englewood Cliffs, NJ: Prentice Hall.

Burgess, A. W., & Dowdell, E. B. (1999, January 25). Forensic nursing and violent school-boys. *Nursing Spectrum, 12*(2), 12–14.

Canty-Mitchell, J. (2001). Life change events, hope, and self-care agency in inner-city adolescents. *Journal of Child and Adolescent Psychiatric Nursing, 14*, 18–31.

Dwyer, K., Osher, D., & Warger, C. (1998). *Early warning, timely response: A guide to safe schools*. Washington, DC: U.S. Department of Education.

Glew, G. M., Fan, M. Y., Katon, W., Rivara, F. P., & Kernic, M. A. (2005). Bullying, psychosocial adjustment, and academic performance in elementary school. *Archives of Pediatric & Adolescent Medicine, 159*(11), 1026–1031.

Herrenkohl, T. I., Hill, K. G., Hawkins, J. D., Chung, I. J., & Nagin, D. S. (2006). Developmental trajectories of family management and risk for violent behavior in adolescence. *Journal of Adolescent Health, 39*(2), 206–213.

Hoffman, A. M., & Summers, R. W. (2001). *Teen violence: A global view*. Westport, CT: Greenwood Press.

Ireland, T., Smith, C., & Thornberry, T. (2002). Developmental issues in the impact of child maltreatment on later delinquency and drug use. *Criminology, 40*, 359–401.

i-SAFE America. (n.d.). Retrieved August 14, 2006, from http://www.isafe.org

Jordan, C., Logan, T. K., & Walker, R. (2003). Stalking: An examination of the criminal justice response. *Journal of Interpersonal Violence, 18*, 148–165.

Litz, B. T. (2004) Introduction. In B. T. Litz (Ed.), *Early intervention for trauma and traumatic loss*. Guilford Press: New York.

North American Nursing Diagnosis Association. (2007). *Nursing diagnosis: Definition and classification, 2007-2008*. Philadelphia: Author.

Pihl, R. O., & Benkelfat, C. (2005). Neuromodulators in the development and expression of inhibition and aggression. In R. E. Tremblay, W. W. Hartup, & J. Archer (Eds.), *Developmental origins of aggression* (pp. 261–280). New York: Guilford Press.

Pollack, W. (2000). *Real boys' voices*. New York: Random House.

Ray, M. M., & Ream, K. A. (2007). The dark side of the job: Violence in the emergency department. *Journal of Emergency Nursing, 33*(3), 257–261.

Riner, M. E., & Flynn, B. C. (1999). Creating violence-free healthy cities for our youth. *Holistic Nursing Practice, 14*(1), 1–11.

Shelton, D. (2000). Health status of young offenders and their families. *Journal of Nursing Scholarship, 32*(2), 173–178.

Simon, R. I. (2004). *Assessing and Managing Suicide Risk*. Washington, DC. American Psychiatric Press.

Skybo, T. (2005). Witnessing violence: Biopsychosocial impact on children. *Pediatric Nursing, 31*(4), 263–270.

U.S. Departmemt of Justice (2005). Crime and victims statistics. Accessed on Feburary 15, 2008, at www.ojp.usdoj.gov/bjs/cvict.htm

Ward, T., & Stewart, C. (2003). The relationship between human needs and criminogenic needs. *Psychology Crime and Law, 9*, 219–225.

Chapter 25
Nursing Management of the Problems Associated With Exposure to Natural Disasters and Terrorism

Contributed by Leslie Rittenmeyer, PsyD, RN

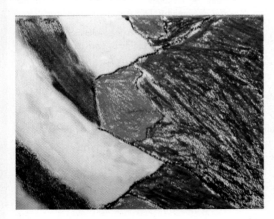

" *In this picture, three volcanoes are erupting.*

My anger is equal to the fury of three volcanoes. "

—Sawyer, Age 14

OBJECTIVES

After reading this chapter, you will be able to:

1. Discuss the development of mental health problems following a natural disaster or terrorism.
2. Outline the process for assessing disaster readiness at the community level.
3. Outline the process for assessing trauma reactions in individuals across the life span.
4. Use the nursing process to develop a comprehensive plan of care for addressing recovery from a natural disaster or terrorism.
5. Develop teaching plans to address recovery from a natural disaster or terrorism.

MediaLink   www.prenhall.com/fontaine

Go to the Pearson Health MediaLink CD-ROM and the Companion Website at www.prenhall.com/fontaine for interactive resources for this chapter.

A traumatic event is defined by its ability to evoke feelings of terror, helplessness, fear, or horror as a response to a threat to life or serious injury (American Psychiatric Association, 2000). The threat of natural disaster and terrorism has been with us long before September 11, 2001. The terror of September 11, 2001, and, more recently, the devastation seen with the natural disaster of hurricane Katrina, have made Americans more aware of their own vulnerabilities. People have always experienced personal traumas—such as accidents, illness, and victimization by crime—that have affected their lives, sometimes profoundly. The difference between these types of events and unanticipated large-scale disasters is the impact on the community. Large-scale trauma such as the Oklahoma City bombing, 9/11, and hurricane Katrina affects the community at many sociocultural levels, and often causes the people of those communities to question their cultural assumptions about safety, cohesiveness, bias, and political effectiveness. In large-scale disasters, even people not directly affected are touched in some way.

Nurses are in the forefront of planning and providing care in the event of mass trauma. They are asked to sit on prevention planning committees, are often first responders, and, as we saw during Katrina, were the ones who stayed behind to nurse those who could not evacuate. Whether at the disaster site, in a community triage area, the emergency room, or a general hospital, nurses should be prepared to provide intervention strategies that address the particular needs of people during different stages of the crisis. This chapter provides information that informs the practice of disaster nursing.

KNOWLEDGE BASE

Types of Traumatic Events

The focus of this chapter is on psychological outcomes of larger community disasters. The models are natural disasters and terrorism.

Events such as tornadoes, hurricanes, earthquakes, tsunamis, floods, fire, and famine are considered to be **natural disasters** because they are not human made and are not intentional. Unlike natural disasters, **human-made disasters** may be accidental or intentional. Examples of accidental disasters are a commercial plane crash or technological accidents. Intentional human-made disasters include sniper attacks, arson, terrorism, and war. Both natural disasters and human-made disasters fall under the category of **adventitious crises**. Adventitious crises come unexpectedly and often without much warning. During this type of crisis, stress levels are very high and the coping resources of individuals as well as communities are challenged.

Motivation of Terrorists

Terrorism is a premeditated, politically motivated violence perpetrated against civilians. The violence is usually intended to influence public opinion. The term **international terrorism** means terrorism involving citizens or the territory of more than one country. A **terrorist group** is any group practicing or having significant subgroups that practice international terrorism (U.S. State Department, 1999).

According to Siegel (2005), the term *terrorism* encompasses an array of behaviors and goals. He defines **revolutionary terrorism** as the type that is meant to frighten those persons who have power and those who support them in order to replace them with an alternative form of government. Kidnappings, assassinations, and bombings are common acts in this form of terrorism. **Political terrorism** is aimed at groups that oppose the terrorists' political or religious ideology. Their goal is not necessarily to take over the government but to influence it. In the United States, political terrorists tend to organize around issues such as white supremacy, with the Ku Klux Klan as an example. **Nationalist terrorism** is meant to push forth the agenda of a minority ethnic group that believes it has been persecuted by the majority and that wants to carve out a piece of the homeland for itself. The Palestinian Liberation Organization (PLO) would be a good example of this type of group. **Environmental terrorism** is perpetrated by extremist environmental groups. "More than 1,500 terrorist acts have been committed by environmental terrorists during the past two decades in an effort to slow down developers who they believe are threatening the environment or harming animals" (Siegel, 2005, pp. 262–263). **State-sponsored terrorism** occurs when an oppressive government terrorizes its citizens into submission and obedience and squashes political dissonance. Political prisoners are being tortured in approximately 100 countries. The "disappearance" of persons who dissent is common. Individuals are often taken off the street or from their homes in the middle of the night and never seen again. Certain terrorist groups fund their cause with money from crime, such as drug dealing, kidnapping, and selling nuclear weapons. This is referred to as **criminal terrorism**. Sometimes groups find this so lucrative that they abandon their original cause. **Cause-based terrorism** occurs when a group directs its activities against individuals or governments who do not agree with it. The acts of Al-Qaeda are an example of this type of terrorism.

Types of Terrorism

The threat of terrorist attack is made more frightening by the fact that there are many ways in which a society can be terrorized. **Bioterrorism** is a terrorist act in which a biological agent is released into the environment to cause fear of exposure or harm to as many as possible. Examples of biological agents that could be used for this purpose are anthrax, botulism, cholera, Ebola virus, typhoid, and plague. **Chemical terrorism** is an act of terror accomplished by the release of toxic chemicals into the environment. Examples of these are blister agents, carbon monoxide, chlorine, chocking pulmonary agents, and nerve agents. **Radiological terrorism** is an act in which radioactive material is released into the environment. One vehicle to accomplish this goal is through a "dirty bomb." Contrary to popular belief, a dirty bomb is not like the atomic bomb but is made of a mixture of explosives, such as dynamite, with radioactive pellets that scatter radioactive dust. **Mass-casualty terrorism** occurs when the goal is to harm large numbers of people and cause large-scale property damage. The vehicles for this are often explosions and blasts.

Individual Responses to the Threat of Terrorism and Disaster

The threat of terrorist attack causes intense feelings of anxiety because of the undefined nature of the threat (Ross, 2006). Complex psychosocial, biological, and cognitive effects come with experiencing any traumatic event (Ursano, 2002; Yahuda, 2002). Schuster et al. (2001) found that, after the 9/11 attacks, 44% of people surveyed reported one or more symptoms of significant stress, and 90% reported at least low levels of stress. For those people that were in the neighborhood directly around the World Trade Center on the day of the attack, it was estimated that 17.3% developed **posttraumatic stress disorder (PTSD)** or depression 1 to 2 months after the attack (Galea et al., 2002). In a national study conducted by Schlenger et al. (2002) of Americans' reactions to 9/11, it was projected that PTSD would develop in 11.2% of the population in New York City, in 2.7% in Washington, DC, in 3.6% in other urban areas, and in 4.0% in the rest of the United States. North et al. (1999) studied the victims of the Oklahoma City bombing and found that PTSD developed within 6 months in 35% of those directly affected.

Symptoms of PTSD usually begin within the first 3 months after trauma, although there may be a delay of months or even years before symptoms appear. Chapter 11 ∞ presents PTSD in greater detail. **Acute stress disorder** develops in many people who experience terrorism or natural disasters. This disorder begins within a month of the traumatic event, lasts at least 2 days, and goes away within 4 weeks. If symptoms persist beyond 4 weeks, PTSD is diagnosed. Other trauma-related diagnoses include panic disorder and major depressive disorder. Additional responses to trauma include anger, sadness, anxiety, fear, irritability, and family conflict (Fullerton and Ursano, 1997; Silver et al., 2002; Ursano, Fullerton, & Norwood, 2003; Williams, 2006).

High-Risk Groups

The risk for development of symptoms of PTSD is higher in those persons who have been directly exposed to the event and experienced a threat to life and feelings of horror (Ursano et al., 2003). Other high-risk groups include those with the most attachment to the primary victims, first responders, and support providers (Wright & Bartone, 1994). Those persons who were vulnerable before the event are at higher risk. For instance, those with a history of PTSD, a prior exposure to trauma, a prior or current psychiatric or medical illness, and those who lack supportive relationships are at higher risk. "Those who were psychologically vulnerable before the terrorist attacks may be also buffeted by the fears and realities of job losses, untenably longer commutes, or eroded interpersonal and community support systems overtaxed now by increased demands" (Ursano, Fullerton, & Norwood, 2003, p. 9).

First responders are particularly vulnerable to the symptoms of PTSD and should not be overlooked. They need opportunities to talk and process the event, ideally with each other. The same holds true for the people who clean up the site after the event. There will always be those workers who are unidentified victims, so it is important that as many as possible be identified and offered support (Ursano et al., 2003).

How individuals cope in the face of severe trauma is dependent on many factors. Data from a national study on coping behavior indicated that, of those experiencing severe to mild stress reactions, 98% talked with others, 90% turned toward religion, 60% got involved in group activities, and 30% gave contributions (Schuster et al., 2001).

Schurfield (2002) identified normal coping behaviors—such as being immersed in the media coverage of the disaster, sometimes to the detriment of other life responsibilities, being in denial about the event, becoming detached from the event, and avoiding discussion about the event. All these responses give the individual a perceived sense of feeling more in control, an ability to maintain daily functioning, and a mechanism to avoid triggering painful memories. Behaviors identified as inappropriate or ineffective were not caring, losing a personal belief system, inappropriate denial, irritability, severe mood swings, difficulty concentrating, or crying all day.

In the end, how individuals cope with disaster depends on an array of factors, such as the extent they or significant others were directly involved in the event, the degree of personal threat, and their ability to ask for and receive support.

Nursing Process

A Client Experiencing Violence

Assessment

Assessment activities occur at many different levels. At the *primary prevention level*, assessment focuses on gathering data pertinent to disaster planning and preparedness. Whether in the hospital or the community setting, good planning for disaster response is essential. It is important to assess the potential impact that different types of disasters will have on individuals and resources. An act of terrorism requires a different response than a catastrophic natural disaster such as a hurricane. It is important to consider who will be affected most by certain types of disaster so that early interventions can be planned that will decrease the long-term psychological effects of the disaster. Predictors include the severity of the event, the degree of life disruption, and the degree of societal disruption. It is also important from a preventative perspective to assess for the psychoeducational needs of the community. Nurses are frequently sought out by others for information. Good information is powerful and helps people feel more in control.

Assessment at the *secondary prevention level* centers on determining the immediate needs of the individuals most affected by disaster. Assessment focuses on anticipating basic human needs, such as shelter, safety, and security. It is vital to determine where resources are most needed. It is also important to determine the type of information necessary and how that information should be disseminated.

Assessment at the *tertiary prevention level* focuses on the long-term needs of individuals, groups, and the larger community. Determining the types of additional interventions required is essential.

Assessment: Across the Life Span

No matter what age, most survivors of disasters experience visual memories of the event, trauma-specific fears, and changed attitudes regarding personal and community safety. Signs of emotional distress are expressed similarly across cultures. There are, however, cultural differences in how trauma is both perceived and processed which must be taken into account during the assessment process. Assessment must also differentiate normal reactions from pathological reactions to the traumatic event.

Assessment of Children and Adolescents

"The empirical literature on the impact of psychological terrorism is sparse; the literature related to children is even more so" (Gurwitch, Pfefferbaum, & Leftwich, 2001, p. 100). The most deadly terrorist incident that affected children in the United States was the Oklahoma City bombing of the Murrah Federal Building in 1995. During that event, 168 people were killed and many more injured. Much of the information on the effect of disaster on American children comes from the work of an array of researchers after the Oklahoma City bombings. "Approximately 3200 middle and high school students were screened seven weeks after the attack and nearly 1200 elementary school students (third through fifth grades) were assessed 8–10 months after the attack" (Gurwitch et al., 2001, p. 104). Also, infants and preschool-age children were assessed using qualitative methods. The sample for this study included the children, parents, and caregivers of children who were enrolled at the YMCA daycare center that was located directly across from the Murrah Center. Although these children experienced the event firsthand, luckily none were killed. Because of the children's ages, this group has been relatively underassessed. The following summarizes the research findings reported by Gurwitch et al. (2001) for infants, 1- to 2-year-old children, 2- to 3-year-old children, preschool children, and school-age children.

Infants

Infants displayed a range of reactions, of which sleep seemed to be the most significant. Parents and daycare center staff both reported that the infants seemed to have greater difficulty falling and staying asleep. While sleeping, the infants were observed twitching, moving restlessly, and grimacing. It was reported that the majority of infants were sleeping in their parent's bed because the parent felt better having them close. These behaviors lasted several months after the bombing. Parents reported that their infants woke up more irritable than they did prior to the bomb. Loud noises seemed to be more disturbing and an increased startle response was noted. Caregivers reported that, before the bombing, children were able to sleep through disturbances but now could not. The infants needed to be calmed and soothed at a high rate. Parents also admitted to increased feelings of stress and fear of separation. Most likely these reactions were transmitted to the infants. Box 25.1 summarizes the psychological responses of infants.

1- to 2-Year-Old Children

In addition, 1- to 2-year-old children also had trouble with sleep and displayed increased clinging behavior. They, too, were disturbed by loud noises. When they experienced a loud noise, the children seemed to freeze and began to cry while looking for a caregiver to offer comfort. These children were also more irritable and engaged in more aggressive play. Regressive behavior was also noted; for example, some toddlers went back to their bottle. Parents admitted to babying their toddlers more and reported experiencing separation anxiety.

BOX 25.1	**Psychological Effects of Disasters on Infants**

- Difficulty falling and staying asleep
- Restlessness while sleeping
- Irritability and fussiness
- Disturbed by loud noises
- Increased startle response

SOURCE: Adapted from Gurwitch, R. H., Pfefferbaum, B., & Leftwich, M. (2002). The impact of terrorism on children: Considerations for a new era. In S. N. Gold & J. Faust (Eds.), *Trauma practice in the wake of September 11, 2001* (pp. 101–124). New York: Haworth Maltreatment & Trauma Press; and Williams, R. (2006). The psychosocial consequences for children and young people who are exposed to terrorism, war, conflict and natural disasters. *Current Opinions in Psychiatry, 19*(4), 337–349.

| BOX 25.2 | **Psychological Effects of Disasters on Children 1 to 2 Years Old** |

- Sleep disturbances
- Increased clinging behavior
- Increased irritability
- Increased aggressive play
- Increased response to loud noise
- Increased startle response

SOURCE: Adapted from Gurwitch, R. H., Pfefferbaum, B., & Leftwich, M. (2002). The impact of terrorism on children: Considerations for a new era. In S. N. Gold & J. Faust (Eds.), *Trauma practice in the wake of September 11, 2001* (pp. 101–124). New York: Haworth Maltreatment & Trauma Press; and Williams, R. (2006). The psychosocial consequences for children and young people who are exposed to terrorism, war, conflict and natural disasters. *Current Opinions in Psychiatry, 19*(4), 337–349.

Like the infants, toddlers were sleeping in their parent's bed. Box 25.2 summarizes the array of psychological responses found in 1- to 2-year-old children.

2- to 3-Year-Old Children

The 2- to 3-year-old children displayed increased irritability and had temper tantrums beyond what would be considered normal for their age. The daycare staff had to mediate the interactions between these children more frequently. Nap and eating times seemed more stressful and crying was frequent during this time. Increased clinging behavior to daycare staff and parents was also noted. Some children experienced regressive behaviors related to toileting, speech, and self-help activities. In response to bright light and noise, this group of children had an increased startle response, with crying that was difficult to comfort.

This age group of children was also observed reenacting the bombing. For example they would build towers with blocks and crash them. The children played with rescue vehicles and costumes of firefighters and policemen more so than before the bombing. As with the parents of the infants and 1- to 2-year-old children, the parents of these children endorsed posttraumatic symptoms related to the event. Please refer to Box 25.3 for a summary of psychological responses found in 2- to 3-year-old children.

Preschool-Age Children

Because this age group is more verbal, these children talked repeatedly about the bombing and asked numerous questions related to the fires, building destruction, and rescue personnel. The children were often heard comparing their own scrapes and injuries. Like the younger children, their play reflected their experiences with the event and focused on the bombing itself and the rescue efforts. The children were observed building and crashing blocks while providing sound effects and narrative. The content of their drawings included bombed buildings, fires, and hurt children.

| BOX 25.3 | **Psychological Effects of Disasters on Children 2 to 3 Years Old** |

- Tantrums greater than what would be expected for developmental age
- Increased need of help in carrying out daily activities
- Regressive behavior
- Increased startle response to noise and bright lights
- Crying that is difficult to soothe
- Increased clinging behavior
- Reenactment of event through play

SOURCE: Adapted from Gurwitch, R. H., Pfefferbaum, B., & Leftwich, M. (2002). The impact of terrorism on children: Considerations for a new era. In S. N. Gold & J. Faust (Eds.), *Trauma practice in the wake of September 11, 2001* (pp. 101–124). New York: Haworth Maltreatment & Trauma Press; and Williams, R. (2006). The psychosocial consequences for children and young people who are exposed to terrorism, war, conflict and natural disasters. *Current Opinions in Psychiatry, 19*(4), 337–349.

Like the younger children, behavioral changes were also noted in this group of children. Nap times were more difficult and sleep disturbances were noted, such as restlessness and crying out during sleep. The children were more irritable with peers and caregivers and an increase in temper tantrums was observed. The children also displayed more clinging behavior and increased startle responses to loud noise and bright lights. Parents of this age group reported experiencing symptoms of stress reaction and sometimes found their preschoolers frequent questions and stories anxiety-producing. Please refer to Box 25.4 for a summary of psychological responses found in preschool children.

School-Age Children and Adolescents

Children who experienced the loss of a family member had more posttraumatic stress symptoms than those who did not. Posttraumatic stress symptoms include recurrent and intru-

| BOX 25.4 | **Psychological Effects of Disasters on Preschool-age Children** |

- Increased verbalization about event
- Compare minor injuries with each other
- Reenactment of event through play
- Artwork reflects the event
- Irritable and more difficult
- Sleep disturbance
- Increased clinging behavior
- Increased response to noise and bright light
- Increased startle behavior

SOURCE: Adapted from Gurwitch, R. H., Pfefferbaum, B., & Leftwich, M. (2002). The impact of terrorism on children: Considerations for a new era. In S. N. Gold & J. Faust (Eds.), *Trauma practice in the wake of September 11, 2001* (pp. 101–124). New York: Haworth Maltreatment & Trauma Press; and Williams, R. (2006). The psychosocial consequences for children and young people who are exposed to terrorism, war, conflict and natural disasters. *Current Opinions in Psychiatry, 19*(4), 337–349.

sive recollections of the event, recurring dreams of the event, flashbacks related to the event, dissociative flashbacks, trauma-specific reenactments, efforts to avoid thoughts and activities that arouse recollections of the trauma, restricted range of affect, difficulty falling or staying asleep, irritability, difficulty concentrating, hypervigilance, and an exaggerated startle response (American Psychiatric Association, 2000). From elementary school through high school, girls experienced more stress symptoms than boys. The older children's retrospective reporting of initial arousal and emotions related to the bombing was significantly correlated to later development of stress symptoms. Approximately 34% of the sample in middle and high school reported feeling worried about their own safety, as well as the safety of their family, 2 months after the attack, and 15% of those children reported not feeling safe at all. One year after the bombing, 33% of the elementary school group remained worried about their safety and 20% reported problems with concentration and anxiety. Refer to Box 25.5 for a summary of the psychological reactions found in school-age children.

Adults

Varying rates of PTSD are reported following exposure to disaster, with the range falling from 20% to 40% depending on the population studied and the degree of exposure. Terrorist events may be one of the most severe disaster stressors. Research on the Oklahoma bombing found high rates of PTSD and major depressive disorder (Ursano et al., 2003). Galea et al. (2002) found increased rates of PTSD in residents of Manhattan after the plane crashes of 9/11, and North et al. (1999) found that women were at higher risk for the development of PTSD, as were those with a history of psychiatric illness. More important, 40% of individuals with no history of psychiatric illness developed PTSD or major depression.

The severity, duration, and proximity of exposure to an event are the most important factors in determining the likelihood of development of PTSD. There is some evidence that

BOX 25.5	Psychological Effects of Disasters on School-age Children and Adolescents

- Increased PTSD symptoms in those that experienced direct loss
- Increased stress reaction by girls
- Long-term worry
- Decreased sense of feelings of safety
- Difficulty concentrating
- Difficulty self-soothing feelings of anxiety

SOURCE: Adapted from Gurwitch, R. H., Pfefferbaum, B., & Leftwich, M. (2002). The impact of terrorism on children: Considerations for a new era. In S. N. Gold & J. Faust (Eds.), *Trauma practice in the wake of September 11, 2001* (pp. 101–124). New York: Haworth Maltreatment & Trauma Press; and Crane, P.A., & Clements, P.T. (2005). Psychological response to disasters: Focus on adolescents. *Journal of Psychosocial Nursing, 43*(8), 31–38.

BOX 25.6	Psychological Effects of Disasters on Adults

- Anxiety
- Tearfulness
- Difficulty sleeping
- Flashbacks
- Nightmares
- Anger
- Guilt
- Feelings of helplessness and powerlessness
- Somatizing of symptoms
- Interpersonal isolation and withdrawal
- Difficulty concentrating
- Profound sadness

SOURCE. Adapted from American Psychiatric Association. (2000). *Diagnostic and statistical manual of mental disorders.* Washington D.C.

availability of social support systems, family history, childhood experiences, and personality styles influence the development of this disorder (American Psychiatric Association, 2000).

All individuals react differently to the experience of disaster. Symptoms such as anxiety and fear about the safety of self and loved ones, mood swings, difficulty concentrating, feeling shocked and numb, smoking and drinking too much, using drugs, having difficulty falling asleep or staying asleep, or experiencing nightmares or obsessive thoughts about the event are common. Sometimes people find themselves feeling angry, guilty, and helpless. In some people, anxiety gets trapped in their bodies and they experience physical reactions, such as headaches, muscle aches, and bowel problems. Withdrawing from others slows the recovery process (Ursano et al., 2003). Early intervention is essential in reducing the chances that these symptoms will become long term. Refer to Box 25.6 for a summary of possible responses of adults experiencing trauma.

DIAGNOSIS

After completing the assessment and appraising the knowledge base, you are ready to analyze and synthesize the information. Nursing diagnostic statements include (North American Nursing Diagnosis Association, 2007):

- Anxiety [specify level]
- Ineffective Community Coping
- Potential for Enhanced Community Coping
- Ineffective Coping
- Ineffective Denial
- Fatigue
- Fear
- Hopelessness

- Posttrauma Syndrome
- Spiritual Distress

OUTCOME IDENTIFICATION AND GOALS

Outcomes are specific behavioral prescriptions that provide a way to evaluate the efficacy of nursing care. The broad outcomes are as follows:

- Prepare communities in response to disasters or terrorism attacks.
- Reduce incidence of PTSD.

More specific goals appropriate to the victims include the following:

- Copes effectively
- Solves problems in a logical manner
- Verbalizes increased feelings of safety

PLANNING

Planning care to decrease the effects of trauma—natural and human made—is a monumental task, particularly in today's world in which the likelihood of some form of disaster is great. An organized approach is needed to provide an effective response. It is important for nurses to be involved in the planning and organization of trauma responses in their communities and places of employment. A common feature of terrorism and disaster is that the event overwhelms local resources and threatens the safety of the community (Fullerton, Ursano, Norwood, & Holloway, 2003). Good planning helps to alleviate the stress on the system.

Using a primary, secondary, and tertiary prevention model can be a useful framework in which to plan and implement a disaster response. Interventions at all stages of the disaster are aimed at decreasing the risk of serious mental illness and disruption of functioning. **Primary prevention** measures are meant to decrease the effect of the disaster. This includes preplanning disaster responses and practicing those responses. **Secondary prevention** measures are meant to meet immediate needs of individuals and communities after an event. **Tertiary prevention** measures include those interventions designed to provide care to those who need it for as long as they need it after the traumatic event.

Different types of prioritization will be needed at different stages of the crisis. The National Center for Post-traumatic Stress Disorder identifies stressors that occur as responses to the initial effect of the event, that have long-term consequences, and that need immediate intervention to prevent serious mental health problems:

- Threat to life and encounter with death
- Feelings of helplessness and powerlessness
- Personal loss of loved one, property, or possessions
- Dislocation from loved ones, home, family, etc.
- Feeling responsible (e.g., feeling that she or he could have done more)
- Inescapable horror (e.g., being trapped or tortured)
- Human malevolence

IMPLEMENTATION

Intervening at the different levels of a crisis can be conceptualized within the primary, secondary, and tertiary prevention framework. As stated before, early intervention is pivotal in preventing longer-term mental health problems.

Primary Prevention

Primary prevention is meant to decrease the severity of a response to a disaster event. It prepares people so that they feel more in control to handle the event.

Providing Community Education

Providing the community with education that teaches them how to best prepare themselves for a possible disaster helps individuals feel more in control if a disaster occurs. Teach families to make a disaster plan that will spell out beforehand how the family members intend to communicate with each other and find each other in the aftermath of an event. Ask them to designate a meeting place that all family members know about. If there are young children, share the plan with their teachers. Parents should familiarize themselves with the disaster plan of their children's daycare center and schools. If affordable, cell phones are a good way to communicate given that the wireless systems are left intact by the disaster. Alternative ways to make contact with significant others should be planned. Individuals who do not have family and live alone should designate at least one person in the community to be their contact. Knowledge of the community disaster plan allows people to know what to expect ahead of time.

The family can prepare a disaster preparedness kit. They can decide what they need in their kit and where they should keep it. Suggest that they have extra medication, eyeglasses, candles, flashlights, bottled water for 3 days, nonperishable food, blankets, and a battery-operated radio with extra batteries on hand. Also, it is wise for families and individuals to keep important documents easily accessible in a place where they are together.

Individuals should be as informed as much as possible about what to expect if they experience a disaster. Teach them about stress reactions and what to expect and how to get help. They should know what symptoms to expect in their children and how to soothe them. They should also be aware of the community resources for social and psychological support. Encourage individuals to maintain strong interpersonal and social networks since a good support system is one of those things that soften the blow of experiencing a disaster.

The desired outcome is that clients (individuals, families, and communities) will develop specific disaster plans, and identify community resources.

Secondary Prevention

Secondary prevention meets immediate needs of individuals and the community during a disaster. Early intervention is essential to decrease the incidence of long-term mental health problems.

Providing for Basic Human Needs

In the initial stages of disaster, individuals experience feelings of insecurity and fear. They ask themselves, "What is happening?" They feel numb, shocked, unsafe, and unsure. It is important to provide places where people affected by the disaster can get shelter, food, information, and support (Fullerton et al., 2003). It is likely the emergency room of the general hospital will be one of the places people will go even if not seriously injured. Because medical personnel will be busy with the seriously injured, it is important that the hospital have a plan to provide supportive care for those in less physical distress. Ideally, this place will be away from the chaos.

The desired outcome will be that client will verbalize feelings of safety.

Providing Psychological Support

One of the goals of providing psychological support is to identify those individuals who are most affected by the disaster and who need immediate intervention. Survivors need to be protected from further harm. It is important to decrease physiological arousal and provide support for those who are most affected (Fullerton et al., 2003). People considered at greatest risk had significant relationships with the primary victims, first responders, and support providers (Wright & Bartone, 1994). First responders, such as police and fire department personnel, need support and a place to process their experiences with each other and support staff. This solidifies group cohesiveness and decreases social isolation. There is no evidence that formal group and critical incidence debriefing is helpful in reducing the development of mental illness or PTSD, as previously thought. Just being able to discuss worries and fears seems to decrease symptoms (Fullerton et al., 2003).

The desired outcome is that client will verbalize a sense of support from others.

Providing Community Education

After the initial effect of the disaster the need for information is great. Client teaching should include the signs and symp-

toms of stress reactions in individuals and family members. Individuals should also be made aware of the community and mental health resources that are available to them and how to access those services. Those with preexisting mental disorders may need assistance in continuing to receive treatment and medications. It is important for the nurse to teach people healthy coping strategies, such as being with friends and family, getting adequate sleep and nutrition, talking to other trauma survivors, joining a survivor's support group, and practicing relaxation techniques.

The desired outcome is that client will use community resources.

Tertiary Prevention

Tertiary intervention is aimed to meet the longer term needs of individuals and the community after the initial effect of the disaster is resolved. There is no predetermined time for people to adjust to the impact of disasters. It is not unusual to find people still experiencing normal stress-related symptoms as long as 2 years after the event.

Providing Long-Term Treatment

Fullerton et al. (2003) identified the need for long-term treatment strategies to reduce psychiatric symptoms and improve functioning. The strategies to achieve this include ensuring adequate resources are available; individual, group, and family therapy; effective pharmacotherapy; short-term and long-term hospital admission; and spiritual support.

The desired outcome is that client will use long-term treatments.

Providing Programs That Foster Healing

The most important activity for mental health professionals is to continue to identify persons in need of psychological services. Providing places where people can come to talk about their feelings with others can be very beneficial to healing. Offering educational programs about stress responses, effective and ineffective coping strategies, and when to seek help is also beneficial to the community. Parents can be helped to feel more in control and therefore better able to assist their children cope with the aftermath of trauma when they participate in parenting classes. It is important for the nurse to help survivors see that, in time, their feelings of anxiety will decrease. Some people find it helpful to volunteer in activities that interest them and help others.

A nurse-designed psychoeducation program entitled Become Empowered: Symptom Management for Abuse and Recovery From Trauma (BE SMART) is being used in inpatient and outpatient group settings. Participants meet in a 3-hour block of time over 12 weeks. The focus is on recovery from trauma and a return to a higher level of wellness (Rice & Moller, 2006).

The desired outcome is that client will attend community programs, and verbalize feelings of control.

EVALUATION

Evaluation occurs on more than one level. All agencies and responders evaluate the effectiveness of their own response. Communities evaluate their effectiveness in meeting the needs of the citizens. Clinicians working with clients evaluate the efficacy of their individual, group, and family interventions during and after treatment. Good evaluation at many levels will lead to improvements in disaster response.

Using Research Evidence   Psychological Responses to 9-11

Silver, R. C., Holman, E. A., McIntosh, D. N., Poulin, M., & Gil-Rivas, V. (2002). Nationwide longitudinal study of psychological responses to September 11. *Journal of the American Medical Association, 288*(10), 1235–1244.

What is the study about?

A national trauma such as the attacks of September 11, 2001, may psychologically affect not only those who directly experienced the attacks but also those who knew them through personal or media contact. Therefore, the purpose of this longitudinal study was to investigate how the September 11 terrorist attacks (hereinafter referred to as "9/11") impacted U.S. residents, measuring posttraumatic stress symptoms (PTSSs), anxiety about future risks, and global distress.

How was the study done?

This quantitative longitudinal study investigated how U.S. adults responded to the 9/11 terrorist attacks. The responses were provided by participants (referred to as panel members) recruited by a research firm called Knowledge Networks, Inc. (KN). KN had obtained self-reported mental and physical histories via a Web survey administered between June 17, 2000, and September 4, 2001. From 9 to 23 days after 9/11, KN collected stress and coping responses (Wave 1) again via the Web. About 2 and 6 months after 9/11, KN again collected data on stress and coping (Waves 2 and 3). The adult sample included 48% males and 52% females; 83% identified themselves as White, the mean age was 48, and they were predominantly married and from the South, with a high-school diploma or equivalent. This study received approval from an institutional review board.

A probability sample of 2,729 adults completed the Wave 1 survey between September 20 and October 4, 2001, yielding data regarding early coping strategies and PTSSs. A Wave 2 survey (n=933) was administered between November 10 and December 3, 2001. A Wave 3 survey (n=787) was completed 6 months after the attacks. In Wave 1, early acute stress symptoms were surveyed through a modified and abbreviated version of the Stanford Acute Stress Reaction Questionnaire (SASRQ); coping was measured via the Brief Cope Survey. Wave 2 and 3 data were obtained using the Impact of Events Scale—Revised and the modified Vaughan Perceived Risk Scale; the Vaughan scale assessed anxiety about future terrorist attacks. The Wave 2 survey assessed global stress via the Hopkins Symptom Checklist (a standardized scale of psychological symptoms). During Wave 2, participants also responded to questions about the occurrence of stressful events in their lives. In Wave 3, the Brief Symptom Inventory assessed participants' history of symptoms of depression, anxiety, and somatization. Participants were also requested to complete several items that focused on their 9/11 experience. These included questions such as hours per day they watched television coverage of the event, their degree of exposure to and loss due to the attacks, physical proximity to the World Trade Center or Pentagon, talks with anyone at the World Trade Center or Pentagon, and so on. Data were analyzed using Stata version 7.0 software. Data were weighted to compensate for differences in the probabilities of selection and nonresponse both within and between households.

What were the results of the study?

Two months after September 11, 17% of these Americans living outside New York City reported 9/11-related PTSSs. After 6 months, PTSSs were reported by 5.8% of the participants. High levels of PTSSs were reported by females, those who were living with marital separation, those who reported pre-9/11 physician-diagnosed anxiety or depression, those who had a physical illness, those with greater exposure to the attacks, and those who had quickly disengaged from coping strategies. Global distress was found in those participants who experienced loss as a direct result of the attacks.

Psychological outcomes over time were significantly related to variations in the use of specific coping strategies directly post-event. The strongest predictors of psychological outcomes over time were coping strategies used shortly after the attacks: acceptance, behavioral disengagement, denial, seeking social support, self-blame, and self-distraction. Significantly more distress was reported by participants who used denial, self-distraction, or self-blame, or who sought social support or disengaged from coping efforts. Six months after the event, significantly lower distress was reported only by those subjects who reported that they began coping actively right after 9/11. More stress and PTSSs were reported by those whose coping strategy after 9/11 was disengagement.

What additional questions might I have?

What PTSSs would be present a year after the trauma of 9/11? Was Web-based survey the best method to collect the data? Could personal interviews or telephone surveys reveal similar data? Is a nonexperimental, quantitative study the best method for studying stress, risk anxiety, and global distress? Were these variables best measured by self-reported data, or would other data sources yield different results? Did the instruments used in this study miss any PTSSs?

How can I use this study?

Nurses need to recognize that the psychological response to a major national trauma is not limited to those who directly experience it. Nor do stress responses expire after 6 months. In addition, degree of response cannot be solely predicted using objective measures only. This study analyzed demographic data regarding those who experienced PTSS, results that may offer a basis for risk assessment in case of further national trauma.

SOURCE: Contributed by Dolores Huffman, PhD, RN, Associate Professor of Nursing, Purdue University Calumet, Hammond, Indiana.

Focus Your Study

OBJECTIVES	KEY CONCEPTS
1. Discuss the development of mental health problems following a natural disaster or terrorism.	<ul><li>People directly exposed to the event are at risk for developing acute stress disorder, posttraumatic stress disorder, panic disorder, or depression.</li><li>In addition to primary victims, first responders and support providers are at increased risk for mental health problems.</li><li>How people cope with disaster depends on many factors such as:<ul><li>The extent they or significant others were directly involved in the event</li><li>The degree of personal threat</li><li>The ability to ask for and receive support</li></ul></li></ul>
2. Outline the process for assessing disaster readiness at the community level.	<ul><li>Plan and practice disaster responses.</li><li>Assess the potential impact that different types of disasters will have on individuals and resources:<ul><li>An act of terrorism requires a different response than a catastrophic natural disaster.</li><li>Plan early interventions to decrease the long-term psychological effects of the event.</li></ul></li><li>Assess the psychoeducational needs of the community.</li></ul>
3. Outline the process for assessing trauma reactions in individuals across the life span.	<ul><li>Stressors that need immediate attention include:<ul><li>Threat to life and encounter with death</li><li>Feelings of helplessness and powerlessness</li><li>Personal loss of loved one, property, or possessions</li><li>Dislocation from loved ones, home, family, etc.</li><li>Feeling responsible (e.g., feeling that she or he could have done more)</li><li>Inescapable horror (e.g., being trapped or tortured)</li><li>Human malevolence</li></ul></li><li>At all ages, people experience sleep disturbances as a result of the event.</li><li>Children demonstrate an increased startle response, irritability, and increased clinging behavior.</li><li>Adolescents experience long-term worries, a decreased sense of security, and difficulty with concentration.</li><li>Adults suffer from feelings such as anxiety, anger, and guilt; they may have flashbacks or nightmares; some withdraw and isolate themselves from others.</li></ul>
4. Use the nursing process to develop a comprehensive plan of care for addressing recovery from a natural disaster or terrorism.	<ul><li>Immediate care includes:<ul><li>Shelter</li><li>Safety</li><li>Security</li><li>The provision of information</li></ul></li><li>Identify and intervene with those individuals who are most affected by the event.</li><li>People also need a place to process their experiences with each other and support staff.</li><li>If appropriate, refer for individual, group, and family therapy.</li><li>Ensure that long-term supportive resources remain available.</li></ul>
5. Develop teaching plans to address recovery from a natural disaster or terrorism.	<ul><li>Teach the family to prepare a disaster preparedness kit.</li><li>Determine what type of information is necessary and how that information should be disseminated.</li><li>Teach clients and families:<ul><li>Potential stress disorders</li><li>Healthy coping strategies</li><li>Available community and mental health resources</li></ul></li><li>Encourage people to maintain strong interpersonal and social networks.</li></ul>

Explore MediaLink

For review questions, case studies, and other resources for this chapter see the Pearson Health MediaLink CD-ROM that accompanies this book and the Companion Website.

CD-ROM
- Audio Glossary
- NCLEX-RN® Review Questions

Companion Website www.prenhall.com/fontaine
- Audio Glossary
- NCLEX-RN® Review Questions
- Case Study
  - Trauma
- Care Plan
  - Care of a Client in Crisis
- Critical Thinking
  - Assessing a Victim of Violence
- MediaLink Application
  - Preparedness in Mental Health and Psychosocial Education
- MediaLinks
  - Books for Clients & Families
  - Community Resources

NCLEX-RN® Review Questions

25-1. A National Guard soldier who returned home from a 1-month tour of disaster-relief duty comes to the mental health clinic with symptoms of insomnia, irritability, and anxiety. The client states, "I just can't get the sight of those dead bodies out of my head. When I was at the disaster, I tried not to think about what I was doing; now I think about it all the time." Which of the following assessment questions would be most relevant for this client?
1. "How many years have you been in the National Guard?"
2. "Do you know when you will be deployed again?"
3. "What more can you tell me about what is happening now?"
4. "How did you cope with the stress while you were there?"

25-2. In response to a recent violent shooting on another university campus, the university leaders are concerned about acts of violence on their campus. These leaders will initiate which of the following primary prevention activities?
1. Request cell phone numbers of all students, faculty, and staff on campus.
2. Arrange for a BE SMART program on campus for affected individuals.
3. Hold a candlelight vigil for victims of the recent campus shooting.
4. Offer psychological counseling for individuals who had friends at the other university.

25-3. A 16-year-old client is having difficulty dealing with the traumatic death of her boyfriend. Which of the following behaviors does the nurse least expect to observe in this adolescent?
1. Recurring dreams of her boyfriend in the casket
2. Failing grades in school
3. Refusing to discuss the death with friends and parents
4. Worrying about increased drug use in her school

25-4. A community nurse assesses a client following a natural disaster. The nurse will intervene first in which area of need?
1. Feelings of helplessness
2. Fear of increased looting activity
3. Concern for the loss of a home
4. Worrying how children will react

25-5. Which of the following community activities is an example of tertiary prevention in a community that experienced a massive fire?
1. A master plan was formulated for what to do in case of another fire.
2. Mental health professionals offered educational programs on effective coping strategies.
3. Hospital personnel reviewed their emergency response plans and made changes.
4. City officials installed warning signals in remote areas where no warning signals were heard.

See Appendix D for answers.

References

American Psychiatric Association. (2000). *Diagnostic and statistical manual of mental disorders* (4th ed.). Washington DC: Author.

Fullerton, C. S., & Ursano, R. J. (Eds.). (1997). *Post traumatic stress disorder: Acute and long term responses to trauma and disaster.* Washington, DC: American Psychiatric Press.

Fullerton, C. S., Ursano, R. J., Norwood, A., & Holloway. H. (2003). Trauma, terrorism and disaster. In R. J. Ursano, C. S. Fullerton, & A. Norwood (Eds), *Terrorism and disaster: Individual and community mental health interventions* (pp. 1–20). Cambridge, MA: Cambridge University Press.

Galea, S., Ahern, J., Resnick, H., Kilpatrick, D., Bucuvalas, M., Gold, J., & Vlahov, D. (2002). Psychological sequelae of the September 11 terrorist attacks in New York City. *New England Journal of Medicine, 346*, 982–987.

Gurwitch, R. H., Pfefferbaum, B., & Leftwich, M. (2001). The impact of terrorism on children: Considerations for a new era. In S. N. Gold & J. Faust (Eds.), *Trauma practice in the wake of September 11, 2001* (pp. 101–124). New York: Haworth Maltreatment & Trauma Press.

National Center for Post-Traumatic Stress Disorder. *Phases of traumatic stress reactions in a disaster.* Retrieved December 26, 2005, from http://www.ncptsd.va.gov

North, C. S., Nixon, S. J., Shariata, S., et al. (1999). Psychiatric disorders among survivors of the Oklahoma City bombing. *Journal of the American Medical Association, 282*, 755–762.

North American Nursing Diagnosis Association. (2007). *Nursing diagnosis: Definition and Classification,* 2007-2008. Philadelphia: Author.

Rice, M. J., & Moller, M. D. (2006). Wellness outcomes of trauma psychoeducation. *Archives of Psychiatric Nursing, 20*(2), 94–102.

Ross, I. (2006). Political terrorism: An interdisciplinary approach. New York: Peter Lang Publishing.

Schlenger, W. E., Caddell, J. M., Ebert, L., Jordan, K., Rourke, K. M., Wilson, D., Thalji, L., et al. (2002). Psychological reactions to terrorist attacks: Findings from the national study of Americans' reactions to September 11. *Journal of the American Medical Association, 288*, 581–588.

Schurfield, R. M. (2002). Commentary about the terrorist acts of September 11, 2001: Posttraumatic reactions and related social and policy issues. *Trauma, Violence and Abuse, 3*, 3–14.

Schuster, M. A., Stein, B. D., Jaycox, L. H., et al. (2001). A national survey of stress reactions after the September 11, 2001 terrorist attacks. *New England Journal of Medicine, 345*, 1507–1512.

Siegel, L. (2005). *Criminology* (2nd ed.). Belmont, CA: Thompson & Wadsworth.

Silver, R. C., Holman, E. A., McIntosh, D. N., Poulin, M., & Gil-Rivas, V. (2002). Nationwide longitudinal study of psychological responses to September 11. *Journal of the American Medical Association, 288*(10), 1235–1244.

Ursano, R. J. (2002). Post traumatic stress disorder. *New England Journal of Medicine, 34*, 130–131.

Ursano, R. J., Fullerton, C., & Norwood, A. E. (2003). Terrorism and disasters: Prevention, intervention and recovery. In R. J. Ursano, C. S. Fullerton, & A. E. Norwood (Eds.), *Terrorism and disaster: Individual and community mental health interventions* (pp. 333–339). Cambridge, MA: Cambridge University Press.

U.S. State Department. (1999). *Title 22 of the United States Code.* Section 2656f(d).

Williams, R. (2006). The psychosocial consequences for children and young people who are exposed to terrorism, war, conflict and natural disasters. *Current Opinions in Psychiatry, 19*(4), 337–349.

Wright, K. M., & Bartone, P. T. (1994). Community responses to disaster: The Gander plane crash. In R. J. Ursano, B. G. McCaughey, & C. S. Fullerton (Eds.), *Individual and community responses to trauma and disaster: The structure of human chaos* (pp. 267–284). Cambridge, MA: Cambridge University Press.

Yahuda, R. (2002). Post-traumatic stress disorder. *New England Journal of Medicine, 34*, 108–114.

Appendix A

DSM-IV-TR CLASSIFICATION*

NOS = Not Otherwise Specified

An *x* appearing in a diagnostic code indicates that a specific code number is required.

An ellipsis (. . .) is used in the names of certain disorders to indicate that the name of a specific mental disorder or general medical condition should be inserted when recording the name (e.g., 293.0 Delirium Due to Hypothyroidism).

If criteria are currently met, one of the following severity specifiers may be noted after the diagnosis:

    Mild
    Moderate
    Severe

If criteria are no longer met, one of the following specifiers may be noted:

    In Partial Remission
    In Full Remission
    Prior History

Disorders Usually First Diagnosed in Infancy, Childhood, or Adolescence

MENTAL RETARDATION

Note: These are coded on Axis II.

317	Mild Mental Retardation
318.0	Moderate Mental Retardation
318.1	Severe Mental Retardation
318.2	Profound Mental Retardation
319	Mental Retardation, Severity Unspecified

LEARNING DISORDERS

315.00	Reading Disorder
315.1	Mathematics Disorder
315.2	Disorder of Written Expression
315.9	Learning Disorder NOS

MOTOR SKILLS DISORDER

315.4	Developmental Coordination Disorder

COMMUNICATION DISORDERS

315.31	Expressive Language Disorder
315.32	Mixed Receptive-Expressive Language Disorder
315.39	Phonological Disorder
307.0	Stuttering
307.9	Communication Disorder NOS

PERVASIVE DEVELOPMENTAL DISORDERS

299.00	Autistic Disorder
299.80	Rett Disorder
299.10	Childhood Disintegrative Disorder
299.80	Asperger Disorder
299.80	Pervasive Developmental Disorder NOS

ATTENTION-DEFICIT AND DISRUPTIVE BEHAVIOR DISORDERS

314.xx	Attention-Deficit/Hyperactivity Disorder
.01	Combined Type
.00	Predominantly Inattentive Type
.01	Predominantly Hyperactive-Impulsive Type
314.9	Attention-Deficit/Hyperactivity Disorder NOS
312.xx	Conduct Disorder
.81	Childhood-Onset Type
.82	Adolescent-Onset Type
.89	Unspecified Onset
313.81	Oppositional Defiant Disorder
312.9	Disruptive Behavior Disorder NOS

FEEDING AND EATING DISORDERS OF INFANCY OR EARLY CHILDHOOD

307.52	Pica
307.53	Rumination Disorder
307.59	Feeding Disorder of Infancy or Early Childhood

TIC DISORDERS

307.23	Tourette Disorder
307.22	Chronic Motor or Vocal Tic Disorder
307.21	Transient Tic Disorder

    Specify if: Single Episode/Recurrent

307.20	Tic Disorder NOS

ELIMINATION DISORDERS

___.__	Encopresis
787.6	With Constipation and Overflow Incontinence
307.7	Without Constipation and Overflow Incontinence
307.6	Enuresis (Not Due to a General Medical Condition)

    Specify type: Nocturnal Only/Diurnal Only/Nocturnal and Diurnal

OTHER DISORDERS OF INFANCY, CHILDHOOD, OR ADOLESCENCE

309.21	Separation Anxiety Disorder

    Specify if: Early Onset

313.23	Selective Mutism
313.89	Reactive Attachment Disorder of Infancy or Early Childhood

    Specify type: Inhibited Type/Disinhibited Type

307.3	Stereotypic Movement Disorder

    Specify if: With Self-Injurious Behavior

313.9	Disorder of Infancy, Childhood, or Adolescence NOS

*Reprinted with permission from the *Diagnostic and Statistical Manual of Mental Disorders, Fourth Edition, Text Revision.* Copyright 2000 American Psychiatric Association.

Delirium, Dementia, and Amnestic and Other Cognitive Disorders

DELIRIUM

293.0   Delirium Due to . . . *[Indicate the General Medical Condition]*

____.__   Substance Intoxication Delirium *(refer to Substance-Related Disorders for substance-specific codes)*

____.__   Substance Withdrawal Delirium *(refer to Substance-Related Disorders for substance-specific codes)*

____.__   Delirium Due to Multiple Etiologies *(code each of the specific etiologies)*

780.09   Delirium NOS

DEMENTIA

294.xx*   Dementia of the Alzheimer Type, With Early Onset *(also code 331.0 Alzheimer disease on Axis III)*

.10   Without Behavioral Disturbance
.11   With Behavioral Disturbance

294.xx*   Dementia of the Alzheimer Type, With Late Onset *(also code 331.0 Alzheimer disease on Axis III)*

.10   Without Behavioral Disturbance
.11   With Behavioral Disturbance

290.xx   Vascular Dementia
.40   Uncomplicated
.41   With Delirium
.42   With Delusions
.43   With Depressed Mood

Specify if: With Behavioral Disturbance

Code presence or absence of a behavioral disturbance in the fifth digit for Dementia Due to a General Medical Condition:

0 = Without Behavioral Disturbance
1 = With Behavioral Disturbance

294.1x*   Dementia Due to HIV Disease *(also code 042 HIV on Axis III)*

294.1x*   Dementia Due to Head Trauma *(also code 042 HIV on Axis III)*

294.1x*   Dementia Due to Head Trauma *(also code 854.00 head injury on Axis III)*

294.1x*   Dementia Due to Parkinson Disease *(also code 332.0 Parkinson disease on Axis III)*

294.1x*   Dementia Due to Huntington Disease *(also code 333.4 Huntington disease on Axis III)*

294.1x*   Dementia Due to Pick Disease *(also code 331.1 Pick disease on Axis III)*

294.1x*   Dementia Due to Creutzfeldt-Jakob Disease *(also code 046.1 Creutzfeldt-Jakob disease on Axis III)*

294.1x*   Dementia Due to . . . *[Indicate the General Medical Condition not listed above] (also code the general medical condition on Axis III)*

____.__   Substance-Induced Persisting Dementia *(refer to Substance-Related Disorders for substance-specific codes)*

____.__   Dementia Due to Multiple Etiologies *(code each of the specific etiologies)*

294.8   Dementia NOS

AMNESTIC DISORDERS

294.0   Amnestic Disorder Due to . . . *[Indicate the General Medical Condition]*

Specify if: Transient/Chronic

____.__   Substance-Induced Persisting Amnestic Disorder *(refer to Substance-Related Disorders for substance-specific codes)*

294.8   Amnestic Disorder NOS

OTHER COGNITIVE DISORDERS

294.9   Cognitive Disorder NOS

Mental Disorders Due to a General Medical Condition Not Elsewhere Classified

293.89   Catatonic Disorder Due to . . . *[Indicate the General Medical Condition]*

310.1   Personality Change Due to . . . *[Indicate the General Medical Condition]*

Specify type: Labile Type/Disinhibited Type/Aggressive Type/Apathetic Type/Paranoid Type/Other Type/Combined Type/Unspecified Type

293.9   Mental Disorder NOS Due to . . . *[Indicate the General Medical Condition]*

Substance-Related Disorders

The following specifiers apply to Substance Dependence as noted:

[a]With Physiological Dependence/Without Physiological Dependence
[b]Early Full Remission/Early Partial Remission/Sustained Full Remission/Sustained Partial Remission
[c]In a Controlled Environment
[d]On Agonist Therapy

The following specifiers apply to Substance-Induced Disorders as noted:

[I]With Onset During Intoxication/With Onset During Withdrawal

ALCOHOL-RELATED DISORDERS

Alcohol Use Disorders

303.90   Alcohol Dependence[a,b,c]
305.00   Alcohol Abuse

Alcohol-Induced Disorders

303.00   Alcohol Intoxication
291.81   Alcohol Withdrawal

Specify if: With Perceptual Disturbances

291.0   Alcohol Intoxication Delirium
291.0   Alcohol Withdrawal Delirium
291.2   Alcohol-Induced Persisting Dementia
291.1   Alcohol-Induced Persisting Amnestic Disorder
291.x   Alcohol-Induced Psychotic Disorder
.5   With Delusions[I,W]
.3   With Hallucinations[I,W]
291.89   Alcohol-Induced Mood Disorder[I,W]
291.89   Alcohol-Induced Anxiety Disorder[I,W]

ICD-9-CM code valid after October 1, 2000.

291.89 Alcohol-Induced Sexual Dysfunction[I]
291.89 Alcohol-Induced Sleep Disorder[I,W]
291.9 Alcohol-Related Disorder NOS

AMPHETAMINE (OR AMPHETAMINE-LIKE)–RELATED DISORDERS

Amphetamine Use Disorders
304.40 Amphetamine Dependence[a,b,c]
305.70 Amphetamine Abuse

Amphetamine-Induced Disorders
292.89 Amphetamine Intoxication

 Specify if: With Perceptual Disturbances

292.0 Amphetamine Withdrawal
292.81 Amphetamine Intoxication Delirium
292.xx Amphetamine-Induced Psychotic Disorder
 .11 With Delusions[I]
 .12 With Hallucinations[I]
292.84 Amphetamine-Induced Mood Disorder[I,W]
292.89 Amphetamine-Induced Anxiety Disorder[I]
292.89 Amphetamine-Induced Sexual Dysfunction[I]
292.89 Amphetamine-Induced Sleep Disorder[I,W]
292.9 Amphetamine-Related Disorder NOS

CAFFEINE-RELATED DISORDERS

Caffeine-Induced Disorders
305.90 Caffeine Intoxication
292.89 Caffeine-Induced Anxiety Disorder[I]
292.89 Caffeine-Induced Sleep Disorder[I]
292.9 Caffeine-Related Disorder NOS

CANNABIS-RELATED DISORDERS

Cannabis Use Disorders
304.30 Cannabis Dependence[a,b,c]
305.20 Cannabis Abuse

Cannabis-Induced Disorders
292.89 Cannabis Intoxication

 Specify if: With Perceptual Disturbance

292.81 Cannabis Intoxication Delirium
292.xx Cannabis-Induced Psychotic Disorder
 .11 With Delusions[I]
 .12 With Hallucinations[I]
292.89 Cannabis-Induced Anxiety Disorder[I]
292.9 Cannabis-Related Disorder NOS

COCAINE-RELATED DISORDERS

Cocaine Use Disorders
304.20 Cocaine Dependence[a,b,c]
305.60 Cocaine Abuse

Cocaine-Induced Disorders
292.89 Cocaine Intoxication

 Specify if: With Perceptual Disturbances

292.0 Cocaine Withdrawal
292.81 Cocaine Intoxication Delirium
292.xx Cocaine-Induced Psychotic Disorder
 .11 With Delusions[I]
 .12 With Hallucinations[I]
292.84 Cocaine-Induced Mood Disorder[I,W]
292.89 Cocaine-Induced Anxiety Disorder[I,W]

292.89 Cocaine-Induced Sexual Dysfunction[I]
292.89 Cocaine-Induced Sleep Disorder[I,W]
292.9 Cocaine-Related Disorder NOS

HALLUCINOGEN-RELATED DISORDERS

Hallucinogen Use Disorders
304.50 Hallucinogen Dependence[b,c]
305.30 Hallucinogen Abuse

Hallucinogen-Induced Disorders
292.89 Hallucinogen Intoxication
292.89 Hallucinogen Persisting Perception Disorder (Flashbacks)
292.81 Hallucinogen Intoxication Delirium
292.xx Hallucinogen-Induced Psychotic Disorder
 .11 With Delusions[I]
 .12 With Hallucinations[I]
292.84 Hallucinogen-Induced Mood Disorder[I]
292.89 Hallucinogen-Induced Anxiety Disorder[I]
292.9 Hallucinogen-Related Disorder NOS

INHALANT-RELATED DISORDERS

Inhalant Use Disorders
304.60 Inhalant Dependence[b,c]
305.90 Inhalant Abuse

Inhalant-Induced Disorders
292.89 Inhalant Intoxication
292.81 Inhalant Intoxication Delirium
292.82 Inhalant-Induced Persisting Dementia
292.xx Inhalant-Induced Psychotic Disorder
 .11 With Delusions[I]
 .12 With Hallucinations[I]
292.84 Inhalant-Induced Mood Disorder[I]
292.89 Inhalant-Induced Anxiety Disorder[I]
292.9 Inhalant-Related Disorder NOS

NICOTINE-RELATED DISORDERS

Nicotine Use Disorder
305.1 Nicotine Dependence[a,b]

Nicotine-Induced Disorder
292.0 Nicotine Withdrawal
292.9 Nicotine-Related Disorder NOS

OPIOID-RELATED DISORDERS

Opioid Use Disorders
304.00 Opioid Dependence[a,b,c,d]
305.50 Opioid Abuse

Opioid-Induced Disorders
292.89 Opioid Intoxication

 Specify if: With Perceptual Disturbances

292.0 Opioid Withdrawal
292.81 Opioid Intoxication Delirium
292.xx Opioid-Induced Psychotic Disorder
 .11 With Delusions[I]
 .12 With Hallucinations[I]
292.84 Opioid-Induced Mood Disorder[I]
292.89 Opioid-Induced Sexual Dysfunction[I]
292.89 Opioid-Induced Sleep Disorder[I,W]
292.9 Opioid-Related Disorder NOS

PHENCYCLIDINE (OR PHENCYCLIDINE-LIKE)–RELATED DISORDERS

Phencyclidine Use Disorders

304.60   Phencyclidine Dependence[b,c]
305.90   Phencyclidine Abuse

Phencyclidine-Induced Disorders

292.89   Phencyclidine Intoxication

    Specify if: With Perceptual Disturbances

292.81   Phencyclidine Intoxication Delirium
292.xx   Phencyclidine-Induced Psychotic Disorder
  .11   With Delusions[I]
  .12   With Hallucinations[I]
292.84   Phencyclidine-Induced Mood Disorder[I]
292.89   Phencyclidine-Induced Anxiety Disorder[I]
292.9   Phencyclidine-Related Disorder NOS

SEDATIVE-, HYPNOTIC-, OR ANXIOLYTIC-RELATED DISORDERS

Sedative, Hypnotic, or Anxiolytic Use Disorders

304.10   Sedative, Hypnotic, or Anxiolytic Dependence[a,b,c]
305.40   Sedative, Hypnotic, or Anxiolytic Abuse

Sedative-, Hypnotic-, or Anxiolytic-Induced Disorders

292.89   Sedative, Hypnotic, or Anxiolytic Intoxication
292.0   Sedative, Hypnotic, or Anxiolytic Withdrawal

    Specify if: With Perceptual Disturbances

292.81   Sedative, Hypnotic, or Anxiolytic Intoxication Delirium
292.81   Sedative, Hypnotic, or Anxiolytic Withdrawal Delirium
292.82   Sedative, Hypnotic, or Anxiolytic-Induced Persisting Dementia
292.83   Sedative-, Hypnotic-, or Anxiolytic-Induced Persisting Amnestic Disorder
292.xx   Sedative-, Hypnotic-, or Anxiolytic-Induced Psychotic Disorder
  .11   With Delusions[I,W]
  .12   With Hallucinations[I,W]
292.84   Sedative-, Hypnotic-, or Anxiolytic-Induced Mood Disorder[I,W]
292.89   Sedative-, Hypnotic-, or Anxiolytic-Induced Anxiety Disorder[W]
292.89   Sedative-, Hypnotic-, or Anxiolytic-Induced Sexual Dysfunction[I]
292.89   Sedative-, Hypnotic, or Anxiolytic-Induced Sleep Disorder[I,W]
292.9   Sedative-, Hypnotic, or Anxiolytic-Related Disorder NOS

POLYSUBSTANCE-RELATED DISORDER

304.80   Polysubstance Dependence[a,b,c,d]

OTHER (OR UNKNOWN) SUBSTANCE-RELATED DISORDERS

Other (or Unknown) Substance Use Disorders

304.90   Other (or Unknown) Substance Dependence[a,b,c,d]
305.90   Other (or Unknown) Substance Abuse

Other (or Unknown) Substance-Induced Disorders

292.89   Other (or Unknown) Substance Intoxication

    Specify if: With Perceptual Disturbances

292.0   Other (or Unknown) Substance Withdrawal

    Specify if: With Perceptual Disturbances

292.81   Other (or Unknown) Substance-Induced Delirium
292.82   Other (or Unknown) Substance-Induced Persisting Dementia

292.83   Other (or Unknown) Substance-Induced Persisting Amnestic Disorder
292.xx   Other (or Unknown) Substance-Induced Psychotic Disorder
  .11   With Delusions[I,W]
  .12   With Hallucinations[I,W]
292.84   Other (or Unknown) Substance-Induced Mood Disorder[I,W]
292.89   Other (or Unknown) Substance-Induced Anxiety Disorder[I,W]
292.89   Other (or Unknown) Substance-Induced Sexual Dysfunction[I]
292.89   Other (or Unknown) Substance-Induced Sleep Disorder[I,W]
292.9   Other (or Unknown) Substance-Related Disorder NOS

POLYSUBSTANCE-RELATED DISORDER

304.80   Polysubstance Dependence[a,b,c,d]

OTHER (OR UNKNOWN) SUBSTANCE-RELATED DISORDERS

Other (or Unknown) Substance Use Disorders

304.90   Other (or Unknown) Substance Dependence[a,b,c,d]
305.90   Other (or Unknown) Substance Abuse

Other (or Unknown) Substance-Induced Disorders

292.89   Other (or Unknown) Substance Intoxication

    Specify if: With Perceptual Disturbances

292.0   Other (or Unknown) Substance Withdrawal

    Specify if: With Perceptual Disturbances

292.81   Other (or Unknown) Substance-Induced Delirium
292.82   Other (or Unknown) Substance-Induced Persisting Dementia
292.83   Other (or Unknown) Substance-Induced Persisting Amnestic Disorder
292.xx   Other (or Unknown) Substance-Induced Psychotic Disorder
  .11   With Delusions[I,W]
  .12   With Hallucinations[I,W]
292.84   Other (or Unknown) Substance-Induced Mood Disorder[I,W]
292.89   Other (or Unknown) Substance-Induced Anxiety Disorder[I,W]
292.89   Other (or Unknown) Substance-Induced Sexual Dysfunction[I]
292.89   Other (or Unknown) Substance-Induced Sleep Disorder[I,W]
292.9   Other (or Unknown) Substance-Related Disorder NOS

Schizophrenia and Other Psychotic Disorders

295.xx   Schizophrenia

The following Classification of Longitudinal Course applies to all subtypes of Schizophrenia:

    Episodic With Interepisode Residual Symptoms (*Specify if:* With Prominent Negative Symptoms)/Episodic With No Interepisode Residual Symptoms
    Continuous (*Specify if:* With Prominent Negative Symptoms)
    Single Episode in Partial Remission (*Specify if:* With Prominent Negative Symptoms)/Single Episode in Full Remission
    Other or Unspecified Pattern

.30	Paranoid Type
.10	Disorganized Type
.20	Catatonic Type
.90	Undifferentiated Type
.60	Residual Type
295.40	Schizophreniform Disorder

Specify if: Without Good Prognostic Features/With Good Prognostic Features

295.70	Schizoaffective Disorder

Specify type: Bipolar Type/Depressive Type

297.1	Delusional Disorder

Specify type: Erotomanic Type/Grandiose Type/Jealous Type/Persecutory Type/Somatic Type/Mixed Type/Unspecified Type

298.8	Brief Psychotic Disorder

Specify if: With Marked Stressor(s)/Without Marked Stressor(s)/With Postpartum Onset

297.3	Shared Psychotic Disorder
293.xx	Psychotic Disorder Due to . . . *[Indicate the General Medical Condition]*
.81	With Delusions
.82	With Hallucinations
___.__	Substance-Induced Psychotic Disorder *(refer to Substance-Related Disorders for substance-specific codes)*

Specify if: With Onset During Intoxication/With Onset During Withdrawal

298.9	Psychotic Disorder NOS

Mood Disorders

Code current state of Major Depressive Disorder or Bipolar I Disorder in fifth digit:

> 1 = Mild
> 2 = Moderate
> 3 = Severe Without Psychotic Features
> 4 = Severe With Psychotic Features
> *Specify:* Mood-Congruent Psychotic Features/
>   Mood-Incongruent Psychotic Features
> 5 = In Partial Remission
> 6 = In Full Remission
> 0 = Unspecified

The following specifiers apply (for current or most recent episode) to Mood Disorders as noted:

> [a]Severity/Psychotic/Remission Specifiers/[b]Chronic/[c]With Catatonic Features/[d]With Melancholic Features/[e]WIth Atypical Features/[f]With Postpartum Onset

The following specifiers apply to Mood Disorders as noted:

> [g]With or Without Full Interepisode Recovery/[h]With Seasonal Pattern/[i]With Rapid Cycling

DEPRESSIVE DISORDERS

296.xx	Major Depressive Disorder
.2x	Single Episode[a,b,c,d,e,f]
.3x	Recurrent[a,b,c,d,e,f,g,h]
300.4	Dysthymic Disorder

Specify if: Early Onset/Late Onset
Specify if: With Atypical Features

311	Depressive Disorder NOS

BIPOLAR DISORDERS

296.xx	Bipolar I Disorder
.0x	Single Manic Episode[a,c,f]

Specify if: Mixed

.40	Most Recent Episode Hypomanic[g,h,i]
.4x	Most Recent Episode Manic[a,c,f,g,h,i]
.6x	Most Recent Episode Mixed[a,c,f,g,h,i]
.5x	Most Recent Episode Depressed[a,b,c,d,e,f,g,h,i]
.7	Most Recent Episode Unspecified[g,h,i]
296.89	Bipolar II Disorder[a,b,c,d,e,f,g,h,i]

Specify (current or most recent episode): Hypomanic/Depressed

301.13	Cyclothymic Disorder
296.80	Bipolar Disorder NOS
293.83	Mood Disorder Due to . . . *[Indicate the General Medical Condition]*

Specify type: With Depressive Features/With Major Depressive-Like Episode/With Manic Features/With Mixed Features

___.__	Substance-Induced Mood Disorder *(refer to Substance-Related Disorders for substance-specific codes)*

Specify type: With Depressive Features/With Manic Features/With Mixed Features
Specify if: With Onset During Intoxication/With Onset During Withdrawal

296.90	Mood Disorder NOS

Anxiety Disorders

300.01	Panic Disorder Without Agoraphobia
300.21	Panic Disorder With Agoraphobia
300.22	Agoraphobia Without History of Panic Disorder
300.29	Specific Phobia

Specify type: Animal Type/Natural Environment Type/Blood-Injection-Injury Type/Situational Type/Other Type

300.23	Social Phobia

Specify if: Generalized

300.3	Obsessive-Compulsive Disorder

Specify if: With Poor Insight

309.81	Posttraumatic Stress Disorder

Specify if: Acute/Chronic
Specify if: With Delayed Onset

308.3	Acute Stress Disorder
300.02	Generalized Anxiety Disorder
293.84	Anxiety Disorder Due to . . . *[Indicate the General Medical Condition]*

Specify if: With Generalized Anxiety/With Panic Attacks/With Obsessive-Compulsive Symptoms

___.__	Substance-Induced Anxiety Disorder *(refer to Substance-Related Disorders for substance-specific codes)*

Specify if: With Generalized Anxiety/With Panic Attacks/With Obsessive-Compulsive Symptoms/With Phobic Symptoms
Specify if: With Onset During Intoxication/With Onset During Withdrawal

300.00	Anxiety Disorder NOS

Somatoform Disorders
300.81   Somatization Disorder
300.82   Undifferentiated Somatoform Disorder
300.11   Conversion Disorder

Specify type: With Motor Symptom or Deficit/With Sensory Symptom or Deficit/With Seizures or Convulsions/With Mixed Presentation

307.xx   Pain Disorder
  .80   Associated With Psychological Factors
  .89   Associated With Both Psychological Factors and a General Medical Condition

Specify if: Acute/Chronic

300.7   Hypochondriasis

Specify if: With Poor Insight

300.7   Body Dysmorphic Disorder
300.82   Somatoform Disorder NOS

Factitious Disorders
300.xx   Factitious Disorder
  .16   With Predominantly Psychological Signs and Symptoms
  .19   With Predominantly Physical Signs and Symptoms
  .19   With Combined Psychological and Physical Signs and Symptoms
300.19   Factitious Disorder NOS

Dissociative Disorders
300.12   Dissociative Amnesia
300.13   Dissociative Fugue
300.14   Dissociative Identity Disorder
300.6   Depersonalization Disorder
300.15   Dissociative Disorder NOS

Sexual and Gender Identity Disorders
SEXUAL DYSFUNCTIONS
The following specifiers apply to all primary Sexual Dysfunctions:

> Lifelong Type/Acquired Type
> Generalized Type/Situational Type
> Due to Psychological Factors/Due to Combined Factors

SEXUAL DESIRE DISORDERS
302.71   Hypoactive Sexual Desire Disorder
302.79   Sexual Aversion Disorder

SEXUAL AROUSAL DISORDERS
302.72   Female Sexual Arousal Disorder
302.72   Male Erectile Disorder

ORGASMIC DISORDERS
302.73   Female Orgasmic Disorder
302.74   Male Orgasmic Disorder
302.75   Premature Ejaculation

SEXUAL PAIN DISORDERS
302.76   Dyspareunia (Not Due to a General Medical Condition)
306.51   Vaginismus (Not Due to a General Medical Condition)

SEXUAL DYSFUNCTION DUE TO A GENERAL MEDICAL CONDITION
625.8   Female Hypoactive Sexual Desire Disorder Due to . . . *[Indicate the General Medical Condition]*

608.89   Male Hypoactive Sexual Desire Disorder Due to . . . *[Indicate the General Medical Condition]*
607.84   Male Erectile Disorder Due to . . . *[Indicate the General Medical Condition]*
625.0   Female Dyspareunia Due to . . . *[Indicate the General Medical Condition]*
608.89   Male Dyspareunia Due to . . . *[Indicate the General Medical Condition]*
625.8   Other Female Sexual Dysfunction Due to . . . *[Indicate the General Medical Condition]*
608.89   Other Male Sexual Dysfunction Due to . . . *[Indicate the General Medical Condition]*
____.__   Substance-Induced Sexual Dysfunction *(refer to Substance-Related Disorders for substance-specific codes)*

Specify if: With Impaired Desire/With Impaired Arousal/With Impaired Orgasm/With Sexual Pain
Specify if: With Onset During Intoxication

302.70   Sexual Dysfunction NOS

PARAPHILIAS
302.4   Exhibitionism
302.81   Fetishism
302.89   Frotteurism
302.2   Pedophilia

Specify if: Sexually Attracted to Males/Sexually Attracted to Females/Sexually Attracted to Both
Specify if: Limited to Incest
Specify type: Exclusive Type/Nonexclusive Type

302.83   Sexual Masochism
302.84   Sexual Sadism
302.3   Transvestic Fetishism

Specify if: With Gender Dysphoria

302.82   Voyeurism
302.9   Paraphilia NOS

GENDER IDENTITY DISORDERS
302.xx   Gender Identity Disorder
  .6   in Children
  .85   in Adolescents or Adults

Specify if: Sexually Attracted to Males/Sexually Attracted to Females/Sexually Attracted to Both/Sexually Attracted to Neither

302.6   Gender Identity Disorder NOS
302.9   Sexual Disorder NOS

Eating Disorders
307.1   Anorexia Nervosa

Specify type: Restricting Type; Binge-Eating/Purging Type

307.51   Bulimia Nervosa

Specify type: Purging Type/Nonpurging Type

307.50   Eating Disorder NOS

Sleep Disorders
PRIMARY SLEEP DISORDERS
Dyssomnias
307.42   Primary Insomnia
307.44   Primary Hypersomnia

Specify if: Recurrent

347	Narcolepsy
780.59	Breathing-Related Sleep Disorder
307.45	Circadian Rhythm Sleep Disorder

Specify type: Delayed Sleep Phase Type/Jet Lag Type/Shift Work Type/Unspecified Type

| 307.47 | Dyssomnia NOS |

Parasomnias
307.47	Nightmare Disorder
307.46	Sleep Terror Disorder
307.46	Sleepwalking Disorder
307.47	Parasomnia NOS

SLEEP DISORDERS RELATED TO ANOTHER MENTAL DISORDER
| 307.42 | Insomnia Related to . . . *[Indicate the Axis I or Axis II Disorder]* |
| 307.44 | Hypersomnia Related to . . . *[Indicate the Axis I or Axis II Disorder]* |

OTHER SLEEP DISORDERS
780.xx	Sleep Disorder Due to . . . *[Indicate the General Medical Condition]*
.52	Insomnia Type
.54	Hypersomnia Type
.59	Parasomnia Type
.59	Mixed Type
___.__	Substance-Induced Sleep Disorder *(refer to Substance-Related Disorders for substance-specific codes)*

Specify type: Insomnia Type/Hypersomnia Type/Parasomnia Type/Mixed Type

Specify if: With Onset During Intoxication/With Onset During Withdrawal

Impulse-Control Disorders Not Elsewhere Classified
312.34	Intermittent Explosive Disorder
312.32	Kleptomania
312.33	Pyromania
312.31	Pathological Gambling
312.39	Trichotillomania
312.30	Impulse-Control Disorder NOS

Adjustment Disorders
309.xx	Adjustment Disorder
.0	With Depressed Mood
.24	With Anxiety
.28	With Mixed Anxiety and Depressed Mood
.3	With Disturbance of Conduct
.4	With Mixed Disturbance of Emotions and Condut
.9	Unspecified

Specify if: Acute/Chronic

Personality Disorders
Note: These are coded on Axis II.
301.0	Paranoid Personality Disorder
301.20	Schizoid Personality Disorder
301.22	Schizotypal Personality Disorder
301.7	Antisocial Personality Disorder
301.83	Borderline Personality Disorder
301.50	Histrionic Personality Disorder
301.81	Narcissistic Personality Disorder
301.82	Avoidant Personality Disorder

301.6	Dependent Personality Disorder
301.4	Obsessive-Compulsive Personality Disorder
301.9	Personality Disorder NOS

Other Conditions That May Be a Focus of Clinical Attention

PSYCHOLOGICAL FACTORS AFFECTING MEDICAL CONDITION
| 316 | . . . *[Specified Psychological Factor] Affecting . . . [Indicate the General Medical Condition]* |

Choose name based on nature of factors:
Mental Disorder Affecting Medical Condition
Psychological Symptoms Affecting Medical Condition
Personality Traits or Coping Style Affecting Medical Condition
Maladaptive Health Behaviors Affecting Medical Condition
Stress-Related Physiological Response Affecting Medical Condition
Other or Unspecified Psychological Factors Affecting Medical Condition

MEDICATION-INDUCED MOVEMENT DISORDERS
332.1	Neuroleptic-Induced Parkinsonism
333.92	Neuroleptic Malignant Syndrome
333.7	Neuroleptic-Induced Acute Dystonia
333.99	Neuroleptic-Induced Acute Akathisia
333.82	Neuroleptic-Induced Tardive Dyskinesia
333.1	Medication-Induced Postural Tremor
333.90	Medication-Induced Movement Disorder NOS

OTHER MEDICATION-INDUCED DISORDER
| 995.2 | Adverse Effects of Medication NOS |

RELATIONAL PROBLEMS
V61.9	Relational Problem Related to a Mental Disorder or General Medical Condition
V61.20	Parent-Child Relational Problem
V61.10	Partner Relational Problem
V61.8	Sibling Relational Problem
V62.81	Relational Problem NOS

PROBLEMS RELATED TO ABUSE OR NEGLECT
V61.21	Physical Abuse of Child *(code 995.54 if focus of attention is on victim)*
V61.21	Sexual Abuse of Child *(code 995.53 if focus of attention is on victim)*
V61.21	Neglect of Child *(code 995.52 if focus of attention is on victim)*
___.__	Physical Abuse of Adult
V61.12	(if by partner)
V62.83	(if by person other than partner) *(code 995.81 if focus of attention is on victim)*
___.__	Sexual Abuse of Adult
V61.12	(if by partner)
V62.83	(if by person other than partner) *(code 995.83 if focus of attention is on victim)*

ADDITIONAL CONDITIONS THAT MAY BE A FOCUS OF CLINICAL ATTENTION
V15.81	Noncompliance With Treatment
V65.2	Malingering
V71.01	Adult Antisocial Behavior
V71.02	Child or Adolescent Antisocial Behavior
V62.89	Borderline Intellectual Functioning

Note: This is coded on Axis II.

780.9   Age-Related Cognitive Decline
V62.82   Bereavement
V62.3   Academic Problem
V62.2   Occupational Problem
313.82   Identity Problem
V62.89   Religious or Spiritual Problem
V62.4   Acculturation Problem
V62.89   Phase of Life Problem

Additional Codes

300.9   Unspecified Mental Disorder (nonpsychotic)
V71.09   No Diagnosis or Condition on Axis I
799.9   Diagnosis or Condition Deferred on Axis I

V71.09   No Diagnosis on Axis II
799.9   Diagnosis Deferred on Axis II

Multiaxial System

Axis I   Clinical Disorders
          Other Conditions That May Be a Focus of Clinical
          Attention
Axis II   Personality Disorders
          Mental Retardation
Axis III General Medical Conditions
Axis IV   Psychosocial and Environmental Problems
Axis V   Global Assessment of Functioning

MULTIAXIAL ASSESSMENT

A multiaxial system involves an assessment on several axes, each of which refers to a different domain of information that may help the clinician plan treatment and predict outcome. There are five axes included in the DSM-IV multiaxial classification:

Axis I   Clinical Disorders
             Other Conditions That May Be a Focus of Clinical Attention
Axis II   Personality Disorders
             Mental Retardation
Axis III   General Medical Conditions
Axis IV   Psychosocial and Environmental Problems
Axis V   Global Assessment of Functioning

The use of the multiaxial system facilitates comprehensive and systematic evaluation with attention to the various mental disorders and general medical conditions, psychosocial and environmental problems, and level of functioning that might be overlooked if the focus were on assessing a single presenting problem. A multiaxial system provides a convenient format for organizing and communicating clinical information, for capturing the complexity of clinical situations, and for describing the heterogeneity of individuals presenting with the same diagnosis. In addition, the multiaxial system promotes the application of the biopsychosocial model in clinical, educational, and research settings.

The rest of this section provides a description of each of the DSM-IV axes. In some settings or situations, clinicians may prefer not to use the multiaxial system. For this reason, guidelines for reporting the results of a DSM-IV assessment without applying the formal multiaxial system are provided at the end of this section.

AXIS I	Clinical Disorders

Other Conditions That May Be a Focus of Clinical Attention

Disorders Usually First Diagnosed in Infancy, Childhood, or Adolescence (*excluding Mental Retardation, which is diagnosed on Axis II*)

Delirium, Dementia, and Amnestic and Other Cognitive Disorders

Mental Disorders Due to a General Medical Condition

Substance-Related Disorders

Schizophrenia and Other Psychotic Disorders

Mood Disorders

Anxiety Disorders

Somatoform Disorders

Factitious Disorders

Dissociative Disorders

Sexual and Gender Identity Disorders

Eating Disorders

Sleep Disorders

Impulse-Control Disorders Not Elsewhere Classified

Adjustment Disorders

Other Conditions That May Be a Focus of Clinical Attention

AXIS I: CLINICAL DISORDERS— OTHER CONDITIONS THAT MAY BE A FOCUS OF CLINICAL ATTENTION

Axis I is for reporting all the various disorders or conditions in the classification except for the Personality Disorders and Mental Retardation (which are reported on Axis II). The major groups of disorders to be reported on Axis I are listed in the box to the right. Also reported on Axis I are Other Conditions That May Be a Focus of Clinical Attention.

When an individual has more than one Axis I disorder, all should be reported. If more than one Axis I disorder is present, the principal diagnosis or the reason for the visit should be indicated by listing it first. When an individual has both an Axis I and an Axis II disorder, the principal diagnosis or the reason for the visit will be assumed to be on Axis I unless the Axis II diagnosis is followed by the qualifying phrase "(Principal Diagnosis)" or "(Reason for Visit)." If no Axis I disorder is present, this should be coded as V71.09. If an Axis I diagnosis is deferred, pending the gathering of additional information, this should be coded as 799.9.

AXIS II: PERSONALITY DISORDERS AND MENTAL RETARDATION

Axis II is for reporting Personality Disorders and Mental Retardation. It may also be used for noting prominent maladaptive personality features and defense mechanisms. The listing of Personality Disorders and Mental Retardation on a separate axis ensures that consideration will be given to the possible presence of Personality Disorders and Mental Retardation that might otherwise be overlooked when attention is directed to the usually more florid Axis I disorders. The coding of Personality Disorders on Axis II should not be taken to imply that their pathogenesis or range of appropriate treatment is fundamentally different from that for the disorders coded on Axis I. The disorders to be reported on Axis II are listed in the box on page 672.

In the common situation in which an individual has more than one Axis II diagnosis, all should be reported. When an individual has both an Axis I and an Axis II diagnosis and the Axis II diagnosis is the principal diagnosis or the reason for the visit, this should be indicated by adding the qualifying phrase

AXIS II	Personality Disorders

Mental Retardation

Paranoid Personality Disorder	Narcissistic Personality Disorder
Schizoid Personality Disorder	Avoidant Personality Disorder
Schizotypal Personality Disorder	Dependent Personality Disorder
Antisocial Personality Disorder	Obsessive Compulsive Personality Disorder
Borderline Personality Disorder	Personality Disorder Not Otherwise Specified
Histrionic Personality Disorder	Mental Retardation

"(Principal Diagnosis)" or "(Reason for Visit)" after the Axis II diagnosis. If no Axis II disorder is present, this should be coded as V71.09. If an Axis II diagnosis is deferred, pending the gathering of additional information, this should be coded as 799.9.

Axis II may also be used to indicate prominent maladaptive personality features that do not meet the threshold for a Personality Disorder (in such instances, no code number should be used). The habitual use of maladaptive defense mechanisms may also be indicated on Axis II.

AXIS III: GENERAL MEDICAL CONDITIONS

Axis III is for reporting current general medical conditions that are potentially relevant to the understanding or management of the individual's mental disorder. These conditions are classified outside the "Mental Disorders" chapter of ICD-9-CM (and outside Chapter V of ICD-10). A listing of the broad categories of general medical conditions is given in the box on page 673.

As discussed in the "Introduction," the multiaxial distinction among Axis I, Axis II, and Axis III disorders does not imply that there are fundamental differences in their conceptualization, that mental disorders are unrelated to physical or biological factors or processes, or that general medical conditions are unrelated to behavioral or psychosocial factors or processes. The purpose of distinguishing general medical conditions is to encourage thoroughness in evaluation and to enhance communication among health care providers.

General medical conditions can be related to mental disorders in a variety of ways. In some cases it is clear that the general medical condition is directly etiological to the development or worsening of mental symptoms and that the mechanism for this effect is physiological. When a mental disorder is judged to be a direct physiological consequence of the general medical condition, a Mental Disorder Due to a General Medical Condition should be diagnosed on Axis I and the general medical condition should be recorded on Axis I and Axis III both. For

example, when hypothyroidism is a direct cause of depressive symptoms, the designation on Axis I is 293.83 Mood Disorder Due to Hypothyroidism, With Depressive Features, and the hypothyroidism is listed again and coded on Axis III as 244.9.

In those instances in which the etiological relationship between the general medical condition and the mental symptoms is insufficiently clear to warrant an Axis I diagnosis of Mental Disorder Due to a General Medical Condition, the appropriate mental disorder (e.g., Major Depressive Disorder) should be listed and coded on Axis I; the general medical condition should only be coded on Axis III.

There are other situations in which general medical conditions are recorded on Axis III because of their importance to the overall understanding or treatment of the individual with the mental disorder. An Axis I disorder may be a psychological reaction to an Axis III general medical condition (e.g., the development of 309.0 Adjustment Disorder With Depressed Mood as a reaction to the diagnosis of carcinoma of the breast). Some general medical conditions may not be directly related to the mental disorder but nonetheless have important prognostic or treatment implications (e.g., when the diagnosis on Axis I is 296.30 Major Depressive Disorder, Recurrent, and on Axis III is 427.9 arrhythmia, the choice of pharmacotherapy is influenced by the general medical condition; or when a person with diabetes mellitus is admitted to the hospital for an exacerbation of Schizophrenia and insulin management must be monitored).

When an individual has more than one clinically relevant Axis III diagnosis, all should be reported. If no Axis III disorder is present, this should be indicated by the notation "Axis III: None." If an Axis III diagnosis is deferred, pending the gathering of additional information, this should be indicated by the notation "Axis III: Deferred."

AXIS IV: PSYCHOSOCIAL AND ENVIRONMENTAL PROBLEMS

Axis IV is for reporting psychosocial and environmental problems that may affect the diagnosis, treatment, and prognosis of mental disorders (Axes I and II). A psychosocial or environmental problem may be a negative life event, an environmental difficulty or deficiency, a familial or other interpersonal stress, an inadequacy of social support or personal resources, or other problem relating to the context in which a person's difficulties have developed. So-called positive stressors, such as job promotion, should be listed only if they constitute or lead to a problem, as when a person has difficulty adapting to the new situation. In addition to playing a role in the initiation or exacerbation of a mental disorder, psychosocial problems may also develop as a consequence of a person's psychopathology or may constitute problems that should be considered in the overall management plan.

When an individual has multiple psychosocial or environmental problems, the clinician may note as many as are judged to be relevant. In general, the clinician should note only those psychosocial and environmental problems that have been present during the year preceding the current evaluation. However,

AXIS III	General Medical Conditions (With ICD-9-CM Codes)

Infectious and Parasitic Diseases (001–139)

Neoplasms (140–239)

Endocrine, Nutritional, and Metabolic Diseases and Immunity Disorders (240–279)

Diseases of the Blood and Blood Forming Organs (280–289)

Diseases of the Nervous System and Sense Organs (320–389)

Diseases of the Circulatory System (390–459)

Diseases of the Respiratory System (460–519)

Diseases of the Digestive System (520–579)

Diseases of the Genitourinary System (580–629)

Complications of Pregnancy, Childbirth, and the Puerperium (630–676)

Diseases of the Skin and Subcutaneous Tissue (680–709)

Diseases of the Musculoskeletal System and Connective Tissue (710–739)

Congenital Anomalies (740–759)

Certain Conditions Originating in the Perinatal Period (760–779)

Symptoms, Signs, and Ill-Defined Conditions (780–799)

Injury and Poisoning (800–999)

the clinician may choose to note psychosocial and environmental problems occurring prior to the previous year if these clearly contribute to the mental disorder or have become a focus of treatment—for example, previous combat experiences leading to Posttraumatic Stress Disorder.

In practice, most psychosocial and environmental problems will be indicated on Axis IV. However, when a psychosocial or environmental problem is the primary focus of clinical attention, it should also be recorded on Axis I, with a code derived from the section "Other Conditions That May Be a Focus of Clinical Attention."

For convenience, the problems are grouped together in the following categories:

- **Problems with primary support group**—e.g., death of a family member; health problems in family; disruption of family by separation, divorce, or estrangement; removal from the home; remarriage of parent; sexual or physical abuse; parental overprotection; neglect of child; inadequate discipline; discord with siblings; birth of a sibling

- **Problems related to the social environment**—e.g., death or loss of friend; inadequate social support; living alone; difficulty with acculturation; discrimination; adjustment of life cycle transition (such as retirement)

- **Educational problems**—e.g., illiteracy; academic problems; discord with teachers or classmates; inadequate school environment

- **Occupational problems**—e.g., unemployment; threat of job loss; stressful work schedule; difficult work conditions; job dissatisfaction; job change; discord with boss or co-workers

- **Housing problems**—e.g., homelessness; inadequate housing; unsafe neighborhood; discord with neighbors or landlord

- **Economic problems**—e.g., extreme poverty; inadequate finances; insufficient welfare support

- **Problems with access to health care services**—e.g., inadequate health care services; transportation to health care facilities unavailable; inadequate health insurance

- **Problems related to interaction with the legal system/crime**—e.g., arrest; incarceration; litigation; victim of crime

- **Other psychosocial and environmental problems**—e.g., exposure to disasters, war, other hostilities; discord with nonfamily caregivers such as counselor, social worker, or physician; unavailability of social service agencies

When using the Multiaxial Evaluation Report Form, the clinician should identify the relevant categories of psychosocial and environmental problems and indicate the specific factors involved. If a recording form with a checklist of problem categories is not used, the clinician may simply list the specific problems on Axis IV.

AXIS V: GLOBAL ASSESSMENT OF FUNCTIONING

Axis V is for reporting the clinician's judgment of the individual's overall level of functioning. This information is useful in planning treatment and measuring its impact, and in predicting outcome.

The reporting of overall functioning on Axis V can be done using the Global Assessment of Functioning (GAF) Scale. The

AXIS IV	Psychosocial and Environmental Problems

Problems With Primary Support Group

Problems Related to the Social Environment

Educational Problems

Occupational Problems

Housing Problems

Economic Problems

Problems With Access to Health Care Services

Problems Related to Interaction with the Legal System/Crime

Other Psychosocial and Environmental Problems

GAF Scale may be particularly useful in tracking the clinical progress of individuals in global terms, using a single measure. The GAF Scale is to be rated with respect only to psychological, social, and occupational functioning. The instructions specify, "Do not include impairment in functioning due to physical (or environmental) limitations."

The GAF Scale is divided into 10 ranges of functioning. Making a GAF rating involves picking a single value that best reflects the individual's overall level of functioning. The description of each 10-point range in the GAF Scale has two components: the first part covers symptom severity, and the second part covers functioning. The GAF rating is within a particular decile if either the symptom severity or the level of functioning falls within the range. For example, the first part of the range 41–50 describes "serious symptoms (e.g., suicidal ideation, severe obsessional rituals, frequent shoplifting)" and the second part includes "any serious impairment in social, occupational, or school functioning (e.g., no friends, unable to keep a job)." It should be noted that in situations where the individual's symptom severity and level of functioning are discordant, the final GAF rating always reflects the worse of the two. For example, the GAF rating for an individual who is a significant danger to self but is otherwise functioning well would be below 20. Similarly, the GAF rating for an individual with minimal psychological symptomatology but significant impairment in functioning (e.g., an individual whose excessive preoccupation with substance use has resulted in loss of job and friends but no other psychopathology) would be 40 or lower.

In most instances, ratings on the GAF Scale should be for the current period (i.e., the level of functioning at the time of the evaluation) because ratings of current functioning will generally reflect the need for treatment or care. In order to account for day-to-day variability in functioning, the GAF rating for the "current period" is sometimes operationalized as the lowest level of functioning for the past week. In some settings, it may be useful to note the GAF Scale rating both at time of admission and at time of discharge. The GAF Scale may also be rated for other time periods (e.g., the highest level of functioning for at least a few months during the past year). The GAF Scale is reported on Axis V as follows: "GAF =," followed by the GAF rating from 0 to 100, followed by the time period reflected by the rating in parentheses—for example, "(current)," "(highest level in past year)," "(at discharge)."

In order to ensure that no elements of the GAF Scale are overlooked when a GAF rating is being made, the following method for determining a GAF rating may be applied:

STEP 1: Starting at the top level, evaluate each range by asking "is either the individual's symptom severity OR level of functioning worse than what is indicated in the range description?"

STEP 2: Keep moving down the scale until the range that best matches the individual's symptom severity OR the level of functioning is reached, **whichever is worse.**

STEP 3: Look at the next lower range as a double-check against having stopped prematurely. This range should be too severe on both symptom severity and level of functioning. If it is, the appropriate range has been reached (continue with step 4). If not, go back to step 2 and continue moving down the scale.

STEP 4: To determine the specific GAF rating within the selected 10-point range, consider whether the individual is functioning at the higher or lower end of the 10-point range. For example, consider an individual who hears voices that do not influence his behavior (e.g., someone with long-standing Schizophrenia who accepts his hallucinations as part of his illness). If the voices occur relatively infrequently (once a week or less), a rating of 39 or 40 might be most appropriate. In contrast, if the individual hears voices almost continuously, a rating of 31 or 32 would be more appropriate.

In some settings, it may be useful to assess social and occupational disability and to track progress in rehabilitation independent of the severity of the psychological symptoms.

Global Assessment of Functioning Scale

Consider psychological, social, and occupational functioning on a hypothetical continuum of mental health-illness. Do not include impairment in functioning due to physical (or environmental) limitations.

TABLE A.1

Code	(Note: Use intermediate codes when appropriate, e.g., 45, 68, 72.)
100/91	Superior functioning in a wide range of activities, life's problems never seem to get out of hand, is sought out by others because of his or her many positive qualities. No symptoms.
90/81	Absent or minimal symptoms (e.g., mild anxiety before an exam), good functioning in all areas, interested and involved in a wide range of activities, socially effective, generally satisfied with life; no more than everyday problems or concerns (e.g., an occasional argument with family members).
80/71	If symptoms are present, they are transient and expectable reactions to psychosocial stressors (e.g., difficulty concentrating after family argument), no more than slight impairment in social, occupational, or school functioning (e.g., temporarily falling behind in schoolwork).
70/61	Some mild symptoms (e.g., depressed mood and mild insomnia) OR some difficulty in social, occupational, or school functioning (e.g., occasional truancy, or theft within the household), but generally functioning pretty well, has some meaningful interpersonal relationships.
60/51	Moderate symptoms (e.g., flat affect and circumstantial speech, occasional panic attacks) OR moderate difficulty in social, occupational, or school functioning (e.g., few friends, conflicts with peers or co-workers).
50/41	Serious symptoms (e.g., suicidal ideation, severe obsessional rituals, frequent shoplifting) OR any serious impairment in social, occupational, or school functioning (e.g., no friends, unable to keep a job).
40/31	Some impairment in reality testing or communication (e.g., speech is at times illogical, obscure, or irrelevant) OR major impairment in several areas, such as work or school, family relations, judgment, thinking, or mood (e.g., depressed man avoids friends, neglects family, and is unable to work; child frequently beats up younger children, is defiant at home, and is failing at school).
30/21	Behavior is considerably influenced by delusions or hallucinations OR serious impairment in communication or judgment (e.g., sometimes incoherent, acts grossly inappropriately, suicidal preoccupation) OR inability to function in almost all areas (e.g., stays in bed all day; no job, home, or friends).
20/11	Some danger of hurting self or others (e.g., suicide attempts without clear expectation of death, frequently violent; manic excitement) OR occasionally fails to maintain minimal personal hygiene (e.g., smears feces) OR gross impairment in communications (e.g., largely incoherent or mute).
10/1	Persistent danger of severely hurting self or others (e.g., recurrent violence) OR persistent inability to maintain minimal personal hygiene OR serious suicidal act with clear expectation of death.
0	Inadequate information.

The rating of overall psychological functioning on a scale of 0–100 was operationalized by Luborsky in the Health-Sickness Rating Scale (Luborsky, (1962). Clinician's judgments of mental health. *Archives of General Psychiatry 7*: 407–417. Spitzer and colleagues developed a revision of the Health-Sickness Rating Scale called the Global Assessment Scale (GAS) (Endicott, I., Spitzer, R. L., Fleiss, J. L., & Cohen, I. (1976). The global assessment scale: A procedure for measuring overall severity of psychiatric disturbance. *Archives of General Psychiatry 33*: 766–771). A modified version of the GAS was included in DSM ILL-R as the Global Assessment of Functioning (GAF) Scale.

Appendix B

Activity Intolerance
Activity Intolerance, Risk for
Airway Clearance, Ineffective
Anxiety
Anxiety, Death
Aspiration, Risk for
Attachment, Parent/Infant/Child, Risk for Impaired
Autonomic Dysreflexia
Autonomic Dysreflexia, Risk for
Blood Glucose, Risk for Unstable
Body Image, Disturbed
Body Temperature: Imbalanced, Risk for
Bowel Incontinence
Breastfeeding, Effective
Breastfeeding, Ineffective
Breastfeeding, Interrupted
Breathing Pattern, Ineffective
Cardiac Output, Decreased
Caregiver Role Strain
Caregiver Role Strain, Risk for
Comfort, Readiness for Enhanced
Communication: Impaired, Verbal
Communication, Readiness for Enhanced
Confusion, Acute
Confusion, Acute, Risk for
Confusion, Chronic
Constipation
Constipation, Perceived
Constipation, Risk for
Contamination
Contamination, Risk for
Coping: Community, Ineffective
Coping: Community, Readiness for Enhanced
Coping, Defensive
Coping: Family, Compromised
Coping: Family, Disabled
Coping: Family, Readiness for Enhanced
Coping (Individual), Readiness for Enhanced
Coping, Ineffective
Decisional Conflict
Decision Making, Readiness for Enhanced
Denial, Ineffective
Dentition, Impaired
Development: Delayed, Risk for
Diarrhea
Disuse Syndrome, Risk for
Diversional Activity, Deficient
Energy Field, Disturbed
Environmental Interpretation Syndrome, Impaired
Failure to Thrive, Adult
Falls, Risk for
Family Processes, Dysfunctional: Alcoholism
Family Processes, Interrupted
Family Processes, Readiness for Enhanced
Fatigue
Fear
Fluid Balance, Readiness for Enhanced
Fluid Volume, Deficient
Fluid Volume, Deficient, Risk for
Fluid Volume, Excess
Fluid Volume, Imbalanced, Risk for
Gas Exchange, Impaired
Grieving
Grieving, Complicated
Grieving, Risk for Complicated
Growth, Disproportionate, Risk for
Growth and Development, Delayed
Health Behavior, Risk-Prone

Health Maintenance, Ineffective
Health-Seeking Behaviors (Specify)
Home Maintenance, Impaired
Hope, Readiness for Enhanced
Hopelessness
Human Dignity, Risk for Compromised
Hyperthermia
Hypothermia
Immunization Status, Readiness for Enhanced
Infant Behavior, Disorganized
Infant Behavior: Disorganized, Risk for
Infant Behavior: Organized, Readiness for Enhanced
Infant Feeding Pattern, Ineffective
Infection, Risk for
Injury, Risk for
Insomnia
Intracranial Adaptive Capacity, Decreased
Knowledge, Deficient (Specify)
Knowledge (Specify), Readiness for Enhanced
Latex Allergy Response
Latex Allergy Response, Risk for
Liver Function, Impaired, Risk for
Loneliness, Risk for
Memory, Impaired
Mobility: Bed, Impaired
Mobility: Physical, Impaired
Mobility: Wheelchair, Impaired
Moral Distress
Nausea
Neurovascular Dysfunction: Peripheral, Risk for
Noncompliance (Specify)
Nutrition, Imbalanced: Less than Body Requirements
Nutrition, Imbalanced: More than Body Requirements
Nutrition, Imbalanced: More than Body Requirements, Risk for
Nutrition, Readiness for Enhanced
Oral Mucous Membrane, Impaired
Pain, Acute
Pain, Chronic
Parenting, Impaired
Parenting, Readiness for Enhanced
Parenting, Risk for Impaired
Perioperative Positioning Injury, Risk for
Personal Identity, Disturbed
Poisoning, Risk for
Post-Trauma Syndrome
Post-Trauma Syndrome, Risk for
Power, Readiness for Enhanced
Powerlessness
Powerlessness, Risk for
Protection, Ineffective
Rape-Trauma Syndrome
Rape-Trauma Syndrome: Compound Reaction
Rape-Trauma Syndrome: Silent Reaction
Religiosity, Impaired
Religiosity, Readiness for Enhanced
Religiosity, Risk for Impaired
Relocation Stress Syndrome
Relocation Stress Syndrome, Risk for
Role Conflict, Parental
Role Performance, Ineffective
Sedentary Lifestyle
Self-Care, Readiness for Enhanced
Self-Care Deficit: Bathing/Hygiene
Self-Care Deficit: Dressing/Grooming
Self-Care Deficit: Feeding

Self-Care Deficit: Toileting
Self-Concept, Readiness for Enhanced
Self-Esteem, Chronic Low
Self-Esteem, Situational Low
Self-Esteem, Risk for Situational Low
Self-Mutilation
Self-Mutilation, Risk for
Sensory Perception, Disturbed (Specify: Auditory, Gustatory, Kinesthetic, Olfactory Tactile, Visual)
Sexual Dysfunction
Sexuality Pattern, Ineffective
Skin Integrity, Impaired
Skin Integrity, Risk for Impaired
Sleep Deprivation
Sleep, Readiness for Enhanced
Social Interaction, Impaired
Social Isolation
Sorrow, Chronic
Spiritual Distress
Spiritual Distress, Risk for
Spiritual Well-Being, Readiness for Enhanced
Spontaneous Ventilation, Impaired
Stress, Overload
Sudden Infant Death Syndrome, Risk for
Suffocation, Risk for
Suicide, Risk for
Surgical Recovery, Delayed
Swallowing, Impaired
Therapeutic Regimen Management: Community, Ineffective
Therapeutic Regimen Management, Effective
Therapeutic Regimen Management: Family, Ineffective
Therapeutic Regimen Management, Ineffective
Therapeutic Regimen Management, Readiness for Enhanced
Thermoregulation, Ineffective
Thought Processes, Disturbed
Tissue Integrity, Impaired
Tissue Perfusion, Ineffective (Specify: Cerebral, Cardiopulmonary, Gastrointestinal, Renal)
Tissue Perfusion, Ineffective, Peripheral
Transfer Ability, Impaired
Trauma, Risk for
Unilateral Neglect
Urinary Elimination, Impaired
Urinary Elimination, Readiness for Enhanced
Urinary Incontinence, Functional
Urinary Incontinence, Overflow
Urinary Incontinence, Reflex
Urinary Incontinence, Stress
Urinary Incontinence, Total
Urinary Incontinence, Urge
Urinary Incontinence, Risk for Urge
Urinary Retention
Ventilatory Weaning Response, Dysfunctional
Violence: Other-Directed, Risk for
Violence: Self-Directed, Risk for
Walking, Impaired
Wandering

SOURCE: NANDA Nursing Diagnoses: Definitions and Classification, 2007–2008. Philadelphia: North American Nursing Diagnosis Association. Used with permission.

Appendix C

ROAD CHAPTER 8 ANSWERS

Below is an example of a completed ROAD feature for chapter 8. It provides an example of how you might answer the ROAD Assessment: Critical Thinking questions and complete the Develop a Care Plan section on the CD-ROM that accompanies this text. For all chapters, you would answer these questions on the CD-ROM that accompanies this textbook as you view the video clips. Then you will complete the nursing care plan on the template provided. Your instructor will have the suggested answers for the ROAD Assessment Critical Thinking questions and care plans.

You will find ROAD features in chapters 8, 11, 12, 13, 14, 15, 16, 17, 21, and 22.

The ROAD to Critical Thinking — A Client Experiencing Bipolar Disorder

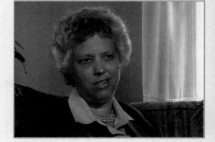

Travel this ROAD to understand Ann and her condition.

Read about Ann below and throughout this chapter.

Observe Ann on the CD-ROM accompanying this book.

Assess Ann by answering the questions at the end of this chapter.

Develop a Care Plan on the CD-ROM to address Ann's condition.

Ann

The onset of Ann's bipolar disorder occurred 6 months after giving birth to her first child. Prior to this, Ann was a successful professional woman with an MBA and a PhD and taught at Harvard Business School. During her manic episode, Ann suffered from paranoid delusions and ideas of reference. With no medical treatment, over the next 6 years she divorced, lost her job, and temporarily lost custody of her daughter.

One woman in a thousand experiences postpartum psychosis. Although the symptoms usually begin shortly after delivery of the infant, the disorder may begin anytime during the first year after the birth. Postpartum psychosis may be accompanied by delusions, which are false beliefs that cannot be changed by logical reasoning or evidence. They may be fixed in the person's mind only for a few weeks or months or may fluctuate over time. Delusions of persecution involve beliefs that someone is trying to harm the person. Delusions can become so intrusive that they disrupt the individual's entire life, with severe consequences for the quality of life.

Ann:

❝ I thought I was under investigation by the CIA and I was getting messages from the TV and the newspaper. I would bring the newspaper into work and read it for a couple of hours a day, trying to decipher the messages. ❞

Ann:

❝ I went to the Dean of the Harvard Business School and I said, 'The place is under electronic surveillance. Please bring the police in.' And it happened to be the same time that the spaceship Challenger exploded. So then I thought I had a role in blowing up the Challenger. ❞

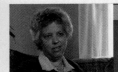

ROAD Assessment: Critical Thinking Questions

Go to the CD-ROM to Assess Ann by answering the following critical thinking questions based on what you have **R**ead about Ann and **O**bserved on the videos.

1. Based on your understanding of what can trigger altered thought processes and mania in bipolar disorder, what would have been important to assess at Ann's postpartum visits after the birth of her daughter? Provide the rationale for your answers. (*Hint*: Refer to chapter 13 ∞ in the textbook for additional information that will help you in formulating your answers.)

2. What type of delusion is Ann describing during her interview on the video clip? Provide the rationale for your answers.

3. When Ann states that she was terrified she would be assassinated by the CIA, what additional assessment questions would it have been important to have asked? Provide the rationale for your answers.

4. Ann has been hospitalized for an increase in delusions that put her at risk for harming others. It is 6 hours after her admission to an open, adult unit. As you are walking out of another client's room, you hear Ann curse a patient. She accuses the client of taking her picture with an invisible camera in a book and working with the CIA to assassinate her while she's in the hospital. During the past 6 hours since admission, Ann has been avoiding contact with staff and clients. Slamming her door, she returns to her room. What phase of escalating aggression is Ann displaying? Give specific examples of nursing and staff responses that can be offered to Ann. Provide the rationale for your answers.

5. Ann's agitated behavior continues. While staff members collaborate to implement nonpharmacological interventions that assist Ann in managing her anxiety and anger, you reflect, wondering whether the physician has ordered the needed medication. Which IM pharmacological agent would you expect to see on the medication sheet and why? Provide the rationale for your answers.

SUGGESTED ANSWERS

Suggested answers to the ROAD Assesment: Critical Thinking questions follow.

1. **SUGGESTED ANSWER:** You would assess **A)** Ann's feelings and thoughts about her new role as a mother, **B)** the routines of activity and sleep for Ann since the birth of her daughter, and **C)** her perceived ability to establish new routines. These include healthy nutrition and activity, and protection of rhythms of activity and sleep. You might ask about the breastfeeding routine, how her sleep was affected, and what support systems were in place to assist her in managing and adapting to her new role as a mother. You would ask about the difficulties Ann perceived or experienced as she strove to adapt and cope with her new role. Educating clients in these matters includes teaching them about the course of illness and how to recognize symptoms of the onset of illness.

   SOURCE: Swann, A., & Ginsberg, D. (2004, August 15). CME Certified Symposium Monograph. An Expert Review of Clinical Challenges in Psychiatry and Neurology: Special Needs of Women with Bipolar Disorder. Sponsored by Intelly Medical Communications and supported through a grant funded by GlaxoSmith Kline, pp. 1–12. Retrieved March 6, 2006, from http://mblcommunications.com/proceed/proceed_08_2004.pdf

2. **SUGGESTED ANSWER:** Ann is experiencing paranoid and persecutory delusions. Her reference to being under investigation by the CIA and her involvement in the Challenger incident are examples of the delusions.

3. **SUGGESTED ANSWER:** It is important to determine whether, in addition to the paranoid and persecutory delusions, there are associated safety risks for Ann or others.

Safety is always the first consideration in mental health assessments. You could ask questions such as: What types of actions do you think about taking when you have those thoughts? When you have that kind of thought, do you ever think about harming yourself or engaging in behaviors that could be harmful to yourself? To others? What sort of pressure do you feel to act on your thoughts? Would you be able to let me know whether you were having an increase in those thoughts?

4. **SUGGESTED ANSWER:** Ann is displaying phase 2, the transition phase. The best nursing response is to not match anger with anger; keep talking; set limits and give directions; negotiate compromise; explore consequences; and get help. **Specifically:** *You may use any combination of the following interventions identified within chapter 8:* Seek out the client and provide an opportunity to discuss what transpired between her and the other client. Provide comfort and reassure the client's safety. After listening and reassuring, refocus the conversation to another topic to provide distraction from the troubling thoughts. Determine whether a behavior triggered the delusion. Focus on the underlying feelings because unexpressed feelings can trigger delusions. Identify beliefs that may be self-harmful or harmful to others to protect the client and others from acting out behaviors that may be harmful. Encourage clients to verbalize delusions to caregivers before impulsively acting on them. Do not attempt to reason, argue, or challenge the delusion because that makes the client defensive. Do not attempt to logically explain the delusion. Once triggers have been identified, assist the client in problem solv-

ing ways to avoid or eliminate stressors that precipitate delusions. Offer recreational and diversional activities that require attention and skill to provide temporary relief from disturbing delusions.

5. **SUGGESTED ANSWER:** Intramuscular lorazepam (Ativan) is frequently used for the immediate control of psychotic disruptive behavior.

Develop a Care Plan

An example of possible nursing care plans for Ann follow and are provided to assist you in developing your own nursing care plans. You will create similar care plans using your CD-ROM, using the same template. Your instructor will evaluate your care plans and provide suggested plans.

Nursing Diagnosis: Altered Thought Process related to persecutory and paranoid delusions

Outcome: Ann will report improved self-restraint of disruption in thoughts during interactions with others.

Intervention	Rationale	Goal
Provide an opportunity for Ann to discuss her delusions.	Delusions are frightening and discussion may lessen the fear.	Ann shares her delusional thoughts.
Discourage long narrations about the delusions.	Lengthy discussions may reinforce her disordered thinking.	Ann talks about other subjects than her delusions.
Implement a stance of reasonable doubt concerning the delusions during interactions with Ann. "I understand that you believe the CIA is trying to assassinate you and that it is a frightening experience to have those thoughts. However, I find those thoughts hard to believe based upon the information I have available."	Gently presents the fact that you do not perceive the delusion as reality.	Ann verbalizes her understanding that your perception is different than hers.
Assist Ann to try to connect the false beliefs to incidents and events that increase feelings of fear, anxiety, and/or insecurity.	Unexpressed feelings can trigger delusions.	Ann identifies the triggers of the delusion.
Provide Ann with assistance in her efforts to verbalize feelings of fear, anxiety, and/or insecurity.	Unexpressed feelings can trigger delusions.	Ann verbalizes her feelings.
Introduce and encourage engagement in distracting activities.	This creates an alternative to constantly focusing on the fixed belief.	Ann participates in diversional activities.
Instruct Ann on thought-interrupting techniques such as snapping a rubberband on her wrist or rubbing a penny she keeps in her pocket.	Increases awareness of feelings that get converted into illogical thoughts.	Ann utilizes techniques to interrupt illogical thoughts.
Provide positive feedback for improvement as it is noticed.	This reinforces positive changes.	Ann acknowledges positive feedback.

Nursing Diagnosis: Potential for Violence Directed at Others related to fear and suspicious, paranoid delusions

Outcome: Ann will not harm others.

Intervention	Rationale	Goal
Encourage Ann to talk about feelings rather than acting upon perceptions and feelings.	This reinforces socially acceptable and safe behavior.	Ann discusses feelings.
Reinforce that talking is a manner in which she can maintain her self-control.	This reinforces health and nondestructive behavior.	Ann remains in control of her behavior.
Explore issues and events in the milieu or in daily life that trigger anxiety, fear, and suspiciousness.	Recognizing triggers improves self-control.	Ann identifies usual triggers.
Offer information to correct misperceptions Ann may develop of interactions and events taking place around her.	This reinforces reality to help Ann interpret what is actually happening.	Ann verbalizes an improved reality perception.
Respect personal space and avoid physical contact during times of increased fear, paranoia, and/or anxiety.	Close proximity and touch may frighten Ann during these times.	Ann's anxiety and agitation is maintained at a manageable level.

Appendix D

ANSWERS TO NCLEX-RN® REVIEW QUESTIONS

CHAPTER 1

1-1.

A nurse has received report on her assigned clients. Which of the following clients should the nurse see first? The client with:

Correct Answer: 3. Schizophrenia and suspicious of staff.
Rationale:
> This is the correct answer. This client has an illness with altered thought and sensory perception. The client is suspicious of others and, due to the inability to think clearly, has the potential of being dangerous to self and others. This client is the most unstable and is the most important client for the nurse to assess.

1-2.

A 57-year-old woman volunteers 3 days a week at a homeless shelter, assists grandmothers raising grandchildren, and reads to clients at a nursing home. According to Erickson's Theories of Personality Development, this woman's behaviors are age appropriate for which developmental crisis?

Correct Answer: 4. Generativity and self-absorption.
Rationale:
> Generativity and self-absorption describes the crises of middle adulthood.

1-3.

A nurse knows that professional nursing care is based on a theoretical framework. Those theories are:

Correct Answer: 4. Ideas that describe and explain phenomena.
Rationale:
> Theories are ideas that describe and explain phenomena.

1-4.

In order for a nurse to effectively use Peplau's theory of interpersonal relations, the nurse must first:

Correct Answer: 4. Deal effectively with personal feelings.
Rationale:
> Peplau's nursing theory on nurse–client relationships begins with the nurse's self-awareness and ability to deal with personal feelings.

1-5.

A registered nurse is asked to serve on a hospital committee that is planning to introduce evidence-based nursing practices. The nurse reads about evidence-based practice and finds that the committee should establish nursing practices based on:

Correct Answer: 4. Research findings.
Rationale:
> Evidence-based nursing practice is the wise use of current evidence to make decisions about nursing care of clients. It is not based on intuition or other unsystematic methods of providing care.

CHAPTER 2

2-1.

An elderly client is admitted to the hospital. He is accompanied by his wife. The client is most tearful and agitated. The client states, "I am fine. I have no worries." The nurse recognizes the client's behavior as:

Correct Answer: 3. Incongruous between his verbal and nonverbal communication.
Rationale:
> Incongruous between his verbal and nonverbal communication is correct because the client is stating one thing but his behavior is exhibiting tearfulness and agitation.

2-2.

What is the first step the nurse should take to assist a family who recently experienced the loss of a family member?

Correct Answer: 1. Assess the family's coping stage.
Rationale:
> Assessment is the first step in helping the family adjust to the loss. The nurse will base interventions on the family's current stage of grief.

2-3.

The family of a client with schizophrenia is struggling to cope with the effects of the clients' illness on family function. Which of the following treatments is the most helpful to the family as it deals with a family member with psychiatric disorder?

Correct Answer: 4. Family education groups.
Rationale:
> Meeting with other families who are experiencing similar situations is most helpful to the client's family. The group is able to discuss the problems that are common to all. The group may serve as a support group.

2-4.

Two married clients and their three children are attending a family therapy group. The 13-year-old son tells the nurse therapist that his father doesn't understand him, and his mother is the only one who cares about him. The father states, "My wife lets him do whatever he wants to do. His grades are poor and when I try to correct him, my wife contradicts everything I tell my son."

Correct Answer: 3. Blurred communication patterns.

Rationale:

Conflicting communication patterns that are blurred in families have unclear boundaries among family members.

2-5.

An advance practice psychiatric nurse and a basic level nurse are caring for families in the mental health clinic. Which of the following nursing interventions can be implemented only by the advanced practice nurse?

Correct Answer: 4. Psychotherapy.

Rationale:

Only the advanced practice nurse is able to provide psychotherapy to families. Psychotherapy is a mode of treatment that focuses on exploring and changing the client's behavior.

2-6.

A psychiatric nurse is conducting a group for couples over 65 years old. The nurse is planning to review successful methods for meeting the developmental tasks using Erikson's eight stages of development. Which of the following psychosocial crises should be the main focus for this group?

Correct Answer: 4. Integrity versus despair.

Rationale:

Integrity versus despair is the last stage in Erikson's Eight Stages of Development. The later years are a time of fulfillment and preparation for death.

CHAPTER 3

3-1.

The psychiatric community nurse is working with clients who have substance abuse issues. Many clients in the group have had relapses. The group is multicultural and comprised of young adults. The most appropriate nursing intervention in dealing with these clients is to:

Correct Answer: 4. Work collaboratively with the clients in developing new coping strategies.

Rationale:

The nurse, in collaboration with the clients, devises a pathway (action) to assist the clients in maintaining abstinence.

3-2.

A nurse is providing secondary crisis care to clients in the community. The nurse recognizes that which of the following clients is experiencing an adventitious crisis?

Correct Answer: 4. A woman attending a rock concert where rioting resulted in many injuries.

Rationale:

An adventitious crisis is a crisis of disaster. Intervening with persons who were at the riot will assist them in dealing with the present crisis. The priority is to assist clients in returning to normal function as soon as they are able.

3-3.

A 17-year-old client comes to the community crisis clinic. She has multiple superficial cuts on her wrists. She is crying uncontrollably and states that her boyfriend has left her and she doesn't want to live without him. The nurse's initial response should be:

Correct Answer: 4. "I know that you are feeling anxious. I will stay with you until you feel better."

Rationale:

The priority is to provide for a safe environment and to use anxiety-reduction techniques to calm the client. The nurse exhibits empathy, calmness, and support in the crisis.

3-4.

The community psychiatric nurse conducts weekly education groups for clients in a senior citizen day care center. The nurse suspects that one of the clients is in an abusive environment. The client has bruises on her body and tells the nurse she often falls in the home. The priority care plan for this client is for the nurse to:

Correct Answer: 1. Make an immediate appointment to visit the home.

Rationale:

Elders are at high risk for abuse and violence in the home because of their cognitive impairment. An immediate visit to the home is recommended.

3-5.

The mobile crisis unit of a large metropolitan city receives an emergency call from a teenage client who states, "My life is worthless. I do not want to live anymore." The mobile crisis unit is on the way to the home. The nurse's first response is to:

Correct Answer: 1. Attempt to calm and support the client.

Rationale:

The priority of need is to calm the client and offer support.

3-6.

A nurse is developing skills to ensure provision of culturally competent care in the community. Which of the following actions is the most important for the nurse?

Correct Answer: 3. Identify the nurse's own attitudes and biases.

Rationale:

> Identifying the nurse's own attitudes and biases is the first step for the nurse who is developing the ability to effectively work with diverse groups of clients in the community. The nurse should first examine personal attitudes and biases in preparation for providing culturally competent care to clients in the community.

CHAPTER 4

4-1.

A nurse therapist conducts group counseling for young homeless women. The leading cause of death for these young women is acquired immunodeficiency syndrome (AIDS). To meet the priority needs for this group the nurse should:

Correct Answer: 1. Determine the women's knowledge level about AIDS and the factors that contribute to the high incidence in this city.

Rationale:

> Assessment is the first step of the nursing process. Determining the women's knowledge of AIDS is the starting point for planning interventions for these clients.

4-2.

A 45-year-old Haitian male is admitted to the hospital with a diagnosis of hypertension. The client lives in a low socioeconomic area of a large metropolitan city. He eats at fast-food restaurants and works two jobs to support his family. This is the client's third admission to the hospital because his hypertension is uncontrolled. What is the priority nursing action for this client?

Correct Answer: 1. Determine the client's level of knowledge about the relationship of hypertension and lifestyle choices.

Rationale:

> The nurse first assesses the client's level of knowledge before beginning a plan of care.

4-3.

The nurse therapist working with minority women teaches a class on acquired immunodeficiency syndrome (AIDS). After four sessions, what would be an indication that the nurse has accomplished the outcome established for the clients?

Correct Answer: 2. The clients have gained an increase of knowledge about the disease and the consequences of the disease.

Rationale:

> 1. The clients' gaining knowledge about the disease gives them power to change their behavior.

4-4.

A group for minority women meets monthly. In one of the sessions, a client tells the group, "My boyfriend tells me I don't love him if he needs to practice safe sex." The response of the nurse should be:

Correct Answer: 3. "Tell me what you mean about not loving him."

Rationale:

> Restating the response allows the nurse to assist the client in exploring her feelings concerning the boyfriend's refusal to practice safe sex.

4-5.

The treatment team conducted a meeting to discuss intervention strategies for a client, an 8-year-old girl who drew a picture of a child in the water alone. The priority strategy for this client is:

Correct Answer: 2. Coax the child to add things to the picture that could help the child.

Rationale:

> Coaxing the child to add positive drawings addresses the child's possible disturbances and other therapeutic strategies to resolve the conflict immediately.

CHAPTER 5

5-1.

A psychiatric treatment team is planning care for a client who was involuntarily admitted for treatment of depression and suicide ideation. One understanding utilized in planning client care is that the client is:

Correct Answer: 1. Able to refuse medication.

Rationale:

> Competent clients have the right to refuse medication. Even though the client has been admitted involuntarily, the client is competent and able to be involved in treatment planning.

5-2.

The health care provider is discussing a new treatment that requires an informed consent with a client. Which of the following does the client receive before signing a statement of informed consent? (Select all that apply.)

Correct Answers:
2. Objective of the treatment.
3. Benefits of the treatment.
4. Risks of the treatment.
6. Any alternatives to the treatment.

Rationale:
2. The health care provider will describe the objective of the treatment.
3. The health care provider will describe the reason the treatment will be beneficial to the client.
4. The health care provider will describe the risks associated with the treatment.
6. The health care provider will describe the alternatives and the outcome of the alternative treatments available to the client.

5-3.

A client with a history of aggression and violence is admitted to the hospital. Which of the following principles guide the health care provider to inform nurses about the client's danger to them?

Correct Answer: 4. Duty to disclose/protect.

Rationale:

> There is a duty to disclose and protect when a client may harm specific individuals or those who provide care to that client.

5-4.

A client was admitted for treatment of the symptoms of bipolar disorder. The court decided that this client was not able to understand the consequences of the decisions that he was making. Which of the following terms describe the status of this client?

Correct Answer: 4. Legally incompetent.

Rationale:

> "Legally incompetent" describes the client who is not able to understand the consequences of decisions. A guardian is appointed for the client who is incompetent.

5-5.

A homeless person with schizophrenia is yelling obscenities at those who pass by. The nurse should first take this client to which of the following locations?

Correct Answer: 2. Crisis center.

Rationale:

> A client with schizophrenia should first receive care at the crisis center. The client should be assessed and assisted in dealing with the events, perceptions, and support system needed in a time of crisis.

5-6.

After three days on the unit a client says to the nurse, "I would like to date you; tell me how I can reach you outside of the hospital." Which response by the nurse is most appropriate?

Correct Answer: 4. "My relationship with you is professional and not social."

Rationale:

> The appropriate response in order to maintain professional boundaries is to tell the client that your relationship with her or him is professional and not social.

CHAPTER 6

6-1.

Executive functions such as reasoning, motivation, and judgment develop differently throughout adolescence. The adolescent's hormones are surging, which contributes to anger and impulsive behavior. The nurse is aware that:

Correct Answer: 2. Boys are less likely to be depressed than girls.

Rationale:

> Girls are more likely to be depressed than boys.

6-2.

The nurse is caring for a 16-year-old client with a history of anorexia nervosa. The nurse is aware of the theories that suggest a specific area of the brain is involved in anorexia nervosa. Which of the following areas of the brain does the nurse know influences a person's eating and drinking?

Correct Answer: 2. Hypothalamus.

Rationale:

> Hormones from the hypothalamus regulate eating and drinking as well as salt balance.

6-3.

The admitting note describes a client on the psychiatric unit as having anhedonia and anergia. The nurse knows that increasing the levels of the neurotransmitter serotonin will have a positive effect on this client. Which of the following activities should the nurse plan to meet the goal of increasing the client's serotonin level?

Correct Answer: 1. Daily exercise.

Rationale:

> Severely depressed clients have anergia (little mental or physical energy). Serotonin from daily exercise elevates mood and self-esteem and induces a sense of calm.

6-4.

Clients with disordered proprioception have the potential for difficulty in:

Correct Answer: 1. Dressing, eating, and drinking in an organized manner.

Rationale:

> Significant functioning of the parietal lobe is proprioception, the ability to know where our bodies are in time and space (position sense). Impairment may contribute to dressing, eating, and drinking in an unorganized manner.

6-5.

An older client has experienced the death of his spouse. They were married for 50 years and the client depended on his wife for simple activities of daily living. The nurse, assessing him for depression, is aware that:

Correct Answer: 1. The client's risk for illness is relatively high.

Rationale:

> Data suggest that acute stress can cause suppression of the immune system. The death of a spouse is a significant stressor for the remaining spouse. This client is at risk for illness because of the suppressed immune system.

6-6.

The nurse is conducting a client education group about the effects of nutrition on healthy daily living. A client asks, "What is one vitamin or mineral I should take to help my mental functioning?" Which vitamin should the nurse suggest that the client take to enhance mental function?

Correct Answer: 2. Vitamin B.

Rationale:

Vitamin B is essential for normal functioning of the nervous system. Larger doses of B vitamins may help to enhance mental functioning.

CHAPTER 7

7-1.

The nurse is caring for a client who attempted suicide 2 weeks ago. The client states, "Sometimes I wish I could die and not feel the pain anymore." Which of the following responses by the nurse demonstrates empathy?

Correct Answer: 2. "It sounds like you're in a lot of pain and you don't have much hope for the future."

Rationale:

The answer "It sounds like you're in a lot of pain and you don't have much hope for the future" is correct because the nurse carefully considered the client's feelings and is seeking to validate that perception.

7-2.

During an interaction with a female client, several of the nurse's nonverbal messages are hindering the conversation. Which of the following nonverbal behaviors by the nurse would effectively facilitate the interaction? (Select all that apply.)

Correct Answers:

1. Make frequent, brief eye contact with the client.
6. Remain seated as the client inches her chair in the opposite direction.

Rationale:

1. Making frequent, brief eye contact with the client is correct because it encourages conversation.
6. Remaining seated as the client inches her chair in the opposite direction shows that the nurse is respecting the client's boundaries and need for personal space.

7-3.

The client is discussing recent marital problems and asks the nurse, "Do you think I should ask for a divorce?" Which of the following questions by the nurse are examples of an effective response? (Select all that apply.)

Correct Answers:

1. "What other options besides asking for a divorce have you considered?"

2. "How would you feel about asking for a divorce?"
4. "Could you explain to me some of the reasons you want a divorce?"

Rationale:

1. Asking, "What other options besides asking for a divorce have you considered?" is correct because it is an open-ended question that asks for more information and encourages problem solving.
2. Asking, "How would you feel about asking for a divorce?" is correct because it leads to a discussion of feelings and encourages the client to develop insight.
4. Asking, "Could you explain to me some of the reasons you want a divorce?" is correct because it is open ended and gives the client some control over the conversation.

7-4.

The client has been attending an anger management workshop and is discussing the changes he has made in his behavior. Which of the following statements demonstrates an effective outcome?

Correct Answer: 3. "I know that I'll feel angry at times, but I can control my response now."

Rationale:

The client's saying, "I know that I'll feel angry at times, but I can control my response now" is correct because it reflects an understanding of anger management principles.

7-5.

Questions that guide the client through the six steps of the problem solving process are provided in the list below. Arrange these questions in the correct sequence. All options must be used.

Correct Order of Answers:

6. "How have you coped with stress in the past?"
5. "What are some other ways you could manage your stress?"
1. "Which of these stress management methods would work best for you?"
4. "Meditation is a good idea. What would happen if you tried it?"
3. "I see you've been practicing meditation this week, haven't you?"
2. "How would you rate your stress level since you've been meditating?"

Rationale:

1. "Which of these stress management methods would work best for you?" is step 3.
2. "How would you rate your stress level since you've been meditating?" is step 6.
3. "I see you've been practicing meditation this week, haven't you?" is step 5.
4. "Meditation is a good idea. What would happen if you tried it?" is step 4.
5. "What are some other ways you could manage your stress?" is step 2.
6. "How have you coped with stress in the past?" is step 1.

CHAPTER 8

8-1.

The nurse is teaching family members about the brain's connection to behaviors commonly seen in psychiatric disabilities. The nurse is using the term "neurotransmitter." The nurse should explain that a neurotransmitter is:

Correct Answer: 2. A chemical that is released in the brain.

Rationale:

> This is correct. Neurotransmitters are chemicals that are stored in the neuron and are released as neural messengers when stimulated by an electrical impulse. Neurotransmitters are involved with functions that affect human emotions and behavior. Neurotransmitters are the target for drugs used to treat psychiatric disabilities.

8-2.

During the initial assessment, the client exhibits pressured speech and launches into a lengthy explanation of her ability to read "the writing on the wall." She points to certain patterns on the wallpaper and says, "This is Hurricane Katrina and this is 9/11. Thousands of people died because I read the writing. I should never have read the writing; it was my fault." When documenting the client's behaviors in the nursing assessment, which of the following words should the nurse use?

Correct Answer: 3. Ideas of reference.

Rationale:

> Ideas of reference is the correct assessment. The client falsely believes that she is responsible for catastrophic events that are unrelated to her. The nurse should document that the client has ideas of reference and quote the client's statements.

8-3.

A client is sitting in the day room and is laughing out loud, shaking his head, and whispering behind his hand. Suddenly he begins banging his head against the wall violently and repeatedly. Which of the following interventions is most appropriate?

Correct Answer: 1. Calmly walk over to the client and say, "Tell me what's going on."

Rationale:

> Calmly walking over to the client and saying, "Tell me what's going on" is correct because it encourages the client to discuss altered perceptions rather than feel guilt or shame. The nurse also supports the client with her or his presence.

8-4.

A female client with a history of being sexually abused is hospitalized for depression after a recent suicide attempt. She states that she often cuts her body in hidden places as punishment. "When I see the blood I feel better because then I know I'm alive." Which of the following nursing diagnoses should have the highest priority?

Correct Answer: 1. Self-Mutilation: Cutting related to feelings of guilt and low self-esteem.

Rationale:

> Self-Mutilation: Cutting related to feelings of guilt and low self-esteem is correct because the client is actually injuring herself as a method to cope with her feelings.

8-5.

A client has been pacing up and down the hallway for the last hour. He stares at others without blinking, clenches his fists, and mutters to himself. Another client walks down the hall and accidentally bumps into the first client. The first client punches the second client in the face and pulls his hair. The team acts quickly to restrain the first client and moves him safely to the seclusion room. During a staff review of this critical incident, several alternatives are discussed. Which of the following actions should be taken to prevent a similar incident? (Select all that apply.)

Correct Answers:

1. Quietly and calmly ask the client if he would rather go to the quiet room or the exercise room.
2. Offer the client a PRN dose of ziprasidone (Geodon) by mouth.
3. Restrict other clients from going down the hallway while the client is pacing.

Rationale:

1. Quietly and calmly asking the client whether he would rather go to the quiet room or the exercise room is correct because it offers the client a choice between two acceptable options.
2. Offering the client a PRN dose of ziprasidone (Geodon) by mouth is correct because it offers an acceptable choice and may help the client gain control of his anger.
3. Restricting other clients from going down the hallway while the client is pacing is correct. This action respects the client's personal space and keeps other clients out of harm's way.

CHAPTER 9

9-1.

Which of the following roles is not within the scope of practice for an advanced practice mental health nurse?

Correct Answer: 3. Administering and interpreting psychological tests.

Rationale:

> 3. Administering and interpreting psychological tests is correct because only psychologists have the education to perform this role.

9-2.

In managing the therapeutic milieu, the nurse is responsible for which of the following activities?

Correct Answer: 2. Providing classes on activities of daily living and social skills to improve healthy lifestyles and communication skills.

Rationale:

> Providing classes on activities of daily living and social skills to improve healthy lifestyles and communication skills is correct because nurses are responsible for nurturing and supporting healthy living and communication within milieu therapy.

9-3.

Which one of the following clients would receive the most benefit from social skills training?

Correct Answer: 3. A 35-year-old homeless man who has a history of chronic paranoid schizophrenia.

Rationale:

> A 35-year-old homeless man who has a history of chronic paranoid schizophrenia is correct because he could learn activities of daily living, communication, and other social skills that are deficits caused by his chronic illness.

9-4.

A 17-year-old high school senior is referred to the outpatient mental health clinic after learning that she is 5 months pregnant. Despite her decision to keep the baby after it is born, she wants to start college next fall. Her parents have offered no financial or emotional support and her boyfriend broke up with her after learning of her pregnancy. Which of the following actions should the nurse take to help the client deal with this crisis?

Correct Answer: 3. Explore with the client different options available to her and possible consequences of each.

Rationale:

> Exploring with the client different options available to her and the possible consequence of each is correct because it encourages the client to begin the problem-solving process during this crisis.

9-5.

The nurse is applying principles of cognitive–behavioral therapy (CBT) in the treatment of a client with depression. Which of the following interventions is an example of CBT?

Correct Answer: 2. Encouraging the client to identify destructive thoughts and practice mindfulness.

Rationale:

> Encouraging the client to identify destructive thoughts and practice mindfulness is correct because the purpose of CBT is to focus on automatic thoughts and schemas.

9-6.

The nurse is leading a medication education group for clients who are taking an antidepressant medication. Which of the following goals is appropriate for this type of group?

Correct Answer: 1. Clients will identify common side effects of selective serotonin reuptake inhibitors.

Rationale:

> Clients will identify common side effects of selective serotonin reuptake inhibitors is correct because SSRIs are the most commonly prescribed antidepressants.

9-7.

The client has been nonresponsive to antidepressant medication and the treatment team has recommended transcranial magnetic stimulation (TMS). An hour after the psychiatrist explained the procedure the client asks, "What exactly does this procedure involve?" Which of the following explanations is correct?

Correct Answer: 3. "You will sit in a lounge chair and a small electromagnet will be placed on your scalp. There will be loud noises for approximately 1 minute so you'll need to wear ear plugs. You will have 5 treatments over 2 to 4 weeks."

Rationale:

> The statements, "You will sit in a lounge chair and a small electromagnet will be placed on your scalp. There will be loud noises for approximately 1 minute so you'll need to wear ear plugs. You will have 5 treatments over 2 to 4 weeks," are correct as this describes this noninvasive procedure.

CHAPTER 10

10-1.

A client has been on antipsychotic medication for 20 years with little control of schizophrenic symptoms. The client was recently switched to clozapine (Clozaril). Which of the following behaviors would indicate a positive therapeutic response to this medication? (Select all that apply.)

Correct Answers:
  4. An increase in motivation.
  5. A decrease in hallucinations.

Rationale:
  4. An increase in motivation is a negative symptom of schizophrenia responsive to second-generation antipsychotic medications.
  5. A decrease in hallucinations is correct, as this is a positive symptom of schizophrenia responsive to both first- and second-generation antipsychotic medications.

10-2.

A client is taking thioridazine (Mellaril) and is exhibiting restlessness, muscle rigidity, involuntary movements, and drooling.

Which of the following medications would be most helpful in treating these side effects?

Correct Answer: 3. Benztropine (Cogentin).

Rationale:

> Benztropine (Cogentin) is correct because these are extrapyramidal side effects that can be effectively treated by an anticholinergic medication.

10-3.

A recent lab report on a client taking olanzapine (Zyprexa) reveals a triglyceride level of 300 mg/dL, high-density lipoprotein (HDL) cholesterol level of 30 mg/dL, and a fasting blood glucose level of 215 mg/dL. In addition, the client has an abdominal girth of 41 inches. Which of the following syndromes does the client exhibit?

Correct Answer: 2. Metabolic syndrome.

Rationale:

> Metabolic syndrome is correct because all laboratory values are elevated and indicate that development of this syndrome is commonly associated with second-generation antipsychotics.

10-4.

A 29-year-old female client is worried that she may be pregnant. She has been taking lithium for the past year and is concerned about the effects of lithium on her unborn child. Which of the following statements is true?

Correct Answer: 3. Lithium should be avoided during the latter part of the first trimester, if possible.

Rationale:

> Avoiding lithium during the latter part of the first trimester will minimize risks to the fetus.

10-5.

A client with bipolar disorder has been taking lithium for the past 2 years. Recently, the client has been experiencing a recurrence of manic symptoms approximately once a month. The psychiatrist has added clonazepam (Klonopin) to help manage the client's mood swings. Which of the following statements should the nurse include in medication teaching?

Correct Answer: 1. "This medication will help to steady your moods by reducing the overstimulation of chemical messengers in your brain."

Rationale:

> 1. The statement, "This medication will help to steady your moods by reducing the overstimulation of chemical messengers in your brain" is correct. This is a simple explanation of how anticonvulsants help to treat manic symptoms in people experiencing rapid mood swings caused by kindling.

CHAPTER 11

11-1.

The nurse in the emergency department (ED) is caring for a client who suffers recurrent panic attacks. The client states, "I want to know what causes these panic attacks so I can do something to keep it from happening again." Which of the following responses by the nurse is correct?

Correct Answer: 2. "One current theory is that panic attacks are caused by high levels of carbon dioxide."

Rationale:

> The response, "One current theory is that panic attacks are caused by high levels of carbon dioxide" is correct. An increase of carbon dioxide (CO_2) in the brain stimulates the fight-or-flight response.

11-2.

Which of the following medications would be used to treat a client who is experiencing ritualistic behavior that interferes with job performance and activities of daily living?

Correct Answer: 2. Fluoxetine (Prozac).

Rationale:

> Fluoxetine (Prozac) is a selective serotonin reuptake inhibitor that effectively corrects the imbalance of serotonin in anxiety disorders such as OCD.

11-3.

A treatment plan is developed for a client diagnosed with dissociative identity disorder (DID). The nurse should object if which of the following was included in the plan for this client?

Correct Answer: 3. Teach the client self-hypnosis.

Rationale:

> Teaching the client self-hypnosis is an inappropriate intervention. A process similar to self-hypnosis already has occurred during the childhood abuses. This is now a self-destructive tool in adulthood. The client uses a trance-like state in an unconscious attempt to manage severe anxiety. A therapist may, however, use hypnosis during therapy to explore the subconscious.

11-4.

A client presents to the emergency department (ED) with a history of chest pain, nausea, and dizziness. These symptoms decreased after talking with the health care provider. Vital signs were T-98.8, P-120, R-20, and BP 140/82. An electrocardiogram (ECG) revealed normal sinus rhythm with a rate of 120/minute. The client was recently fired and is worried about paying his bills. The client was driving to file for bankruptcy when the symptoms occurred. After assessing the client, the nurse would decide that which of the following nursing diagnoses is most important for this client?

Correct Answer: 3. Panic and Anxiety related to loss of job and financial changes.

Rationale:

> Panic and Anxiety related to loss of job and financial changes is the correct nursing diagnosis. The client displays signs of a sudden panic attack, which may be an unconscious reaction to the current situation.

11-5.

The nurse is leading a group for clients who have returned from fighting in Iraq. Which of the following client statements indicates the need for further interventions?

Correct Answer: 3. "I need to forget the war and get used to my life at home again."

Rationale:

> The statement, "I need to forget the war and get used to my life at home again" is correct. The client is denying the need to verbalize trauma and cope with the adverse effects of the experience.

11-6.

A nurse is teaching clients about various techniques for stress management. Which of the following client statements indicates the correct use of a stress management technique?

Correct Answer: 4. "Imagining myself on a beach and listening to the waves makes me fall asleep at night."

Rationale:

> The response, "Imagining myself on a beach and listening to the waves makes me fall asleep at night" is correct. The use of imagery is a distraction technique that promotes relaxation.

11-7.

The client is a 25-year-old pregnant mother of two children under the age of 6. She is a very protective mother and will not allow her children to play outdoors for fear of tick bites. She is worn out from cleaning the house from top to bottom everyday. She asks the nurse how she can stop worrying so much. What is the most appropriate response for the nurse?

Correct Answer: 3. "Tell me your concerns about the children playing in your backyard."

Rationale:

> The response, "Tell me your concerns about the children playing in your backyard" assists the client in identifying thoughts that are improbable. This is the beginning of the process of restructuring her cognitive thoughts and reducing anxiety.

CHAPTER 12

12-1.

A client with bulimia asks the nurse, "I wish I knew more about what causes bulimia. I read on the Internet that some people with bulimia have trouble knowing when they're full and that's why they keep bingeing." Which of the following responses by the nurse would be most appropriate?

Correct Answer: 1. "That's right. Some people with bulimia have a low level of serotonin, the neurotransmitter that lets you know when you're full."

Rationale:

> The response, "That's right. Some people with bulimia have a low level of serotonin, the neurotransmitter that lets you know when you're full" is correct. Recent research has shown that a neurobiological deficit of serotonin can decrease satiety and increase food intake.

12-2.

A high school wrestler fasts before every wrestling meet and then binges immediately after the meet. On the way to each meet, he walks rapidly up and down the bus aisle and spits repeatedly into a cup. Which of the following is the best intervention for this client?

Correct Answer: 1. Discuss secondary gains that are unconsciously driving the client's behavior.

Rationale:

> Discussing secondary gains that are unconsciously driving the client's behavior is correct. The client and his family need assistance to examine motives for this behavior. The client first needs to discuss the altered behaviors and deal with the issue openly.

12-3.

A female Asian American client who has a BMI of 25 kg/m² is referred to the outpatient clinic by her primary care provider to be assessed and treated for an eating disorder. Which of the following signs and symptoms would the nurse recognize as supporting the diagnosis of bulimia? (Select all that apply.)

Correct Answers:

1. The client has become socially withdrawn and never eats out with friends.
3. The client has a callous on the back of her hand.
4. The client has an obsession with fad diets in order to lose weight.
5. The client expresses a fear of her inability to maintain her normal body weight.

Rationale:

1. Clients with bulimia (and anorexia) usually seek privacy when eating to avoid detection.
3. This sign (known as Russell's sign) is caused by repeated trauma from the teeth when forcing vomiting.

4. Clients with bulimia exhibit a preoccupation with body image and commonly diet to lose weight.

5. Clients with bulimia are often perfectionists and fear gaining weight.

12-4.

A 30-year-old female client has been admitted to the intensive care unit (ICU) with metabolic alkalosis. She was diagnosed with anorexia nervosa 10 years ago and says that she is "too fat" even though she weighs 70 pounds and is 5 feet 4 inches. Her primary nursing diagnosis is Imbalanced Nutrition: Less Than Body Requirements related to reduced food intake and self-induced vomiting. Which of the following nursing diagnoses is the greatest priority immediately after she is medically stable in the ICU?

Correct Answer: 3. Body Image Disturbance related to delusional perception of body.

Rationale:

The client is still struggling with cognitive distortions that led to her metabolic alkalosis.

12-5.

A nurse is teaching clients with anorexia nervosa methods of normalizing eating behaviors. Which of the following statements by a client indicates to the nurse that the client needs further teaching?

Correct Answer: 2. "I will eat a diet high in protein, fiber, and fat."

Rationale:

This client needs further teaching about types of foods to eat. Because of starvation, the client will have insufficient bowel enzymes to digest foods high in fat.

12-6.

Which of the following statements made by a client with anorexia require the nurse's counsel to address the client's distorted cognitive views?

Correct Answer: 1. "If I stick to my diet and eat the right foods, I will be able to live a normal life."

Rationale:

This statement shows an unrealistic view of the client's illness. The nurse should use therapeutic communication techniques to assist the client to address the magical thinking and the all-or-none attitude this statement demonstrates.

CHAPTER 13

13-1.

The daughter of an 82-year-old depressed client asks the nurse why her mother has developed depression so late in life without a previous history of depression. Which of the following responses by the nurse is most appropriate?

Correct Answer: 1. "Women and older adults have higher levels of an enzyme called monoamine oxidase that results in slower signals in the brain, causing depression."

Rationale:

Compared with men or younger adults, women and older adults have higher levels of MAO, which deactivates neurotransmitters resulting in decreased impulse transmission.

13-2.

Which of the following outcomes indicates that a client taking lithium is responding effectively to therapy?

Correct Answer: 3. The client completes a crossword puzzle in the daily newspaper.

Rationale:

This complicated activity requires intense concentration and a longer attention span.

13-3.

A female client who has recently moved into a basement apartment asks the nurse what she can do to cope with her depressed mood, craving for carbohydrates, and increased appetite. Which of the following treatment modalities is most effective to recommend?

Correct Answer: 1. Phototherapy.

Rationale:

The client's symptoms are typical of seasonal affective disorder brought on by her recent move to a darker environment. Exposure to light each day will increase melatonin production, a hormone that affects mood.

13-4.

Which of the following symptoms can be assessed in clients with bipolar disorder during a hypomanic phase? (Select all that apply.)

Correct Answers:

3. Lack of sleep.
4. Preoccupation with sex.
5. Rapid speech.

Rationale:

3. People in a hypomanic state experience a dramatically decreased need for sleep and may sleep only 1 or 2 hours a night.

4. Clients in a hypomanic state develop emotional attachments rapidly and may engage in impulsive or simultaneous sexual relationships.

5. People in a hypomanic state have increased neurotransmission, which leads to racing thoughts and pressured or rapid speech.

13-5.

A 17-year-old client gave birth to her first child 2 months ago and tells the nurse in her obstetrician's office that she fears she's a terrible mother because she doesn't know what to do when her baby continues to cry after feeding and changing him. Which of the following nursing diagnoses is most appropriate for a single, new mother experiencing insomnia, lack of energy, poor concentration, and anxiety?

Correct Answer: 4. Ineffective Coping related to feeling overwhelmed by parenting tasks.

Rationale:
> The client is exhibiting signs of postpartum depression that has affected her ability to cope with the stressful situation of caring for a new baby on her own.

13-6.

A client with bipolar disorder has been experiencing more frequent mood swings even though his serum lithium level is 1.3 mEq/dL. Which of the following statements by the nurse would assist the client's understanding of bipolar disorder?

Correct Answer: 1. "The part of your brain that controls emotion becomes supersensitive to stress over time and it releases extra neurotransmitters, causing more rapid mood swings."

Rationale:
> A defective feedback mechanism in the limbic system (known as kindling) can occur causing excessive release of neurotransmitters and increased transmission of impulses.

13-7.

A client is admitted with a diagnosis of major depression. The client expresses feelings of worthlessness and a feeling of being abandoned by significant persons in her life. Which of the following replies by the nurse conveys empathy to this client?

Correct Answer: 4. "This must really be a difficult time for you."

Rationale:
> This is an empathetic response. The response signifies that the nurse understands the ideas and the feelings that are present in the client.

CHAPTER 14

14-1.

A 45-year-old client with a diagnosis of paranoid schizophrenia, with auditory hallucinations, is in her third day on the unit and has refused all personal contact. She is sitting on her bed with her knees drawn to her chest and informs the staff nurse that she wants to call the FBI. The client states, "The FBI knows me and they will get me out of here." What would be the nurse's most appropriate therapeutic communication when talking to this client?

Correct Answer: 4. Ask the client directly, "What do you want to talk to the FBI about?"

Rationale:
> This question is clear, direct, and productive. It will produce information relative to the stressors that the client is experiencing.

14-2.

The therapeutic team has identified the need to formulate strategies for a client's inappropriate behavior and how to maintain a safe environment for the clients on the unit. Of the following intervention strategies, which strategy must be initiated immediately?

Correct Answer: 1. Monitor the client's behavior.

Rationale:
> The unit must be maintained as a safe environment for the client and the other clients; therefore, the client should never have unsupervised time on the unit.

14-3.

Select the response which accurately describes genetics and schizophrenia.

Correct Answer: 4. A person has an 8% to 13% chance of being diagnosed with schizophrenia if a sibling or parent has the disorder.

Rationale:
> A person has an 8% to 13% chance of being diagnosed with schizophrenia if a sibling or parent has the disorder.

14-4.

Which of the following aspects of family communication patterns may be problematic for the client with schizophrenia? Select all that apply.

Correct Answers:
1. Family members appear to use language patterns that appear to be characteristic of the client's family only.
3. Family members appear to be enmeshed or over-involved with each other.
5. Family members talk loudly at the same time and do not listen while others are talking.

Rationale:
1. Language patterns that appear to be characteristic of the client's family only may indicate a lack of communication skills in social settings outside the family.
3. If family members appear to be enmeshed or over-involved with each other, they are less likely to be communicating in a healthy manner.
5. Loud, confusing group interactions are difficult for clients with schizophrenia to handle.

14-5.

An 18-year-old client is admitted with a diagnosis of paranoid-type schizophrenia. The student nurse asks the charge nurse about the approach to take with the client. The client has been exhibiting behavior of hostility and isolation. The best approach would be to:

Correct Answer: 3. Respect the client's need for personal space and avoid physical contact with the client.

Rationale:

> A newly admitted client with a diagnosis of paranoid schizophrenia needs to have a sense of trust before the nurse attempts to touch the client.

CHAPTER 15

15-1.

An intoxicated client, with injuries sustained from a motor vehicle accident, is admitted to the hospital at 10:00 p.m. What time of the following day will the nurse expect signs and symptoms of withdrawal?

Correct Answer: 1. 5:00 a.m.

Rationale:

> The symptoms of alcohol withdrawal begin 6–8 hours after the last drink. Coarse tremors, elevated BP, and tachycardia are symptoms of withdrawal from the prolonged alcohol use.

15-2.

A nurse is teaching an adolescent group about substance abuse. Which of the following statements indicates that further teaching is necessary?

Correct Answer: 3. "Women become addicted more easily than men."

Rationale:

> This is incorrect. Women have a lower rate of diagnosed substance use than men.

15-3.

Health care providers in Europe and Australia routinely prescribe the narcotic antagonist naltrexone (Trexan, ReVia) to help clients manage alcohol craving. Only 5% of clients in the United States are given naltrexone. The efforts to treat addiction with medications in the United States are hampered by:

Correct Answer: 3. Public view of addiction.

Rationale:

> This is correct. The drug is not used in the United States due to biases about substance abuse and the public view of addiction.

15-4.

A client with a long history of cocaine abuse and frequent relapse episodes is hospitalized. Which of the following goals is a priority for this client?

Correct Answer: 1. Acknowledge association between substance use and personal problems.

Rationale:

> The priority problem for the client with a substance-related disorder is ineffective denial.

15-5.

A client drank a liter of wine every day for the past year. The client has been arrested three times for driving while impaired. Which of the following terms should the nurse use to describe this client's behavior?

Correct Answer: 3. Abuse.

Rationale:

> Abuse describes this client's maladaptive behavior. The client continues to use the substance despite repeated legal problems.

15-6.

A client is admitted to the emergency department with needle marks on both arms. The spouse states that the client only uses heroin when feeling a great deal of stress at work. The spouse tells the nurse that the client only uses drugs on the weekend and can handle them. Which of the following assessments will the nurse make about the client and spouse?

Correct Answer: 3. Codependent behavior.

Rationale:

> The spouse is enabling the client by excusing behaviors and by not acknowledging that cocaine use is a problem. This spouse is permitting the client to have self-destructed behavior.

15-7.

The nurse should initially focus on which of the following interventions when caring for a pregnant client with a substance abuse disorder?

Correct Answer: 1. Accept client unconditionally.

Rationale:

> Treatment programs designed for women require gender-specific approaches. It is believed that women's substance abuse is based on poor self-esteem, depression, relationships, and a history of substance abuse. Unconditional acceptance will assist the nurse and client to form a therapeutic relationship.

CHAPTER 16

16-1.

A client who has paranoid personality disorder is participating in a treatment group. Which behavior should the nurse be most aware of as the client participates in the group?

Correct Answer: 1. Hypervigilance.
Rationale:

> The client with a paranoid personality disorder is suspicious of others. The client is extremely sensitive and may misinterpret cues from other clients in the group.

16-2.

A psychiatric nurse is providing education about clients with personality disorders to medical–surgical nurses. One nurse asks, "What is the cause of personality disorders?" The nurse knows there is a need for further teaching if she hears which of the following statements?

Correct Answer: 1. "It is a brain disorder in which there is not enough serotonin."
Rationale:

> This is incorrect. Personality disorders are thought to be a combination of psychosocial and biological factors. The neurotransmitter serotonin is responsible for sleep regulation, hunger, and mood states but is not linked to personality disorders.

16-3.

A 19-year-old client is diagnosed with borderline personality disorder (BPD). The client has an eating disorder behavior consisting of eating and then purging. Which of the following is the best question to assess the client's nutritional status?

Correct Answer: 4. "What do you eat in a day?"
Rationale:

> This is the best way to assess the client's usual food intake. The nurse can ask questions and learn about the client's usual eating patterns.

16-4.

A client with a borderline personality disorder tells the nurse: "Everything bad happens to me. It is entirely my fault." What is the best response by the nurse to assist the client to reframe this negative thought?

Correct Answer: 2. "Let us examine what you mean by bad things."
Rationale:

> By reframing the belief by the client, the nurse can help the client's perception of himself and his environment.

16-5.

In what phase of the nurse–client relationship should the nurse introduce the issue of termination to the client?

Correct Answer: 2. The orientation phase.
Rationale:

> The nurse must inform the client at the orientation phase that the nurse–client relationship has a time limit.

16-6.

The nurse is teaching assertiveness techniques to a group of clients diagnosed with a dependent personality disorder. Which of the following statements indicates that the teaching was not successful?

Correct Answer: 3. "I learned so much that I didn't know before."
Rationale:

> This is not a successful outcome. The client is underplaying personal abilities and attributing the learning to the teacher. Clients with a dependent personality disorder will demean themselves to gain acceptance.

CHAPTER 17

17-1.

An adolescent is admitted to the hospital with a diagnosis of conduct disorder. The parent asks why the adolescent gets into so much trouble. The nurse informs the parent that there are several thoughts about the cause of this disorder. Which of the following statements indicates that the parent needs more information about the causative factors of conduct disorder?

Correct Answer: 1. "Yes, my child fits in with the group so well."
Rationale:

> The parent needs more teaching about the role of peer relationships and the diagnosis of conduct disorder. It is thought that difficulty in peer relationships are implicated in the development of conduct disorder.

17-2.

A child diagnosed with attention deficit hyperactivity disorder (ADHD) is receiving methylphenidate (Ritalin, Concerta). The nurse recognizes which of the following behaviors as a therapeutic outcome of this medication?

Correct Answer: 2. Increased ability to concentrate.
Rationale:

> Methylphenidate does improve focus and concentration by lessening the symptoms of hyperactivity, impulsiveness, and aggression. Improved concentration will give the child new opportunities to learn.

17-3.

A school nurse is assessing a 5-year-old child. Which assessment finding should the nurse report to the child protection agency?

Correct Answer: 3. Unexplained bruises on the child.
Rationale:

> The nurse should report unexplained bruises on the child to the local Child Protection Agency. Unexplained bruises are the most obvious sign of child maltreatment. The nurse should further assess for behavioral indicators of abuse.

17-4.

A nurse is providing counseling to a group of teenagers who have lost two friends in an automobile accident. One of the teenagers walks out of the group and states, "I don't want to talk about this, there is no fairness in life." The nurse recognizes this behavior as:

Correct Answer: 4. Depression.

Rationale:

> The behavior the client is exhibiting is depression, by grieving over the loss and the inability to accept what can never be.

17-5.

A 6-year-old boy with attention deficit hyperactivity disorder (ADHD) is acting aggressively toward the other children in a day care center. The best action for the nurse is to:

Correct Answer: 4. Take him to another room to play out his feelings.

Rationale:

> The use of play is an important cognitive and emotional tool to assist the child to express his feelings.

17-6.

A teen, attending a substance abuse group, threatens other clients and swears at the nurse. Which response by the nurse is the most helpful to the client?

Correct Answer: 3. "Sit down and join the group."

Rationale:

> Setting limits and telling the client the expectations of his behavior gives the client the information about acceptable behavior in this group.

17-7.

A nurse is counseling a teenager with depression whose parent died 2 months ago. Before teaching the steps of the grief process to the client, the nurse should assess the client's current stage of grief. Which of the following statements indicates guilt?

Correct Answer: 2. "I wish I had been nicer."

Rationale:

> "I wish I had been nicer." This statement indicates guilt. The client may feel as if a behavior may be responsible for the parent's death. The teaching should focus on identifying the guilt and recognizing that the adolescent's actions had nothing to do with the parent's death.

CHAPTER 18

18-1.

A client is upset after learning that a family member is arrested for exhibitionism. The nurse informs the client about the current theories related to the cause for this paraphilia. Which of the following statements indicates that the client requires more information?

Correct Answer: 4. "This must be done by a person with a sexual dysfunction."

Rationale:

> This is the correct answer. Sexual dysfunction is not thought to be a causative factor for paraphilias. The person with a sexual dysfunction has a disturbance in any of the phases of the sexual response cycle. Interventions assist the client to identify the stressors that interfere with a normal sexual response cycle.

18-2.

A client with a sexual arousal disorder asks the nurse if taking sildenafil (Viagra) is the only method to treat erectile dysfunction. What is the best response by the nurse?

Correct Answer: 3. "Group therapy reduces the anxiety connected with erectile difficulties."

Rationale:

> This is correct. Group therapy is a successful treatment to reduce the anxiety connected with erectile dysfunction.

18-3.

A 70-year-old client who has had numerous affairs throughout his marriage tells the nurse, "The affairs helped me to have better sex with my spouse." What defense mechanism is this client using?

Correct Answer: 3. Rationalization.

Rationale:

> Rationalization is the correct answer. Rationalization is the use of logical reasons to justify the unacceptable behavior. The client is making a logical statement to excuse the affairs.

18-4.

The nurse uses the PLISSIT model to help clients with gender issues or sexual problems. Which of the following are the four progressive levels? (Select all that apply.)

Correct Answers:
1. Permission giving.
2. Limited information.
4. Specific suggestions.
5. Intensive therapy.

Rationale:
1. The model involves four progressive levels represented by the acronym PLISSIT. The goal is to gather information about the client's sexuality. Permission from the client to begin the discussion is the first level.
2. The second level in PLISSIT is providing the limited information needed to assess function.

4. Giving specific suggestions for the individual to proceed with sexual relations is the third level in PLISSIT.
5. Providing intensive therapy about the issues of sexuality is the last level of PLISSIT.

18-5.

A client tells the nurse that he has lost the desire to have sex with his wife. Further assessment reveals that the client is taking antihypertensive and antidepressant medication. Which of the following nursing diagnoses will the nurse select to identify the problem the client is experiencing?

Correct Answer: 1. Sexual Dysfunction.
Rationale:
> This is the correct nursing diagnosis. The client has a change in sexual functioning that is not satisfying. The nurse should set the goal of identifying the cause of the dysfunction.

18-6.

A nurse is conducting a sexual awareness group of known pedophiles. What will the nurse emphasize as the primary focus of this group?

Correct Answer: 2. Cognitive restructuring.
Rationale:
> This is the correct answer. The nurse's focus should be on education. The first priority is to gain an awareness of the sexual behaviors and the consequences. Cognitive restructuring is used in an effort to change the individual's maladaptive behaviors.

CHAPTER 19

19-1.

A client who developed delirium following surgery asks if having delirium is the beginning of Alzheimer disease. The nurse explains the differences between delirium and dementia. Which of the following statements by the client requires further teaching?

Correct Answer: 3. "In dementia, there are quick changes in the levels of consciousness, too."
Rationale:
> This is an incorrect answer. While a client with delirium has fluctuating changes in levels of consciousness, the client with dementia does not.

19-2.

A client is diagnosed with vascular dementia. Which of the following explanations will assist the family to understand the cause of this type of dementia?

Correct Answer: 1. Blood vessels in the brain are bleeding.

Rationale:
> Vascular dementia is caused by bleeding and ischemia in the brain. Risk factors for vascular dementia are similar to those for cerebral vascular accident (CVA).

19-3.

Clients on the unit avoid the client with HIV dementia. Which of the following is an appropriate intervention for this group of clients?

Correct Answer: 1. Form an educational focus group on the unit.
Rationale:
> Forming an educational group on the unit assists the clients to verbalize their thoughts, gain knowledge, recognize their biases and value system, and change their behavior.

19-4.

An 80-year-old client who lives with her daughter tells the nurse, "No one lets me eat with them. I have to hide my food under the bed." The nurse plans a family meeting to discuss:

Correct Answer: 1. Family eating patterns.
Rationale:
> People with dementia may make paranoid accusations against family members. The initial assessment should include asking the family if the mother is a member at each meal and if there is a schedule for meals.

19-5.

The family is caring for their parent with Alzheimer disease. Which of the following topics should the nurse include in the family education? (Select all that apply.)

Correct Answers:
1. Management of the illness.
3. Nature of cognitive impairment.
5. Support services.
Rationale:
1. This is an important topic for the family. Key ideas include client safety, nutrition, medication administration, and daily activities.
3. This is an important topic for the family. It is helpful to them to know the causes and symptoms of the illness.
5. The family may need assistance with financial, legal, and home health services. The availability of respite care is also helpful information.

19-6.

A client with dementia has a disturbed sleep pattern. Which of the following interventions should the nurse utilize for the client?

Correct Answer: 3. Promote mild exercise.
Rationale:
> Mild exercise is therapeutic and stimulates the client.

19-7.

The nurse is working with families of clients with Alzheimer disease. One of the members says, "I feel so sad because my loved one is lost." The nurse can best facilitate group discussion on this issue by saying:

Correct Answer: 3. "How have others in the family dealt with these feelings?"

Rationale:

> Asking the group to share their experiences facilitates discussion of the topic of loss. Group participation facilitates a sense of universality for the families.

CHAPTER 20

20-1.

Which of the following assessment results would the nurse expect to find in a client with Pick disease?

Correct Answer: 1. Poor insight and lack of judgment.

Rationale:

> Poor insight and lack of judgment are significant symptoms of Pick disease.

20-2.

A client is in the late stages of Parkinson disease. He states that he wants to be left alone and does not want visitors. In planning for treatment strategies the nurse should focus on:

Correct Answer: 4. Respecting the client's decision.

Rationale:

> Respecting the client's decision is valuing the uniqueness of the client. As the client becomes further engulfed into his illness, he is tired and interactions become burdensome.

20-3.

What distinctive symptoms do clients with Huntington disease manifest? (Select all that apply.)

Correct Answers:
1. Cognitive changes.
2. Severe irritability.
3. Inability to tolerate frustration.
5. Ability to remember words and stories.

Rationale:
1. Cognitive changes are symptoms of Huntington disease.
2. Severe irritability is a symptom of Huntington disease.
3. Inability to tolerate frustration is a symptom of Huntington disease.
5. Ability to remember words and stories is present in clients with Huntington disease.

20-4.

A delirious client is physically restrained. The restraining intervention and the safety of the client is the responsibility of the:

Correct Answer: 1. Nurse who is assigned to care for the client.

Rationale:

> The nurse has the primary responsibility for continued assessment, interventions, and evaluation of the client in restraints.

20-5.

During a family education session, the nurse focuses on the care of the client diagnosed with dementia. The nurse should counsel the family on the need to:

Correct Answer: 1. Understand the potential for the client wandering from the home.

Rationale:

> The priority of care for a client with dementia is wandering from the home. The components of dementia are loss of short- and long-term memory and lack of the ability to focus, which can lead to the client wandering away from home.

CHAPTER 21

21-1.

A client who attempted suicide 5 years ago with an overdose was brought to the emergency department (ED) by a friend. The client states, "I just don't feel like living anymore. No one would care if I lived or died." What question should the nurse ask next?

Correct Answer: 1. "Do you have a plan for suicide at this time?"

Rationale:

> The correct answer is "Do you have a plan for suicide at this time?" This question ascertains whether the client is planning another suicide attempt. The best clinical predictors for suicide risk are previous attempts and a sense of hopelessness or desperation.

21-2.

The mental health nurse is giving a presentation in a rural community to increase the awareness of suicide risks. Which of the following population groups has a high risk for suicide and is an appropriate target audience? (Select all that apply.)

Correct Answers:
2. Elderly men with a terminal disease.
4. Nurses who work on a pediatric oncology unit.

Rationale:
2. Elderly men with a terminal disease is correct because men, especially older adult males living in a rural area, have a higher suicide completion rate than women due to use of firearms in a suicide attempt and social isolation.
4. Nurses who work on a pediatric oncology unit is correct because the daily stress of caring for children with a terminal disease could be a contributing factor. Nurses also have easier access to drugs and knowledge regarding lethal doses of medications.

21-3.

The guardian of a client diagnosed with paranoid schizophrenia is concerned that the client is at risk for suicide. The nurse should assess which of the following behaviors as a significant sign that the client is contemplating suicide?

Correct Answer: 4. The client has been asking how to load a gun.
Rationale:
> The client has been asking how to load a gun is the correct answer. A sudden interest in firearms is a strong indicator of impending suicide.

21-4.

Which of the following client statements indicates a positive outcome to treatment for suicidal behavior?

Correct Answer: 1. "I am thankful for my husband and children."
Rationale:
> The statement, "I am thankful for my husband and children" is correct because the client is able to list reasons to live.

21-5.

A client admitted to the hospital for a recent suicide attempt has been taking antidepressants as prescribed and attending group therapy. The client is sleeping 6 hours per night and reports a significant improvement in mood. The client states, "I have lots of things to do when I get home and I don't really need to be in the hospital anymore." Which of the following responses by the nurse would be most appropriate?

Correct Answer: 1. "Are you still having thoughts of suicide?"
Rationale:
> The question, "Are you still having thoughts of suicide?" is correct because the client may have more energy and capacity to act on suicidal thoughts. The client remains at risk. It is necessary to assess the client's continued risk for suicide before discharge is considered.

21-6.

The nurse is leading a group for depressed clients who have attempted suicide in the past. Which of the following topics is not appropriate to discuss in this group?

Correct Answer: 3. Movies that dramatize suicidal behavior.
Rationale:
> Movies that dramatize suicidal behavior is correct because fictional portrayals of suicide can glamorize the event and present an unrealistic or attractive picture of suicidal behavior.

CHAPTER 22

22-1.

Which of the following individuals is at highest risk for physical abuse?

Correct Answer: 4. A 17-year-old pregnant woman who did not seek prenatal care until her seventh month.
Rationale:
> A 17-year-old pregnant woman who did not seek prenatal care until her seventh month is correct. Pregnant teens are at higher risk for physical abuse than other pregnant women. Delaying prenatal care until the third trimester is also more common in abused women.

22-2.

Which of the following behaviors does the school nurse recognize is an indicator that a school-age child has been physically abused?

Correct Answer: 3. The child bullies other children and threatens them to "keep quiet about it or else."
Rationale:
> The child bullies other children and threatens them to "keep quiet about it or else" is correct. Abused children frequently act out with aggressive behavior, especially toward someone who is smaller and weaker.

22-3.

A client who has been physically abused asks the nurse, "What makes people so violent toward others?" Which of the following is the best response to this question?

Correct Answer: 1. "It is difficult to give one specific reason for violent behavior."
Rationale:
> This is the correct answer. There is no single cause of interpersonal violence. It is a result of the interaction of biology, personality, relationships, and societal factors that impact individuals and families.

22-4.

A 63-year-old man with Alzheimer disease is brought to the emergency department (ED) with pressure sores and severe dehydration. Upon further assessment, the nurse notices bruises on the client's neck, arms, and legs. Which of the following questions should the nurse ask the client's wife?

Correct Answer: 1. "What kind of support do you have at home to care for your husband?"
Rationale:
> The question, "What kind of support do you have at home to care for your husband?" is correct because it will assess the wife's support system and ability to care for her husband in a safe manner. This question also indicates that the nurse is aware of possible stress on the caregiver without accusing the wife of abuse.

22-5.

Which of the following nursing diagnoses is the most important for a homosexual client who has been repeatedly physically assaulted by his partner?

Correct Answer: 2. Risk for Injury related to history of abuse by significant other.

Rationale:

Risk for Injury related to history of abuse by significant other is correct. The safety of the client is the priority diagnosis. The greatest predictor of continued violence is the previous history of violence by the partner.

22-6.

A student health nurse employed by a university is concerned about the increase of dating violence reported on campus. The nurse should be concerned if which preventive measure was included in a safety presentation for women in the dormitory?

Correct Answer: 3. If you are uncomfortable in a situation, always ask a male student to drive you home.

Rationale:

If you are uncomfortable in a situation, always ask a male student to drive you home is the correct answer. The nurse should be concerned that the male student could take advantage of a female who is alone. It would be wiser to ask another female student to drive you home or call a taxi.

22-7.

A nurse came to work with a black eye and swollen lip. Her coworkers have noticed that her boyfriend calls her at least 10 times during her 12-hour shift. She has refused all invitations to go out with her coworkers, saying that her boyfriend will be there to pick her up and he doesn't like to wait for her. What is the most helpful response by the coworkers?

Correct Answer: 4. Encourage the nurse to talk to a professional.

Rationale:

Encouraging the nurse to talk to a professional is correct. The abused adult needs to be her own rescuer. Her friends should encourage her to ask for help directly.

CHAPTER 23

23-1.

A high school teacher offers a 15-year-old student a ride home from an extracurricular activity. The teacher turns onto a deserted rural road and begins to manipulate the student's penis until he ejaculates. The student is embarrassed by his inability to stop his response and asks the teacher to take him home. He does not report the incident because of his feelings of shame and guilt. Which of the following types of rape is described in the above scenario?

Correct Answer: 4. Acquaintance rape.

Rationale:

Acquaintance rape is correct because forced sexual activity was perpetrated by someone known to the victim.

23-2.

Which of the following behaviors would lead a nurse to suspect that a child has been sexually abused?

Correct Answer: 3. The child continues to masturbate at school when told it is not appropriate to do so.

Rationale:

The child continues to masturbate at school when told it is not appropriate to do so is the correct answer. The child may be imitating what an adult has done to him or her and does not realize that this is inappropriate behavior.

23-3.

A 40-year-old male is accused of sexually abusing his 6-year-old niece while helping her out of the swimming pool. The man denies touching his niece in a sexual way. Which of the following factors is present if no sexual abuse occurred?

Correct Answer: 2. The niece was confused because she had been told that no one should ever touch her between the legs without her permission.

Rationale:

The niece was confused because she had been told that no one should ever touch her between the legs without her permission is correct. The instructions given to her were not explicit enough for her to identify whether or not this incidence was sexual abuse.

23-4.

The nurse notified child protective services about the sexual abuse of a 10-year-old child by an unidentified family member. Which of the following options would best ensure the safety of this victim?

Correct Answer: 1. The victim is removed from the home and placed in foster care.

Rationale:

The victim is removed from the home and placed in foster care is correct. This is the only option that would prevent the child from further sexual, emotional, or physical abuse.

23-5.

A nurse is teaching victims of sexual violence and their families about available community resources. The nurse recognizes that more education is needed if a member of this class asks about joining which of the following organizations?

Correct Answer: 3. Safer Society Foundation.

Rationale:

Safer Society Foundation is the correct answer. This is an organization that provides education for perpetrators and referrals to sex offender treatment programs.

CHAPTER 24

24-1.

The nurse is aware that changing levels of hormones and neurotransmitters may contribute to violent behavior. The nurse is most concerned about a potential for violence if a client has elevated levels of which of the following?

Correct Answer: 2. Testosterone.

Rationale:

> Testosterone is correct because higher testosterone levels may cause a deficit in serotonin levels which, in turn, causes men to react more aggressively to annoying situations.

24-2.

Which of the following population groups are most likely to be victims of murder, rape, robbery, or aggravated assault?

Correct Answer: 4. Young adult male gang members.

Rationale:

> Young adult male gang members is the correct answer. Males age 18–24 are the chief perpetrators and victims of violent crime.

24-3.

A high school freshman has been teased and taunted about his small size by senior class members. He has no close friends and usually sits alone when eating lunch in the cafeteria. When he fell down in physical education class, the other students laughed and called him "klutz." The school nurse should provide further teaching if the nursing student selected which of the following nursing diagnoses for this student?

Correct Answer: 2. Risk for Other-Directed Violence related to history of violent behaviors.

Rationale:

> Risk for Other-Directed Violence related to history of violent behavior is the correct answer. There is no data to support this nursing diagnosis. The student has not made any violent threats, exhibited signs of uncontrolled anger, or brandished a firearm.

24-4.

The nurse plans to teach employees in the community about methods of preventing workplace violence. The nurse will begin teaching the groups of employees who are at highest risk. Which of the following groups should the nurse teach first? (Select all that apply.)

Correct Answers:
1. Court judges.
4. Gas station attendants.
5. Taxi drivers.

Rationale:
1. Court judges is correct because individuals who have positions of authority such as in law enforcement and government service are at highest risk for workplace violence.
4. Gas station attendants is a correct answer. These employees often work alone and during the night when most violent crimes are likely to occur.
5. Taxi drivers is a correct answer. Taxi drivers work alone, are constantly interacting with strangers, and drive in unfamiliar and possibly unsafe areas at all times of the day and night.

24-5.

An adult client is pacing and yelling. Which of the following is the best response by the nurse?

Correct Answer: 4. "When did this feeling begin?"

Rationale:

> This is the correct answer. When a client is angry, use open-ended questions to clarify the client's behavior. Use an empathetic approach to assist the client to discover the source of the anger.

CHAPTER 25

25-1.

A National Guard soldier who returned home from a 1-month tour of disaster-relief duty comes to the mental health clinic with symptoms of insomnia, irritability, and anxiety. The client states, "I just can't get the sight of those dead bodies out of my head. When I was at the disaster, I tried not to think about what I was doing; now I think about it all the time." Which of the following assessment questions would be most relevant for this client?

Correct Answer: 3. "What more can you tell me about what is happening now?"

Rationale:

> The question, "What more can you tell me about what is happening now?" is correct. A client who has experienced an adventitious crisis should be allowed to talk without feeling pushed. An open-ended question allows the client to continue to talk about the current personal responses to the disaster, rather than focus on events in the past.

25-2.

In response to a recent violent shooting on another university campus, the university leaders are concerned about acts of violence on their campus. These leaders will initiate which of the following primary prevention activities?

Correct Answer: 1. Request cell phone numbers of all students, faculty, and staff on campus.

Rationale:

Requesting cell phone numbers of all students, faculty, and staff on campus is correct. Primary prevention involves the development of a disaster-preparedness plan. An effective communication system is an example of one aspect of this plan.

25-3.

A 16-year-old client is having difficulty dealing with the traumatic death of her boyfriend. Which of the following behaviors does the nurse least expect to observe in this adolescent?

Correct Answer: 4. Worrying about increased drug use in her school.

Rationale:

Worrying about increased drug use in her school is correct. Although adolescents will typically experience long-term worries about their safety and security, drug use in the school is an ongoing issue that is not necessarily a response to the death of her boyfriend.

25-4.

A community nurse assesses a client following a natural disaster. The nurse will intervene first in which area of need?

Correct Answer: 3. Concern for the loss of a home.

Rationale:

Concern for the loss of a home is correct. The provision of food, shelter, water, and clothing is the priority for the victim of a natural disaster. Physical needs are met first; psychological needs are addressed as basic needs are provided.

25-5.

Which of the following community activities is an example of tertiary prevention in a community that experienced a massive fire?

Correct Answer: 2. Mental health professionals offering educational programs on effective coping strategies.

Rationale:

Mental health professionals offering educational programs on effective coping strategies is correct. Tertiary prevention is aimed at meeting the long-term needs of a community or individual after the initial effect of the disaster is resolved. Teaching coping skills is an effective tool to assist those who have experienced disaster to cope with the long-term effects of the disaster.

abstinence   Stopping the intake of alcohol or drugs.

abuse   A pattern of behavior that dominates, controls, lowers self-esteem, or takes away freedom of choice of the victim.

acquaintance rape   Rape committed by someone known to the victim.

acute stress disorder   A DSM-IV diagnosis for the initial symptoms of severe stress; A numbing and emotionally nonresponsive reaction to an extreme trauma.

advance directive   The client's formulation of a plan of care to assist family and caregivers who must make decisions for the client when she or he is unable to make decisions for herself or himself.

advanced practice registered nurses (APRNs)   Nurses with a doctorate or master's degree who focus on health promotion, illness prevention, education, psychotherapy, consultation, and research.

adventitious crisis   An unexpected crisis, such as a natural disaster.

advocacy   Supporting and defending people's rights to their beliefs, attitudes, and values.

affect   Immediate emotional expression; what others observe.

affective style (AS)   The emotional climate of the family; high AS families are intrusive and make guilt-inducing remarks to one another.

affective violence   The verbal expression of intense anger and emotions; bullying, ugly taunts, disrespect, alienation, scapegoating, and physical threats.

aggression   Any verbal or nonverbal force meant to harm or abuse another person.

agnosia   An inability to recognize familiar situations, people, or stimuli; not related to impairment in sensory organs.

agonists   Substance that binds to and activates receptors; may have weak or strong potency.

agoraphobia   A phobic disorder characterized by fear of being away from home and of being alone in public places when assistance might be needed.

agraphia   An inability to read or write.

akathisia   The inability to sit or stand still, along with a feeling of anxiety. It is the result of extrapyramidal side effects of antipsychotic medication.

akinesia   Muscular weakness or the partial loss of movement as the result of extrapyramidal side effects of antipsychotic medication.

alcohol withdrawal delirium   A complication of withdrawal from alcohol occurring between 2 and 14 days after the last drink; marked by confusion, disorientation, hallucinations, tachycardia, tremors, agitation, diaphoresis, and fever.

alcohol-related birth defects (ARBDs)   Abnormalities ranging from subtle cognitive–behavioral impairments to heart defects and malformed facial features.

alexia   Inability to identify objects or their use by sight; also called visual agnosia.

alexithymia   Inability to analyze, interpret, and name physical feelings and sensations.

Alzheimer disease (AD)   A disease characterized by progressive dementia with atrophy of the central nervous system.

androgyny   Flexibility in gender-stereotypic behaviors and roles; neither specifically masculine or feminine; having traditional male and female roles reversed or obscured.

anger rape   Rape distinguished by physical violence and cruelty to the victim.

anhedonic   The state in which a person is unable to experience pleasure.

anorexia nervosa   An eating disorder in which a person attempts to lose weight by dramatically decreasing food intake and increasing physical exercise.

antagonists   Substances that bind to receptors, preventing agonists from binding, creating a blockage.

anticholinergic side effects   Side effects that occur when medication blocks the acetylcholine receptors, resulting in the inhibition of the transmission of parasympathetic nerve impulses.

antioxidants   Enzymes that search out and neutralize dangerous oxygen free radicals.

antisocial behavior   Behavior that is against the norms of other individuals and society.

antisocial personality disorder (ASPD)   A disorder beginning in childhood and continuing into adulthood, characterized by a pattern of irresponsible and antisocial behavior.

anxiety   (1) A feeling of tension, distress, and discomfort produced by a perceived or threatened loss of inner control rather than from external danger. (2) Emotion in response to the fear of being hurt or losing something valued.

aphasia   Loss of the ability to understand or use language.

apraxia   Inability to carry out skilled and purposeful movement; the inability to use objects properly.

Asperger disorder   Severe impairment in social interactions as well as repetitive patterns of behavior and activities.

assisted suicide   A person commits suicide with the help of a physician or nurse, who only provides the means for the suicide.

astereognosia   Inability to identify familiar objects placed in one's hand; also called tactile agnosia.

attention deficit/hyperactivity disorder (ADHD)   A disorder characterized by inattention, hyperactivity, and impulsivity.

authority killing   Retaliation for real or imagined offenses; targets may be individuals or a building or structure that symbolizes the authority.

autistic disorder   A disorder characterized by social isolation, communication impairment, and strange repetitive behaviors.

autoerotic asphyxia   Use of a tourniquet-like device that constricts the neck, decreasing the blood and oxygen supply to the brain, followed by masturbation, and, at the point of orgasm, releasing the bonds to enhance the sensation or sexual high.

autonomy   The freedom to choose and the ability to assume responsibility for one's acts.

avoidant personality disorder (AVPD)   A disorder characterized by timidity, fear of negative evaluation, and social discomfort.

behavioral therapy   Therapy based on the principle that all behavior has specific consequences that lead to an increase or decrease of a particular behavior.

bereavement   The feelings, thoughts, and responses that loved ones experience after the death of a person with whom they have shared a significant relationship.

binge eating disorder   Overeating and feeling out of control; occurs at least twice a week for 6 months.

biological rhythms   Regular fluctuations of a variety of physiological factors over a set period of time.

bioterrorism   Terrorism committed with biological weapons.

bipolar disorder   A mood disorder characterized by alternating depression and elation, with periods of normal mood in between; also called manic–depressive disorder.

blood–brain barrier   A membrane between circulating blood and the brain that protects the brain against potential toxins and exports waste products.

body dysmorphic disorder   A preoccupation with an imagined or slight defect in physical appearance.

body image   The integration of a person's perceptions, thoughts, and feelings about her or his own body.

body language   Nonverbal communication conveyed by a person's position, posture, and movements.

borderline personality disorder (BPD)   A disorder characterized by a pattern of instability in self-image, interpersonal relationships, and mood.

boundaries   The invisible lines that define the amount and kind of contact allowable between members of the family and between the family and outside systems.

brain attack   Also called a stroke; may be the result of a thrombus, emboli, or hemorrhage in the brain.

brief psychotic disorder   Rapid onset of at least one of the following psychotic symptoms: delusions, hallucinations, disorganized speech, or disorganized behavior. The episode lasts at least 1 day but less than 1 month, after which the person returns to the premorbid level of functioning.

bulimia nervosa   An eating disorder in which a person attempts to manage weight through dieting, binge eating, and purging.

caring   A commitment and binding together of individuals in interpersonal connections.

catastrophizing   A distorted thinking process that exaggerates failures in one's life.

catatonic excitement   Hyperactivity and bizarre behavior; would be described as a positive symptom of schizophrenia.

catatonic inhibition   Decreased activity level, limited speech, minimal self-care, and at times, a trancelike state; would be described as a negative symptom of schizophrenia.

cause-based terrorism   Terrorism based on a cause embracing a particular ideology.

chemical terrorism   Terrorism committed with chemical agents.

childhood sexual abuse   Inappropriate sexual behavior with a child instigated by a perpetrator for purposes of the perpetrator's sexual pleasure or for economic gain through child prostitution or pornography.

circadian rhythms   Regular fluctuations of a variety of physiological factors over a period of 24 hours.

civil rights protection   A person's legal rights to political, economic, and social equality.

Cluster A personality disorders   A category of personality disorders characterized by eccentric behavior and social withdrawal.

Cluster B personality disorders   A category of personality disorders characterized by dramatic, emotional, or erratic behavior; disorders are antisocial, borderline, histrionic, and narcissistic.

Cluster C personality disorders   A category of personality disorders characterized by anxious and fearful behavior; disorders are avoidant, dependent, and obsessive–compulsive.

codependency   A psychological condition or a relationship in which a person is controlled or manipulated by another affected with a pathological condition (as an addiction to alcohol or heroin); dependence on the needs of or control by another. Non–substance-abusing partners enable their partners to continue to abuse alcohol or drugs.

cognitive distortions   Errors in thinking that continue even when there is obvious contradictory evidence.

cognitive processes   In Sullivan's social–interpersonal theory, the development of thinking progresses from unconnected to causal to symbolic.

cognitive schemas   Personal controlling beliefs that influence the way people process data about themselves and others.

cognitive-behavioral therapy   The behavioral aspect helps people identify habitual reactions to troublesome situations. It also teaches people how to relax and calm their bodies. The cognitive aspect focuses on distorted thinking patterns that cause unpleasant feelings or symptoms of mental disorders.

collaboration   The involvement of clients, family members, and professionals working together to improve quality of life and the highest level of functioning.

commitment   Detaining a client in a psychiatric facility against his or her will, requested on the basis of dangerousness to self or others; also called involuntary admission.

competency   A legal determination affirming that a client can make reasonable judgments and decisions about treatment and other significant personal issues.

competency model   The belief that all families are resourceful and have the capacity to grow and change.

complementary/alternative therapies   The umbrella term for hundreds of therapies from all over the world that are not based on a biomedical model.

complicated grief   Grief that includes symptoms such as intrusive images, severe feelings of emptiness, neglect of activities at home and at work, preoccupation with thoughts of the deceased person, yearning and searching for her or him, inability to accept the death, auditory and visual hallucinations of the person, bitterness, and survivor guilt over the death.

compulsion   A repetitive behavior or thought used to decrease the fear or guilt associated with an obsession; A preoccupation with an imagined or slight defect in physical appearance.

conduct disorder (CD)   A disorder characterized by a persistent pattern of aggressive and destructive behavior with disregard for the rights of others and the norms of society.

confabulation   Filling in memory gaps with imaginary information.

confidentiality   The legal and ethical duty to not share information about clients.

conscious   The aspect of consciousness, which is the quality or state of being aware, especially of something within oneself or of being conscious of an external object, state, or fact, that encompasses all things that are easily remembered.

consumers   Individuals who utilize mental health services.

contextual sensitivity hypothesis   The belief that human behavior is highly sensitive to social contexts.

contextualization   Maintaining clients in their usual surroundings, both geographic and interpersonal.

control   The exercise of authority or domination of another person.

conversion disorder   A somatoform disorder characterized by sensorimotor symptoms.

coping behaviors   A conscious attempt to manage stress and anxiety; may be physical, cognitive, or affective.

coprolalia   Use of obscene words, often involuntary; related to Tourette's syndrome.

copycat suicide   Suicide that is inspired by reports of suicides in the media; an adolescent phenomenon.

countertransference   A nurse's emotional reaction to a client based on significant relationships in the nurse's past; the process may be conscious or unconscious, and the feelings may be positive or negative.

covert messages   The modification of spoken words through tone of voice, rate of speech, body posture, gestures, eye contact, and facial expression.

Creutzfeldt–Jakob disease (CJD)   A degenerative brain disorder resulting in dementia.

criminal terrorism   Terrorists that fund their cause by criminal behavior.

crisis   A turning point in a person's life at which usual resources and coping skills are no longer effective and the person enters a state of disequilibrium.

crisis intervention   Assisting people to resolve the immediate problem and regain emotional equilibrium.

critical thinking   An analytic process used to make reliable observations, draw sound conclusions, create new ideas, solve problems, evaluate lines of reasoning, and improve self-knowledge.

cross-dressers   People, typically males, who wear clothes designed for the opposite sex to express the feminine side of their personality. In most instances cross-dressers are not interested in permanently altering their bodies through surgical means, especially since the majority of them are comfortable with their original birth gender.

cultural competence   Understanding and respecting cultural diversity in the practice of nursing; based on cultural knowledge and sensitivity, appropriate communication skills, and client advocacy.

culture   Pattern of learned behavior based on values, beliefs, and perceptions of the world; culture is taught and shared by members of a group.

cyberstalking   The use of the Internet, e-mail, or other electronic communications to stalk another person.

cycle of violence   The pattern of abuse when conflict escalates into violence followed by a begging of forgiveness, a period of calm, and then another violent outbreak.

cyclothymic disorder   A mood disorder characterized by a mood range from moderate depression to hypomania, which may or may not include periods of normal mood.

date rape   Verbal coercion and deception to pressure a date into having sex.

deep brain stimulation (DBS)   The surgical implant of electrodes in deep subcortical nuclei to provide intermittent stimulation.

defense mechanism   An unconscious attempt to deny, misinterpret, or distort reality to alleviate anxiety.

delirium   An acute, usually reversible brain disorder characterized by clouding of the consciousness (decreased awareness of the environment) and a reduced ability to focus and maintain attention.

delusion   False belief that cannot be changed by logical reasoning or evidence.

dementia   A chronic, irreversible brain disorder characterized by impairments in memory, abstract thinking, and judgment, as well as changes in personality.

dependent personality disorder (DPD)   A disorder characterized by an inability to make everyday decisions without an excessive amount of advice and reassurance from others.

depersonalization disorder   Persistent or recurrent feelings of being detached from one's body or thoughts.

depressive personality disorder   A disorder characterized by persistent gloom and inability to experience pleasure, joy, or humor.

diathesis-stress model An etiological theory that proposes that stress can trigger symptoms in individuals with biological predisposition to severe mental illness.

dichotomous thinking Distorted, all-or-none reasoning involving opposite and mutually exclusive categories.

discontinuation syndrome Flu-like symptoms, gastrointestinal problems, fatigue, headaches, and anxiety may occur when psychotropic drugs are stopped suddenly.

discrimination Prejudice expressed behaviorally; the isms are forms of discrimination.

disempowerment Individuals have little voice or power in what happens to them leading to feelings of inadequacy or helplessness.

disenfranchised grief Grief in which the loss cannot be openly acknowledged, socially validated, or publicly mourned.

dissociation A disruption in the usually integrated functions of consciousness, memory, identity, and perception of the environment.

dissociative amnesia Loss of memory in response to trauma; may be localized, selective, generalized, or continuous.

dissociative disorders A category of anxiety disorders characterized by an alteration in conscious awareness of behavior, affect, thoughts, and memories, and an alteration in identity, particularly in the consistency of personality.

dissociative fugue A rare dissociative disorder in which people, while either maintaining their identity or adopting a new identity, wander or take unexpected trips.

dissociative identity disorder (DID) A dissociative disorder characterized by the existence of two or more personalities in the same individual.

diversity Variation among people.

double depression Occurs when a person with dysthymic disorder also experiences an episode of major depressive disorder.

dual diagnosis The concurrent presence of a major psychiatric disorder and chemical dependence.

duty to disclose/protect A health care professional's obligation to warn identified individuals if a client has made a credible threat of violence or death.

dysthymic disorder A mood disorder similar to major depression but remaining mild or moderate.

dystonia An impairment of muscle tone of the head, neck, and tongue resulting from extrapyramidal side effects of antipsychotic medications.

ecomap Based on the genogram, a diagram outlining the history of the behavior patterns within a family, the ecomap identifies interaction between the family and the larger community.

ego In intrapersonal theory, the component of the personality that mediates the drives of the id with objective reality in a way that promotes well-being and survival.

egocentric self Exhibits characteristics such as individualism, separateness, autonomy, competition, and mastery of and control over one's environment.

ego-dystonic behavior Behavior that is inconsistent with one's thoughts, wishes, and values.

ego-syntonic behavior Behavior that conforms to one's thoughts, wishes, and values.

electroconvulsive therapy (ECT) The application of electricity through the temples, which artificially induces a grand mal seizure; used to treat depression.

elopement Leaving a psychiatric facility against medical advice.

emotional availability Describes the quality of the parent–child relationship in terms of sensitivity, structuring, nonintrusiveness, and nonhostility.

emotions Responses evoked by environmental stimuli, which may be negative (fear) or positive (joy).

empowerment Helping people recover their sense of own value, strength, and the ability to cope with life.

enabling behavior Any action by a person, called a codependent, that consciously or unconsciously facilitates substance dependence.

environmental terrorism Terrorism based on environmental activism.

epilepsy Recurring seizures caused by sporadic electrical discharge of cortex neurons.

ethics A system of morals or rules of behavior.

ethnicity Belonging to a particular cultural group or relating to large groups of people classed according to common racial, national, tribal, religious, linguistic, or cultural origin or background.

ethnocentrism The belief that one's own culture is more important than and preferable to any other culture.

ethnopharmacology The study of medications in the context of culture and ethnicity.

evidence-based practice The use of critical thinking skills and relevant research to improve the quality of client care and promote clinical judgment.

excitotoxicity The process of killing neurons by overexciting them; usually from the release of toxic levels of glu when neurons are damaged.

executive function Ability to set goals, plan ahead, carry out plans, and adapt as necessary.

expressed emotion (EE) The emotional climate of the family; high EE families are hostile, critical, enmeshed, with minimal tolerance, flexibility, empathy, and achievement.

external locus of control The belief that personal events and behavior are imposed from the outside and the individual is not responsible for the cause or the cure.

extrapyramidal side effects (EPS) Side effects caused by antipsychotic medications, which include dystonia, pseudoparkinsonism, neuroleptic malignant syndrome (NMS), and tardive dyskinesia.

eye contact Looking directly into another person's eyes during the process of interpersonal communication.

factitious disorder The intentional simulation or production of physical or psychological symptoms in order to assume the sick role.

family Two or more persons related by birth, marriage, formal or informal adoption, or choice.

family cohesion The emotional bond that family members have between one another.

family communication The manner in which families listen, speak, self-disclose, and track with one another.

family flexibility The amount of change in a family's leadership, role relationships, and relationship rules.

family systems theory The consideration of the structure, cohesion, adaptability, and communication patterns of families.

family therapy The family system is treated as a unit, with a focus on family dynamics and problem solving.

feedback Internal information that allows for a modification of a behavior while it is in progress.

feedforward Internal information that predicts what is about to occur.

fetal alcohol spectrum disorder A syndrome evidenced by low birth weight, slow growth rate, hyperactivity, maladaptive behavior, learning disabilities, heart defects, and malformed facial features. Also known as fetal alcohol syndrome (FAS).

fetishism A fetish is the sexualization of a body part, such as feet or hair, or an inanimate object, such as shoes, leather, or rubber that is not typical for the culture. Fetishism is the pathological displacement of erotic interest and satisfaction to a fetish.

frontal lobe dementia Degenerative brain disease resulting in chronic dementia.

gang A group of people, often young, who band together, often for the purpose of conducting illegal or antisocial activities.

gang rape Rape by a number of perpetrators against the same victim.

gender identity An individual's personal or private sense of identity as female or male.

gender identity disorder Strong and persistent feelings of discomfort with one's assigned sex or gender.

gender roles The roles a person is expected to perform as a result of being male or female in a particular culture.

gene therapy The transfer of genes that will have a therapeutic effect on cellular function.

generalizations The drawing of inferences to process information.

generalized anxiety disorder (GAD) A chronic disorder characterized by persistent anxiety without phobias or panic attacks.

genetics The study of single genes and their effects.

genogram   A three-generational family tree of structures and relationships of family members.

genome   The full complement of genetic information.

genomics   The study of function, interaction, and role in disease of all genes.

grief   The active process of learning to adapt to a loved one's death.

grooming behaviors   Behaviors used to gain the trust of children or family members before sexual abuse begins. The purpose is to persuade the victim to comply with the abuse.

group therapy   Therapy in which group members and the group therapist help people manage their symptoms and cope more effectively.

hallucination   The occurrence of a sight, sound, touch, smell, or taste without any external stimulus to the corresponding sensory organ; the experience is real to the person.

hate crimes   Crimes motivated by bias and hatred of minority groups.

histrionic personality disorder (HPD)   A disorder characterized by showing excessive emotion for the purpose of gaining attention.

HIV/AIDS encephalopathy   Infection of the central nervous system from the direct effect of HIV or from secondary opportunistic infections and malignancies.

hoarding compulsions   Acquisition of and inability to discard worthless items.

homeless   Living on the streets and in emergency shelters.

homeless population   The population of people living on the streets and in shelters; one third suffers from psychiatric disabilities.

homicide   The killing of one person by another.

Huntington disease (HD)   A hereditary neurodegenerative disorder characterized by undesired movements and lack of muscle tone.

hyperactive behavior   Excessive activity as well as an inability to stop being active when appropriate.

hyperetamorphosis   The need to compulsively touch and examine every object in the environment.

hyperorality   The need to taste, chew, and examine any object small enough to be placed in the mouth.

hypertonia   An increase in muscle tone that results in muscular twitching.

hypoactive behavior   A behavior seen in people who move less than other people and may even seem lethargic.

hypochondriasis   A somatoform disorder characterized by the belief of having a serious disease despite all medical evidence to the contrary.

id   In intrapersonal theory, the biological and psychological drives with which a person is born; its major concern is the instant gratification of needs.

ideas of reference   A cognitive distortion in which a person believes that what is in the environment is related to him or her, even when no obvious relationship exists; also called personalization.

idioms of distress   Stressful life events that make people susceptible to a wide variety of physical and mental illnesses.

illnesses of attribution   Culture-specific syndromes that have a presumed cause but no specific signs and symptoms.

illusions   A sensory misperception of environmental stimuli.

impulsivity   Failure to resist an impulse or urge or to respond with reflection.

inattention   Inability to regulate attention or concentration during the performance of a task.

individual psychotherapy   A therapeutic relationship between a client and therapist with a goal of solving problems through identifying feelings, thoughts, and behaviors and the gaining of insight.

informed consent   A client's right to receive enough information to make a decision about treatment and to communicate the decision to others.

intermittent explosive disorder   A disorder in which episodes of aggression result in serious assaultive acts or destruction of property.

internal locus of control   The recognition that one is responsible for his or her behaviors, thoughts, and feelings as well as his or her own movement toward health or illness.

intersex   Gender of the infant is ambiguous since there are contradictions among chromosomal gender, gonadal gender, internal organs, and external genital appearance.

involuntary admission   Detaining a client in a psychiatric facility against his or her will, requested on the basis of dangerousness to self or others; also called commitment.

least restrictive environment   A therapeutic setting that will provide safe care while allowing maximum freedom. The least restrictive environment ranges from clients living on their own to being hospitalized in a locked unit. The determination is always made based on the level of protection needed to keep the client safe at that moment in time.

lethality   The degree to which a suicide plan is capable of causing death.

ligand   Any substance that binds to receptors.

listening   Entering into the experience of another person by paying attention to their words as well as the meaning of their communication.

loose association   Thinking in which there is no apparent relationship between thoughts.

loss   To be deprived of in terms of a person, object, self-esteem, or control.

Lyme disease   A tick-borne infection that may affect the central nervous system.

magnetic seizure therapy (MST)   Use of very-high-frequency rTMS to induce a controlled seizure in selected areas of the brain; it is a substitute for ECT.

magnification   A cognitive distortion in which much importance is attributed to unpleasant occurrences.

major depressive disorder   A mood disorder characterized by loss of interest in life and unresponsiveness, moving from mild to severe, severe lasting at least 2 weeks; also called unipolar disorder.

malingering   The intentional production of false physical or psychological symptoms for external incentives such as sick leave, financial compensation, or obtaining drugs.

marital rape   Rape in which the victim and perpetrator are in an intimate relationship.

mass-casualty terrorism   Large-scale terrorism meant to cause large-scale damage.

memory   The retention of knowledge for future use.

mental health   A lifelong process that includes a sense of harmony and balance for the individual, family, friends, and community; a growth toward potential; an inner feeling of aliveness.

mental illness   A sense of disharmony with aspects of living that may be distressing to the individual, family, friends, or community.

metabolic syndrome   A side effect of second generation antipsychotic medications resulting in abdominal obesity, and elevated levels of triglycerides, cholesterol, blood glucose, and blood pressure.

milieu   The entire social structure of the unit or residence that is designed to be part of the helping process.

mind   A property of brain activity; the mind grows in response to experience and is influenced by interpersonal relationships.

mirroring   Using verbal communication and body language similar to a clients' as a way to build rapport.

misidentification syndrome   Syndrome in which familiar people are seen as unfamiliar and vice versa; may even believe people on television are really present.

mood   A pervasive and sustained quality of a person's emotional tone.

motivation   An inner state that energizes people to create goals and guides their goal-directed behavior.

motor tics   Involuntary movements.

multiple sclerosis (MS)   A chronic disorder caused by destruction of the myelin sheath.

Munchausen syndrome by proxy (MSBP)   A disorder in which the parent persistently fabricates or induces illness in a child with the intent of keeping in contact with health care providers and hospitals.

NANDA nursing diagnoses   Standardized labels applied to clients' problems and responses to disorders.

narcissistic personality disorder (NPD)   A disorder characterized by a pattern of grandiosity, hypersensitivity to evaluation by others, and lack of empathy.

nationalist terrorism   Terrorism that pushes forth the agenda of a particular ethnic group.

natural bias   How a person's point of view influences what is noticed and not noticed.

natural disaster   Unanticipated disaster, such as hurricanes and tornadoes.

negative bias   Refusal to recognize that there are points of view other than one's own.

negative reinforcement The rebound dysphoria that occurs after the drug high.

negative symptoms Loss of normal function that is usually seen in mentally healthy adults.

neglect Acts of omission; a failure to provide adequate care.

neurobiologic theory The focus on genetic factors, neuroanatomy, neurophysiology, and biological rhythms as they relate to the cause, course, and prognosis of mental disorders.

neuroleptic malignant syndrome (NMS) A potentially fatal side effect of antipsychotic drugs related to sympathetic nervous system hyperactivity.

neuromodulator Chemical that alters the threshold to the flow of information but does not necessarily alter the nature of the signal.

neuropeptides Large molecules stored in and released from axons; they serve as neurotransmitters and neuromodulators.

neuroplasticity The brain's ability to improve itself, refine structures, and respond to internal and external changes.

neurotransmitter Brain chemical that carries an inhibiting or stimulating message from one brain cell to another across the synapse. Examples are dopamine, serotonin, norepinephrine, and gamma-aminobutyric acid (GABA).

nicotinic dysregulation Problems with the nicotinic acetylcholine (ACh) receptors during neurotransmission.

nicotinic receptors Subtype of acetylcholine receptors in the hippocampus.

nonspecific homicide Homicide in which only the perpetrator knows the motive.

normalization Achievement of valued social roles for consumers of mental health care; a guiding principle of psychiatric rehabilitation.

no-suicide contract An agreement the client makes with the staff that spells out the intent to remain safe.

nursing informatics Integration of nursing science, computer science, and information science to manage and communicate data, information, and knowledge in nursing practice.

Nursing Interventions Classification (NIC) A comprehensive standardized classification of nursing interventions.

Nursing Outcomes Classification (NOC) A comprehensive standardized classification of nursing outcomes.

nursing process The organization of scientific data to prescribe practice criteria.

obesity State of being overweight; the most common form of malnourishment in the United States.

objective family burden The actual, identifiable family problems associated with the person's mental illness.

obsession An unwanted, recurrent persistent idea, thought, image, or impulse.

obsessive–compulsive disorder (OCD) An anxiety disorder characterized by unwanted, repetitious thoughts and behaviors.

obsessive–compulsive personality disorder (OCPD) A disorder characterized by perfectionism and inflexibility.

oppositional defiant disorder (ODD) A recurrent pattern of disobedient and hostile behavior toward authority figures.

overgeneralization A cognitive distortion in which information is taken from one situation and applied to a wide variety of situations.

overt messages The part of communication consisting of spoken words.

pain disorder A disorder in which the primary symptom is pain that cannot be explained organically.

panic attack The highest level of anxiety, characterized by disorganized thinking, feelings of terror and helplessness, and nonpurposeful behavior.

panic disorder A progressive anxiety disorder characterized by sudden and unexpected panic attacks; may or may not be accompanied by agoraphobia.

paralanguage Nonword sounds that provide additional information about the message being communicated.

paranoid personality disorder (PPD) A disorder characterized by a tendency to interpret the actions of others as deliberately demeaning or threatening.

paraphilias A group of psychosexual disorders characterized by unconventional sexual behaviors.

Parkinson disease (PD) A degenerative disease of the brain caused by a deficit of dopamine.

parkinsonism A type of extrapyramidal side effect of antipsychotic drugs that results in stooped posture, shuffling gait, tremors, and stiff facial expression.

passive–aggressive personality disorder A disorder in which a person opposes and resists others' expectations and demands by procrastination, forgetfulness, and chronic lateness.

patricide/matricide homicide Killing of one or both parents, often after many years of physical and sexual abuse.

pediatric autoimmune neuropsychiatric disorders (PANDAS) A neurological complication of streptococcal infections in some children.

pedigree analysis Three-generational family tree specifying biologic and medical histories.

perseveration phenomena Continuous, repetitive behaviors that have no meaning or direction.

personal space Culturally determined boundaries that dictate how physically close other people may get to the individual.

personality The individual qualities, including habitual behavior patterns, that make a person unique; refers to stable patterns of thoughts, feelings, behaviors, and motivation.

personalization A cognitive distortion in which a person believes that what is in the environment is related to him or her, even when no obvious relationship exists; also called ideas of reference.

pervasive developmental disorder (PDD) not otherwise specified (NOS) Severe impairment in social interaction and very limited verbal communication.

pharmacodynamics What the drug does to the body.

pharmacogenomics The customization of medications based on knowledge from genomics. The identification of genes that affect individuals' responses to medications.

pharmacokinetics What the body does to the drug.

phobic disorders An anxiety disorder characterized by a persistent disabling fear of an object or situation; when the object or situation cannot be avoided, the person responds with panic.

photosensitivity Increased sensitivity of the skin and the eyes to sunlight.

Pick disease A rare form of a progressive dementia affecting the frontal and temporal lobes in which cerebral atrophy is present in the frontal and/or temporal lobes. The temporal patterns of behavior include talkativeness, lightheartedness, gaiety, anxiety, and hyperattentiveness; the frontal patterns include inertia, emotional dullness, and lack of initiative.

positive reinforcement The mood altering effects of some drugs, such as euphoria, energy, mental alertness, self-confidence, and sexual arousal. A reward for desired behavior. An environmental event that rewards, and thus increases the probability of, a behavioral response. Positive reinforcement with smoking behaviors could be the satisfaction of the nicotine craving or filling up time with an activity labeled by the client as enjoyable.

positive symptoms Excessive or added behaviors not normally seen in mentally healthy adults. An excess or distortion of normal functioning, or an aberrant response; typically refers to hallucinations, delusions, and disorganized thinking and behavior.

posttraumatic stress disorder (PTSD) An anxiety disorder characterized by a constant anticipation of danger and a phobic avoidance of triggers that remind the person of the original trauma; other characteristics include irritability, aggression, and flashbacks.

potency The power to produce the desired effects per milligram of medication.

power The ability to exercise control over another person.

power rape Rape in which the intent of the rapist is to command and master the victim sexually.

Prader-Willi syndrome (PWS) A congenital disorder causing morbid obesity by age 2 or 3.

preconscious The aspect of consciousness that encompasses thoughts, feelings, and experiences that have been forgotten but that can easily be recalled to consciousness; sometimes called the subconscious.

predatory violence Violence in which individuals are attacked who have done nothing to provoke the attack.

prejudice A negative feeling about people who are different from us; beliefs, opinions, or points of view that are formed before the facts are known or in spite of them.

primary prevention Interventions aimed at decreasing the severity of a response.

prions   A pathogen that transforms normal protein molecules into infectious ones; thought to be responsible for Creutzfeldt–Jakob disease.

proprioception   The ability to know where one's body is in time and space, and the ability to recognize objects and their functions.

pseudodelirium   Symptoms of delirium without any identifiable organic cause.

pseudodementia   A disorder, frequently depression, that simulates dementia. The reversible cognitive impairments seen in depression such as impaired attention and memory, apathy, self-neglect, and no complaints of depression.

psychiatric consultation liaison nursing (PCLN)   Nursing discipline in which the focus of practice is with clients who are physically ill or disabled and their families; care is provided in nonpsychiatric care settings such as hospitals, rehabilitation centers, extended-care facilities, clinics, and home settings.

psychiatric/psychosocial rehabilitation   Development of skills and support necessary for successful living, learning, and working in the community.

psychoneuroimmunology   The study of the relationship between environment, the hormonal system, the immune system, and the central nervous system.

psychosis   A state in which a person is unable to comprehend reality and has difficulty communicating and relating to others; often accompanied by hallucinations and delusions.

psychosocial rehabilitation   The development of skills and supports necessary for successful living, learning, and working in the community.

psychosurgery   Surgical interruption of brain tissue; considered a last-ditch option for people whose conditions have not responded to other treatments.

purging disorder   A disorder in which the individual does not binge eat but frequently self-induces vomiting or uses large doses of laxatives, enemas, or diuretics aimed at ridding the body of food consumed.

racism   Excessive and irrational beliefs regarding the superiority of a given group.

radiological terrorism   Terrorism committed with radiological agents.

rape   Any forced sexual activity, the key factor being the absence of consent.

rape-trauma syndrome   Symptoms of, or specific responses to, the experience of being raped; also, a nursing diagnosis.

rapport   A sense of harmony and understanding between nurse and client.

reactive attachment disorder   A disorder in which children either avoid interaction with others or have few boundaries and quickly attach to others.

receptors   Docking sites for neurotransmitters on the dendrites of the postsynaptic cells.

recovery   A facet of rehabilitation; incorporating one's disability as part of reality and adapting to one's disorder.

recovery model   A lifelong, day-to-day process of recovery from chemical addiction.

repetitive transcranial magnetic stimulation (rTMS)   Use of a magnetic field that passes through the skull, which causes cells in the cerebral cortex to fire.

resilience   The ability to emerge relatively unscathed from negative life events, to not only survive and bounce back from difficult and traumatic experiences, but also to continue to grow and develop emotionally and psychologically; resilience is the rule, not the exception.

revenge homicide   Homicide in retaliation for real or imagined offenses.

revolutionary terrorism   Terrorism meant to frighten those persons that have power and those who support them in order to replace them with an alternative form of government.

reward deficiency syndrome   The decreased ability to experience pleasure that drives a person to seek external forms of gratification through the use of high-risk behaviors.

Russell's sign   A callus on the back of the hand, caused by forcing vomiting.

sadistic rape   Forced sexual activity in which brutality is used for sexual excitement for the perpetrator.

schizoaffective disorder   A disorder characterized by symptoms that appear to be a mixture of schizophrenia and mood disorders.

schizoid personality disorder (SZPD)   A disorder characterized by a pattern of indifference to social relationships and a restricted range of emotional experience and expression.

schizophrenia   Disabling major mental disorder characterized by distortions in thinking, perceiving, and expressing feelings.

schizophreniform disorder   A disorder with rapid onset of psychotic symptoms, very similar to schizophrenia, lasting less than 6 months.

schizotypal personality disorder (STPD)   A disorder characterized by peculiarities of ideation, appearance, and behavior that are not severe enough to meet the criteria for schizophrenia.

school violence   Injury or death of students or staff that occur in or around school property.

seasonal affective disorder (SAD)   A mood disorder characterized by depression during fall and winter and normal mood or hypomania during spring and summer.

secondary gain   An advantage from, or reward for, being ill that is outside conscious awareness.

secondary prevention   Interventions aimed to meet the immediate needs of individuals and the community.

selective abstraction   A cognitive distortion that focuses on certain information while ignoring contradictory information.

selective mutism   A form of social phobia in which the person is unable to speak in specific social situations, despite being able to speak in other situations.

selective perception   Process of filtering out unnecessary and distracting information in order to focus on what is important at any given moment.

self-advocacy   The concept that people who are most impacted by health care decisions should have the most power in the decision-making process.

self-mutilation   The deliberate destruction of body tissue without conscious intent of suicide; Injuring oneself physically by cutting, burning, pulling out hair, biting fingernails into the cuticle to deal with anxiety and stress.

separation anxiety disorder   A disorder in which a child needs proximity to caregivers, worries excessively, and has physical symptoms; developmentally inappropriate and excessive anxiety about separation from home or from parents or other attachment figures.

serotonin syndrome (SS)   A potentially fatal side effect of antidepressant drugs caused by excess serotonin.

sexual addiction   A disorder in which the central focus of life is sex. People with this addiction spend 50% or more of all waking hours dealing with sex, from fantasy to acting-out behavior.

sexual dysfunctions   Problems or difficulties with sexual expression.

sexual harassment   Unwanted and unwelcome sexual behavior that interferes with everyday life; a form of sexual violence.

sexual healing   An empowering process that enables survivors of sexual abuse to reclaim their sexuality as positive and pleasurable.

sexual violence   The use of threat, intimidation, force, and exploitation of authority with the goal of imposing one's will on a nonconsenting person for the purpose of personal gratification that may or may not be predominantly sexual in nature.

shaken baby syndrome   A form of child abuse that involves the vigorous shaking of infants, which causes intracranial and intraocular bleeding.

shared psychotic disorder   Disorder in which delusional beliefs of a person who is in a close relationship are shared with another person who is delusional.

sibling incest   Sexual abuse in which the victim and perpetrator are siblings.

sobriety   Abstinence from drug use as well as psychological growth and balance.

social network interventions   A plan to improve the relationships of clients within their social network.

social skills training   Teaching basic coping skills necessary to live as autonomously as possible in the community; skills include ADLS, vocational, leisure time, communication, and conflict management skills.

social-emotional intelligence   The ability to recognize emotions in oneself and others, the ability to manage one's own emotions, and the ability to handle interpersonal relationships.

sociocentric self   Cultural value of interdependence among people with stress on cooperation, cohesion, and group identity.

somatization disorder   A somatoform disorder characterized by multiple physical complaints involving several body systems, with no evidence of physiologic impairment.

somatization   Process by which psychological distress is experienced and communicated in the form of somatic (bodily) symptoms.

somatoform disorder   An anxiety disorder characterized by physical symptoms that have no underlying organic basis; formerly referred to as psychosomatic disorders.

spiritual recovery   Regaining a sense of purpose in life, finding meaning in trauma, and learning to trust others once again.

spirituality The part of a person that deals with relationships and values and addresses the questions of purpose and meaning in life; the search for meaning and purpose in life through a connection with others, nature, and/or a belief in a higher power.

Stages of Change model A framework for understanding the process of behavior change; the stages are precontemplation, contemplation, preparation, action, and maintenance.

stalking The act of following, viewing, communicating with, or moving threateningly toward another person. May be accompanied by property damage and assault.

state-sponsored terrorism Terrorism that occurs when an oppressive government terrorizes its citizens into submission and obedience and squashes political dissonance.

stereotypes A standardized mental picture held in common by members of a group and that represents an oversimplified opinion, prejudiced attitude, or uncritical judgment; images frozen in time that cause us to see what we expect to see; arise out of negative biases.

Stevens–Johnson syndrome A severe and sometimes fatal allergic reaction that attacks the skin, mucous membranes, lungs, and kidneys. It can be caused by sulfa drugs, penicillin, Dilantin, and Lamictal, especially when Lamictal is combined with Depakote.

stigma A collection of negative attitudes and beliefs that lead people to fear, reject, avoid, and discriminate against people with mental illness.

street violence Injury or death of people in their neighborhoods or other community settings.

stress An aversive state of arousal triggered by the perception that an event threatens a person's ability to cope effectively; a broad class of experiences in which a demanding situation taxes a person's resources or capabilities, causing a negative effect.

subculture A smaller group within a larger cultural group.

subjective family burden The psychological distress of the family members in relation to the objective burden.

substance abuse The purposeful use, for at least 1 month, of a drug that results in adverse effects to oneself or others; does not meet the criteria for substance dependence.

substance dependence The habitual use of a drug that continues despite adverse effects.

suicidal behavior The behavior and thoughts leading up to the act of suicide.

suicide The act of taking one's own life; a person who takes his or her own life; the end result—survival or death—described as either attempted or completed suicide.

sundown syndrome The intensification of behavioral symptoms during the late afternoon or early evening hours; seen in dementia and delirium.

superego In intrapersonal theory, the component of personality that is concerned with moral behavior.

superstitious thinking A cognitive distortion in which a person believes that some unrelated action would magically influence the course of events.

tardive dyskinesia An irreversible form of extrapyramidal side effects of antipsychotic medications that can be socially disfiguring, with spastic facial distortions and abnormal movements of the arms and legs.

telehealth Network of electronic information and telecommunications technologies to support long-distance clinical health care and client and professional health-related education.

terrorism Premeditated, politically motivated violence perpetrated against noncombatant targets by subnational groups or clandestine agents, usually intended to influence an audience.

terrorist group Any group practicing or having significant subgroups that practice international terrorism.

tertiary prevention Interventions aimed to meet the care goals of individuals and communities on a long-term basis.

therapeutic alliance The conscious process of nurse and client working together toward mutually established goals.

therapeutic milieu An active part of the treatment plan, which includes the physical environment as well as all interactions with staff members and other clients.

touch Physical contact between two or more persons.

Tourette's disorder (TD) Multiple motor and vocal tics that occur many times a day nearly every day for more than a year; appears to be attention-deficit/hyperactivity disorder (ADHD) with chronic motor and vocal tics.

transference A client's unconscious displacement of feelings for a significant person in the past onto the nurse in the current relationship; the feelings may be positive or negative.

transgender A person who identifies with the other sex; the many gradations of gender running from female to male; in opposition to the belief that there are only two genders.

transsexual A person who identifies with the other sex and who usually seeks to transition to the other sex by means of hormone treatment and sex reassignment surgery; a person whose sexual anatomy is not consistent with gender identity.

traumatic brain injury Disruption of the central nervous system through internal processes or external assaults.

true syndromes Culture-specific syndromes that are illnesses with specific symptoms.

twelve-step programs A spiritual plan for recovery consisting of prescribed beliefs, values, and behaviors.

unconscious The aspect of consciousness that encompasses thoughts, feelings, experiences, and dreams that cannot be brought to conscious thought or remembered.

unipolar disorder A mood disorder characterized by loss of interest in life and unresponsiveness, moving from mild to severe, severe lasting at least 2 weeks; also called major depressive disorder.

vagus nerve stimulation (VNS) Involves the surgical implant of a small generator to provide intermittent stimulation to the vagus nerve; for treatment resistant depression.

vocal tics Involuntary vocalizations.

voluntary admission The process through which a person consents to confinement for the purpose of assessment and treatment of a mental disorder.

withdrawal Symptoms that occur after long-term use of a drug is reduced or stopped.

workplace violence Injury or death of individuals occurring at their place of employment.

Page numbers followed by *f* indicate figures and those followed by *t* indicate tables, boxes, or special features. The titles of special features (e.g., Clinical Interactions; Using Research Evidence) are also capitalized.